SLEEP
MEDICINE
PEARLS

SLEEP MEDICINE PEARLS

THIRD EDITION

Richard B. Berry, MD

Professor of Medicine
Division of Pulmonary, Critical Care, and Sleep Medicine
University of Florida College of Medicine;
Medical Director
UF Health Sleep Disorder Center
Gainesville, Florida

Mary H. Wagner, MD

Associate Professor of Pediatrics
Division of Pediatric Pulmonary
University of Florida College of Medicine;
Director, Pediatric Sleep Program
UF Health Sleep Disorder Center
Gainesville, Florida

ELSEVIER
SAUNDERS

SAUNDERS

1600 John F. Kennedy Blvd.
Ste 1800
Philadelphia, PA 19103-2899

Sleep Medicine Pearls   ISBN: 978-1-4557-7051-9

Notices

Knowledge and best practice in this field are constantly changing. As new research and experience broaden our understanding, changes in research methods, professional practices, or medical treatment may become necessary.

Practitioners and researchers must always rely on their own experience and knowledge in evaluating and using any information, methods, compounds, or experiments described herein. In using such information or methods they should be mindful of their own safety and the safety of others, including parties for whom they have a professional responsibility.

With respect to any drug or pharmaceutical products identified, readers are advised to check the most current information provided (i) on procedures featured or (ii) by the manufacturer of each product to be administered, to verify the recommended dose or formula, the method and duration of administration, and contraindications. It is the responsibility of practitioners, relying on their own experience and knowledge of their patients, to make diagnoses, to determine dosages and the best treatment for each individual patient, and to take all appropriate safety precautions.

To the fullest extent of the law, neither the Publisher nor the authors, contributors, or editors, assume any liability for any injury and/or damage to persons or property as a matter of products liability, negligence or otherwise, or from any use or operation of any methods, products, instructions, or ideas contained in the material herein.

Library of Congress Cataloging-in-Publication Data
Berry, Richard B., 1947- author.
    Sleep medicine pearls / Richard B. Berry, Mary H. Wagner. – Third edition.
        p. ; cm.
    Includes bibliographical references and index.
    ISBN 978-1-4557-7051-9 (hardcover : alk. paper)
    I. Wagner, Mary H., author. II. Title.
    [DNLM: 1. Sleep Disorders–diagnosis–Case Reports. 2. Sleep Disorders–therapy–Case Reports. 3. Polysomnography–Case Reports. WL 108] RC547
    616.8'498–dc23
                                         2014016503

Content Strategist: Helene T. Caprari
Senior Content Development Specialist: Dee Simpson
Publishing Services Manager: Catherine Jackson
Senior Project Manager: Rachel E. McMullen
Design Direction: Steven Stave

Printed in India

Last digit is the print number: 10

  Working together to grow libraries in developing countries

www.elsevier.com • www.bookaid.org

This book is dedicated to our families:
David, Sarah, and Catherine Berry
Daniel, Analiese, and Barry Wagner

And to our past and present sleep fellows:
Eric Friskel, MD
Prakash Patel, MD
Kapil Dhawan, MD
Michael Maraist, MD
Sreekala Prabhakaran, MD
Klark Turpen, MD
Ashish Prasad, MD
Emily Beck, MD
Anil Puri, MD
Robert Tilley, MD
Lubna Al Hourani, MD
Holly Skinner, DO
Malini Dondapati, DO

Preface

It has been 10 years since the 2nd edition of Sleep Medicine Pearls was published. Since that time the field of Sleep Medicine has changed tremendously. Digital polysomnography has completely replaced recording on paper, the American Academy of Sleep Medicine Manual for the Scoring of Sleep and Associated Events has been published and revised. The International Classification of Sleep Disorders, 2nd edition was published and publication of the third edition by early 2014 is planned. Board certification in Sleep Medicine is now available through member boards of the American Board of Medical Specialties. Limited channel sleep testing outside of sleep centers (Out of Center Sleep Testing) is now acceptable for the diagnosis of obstructive sleep apnea in adults. New modes of positive airway pressure treatment are available to treat patients with hypoventilation or central apnea due to Cheyne-Stokes breathing or opioids. New treatments for the restless legs syndrome have appeared and the importance of augmentation with dopaminergic medications has been recognized. Our knowledge of the causes of narcolepsy and circadian sleep wake rhythm disorders has increased and use of actigraphy is a growing part of most sleep medicine practices. The behavioral treatment of insomnia has been established as an effective method for treatment of insomnia and is now an integral part of a growing number of sleep centers. These and many other changes provide more that ample justification for updating the previous edition of Sleep Medicine Pearls. The basic format has been very popular with readers and case based instruction is now used in many sleep medicine texts.

We have been encouraged by numerous readers of the previous editions to update the text. There are many fine textbooks on sleep medicine. The goal of Sleep Medicine Pearls is to concisely introduce the basic knowledge needed to take care of patients with sleep disorders using short didactic fundamentals chapters followed by case presentations illustrating use of the information provided. It is beyond the scope of this textbook to cover every aspect of sleep medicine. Topics thought to be most relevant to clinical practice are included. Updating all of the chapters to reflect the explosion of knowledge in sleep medicine has been a formidable task. In addition nearly all of the figures in the previous text have been updated to contain the new montages and sensors recommended for sleep recording. Many new figures have been added. It is hoped that the reader will find the new edition informative and useful.

Richard B. Berry, MD

Contents

FUNDAMENTALS **41**
Psychiatry and Sleep,   654

BONUS ONLINE CONTENT*

---

*To access your account, look for your activation instructions on the inside front cover of this book.

Video Contents

Sleep Stage Nomenclature and Basic Monitoring of Sleep

Sleep is divided into non–rapid eye movement (NREM) and rapid eye movement (REM) sleep. From 1968 until 2007, sleep was usually staged according to *A Manual of Standardized Terminology, Techniques, and Scoring System for Sleep Stages of Human Subjects*, edited by Rechtschaffen and Kales (R&K).[1] In the *R&K Scoring Manual*, *NREM sleep* was divided in stages 1, 2, 3, and 4. *REM sleep* was referred to as *stage REM*. Sleep stage nomenclature has changed following the publication of the *American Academy of Sleep Medicine (AASM) Manual for the Scoring of Sleep and Associated Events* (hereafter referred to as the *AASM Scoring Manual*) in 2007.[2,3] To denote sleep staging by new criteria, sleep stage nomenclature has changed. The old and new nomenclatures are shown in Table F1-1. Stages 3 and stage 4 are combined into stage N3. REM sleep is referred as *stage R*. An update of the *AASM Scoring Manual* has recently been published, but sleep stage nomenclature remains unchanged.[4]

Sleep staging is based on electroencephalography (EEG), electrooculography (EOG), and submental (chin) electromyography (EMG) criteria. EOG (eye movement recording) and chin EMG recordings are used to detect stage R, which is characterized by rapid eye movements (REMs) and reduced muscle tone.

TIME WINDOW FOR STAGING SLEEP

Digital polysomnography (sleep recording) allows visualization of the waveforms in multiple time windows (10, 15, 30, 60, 90, 120, and 240 seconds) (Table F1-2). A 30-second window is used to stage sleep (known as an *epoch*), whereas a 10-second window is used for clinical electroencephalography (EEG) monitoring. A 10-second window allows for detailed visualization of waveforms to determine frequency. The convention of using a 30-second window for sleep staging is based on paper recording using ink pens during the early days of sleep monitoring. At a page speed of 10 millimeters per second (mm/s), a standard 30-centimeter (cm) page of recording paper represented 30 seconds. Each page represented one epoch. Sleep is still staged today in sequential 30-second epochs, although digital polysomnography allows for use of different time windows for scoring respiratory and other events.

Electroencephalography Monitoring

EEG monitoring to detect and stage sleep requires only a portion of the electrodes used for clinical EEG monitoring. The nomenclature for EEG

TABLE F1-1	Sleep Stage Nomenclature	
	R&K	**AASM**
Wake	Stage W	Stage W
NREM	Stage 1	Stage N1
	Stage 2	Stage N2
	Stage 3	Stage N3
	Stage 4	
REM	Stage REM	Stage R

AASM, American Academy of Sleep Medicine; *NREM*, non–rapid eye movement; *REM*, rapid eye movement; *R&K*, Rechtschaffen and Kales.

TABLE F1-2	Optimal Window Duration for Viewing Events in Polysomnography
Window Duration	**Use**
30 seconds (an epoch)	Sleep staging
60–120 seconds	Respiratory Events
15 seconds	Clinical EEG
10 seconds	ECG rhythms Identifying wave form frequency

ECG, Electrocardiography; *EEG*, electroencephalography.

electrodes follows the International 10-20 system.[5] In this system, **even-numbered** subscripts refer to the **right** side of the head and **odd-numbered** subscripts to the **left**. Electrodes are named for the part of the brain they cover: *F* for frontal, *C* for central, and *O* for occipital (Figure F1-1). The central midline (vertex) electrodes (Cz) and the frontopolar midline electrode (Fpz) are also of interest. The Fpz position is often used for the ground electrode and the Cz position for the reference electrode. Note that before publication of the *AASM Scoring Manual*, electrodes M1 and M2 were referred to as *A1* and *A2*, respectively. In clinical EEG monitoring, A1 and A2 are, in fact, referred to as *earlobe electrodes*.

The "10-20" in the International 10-20 system of nomenclature for EEG electrodes refers to the fact that the electrodes are positioned at either 10% or 20% of the distance between landmarks.[5] The major landmarks include the nasion (bridge of the nose), inion (prominence at base of the occiput), and preauricular points (Figure F1-2).

Electroencephalography Derivations

EEG recording uses differential alternating current (AC) amplifiers, which are designed to amplify the difference in voltage between electrodes. There is cancellation of signals common to both electrodes (common mode rejection). (Figure F1-3), this type of AC amplifier allows the recording of relatively low-voltage EEG activity superimposed on a background of higher-voltage electrical noise. The term *derivation* describes a pair of electrodes and the voltage difference between them (e.g., Input-1 − Input-2). By convention, a change in the voltage difference between Input-1 and Input-2 results in an upward deflection if Input-1 is NEGATIVE with respect to Input-2 (see Figure F1-3). Of note, the term *channel* is used to describe each horizontal display of a given signal versus time (each line of the display). Sometimes, an EEG derivation is referred to as a *channel*. However, a given channel may display other signals, for example, the air flow channel or the chest effort channel.

Recommended Electroencephalography Derivations

The EEG derivations and backup derivations recommended by the *AASM Scoring Manual* are presented in Table F1-3. All of the electrodes—F3, F4, C4, C3, O1, O2, M1, M2—are recorded, although display of only the recommended derivations is required for sleep staging. Of historical interest, in the *R&K Scoring Manual*, only central derivations were used to stage sleep. Note that each of the recommended derivations uses a frontal, central, or occipital electrode and the **opposite mastoid electrode**. If the electrode F4 is faulty, the derivation F3-M2 is used. The derivations C4-M1 and O2-M1 are used along with F3-M2. The group of electrodes chosen for visualization is called the *montage*. Digital polysomnography allows for display of all or only a subset of the possible derivations using the electrodes that are recorded.

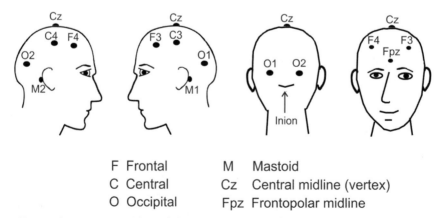

F Frontal   M Mastoid
C Central   Cz Central midline (vertex)
O Occipital Fpz Frontopolar midline

FIGURE F1-1 ■ Nomenclature and position of the basic electrodes for sleep monitoring. *C*, Central; *F*, frontal; *O*, occipital. Even numbers on the right and odd on the left. (Adapted from Berry RB: *Fundamentals of sleep medicine*, Philadelphia, 2012, Saunders, pp. 2-3.)

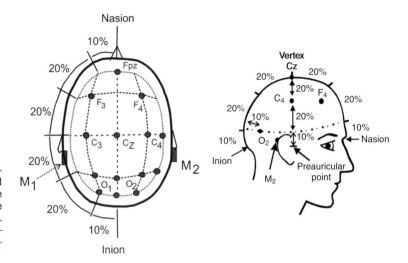

FIGURE F1-2 ■ Electrode positions using the international 10-20 system. Electrodes are placed at 10% or 20% of the distance between landmarks. (Adapted from Berry RB: *Fundamentals of sleep medicine*, Philadelphia, 2012, Saunders, pp. 2-3.)

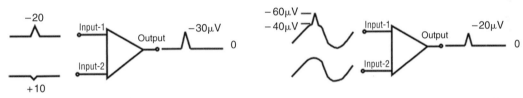

FIGURE F1-3 ■ Differential alternating current (AC) amplifiers amplify the difference in signals at the inputs. Common signals are not amplified as they cancel (common mode rejection). In the figure, the gain or amplification factor is ×1 for simplicity. By convention, if Input-1 is negative with respect to Input-2, the deflection is upward. (Adapted from Berry RB: *Fundamentals of sleep medicine*, Philadelphia, 2012, Saunders, p. 14.)

TABLE F1-3	Recommended and Backup Electroencephalography Derivations	
Recommended	**Backup**
F4-M1	F3-M2
C4-M1	C3-M2
O2-M1	O1-M2

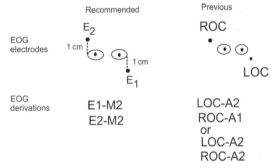

FIGURE F1-4 ■ Placement of recommended electrooculography (EOG) electrodes and EOG derivations. For comparison, previous typical locations and derivations are presented on the right. A1 and A2 are older terminology for left and right mastoid electrodes. (Adapted from Berry RB: *Fundamentals of sleep medicine*, Philadelphia, 2012, Saunders, p. 7.)

ELECTROOCULOGRAPHY MONITORING OF SLEEP

Recording of eye movements is possible because a potential difference exists across the eyeball with the front (cornea) positive (+) and back (retina) negative (−). Eye movements are detected by EOG recording of voltage changes associated with eye movement by using electrodes positioned near the eyes. The recommended EOG electrodes in the *AASM Scoring Manual*[2] are illustrated in Figure F1-4. E1 and E2 refer to the left and right eye electrodes, respectively.

Previously, eye electrodes were named *right outer canthus (ROC)* and *left outer canthus (LOC)*.[1,6,7] Note that E1 is placed *below* the left outer canthus and E2 is placed *above* right outer canthus, whereas LOC and ROC were placed slightly lateral to the respective outer canthus. Because E1 is below the eyes and E2 is above the eyes, vertical as well as horizontal movements can be detected. The *AASM Scoring Manual* recommends the EOG derivations E1-M2 and E2-M2 (see Figure F1-4). Note that both eye derivations use the right mastoid electrode (M2) as the reference electrode.

When the eyes move toward an electrode, a positive voltage is recorded. Recall that, by convention, if Input-1 is positive with respect to Input-2, then a **downward** deflection occurs in the derivation Input-1 − Input-2. Thus, eye movement (cornea +) **toward an eye electrode** referenced to another electrode further away from the eyes results in a **downward** deflection. Using the recommended EOG derivations, eye movements result in **out of phase deflections in the two derivations.** This is because eye movements are conjugate, and when both eyes move laterally or vertically, they both move toward one EOG electrode and away from the other EOG electrode. The polarity of the eye electrodes determines the net voltage difference of the EOG derivations, as the electrodes are much closer to the eyes than M2. The schematic in Figure F1-5 illustrates lateral eye movements and the resulting deflections. This assumes that both eye derivation tracings are displayed with negative polarity upward (standard).

During eyes-open wakefulness and REM sleep, the associated eye movements are characterized by narrow (sharp) EOG deflections, and are called *rapid eye movements (REMs).* The slow undulating eye movements of drowsiness (eyes-closed wakefulness) and stage N1 are called *slow eye movements (SEMs).* Eye movement patterns

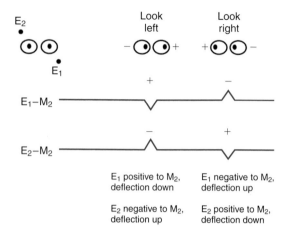

FIGURE F1-5 ■ Lateral eye movement with the resulting deflections in the recommended electrooculography (EOG) derivations. When the eyes move toward the EOG electrodes, the deflection is downward. (Adapted from Berry RB: *Fundamentals of sleep medicine*, Philadelphia, 2012, Saunders, p. 7.)

are discussed in more detail in Fundamentals 2. The recommended eye derivations make it easier to recognize artifacts or EEG activity transmitted to the eye derivations, as these cause **in-phase deflections,** whereas eye movements cause out-of-phase deflections. In Figure F1-6, a large-amplitude EEG wave (K-complex [KC]) causes in-phase deflections in the EOG derivations, whereas REM results in out-of-phase deflections. KC and other wave forms important for sleep staging are discussed in Fundamentals 2.

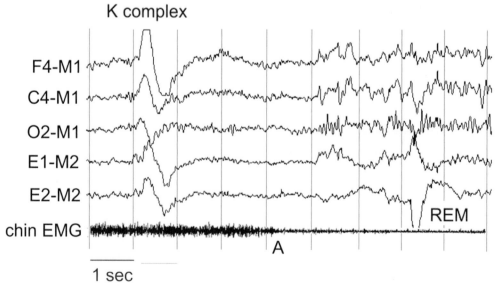

FIGURE F1-6 ■ A K-complex (KC) causes in-phase deflections in the derivations E1-M2 and E2-M2, whereas a rapid eye movement (REM) causes an out-of-phase deflection. The chin electromyography (EMG) activity falls just before an REM is noted and a transition from NREM to REM sleep occurs.

CHIN (SUBMENTAL) ELECTROMYOGRAPHY MONITORING

The placement of EMG electrodes recommended by the *AASM Scoring Manual* is illustrated in Figure F1-7. The revised AASM Scoring manual defines the position and nomenclature of the chin electrodes (Figure F1-7). ChinZ refers to the midline electrode above the mandible and Chin1 and Chin2 refer to the electrodes below the mandible on the patient's left (Chin1) and right (Chin2). The recommended derivations are either Chin1-ChinZ or Chin2-ChinZ. The electrode not used in the displayed derivation is placed as a backup. For example, if the Chin1 electrode is faulty the derivation Chin2-ChinZ is used for staging. If ChinZ is faulty, ideally it should be replaced. If this is not feasible, the derivation Chin1-Chin2 can be used.

The monitoring of chin EMG activity is *an essential element only for identifying stage R (REM sleep)*. In stage R, chin EMG is relatively reduced, that is, the amplitude is equal to or lower than the lowest chin EMG amplitude during NREM sleep. Chin EMG amplitude during other sleep stages is variable. Depending on the EMG gain, a reduction in EMG amplitude from wakefulness to sleep and often a further reduction on transition from stage N1 to stage N2 to stage N3 may be seen. A further drop may be seen on transition from NREM to REM sleep. In Figure F1-6, a fall in chin EMG amplitude

(point A) at the transition to Stage R (just before REMs occur) is shown. However, chin EMG often reaches the REM level during NREM sleep well before the transition to stage R. Of note, the reduction in chin EMG amplitude during REM sleep is a reflection of the generalized skeletal muscle hypotonia present in this sleep stage.

REVIEW QUESTIONS

1. If electrode C4 fails in the recommended EEG derivations F4-M1, C4-M1, and O2-M1 what EEG derivations should be used?
   A. F4-M1, C3-M1, O2-M1
   B. F4-M1, C3-M2, O2-M1
   C. F3-M2, C3-M2, O1-M2
   D. F4-M2, C3-M2, O2-M2

2. The deflection in the derivation F4-M1 is downward. This means:
   A. F4 is positive with respect to M1
   B. F4 is negative with respect to M1

3. When the eyes move toward the right, this causes:
   A. An upward deflection in E2-M2
   B. A downward deflection in E2-M2

ANSWERS

1. B

2. A

3. B

Three electrodes are recommended to record the chin EMG

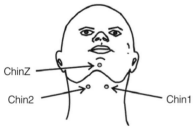

ChinZ Electrode	Midline 1 cm above inferior edge of mandible
Chin2 Electrode	2 cm below inferior edge of the mandible and 2 cm to the right of the midline
Chin1 Electrode	2 cm below inferior edge of mandible and 2 cm to the left of the midline

Standard chin EMG derivations   Chin1 – ChinZ or Chin2 – ChinZ

FIGURE F1-7 ■ Positions of the recommended chin electrodes as specified in the *American Academy of Sleep Medicine (AASM) Manual for the Scoring of Sleep and Associated Events*. The standard chin derivation is either of the electrodes below the mandible referred to the midline electrode above the manual. (Adapted from Berry RB: *Fundamentals of sleep medicine*, Philadelphia, 2012, Saunders, p. 9.)

REFERENCES

1. Rechtschaffen A, Kales A (eds): *A manual of standardized terminology techniques and scoring system for sleep stages of human sleep*, Los Angeles, 1968, Brain Information Service/Brain Research Institute, University of California, Los Angeles.
2. Iber C, Ancoli-Israel S, Chesson A, Quan SF, for the American Academy of Sleep Medicine: *The AASM manual for scoring of sleep and associated events: rules, terminology and technical specifications*, ed 1, Westchester, IL, 2007, American Academy of Sleep Medicine.
3. Silber MH, Ancoli-Israel S, Bonnet MH, et al: The visual scoring of sleep in adults, *J Clin Sleep Med* 15:121–131, 2007.
4. Berry RB, Brooks R, Gamaldo CE, et al., for the American Academy of Sleep Medicine: *The AASM manual for the scoring of sleep and associated events: rules, terminology and technical specifications*, Version 2.0, Darien, IL, 2012, American Academy of Sleep Medicine Accessed June 1, 2014.

5. International Federation of Societies for Electroencephalography and Clinical Neurophysiology: Ten-twenty electrode system, *Electroencephalogr Clin Neurophysiol* 10:371–375, 1958.
6. Berry RB: *Fundamentals of sleep medicine*, Philadelphia, PA, 2012, Elsevier, pp. 1–26.

7. Caraskadon MA, Rechtschaffen A: Monitoring and staging human sleep. In Kryger MH, Roth T, Dement WC (eds): *Principles and practice of sleep medicine*, Philadelphia, 2005, Saunders, p. 1.

PATIENT 1

EEG Derivations and Eye Movements

A 15-second tracing of a patient undergoing sleep monitoring is shown in Figure P1-1. The two questions refer to the figure.

QUESTIONS

1. The eye movements at **A** and **B** (rapid eye movements) in Figure P1-1 result in out of phase deflections in the two electrooculography (EOG) derivations (one up–one down). Assuming that the eye movement at **B** is a *vertical* eye movement, is the direction up or down?

2. What is the deflection at **C** in Figure P1-1 called?

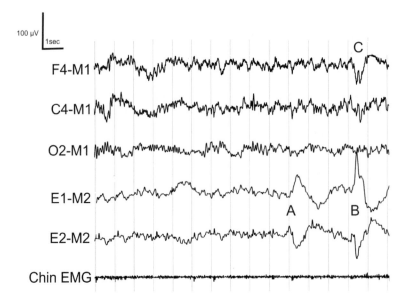

FIGURE P1-1 ■ A 15-second tracing. Rapid eye movements are noted at **A** and **B**.

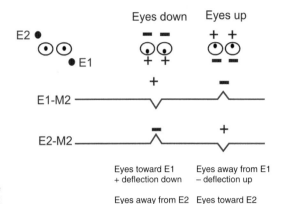

FIGURE P1-2 ■ Vertical eye movements cause out-of-phase deflections in the recommended EOG derivations (E1-M2 and E2-M2).

ANSWERS

1. Assuming A and B are vertical eye movements, the eye movement is upward.

   Discussion: In Figure P1-1 an upward deflection in E1-M2 means that the eyes are moving away from E1, for example, in an upward direction (see Fundamentals 1). The downward deflection in E2-M2 means the eyes are moving toward E2 (upward). The effect of vertical eye movements on tracings in the recommended EOG derivations is illustrated in Figure P1-2. Recall that the cornea of the eye is positive with respect to the retina. When the eyes move toward an EOG electrode, the deflection is downward. Because eye movements are conjugate (both eyes move in the same direction horizontally or vertically), both eyes move toward one EOG electrode and away from the other using the recommended derivations E1-M2 and E2-M2. Therefore, both horizontal and vertical movements result in out-of-phase deflections. As a consequence, it is not possible to tell if the eyes are moving vertically or horizontally.

2. The deflection at C is called *eye movement artifact* but is simply the recording of voltage changes associated with the vertical eye movements in F4-M1.

   Discussion: The deflection in F4-M1 at C in Figure P1-1 is associated with the rapid eye movement at B. The deflection at C is sometimes called *eye movement artifact* but is not really an artifact as the voltage change associated with the eye movement is recorded in a derivation using F4, which is located near the eyes. Such deflections may be quite large, especially with voluntary eye movements. Note that the minimal deflection in C4-M1 and none in O2-M1 are associated with the eye movement (C4 and O2 are more distant from the eyes). If both F4-M1 and F3-M2 derivations are displayed (Figure P1-3), it is possible to detect the direction of eye movements. As both frontal electrodes are above the eyes, vertical eye movements result in in-phase deflections in F3-M2 and F4-M1. Out-of-phase deflections in the frontal derivations mean that the eye movements are horizontal. The tracing if Figure P1-3 shows in-phase deflections in the two frontal derivations, that is, the eye movement is vertical. Downward deflections in F4-M1 and F3-M2 document that both eyes move toward both frontal electrodes (upward movement). Note that minimal to no deflection in the frontal derivations was associated with the rapid eye movement at A. This could be because the eye movement was downward (further away from the frontal electrodes) or resulted in only a small voltage change in the frontal derivations. Not all movements are associated with distinct deflections in the frontal derivations.

   The AASM scoring manual[2-4] provides *an acceptable set of EOG electrode locations and derivations* (Figure P1-4). Note that the nomenclature of the acceptable electrodes is the same as the recommended electrodes (E1, E2) *but the locations for acceptable E1 and E2 are different*, and both electrodes are below the eyes and slightly lateral to the respective outer canthus. Both electrodes are referred to

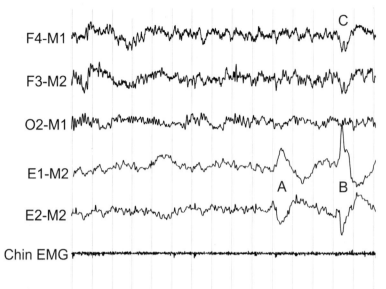

FIGURE P1-3 ■ A 15-second tracing of the patient in the previous figure with F3-M2 substituted for C4-M1. As the deflections (**C**) in both frontal derivations associated with the eye movement (**B**) are in phase this means that the eye movement is vertical. A downward deflection means the eyes are moving toward the electrodes F3 and F4 (upward).

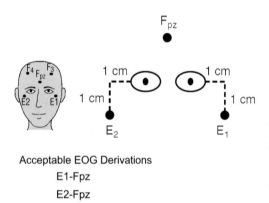

Acceptable EOG Derivations

    E1-Fpz

    E2-Fpz

FIGURE P1-4 ■ Acceptable electrooculography (EOG) electrodes and EOG derivations. (*AASM Scoring Manual*). Note that although the same nomenclature (E1 and E2) is used to refer to EOG electrodes in both the recommended and acceptable EOG derivations, the positions of the acceptable EOG electrodes are different. Acceptable E1 and E2 electrodes are located below and slightly lateral to the left and right outer canthus, respectively.

TABLE P1-1	Eye Movements in the Recommended and Acceptable Derivations[1,3]			
EOG Derivations		**Vertical Eye Movements**	**Horizontal Eye Movements**	**K-Complex**
Recommended	E1-M2 E2-M2	Out-of-phase deflections	Out-of-phase deflections	In-phase deflections
Acceptable	E1-Fpz E2-Fpz	In-phase deflections	Out-of-phase deflections	In-phase deflections

the frontopolar midline electrode Fpz. In these EOG derivations (E1-Fpz, E2-Fpz) vertical eye movements are associated with in-phase deflections and horizontal eye movements with out-of-phase deflections (Table P1-1). With vertical eye movements, the eyes move toward or away from both EOG electrodes. With horizontal eye movements the eyes move away from one EOG electrode and toward the other EOG electrode, resulting in out-of-phase deflections.

An advantage of the acceptable EOG derivations (E1-Fpz, E2-FPz) is that they are more sensitive for detecting vertical eye movements such as blinks compared with the recommended EOG derivations. The vertical distance separating the recommended E1 (or E2) electrode from

M2 is much smaller than that between the acceptable E1 (or E2) and electrode and Fpz. Hence vertical eye movements are associated with larger deflections in E1-Fpz and E2-Fpz compared with the recommended EOG derivations.

CLINICAL PEARLS

1. Conjugate eye movements (both eyes move left or right or up or down) result in out-of-phase deflections in the recommended EOG derivations E1-M2 and E2-M2.

2. Eye movements may cause deflections in the frontal derivations ("eye movement artifact").

3. The *American Academy of Sleep Medicine (AASM) Scoring Manual* also defines acceptable EOG derivations with both E1 and E2 below and lateral to the respective outer canthus. Using E1-Fpz and E2-Fpz, vertical eye movements are characterized by in-phase deflections and horizontal movements by out-of-phase deflections (see Table P1-1).

REFERENCES

1. Iber C, Ancoli-Israel S, Chesson A, Quan SF, for the American Academy of Sleep Medicine: *The AASM manual for scoring of sleep and associated events: rules, terminology and technical specifications*, ed 1, Westchester, IL, 2007, American Academy of Sleep Medicine.
2. Silber MH, Ancoli-Israel S, Bonnet MH, et al: The visual scoring of sleep in adults, *J Clin Sleep Med* 15:121–131, 2007.
3. Berry RB, Brooks R, Gamaldo CE, et al: for the American Academy of Sleep Medicine: *The AASM manual for the scoring of sleep and associated events: rules, terminology and technical specifications*, *Version 2.1*, Darien, IL, 2012, American Academy of Sleep Medicine. www.aasmnet.org, Accessed June 1, 2014.
4. Berry RB: *Fundamentals of sleep medicine*, Philadelphia, 2012, Saunders.

FUNDAMENTALS 2

Electroencephalography and Electrooculography Patterns of Interest for Staging Sleep

Recognition of certain characteristic electroencephalography (EEG) patterns is essential for sleep staging (Figure F2-1; Table F2-1).[1-3] EEG activity is described by frequency in cycles per second (hertz [Hz]), amplitude (microvolts [μV]), and shape. Activity with a higher frequency results in narrower deflections, and slower frequency results in wider deflections. The classically described EEG frequency ranges are delta (0–4 Hz), theta (4–8 Hz), alpha (8–13 Hz), and beta (>13 Hz). **Sharp waves** are narrow waves of 70 to 200 milliseconds (msec) duration, and **spikes** have a shorter duration of 20 to 70 msec. The distribution of EEG activity (the derivations in which the activity is most prominent) and the effects of eye opening or closure are also important for some types of EEG activity.

The term *alpha activity* is used to describe any EEG activity with a frequency in the alpha range (8–13 Hz). However, **alpha rhythm** consists of alpha activity that is most prominent in occipital derivations (see Figure F2-1) and is attenuated by eye opening (increased by eye closure). Another term for alpha rhythm is *posterior dominant rhythm (PDR)*. Alpha rhythm is characteristic of eyes closed stage W. Alpha activity may be noted during stage R and is often associated with brief awakenings (arousals). Bursts of alpha activity are common in stage R.

Sleep spindles and K complexes (KCs) are defining characteristics of stage N2 sleep. **Sleep spindles**[1-3] are bursts of activity with a frequency range of 11 to 16 Hz (usually 12–14 Hz) with a duration of 0.5 seconds or greater (usually 0.5–1.5 seconds). The term *spindle* is used because the shape of sleep spindle burst is often like that of a yarn spindle. If uncertainty exists about whether activity is a burst of alpha activity or a sleep spindle, a 10-second window may be displayed and the deflections (waves) per second actually counted.

Sleep spindles arise from thalamocortical oscillations. The **reticular nucleus** of the thalamus is responsible for generating sleep spindles.

A **K-complex (KC)** is a high-amplitude biphasic wave composed of an initial negative sharp wave (deflection up) followed by a slow wave. A burst of spindle activity is often superimposed on a KC. The KC *stands out from the lower voltage background*. KC activity is greatest in frontal derivations (also central > occipital). A KC is said to be associated with an arousal if the arousal commences no more than 1 second after the KC. An arousal during sleep stages N1, N2, and N3 is scored if an abrupt shift of EEG frequency occurs, including alpha, theta, and/or frequencies greater than 16 Hz (but not spindles) that lasts *at least 3 seconds*, with at least 10 seconds of stable sleep preceding the change. Arousals are discussed in more detail in Fundamentals 5. Note that the KC is seen in the EOG derivations E1–M2 and E2–M2 as an **in-phase deflection** (see Fundamentals 1, Figure F1-6).

Slow wave activity is a defining characteristic of stage N3 sleep. As noted previously, the frequency of delta activity is 0 to 4 Hz. EEG activity in this range produces relatively wide duration deflections, often called *delta* or *slow waves* (see Figure F2-1). However, for sleep staging, the designation **slow wave activity (SWA)**[2] specifically refers to waves with a frequency range of 0.5 to 2 Hz (2- to 0.5-second duration) and a peak-to-peak amplitude *greater than 75 μV in the frontal derivations* (see Figure F2-1). When SWA is 20% of an epoch stage or greater, N3 is scored. Slow waves have the greatest amplitude over frontal areas. In the Rechtschaffen and Kales (R&K) definitions, only central derivations were utilized for sleep staging. Because slow wave amplitude is higher over the frontal areas compared with central areas, a given epoch of EEG activity would potentially have greater SWA

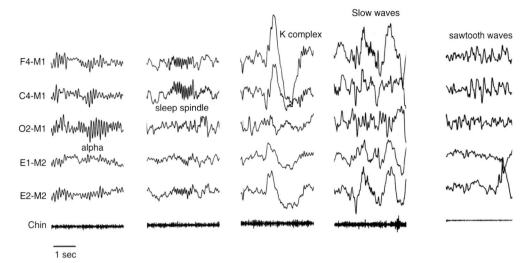

FIGURE F2-1 ■ Electroencephalography (EEG) waveforms used to stage sleep.

TABLE F2-1   **Summary of Important Wave Forms for Sleep Staging**

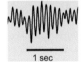

Alpha Activity (Alpha Rhythm)
8–13 hertz (Hz).
Most prominent over the occipital areas (alpha rhythm).
Activity increased by eye closure and attenuated by eye opening (alpha rhythm).
Characteristic electroencephalography (EEG) activity in drowsy, eyes-closed stage W
  (alpha rhythm).
Common in rapid eye movement (REM) sleep (1–2 Hz slower than during stage W).
May occur with arousals (brief awakenings).
10% of persons do not produce alpha rhythm with eye closure.

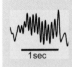

Sleep Spindle
11–16 Hz (classically 12–14 Hz).
Maximal over central areas.
Duration ≥0.5 sec (0.5–1.5 sec).
One of the defining characteristics of stage N2.
Thalamocortical oscillations (reticular thalamic nucleus).
May be seen in stage N3 sleep.
Drug spindles (benzodiazepines) may have a slightly faster frequency.

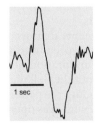

K-Complex (KC)
High amplitude–biphasic deflection.
A well-delineated negative sharp wave (upward) followed by a positive (downward) slow wave.
Stands out from the lower voltage background.
Duration ≥0.5 sec.
Characteristic of stage N2 sleep.
Maximal over frontal areas (frontal > central > occipital).
KC–associated arousal requires arousal to start no more than 1 second after KC termination.

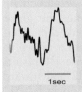

Slow Waves (Slow Wave Activity [SWA])
Frequency 0.5–2 Hz and >75 microvolts (μV) peak-to-peak amplitude in the frontal
  derivations.
Used to define stage N3 sleep.
Stage N2 <20% SWA (<6 sec).
Stage N3 ≥20% SWA (≥6 sec).
SWA is usually transmitted to eye derivations.

Continued

TABLE F2-1	**Summary of Important Wave Forms for Sleep Staging—Cont'd**
1 sec	**Sawtooth Waves** Trains of triangular waves, often serrated. 2–6 Hz waves. Maximal in amplitude in central derivations. Often, but not always, preceding a burst of REMs. Characteristic of stage R but not required for scoring stage R.
1 sec	**Vertex Sharp Wave** Sharply contoured waves. Duration <0.5 sec. Maximal over the central region (derivations containing C3, C4, Cz) and distinguishable from the background activity (higher amplitude). Occurs in stage N1 often near transition to stage N2 (and also in stage N2).

(longer duration meeting amplitude criteria) using the *American Academy of Sleep Medicine (AASM) Scoring Manual* definition[2] (frontal derivations) compared with the R&K definition (using central derivations). It is not surprising that sleep staging using the *AASM Scoring Manual* shows a result of slightly more stage N3 sleep (as a percentage of total sleep time).

Vertex sharp waves are narrow duration waves (<500 msec according to the *AASM Scoring Manual*[2]) prominent in derivations containing electrodes near the vertex (Cz, C3, C4). They are often seen near the transition between stage N1 and stage N2 sleep. **Sawtooth waves** (see Figure F2-1) occur during rapid eye movement (REM) sleep, although they are not always present during this sleep stage. They are triangular waves of 2 to 6 Hz of highest amplitude in the central derivations. The presence of sawtooth waves is *not required* to score stage R. However, the presence of sawtooth waves, when they occur, is very helpful.

The key points concerning EEG waveforms used to stage sleep are summarized in Table F2-1.

EYE MOVEMENT ELECTROOCULOGRAPHY PATTERNS

Typical eye movement patterns (Box F2-1; Figure F2-2) include blinks, slow eye movements (SEMs), rapid eye movements (REMs), and reading eye movements. Slow eye movements are typical of eyes-closed drowsiness and wakefulness and also may occur in stage N1 sleep. REMs are seen in eyes-open wakefulness and stage R sleep. SEMs typically **disappear** with the onset of stage N2 sleep. However, patients on selective serotonin reuptake inhibitors (SSRIs) may have

BOX F2-1	Eye Movements Pattern Definitions

Eye blinks: Conjugate vertical eye movements at a frequency of 0.5 to 2 hertz (Hz) present in wakefulness with the eyes open or closed.
Reading eye movements: Trains of conjugate eye movements consisting of a slow phase followed by a rapid phase in the opposite direction as the subject reads.
Slow eye movements: Conjugate, fairly regular, sinusoidal eye movements with an initial deflection lasting >500 milliseconds (msec).
Rapid eye movements (REM): Conjugate, irregular, sharply peaked eye movements with an initial deflection usually lasting <500 msec. While rapid eye movements are characteristic of stage R sleep, *they may also be seen in wakefulness with eyes open* (as patients look around the room).

Adapted from the AASM Scoring Manual.[1,3]

eye movements that are a mixture of slow and more rapid activity that persists into stage N2.[4,5] This pattern is called *Prozac eyes* but may occur with any of the SSRIs.

Blinks are vertical eye movements that occur usually during wakefulness but may occur during sleep. They are typically short in duration, less than 0.5 seconds. Knowledge about the Bell phenomenon is helpful in understanding the pattern of blinks or changes in the EOG with eyes opening or closing. The Bell phenomenon consists of a reflex upward movement of the eye globe with eye lid closure. With eye opening, the globe returns to a neutral position. A blink, then, consists of eye movement upward with a return to neutral. The movement away from E1 results in an upward deflection in E1-M2 and toward E2 results in a downward deflection in E2-M2 (Figure F2-3). As an upward deflection causes

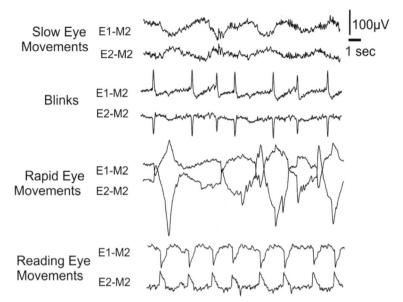

FIGURE F2-2 ■ Eye movement patterns—15 second tracings. (Adapted from Berry RB: *Fundamentals of sleep medicine*, Philadelphia, 2012, Saunders, p. 9.)

the eyes to be closer to E2, blinks may be of a greater amplitude in E2-M2 than in E1-M2 and may also cause deflections in the frontal derivations.

Recognition of the pattern of reading eye movements (Figure F2-4) is assisted by observation of the patient reading on the synchronized video recorded with the sleep study. Reading eye movements display a pattern of a slow gaze to the right (reading from left to right) followed by a fast deflection to the left (to begin reading the next line of print). The resulting

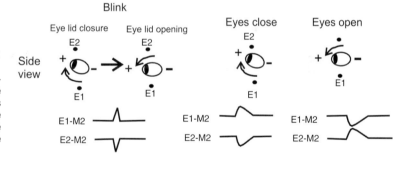

FIGURE F2-3 ■ The electrooculography (EOG) pattern of blinks, eye closure, and eye opening is understood by knowledge of the Bell phenomenon. When the eye lids close, the eye globe turns upward.

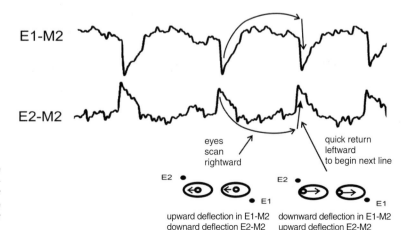

FIGURE F2-4 ■ The etiology of the pattern of reading eye movements. The eyes move slowly to the right while reading a line of print and then move rapidly leftward to start a new line.

pattern is predictable, based on slow eye movement to the right (reading from left to right) and then rapid eye movement leftward to begin a new line.

REFERENCES

1. Iber C, Ancoli-Israel S, Chesson A, Quan SF, for the American Academy of Sleep Medicine: *The AASM manual for scoring of sleep and associated events: rules, terminology and technical specifications*, ed 1, Westchester, IL, 2007, American Academy of Sleep Medicine.
2. Silber MH, Ancoli-Israel S, Bonnet MH, et al: The visual scoring of sleep in adults, *J Clin Sleep Med* 15:121–131, 2007.
3. Berry RB, Brooks R, Gamaldo CE, et al: for the American Academy of Sleep Medicine: *The AASM manual for the scoring of sleep and associated events: rules, terminology and technical specifications*, Version 2.3, Darien, IL, 2012, American Academy of Sleep Medicine. Accessed June 1, 2014.
4. Schenck CH, Mahowlad MW, Kim SW, et al: Prominent eye movements during NREM sleep and REM sleep behavior disorder associated with fluoxetine treatment of obsessive-compulsive disorder, *Sleep* 15:226–235, 1992.
5. Armitage R, Trivedi M, Rush AJ: Fluoxetine and oculomotor activity during sleep in depressed patients, *Neuropsychopharmacology* 12:159–165, 1995.

PATIENT 2

Eye Movements, Alpha Rhythm, and Sleep Spindles in a 20-Year-Old Man

A 20-year-old man undergoes a sleep study for a history of daytime sleepiness and snoring. Figures P2-1 and P2-2 are 15-second and 6-second tracings, respectively.

QUESTIONS

1. Biocalibrations are a series of maneuvers that a patient performs while awake, before lights out, in response to technologist instructions. At "A" in Figure P2-1, was the command "eyes open" or "eyes closed"?

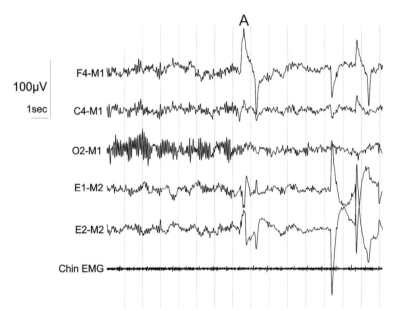

FIGURE P2-1 ■ A 15-second tracing during biocalibration.

2. What are the names of the waveforms A and B in Figure P2-2? The short black lines are 1-second long.

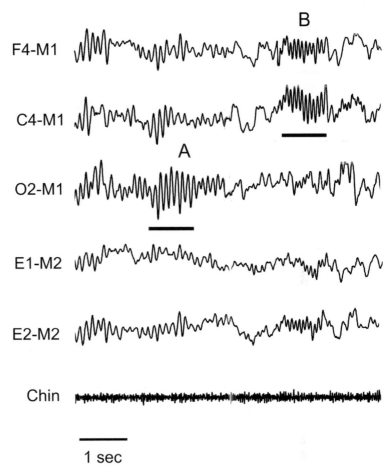

FIGURE P2-2 ■ A 6 second tracing is shown. The short dark lines are 1 second in duration.

ANSWERS

1. **Answer:** "Eyes open"

   Discussion: To the left of "A," the eyes were closed with prominent alpha rhythm. Alpha rhythm has a frequency of 8 to 13 Hz, is most prominent in occipital derivations, and is attenuated with eye opening. After "A" alpha rhythm is attenuated and you can also see rapid eye movements (REMs) consistent with eyes-open stage W. A more general term for a rhythm that is most prominent in occipital areas and attenuated by eye opening is *posterior dominant rhythm*. It is important to review the biocalibrations to determine if the individual generates alpha rhythm with eye closure. As will be discussed in Fundamentals 3, the rules for scoring stage W and stage N1 are different if an individual does not generate alpha rhythm with eye closure. Note that at "A," a large upward deflection occurs in F4-M1 derivation. Recall that when the eyes lids are closed, the globe turns upward. With eye opening, the eye moves downward (away from F4), and this results in a positive deflection in F4-M1.

2. **Answer:** The activity at A is *alpha rhythm*. The activity at B is a *sleep spindle*.

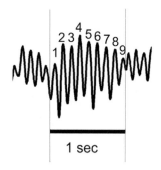

FIGURE P2-3 ■ A 10-second window allows counting of the deflections in a wave form in 1 second to determine the frequency.

Discussion: At times, distinguishing alpha rhythm from sleep spindles may be challenging. Some overlap exists in the frequency range (alpha 8 to 13 hertz [Hz] and sleep spindles 11 to 16 Hz). Although alpha rhythm is typically present at the transition from wake to sleep, bursts of alpha activity may occur during epochs of sleep. Bursts of alpha activity are especially common during stage R, and the frequency is often 1 to 2 Hz slower than during wakefulness. Bursts of alpha activity also commonly occur during arousal from sleep (brief awakenings). Sleep spindles are characteristic of stage N2 but may also be noted in stage N3. Although the sleep spindle frequency range is 11 to 16 Hz, the activity is usually 12 to 14 Hz. Sleep spindle activity may also be superimposed on a K-complex (KC). A KC with sleep spindle activity may be mistaken for a KC associated with an arousal (with associated alpha activity). It is helpful to remember that alpha rhythm is most prominent in the occipital derivations, whereas sleep spindle activity is more prominent in central or frontal derivations.

In Figure P2-2, the activity at A is most prominent in the occipital derivation and has a frequency of 8 to 9 Hz (within the 8 to 13 Hz alpha range) consistent with alpha rhythm. The activity at B is a sleep spindle. This activity is faster 12 to 13 Hz (within the 11 to 16 Hz sleep spindle range) and most prominent in the central derivation (also prominent in frontal derivation).[1-3]

If the frequency of the activity of a waveform is in doubt change to a 10-second page with the 1-second lines visible.[4] The number of oscillations in 1 second may be counted (Figure P2-3). In Figure P2-3, the waveform frequency is 9 Hz and therefore consistent with alpha activity (8 to 13 Hz).

CLINICAL PEARLS

1. To determine the frequency of a waveform, switch to a 10-second view with 1-second lines visible, and count the oscillations in 1 second.
2. The frequency range of alpha rhythm and sleep spindles overlap. Alpha rhythm is most prominent in the occipital areas and attenuated by eye opening. Sleep spindles are most prominent in the central or frontal derivations and occur in short bursts.
3. Alpha rhythm is a specific type of alpha activity most prominent in occipital derivations and attenuated by eye opening.
4. Review of biocalibrations prior to reading a sleep study is important to determine if the individual generates alpha rhythm with eye closure.

REFERENCES

1. Iber C, Ancoli-Israel S, Chesson A, Quan SF, for the American Academy of Sleep Medicine: *The AASM manual for scoring of sleep and associated events: rules, terminology and technical specifications*, ed 1, Westchester, IL, 2007, American Academy of Sleep Medicine.
2. Berry RB, Brooks R, Gamaldo CE, et al., for the American Academy of Sleep Medicine: *The AASM manual for the scoring of sleep and associated events: rules, terminology and technical specifications*, Version 2.1, Darien, IL, 2012, American Academy of Sleep Medicine. www.aasmnet.org, Accessed July 3, 2014.
3. DeGennaro L, Ferrara M: Sleep spindles: an overview, *Sleep Med Rev* 7:423–440, 2003.
4. Berry RB: *Fundamentals of sleep medicine*, Philadelphia, 2012, Saunders, pp. 1–26.

Sleep Staging in Adults I

The *American Academy of Sleep Medicine (AASM) Manual for the Scoring of Sleep and Associated Events*[1,2] was published in 2007 (subsequently referred to as the *AASM Scoring Manual*). This manual changed the rules of staging sleep and made recommendations about the methods used to monitor sleep. Previously, sleep was staged according to the manual edited by Rechtschaffen and Kales (R&K).[3] A recent update to the scoring manual has been published, but relatively few changes have been made in the rules for scoring sleep.[4] The manual is on-line and periodically revised. The reader should review the latest version. The definitions of the electroencephalography (EEG) and eye movement patterns used for staging sleep are discussed in Fundamentals 2. This chapter provides an overview of sleep stages and specific rules for scoring stage W, N1, N2, and N3. See Fundamentals 4 for scoring stage R.

SLEEP CYCLES

In staging sleep, it is important to keep in mind that sleep occurs in cycles of non–rapid eye movement (NREM) and rapid eye movement (REM) sleep (Figure F3-1). The first epoch of sleep in adults is typically stage N1. As the night progresses, less stage N3 occurs, and the duration of stage R episodes increases. The number of REMs per epoch of stage R (REM density) also increases in the second part of the night. Brief episodes of wakefulness also occur during the night.

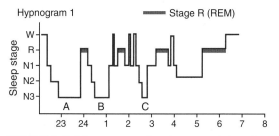

FIGURE F3-1 ■ A hypnogram showing normal sleep in a young adult is shown.

OVERVIEW OF SLEEP STAGES

The rules of scoring sleep are detailed and a brief overview is helpful (Table F3-1). During wakefulness, individuals make the transition from full alertness to the early stages of drowsiness. The characteristics of **stage W** depend on whether an individual has the eyes open or closed. During eyes-open wakefulness, the EEG consists of alpha (8–13 Hz) and beta (>13 hertz [Hz]) frequencies, and the electrooculography (EOG) may demonstrate blinks, voluntary REMs, or reading eye movements (Figure F3-2). Chin electromyography (EMG) activity is usually relatively high compared with sleep. As individuals become drowsy, blink frequency decreases, and the eyes close. Following eye closure, alpha rhythm is the predominant pattern (>50% of the epoch) and slow eye movements (SEMs) may be present (Figure F3-3).

On transition to stage N1, low-amplitude mixed-frequency (LAMF) EEG activity replaces alpha rhythm for the majority of the epoch. **LAMF** activity is characterized by predominantly 4 to 7 Hz activity. The SEMs that may be present in stage W often persist into stage N1. Chin EMG in stage N1 is variable but usually lower than stage W. Stage N1 is usually brief, as the transition from stage N1 to stage N2 occurs quickly after sleep onset unless sleep is disturbed by frequent brief awakenings (arousals). Episodes of stage N1 may also occur following periods of wakefulness during the night (see Figure F3-1).

About 10% of individuals do not generate alpha rhythm on eye closure, and a further 10% may generate limited alpha rhythm. The scoring of stage W and stage N1 sleep in these individuals is different compared with alpha generators and is discussed in detail below. The onset of **stage N2** is characterized by the presence of sleep spindles, K-complexes (KCs), or both, but these waveforms may not be present in every epoch of this sleep stage. As noted in the scoring rules, once an epoch of stage N2 is scored, this sleep stage is considered to continue until evidence of a transition to another stage of

TABLE F3-1 **Overview of Sleep Stage Characteristics**

	EEG	EOG	Chin EMG
Stage W (eyes open)	Alpha+beta	REMs, blinks, reading EM	Relatively high
Stage W (eyes closed)	>50% alpha	±SEMs	Variable
Stage N1	<50% alpha >50% LAMF	±SEMs	Variable, usually <wake
Stage N2	SS, KC*	None	Variable
Stage N3	SWA ≥ 20% (6 sec) SS may occur	None	Variable
Stage R	LAMF, no SS or KC	REMs*	Lowest of night

KC, K complex; *LAMF,* low amplitude mixed frequency; *REM,* rapid eye movement; *Reading EM,* reading eye movements; ±, may or may not be present; *SS,* sleep spindle; *SEM,* slow eye movement; *SWA,* slow wave activity.
*Characteristic but not in all epochs

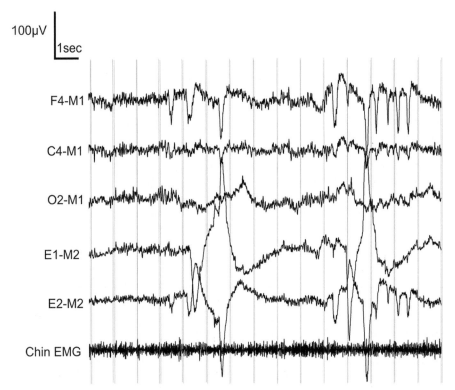

FIGURE F3-2 ■ A 15-second tracing of eyes-open wakefulness with rapid eye movements (REMs) and blinks. Note that electroencephalography (EEG) shows high-frequency activity. In this individual, blinks are noted in F4-M1 and E2-M2, but not in E1-M2. As the eyes turn upward during blinks (Bell phenomenon), they are closer to E2 and F4 than E1. (see Fundamentals 2).

sleep or a brief awakening (arousal) is seen. As stage N2 continues, an increasing amount of slow wave activity (SWA) is usually noted (0.5–2 Hz, peak to peak amplitude >75 microvolts [µv] **over the frontal areas**) but occupies less than 20% of the epoch (6 seconds). Eye movement activity has usually ceased during stage N2, and chin EMG is variable in amplitude. Stage N3 is scored when SWA activity occupies 20% or more of an epoch (≥6 seconds). SWA is noted in the EOG derivations, and sleep spindles may be superimposed on the slow waves. An abrupt transition from stage N3 to stage R may occur, or the SWA (and EEG amplitude) may decrease sufficiently so that stage N3 transitions briefly into stage N2 before the onset of stage R. A reduction in SWA, chin EMG activity, or both is a clue that stage R may soon occur.

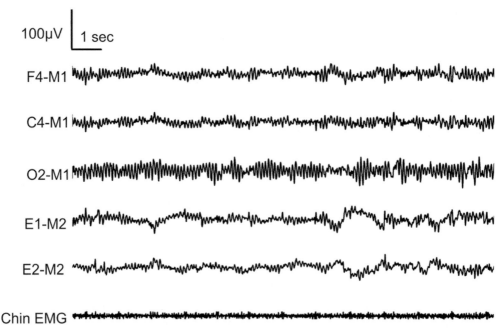

FIGURE F3-3 ■ A 15-second tracing of stage W (eyes closed) in an individual generating alpha rhythm with eye closure. Note that the alpha rhythm is most prominent in the occipital derivation and present for the entire 15 seconds. Subtle slow eye movements are also noted.

Epochs of definite stage R are characterized by the absence of sleep spindles or K complexes and the presence of REMs and low chin EMG activity. However, REMs do not occur in every epoch, and chin EMG may reach REM levels during NREM sleep before REMs appears. Specific rules exist for the start and continuation of stage R. Also, scoring rules exist to deal with the occurrence of arousals (brief awakenings) that interrupt an episode of REM sleep.

SCORING BY EPOCHS

Sleep is staged in sequential 30 second epochs. Each epoch is assigned a sleep stage. If two or more stages coexist during a single epoch, the epoch is assigned the stage comprising the greatest portion of the epoch. *Note that any time the individual being monitored is unhooked from the monitoring equipment during the night (e.g., trips to the bathroom), this time is considered to be stage W.*

STAGE W (WAKEFULNESS) RULES

The EEG of eyes-open stage W in alpha generators consists of a low amplitude mixture of alpha and higher frequencies (see Figure F3-2). The EEG of eyes-closed wakefulness is characterized by alpha rhythm most prominent in the occipital derivations (see Figure F3-3). Stage W is scored when rhythmic alpha activity is present in the occipital derivations for more than 50% of the epoch (Table F3-2). SEMs **may** be present, and chin EMG activity is variable but usually with a higher amplitude than during sleep.

In individuals who do not generate alpha rhythm with eye closure, the occipital EEG activity is similar during eye opening and eye closure. The EEG of stage W in non–alpha generators (both eyes open and closed) consists of a low amplitude mixture of alpha and higher frequencies (similar to eyes-open wakefulness in alpha generators). In non–alpha generators, stage W is scored with evidence of wakefulness based on

TABLE F3-2   Rules for Scoring Stage W
Score epochs as stage W when more than 50% of the epoch contains EITHER (a) or (b) or BOTH:
a. Alpha rhythm (posterior dominant rhythm) over the occipital region (individuals generating alpha rhythm with eye closure)

b. Other findings consistent with stage W (all individuals)
   i. Eye blinks (0.5 to 2 Hz)
   ii. Rapid eye movements associated with normal or high chin muscle tone
   iii. Reading eye movements

eye movements associated with eyes-open wakefulness, including blinks, reading eye movements, or REMs in association with normal or increased chin EMG activity (Table F3-2).

The current version of the AASM scoring manual addresses epochs containing a mixture of alpha rhythm and eye movement patterns of wakefulness. An epoch is scored as stage W if more than 50% contains alpha, eye movements associated with wakefulness or both.

STAGE N1

In individuals who generate alpha rhythm on eye closure, stage N1 is scored when the alpha rhythm in the EEG is attenuated for more than 50% of the epoch and replaced by LAMF (4–7 Hz) activity (N1 rules Table F3-3) (Figures F3-4 and F3-5). SEMs may occur. Chin EMG is variable but usually lower than during wakefulness. In general, sleep spindles (SS) and KCs not associated with arousals are absent. The exception is at the transition between stage N1 and stage N2. The final epoch of stage N1 may contain KCs or SSs in the last half of the epoch. At the transition to stage N2, vertex sharp waves may appear in stage N1 and continue during early stage N2.

In individuals who do not produce alpha activity with eye closure, sleep onset (typically stage N1) is more difficult to determine. The *AASM*

Scoring Manual states that stage N1 occurs at the earliest occurrence of any of the following: SEMs, an EEG with LAMF activity showing a slowing of the background EEG frequencies by 1 Hz or greater from that in stage W, or the presence of vertex sharp waves (Table F3-3). If SEMs start in the last half of an epoch, then the epoch would be scored as stage W, but the next epoch would be staged N1 (assuming no evidence of N2 exists). As noted in the *AASM Scoring Manual*, as SEMs may occur before alpha attenuation in subjects who make alpha activity, the onset of stage N1 may be scored somewhat earlier (based on the appearance of SEMs) in individuals who do not produce alpha activity with eye closure compared with those that do so. As stage N1 is usually the first stage of sleep in adults, this means that the sleep latency (lights out to the first sleep) is shorter in non–alpha generators. No specific rules exist for the end of stage N1, as this stage ends when epochs meet criteria for other sleep stages W, N2, N3, or stage R.

STAGE N2

In scoring stage N2, KC with (KC+A) and without (KC-A) an associated arousal are treated very differently. Arousal rules are discussed in detail in Fundamentals 5. *An arousal is scored during NREM sleep if an abrupt shift of EEG frequency, including alpha, theta, and frequencies greater than 16 Hz (but not spindles), lasts at least 3 seconds, with at least 10 seconds of stable sleep preceding the change* (Figure F3-6). A KC is said to be associated with an arousal if the arousal commences no more than 1 second after the termination of the KC. For simplicity, in the discussion below, *KC will be used to denote a K-complex not associated with an arousal.*

Start of Stage N2

Start scoring stage N2 when one or more KCs (not associated with an arousal) or trains of sleep spindles (SS) occur in the first half of the **current epoch** or the **last half of the previous epoch** (Figure F3-7). This assumes that the epoch does not meet criteria for stage N3. Epochs of stage N2 contain less than 20% of slow wave activity (0.5–2 Hz, >75 μV peak-to-peak in frontal derivations). Most digital polysomnography (PSG) systems allow display of amplitude grid lines and placing lines at -37.5 μv $+37.5$ μv in F4-M1 or F3-M2 allows one to easily note greater than 75 μv peak-to-peak activity in F4-M1 (Figure F3-8; Table F3-4).

TABLE F3-3 Stage N1 Rules

1. **In individuals who generate alpha rhythm, score stage N1 if the alpha rhythm is attenuated and replaced by low-amplitude, mixed-frequency activity for more than 50% of the epoch.**

2. **In individuals who do not generate alpha rhythm, score stage N1 commencing with the earliest of ANY of the following phenomena:**

   a. EEG activity in range of 4–7 Hz with slowing of background frequencies by ≥1 Hz from those of stage W
   b. Vertex sharp waves
   c. Slow eye movements

Notes:
1. Slow eye movements may occur in stage N1 but are not required for scoring stage N1
2. Slow eye movements are evidence for stage N1 in non-alpha generators
3. The chin EMG tone in stage N1 is variable but usually lower than stage W
4. Low amplitude mixed frequency activity (LAMF) is low amplitude EEG activity with frequencies of 4 to 7 Hz

Adapted from the *AASM Scoring Manual*.

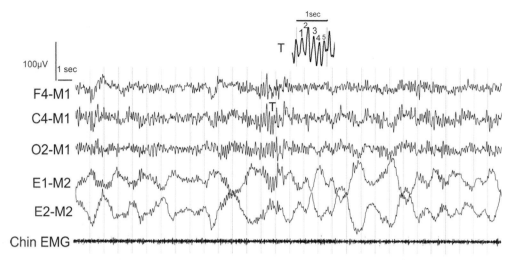

FIGURE F3-4 ■ Stage N1. A 30 second epoch of stage N1 showing low-amplitude, mixed-frequency electroencephalography (EEG) output without K-complexes or sleep spindles. Slow eye movements (SEMs) are prominent here but are not required for scoring stage N1. In individuals who do not generate alpha on eye closure, the presence of slow eye movements is a criteria for scoring stage N1. Note the activity at (T) is theta activity of 5 hertz (Hz) (theta is 4–8 Hz).

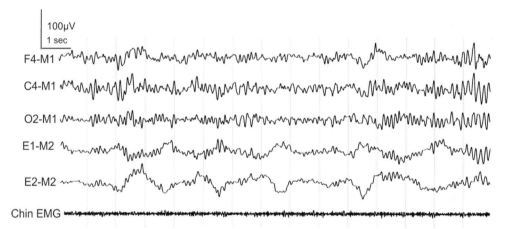

FIGURE F3-5 ■ The first 15 seconds of the epoch in F3-F4 is shown here. The electroencephalography (EEG) activity in the last second is theta activity. This figure shows the appearance of stage N1 as seen on a large screen monitor.

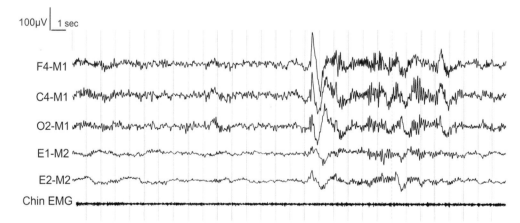

FIGURE F3-6 ■ A K-complex associated with an arousal. An arousal is scored during non–rapid eye movement (NREM) sleep if an abrupt shift of EEG frequency, including alpha, theta, and or frequencies greater than 16 Hz (but not spindles), lasts at least 3 seconds, with at least 10 seconds of stable sleep preceding the change.

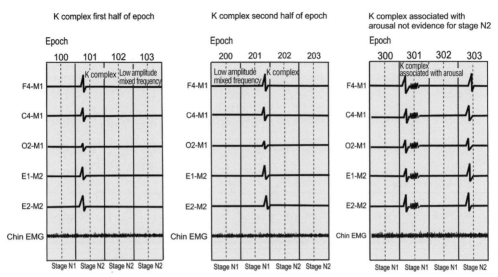

FIGURE F3-7 ■ Start of stage N2: Schematics show the start and continuation of stage N2. A K complex associated with an arousal does not signal the start or the presence of stage N2.

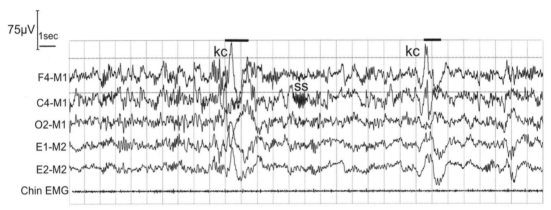

FIGURE F3-8 ■ Stage N2: A 30-second epoch with sleep spindles (SS) and K-complexes (KCs). The dark horizontal bars at the top denote the presence of slow wave activity (>75 microvolts [μV] peak to peak, 0.5–2.0 hertz [Hz] in frontal areas). The total duration of slow wave activity is less than 6 seconds. The dotted lines in F4-M1 are 75 μV apart.

Continuation and End of Stage N2

Stage N2 continues until it is necessary to score an end of a period of stage N2 sleep. Epochs with LAMF EEG activity (without KC or SS) that follow an epoch with sleep spindles or KCs (not associated with arousal) continue to be scored as stage N2 (Table F3-4). If an arousal occurs, a major body movement (MBM) is *followed by SEMs* (signaling a transition to stage N1), or the epoch meets criteria for stages W, N3, or R, then stage N2 ends. MBMs in Fundamentals 5.

End of Stage N2: Effects of Arousals

When an arousal occurs in stage N2 sleep, this signals a transition of sleep stage (Figure F3-9). The scoring of the epoch containing the arousal depends on whether the arousal occurs in the first or second half of an epoch. In Figure F3-9, an arousal occurs in epoch 201. As the arousal occurs in the last half of the epoch, the current epoch remains as stage N2, but the next epoch is scored as stage N1. Stage N2 resumes only in the presence of a KC not associated with an arousal or sleep spindle (using rules for the start of stage N2, rule N2-A).

End of Stage N2: Effect of Major Body Movement

A **major body movement (MBM)** is defined as movement and muscle artifact obscuring the EEG for more than half an epoch to the extent that the sleep stage cannot be determined. If an

TABLE F3-4 Stage N2 Rules

N2-A	Rule defining the **start** of N2 sleep: EEG: Begin Scoring stage N2 (in the absence of evidence of N3, SWA is <6 seconds) if **either or both** of the following occur during the **first half of the current epoch** or the **last half of the previous epoch**: One or more K complexes **unassociated with arousals, or** One or more trains of sleep spindles. EEG: If the only K-complexes present are associated with arousal continue to score Stage N1. EOG: Usually no eye movements, slow eye movements have ended. Chin EMG: Variable usually less than wakefulness. *Note:* Slow wave activity (SWA) = EEG activity 0.5 to 2 hertz (Hz) with >75 μv peak-to-peak amplitude in the frontal areas. If SWA >20% of the epoch (≥6 seconds), score stage N3.
N2-B	Rule defining the **continuation** of stage N2 sleep: Continue to score epochs with low-amplitude, mixed-frequency (LAMF) EEG activity without K-complexes or sleep spindles as stage N2 if they are preceded by an epoch containing **either** of the following: a. K-complexes unassociated with arousals. b. Sleep spindles.
N2-C	Rule defining the **end** of a period of stage N2 sleep: End stage N2 sleep when one of the following events occurs: a. Transition to stage W, stage N3, or stage R. b. An **arousal** (change to stage N1 until a K-complex unassociated with an arousal, or a sleep spindle occurs). c. A **major body movement** is followed by **slow eye movements** and LAMF EEG without non-arousal associated K-complexes or sleep spindles, then score epochs following the major body movement as stage N1. If no slow eye movements follow the major body movement, score the epoch as stage N2. The epoch containing the body movement is scored using criteria for major body movements.

Adapted from AASM scoring manual. See later rules for arousal and major body movement rules.
EEG, Electroencephalography; *EOG,* electrooculography.

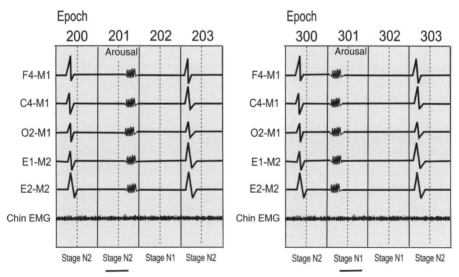

FIGURE F3-9 ■ An arousal interrupts stage N2. The epoch containing the arousal is scored, based on the position of the arousal. Compare epochs 201 and 301.

episode of stage N2 is interrupted by an MBM epoch, the scoring of subsequent epochs depend on the MBM rules (see Fundamentals 5) and stage N2 rules (N2-C-c) (Figure F3-10). If the epoch with the MBM has any alpha activity,

the MBM epoch is scored as stage W, and stage N2 ends. If the MBM epoch is followed by an SEM (evidence of transition to a lighter stage of sleep), then a transition to stage N1 is scored. If the MBM is not followed by an SEM, stage N2

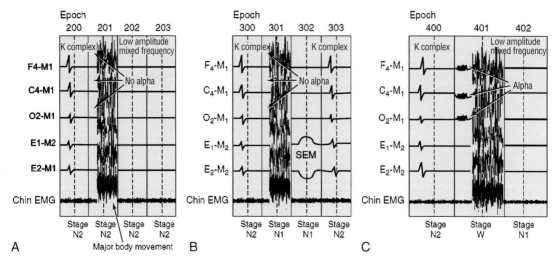

FIGURE F3-10 ■ A major body movement (MBM) interrupts stage N2 (Stage N2 Rule C.1.c). If the epoch containing the MBM has no alpha and no slow eye movements (SEMs) occur in the subsequent epoch, stage N2 continues (Epochs 202-203). However, if SEMs follow the MBM, a transition to stage N1 is scored (Epochs 302). If the MBM epoch contains alpha, the epoch is scored as stage W (see MBM rules). In this case, stage N2 ends. The next epoch of sleep without K-complexes or sleep spindles is scored as stage N1 (unless there is evidence of another sleep stage).

continues. The scoring of the MBM epoch itself is as follows: As noted above, the MBM epoch is scored as stage W if it contains any alpha activity. If the epochs preceding or following the MBM are scored as stage W, then the MBM epoch is scored as stage W. If the MBM epoch does *not* contain alpha activity and is not preceded or followed by an epoch of stage W, the MBM epoch is scored as having the sleep stage of the epoch that follows it.

A recent revision of stage N3 rules states that epochs following an epoch of stage N3 that do not meet criteria for stage N3 are scored as stage N2 if there is no intervening arousal and the epoch does not meet criteria for stage W or stage R. The scoring rules for stage N2 are summarized in Table F3-5.

STAGE N3

Stage N3 is scored when the amount of SWA is 20% of an epoch or greater (≥6 seconds) over the **frontal regions**. Note that the SWA is also recorded in the EOG derivations but SEMs or REMs are not present (Table F3-6; Figure F3-11). Chin EMG is variable but typically less than wakefulness. The amount of stage N3 decreases in adult men but not in women with

TABLE F3-5 Summary of Scoring Rules for Stage N2

Start N2	Continue N2	Stop N2
KC-nonA or SS in **first half** of current epoch or last half of the previous epoch	EEG with LAMF **without** KC or SS **If** the epoch (or a group of epochs) is preceded by an epoch with a non-arousal KC or SS	Transition to stages W, N3, or R Arousal Major body movement followed by a **slow eye movement**

KC-nonA, K-complex not associated with arousal; *LAMF*, low-amplitude mixed-frequency; *SS*, sleep spindle.

TABLE F3-6 Scoring Rules of Stage N3

N3-A   Score stage N3 when **20% or more** of an epoch consists of slow wave activity, irrespective of age. *(20% of 30 second epoch = 6 seconds)*

EEG: SWA ≥20% of the epoch (≥6 seconds), sleep spindles may be present in stage N3.
EOG: Eye movements are not typically seen during stage N3 sleep.
EMG: In stage N3, chin EMG is of variable amplitude, often lower than in stage N2 sleep and sometimes as low as in stage R sleep.

EEG, Electroencephalography; *EMG*, electromyography; *EOG*, electrooculography.
Note: SWA = EEG activity 0.5 to 2 Hz with peak-to-peak amplitude >75 μv measured over the frontal areas. SWA may be seen in the EOG derivations.

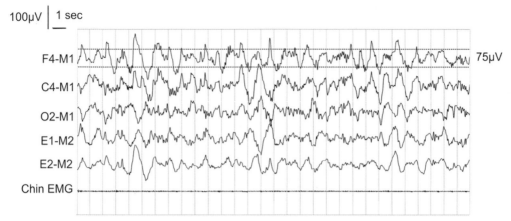

FIGURE F3-11 ■ Stage N3 sleep (30-second epoch). The horizontal *amplitude grid lines* in F4-M1 are 75 microvolts (μV) apart. The vertical time lines are 1 second apart. Slow wave activity is present for 6 seconds or greater. Note that slow wave activity is also present in the electromyography (EOG) derivations.

increasing age. This is primarily caused by a decrease in the amplitude of slow waves that occurs in men with aging. Sleep staging based on the criteria of the *R&K Manual* used central derivations to detect the amount of stage 3 and 4 sleep. As slow waves have a greater amplitude in the frontal regions, the amount of stage N3 exceeds the amount of stage 3 and stage 4 using R&K rules with central derivations.

REFERENCES

1. Iber C, Ancoli-Israel S, Chesson A, Quan SF: for the American Academy of Sleep Medicine: *The AASM manual for scoring of sleep and associated events: rules, terminology and technical specifications*, ed 1, Westchester, IL, 2007, American Academy of Sleep Medicine.
2. Silber MH, Ancoli-Israel S, Bonnet MH, et al: The visual scoring of sleep in adults, *J Clin Sleep Med* 15:121–131, 2007.
3. Rechtschaffen A, Kales A (eds) *A manual of standardized terminology techniques and scoring system for sleep stages of human sleep*, Los Angeles, 1968, Brain Information Service/Brain Research Institute, UCLA.
4. Berry RB, Brooks R, Gamaldo CE, et al: for the American Academy of Sleep Medicine: *The AASM manual for the scoring of sleep and associated events: rules, terminology and technical specifications*, Version 2.0, Darien, IL, 2012, American Academy of Sleep Medicine. www.aasmnet.org, Accessed June 1, 2014.

A 35-Year-Old Woman Who is Taking Fluoxetine and a Benzodiazepine

Patient A: Thirty second tracing of stage N2 from a sleep study of a patient with depression and daytime sleepiness is shown in Figure P3-1. The patient is taking fluoxetine and clonazepam.

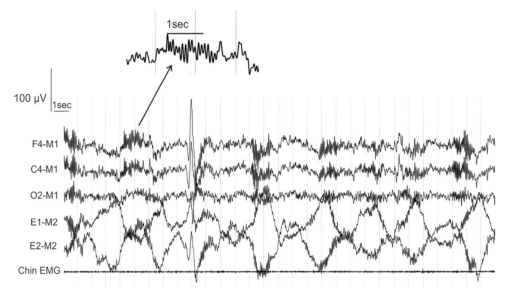

FIGURE P3-1 ■ A 30-second tracing, with magnification of a waveform present in frequent bursts of activity.

QUESTIONS

1. What is the pattern of the eye movements shown in Figure P3-1 called?

2. Why are the bursts of the waveform shown in the blow-up in Figure P3-1 so frequent?

3. Figure P3-2 is a 30-second tracing of the patient undergoing biocalibration. During this procedure, the patient is asked to open and close the eyes and to look up, down, left, and right. Consider the first commands. In what order were the commands "eyes open" and "eyes closed" given?

ANSWERS

1. **Answer:** The eye movement pattern is called *Prozac eyes*.

   Discussion: Such eye movements were first described in patients taking fluoxetine, but the pattern is common in patients taking any selective serotonin reuptake inhibitor (SSRI). Slow eye movement may be seen in eyes-closed wakefulness and stage N1 sleep. Normally, eye movements cease during stage N2 sleep. However, SSRI eyes are often present during stage N2. Of note, the pattern of SSRI

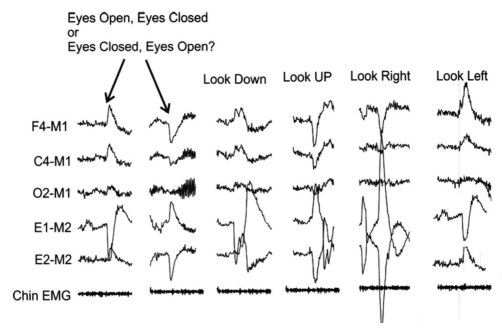

FIGURE P3-2 ■ Tracings during biocalibration. The patient performed eye movements at the commands (Look down, Look up, Look right, Look left) from the sleep technologist.

eyes may be a mixture of slow eye movements (SEMs) and more rapid eye movements (REMs).[2,3] SSRI eye movements are not thought to have special significance but may make staging sleep more challenging (specifically scoring stage N2 and stage R).

2. **Answer:** Sleep spindle bursts are frequent, which is consistent with the use of clonazepam.

    Discussion: Sleep spindle activity is pronounced, which suggests that the patient is taking a benzodiazepine receptor agonist (BZRA)[4,5] (e.g., a benzodiazepine or non-benzodiazepine hypnotic such as zolpidem, eszopiclone, or zaleplon). Frequent spindles in patients taking BZRAs are sometimes called *drug spindles*. They tend to be faster, but in this patient, spindle activity is 12 to 13 Hz. Recall that sleep spindles may range from 11 to 16 Hz. How many sleep spindle bursts per epoch is abnormal? In general, the number of sleep spindle bursts per epoch decreases with age. For patients of age greater than 20 years, more than 4 to 5 sleep spindles bursts per epoch suggests the possibility of a BZRA medication effect. Benzodiazepines increase sleep spindle activity and decrease the amplitude of slow waves and therefore tend to reduce the amount of stage N3. The non-benzodiazepine BZRAs also increase sleep spindles bursts but have much less effect of slow wave amplitude. Hence they do not reduce the amount of stage N3. In this patient, the benzodiazepine clonazepam is causing the frequent bursts of sleep spindles. Clonazepam is a benzodiazepine with a long duration of action that is used for its antianxiety activity. Although not approved by the U.S. Food and Drug Administration (FDA) as a hypnotic, it is often used for this indication in patients with both anxiety and insomnia.

3. **Answer:** "Eyes open," "eyes closed"

    Discussion: When the eyes are closed, the globe is turned upward (Bell phenomenon). With eye opening, the globe turns downward. As the cornea is positive, this makes E1 more positive and E2 more negative, which results in a downward deflection in E1-M2 and an upward deflection in E2-M2. For eye closure, the globe turns upward, and the deflections in E1 and E2 are the opposite. Deflections in the frontal derivations may also be seen and are parallel to changes in E2-M2, as E2, F3, and F4 are located above the eyes. Note the upward deflection in F4-M1 with eye opening in parallel with E2-M2. For lateral eye movements, remember that the rightward movement makes E2 more positive (downward deflection) and E1 more negative (upward deflection). As F4 is on the right side, deflections with lateral movements are similar to E2 and for F3 similar to E1. In Figure P3-1, note the upward deflection in E2-M2 and F4-M1 with eye opening and the downward deflection in E-M1 and F4-M1 with lateral eye movement to the right.

CLINICAL PEARLS

1. It is important to review a patient's history for drugs that may affect the PSG waveforms, sleep architecture, or both.

2. Patients taking SSRIs may have persistent eye movements in stage N2. Normally, eye movements have ceased with transition to stage N2. Recall that SEMs may be seen both in stage W and stage N1.

3. BZRAs may increase the frequency of sleep spindle bursts per epoch.

4. Eye opening is associated with a downward deflection of the globe and eye closure with an upward deflection (Bell phenomenon). F4-M1 has upward deflections with eye opening and downward with eye closure. Deflections in F4-M1 parallel deflections in E2-M2 as both electrodes are above the eyes on the right side of the body.

REFERENCES

1. Berry RB, Brooks R, Gamaldo CE, et al: for the American Academy of Sleep Medicine: *The AASM manual for the scoring of sleep and associated events: rules, terminology and technical specifications*, Version 2.0, Darien, IL, 2012, American Academy of Sleep Medicine. www.aasmnet.org, Accessed June 1, 2014.
2. Schenck CH, Mahowald MW, Kim SW, et al: Prominent eye movements during NREM sleep and REM sleep behavior disorder associated with fluoxetine treatment of obsessive-compulsive disorder, *Sleep* 15:226–235, 1992.
3. Armitage R, Trivedi M, Rush AJ: Fluoxetine and oculomotor activity during sleep in depressed patients, *Neuropsychopharmacology* 12:159–165, 1995.
4. Nicolas A, Petit D, Rompré S, Montplaisir J: Sleep spindle characteristics in healthy subjects of different age groups, *Clin Neurophysiol* 112:521–527, 2001.
5. Johnson LC, Spinweber CL, Seidel WF, et al: Sleep spindle and delta changes during chronic use of a short acting and a long acting benzodiazepine hypnotic, *Electroencephalogr Clin Neurophysiol* 55:662–667, 1983.
6. Libenson MH: *Practical approach to electroencephalography*, Philadelphia, 2010, Saunders pp. 27–20, 126–129.
7. Berry RB: *Fundamentals of sleep medicine*, Philadelphia, 2012, Saunders, pp. 48–52.

PATIENT 4

Scoring Stage N1 versus Stage W in Two Patients

Patient A: A 30-second epoch soon after lights out is shown in Figure P4-1.

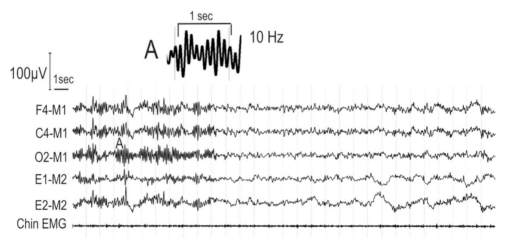

FIGURE P4-1 ■ A 30-second epoch soon after the start of the sleep study.

Patient B: A 30-second epoch in a patient who does not generate alpha rhythm with eye closure is shown in Figure P4-2. Assume the previous epoch is stage W.

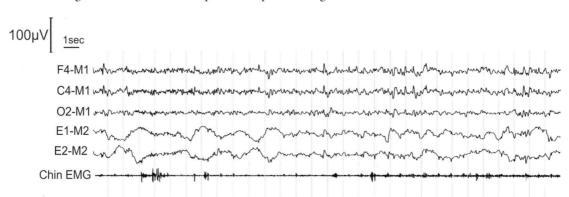

FIGURE P4-2 ■ A 30-second epoch following an epoch of stage W. This patient does not generate alpha rhythm with eye closure.

QUESTIONS

1. What sleep stage is shown in Figure P4-1?

2. What sleep stage is shown in Figure P4-2?

ANSWERS

1. **Answer:** Stage N1

   Discussion: Alpha rhythm is present in the first third of the epoch (A) but is attenuated for the majority of the epoch and replaced by low amplitude mixed frequency activity. No sleep spindles or K-complexes are present. Thus, the epoch meets criteria for stage N1. The EEG of stage N1 is low-amplitude mixed-frequency (LAMF) with predominant activity in the 4 to 8 Hz range. Stage N1 may contain slow eye movements (SEMs). Vertex sharp waves often occur at the transition to stage N2.

2. **Answer:** Stage N1

   Discussion: In individuals who do not generate alpha rhythm with eye closure, the occipital electroencephalography (EEG) stage W with eyes open and eyes closed, appear much the same. The EEG shows low amplitude activity with a mixture of alpha and beta frequencies without the rhythmicity of alpha rhythm. Electrooculographic derivations may show REMs, blinks, or reading eye movements. Chin electromyography (EMG) tone is variable but usually higher than during sleep. In individuals who do not generate alpha rhythm with eye closure, the *AASM Scoring Manual*[1,2] states that stage W should be scored if the majority of the epoch contains *any* of the following: rapid eye movements (REMs) with normal or high muscle tone, eye blinks, or reading eye movements. The requirement of normal or high muscle tone with REMs is to differentiate stage W with REMs from stage R (low muscle tone). The *AASM Scoring Manual* states that stage N1 should be scored in patients who do not generate alpha rhythm at the earliest occurrence of SEMs, vertex sharp waves, or the presence of LAMF activity with a slowing of the EEG by 1 Hz or greater compared with stage W. The *AASM Scoring Manual* does not directly address the position in the epoch where SEMs, vertex sharp waves, or slowing of the EEG first occur. However, by convention, the sleep stage occupying the majority of the epoch names the epoch. If these phenomenon occur in the first half of the epoch then stage N1 is scored (unless there is evidence for another sleep stage). In Figure P4-2, SEMs are noted in the first half of the epoch, so stage N1 is scored. If the first

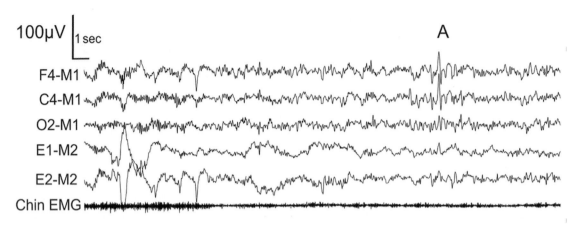

FIGURE P4-3 ■ A 30-second epoch following an epoch of stage W in a patient who does not generate alpha rhythm with eye closure. This is stage N1 as the slow eye movements appear in the first half of the epoch. A vertex sharp wave is noted at A.

evidence of stage N1 was in the last half of the epoch, then the current epoch would be stage W and the next epoch stage N1. This assumes that no evidence for another sleep stage (e.g., stage N2) exists in the following epoch.

In Figure P4-3, another example of an epoch at sleep onset in a patient who does not generate alpha activity is shown. The first part of the epoch has REMs associated with higher EMG tone than is present for the rest of the epoch (consistent with stage W). However, the chin EMG falls during the first half of the epoch, REMs cease, the EEG slows, and slow eye movements are noted. As the slow eye movements and EEG slowing begin in the first half of the epoch, the majority of the epoch meets criteria for stage N1. Therefore, the epoch is scored as stage N1. A vertex sharp wave is also seen in the last half of the epoch (A).

CLINICAL PEARLS

1. The scoring rules for stage W and N1 are different for patients who do not generate alpha rhythm with eye closure.

2. In individuals who do not generate alpha rhythm with eye closure, stage W is scored if REMs with normal or high muscle tone, eye blinks, or reading eye movements are present for the majority of the epoch.

3. In patients who do not generate alpha rhythm with eye closure, stage N1 is scored at the earliest occurrence of any of the following phenomenon: SEMs, vertex sharp waves, or the presence of LAMF EEG activity with a slowing of the frequency by 1 Hz or greater compared with stage W.

REFERENCES

1. Iber C, Ancoli-Israel S, Chesson A, Quan SF, for the American Academy of Sleep Medicine: *The AASM manual for scoring of sleep and associated events: rules, terminology and technical specifications,* ed 1, Westchester, IL, 2007, American Academy of Sleep Medicine.
2. Berry RB, Brooks R, Gamaldo CE, et al: *for the American Academy of Sleep Medicine: The AASM manual for the scoring of sleep and associated events: rules, terminology, and technical specifications,* Version 2.0, Darien, IL, 2012, American Academy of Sleep Medicine, www.aasmnet.org, Accessed June 1, 2014.

Recognizing Stages N1 and N2

QUESTIONS

1. What is the sleep stage in Figure P5-1? Assume the previous epoch was stage N1.

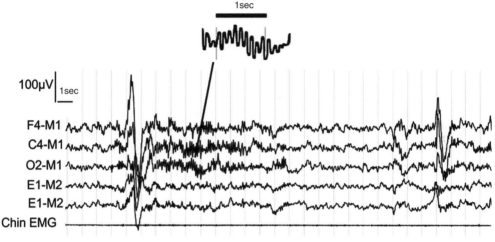

FIGURE P5-1 ■ A 30-second tracing. Assume the previous epoch was stage N1.

2. What sleep stage is shown in Figure P5-2?

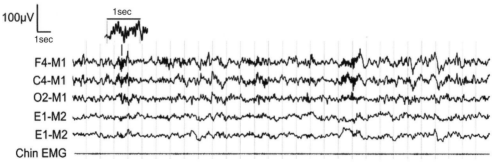

FIGURE P5-2 ■ A 30-second tracing with a blow up of waveform activity.

3. Figures P5-3 and P5-4 are two consecutive epochs. What sleep stage are these epochs?

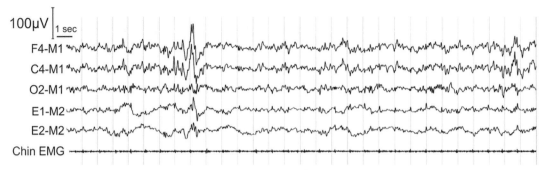

FIGURE P5-3 ▦ A 30-second tracing. Figure P5-4 is the next epoch.

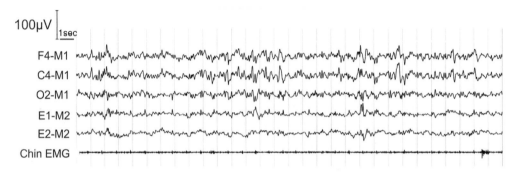

FIGURE P5-4 ▦ A 30-second tracing of the epoch following the one in Figure P5-3.

ANSWERS

1. **Answer:** Stage N1

   Discussion: The K-complex (KC) in the first part of the figure is associated with an arousal (note alpha activity) and therefore the epoch should not be scored as stage N2. A KC not associated with an arousal is present in the second half of the epoch. The next epoch would be scored as stage N2 if electroencephalography (EEG) continued to demonstrate low-amplitude mixed-frequency (LAMF) activity even if another KC or sleep spindle was not present in that epoch. Although the arousal occupies a considerable amount of the time, majority of the epoch in Figure P5-1 was sleep. Arousal scoring is discussed in Fundamentals 5. Score an arousal during sleep stages N1, N2, and N3 if an abrupt shift of EEG frequency, including alpha, theta, and frequencies greater than 16 Hz (but not spindles), lasts *at least 3 seconds*, with at least 10 seconds of stable sleep preceding the change. Scoring of an arousal during stage R requires a concurrent increase in the submental (chin) electromyography (EMG) tone, lasting at least 1 second.[1-3] KCs may be associated with sleep spindles. Therefore, it is important to avoid incorrectly identifying a KC associated with sleep spindles as a KC associated with an arousal. If necessary, go to a 10-second window, and count oscillations to determine the wave form frequency. In Figure P5-1, a blow-up shows the frequency to be 8 to 9 hertz (Hz).

2. **Answer:** Stage N2

   Discussion: Sleep spindles are noted in the first half of the epoch, and not enough slow wave activity is present to score stage N3. The sleep spindle shown in the blow-up has a frequency of 14 Hz.

3. **Answer:** Both epochs are stage N2

   Discussion: The first epoch has a KC (not associated with an arousal) in the first half and is stage N2. The second epoch does not have KCs or sleep spindles but is still stage N2, according to the stage N2 continuation rule. Epochs with LAMF EEG activity without KCs or sleep spindles are scored as stage N2 if they follow epochs with sleep spindles of KCs. This assumes that there is no intervening arousal or intervening major body movements followed by slow eye movements.

CLINICAL PEARLS

1. A K complex (KC) associated with an arousal does not indicate the presence of stage N2 sleep. The KC arousal event affects sleep staging in the same way as an arousal without a KC. It is important not to confuse a KC associated with spindles with a KC arousal.

2. Epochs following an epoch of definite stage N2 (one or more KCs or sleep spindles in first half of the epoch or last half of previous epoch) continue to be scored as stage N2, even if the epochs in question do not contain KCs or sleep spindles. This assumes that no intervening arousal or a transition to stage W, stage N3, or stage R exists.

REFERENCES

1. Iber C, Ancoli-Israel S, Chesson A, Quan SF: for the American Academy of Sleep Medicine: *The AASM manual for scoring of sleep and associated events: rules, terminology and technical specifications,* ed 1, Westchester, IL, 2007, American Academy of Sleep Medicine.
2. Silber MH, Ancoli-Israel S, Bonnet MH, et al: The Visual scoring of sleep in adults, *J Clin Sleep Med* 15:121–131, 2007.
3. Berry RB, Brooks R, Gamaldo CE, et al., for the American Academy of Sleep Medicine: *The AASM manual for the scoring of sleep and associated events: rules, terminology and technical specifications,* Version 2.0, Darien, IL, 2012, American Academy of Sleep Medicine. www.aasmnet.org, Accessed June 1, 2014.

PATIENT 6

Recognizing Stage N3 in a Normal Individual and a Patient with Chronic Pain

QUESTIONS

1. What sleep stage is shown in the 30-second tracing in Figure P6-1? Amplitude gridlines of +37.5 and −37.5 microvolts (µV) are shown for derivation F4-M1.

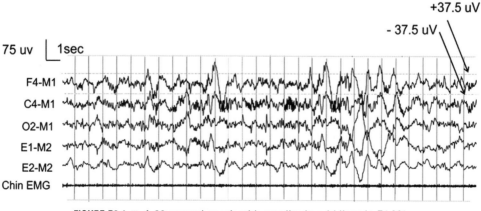

FIGURE P6-1 ■ A 30-second epoch with amplitude grid lines in F4-M1.

2. What is the sleep stage shown in Figure P6-2 with a blow-up in Figure P6-3? What is the name of this particular pattern of this sleep stage? Assume the second 15 seconds has the same characteristics as the 15 seconds shown.

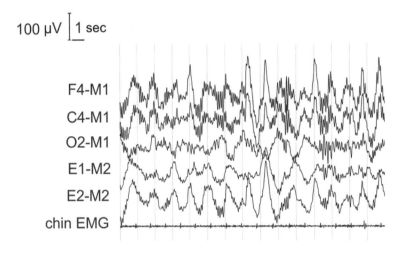

FIGURE P6-2 ■ A 15-second tracing.

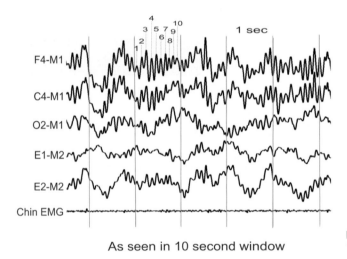

As seen in 10 second window

FIGURE P6-3 ■ A 6-second tracing (as seen in a 10-second window) of Figure P6-2.

ANSWERS

1. **Answer:** Stage N3

   Discussion: Just enough slow wave activity (SWA) is present to meet the criteria for stage N3—about 8 seconds (≥6 seconds required) (Figure P6-4). The dark bars at the top of Figure P6-4 indicate portions meeting the criteria for SWA (0.5 to 2 hertz [Hz] with >75 μV peak-to-peak amplitude of the electroencephalography (EEG) frequency in F4-M1). It is sometimes difficult to see the background of 0.5 to 2 Hz and to determine if amplitude criteria are met. In Figure P6-5, a schematic shows the appearance of waves with frequencies of 0.5, 1, and 2 Hz.

2: **Answer:** Studies have shown that for epochs on the borderline between stage N2 and N3 that scorer agreement is often as low as 50%.[1] Stage N3, as slow wave activity is present for the entire epoch. The patient has alpha–delta sleep. Alpha waves are superimposed on the slow waves.

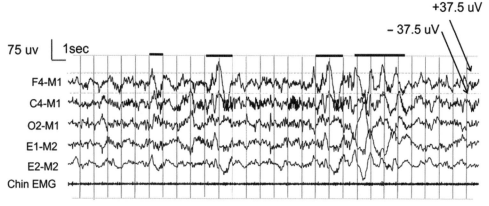

FIGURE P6-4 ■ Stage N3 with slow wave activity (SWA) shown by dark horizontal bars on the top of the tracing. Amplitude grid lines of −37.5 and +37.5 μV allow one to determine if amplitude criteria are met.

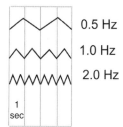

FIGURE P6-5 ■ Illustration of the frequency range 0.5 to 2 hertz (Hz) used to determine slow wave activity.

Discussion: The finding of prominent alpha activity (8–13 Hz) during non–rapid eye movement (NREM) sleep is often called *alpha anomaly, alpha sleep, alpha intrusion,* or *alpha–delta sleep* (if noted in association with stage N3). Prominent alpha activity makes sleep staging more challenging. Of interest, the alpha activity may be more prominent in the frontal regions than in the occipital regions in contrast to the typical alpha rhythm. When viewing a tracing of alpha–delta sleep in a 30-second window (see Figure P6-2), a background of diffuse higher-frequency activity is felt to be superimposed on the slow waves. By switching to a 10-second window (see Figure P6-3), the smaller wave forms that are superimposed on slower activity (alpha 8–13 Hz) can be counted in 1 second.

First described in 1973 by Hauri and Hawkings,[2] alpha–delta sleep was once thought to be a characteristic finding associated with fibromyalgia (FM).[3] However, alpha sleep is not seen in all patients with FM and may occur in patients with psychiatric and chronic pain disorders. Mahowald and Mahowald[4] concluded that alpha sleep was not specific for FM and was not necessarily associated with symptoms of myalgia. It was present in 15% of normal subjects in undisturbed sleep.

Roizenblatt and coworkers[5] also studied patients with FM who were off medications and normal controls. Alpha rhythm was noted during sleep in 70% of patients with FM and 16% of normal individuals. Three distinct patterns were noted: (1) phasic alpha patterns—episodic alpha occurring simultaneously with delta activity (70% FM, 7% controls); (2) tonic alpha continuously present throughout NREM sleep (20% of FM and 9% of controls); and (3) low alpha pattern seen in 30% of FM patients and 84% of controls. The phasic pattern was associated with lower sleep efficiency, decreased slow wave sleep, longer morning pain, and subjective feeling of superficial sleep. Further research is needed to confirm these findings.

CLINICAL PEARLS

1. To determine slow wave activity, place amplitude grid lines $-37.5 + 37.5 \, \mu V$ to identify slow activity with greater than 75 μV peak-to-peak activity in F4-M1 (or F3-M2).
2. If a fast frequency appears to be superimposed on slow waves, switch to a 10-second window to determine if fast activity is in the alpha range. This may help identify alpha–delta sleep.
3. Alpha sleep is nonspecific but is present in many patients with psychiatric disorders and chronic pain syndromes. It may be a normal variant. One study suggests that when alpha activity is restricted to stage N3 sleep (versus all stages of sleep), it may be more specific for disorders associated with chronic pain. However, the pattern may still be a normal variant.

REFERENCES

1. Rosenberg RS, Van Hout S: The American Academy of Sleep Medicine inter-scorer reliability program: sleep stage scoring, *J Clin Sleep Med* 9:81–87, 2013.
2. Hauri P, Hawkins DR: Alpha-delta sleep, *Electroenceph Clin Neurophysiol* 34:233–237, 1973.
3. Moldofsky H, Scarisbrick P, England R, Smythe H: Musculoskeletal symptoms and non-REM sleep disturbance in patients with "fibrositis syndrome" and healthy subjects, *Psychosom Med* 37:341–351, 1975.
4. Mahowald ML, Mahowald MW: Nighttime sleep and daytime functioning (sleepiness and fatigue) in less well defined chronic rheumatic disease with particular reference to "alpha-delta NREM sleep anomaly," *Sleep Med* 1:195–207, 2000.
5. Roizenblatt S, Moldofsky H, Benedito-Silva AA, Tufik S: Alpha sleep characteristics in fibromyalgia, *Arthritis Rheum* 44:222–230, 2001.

Scoring Stage R

The electroencephalographic (EEG) activity in stage R resembles that of stage N1 and generally contains low-amplitude mixed-frequency (LAMF) activity (frequencies 4 to 7 hertz [Hz]). However, alpha activity in also commonly present in stage R and usually has a frequency 1 to 2 Hz lower than during wakefulness.[1-4] Because rapid eye movements (REMs) may occur during eyes-open wakefulness, the presence of low chin electromyographic (EMG) tone is essential for identification of stage R (versus stage W with REMs). In the *AASM Scoring Manual*,[1-4] *low chin EMG tone* is defined as baseline EMG activity in the chin derivation no higher than in any other sleep stage and usually at the lowest level of the entire night.

Sawtooth waves in the EEG (see Fundamentals 2) and brief transient muscle activity (TMA) in the chin EMG (see Patient 9) are often present during stage R but are not part of the criteria for scoring stage R. However, the presence of sawtooth waves or TMA is supportive that stage R is present. Sawtooth waves are characterized by triangular waves with serrated edges and a frequency of 2 to 6 Hz maximal over central

regions. TMA is characterized by short irregular bursts of EMG activity (<0.25 seconds) in the chin derivations superimposed on low chin activity. TMA may also occur in leg derivations often associated with bursts of REMs.

The three components of stage R include (1) LAMF EEG without K-complexes (KCs) or sleep spindles, (2) rapid eye movements (REMs), and (3) low chin EMG tone (Figure F4-1). An epoch containing all three characteristics of stage R is referred to as definite or *unambiguous stage R*.

The three components of stage R may not all start and stop at the same time. In addition, REMs are episodic, and not all epochs of stage R contain REMs. Therefore, special rules are needed for the start, continuation, and end of stage R as well as transitions from other sleep stages to REM sleep. During periods of REM sleep early in the night, segments of sleep may have a mixture of KCs or sleep spindles and REMs. Rules for scoring segments of the record with a mixture of REMs, low chin muscle tone, and KCs, or sleep spindles, or a combination of all of these; these are also discussed in this chapter.

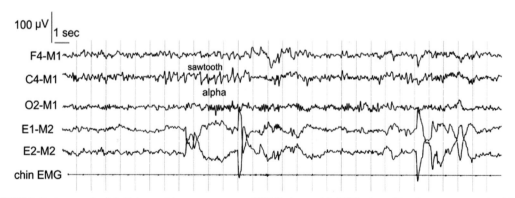

FIGURE F4-1 ■ An epoch of definite rapid eye movement (REM) sleep with REMs, low chin electromyography (EMG) tone, and an electroencephalography (EEG) with low amplitude mixed frequency activity without K- complexes or sleep spindles. Sawtooth waves (C4-M1) and a burst of alpha activity (O2-M1) are also present in this epoch and are often present during stage R. However sawtooth waves are not required for scoring stage R. Alpha activity during stage R is often 1 to 2 Hz lower in frequency than the alpha activity during stage W.

RULES FOR SCORING STAGE R

Rules for scoring stage R are displayed in Tables F4-1, F4-2, and F4-3 (adapted from the *AASM Scoring Manual*[1–4]).

DEFINITE STAGE R

Score stage R sleep (definite stage R) in epochs with ALL of the following phenomena (REM rule 1, Table F4-1):

a. LAMF EEG activity without KCs or sleep spindles
b. Low chin EMG tone for the majority of the epoch and concurrent with REMs
c. REMs at any position within the epoch

An example of an epoch of definite stage R is shown in Figure F4-1.

START OF STAGE R

Segments of sleep *that precede and are contiguous with an epoch of definite stage R* (REM rule 1, Table F4-1) are scored as stage R if the EEG shows LAMF activity without KCs or sleep spindles, the chin EMG activity is at the REM level, and no intervening arousal occurs (REM rule 2, Table F4-1). The segments of sleep must also not contain slow eye movements (SEMs) that follow an arousal or stage W. SEMs may sometimes be seen in stage R (usually mixed with REMs). However, SEMs following an arousal or stage W are evidence for a transition to stage N1.

If the *majority* of an epoch meets all the above criteria (REM rules 2a to 2d, Table F4-1), the epoch is scored as stage R. *If a conflict with a stage N2 rule exists, REM rules take precedence.*

TABLE F4-1   Stage R Rules: Part 1

1. Score stage R sleep in epochs with ALL of the following phenomena (definite stage R):
   a. Low-amplitude, mixed-frequency (LAMF) EEG activity without K-complexes or sleep spindles
   b. Low chin EMG tone for the majority of the epoch and concurrent with REMs
   c. Rapid eye movements (REMs) at any position within the epoch

2. Begin scoring stage R according to the following rule: Score segments of sleep preceding and contiguous with an epoch of definite stage R in the *absence of rapid eye movements*, as stage R IF all of the following are present:
   a. The EEG shows LAMF activity without K-complexes or sleep spindles
   b. The chin EMG tone is low (at the stage R level)
   c. No intervening arousal is present
   d. Slow eye movements following an arousal or stage W are absent
   If the majority of an epoch meets all the criteria (2a to 2d), the epoch is scored as stage R. If there is a conflict with a stage N2 rule, REM rules takes precedence.

3. Continue to score segments of sleep that follow one or more epochs of definite stage R as defined in rule 1, in the absence of rapid eye movements, as stage R if ALL of the following are present:
   a. The EEG shows LAMF EEG activity without K-complexes or sleep spindles
   b. The chin EMG tone is low (at the stage R level) for the majority of the epoch
   c. There is no intervening arousal
   If the majority of an epoch meets these criteria, the epoch is scored as stage R.

Adapted from references 1 and 4.
EEG, Electroencephalography; *EMG*, electromyography.

TABLE F4-2   REM Rules: Part 2

4. End scoring stage R sleep when ONE OR MORE of the following occur:
   a. Transition to stage W or N3 has occurred.
   b. An increase in chin electromyography (EMG) tone above the level of stage R is seen for the majority of the epoch and criteria for stage N1 are met.
   c. Arousal occurs and is followed by low-amplitude, mixed-frequency (LAMF) electroencephalography (EEG) and the EMG tone remains low. If slow eye movements (SEMs) follow the arousal, score the segment containing them as stage N1, and continue to score stage N1 until evidence for another stage of sleep is present. If no SEMs follow the arousal and chin EMG tone remains low, continue to score as stage R.
   d. A major body movement followed by SEMs and LAMF EEG without K-complexes (KCs) or sleep spindles (SS), score stage N1 until evidence for another sleep stage. (If no SEMs are present, and chin tone remains low, continue to score stage R).*
   e. One or more K complexes or sleep spindles are present in the first half of the epoch in the absence of rapid eye movements, even if chin EMG tone remains low. (Score the epoch as stage N2.)

Adapted from references 1 and 4.
*Score epoch containing major body movement (MBM) by MBM rules (see Fundamentals 5).

TABLE F4-3 Stage R Rules Part 3

5. Score segments of the record with low chin (EMG) activity (at the stage R level) and a mixture of rapid eye movements (REMs) and sleep spindles, and/or K-complexes as follows:
a. Segments between two K-complexes, two sleep spindles, or a K-complex and sleep spindle without intervening REMs are considered stage N2.
b. Segments of the record containing REMs without K-complexes or sleep spindles and chin EMG tone at the REM level are considered stage R.
c. If the majority of an epoch contains a segment(s) considered stage N2, it is scored as stage N2. If the majority of an epoch contains a segment (s) considered stage R, it is scored as stage R.

Adapted from references 1 and 4.

Stage R most commonly starts following a transition from stage N2 (Figures F4-2 and F4-3). However, transitions to stage R from other sleep stages (e.g., N1, N3) or wake may occur (Figure F4-4).

CONTINUATION OF STAGE R

Continue to score segments of sleep that follow one or more epochs of definite stage R, *in the absence of rapid eye movements,* as stage R if ALL

FIGURE F4-2 ■ Transition from stage N2 to definite stage R (Epochs 103 and 203). Epochs 101, 102, and 202 are scored as stage R, as the chin EMG tone is low for the majority of the epoch, no sleep spindles or K complexes are present, and the epochs are contiguous with an epoch of definite stage R (REM rule 2, Table F4-1). In Epoch 201, chin EMG does not drop to the rapid eye movement (REM) level until the last part of the epoch (scored as stage N2).

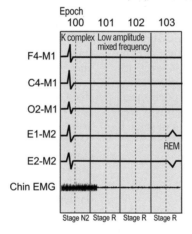

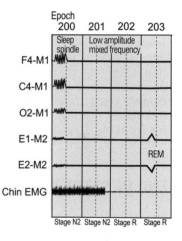

FIGURE F4-3 ■ Transition between stage N2 and definite R. Stage N2 is considered to be present until the last K complex or sleep spindle. Epoch 102 is scored as stage N2, even if the chin EMG is at the REM level. Epoch 201 could be considered an epoch of definite stage N2 by the Stage N2 rules. However, the REM rules take precedence. Epoch 201 is scored as stage R by REM rule 2 (see Table F4-1). (Reproduced from Berry RB: *Fundamentals of sleep medicine,* Philadelphia, 2012, Saunders, p 40.)

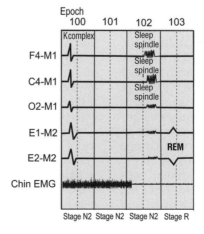

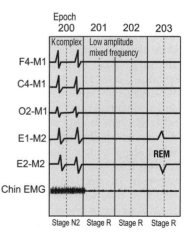

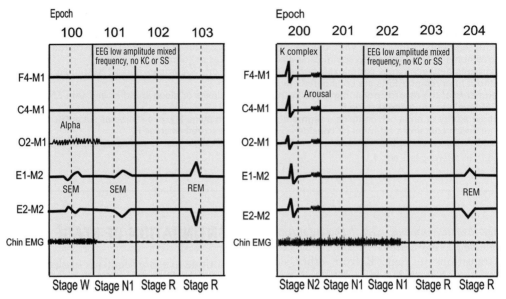

FIGURE F4-4 ■ Transition from stage N1 to definite stage R. Epoch 102 is scored as stage R using REM rule 2 (see Table F4-1). Epoch 101 contains SEMs and is scored as stage N1 even though the chin EMG is at the stage R level. Epoch 203 also meets the criteria in REM rule 2 and is scored as stage R.

of the following are present (REM rule 3, Table F4-1): (a) The EEG shows LAMF EEG activity without KCs or sleep spindles; (b) the chin EMG tone is low (at the stage R level) for the majority of the epoch, and (c) no intervening arousal occurs. If the *majority* of an epoch meets these criteria, (3 a, b, and c), the epoch is scored as stage R. An example of continuation of stage R is shown in Figure F4-5.

END OF STAGE R

Stage R ends if a transition to stage W or N3 occurs (REM rule 4a). A transition to stage N3 is very rare. If chin EMG level increases above the REM level for the majority of the epoch, stage R also ends (see Figure F4-5; REM rule 4b). Stage R may be interrupted by an arousal. An arousal is scored during stage R if an abrupt shift of EEG frequency, including alpha, theta, and or frequencies greater than 16 Hz (but not spindles), lasts at least 3 seconds, with at least 10 seconds of stable sleep preceding the change and a concurrent increase occurs in the submental EMG level lasting at least 1 second (see Fundamentals 5). Bursts of alpha are common in REM sleep and, without a concurrent change in chin EMG, do not indicate an arousal. If the segments of sleep following the arousal continues to have low chin tone and the EEG has LAMF activity without sleep spindles or KCs in the absence of the appearance of SEMs, stage R

continues to be scored (Figure F4-6; REM rule 4c, Table F4-2) until evidence for another sleep stage is present. On the other hand, the appearance of SEM(s) following the arousal suggests a sleep stage transition, and the segment of sleep following the arousal is scored as stage N1. If the majority of the epochs following the arousal contain segments of sleep scored as stage N1, the epochs are scored as stage N1. Stage N1 continues until evidence for another sleep stage is present.

If a major body movement (MBM; see Fundamentals 5) interrupts stage R, the epoch following the MBM epoch continues to be scored as stage R, even in the absence of REMs, if the chin EMG tone remains low for the majority of the epoch and the EEG has LAMF activity without KCs or sleep spindles (Figure F4-7; REM rule 4d, Table F4-2). However, if an SEM is noted following the MBM, this is evidence for a stage shift. The segment of sleep is scored as stage N1 (in the absence of evidence for stage N2). Stage N1 continues until evidence for another sleep stage is present. If the MBM epoch is scored as stage W, stage R ends (REM rule 4a). Of note, the MBM epoch is scored as stage W if it contains any alpha activity. The MBM scoring rules are discussed in Fundamentals 5.

Stage R ends if evidence for stage N2 is present. If a KC or sleep spindle occurs in the first half of an epoch without REMs, stage N2 is scored even if the chin EMG remains at the

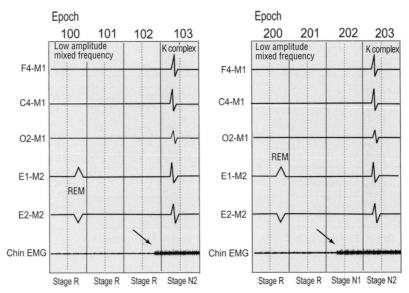

FIGURE F4-5 ■ Continuation of stage R and end of stage R because of an increase in chin EMG tone. Following an epoch of definite stage R (epochs 100 and 200), stage R continues if the chin EMG tone remains low for the majority of the epoch and the electroencephalography (EEG) level has low-amplitude mixed-frequency (LAMF) activity with an absence of K-complexes or sleep spindles (Epochs 101,102, 201). These epochs illustrate REM rule 3 (see Table F4-1). In Epoch 202, the chin EMG tone increases above the rapid eye movement (REM) level for the majority of the epoch. Epoch 202 is scored as stage N1. This epoch illustrates REM Rule 4.b (From Berry RB: *Fundamentals of sleep medicine*, Philadelphia, 2012, Saunders, p 38.)

FIGURE F4-6 ■ Stage R and Arousal. Stage R continues (even if rapid eye movements are absent) following an arousal if the chin EMG tone remains low for the majority of the epoch, the EEG shows low-amplitude mixed-frequency activity without K-complexes or sleep spindles, and SEMs are absent. However, if slow eye movements are present following the arousal, this suggests a stage shift, and stage N1 is scored (REM Rule 4.c, see Table F4-2). (Reproduced from Berry RB: *Fundamentals of sleep medicine*, Philadelphia, 2012, Saunders, p 39.)

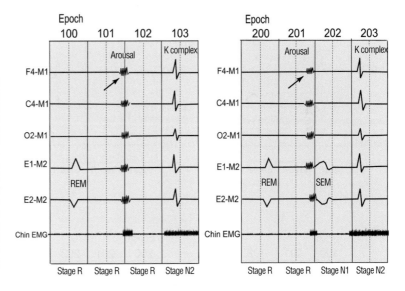

REM level (Figure F4-8; REM rule 4e, Table F4-2).

SCORING SLEEP WITH A MIXTURE OF K-COMPLEXES OR SLEEP SPINDLES AND RAPID EYE MOVEMENTS

Some epochs would otherwise be unambiguous epochs of stage R except that they contain either a KC or a sleep spindle. That is, the epochs

have low chin EMG (at the REM level) and at least one REM. The phenomenon tends to occur in the initial REM period of the night. Sleep is staged according to the rules in Table F4-3. Application of the rules is illustrated in Figure F4-9. Segments of sleep containing REMs, low chin EMG activity, and an EEG without KCs or sleep spindles are considered stage R. Segments of sleep between two KCs, two sleep spindles, or a KC and a sleep spindle without intervening REMs are considered stage N2. A given epoch is scored as stage N2 or R, depending on which sleep stage comprises the majority of the epoch.

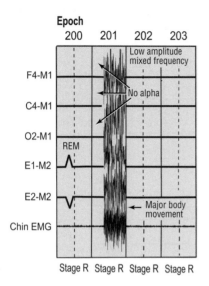

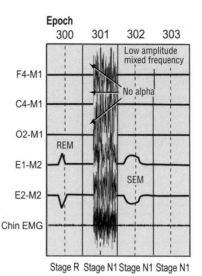

FIGURE F4-7 ■ Stage R interrupted by a major body movement (MBM). If the EEG following the MBM has low-amplitude mixed-frequency activity without a K-complex or sleep spindle and chin EMG remains low for the majority of the epoch, Stage R continues, even if REMs are absent. However, if a slow eye movement follows the MBM, a stage transition is assumed to have occurred and stage N1 is scored (REM Rule 4d, see Table F4-2). (Reproduced from Berry RB: *Fundamentals of sleep medicine*, Philadelphia, 2012, Saunders, p 39.)

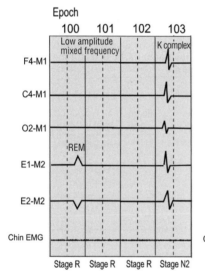

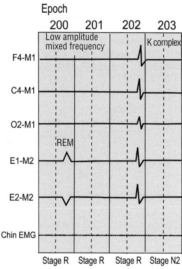

FIGURE F4-8 ■ End of REM sleep because of transition to stage N2. If a K complex (KC) or sleep spindle occurs in the first half of the epoch, stage N2 is scored (in the absence of REMs), even if the chin EMG tone remains low (REM rule 4.e, see Table F4-2). In Epoch 202, the KC does not occur until the last half of the epoch, and the epoch is scored as stage R. The following epoch will be scored as stage N2, even if chin EMG remains at the REM level (assuming no REMs are present).

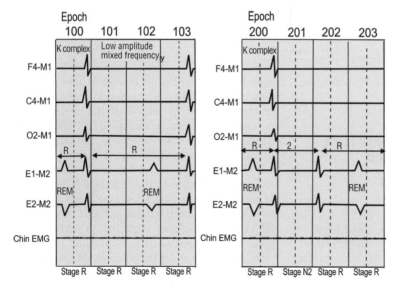

FIGURE F4-9 ■ Scoring of segments of sleep containing a mixture of K complexes and REMs. Segments of sleep containing REMs and low chin EMG without K complexes or sleep spindles are considered stage R. Segments of sleep between two K complexes without intervening REMs are considered stage N2. Epochs are scored based on whether stage N2 or Stage R composes the majority of the epoch (see Table F4-3).

REFERENCES

1. Rechtschaffen A, Kales A, editors: *A manual of standardized terminology techniques and scoring system for sleep stages of human sleep*, Los Angeles, CA, 1968, Brain Information Service/Brain Research Institute, UCLA.
2. Iber C, Ancoli-Israel S, Chesson A, Quan SF: for the American Academy of Sleep Medicine: *The AASM manual for scoring of sleep and associated events: rules, terminology and technical specifications*, ed 1, Westchester, IL, 2007, American Academy of Sleep Medicine.
3. Silber MH, Ancoli-Israel S, Bonnet MH, et al: The visual scoring of sleep in adults, *J Clin Sleep Med* 15:121–131, 2007.
4. Berry RB, Brooks R, Gamaldo CE, et al, for the American Academy of Sleep Medicine: *The AASM manual for the scoring of sleep and associated events: rules, terminology and technical specifications*, Version 2.1, Darien, IL, 2014, American Academy of Sleep Medicine. www.aasmnet.org.

PATIENT 7

An Arousal Interrupts Stage N2 and Stage R Sleep

QUESTIONS

1. Figures P7-1 and P7-2 show consecutive Epochs 100 and 101. What are the sleep stages?

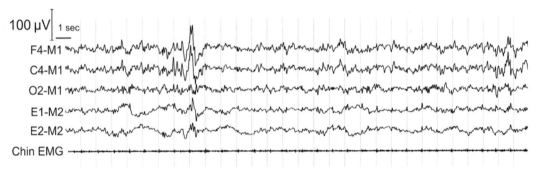

FIGURE P7-1 ■ A 30-second tracing.

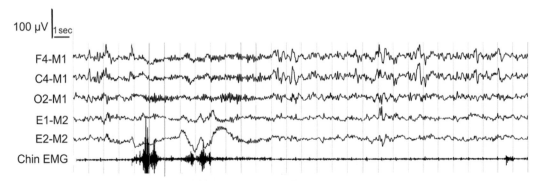

FIGURE P7-2 ■ A 30-second tracing.

2. Figure P7-3 is a 60-second tracing of Epochs 300 and 301. What are the sleep stages?

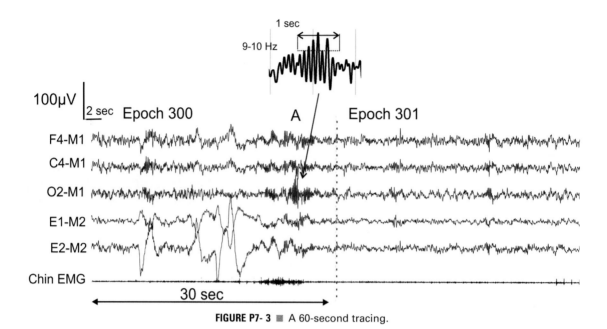

FIGURE P7- 3 ■ A 60-second tracing.

3. What sleep stage in Epoch 202 and 203 is shown in Figure P7-4?

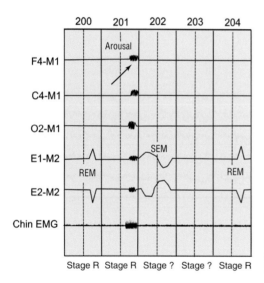

FIGURE P7-4 ■ Schematic of interruption of stage R by an arousal. Assume that electroencephalography (EEG) shows low-amplitude mixed-frequency activity unless otherwise stated. (Adapted from Berry RB: *Fundamentals of sleep medicine*, Philadelphia, 2012, Saunders.)

ANSWERS

1. **Answer:** Epoch 100 is stage N2; Epoch 101 is stage N1.

Discussion: A K-complex (KC) is present in the first half of Epoch 100, and the epoch meets criteria for stage N2. An arousal occurs at the start of Epoch 101. The rules for staging N2 sleep (Fundamentals 3) state that stage N2 ends following an arousal. The subsequent epoch meets criteria for stage N1 with low-amplitude mixed-frequency (LAMF) electroencephalography (EEG) activity. As the arousal was noted in the first third of Epoch 101, the epoch is stage N1. However, had the arousal occurred in the last half of the epoch, most of Epoch 101 would be a continuation of N2 from the previous epoch. In that case, the epoch would be scored as stage N2.

2. **Answer:** Epochs 300 and 301 are stage R.

   Discussion: Although an arousal (A) occurs at the end of Epoch 300, the rules for scoring stage R state that following arousal, if no slow eye movements (SEMs) are present, the chin electromyography (EMG) tone remains low (at the rapid eye movement [REM] level), and the EEG shows LAMF activity without sleep spindles or KCs, then stage R continues. If SEMs are noted following arousal, even if the chin EMG tone returns quickly to the REM level, then stage R ends. The sleep following the arousal would be scored as stage N1 unless evidence for scoring another sleep stage exists.

3. **Answer:** Epoch 202 is scored as stage N1 and epoch 203 as stage R.

   Discussion: If stage R is interrupted by an arousal and the following segment of sleep containing contains SEMs, the segment of sleep containing the SEMs is scored as stage N1, even if the EEG has LAMF activity and the chin EMG tone returns to the REM level for most of the epoch (see Fundamentals 4). Stage N1 continues until there is evidence for another stage of sleep. The last part of epoch 202 (following the SEMs) and all of epoch 203 is scored as stage R as the epoch has LAMF EEG activity and a chin EMG at the REM level even if no REMs are present. Stage R is scored because the epoch 203 is contiguous with an epoch of definite stage R. Note that the majority of epoch 202 is stage N1 and therefore is scored as stage N1.

CLINICAL PEARLS

1. The scoring rules for stage N2 and stage R concerning the effect of an arousal differ (Table P7-1). Unless evidence of a stage shift (SEMs following arousal, increased chin EMG tone, a KC or sleep spindle in the EEG) exists, stage R continues. In contrast, an arousal ends stage N2 (with or without following SEMs). Stage N2 does not start again until a KC or sleep spindle is noted.

2. If an arousal interrupts stage R and is followed by SEMs, stage N1 is scored even if the chin tone quickly reverts to the REM level and the EEG contains low amplitude mixed frequency EEG activity without KC or spindles. Stage N1 is scored until there is evidence for another stage of sleep.

TABLE P7-1 Scoring Rules for Stage N2 and Stage R When Interrupted by an Arousal

	Arousal	Arousal and SEM	Comments
Stage N2	Ends	Ends	This assumes that the epoch following the arousal does not have a KC or SS in the first half of the epoch. The epoch is scored as stage N1 if it has LAMF activity.
Stage R	Continues	Ends	This assumes that the epoch following the arousals has: 1. No SEM 2. LAMF EEG with no KC, SS 3. Chin EMG returns to REM level for the majority of the epoch 4. No REMs (if REMs were present it would be an epoch of definite stage R).

EEG, Electroencephalography; *EMG*, electromyography; *KC*, K-complex without associated arousal; *LAMF*, low-amplitude mixed-frequency electroencephalography activity; REM, rapid eye movement; *SEM*, slow eye movement; *SS*, sleep spindle.

FUNDAMENTALS 5

Arousals and Major Body Movements

AROUSAL RULES

Arousals are transient phenomena that may lead to wakefulness or only briefly interrupt sleep[1–5]. They are important to score, as patients with frequent arousals may have daytime sleepiness, even if the total sleep duration is normal (Box F5-1).

BOX F5-1 | **Arousal Rule**

Score an arousal during sleep stages N1, N2, N3, or R if there is an abrupt shift of EEG frequency including alpha, theta and/or frequencies greater than 16 Hz (but not spindles) that lasts at least 3 seconds, with at least 10 seconds of stable sleep preceding the change. Scoring of arousal during REM requires a concurrent increase in submental EMG lasting at least 1 second.

EEG, Electroencephalography; *EMG,* electromyography; *Hz,* hertz.
From the *AASM Scoring Manual.*

Scoring an arousal during non–rapid eye movement (NREM) sleep **does not depend on an increase in chin electromyography (EMG) activity,** although an increase is often noted along with the shift in electroencephalography (EEG) frequencies. Although a K-complex (KC) or several delta waves may appear concurrently with a change in EEG frequency, these waveforms are not considered evidence for an arousal. As alpha bursts are common during stage R, a concurrent increase in chin EMG activity is required to score an arousal during stage R. Also, note that at least 10 seconds of sleep must be present prior to an event scored as an arousal. The 10 seconds of stable sleep required prior to scoring an arousal may begin in the preceding epoch, including a preceding epoch that is scored as stage W.[5]

In Figure F5-1, an epoch of stage R is illustrated with a burst of alpha at A. The alpha activity during

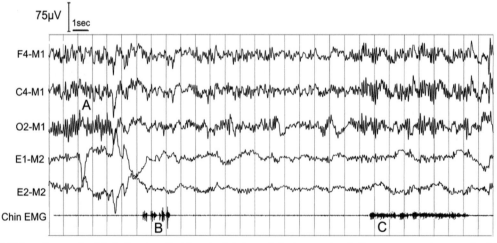

FIGURE F5-1 ■ An epoch of definite stage R. A burst of alpha activity is noted at A. No concurrent increase in the chin electromyography (EMG) is seen, so this is not an arousal. Bursts of alpha activity are common in stage R. A brief period of increased activity in chin EMG activity is noted at B (transient muscle activity). However, no concurrent shift in electroencephalography (EEG) frequency is observed, so no arousal is seen at B. An arousal is noted at C. An abrupt change in EEG frequency (≥3 seconds) and a concurrent increase in the chin EMG (≥1 second) are noted. The majority of the epoch meets criteria for stage R, so the epoch is scored as stage R.

REM sleep is often about 1 hertz (Hz) slower than during wakefulness. No concurrent chin EMG change occurs, so this is not an arousal. A burst of chin EMG activity (transient muscle activity) is seen at B, but no associated abrupt change is seen in the EEG frequency for 3 or more seconds (not an arousal). At C, an abrupt shift in EEG frequency occurs, with a concurrent increase in chin EMG. Thus, an arousal has occurred at C in the last portion of an epoch of stage R sleep.

Although the choice of a 3-second EEG change for scoring an arousal appears arbitrary, studies have shown that reliability of scoring arousals is better with a 3-second EEG change than shorter durations of required EEG change.[3,4] Of note, arousal scoring should incorporate information from both the occipital and central derivations. Controversy exists about whether bursts of slow waves, KCs, or both associated with increased chin EMG should be considered evidence for arousal. At the current time, these are not considered evidence of arousal by the *AASM Scoring Manual*.

MAJOR BODY MOVEMENTS

A **major body movement (MBM)** is defined as movement and muscle artifact obscuring the EEG for more than half an epoch to the extent that the sleep stage cannot be determined. Three scoring rules govern MBM (Box F5-2). First, if the MBM epoch contains any alpha activity, it is scored as stage W. Second, the MBM epoch is scored as stage W if either the preceding or following epochs are definite stage W. Third, if neither of these rules applies, the epoch is scored as the same stage as the epoch that follows it. The scoring rules for MBMs are illustrated in Figure F5-2.

BOX F5-2	**Scoring Rules for Major Body Movements**

A. Score stage W if alpha rhythm is present for part of the epoch (even if <15 seconds in duration).
B. Score stage W in the absence of alpha rhythm if an epoch scorable as stage W either precedes or follows the epoch with the major body movement.
C. If neither A or B apply, score an epoch with a major body movement as the same stage as the epoch that follows it.

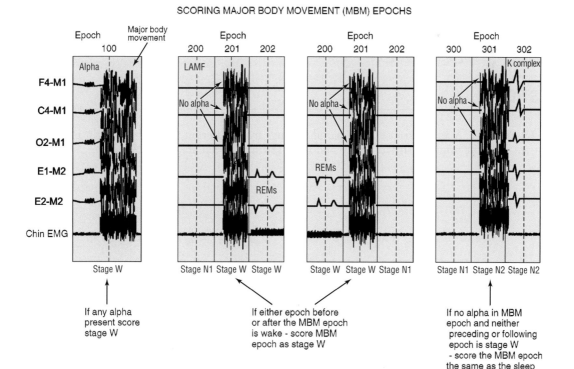

SCORING MAJOR BODY MOVEMENT (MBM) EPOCHS

FIGURE F5-2 ■ Schematic illustrating the scoring of epochs with major body movements and contiguous epochs. (Adapted from Berry RB: *Fundamentals of sleep medicine*, Philadelphia, 2012, Saunders, p. 44.)

CLINICAL PEARLS

1. MBM epochs are scored as stage W if they contain any duration of alpha activity.

2. Arousals cannot be scored on the basis of changes in submental EMG alone.

3. Slow wave activity (delta bursts), when not accompanied by other changes required for an arousal, does not meet the criteria for scoring an arousal.

4. Scoring an arousal during NREM sleep is based on EEG criteria. Scoring an arousal during REM sleep is based on *both* EEG and chin EMG criteria.

5. The duration of changes required for arousal scoring during stage R are EEG frequency changes 3 seconds or greater and increase in chin EMG 1 second or greater. The increase in chin EMG must be concurrent with the abrupt shift in EEG frequency.

6. Transitions from one stage of sleep to another are not scored as arousals unless they meet the criteria indicated above.

REFERENCES

1. Iber C, Ancoli-Israel S, Chesson A, Quan SF, for the American Academy of Sleep Medicine: *The AASM manual for scoring of sleep and associated events: rules, terminology and technical specifications*, ed 1, Westchester, IL, 2007, American Academy of Sleep Medicine.
2. Silber MH, Ancoli-Israel S, Bonnet MH, et al: The visual scoring of sleep in adults, *J Clin Sleep Med* 15:121–131, 2007.
3. Bonnet MH, Doghrqamji K, Roehrs T, et al: The scoring of arousals in sleep: reliability, validity, and alternatives, *J Clin Sleep Med* 147–154, 2007.
4. American Sleep Disorders Association—The Atlas Task Force: EEG arousals: scoring rules and examples, *Sleep* 15:174–184, 1992.
5. Berry RB, Brooks R, Gamaldo CE, et al: for the American Academy of Sleep Medicine: *The AASM manual for the scoring of sleep and associated events: rules, terminology and technical specifications*, Version 2.0, Darien, IL, 2012, American Academy of Sleep Medicine. www.aasmnet.org, Accessed June 1, 2014.

PATIENT 8

Scoring Stage R

QUESTION

1. In Figure P8-1, **A** and **B** are two 15-second tracings from different parts of the night in the same patient with the same sensitivity (gain) and filter settings. What stages are A and B?

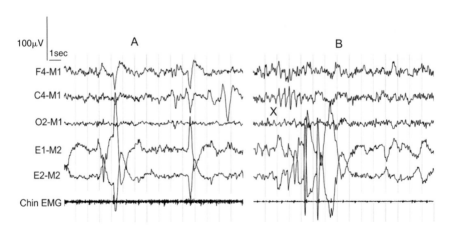

FIGURE P8-1 ■ Two 15-second segments in different parts of the night that both contain rapid eye movements (REMs).

ANSWER

1. **Answer:** Segment A is stage W with the eyes open and segment B is stage R.

   Discussion: Because rapid eye movements (REMs) may occur in both stage W (eyes open) and stage R, correctly identifying these stages depends on chin electromyography (EMG) activity. Chin EMG activity during REM is no higher than any other sleep stage and is often lower than any other sleep stage (the lowest of the night). In stage W, chin activity is usually higher than stage R, and the background electroencephalography (EEG) also typically shows higher-frequency activity. However, in some epochs, differentiating stage R from stage W with REMs and low chin EMG activity may be difficult.

   A drop in chin EMG tone from stage W to stage R cannot be detected if the sensitivity (gain) is not adjusted to see some activity during stage W. An important clue that helps identify stage R is the presence of sawtooth waves[1]. Sawtooth waves are triangular waves in the theta frequency range and are most prominent in the central and frontal derivations (X in segment B of Figure P8-1). Although sawtooth waves are not required to score stage R, their presence may be helpful. Alpha bursts are common in stage R, but the frequency is often 1 to 2 hertz (Hz) lower than during wakefulness. The presence of alpha bursts should *not* eliminate the possibility that stage R is present. Transient muscle activity (TMA) consists of short bursts of activity in chin or leg EMG during stage R. TMA may also provide a clue that an epoch is stage R. The pattern of TMA has a "spiky appearance" (see Patient 9). Although not included in the scoring stage R rules, noting irregular respiration during bursts of REMs or using video to visualize the patient's face during a given epoch is helpful. During stage R, the eyes are closed and obviously open during eyes-open stage W.

   The first episode of stage R during the night is often the most challenging. This REM episode is usually of a short duration, and the REM density (number of REMs per epoch) is lower in the first part of the night. Comparison with unambiguous stage R during later parts of the night may be helpful. Looking at the appearance of eyes-open stage W during calibrations is also helpful in identifying eyes-open wakefulness.

   In the current patient, segment B can be identified as stage R, as the segment has a lower chin EMG tone than segment A and sawtooth waves are present. Segment A has REMs, but the chin EMG tone is above the REM level.

CLINICAL PEARLS

1. Differentiating between stage W with REMs and stage R can be difficult in some individuals. It is important to adjust the chin EMG so some activity is present during eyes-open stage W to see lower amplitude chin EMG activity during stage R.

2. Sawtooth waves are helpful for identification of stage R, even though they are not required for scoring stage R. These waves are most prominent in the central derivations and have a triangular shape with serrated edges.

3. Scoring difficult epochs with REMs is aided by looking at the pattern of eyes-open stage W during biocalibrations and epochs of unambiguous stage R late in the night when the REM density is higher (more REMs per epoch).

REFERENCE

1. Berry RB, Brooks R, Gamaldo CE, et al: for the American Academy of Sleep Medicine: *The AASM manual for the scoring of sleep and associated events: rules, terminology and technical specifications,* Version 2.0, Darien, IL, 2012, American Academy of Sleep Medicine. www.aasmnet.org, Accessed April 5, 2014.

Identifying Stage R in a Woman with Violent Behavior During Sleep

A 70-year-old woman undergoes a sleep study to evaluate snoring and violent behavior at night. Figure P9-1 shows two 15 second tracings recorded during different times during the night.

QUESTION

1. What is the sleep stage of the two tracings in Figure P9-1?

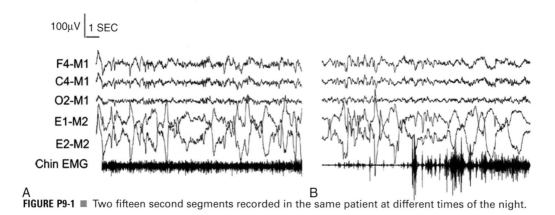

FIGURE P9-1 ■ Two fifteen second segments recorded in the same patient at different times of the night.

ANSWER

1. **Answer:** Epoch A is stage W, and Epoch B is stage R in a patient with REM sleep without atonia.

   Discussion: Both stage W and stage R may have rapid eye movements (REMs) and electroencephalography (EEG) generally shows low-amplitude mixed-frequency (LAMF) activity. The main difference is that the chin electromyography (EMG) tone is at the REM level (no higher than any other sleep stage and usually the lowest of the night) during stage R and is usually higher during stage W. However, telling the difference between stage W and stage R may be very difficult at times (Table P9-1), for example, if the chin EMG tone is actually already quite low during stage W. Another situation is when the patient has REM sleep without atonia as in Figure P9-1. In these patients, sustained chin EMG activity or transient muscle activity (phasic activity) in the chin or leg EMG may be present. Sustained muscle activity (tonic activity) in stage R is defined as a stage R epoch with greater than 50% of the epoch duration with chin EMG amplitude greater than the minimum chin EMG amplitude during non-REM (NREM) sleep. Transient muscle activity (TMA; formerly called "phasic activity") consists of short irregular bursts of EMG activity (usually <0.25 seconds) that has a "spiky" appearance that is distinctive. If TMA is present in either chin EMG or leg EMG, this finding may be helpful in identifying stage R (Figure P9-2). TMA is termed excessive TMA in REM sleep when more than 50% of 10 sequential 3-second mini-epochs contain such EMG activity. Excessive TMA (or an increase in tonic EMG activity during stage R) is said to represent REM sleep without atonia.

TABLE P9-1   Differences between Stage W with REMs and Stage R

	Eyes-Open Wakefulness	Stage R
REMs	Yes	Yes, often in bursts of many eye movements
EEG	Mixture of alpha and beta frequencies	Low-amplitude mixed-frequency (predominantly 4 to 7 hertz [Hz]) Higher frequencies present if patient moving or muscle artifact present
Eyes	Open	Closed
Chin EMG	variable	Usually lowest of the night If REM sleep without atonia: A. sustained EMG activity B. Transient muscle activity
Respiration	Regular	Irregular

EEG, Electroencephalography; *EMG,* Electromyography; *REM,* rapid eye movement.

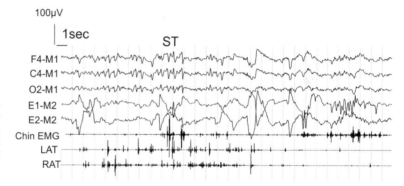

FIGURE P9-2 ■ An epoch of stage R with transient muscle activity in both chin EMG and leg EMG. *EMG,* Electromyography; *LAT,* left anterior tibial EMG; *RAT,* right anterior tibial EMG; *ST,* sawtooth waves.

If REM sleep without atonia is combined with abnormal dream-enacting behavior documented at the time of polysomnography (PSG) (ideally video PSG) or by history, this is consistent with the presence of the REM sleep behavior disorder. The EMG findings alone do *not* allow a diagnosis of REM sleep behavior disorder. Patients on selective serotonin reuptake inhibitors (SSRIs) are especially likely to show TMA, although they usually do not meet criteria for excessive TMA. Winkelman and James[4] determined the number of 2-second bins during REM sleep that contained phasic chin (defined as EMG activity lasting 0.1 to 5 seconds with an amplitude four times the background EMG activity). The mean percentages of 2-second REM sleep bins containing phasic activity in the control group and SSRI groups were 2.36% and 9.54%, respectively ($p = 0.07$).

In stage W with REMs, the eyes are open, and in stage R, the eyes are closed. Therefore, looking at the synchronized video might be helpful if a good view of the eyes is available. In patients with REM sleep without atonia, jerky body movement or overt violent behavior with arms and legs moving (REM sleep behavior disorder) may be present. If overt movement is present, EMG artifact or movement artifact may obscure the EEG reading. Some other clues may be helpful in identifying stage R. During stage R, EEG may show sawtooth waves (ST in Figure P9-2). In EEG, stage W also tends to have higher-frequency activity than stage R. Bursts of eye movements during stage R may be associated with periods of decreased tidal volume.

In the current patient, both segments **A** and **B** in Figure P9-1 have REMs and high chin EMG activity during at least part of the epoch. The epoch in A was taken during biocalibrations, and the video shows open eyes. The epoch in B is an example of REM sleep without atonia, making it difficult to score stage R according to the usual rules. However, note that parts of the epoch in B do have low chin tone as well as a spiky pattern on chin EMG. In at least the first part of the epoch in B, the background EEG frequency is lower than in epoch A. For epochs with movement artifact, it may be impossible to apply the scoring rules to score stage R, and one must depend on the video and the type of behavior noted.

CLINICAL PEARLS

1. In some patients, identification of stage R versus stage W with REMs may be difficult. The chin EMG tone during stage R is at least as low as any other stage and usually the lowest of the night.

2. Correct identification of stage W with REMs versus stage R may be very difficult in patients with REM sleep without atonia. On the other hand, normal individuals may show a limited amount of TMA, and this may be helpful in identifying stage R.

3. Patients taking SSRIs have an increased amount of TMA compared with patients not taking this medication.

4. Synchronized video or audio, although not part of the staging criteria, may be very useful in identifying stage R during periods without atonia.

REFERENCES

1. Iber C, Ancoli-Israel S, Chesson A, Quan SF: for the American Academy of Sleep Medicine: *The AASM manual for scoring of sleep and associated events: rules, terminology and technical specifications*, ed 1, Westchester, IL, 2007, American Academy of Sleep Medicine.
2. Silber MH, Ancoli-Israel S, Bonnet MH, et al: The visual scoring of sleep in adults, *J Clin Sleep Med* 15:121–131, 2007.
3. Berry RB, Brooks R, Gamaldo CE, et al: for the American Academy of Sleep Medicine: *The AASM manual for the scoring of sleep and associated events: rules, terminology and technical specifications*, Version 2.0, Darien, IL, 2012, American Academy of Sleep Medicine. www.aasmnet.org, Accessed April 5, 2014.
4. Winkelman JW, James L: Serotonergic antidepressants are associated with REM sleep without atonia, *Sleep* 15:317–321, 2004.

A Patient with a Major Body Movement During Sleep

QUESTIONS

1. What stage are Epochs 100, 101, and 102 in Figure P10-1? Assume that Epoch 101 has no alpha activity.

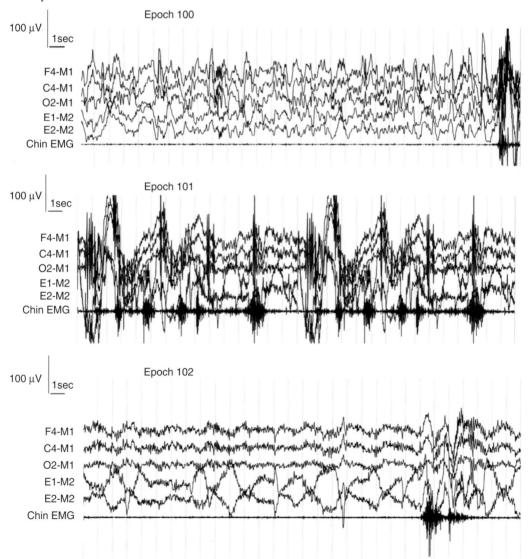

FIGURE P10-1 ■ Three consecutive epochs. Assume no alpha is present in epoch 101.

TABLE P10-1	Three Consecutive Epochs in a Patient with a Major Body Movement		
Epoch	**101**	**102**	**103**
Stage	Stage R	MBM Epoch (? stage)	Stage N1

2. How should epoch 102 in Table P10-1 be staged? Epoch 102 has a major body movement (MBM) but contains no alpha activity.

ANSWERS

1. **Answer:** The epochs are stage N3, stage W, and stage W.

   Discussion: A *major body movement (MBM)* is defined as movement and muscle artifact obscuring electroencephalography (EEG) for more than half an epoch to the extent that the sleep stage cannot be determined.[1-3] The rules for MBM are detailed in Fundamentals 5. In epoch 101 a major body movement obscures the EEG. Epoch 100 is stage N3, given that slow wave activity is present for nearly all of the epoch duration. Epoch 102 is stage W, given the REMs and relatively high chin electromyography (EMG) activity. Note that the chin EMG tone in epoch 100 is actually lower, and therefore epoch 102 cannot be stage R (equal to or lower than the chin EMG activity in NREM sleep and wakefulness). If either the epoch preceding or following an MBM epoch is stage W, then the MBM epoch is stage W.

2. **Answer:** Epoch 102 is stage N1.

   Discussion: If an MBM epoch contains no alpha activity and if the epoch preceding or following the MBM epoch is not stage W, then the MBM epoch is scored as the same stage as the following epoch (in this case stage N1).

REFERENCES

1. Iber C, Ancoli-Israel S, Chesson A, Quan SF: for the American Academy of Sleep Medicine: *The AASM manual for scoring of sleep and associated events: rules, terminology and technical specifications*, ed 1, Westchester, IL, 2007, American Academy of Sleep Medicine.
2. Silber MH, Ancoli-Israel S, Bonnet MH, et al: The visual scoring of sleep in adults, *J Clin Sleep Med* 15:121–131, 2007.
3. Berry RB, Brooks R, Gamaldo CE, et al: for the American Academy of Sleep Medicine: *The AASM manual for the scoring of sleep and associated events: rules, terminology and technical specifications*, Version 2.1, Darien, IL, 2012, American Academy of Sleep Medicine. www.aasmnet.org, Accessed July 3, 2014.

Sleep Staging in Infants and Children

SLEEP STAGING IN INFANTS AND CHILDREN

The *American Academy of Sleep Medicine (AASM) Scoring Manual*[1,2] provides scoring rules for infants older than 2 months and for children. For younger infants, non–rapid eye movement (NREM) sleep is referred to as *quiet sleep* (QS) and stage R as *active sleep* (AS). Rules for scoring the sleep in infants aged 2 months of age or younger are not including in the current AASM scoring manual but are usually based on the Atlas of Anders, Emde, and Parmelee.[3,4]

By 6 months of age, electroencephalography (EEG) in of most infants during sleep shows the familiar wave forms that are used to stage adults sleep (Table F6-1). Behavioral correlates are important for scoring sleep in children 6 months postterm or younger. NREM sleep is characterized by regular respiration, no or rare vertical eye movements, and preserved chin electromyography (EMG) tone. Stage R is characterized by irregular respiration, chin EMG atonia, REMs, and muscle twitching. Spontaneous eye closure in an infant indicates drowsiness.

AGES FOR WHICH AASM PEDIATRIC SLEEP SCORING APPLY

Pediatric sleep scoring rules outlined in the AASM scoring manual may be used to score sleep and wakefulness in children 2 months postterm or older. There is currently no upper age boundary for using the pediatric sleep staging rules.

1. *Postterm* means at least 40 weeks after conception (2 months postterm = 48 weeks conceptional age). For example, for an infant born at 36 weeks post-conception, the scoring rules apply 3 months after birth.
2. No precise upper age limit exists for pediatric rules.

TERMINOLOGY OF SLEEP STAGES

Terminology in children is similar to that in adults except that *stage N* is used to refer to NREM sleep in the absence of characteristic waveforms (sleep spindles, K-complexes [KCs], or slow wave activity [SWA]) (Table F6-2). That is, *stage N* is used for NREM sleep that does not meet the usual criteria for stage N2 or stage N3. Figure F6-1 shows sleep in a 3-month-old infant without development of either sleep spindles or KCs.

TABLE F6-1	Age of Onset of Electroencephalography Activity Used for Staging Sleep
Wave Form	**Age First Seen**
Sleep spindles	2 weeks to 3 months postterm
Slow wave activity	2 to 5 months postterm
K-complexes	3 to 6 months postterm

TABLE F6-2	Nomenclature for Scoring Pediatric Sleep[1,2]
Stages scored	**Waveforms**
Stage N, R	SS, KC, SWA ≥ 6 sec are absent
Stage N, N3, R	KC and SS absent, SWA ≥ 6 sec present
Stage N2, N, R	KC or SS present, SWA ≥ 6 sec absent
Stage N1, N2, N3, R	SS or KC, SWA present

KC, K complex; *SS*, sleep spindles; *SW*, slow wave activity.

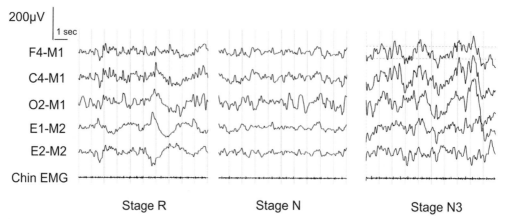

FIGURE F6-1 ■ Three 10-second segments of different stages in a 3-month-old infant. No sleep spindles or K-complexes were present. However, slow wave activity was present. The epochs that were not stage R or stage N3 (non–rapid eye movement [NREM] 3) were scored as stage N.

POSTERIOR DOMINANT RHYTHM

Posterior dominant rhythm (PDR) in both adults and children is defined as the predominant rhythm seen over occipital derivations during eyes-closed wakefulness that is reactive. (The term *reactive* refers to activity that blocks or attenuates with eye opening and appears with eye closure). PDR in adults is often called "alpha rhythm" and consists of 8 to 13 Hz activity most prominent over occipital derivations and is reactive to eye opening (decreased amplitude).

PDR in infants and children changes with age. In Table F6-3 the characteristic changes are noted. A simple rule to remember is "greater than 8 by age 8," that is, in normal awake children older than 8 years of age, the PDR is greater than 8 hertz (Hz; 8–13 Hz). However, a PDR of 8 Hz is typically reached in children much younger than 8 years. Another useful fact is that at age 9 years

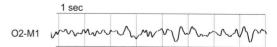

FIGURE F6-2 ■ Posterior dominant rhythm of 4 to 5 hertz (Hz) in a 3-month-old infant decreases in frequency on transition to sleep. The PDR is seen in the seconds 1 and 2 and slowing in seconds 3-8.

the mean PDR frequency is 9 Hz. Figure F6-2 provides an example of PDR that decreases in frequency with sleep onset.

ADDITIONAL WAVEFORMS OF WAKEFULNESS

1. *Posterior slow waves of youth (PSW):* This waveform occurs in children ages 8 to 14 years and has a frequency of 2.5 to 4.5 Hz. PSW usually occurs at the same time as PDR with eyes-closed wakefulness and disappears with drowsiness or transition to stage N1 sleep. Maximal incidence is 8 to 14 years of age and is rare in children younger than 2 years or in adults older than 21 years. (Figure F6-3).
2. *Blinks:* Eye blinks in children, as in adults, are associated with the eye ball turning upward (Bell phenomenon). In children, they cause *occipital sharp waves* that are monophasic or biphasic (200–400 milliseconds [msec]) and less than 200 microvolts (μV) that follow eye blinks.
3. *Slow eye movements (SEMs) or rapid eye movements (REMs):* These have the same definitions as in adults.

TABLE F6-3	**Changes in Dominant Posterior Rhythm by Age**[1]	
	Frequency (hertz [Hz])	**% of Children Showing the Pattern at This Age**
<3–4 months	Slow	100%
3–4 months	3.5–4.5	75%
5–6 months	5–6	70% by 12 months
3 years	7.5–9.5	82%
6–9 years	8–13	About 88%
>9 years	8–13	90%

From the *AASM Scoring Manual.*
Dominant posterior rhythm (DPR) is sinusoidal except for age <3–4 months.
PDR has occipital predominance.

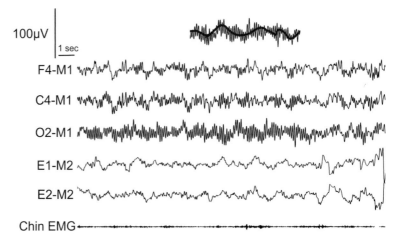

FIGURE F6-3 ◼ An example of posterior slow waves (PSW) of youth. The usual posterior dominant rhythm is superimposed on underlying slow wave activity. PSW is only present with the eyes closed and disappears with drowsiness and the onset of sleep.

PEDIATRIC STAGE W RULES (ADAPTED FROM *AASM SCORING MANUAL*)[1]

A. PDR in children is the same as alpha rhythm in adults for scoring sleep and wakefulness.

B. Score stage W when age appropriate PDR or alpha rhythm occupies more than 50% of the epoch over the occipital region.

C. If no discernable reactive alpha rhythm or age-appropriate PDR exist, score stage W when any of the following is present:
  1. Eye blinks at a frequent of 0.5–2 Hz
  2. Reading eye movements
  3. Irregular conjugate REM associated with normal or high chin muscle tone.

D. If epochs have a mixture of PDR and eye movement activity defined in C, score stage W when these occupy greater than 50% of the epoch.

PEDIATRIC STAGE N1

In staging N1, the presence or absence of certain waveforms is important (Table F6-4; Figure F6-4).

1. Rhythmic anterior theta (RAT) activity consists of runs of moderate voltage 5 to 7 Hz activity that is largest over the frontal regions. RAT is common in adolescents and young adults during drowsiness and first appears around 5 years of age.

2. Hypnagogic hypersynchrony (HH) is characterized by bursts of very high amplitude 3- to 4.5-Hz sinusoidal waves that are maximal in frontal and central derivations and smallest in the occipital derivation (widely distributed).

3. Low-amplitude mixed-frequency (LAMF) has low amplitude and predominantly 4 to 7 Hz activity.

4. Vertex sharp waves and slow eye movements (SEMs) are the same as in adults.

TABLE F6-4 Waveforms Important for Scoring Pediatric Stage N1

	Frequency/ Duration	Distribution	Amplitude	Age of Onset
Low-amplitude mixed-frequency (LAMF)	4–7 hertz (Hz)	All regions	Low	—
Vertex sharp waves	<0.5 seconds	Central, vertex	Stands out from background	
Rhythmic anterior theta (RAT) activity	5–7 Hz	Frontal regions	Not a criterion – generally low	Starts around age 5 years. Common in children and adolescents.
Hypnagogic hypersynchrony (HH)	3–4.5 Hz	Frontal and central	Very large 75–350 microvolts (µV)	Appears around age 3 months. Common in children ages 6–8 years. Rare in children ages >12 years.

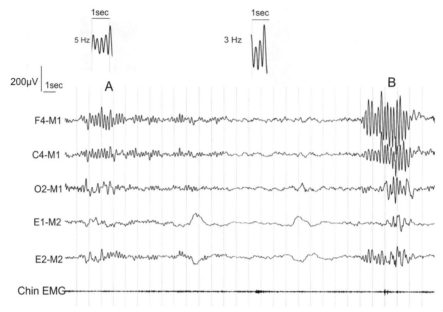

FIGURE F6-4 ■ A 30-second tracing (stage N1) in a 5-year-old child. **A,** An example of rhythmic anterior theta (RAT) activity (5 hertz [Hz]) that is more prominent in the frontal and central derivations. B, An example of hypnagogic hypersynchrony. This is a high-amplitude waveform 3 to 4.5 Hz that is prominent in the frontal and central derivations but also seen in the occipital derivations.

PEDIATRIC STAGE N1 RULES (ADAPTED FROM *AASM SCORING MANUAL*)

A. If alpha rhythm or PDR is generated, score stage N1 if the posterior rhythm is attenuated or replaced by LAMF for more than 50% of the epoch.

B. If alpha rhythm or PDR is not present with eye closure, score stage N1, commencing with the earliest of any of the following phenomena (see Table F6-4):
1. Activity in the range of 4 to 7 Hz, with slowing of background frequencies by 1 to 2 Hz or greater from stage W (e.g., 5 Hz, and stage W had 7 Hz)
2. SEMs
3. Vertex sharp waves
4. RAT activity
5. HH
6. Diffuse or occipital predominant high-amplitude rhythmic activity (3 to 5 Hz)

PEDIATRIC STAGE N2

This stage is scored per adult rules (Figure F6-5).

Sleep spindles in children differ somewhat from adults. In infants, sleep spindles are often asynchronous (spindles on the right but not on the left, and then vice versa) until age 1 to 2 years.[3] Sleep spindles occur independently at two different locations and frequencies in children and adolescents. Frontal spindles typically are 11 to 12.5 Hz compared with 12.5 to 14.5 Hz in the centroparietal regions. Centeroparietal spindles show little change with ages 4 to 24 years, but frontal spindles decrease dramatically in power and become stable about age 13 years.[1]

PEDIATRIC STAGE N3

This stage is scored per adult rules (Box F6-1).

SWA for sleep staging is defined as greater than 75 µV peak to peak in the frontal derivation with a frequency 0.5 to 2 Hz (2-second to 0.5-second width). Slow waves in children are often 100 to 400 µV (Figure F6-6). Slow waves appear as early as 2 months but more often about 3 to 4.5 months postterm. In scoring adult sleep, the major question for epochs containing low-frequency activity is: "Are amplitude criteria met for at least 6 seconds?" In children, nearly all EEG activity in the 0.5 to 2 Hz range exceeds 75 µV peak to peak.

PEDIATRIC STAGE R

This stage is scored per adult rules.

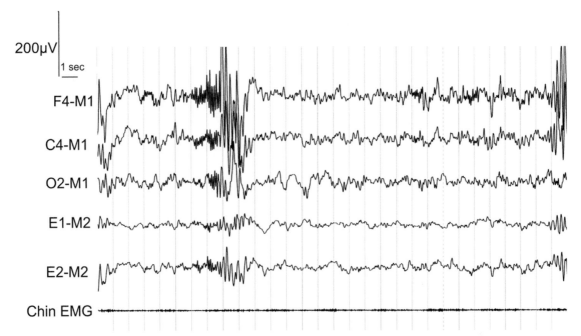

FIGURE F6-5 ■ Stage N2 in a 5-year-old child. A spindle occurs next to a theta burst (hypnogogic hypersynchrony) in the first half of the epoch. Note that sleep spindle activity has the highest amplitude in the frontal derivation.

BOX F6-1	Pediatric Stage N3

SCORE STAGE N3 CRITERIA

1. Slow wave activity (SWA) (≥20% of epoch) (≥6 seconds)
2. SWA >75 microvolts (μV) peak to peak in frontal derivation and frequency 0.5 to 2 hertz (Hz)
3. Sleep spindles may or may not be present
4. Usually no eye movements in stage N3
5. Chin electromyography (EMG) tone is variable and not part of the scoring criteria

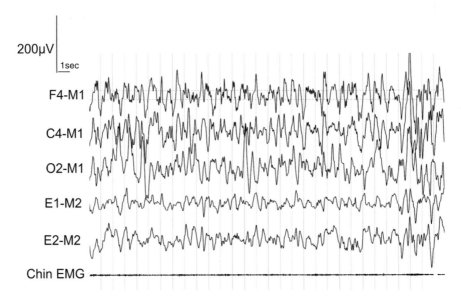

FIGURE F6-6 ■ A 30-second epoch of stage N3 sleep in a 5-year-old child. Nearly all of the epoch meets amplitude criteria for slow wave activity.

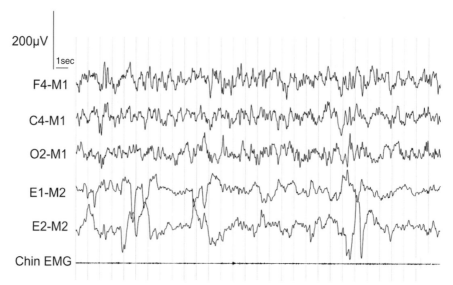

FIGURE F6-7   ■   A 30-second epoch of stage R in a 5-year-old child. The background activity may have higher amplitude than is typical in adults.

The stage R of pediatric sleep differs from that in adults only in that the background activity may not look as familiar. The background rhythm varies somewhat and may have some SWA (Figure F6-7). Sawtooth waves appear around 5 months.

PEDIATRIC AROUSAL RULES

These are the same as for adults.

REFERENCES

1. Grigg-Damberger M, Gozal D, Marcus CL, et al: The visual scoring of sleep and arousal in infants and children, *J Clin Sleep Med* 3:201–240, 2007.
2. Iber C, Ancoli-Israel S, Chesson AJ, Quan S: *The AASM manual for the scoring of sleep and associated events: rules, terminology and technical specification*, Westchester, IL, 2007, American Academy of Sleep Medicine.
3. Anders T, Emde R, Parmelee A: *A manual of standardized terminology, techniques and criteria for scoring of stages of sleep and wakefulness in newborn infants*, Los Angeles, 1971, Brain Information Service, UCLA.
4. Libenson MH: *Practical approach to electroencephalography*, Philadelphia, 2010, Saunders, p 321.

A 3-Year-Old Male Undergoes a Sleep Study

QUESTIONS

1. Two sequential 30-second epochs (Figures P11-1 and P11-2) from a sleep study on a 3-year-old male are shown below. During stage R, the chin electromyography (EMG) activity was *lower* than noted in Figure P11-1. The sinusoidal occipital activity shown in the blow-up above Figure P11-2 is 6 hertz (Hz). What sleep stages are shown?

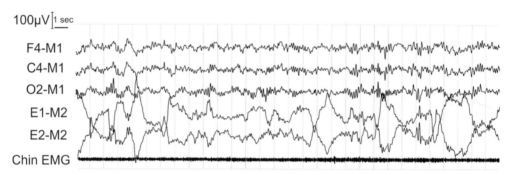

FIGURE P11-1 ■ 30-second tracing in a 3-year-old.

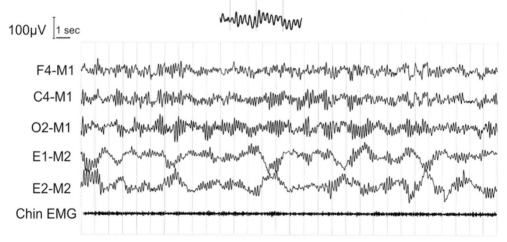

FIGURE P11-2 ■ A 30-second tracing of the epoch following the one Figure shown in P11-1.

2. The 30-second tracing in Figure P11-3 was recorded in a 5-year-old child, who does not generate a posterior dominant rhythm with eye closure. The preceding epoch was stage W. The blow-up shows 4 Hz activity. What sleep stage is shown?

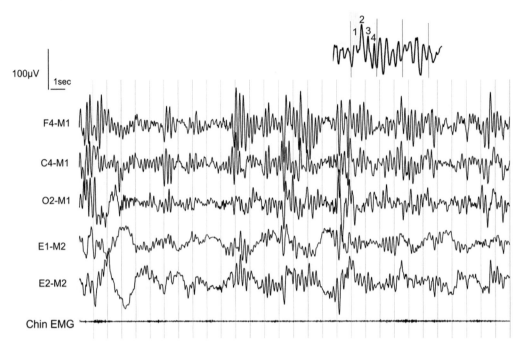

FIGURE P11-3 ■ A 30-second epoch with a blow-up of EEG activity. The preceding epoch was stage W. The patient did not generate posterior dominant rhythm with eye closure.

3. The 30-second tracing in Figure P11-4 was recorded in a 5-year-old child. The preceding epoch was stage W. The child did not generate a posterior dominant rhythm with eye closure. What sleep stage is shown?

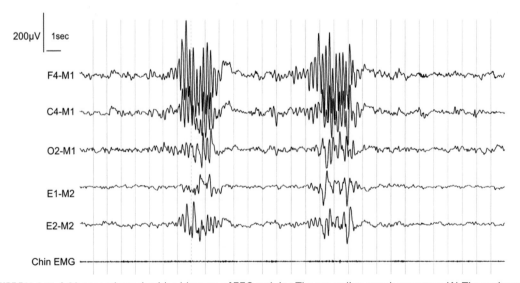

FIGURE P11-4 ■ A 30-second epoch with a blow-up of EEG activity. The preceding epoch was stage W. The patient did not generate posterior dominant rhythm with eye closure.

ANSWERS

1. **Answer:** Stage W.

   Discussion: The 6 Hz is the posterior dominant rhythm (PDR) in this patient and is normal for a patient 3 years of age[1-4]. In Figure P11-1, rapid eye movements (REMs) are present (eyes open), and the PDR activity is suppressed. In Figure P11-2, the activity is most prominent in the occipital derivation. By age 8 years, most children will have a PDR of 8 Hz or more. Many have a PDR of 8 Hz several years before age 8 years.

2. **Answer:** Stage N1.

   Discussion: The epoch shows diffuse high amplitude theta activity (4 Hz) and is consistent with stage N1 in an individual who does not generate a PDR with eye closure (see below).

3. **Answer:** Stage N1.

   Discussion: Two bursts of hypnagogic hypersynchrony (HH) are noted in the epoch (Figure P11-4); the first is in the first half of the epoch. No sleep spindles or K-complexes are present. Therefore, the epoch is stage N1. Hypnagogic hypersynchrony (HH) is characterized by bursts of very high amplitude 3- to 4.5-Hz sinusoidal waves that are maximal in frontal and central derivations and smallest in the occipital derivation. Of note, HH may be seen in both stage N1 and stage N2[1-4].

CLINICAL PEARLS

1. The posterior dominant rhythm may be slower that 8 Hz in normal children less than 8 years of age. However, many children have a PDR of 8 Hz or greater at an age younger than 8 years. PDR is an occipital sinusoidal rhythm that is attenuated with eye opening and enhanced with eye closure (See Fundamental 6).

2. The *AASM Scoring Manual*[1,4] states that in children who do not generate a posterior dominant rhythm, stage N1 is scored commencing with the earliest of any of the following phenomenon:
   a. Activity in the range of 4 to 7 Hz with slowing of the background frequencies by 1 to 2 Hz or greater from those of stage W
   b. Slow eye movements (SEMs)
   c. Vertex sharp waves
   d. Rhythmic anterior theta (RAT) activity
   e. Hypnagogic hypersynchrony (HH)
   f. Diffuse or occipital predominant, high amplitude, rhythmic 3 to 5 Hz activity

---

REFERENCES

1. Iber C, Ancoli-Israel S, Chesson A, Quan SF, for the American Academy of Sleep Medicine: *The AASM manual for scoring of sleep and associated events: rules, terminology and technical specifications*, ed 1, Westchester, IL, 2007, American Academy of Sleep Medicine.
2. Silber MH, Ancoli-Israel S, Bonnet MH, et al: The visual scoring of sleep in adults, *J Clin Sleep Med* 15:121–131, 2007.
3. Grigg-Damberger M, Gozal D, Marcus CL, et al: The visual scoring of sleep and arousal in infants and children, *J Clin Sleep Med* 3(2):201–240, 2007.
4. Berry RB, Brooks R, Gamaldo CE, et al: *for the American Academy of Sleep Medicine: The AASM manual for the scoring of sleep and associated events: rules, terminology and technical specifications*, Version 2.0.3, Darien, IL, 2012, American Academy of Sleep Medicine. www.aasmnet.org, Accessed July 3, 2014.

FUNDAMENTALS 7

Sleep Architecture Terminology and Normal Patterns

SLEEP ARCHITECTURE PARAMETERS

A number of parameters concerning the quantity and quality of sleep are usually reported in polysomnography (PSG) reports[1-3] (Table F7-1). Typically, PSG data recording starts before lights-out to verify that the electrodes and monitoring equipment are providing adequate signals. In addition, calibrations (to verify amplifier function) and biocalibrations are recorded as described in Fundamentals 10. **Lights-out time** is the time at which the patient is allowed to fall asleep and marks the start of data that will be staged and analyzed. **Lights-on** is the time that recording of sleep is terminated. **Total recording time** (TRT) is the time from lights-out to lights-on. **Sleep latency** is the time from lights-out to the start of the first epoch of sleep. **Wake after sleep onset (WASO)** includes all stage W after sleep onset (from the *start of the first epoch of sleep*)

until lights-on. It also includes out-of-bed wake time during the period from sleep onset until lights-on. The total amount of stage W (during TRT) = sleep latency + WASO. **REM latency** is the time from the *start of the first epoch of sleep* until the start of the first epoch of stage R. It is *not* the time from lights-out to the first epoch of stage R. **Total sleep time** (TST) comprises the minutes of stages of sleep (N1, N2, N3, R). **Sleep efficiency** (as a percent) is the total sleep time in minutes $\times 100 \div$ TRT in minutes. It is common practice to present the time spent in each of stages N1, N2, N3, and stage R in minutes and as a percentage of the TST. See Appendix 2 for normative values of sleep architecture in children and adults.

NORMAL SLEEP IN ADULTS

Sleep occurs in cycles, each usually composed of a period of non–rapid eye movement (NREM) sleep

TABLE F7-1 Parameters Reported in Polysomnography Reports

Term	Abbreviation	Definition
Lights-out time (hr : min)	LOUT	Time of the start of the recording.
Lights-on time (hr : min)	LON	Time of the end of the recording.
Total recording time (min)	TRT	Time from lights-out to lights-on. TRT = SL + WASO + TST
Total sleep time (min)	TST	Time spent in stages N1, N2, N3, and R.
Sleep latency (min)	SL	Time from lights-out until the start of the first epoch of sleep (stages N1, N2, N3, or R).
Stage R latency or (REM latency) (min)	RL	Time from start of first epoch of sleep until the start of the first epoch of stage R.
Sleep efficiency (%)		= TST × 100/TRT.
Stage wake (min)	Stage W	All minutes of stage W during TRT.
Wake after sleep onset	WASO	Stage W recorded after sleep onset until lights-on time. =Stage W-SL
Time in each sleep stage (min)	N1, N2, N3, R	Minutes of stages N1, N2, N3, R.
Time in each sleep stage as a % of TST	N1%TST, etc.	Minutes or each sleep stage × 100/TST.
Arousal (number)	Ar#	Total number of arousals.
Arousal index (#/hr)	ArI	Total number of arousals × 60/TST (min).

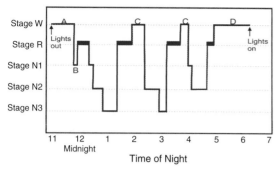

FIGURE F7-1 ■ A hypnogram of a patient with depression. This hypnogram shows a long sleep latency (**A**), short REM latency (**B**), awakening during the night (**C**), and early morning awakening (**D**).

followed by a period of stage R (REM) sleep. Usually, three to five NREM/REM cycles occur per night. A hypnogram is a plot of sleep stage versus time of night (Figure F7-1). Although the sleep architecture parameters listed previously are useful, a hypnogram often provides more useful information about the pattern of sleep over the night.

SLEEP ARCHITECTURE

Sleep architecture is a term used to denote the structure of sleep. In young adults, stage N1 usually occupies approximately 5% to 10% of the TST.[3–6] It is a transitional state between wakefulness and the other stages of sleep. Stage N2 occupies the greatest proportion of the TST and accounts for approximately 50% to 60% of sleep. Stage N3 occupies approximately 15% to 20% of the TST in young adults. The amplitude of the slow waves and amount of stage N3 is greatest in the first sleep cycle. The amount of stage N3 decreases with age in men but not in women. The episodes of stage R occur about every 90 to 100 minutes, and they are of longer duration as the night progresses. The REM density is the number of eye movements per time. The REM density tends to be the highest in the later REM periods. In fact, the initial REM period of the night which is typically short is often difficult to score because of infrequent REMs.

CHANGES IN SLEEP ARCHITECTURE WITH AGE IN ADULTS

The most comprehensive studies of the effects of age on sleep parameters were published before 2007 and used Rechtschaffen and Kales (R&K) scoring rules. Ohayon et al.[6] published a meta-analysis combining data from men and women

(although analysis for gender effects was performed) and looked at the age range from childhood to old age. Redline et al.[7] analyzed the data from both genders separately and only evaluated individuals over age 45 years. Ambulatory rather than in lab PSG was used. Sleep gets shorter and lighter with increasing age (Tables F7-2 and F7-3). *Sleep latency increases with age, and the REM latency and amount of stage R both decrease.*

TST and Sleep Efficiency

TST decreases with age (Figure F7-2) as does sleep efficiency. Decrease in TST tends to be more rapid from childhood to adolescence and slows during ages 20 to 80 years. Sleep efficiency decreases with age, especially after age 50 years.[6]

TABLE F7-2 Changes in Sleep Architecture with Age

Increasing with Age	Decreasing with Age
Sleep latency	TST
WASO (most change after 40 years)	Sleep efficiency
Stage N1 (%TST)[1]	REM latency
Stage N1 (%TST) men only[2]	Stage N3 (%TST)[1]
Stage N2 (%TST)[1]	Stage N3 (% TST) men only[2]
Stage N2 (%TST) men only[2]	Stage R (%TST)

From (1) Ohayon MM, Carskadon MA, Guilleminault C, Viteiello MV: Meta-analysis of quantitative sleep parameters from childhood to old age in healthy individuals: developing normative sleep values across the human lifespan, *Sleep* 27:1255-1273, 2004; (2) Redline S, Kirchner L, Quan SF, et al: The effects of age, sex, ethnicity, and sleep-disordered breathing on sleep architecture, *Arch Intern Med* 164:406-418, 2004.
REM, Rapid eye movement; *TST*, total sleep time; *WASO*, wake after sleep onset.

TABLE F7-3 Typical Sleep Architecture in Men at Ages 20 and 60 Years

	Age 20	Age 60
Total sleep time (TST; min)	450	380
Sleep efficiency (%)	95	85
Sleep latency (min)	10	15
REM latency (min)	90	70
Wake after sleep onset (WASO) (min)	15	30
Stage N1 (%TST)	5	15
Stage N2 (%TST)	45	55
Stage N3 (%TST)	20	10
Stage R (%TST)	25	20
Arousal index (#/hour)	5–10	15–20

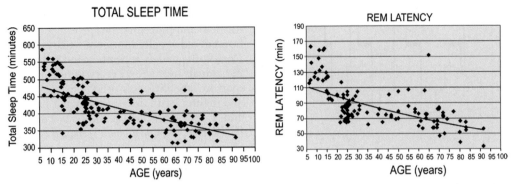

FIGURE F7-2 ■ Plots of total sleep time and rapid eye movement (REM) latency versus age. Both of these decrease with increasing age. (From Ohayon MM, Carskadon MA, Guilleminault C, Viteiello MV: Meta-analysis of quantitative sleep parameters from childhood to old age in healthy individuals: developing normative sleep values across the human lifespan, *Sleep* 27:1255-1273, 2004.)

Sleep Latency

Sleep latency increases slightly with age but should be less than 30 minutes. Patients with sleep-onset insomnia typically have sleep latency longer than 30 minutes.

REM Latency

REM latency decreases with age (see Figure F7-2). A number of sleep disorders affect REM latency. These are discussed in Fundamentals 8.

WASO and Stage N1 (as a Percentage of TST)

In the meta-analysis by Ohayon and coworkers,[6] WASO and stage N1 (as %TST) increased during ages 20 to 60 years. In the analysis of Redline and colleagues,[7] the amount of stage N1 increased over the four age quartiles for men but not for women.

Stage N2 (as a Percentage of TST)

In the meta-analysis of Ohayon and coworkers,[6] the amount of stage N2 increased with age. Redline and colleagues[7] found stage N2 to increase with age in men but not in women. This is consistent with the findings of a decrease in stage N3 in men (see later). The amount of stage N2 was higher in men than in women when all age groups were considered.

Stage N3 (as a Percentage of TST)

In the large meta-analysis by Ohayon and coworkers,[6] the amount of stage N3 decreased with age. The effect size was greater in men than in women. In the study by Redline and

colleagues,[7] the amount of stage N3 (%TST) decreased with age only in men. The decrease in stage N3 in men with age was associated with an increase in stages N1 and N2. For the entire group of women (all ages), the amount of stage N3 was higher compared with men.

Stage R (as a Percentage of TST)

Ohayon and coworkers[6] found a decrease in stage R between 20 and 60 years of age. Most of the decrease in REM as a percentage of TST was noted during ages 10 to 35 years. In the study of Redline and colleagues,[7] a small but statistically significant decrease was seen in stage R with age for both men and women. The amount of REM sleep decreases slightly with age from around 20% to 25% (%TST) in younger adults to 15% to 20% in older adults. Factors that increase in REM latency tend to decrease the amount of REM sleep.

Changes in Arousal Index with Age

Scoring of arousals is important because frequent arousals result in nonrestorative sleep and may cause daytime sleepiness even in the absence of a decrement in TST. The arousal index (ArI, number of arousals per hour of sleep) in normal individuals increases with age (Figure F7-3). The ArI in older adults may be considerably higher than in younger individuals. Bonnet and Arand[8] found the ArI in 51- to 60-year-old individuals and 61- to 70-year-old individuals to be 21.9 ± 8.9/hour (hr) and 22.3 ± 6.8/hr, respectively (mean ± standard deviation [SD]). Therefore, the 95% confidence limits may approach 35/hr in older age groups. Conversely, an ArI of 25/hr would be high for a young adult.

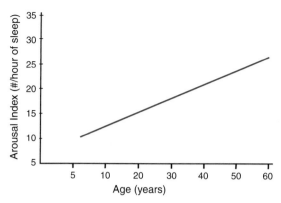

FIGURE F7-3 ■ Effect of age on the arousal index in normal individuals. (Redrawn from data in Bonnet M, Arand DL: EEG arousal norms by age, *J Clin Sleep Med* 3:271-274, 2007.)

First-Night Effect

The first-night effect was described by Agnew and coworkers[9] and Webb and Campbell[10] from analysis of individuals undergoing multiple sleep studies. The phenomenon consists of lower sleep efficiency, lower amount of REM sleep, and longer REM latency on the first night in the sleep center.

COMPARISON OF NORMATIVE VALUES USING THE *AASM SCORING MANUAL* VERSUS THE MANUAL OF RECHTSCHAFFEN AND KALES

Moser and colleagues[11] found that sleep latency, REM latency, TST, and sleep efficiency were similar using the *AASM Scoring Manual* or the manual of Rechtschaffen and Kales (R&K). An increase was seen in stage N1 (absolute duration and % TST) with AASM scoring rules compared with R&K. Stage N2 decreased (absolute duration and %TST) with AASM criteria compared with those of R&K. Stage R also differed but was age dependent, being slightly higher with AASM criteria in older individuals. The amount of stage N3 was higher according to the *AASM Scoring Manual* as expected with use of frontal rather than central derivations to assess slow wave activity (slow waves have the higher amplitude in frontal derivations compared with central derivations).

NORMAL SLEEP IN INFANTS AND CHILDREN

The major points regarding normal sleep in infants and children are listed in Tables F7-4 and F7-5. When discussing sleep architecture, findings are usually categorized as those for infants, children, and adolescents.[6,12–15]

TABLE F7-4 Normal Sleep in Infants and Children

Infants < 3 months
- Stage R (REM sleep, active sleep) at sleep onset is common.
- Total sleep time 16–18 hours.
- Sleep episodes of 3–4 hours duration interrupted by feeding.
- Sleep cycles 45 to 60 minutes (90–100 minutes in adults).
- Stage R about 50% of sleep.

Infants > 3 months
- Percentage of REM sleep starts to decrease.
- Entering sleep through NREM sleep instead of stage R.
- Sleep consolidates into major episodes at night with daytime naps.

Children
- Sleep cycle period does not reach adult values until adolescence.

Changes in Sleep Childhood to Adolescence

No Change	Decrease	Increase
TST (recording on nonschool days)	Stage N3 as % TST	Stage N2
Sleep efficiency	REM sleep as %TST	
Sleep latency	TST (recording on school days)	

From Kahn A, Dan B, Grosswasser J, Franco P, Sottiaux M: Normal sleep architecture in infants and children, *J Clin Neurophysiol* 13:184-197, 1996.
NREM, Non–rapid eye movement; *REM*, rapid eye movement; *TST*, total sleep time.

TABLE F7-5 Typical Sleep Architecture Values for Normal Children Aged 1–18 Years

Parameter	Usual Values
Sleep efficiency (%)	89%, large variability
Sleep latency (minutes)	23 minutes, large variability
REM latency (minutes)	85–155 (<10 years) 136–156 (> 10 years) large variability
Arousal index (#/hour)	9–16
Stage N1 (%TST)	4–5
Stage N2 (%TST)	44–56
Stage N3 (%TST)	29–32 (<10 years) 20–32 (>10 years)
Stage R (%TST)	17–21 (can be higher in younger children)

Adapted From Beck SE, Marcus CL: Pediatric polysomnography, *Sleep Med Clin* 4:393-406, 2009.
REM, Rapid eye movement; *TST*, total sleep time.

Infants

For infants less than 2 months of age, stage R is often referred to as *active sleep* and NREM as *quiet sleep*. Infants normally enter sleep via stage R (active sleep) and spend approximately 50% of the TST in this sleep stage. Infants have shorter sleep cycles of approximately 45 to 60 minutes (in contrast to adult cycles of 90–100 minutes).[12-15] By age 3 months, the amount of REM sleep starts to decrease. Infants have cycles of sleep interrupted by episodes of feeding around the clock. Sleep begins to consolidate into longer nocturnal sleep periods with shorter naps during the day. Iglowstein et al. found daily napping to be uncommon at 5 years or older and any napping to be uncommon at 7 years of age.[13]

Children

In children, the percentage of REM sleep decreases to approximately 30% at ages 1 to 2 years and 20% to 25% at 3 to 5 years. As in adults, the duration of REM periods increases across the night (longer in the second part of the night). Montgomery-Downs et al.[14] found a higher REM latency of 132 minutes in 6- to 7-year-olds compared with 87.8 minutes in 3- to 5-year-olds, but a large degree of variability existed. As children move toward adolescence, a decrease tends to occur in stage N3 sleep and stage R and an increase in stage N2. TST decreases from early childhood to adolescence from 14 hours at age 1 down to 9 hours in early adolescence.[13] Typical values for sleep parameters in children are listed in Appendix 2.

CLINICAL PEARLS

1. Sleep in adults is characterized by of three to five cycles of NREM/REM sleep, each lasting about 90 to 100 minutes. In children, sleep cycle duration is 45 to 60 minutes with a greater number of NREM/REM cycles per night compared to adults.

2. In adults, entry into sleep from wakefulness is via NREM sleep (usually stage N1). In infants, entry via REM sleep (active sleep) is common.

3. The amount of stage R in each cycle is longer in the second part of the night. The REM density (number of eye movements ÷ time) is greater in the second part of the night.

4. Most stage N3 occurs in the first part of the night. The greatest slow wave activity is typically in the first episode of stage N3 sleep.

4. In adults, total sleep time and sleep efficiency decrease and the amount of wake increases with age. A modest increase in the sleep latency also occurs.

5. In men, the amount of stage N3 decreases with age, and the amount of stage N1 and N2 increases. In women, the amount of stage N3 does not decrease with age.

6. In adults, the amount of stage R and the REM latency both decrease slightly with age.

7. The normal arousal index increases with age.

8. Napping in children is uncommon at age 7 years or older (daily napping uncommon after age 5 years).

REFERENCES

1. Kushida CA, Littner MR, Morgenthaler T, et al: Practice parameters for the indications for polysomnography and related procedures: an update for 2005, *Sleep* 28:499–521, 2005.

2. Iber C, Ancoli-Israel S, Chesson A, Quan SF: for the American Academy of Sleep Medicine: *The AASM manual for scoring of sleep and associated events: rules, terminology and technical specifications*, ed 1, Westchester, IL, 2007, American Academy of Sleep Medicine.

3. Berry RB, Brooks R, Gamaldo CE, et al: for the American Academy of Sleep Medicine: *The AASM manual for the scoring of sleep and associated events: rules, terminology and technical specifications*, Version 2.1, Darien, IL, 2012, American Academy of Sleep Medicine. www.aasmnet.org, Accessed July 3, 2014.

4. Rechtschaffen A, Kales A, editors: *A manual of standardized terminology techniques and scoring system for sleep stages of human subjects*, Los Angeles, 1968, Brain Information Service/Brain Research Institute, UCLA.

5. Bliwise DL: Normal aging. In Kryger M, Roth T, Dement W, editors: *Principles and practice of sleep medicine*, Philadelphia, 2005, Saunders, pp 24–38.

6. Ohayon MM, Carskadon MA, Guilleminault C, Viteiello MV: Meta-analysis of quantitative sleep parameters from childhood to old age in healthy individuals: developing normative sleep values across the human lifespan, *Sleep* 27:1255–1273, 2004.

7. Redline S, Kirchner L, Quan SF, et al: The effects of age, sex, ethnicity, and sleep-disordered breathing on sleep architecture, *Arch Intern Med* 164:406–418, 2004.

8. Bonnet M, Arand DL: EEG arousal norms by age, *J Clin Sleep Med* 3:271–274, 2007.

9. Agnew HW Jr., Webb WB, Williams RL: The first night effect: an EEG study of sleep, *Psychophysiology* 2:263–266, 1966.

10. Webb WB, Campbell S: The first night effect revisited with age as a variable, *Waking Sleeping* 3:319–324, 1979.

11. Moser D, Anderer P, Gruber G, et al: Sleep classification according to AASM and Rechtschaffen & Kales: effects of sleep scoring parameters, *Sleep* 32:139–149, 2009.

12. Kahn A, Dan B, Groswasser J, et al: Normal sleep architecture in infants and children, *J Clin Neurophysiol* 13:184–197, 1996.

13. Iglowstein I, Jenni OG, Molinari L, Largo RH: Sleep duration from infancy to adolescence: reference values and generational trends, *Pediatrics* 111:302–307, 2003.

14. Montgomery-Downs HE, O'Brien LM, Gulliver TE, et al: Polysomnographic characteristics in normal preschool children, *Pediatrics* 117:741–753, 2006.

15. Beck SE, Marcus CL: Pediatric polysomnography, *Sleep Med Clin* 4:393–406, 2009.

Sleep in a 20-Year-Old Man, a 2-Month-Old Infant, and a 6-Month-Old Child

QUESTIONS

1. Which statement is true about sleep in a 2-month-old infant?
   A. In infants less than 2 months old, non–rapid eye movement (NREM) sleep is often called *active sleep*.
   B. In infants, entry into sleep through stage R is normal.
   C. The typical sleep cycle duration in infants is 20 to 30 minutes.
   D. Typical total sleep time in infants is 10 hours.

2. A 7-year-old child is evaluated for problems with attention in school. Which of the following statements is true?
   A. He should be getting 8 hours of sleep at night.
   B. Taking naps during the day is common in a 7-year-old.
   C. The amount of REM sleep (%TST [total sleep time]) is less than in an adult.
   D. An REM latency less than 15 minutes would be abnormal.

3. A 20-year-old man is monitored for complaints of excessive daytime sleepiness. His sleep architecture was found to be normal. Which statement is true about the sleep of this young man in comparison with a normal 60-year-old man?
   A. The REM latency will be longer than in a normal 60-year-old man.
   B. Stage N3 (%TST) will be less than in a normal 60-year-old man.
   C. The amount of stage R (%TST) will be about the same.
   D. Stage N2 (%TST) will be more than in a normal 60-year-old man.

ANSWERS

1. **Answer:** B.

   Discussion: In infants, entry into sleep via active sleep is normal.[1–4] Stage R (active sleep) makes up about 50% of the total sleep time. Stage R is often called *active sleep* in infants; therefore, answer A is incorrect. Active sleep characterized by irregular respiration and muscle twitching during this sleep stage in infants is normal. The typical sleep cycle in infants is 45 to 60 minutes in contrast to 90 to 120 minutes in adults. Therefore, answer C is incorrect. The sleep duration in infants is typically around 14 hours, with periods of sleep alternating with periods of wakefulness for feeding. Therefore, answer D in incorrect. As infants mature the sleep episodes consolidate into a longer period at night with shorter naps during the day.[3,4]

2. **Answer:** D.

   Discussion: Although entry into REM sleep in an infant would be normal (very short REM latency), by age 6 years, such a short REM latency would be distinctly abnormal. See Appendix II Table 2 for the typical sleep durations by age in normal children. A child of age 7 years should be getting at least 10 hours of sleep at night (see Fundamentals 7 and 18). Therefore, answer A is incorrect. If the family must wake up at 6 AM, this would translate into a bedtime around 8 PM. In the digital entertainment age, enforcing an adequate bedtime is essential for children to obtain a normal amount of sleep. Taking a nap would be normal in young preschool children, but after age 7 years, daytime napping is unusual. Therefore, answer B is incorrect. Napping in an individual of this age may indicate a sleep disorder or inadequate sleep. The amount of stage R (%TST) decreases with age and would be greater in a 6-year-old than in an adult. Therefore, answer C is incorrect.

3. **Answer:** A.

   Discussion: REM latency decreases slightly with age in both men and women. In men, the amount of stage N3 decreases with age; therefore, answer B is incorrect. A younger man would be expected to have more stage N3 sleep. The amount of stage R decreases slightly in both men and women as they age. Therefore, answer C is incorrect. In older men, the amount of stage N1 and N2 tends to be higher than in younger men to correspond to the lower amount of stage N3. Therefore, stage N2 (%TST) would be less in a 20-year-old man. Therefore, answer D is incorrect.

REFERENCES

1. Ohayon MM, Carskadon MA, Guilleminault C, Viteiello MV: Meta-analysis of quantitative sleep parameters from childhood to old age in healthy individuals: developing normative sleep values across the human lifespan, *Sleep* 27:1255–1273, 2004.
2. Kahn A, Dan B, Groswasser J, et al: Normal sleep architecture in infants and children, *J Clin Neurophysiol* 13:184–197, 1996.
3. Iglowstein I, Jenni OG, Molinari L, Largo RH: Sleep duration from infancy to adolescence: reference values and generational trends, *Pediatrics* 111:302–307, 2003.
4. Montgomery-Downs HE, O'Brien LM, Gulliver TE, et al: Polysomnographic characteristics in normal preschool children, *Pediatrics* 117:741–753, 2006.

PATIENT 13

Short REM Latency

Information on Patients A and B is presented below followed by questions.

   Patient A: A 40-year-old woman complained of snoring, fatigue, and daytime sleepiness (but the Epworth sleepiness scale was 8, normal is 10 or less). The patient denied cataplexy (weakness triggered by emotion). A sleep study was performed (Table P13-1). The patient had a final awakening at 5:20 AM. Figure P13-1 shows an epoch 15 minutes after sleep onset.

TABLE P13-1	**Lights-Out (10:30 PM) and Lights-On (6:00 AM)**		
Sleep Architecture		**Total Night**	**Range**
Total recording time	(min)	450	(425–462)
Total sleep time	(min)	340	(394–457)
Sleep efficiency	(%)	75	(90–100)
Sleep latency	(min)	25.0	(0–19)
REM latency	(min)	10.0	(69–88)
Sleep Stages			
Awake (WASO):	(min)	85.0	(0–26) min
		%TST	
Stage N1:	(min)	34.0	10.0	(3–6) (%)
Stage N2:	(min)	275.5	67.5	(46–62) (%)
Stage N3:	(min)	20.5	5.4	(10–21) (%)
Stage R:	(min)	64.5	19.8	(21–31) (%)
AHI	3/hour		

AHI, Apnea–hypopnea index; *min*, minutes; *REM*, rapid eye movement; *%TST*, percentage of total sleep time; *WASO*, wake after sleep onset.

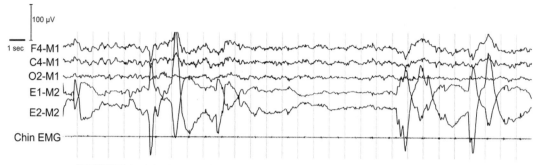

FIGURE P13-1 ■ A 30-second epoch that was noted 15 minutes after sleep onset.

QUESTIONS

1. What is the most notable finding in the sleep architecture (Table P13-1)? What causes should be considered? Would Figure P13-1 provide a clue?
   Patient B: A 45-year-old man with loud snoring and breathing pauses has not been evaluated or treated for sleep apnea and undergoes abdominal surgery. In the postoperative period, the patient developed the most severe nocturnal hypoxemia on nights 3 and 4 not the first of second postoperative night.

2. Considering that patient B received the most pain medication in the immediate postoperative period, how do you explain the more severe hypoxemia on nights 3 and 4? Consider the fact that patients with obstructive sleep apnea have the most severe arterial oxygen desaturation during REM sleep.
   Patient C. The hypnogram shown in Figure P13-2 is from a 2-month-old infant. As features of stage N1, N2, and N3 were not yet developed, sleep was staged as stage W, stage N, and stage R.

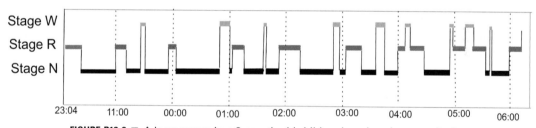

FIGURE P13-2 ■ A hypnogram in a 3-month-old child undergoing sleep monitoring.

3. Name two things about the timing of the sleep stages that differs from that in adults?

ANSWERS

1. **Answer:** Short REM latency on polysomnography PSG (short nocturnal REM latency). High REM density for an early REM period. Consider depression.

   Discussion: A short REM latency on a **nocturnal** study should prompt consideration of a number of possible explanations.[1,2] Sleep-onset REM periods (SOREMPs) are defined as REM sleep within 15 minutes of sleep onset. A nocturnal sleep study with sleep onset REM occurs in 20% to 50% of patients with narcolepsy, depending on the study and patient population.[1] The finding has a high positive predictive value for narcolepsy if other causes are eliminated. Aldrich found a nocturnal SOREMP in only 1% of patients with sleep related breathing disorders.[1] The sleep of patients with narcolepsy may show an increase in stage N1 and decreased sleep efficiency. The amount of REM sleep is usually normal.[2,3] The sleep latency is usually short. In **untreated** patients with depression, the REM latency is reduced, although usually not as short as in patients with narcolepsy (e.g., 40 minutes). However, sleep onset REM may be noted. Often, the first REM period is relatively long, and the REM density (eye movements per epoch) is often increased in the first REM period. Recall that the REM density is typically low in the first REM period (often 0 to 2 REMs per epoch). Other PSG findings in depression include a reduced total sleep time (TST), sleep efficiency, and amount of stage N3. The amount of REM sleep as a percentage of TST is usually normal or increased. Early awakening is common. Of note, the PSG findings are interesting but not specific enough to be useful for diagnosis of depression. On the other hand, they may be clues to consider a diagnosis of depression.

If patients with depression are taking an antidepressant, the REM latency is usually prolonged, and the amount of REM sleep reduced (exception nefazodone, which may increase the amount of REM sleep, or mirtazapine which usually has minimal effect). The sleep complaint in depression is often insomnia in about two thirds of patients, but up to one third may complain of hypersomnia. For some of these patients, fatigue may be a better description of the symptom. The mean sleep latency on a multiple sleep latency test (MSLT) is usually **normal (no objective sleepiness**; see Fundamentals 17 and 41). If insomnia is present in depression, sleep latency will be prolonged unless a sedating antidepressant is being taken (e.g., mirtazapine, trazodone). Untreated OSA may reduce REM latency on a nocturnal PSG, although this is very uncommon (1% or less).

Recent withdrawal of an REM-suppressing medication (selective serotonin reuptake inhibitor [SSRI], serotonin–norepinephrine reuptake inhibitor [SNRI]) may result in a short nocturnal REM latency. An increase in the duration of REM sleep may also occur. Withdrawal of other REM-suppressing medications may also cause a short nocturnal REM latency (e.g., stimulants). Recovery from prior sleep restriction usually is associated with a rebound in stage N3 the first night and an increase in stage R the second night. In summary, a careful history of sleep in the preceding week before the study, medications taken (or withdrawn), symptoms of cataplexy (narcolepsy), and depression are useful in determining the reason for a short nocturnal REM latency.

In the current patient, no evidence of significant sleep apnea was present. The sleep latency was mildly increased. In most patients with narcolepsy, the sleep latency is short. Also no history of cataplexy is present. Wakefulness after sleep onset was increased, and sleep efficiency was quite low. Of note, the patient did have an early morning awakening. The epoch of REM sleep (see Figure P13-1) shows a higher REM density than expected for the first period of REM sleep during the night. On further questioning, the patient reported never falling asleep during the day but really experienced fatigue. She reported feeling down and to have no real pleasure in any of her recent activities. The picture was most consistent with depression, and the patient was referred for psychiatric treatment (see Fundamentals 41 for more discussion on depression).

2. **Answer:** REM rebound on the third or fourth night.

Discussion: A rebound in REM sleep may occur after prior sleep deprivation, although the first recovery night stage N3 rebound is predominantly noted at least in younger individuals.[4] Among patients with sleep apnea, some show a rebound in REM sleep when first placed on continuous positive airway pressure (CPAP).[5] They may also have a rebound in stage N3 sleep. One study suggests that patients with REM rebound (but no stage N3 rebound) may have better CPAP adherence.

REM rebound may have important consequences in patients with sleep disordered breathing (not on CPAP). The worst nocturnal oxygenation in patient with untreated OSA or lung disease (chronic obstructive pulmonary disease [COPD]) usually occurs during periods of REM sleep. An example of an important consequence is the effect on nocturnal oxygenation after surgery. Studies have shown that REM sleep is usually absent on postoperative nights 1 and 2 after abdominal surgery.[6] Stress from surgery, anesthesia, and medications are thought to be causative factors. This is usually followed by a profound increase in the amount and density of REM sleep (REM sleep rebound) during recovery nights 3 to 5. These may be associated with severe and unanticipated nocturnal hypoxemia.[8,9]

3. **Answer:** Entry into sleep via stage R, sleep cycles shorter (often 45 to 60 minutes).

Discussion: The sleep of infants is typically 16 to 18 hours per day with sleep episodes of 3 to 4 hours interrupted by feeding.[10-12] Entry into sleep via stage R is normal. The sleep cycles are shorter than in adults (45 to 60 minutes versus 90 to 100 minutes).

CLINICAL PEARLS

1. A number of causes of a short **nocturnal** REM latency exist. Major causes to consider are OSA (uncommon), depression, narcolepsy, prior sleep loss, and withdrawal of a REM suppressing medication.

2. After sleep loss, rebound in stage N3 is more common on the first recovery night with REM rebound to follow.

3. On the first night of CPAP, some patients with OSA have a large amount of REM sleep (REM rebound).

4. Patients with depression have a number of REM sleep abnormalities, including a short REM latency, a long first REM period, and high REM density.

5. REM rebound occurs on postoperative nights 3 to 5 and may be associated with significant arterial oxygen desaturation.

6. Entry into sleep via stage R is normal in infants. Sleep cycles (REM-NREM) are shorter than in adults (often 45 to 60 minutes).

REFERENCES

1. Aldrich MS, Chervin RD, Malow BA: Value of the multiple sleep latency test (MSLT) for the diagnosis of narcolepsy, *Sleep* 20(8):620–629, 1997.
2. Benca RM, Obermeyer WH, Thisted RA, et al: Sleep and psychiatric disorders: a meta-analysis, *Arch Gen Psychiatry* 49:651–668, 1992.
3. Kupfer DJ: Sleep research in depressive illness: clinical implications—a tasting menu, *Biol Psychiatry* 38:391–403, 1995.
4. Bonnet MH, Arand DL: Clinical effects of sleep fragmentation versus sleep deprivation, *Sleep Med Rev* 7(4):297–310, 2003.
5. Koo BB, Wiggins R, Molina C: REM rebound and CPAP compliance, *Sleep Med* 13(7):864–868, 2012.
6. Knill RL, Moote CA, Skinner MI, et al: Anesthesia with abdominal surgery leads to intense REM sleep during the first post-operative week, *Anesthesiology* 73:52–61, 1990.
7. Deleted in proof.
8. Rosenberg JF, Ullstad TF, Rasmussen J, et al: Time course of postoperative hypoxaemia, *Eur J Surg* 160:137–143, 1994.
9. Rosenberg JF, Wildschiodtz G, Pedersen MH, et al: Late postoperative nocturnal episodic hypoxaemia and associated sleep pattern, *Br J Anaesth* 72:145–150, 1994.
10. Kahn A, Dan B, Groswasser J, et al: Normal sleep architecture in infants and children, *J Clin Neurophysiol* 13:184–197, 1996.
11. Seldon S: Polysomnography in infants and children. In Sheldon SH, Ferber R, Kryger MH, editors: *Principles and practice of pediatric sleep medicine*, Philadelphia, 2005, Saunders, pp 49–71.
12. Iglowstein I, Jenni OG, Molinari L, Largo RH: Sleep duration from infancy to adolescence: reference values and generational trends, *Pediatrics* 111:302–307, 2003.

FUNDAMENTALS 8

Effects of Sleep Disorders and Medications on Sleep Architecture

A number of sleep disorders and medications may alter the amount of sleep or sleep architecture.[1-4] This section is not meant to be comprehensive but to cover some of the more commonly encountered disorders and circumstances. Recall that the sleep latency is the time from lights-out until the first epoch of sleep. The rapid eye movement (REM) latency is the time from sleep onset until the first stage of stage R. Frequent alternations in nocturnal sleep architecture include an increase in sleep latency, increase or decrease in REM latency, and increases or decreases of the amount of wake after sleep onset (WASO; minutes) or stages N1, N2, N3, and R (as a percentage of total sleep time [TST]). Typical sleep complaints include increased time to fall asleep (increased sleep latency, sleep onset insomnia), difficulty staying asleep (increased WASO, sleep maintenance insomnia), early morning awakening, or nonrestorative sleep.

MEDICATIONS AND SLEEP

A number of medications and substances may impair sleep (Table F8-1). The history of the onset of a sleep complaint with starting a particular medication or an increase in the dose of a current medication is an important element for identification of the medication as a cause of sleep disturbance. The medication might not be suspected by the patient as causing his or her problem (e.g., a medication for blood

TABLE F8-1 Medications Commonly Associated with Insomnia and Long Sleep Latency

Class	Examples	Comments
Stimulants	Methylphenidate Dextroamphetamine Atomoxetine (adults > children)	Especially sustained release medications if taken too late
Xanthines	Caffeine, theophylline	
Anticholinergic medications	Donepezil (Aricept)	2% to 14% incidence of insomnia, if so take in the morning
Beta-blockers	Propranolol, metoprolol	Atenolol lower risk
Ethanol	Ethanol	May shorten sleep latency but fragments sleep
Drugs for hyperlipidemia	Atorvastatin	(Not Simvastatin)
Selective serotonin reuptake inhibitors	Fluoxetine, sertraline, paroxetine, citalopram, escitalopram	Take in the morning (unless sedating)
Nonsedating tricyclic antidepressants	Nortriptyline	Amitryptyline and doxepin are sedating
Other antidepressants	Bupropion, venlafaxine, duloxetine	Mirtazapine is sedating
Angiotensin-converting enzyme inhibitors	Enalapril	Rare nightmares and insomnia

pressure causing insomnia). In some patients, a trial of withdrawal of the suspected medication is indicated. When continuing a medication known to cause sleep problems is essential, interventions for the sleep complaint or a search for an alternative medication is indicated. Of note, different medications in the same drug class may **not** be associated with the complaint. For example, nightmares with one dopamine agonist (pramipexole) might not occur with another (ropinirole). Alteration of the timing of the dose may be helpful. If an antidepressant causes an alert state, it may be taken in the morning. If a once-a-day medication that is often taken at bedtime, for example, donepezil (Aricept) causes insomnia, it may be taken in the morning.

SLEEP LATENCY AND INSOMNIA

Sleep latency may be prolonged because of the first-night effect, chronic insomnia disorder (sleep onset insomnia), co-morbid insomnia (depression), stimulant medications, nonsedating antidepressants, and bronchodilators (see Table F8-1). Beta-blockers may cause insomnia,[5] with propranolol carrying the highest risk. Beta-blockers with higher lipidophilicity (propranolol, metoprolol, carvedilol, labetalol) are associated with a greater incidence of insomnia compared with less lipophilic medications (atenolol, naldolol). Sedating antidepressants may decrease sleep latency (compared with the untreated state). Depression and medical disorders associated with pain can increase the sleep latency and amount of wake after sleep onset. Sleep disorders such as the restless legs

syndrome and the delayed sleep phase disorder can increase the sleep latency.

REM LATENCY

Circumstances that prolong or shorten the REM latency are listed in Table F8-2. A short REM latency (typically <70 minutes) may be associated with untreated obstructive sleep apnea (5% to 7%),[6] depression, withdrawal of an REM-suppressing medication, and narcolepsy. REM latency of 0 to 15 minutes is often referred to as *sleep-onset REM*. Sleep-onset REM is a defining characteristic of narcolepsy. In depression, REM latencies in the order of 40 minutes are typical but may be as short as those seen in patients with narcolepsy. In depression, the first episode of REM sleep is often prolonged with a higher REM density (number of eye movements per epoch) than usual. In normal sleep, the first REM period is short with infrequent REMs (low REM density).

A number of sleep disorders and medications may prolong REM latency (see Table F8-2). Untreated sleep apnea may be associated with a long REM latency (rarely a short REM latency). Medications known to prolong REM latency include tricyclic antidepressants, selective serotonin reuptake inhibitors (SSRIs), monoamine oxidase inhibitors (MAOIs), and lithium. MAOIs are said to be the most potent suppressors of REM sleep. Some substances such as alcohol may also increase REM latency. Bupropion, often classified as an atypical antidepressant, was reported to decrease the REM latency in a group of depressed patients in one study but was observed to increase REM latency in another

TABLE F8-2 **Causes of Changes in the REM Latency**		
Short REM Latency	**Long REM Latency**	**No/Minimal Change**
Narcolepsy	SSRIs, SNRIs	Mirtazapine
Depression	Tricyclic antidepressants	
Withdrawal of REM-suppressing medication	Trazodone	
Untreated sleep apnea (uncommon)	MAIOs? (minimal data)	
Previous REM sleep deprivation	Ethanol	
Nefazodone (or no change)	Lithium	
Bupropion*?	First-night effect	
	Bupropion*?	

MAIO, Monoamine oxidase inhibitors; *REM*, rapid eye movement; *SNRIs*, selective serotonin norepinephrine uptake inhibitors; *SSRIs*, selective serotonin reuptake inhibitors.
*Bupropion conflicting data.

study.[7,8] Rye et al.[9] found bupropion to decrease sleep onset REM periods in a patient with narcolepsy, with an increase occurring after withdrawal of the medication. In many textbooks, bupropion is listed as decreasing the REM latency.

AMOUNT OF REM SLEEP

The amount of REM sleep may increase after prior REM sleep deprivation, during the first night of treatment of obstructive sleep apnea (REM rebound) and after withdrawal of REM suppressing medications (Table F8-3). Factors that shorten REM latency also typically increase the duration of REM sleep. However, a number of exceptions exist. For example, patients with narcolepsy may exhibit a short nocturnal REM latency (about 20% to 50% of patients) but have a normal amount of REM sleep. Of note, the first night of recovery sleep after sleep loss is often characterized by a rebound in stage N3 with an increase in stage R on the second recovery night.

AMOUNT OF STAGE N3

A number of medications may decrease or increased stage N3 (Table F8-4). Benzodiazepines tend to decrease stage N3 because of a decrease in the amplitude of sleep waves. Non-benzodiazepine receptor agonist hypnotics (zaleplon, zolpidem, eszopiclone) do not decrease stage N3. Caffeine and theophylline may decrease stage N3.[10] Medications that may increase stage N3 include

TABLE F8-4	Medications Affecting the Duration of Stage N3 Sleep	
Increased	**Decreased**
Trazodone	Benzodiazepine*
Mirtazapine	Caffeine
Lithium	Theophylline
Pregablin	Stimulants
Gabapentin	(amphetamines)
Phenytoin	
Carbamazepine	
Sodium oxybate	
Levitiracetam	
Sedating tricyclic	
antidepressants	

*Benzodiazepine receptor agonist hypnotics that are not benzodiazepines (zolpidem, zaleplon, eszopiclone) do not decrease stage N3 sleep.

trazodone, gabapentin, pregablin, lithium, phenytoin, levitiracetam, carbamazepine, and some sedating antidepressants. Sodium oxybate increases stage N3 in patients with narcolepsy,[11] and this may be one mode of its beneficial action.

MEDICATIONS AND NIGHTMARES

Nightmares are unpleasant dreams that occur predominantly during REM sleep. A number of medications have been reported to cause nightmares (Table F8-5). Medications such as varenicline (Chantix), pramipexole, and efavirenez are notorious for causing vivid or unpleasant dreams. Melatonin, often used as a hypnotic, may also cause unpleasant dreams in some people.

TABLE F8-3	Factors Affecting the Duration of REM Sleep	
Decreased REM Sleep	**Increased REM Sleep**	**Minimal Change or Increase/Decrease in REM Sleep**
SSRIs	Withdrawal of REM suppressant medication	Mirtazapine
Tricyclic antidepressants	Prior REM sleep deprivation	Bupropion (or increase)
MAOIs	REM rebound on first night of PAP treatment	
Trazodone	Nefazodone	
Morphine		
Lithium		
Benzodiazepines (slight)		
First-night effect		

MAIO, Monoamine oxidase inhibitors; *PAP*, positive airway pressure; *REM*, rapid eye movement; *SSRIs*, selective serotonin reuptake inhibitors, *TCA*, tricyclic antidepressants.

TABLE F8-5 **Medications Commonly Associated with Nightmares**

Class of Agent	Examples	Comments
Amphetamines/amphetamine-like agents	Dextroamphetamine	Chronic use
Cholinergic medications	Donezepril (Aricept)	Chronic use
Benzodiazepines, BZRAS	Alprazolam, Zolpidem	Chronic use and withdrawal
Melatonin	Melatonin	Chronic use
Ethanol	Ethanol	REM rebound on withdrawal
Tricyclic antidepressants	Amitryptyline, doxepin, imipramine, nortriptyline	Chronic use
SSRIs	Fluoxetine, sertraline, paroxetine, citalopram, escitalopram	Insomnia, nightmares
Other antidepressants	Bupropion, Venlafaxine, Duloxetine	Insomnia, nightmares
Antiviral	Amantadine, oseltamivir	
Antiretroviral medications	Efavirenez (Sustiva) Tenofovir	Chronic use
Beta-blockers	Propanolol, metoprolol, carvedilol > atenolol	Chronic use
Beta-agonists	Albuterol	
Alpha-agonists	Methyldopa, clonidine	
Dopaminergic agents	Levadopa, pramipexole (up to 11%), ropinirole	Acute or chronic use
Agents for smoking cessation	Varenicline (Chantix)	10% to 13%
Calcium channel blockers	Verapamil, amlodipine	
Antibiotics	Erythromycin, levofloxacin, ciprofloxacin	
Angiotensin-converting enzyme	Enalapril	Rare nightmares and insomnia
Agents for hyperlipidemia	Atorvastatin	

BZRAs, benzodiazepine receptor agonists; *REM,* rapid eye movement; *SSRIs,* selective serotonin reuptake inhibitors.

REFERENCES

1. Schweitzer P, Dodson ER: Effects of drugs on sleep. In Avidan A, Barkoukis T, editors: *Review of sleep medicine,* ed 3, Philadelphia, 2012, Saunders, pp 272–291.
2. Roux FJ, Kryger MH: Medication effects on sleep, *Clin Chest Med* 31(2):397–405, 2010.
3. Winokur A, Gary KA, Rodner S, et al: Depression, sleep physiology, and antidepressant drugs, *Depress Anxiety* 14:19–28, 2001.
4. Gursky JT, Krahn LE: The effects of antidepressants on sleep: a review, *Harvard Rev Psychiat* 8:298–306, 2000.
5. Chang CH, Yang YH, Lin SJ, et al: Risk of insomnia attributable to β-blockers in elderly patients with newly diagnosed hypertension, *Drug Metab Pharmacokinet* 28 (1):53–58, 2013.
6. Chervin RD, Aldrich MS: Sleep onset REM periods during multiple sleep latency tests in patients evaluated for sleep apnea, *Am J Respir Crit Care Med* 161:426–431, 2000.
7. Nofzinger EA, Reynolds CF 3rd., Thase ME, et al: REM sleep enhancement by bupropion in depressed men, *Am J Psychiatry* 152(2):274–276, 1995.
8. Ott GE, Rao U, Lin KM, et al: Effect of treatment with bupropion on EEG sleep: relationship to antidepressant response, *Int J Neuropsychopharmacol* 7 (3):275–281, 2004.
9. Rye DB, Dihenia B, Bliwise DL: Reversal of atypical depression, sleepiness, and REM-sleep propensity in narcolepsy with bupropion, *Depress Anxiety* 7:92–95, 1998.
10. Drake CL, Jefferson C, Roehrs T, et al: Stress-related sleep disturbance and polysomnographic response to caffeine, *Sleep Med* 7:567–572, 2006.
11. Mamelak M, Black J, Montplaisir J, Ristanovic R: A pilot study on the effects of sodium oxybate on sleep architecture and daytime alertness in narcolepsy, *Sleep* 27:1327–1334, 2004.

Medications and Sleep

A 32-year-old woman is being evaluated for loud snoring and fatigue. Her medical problems include depression and hypertension. Her medications include fluoxetine, metoprolol, and lisinopril. The patient is also taking pramipexole for restless legs syndrome and clonazepam for insomnia. Lights out was at the patient's usual bedtime of 10:00 PM. The sleep architecture is summarized in Table P14-1.

TABLE P14-1 Sleep Architecture

Sleep Architecture		Total Night		Normal Range
Total recording time	(min)	450		(425–462)
Total sleep time	(min)	380		(394–457)
Sleep efficiency	(%)	84		(90–100)
Sleep latency	(min)	35.0		(0–19)
REM latency	(min)	200.0		(69–88)
Sleep Stages				
Awake (WASO):	(min)	35.0	%TST	(0–26) min
Stage N1:	(min)	24.0	6.3	(3–6) (%)
Stage N2:	(min)	275.5	72.5	(46–62) (%)
Stage N3:	(min)	20.5	5.4	(10–21) (%)
Stage R:	(min)	60.0	15.8	(21–31) (%)

min, Minutes; *REM*, rapid eye movement; *TST*, total sleep time; *WASO*, wake after sleep onset.

QUESTIONS

1. What is abnormal about the sleep architecture?

2. Which of the patient's medication is most likely to increase the rapid eye movement (REM) latency?

3. Which of the medications have been associated with disturbing dreams?

4. Which of the patient's medications may affect the amount of stage N3?

5. What medications may have decreased the amount of REM sleep?

ANSWERS

1. **Answer:** REM latency is very prolonged. The sleep latency is prolonged, and the total sleep time (TST) is decreased. The amount of stage N3 is decreased, and stage N2 is increased. The amount of REM sleep is also mildly decreased.

2. **Answer:** Fluoxetine

   Discussion: Nearly all antidepressants may increase REM latency (Table P14-2).[1-3] The limited data on bupropion is conflicting. Nefazodone may decrease REM latency. Mirtazapine is said to have minimal effect on the REM latency. Both depression and nonsedating antidepressants tend to increase sleep latency and decrease TST. Mirtazapine, trazodone, and nefazodone are sedating

TABLE P14-2	**Effects of Antidepressant Medications on Sleep**			
	Continuity	**Stage N3**	**REM Sleep (%TST)**	**REM Latency**
TCAs	Decreased (increased if sedating)	Unchanged	Decreased	Increased
SSRIs	Decreased	Unchanged	Decreased	Increased
Bupropion	Unchanged or decreased	Unchanged	?Conflicting data	? Conflicting data
Venlafaxine	Decreased	Unchanged	Decreased	Increased
Nefazodone	Increased	Unchanged	Increased?	Decreased
Mirtazapine	Increased	Increased?	Unchanged	No change
Trazodone	Increased	Increased	Decreased	Increased

Adapted from Gursky JT, Krahn LE: The effects of antidepressants on sleep: a review, *Harvard Rev Psychiatry* 8:298-306, 2000.
REM, Rapid eye movement; *SSRI*, selective serotonin reuptake inhibitor; *TCA*, tricyclic antidepressant; *TST*, total sleep time.

antidepressants, which may reduce the sleep latency. Mirtazapine and trazodone are often used in low doses at bedtime to improve the sleep in patients taking other antidepressants. Nefazodone may also improve sleep quality. Data about bupropion is conflicting, with one study showing a decrease, and another reported an increase in REM latency. The first-night effect (sleep in a new environment) or ethanol consumption near bedtime may also prolong REM latency.

3. **Answer:** Both metoprolol (a beta blocker) and pramipexole may cause disturbing dreams.

 Discussion: Pramipexole is commonly associated with nightmares (up to 11% in some reports).[1,2] See Fundamentals 8 for other medications associated with nightmares.

4. **Answer:** Clonazepam

 Discussion: Benzodiazepines tend to decrease the amount of stage N3 and increase stage N2. They may also cause small decreases in REM sleep. Clonazepam is a benzodiazepine with a long duration of action and is sometimes used off-label as a hypnotic, especially in patients with anxiety. Note that in this patient, sleep latency remained prolonged. The nonbenzodiazepine benzodiazepine receptor agonists zolpidem, zaleplon, and eszopiclone do not reduce the amount of stage N3 sleep.

5. **Answer:** Fluoxetine, possibly clonazepam

 Discussion: Most antidepressants reduce the amount of REM sleep.[3] Exceptions include mirtazapine, which has little effect on REM sleep, and nefazodone, which may actually increase the amount of REM sleep (see Table P14-2). Nefazodone is rarely used today due to concerns about liver toxicity and the availability of many alternative medications. Benzodiazepines may cause mild reductions in the amount of REM sleep (as a percentage of TST).

CLINICAL PEARLS

1. Medications are a common etiology of abnormal sleep architecture. It is essential to know what medications the patient has been taking, what medications were recently stopped, and if a hypnotic was taken at bedtime before the sleep study.
2. Most antidepressants prolong the REM latency. Exceptions include mirtazapine (no change) and nefazodone (decrease). Data about bupropion is conflicting.
3. Benzodiazepines tend to reduce stage N3 and increase stage N2. They may also induce a mild reduction in the amount REM sleep. Nonbenzodiazepine benzodiazepine receptor agonists do not decrease stage N3.
4. A number of medications may cause nightmares, including beta-blockers, varenicline, and pramipexole.

REFERENCES

1. Schweitzer P, Dodson ER: Effects of drugs on sleep. In Avidan A, Barkoukis T, editors: *Review of sleep medicine*, ed 3, Philadelphia, 2012, Saunders, pp 272–291.
2. Roux FJ, Kryger MH: Medication effects on sleep, *Clin Chest Med* 31(2):397–405, 2010.
3. Gursky JT, Krahn LE: The effects of antidepressants on sleep: a review, *Harvard Rev Psychiat* 8:298–306, 2000.

FUNDAMENTALS 9

Polysomnography I

Polysomnography (PSG) is the comprehensive monitoring of sleep. Digital PSG systems provide the ability to recorded many more parameters (signals) compared with paper recording. In Table F9-1 the commonly recorded parameters and purposes are displayed. Digital PSG systems allow one to view all or a portion of the parameters recorded. A *channel* is a horizontal display of a recorded parameter versus time. The number of channels displayed may be customized. Display windows of 5, 10, 15, 30, 60, 90, 180, and 240 minutes are typically available. The current epoch number, body position, and level of positive airway pressure (PAP), if applicable, are displayed along with the selected tracings.

A graphic display and summary of parameter values over the night is also available. Typically, body position and the values of PAP may also be displayed. By clicking on a portion of the all-night display, the epoch display view will instantly move to the time of night selected (Figure F9-1). It is easy to move to areas of interest, for example, a time when supine REM sleep occurred.

TABLE F9-1 Polysomnography

Parameter	Sensors	Purpose
EEG derivations	F4-M1, C4-M1, O2-M1 (Frontal, central, occipital)	Staging of sleep
EOG derivations	E1-M2, E2-M2	
Chin EMG	Chin1, Chin2, ChinZ	
ECG	ECG	Cardiac rate and rhythm
Air flow (diagnostic study)	Nasal pressure	Detection of hypopnea
	Oronasal thermal flow	Detection of apnea
Air flow (PAP titration)	PAP device flow	Detection of apnea, hypopnea
Snoring	Microphone, piezoelectric sensor	Detection of snoring
Respiratory effort	Chest and abdominal RIP bands	Classify apneas as obstructive, mixed, or central
Arterial oxygen saturation (SpO$_2$)	Pulse oximetry	Detect arterial oxygen desaturation
Left anterior tibial (LAT) EMG	EMG surface electrodes	Detect periodic limb movements in sleep
Right anterior tibial (RAT) EMG	EMG surface electrodes	
Optional:		
Heart rate (HR)	Oximeter output	Moving time average estimate of HR
Estimate of tidal volume	RIP sum	Alternate sensor for apnea and hypopnea detection
Estimate of air flow	RIP flow	Alternate sensor for apnea and hypopnea
Intercostal EMG	Right costal EMG electrodes	Detect inspiratory muscle firing (respiratory effort)
End-tidal PCO$_2$	Diagnostic study	Detect hypoventilation
Transcutaneous PCO$_2$	Diagnostic and PAP titration	
PAP device pressure, leak, tidal volume	PAP device flow and pressure sensors	Monitor delivered pressure, leak, tidal volume

ECG, Electrocardiography; *EEG,* electroencephalography; *EMG,* electromyography; *EOG,* electrooculography; *LAT,* left anterior tibial; *PAP,* positive airway pressure; *PCO$_2$,* partial pressure of carbon dioxide; *RAT,* right anterior tibial; *RIP,* respiratory inductance (inductive) plethysmography; *SpO$_2$,* arterial oxygen saturation by pulse oximetry.

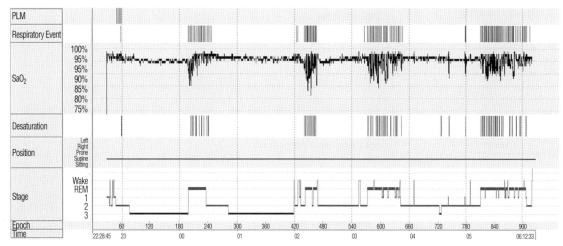

FIGURE F9-1 ■ A typical entire night summary plot showing sleep stage, body position, respiratory events, arterial oxygen saturation (SaO₂), and desaturations. The time of night is also displayed.

REFERENTIAL AND BIPOLAR RECORDING

Most digital PSG systems use a combination of referential, true bipolar, and direct current (DC) recording (Table F9-2).[1,2] Electroencephalography (EEG), electrooculography (EOG), and mastoid and chin electromyography (EMG) electrodes are recorded referentially (see Table F9-2). In **referential** recording, multiple electrodes are recorded against a common electrical reference (often located at Cz, central vertex). A **display** of any derivation using two referentially recorded electrodes may then obtained by digital subtraction:

[electrode A-electrode B = (electrode A-reference) − (electrode B-reference)]

either during acquisition or during review (Figure F9-2). The digital subtraction for display of derivations does *not* change the recorded data.

TABLE F9-2	Types of Recording
Referential recording	EEG: F4, F3, C4, C3, O2, O1, M1, M2 EOG: E1,E2 M1, M2 Chin1, Chin2, ChinZ REF (Reference electrode)
True bipolar (2 inputs each)	ECG, oronasal thermal flow, thorax and abdominal effort belts, right and left anterior tibial EMG
Direct current (DC)	Nasal pressure, SpO2, positive airway pressure device (flow, leak, pressure), end-tidal or transcutaneous PCO2

ECG, Electrocardiography; *EEG*, electroencephalography; *EMG*, electromyography; *EOG*, electrooculography; *PCO₂*, partial pressure of carbon dioxide; *SpO₂*, arterial oxygen saturation by pulse oximetry.

For example, both F3 and F4 are recorded (against the reference electrode) even though only F4-M1 may be displayed in the default display view (montage). If the sleep technologist failed to observe that the electrode F4 fails during the recording, the reviewer may change the viewed frontal derivation to F3-M1 or F3-M2 (recommended backup derivation).[3,4]

In true bipolar recording, each amplifier records the difference between two electrodes of interest (A-B, C-D). However, changing the derivation once the signal is recorded (e.g., A-D) is not possible. True bipolar recording is used for inputs that one would usually not desire to change in review. For example, the two inputs of the oronasal thermal flow sensor, respiratory effort bands (two each: thorax and abdomen), leg EMG inputs (two inputs or electrodes for each leg), and two electrocardiography (ECG) inputs. DC recording is used for nasal pressure, pulse oximetry, and other DC signals such as those from the PAP device (flow, leak, tidal volume, delivered pressure), end-tidal or transcutaneous partial pressure of carbon dioxide (PCO₂) devices.

PSG CHANNELS

Digital PSG systems allow for the display of the desired number of channels, each with the desired parameter to be displayed. Typically, preset default display views are predefined, each with a unique name stored in the computer (sometimes called *montages*) containing the desired parameters and display characteristics for each channel. It is possible to set a default tracing color, channel width, low and high filter settings, sensitivity (peak-to-peak voltage visible in channel window), and polarity for each

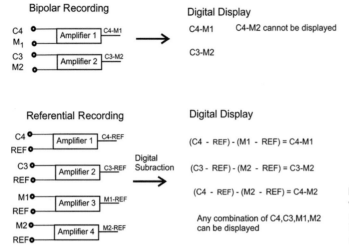

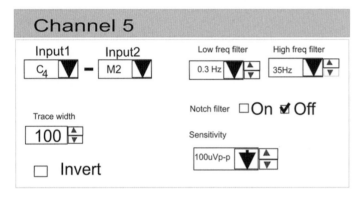

FIGURE F9-2 ■ Display of differences between true bipolar recording and referential recording. In referential recording, the two inputs are the electrode of interest and the reference electrode.

FIGURE F9-3 ■ Typical referential channel controls. For simplicity, color adjustment was not included. 100 microvolts (μV); *p-p* refers to the peak-to-peak voltage range displayed within the channel width, which is 100 μV.

channel. In referential channels, the default is negative polarity up (deflection upward in voltage from Input1 minus voltage from Input2, if Input 1 is negative with respect to Input2). The 60-hertz (Hz) notch filter may be turned on or off. It is possible to access each channel's controls, as shown in Figure F9-3, to adjust the settings. It is also possible to change between different displays, for example, between one display view suitable for diagnostic study and another for a PAP titration. Sample display views are shown in Table F9-3.

IMPEDANCE CHECKING, CALIBRATION, AND BIOCALIBRATIONS

The impedance of all EEG, EOG, ECG, and EMG electrodes should be checked prior to recording. In some systems, the head box is connected to an impedance device. In others, the amplifier sends a signal via the electrodes to measure the impedance. *The ideal electrode impedance is 5 kilo ohms or less (<10 acceptable).* Many PSG systems have the ability to recheck impedance values

during the study. A **calibration signal** is also usually sent to all alternating current (AC) channels either as a step voltage or a sine wave. The amplifier in digital PSG systems typically has a fixed gain, but scaling factors may be applied by the PSG computer program to the amplifier output for each parameter being recorded. For example, a 5-volt (V) signal is sent to F4-REF and M1-REF. If the former reads 5.1 V and the later 4.9 V, these outputs are scaled by the computer program to be equal to 5 V. Then the display F4-M1 is equal to 0 rather than 0.2 V.

Biocalibration (Table F9-4; Fig. F9-4) is an important part of every PSG recording, but the information gained is often under utilized. During the biocalibration procedure, signals are recorded, while the patient performs maneuvers, to verify that the monitoring equipment, electrodes, and sensors are working properly. The reviewer notes the patient's EEG, EOG, and EMG pattern of eyes-open wakefulness. It is especially important to know whether the person being monitored generates alpha rhythm activity with eye closure because this affects the scoring criteria for stage W and stage N1 (see Fundamentals 3 and 4).

TABLE F9-3 Sample Polysomnography Display Views (Montages)

Channel	Diagnostic 1	Diagnostic 2	PAP Titration
1	F4-M1	E1-M2	F4-M1
2	C4-M1	E2-M2	C4-M1
3	O2-M1	F4-M1	O2-M1
4	E1-M2	F3-M2	E1-M2
5	E2-M2	C4-M1	E2-M2
6	Chin EMG	C3-M2	Chin EMG
7	ECG	O2-M1	ECG
8	Heart rate	O1-M2	Heart rate
9	Nasal pressure	Chin EMG	PAP flow
10	Oronasal thermal flow	ECG	Chest
11	Chest	Heart rate	Abdomen
12	Abdomen	Nasal pressure	SpO_2
13	SpO_2	On therm	LAT
14	LAT	Chest	RAT
15	RAT	Abdomen	PAP leak
16	Exhaled PCO_2	SpO_2	PAP pressure
17		LAT	PAP tidal volume
18		RAT	$PtcCO_2$

ECG, Electrocardiographic; *EMG*, electromyographic; *LAT*, left anterior tibial; *On therm*, oronasal thermal flow; *PAP*, positive airway pressure; *PCO₂*, partial pressure of carbon dioxide; *PtcCO₂*, transcutaneous carbon dioxide tension; *RAT*, right anterior tibial; *SpO₂*, arterial oxygen saturation by pulse oximetry.

TABLE F9-4 Biocalibration Procedure

Command	What to Check and Observe
While looking straight ahead, close your eyes.	Is alpha rhythm generated with eye closure? Slow eye movements
Open your eyes.	Attenuation of alpha rhythm. EEG and eye movement pattern of wakefulness. (REMs during wakefulness)
Look up. Look down. Look right. Look left. Blink eyes.	Integrity of eye electrodes. Pattern of the patient's REMs and blinks. Ability to detect horizontal and vertical eye movements.
Grit teeth.	Function of chin EMG. (Sensitivity should be adjusted so that some activity is present during relaxed wakefulness).
Breath in, breathe out.	Ensure air flow sensors show are working properly; adjust sensitivity. Ensure proper polarity and function for all respiratory sensors (air flow sensors and respiratory effort belts). That is, during inspiration, all deflections are upward or downward (depending on sleep center protocol). Adjust sensitivity of chest and abdomen tracings.
Hold your breath.	Ability to detect apnea.
Wiggle your right toe. Wiggle your left toe.	Ability to detect leg movements. Adjust leg derivation sensitivity so that movements can be easily seen in both legs.

EEG, Electroencephalography; *EMG*, electromyography; *REM*, rapid eye movement.

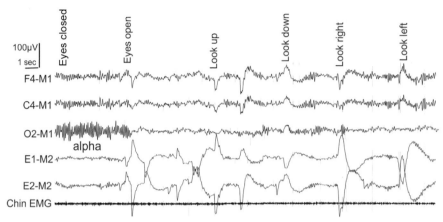

FIGURE F9-4 ■ Biocalibration for the electroencephalography (EEG) and electrooculography (EOG) derivations. In this patient, eye closure generated alpha rhythm.

INFORMATION FLOW DURING DIGITAL PSG

Although PSG digital systems vary, what follows generally applies to all systems (Figure F9-5). The signals are input to the amplifier at the bedside via a head box where electrodes are inserted. Some PSG systems input all signals via the head box, but others have a separate DC input box or separate DC inputs on the amplifier (e.g., input from external devices such as signals from the PAP device). The amplifiers used in modern digital PSG systems both amplify the signal and process the signal with a default low filter (typically 0.1 Hz or lower) and a default high filter (anti-aliasing filter, typically half the sampling rate).[5] Thus, signals over a wide frequency range (band pass) are recorded. After wide band pass filtering by the amplifier, the analog signal is then converted to a digital signal by using an analog to digital converter usually located inside the amplifier case. In digital form, the data may be sent by network cable to an acquisition computer without any degradation of signal. The digital information is then recorded by the computer. Further filtering may be applied before the recorded (stored) signals are displayed during acquisition or review, *but this filtering does not change the recorded data.* Similarly, the data may be scaled to an appropriate size to fit in the chosen channel window. Again,

the recorded data are not changed, but the display is simply scaled. For example, a 50-microvolt (μV) peak-to-peak waveform when displayed in a 100-μV peak-to-peak window will take up half the channel width.

SAMPLING RATE AND DIGITAL RESOLUTION

Most digital recording systems use analog amplifiers that produce a continuous signal output. The signal is then sampled by an analog to digital (A/D) conversion board, which converts the signal to a digital form that can be stored and manipulated by a computer. The sampling rate must be more than twice the frequencies being recorded to avoid signal distortion (Nyquist theorem). If lower sampling rates are used, the signal may be extremely distorted, and the addition of frequencies lower that the original signal sampled may be introduced (Figure F9-6). For this reason, signals with a frequency higher than half the sampling rate must be filtered out, as they can cause aliasing distortion. For example, *if the sampling rate is 200 samples per second, the amplifier output must be filtered with a high filter of 100 Hz or lower before being digitized.* The required sampling rate depends on the frequency of the signal to be recorded. Slower varying signals require a lower sampling rate.

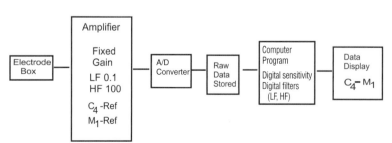

FIGURE F9-5 ■ Information flow for digital polysomnography (PSG). The signals are filtered by a wide band pass (0.1 to 100 hertz [Hz]) before the signal is digitized. Further filtering may be performed before signals are displayed, but this does not change the stored data. *HF,* High filters; *LF,* low filters.

FUNDAMENTALS 9 POLYSOMNOGRAPHY I   **85**

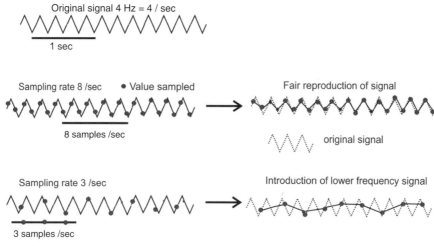

FIGURE F9-6 ■ Sampling (*dots represent value sampled*) with a frequency less than the signal of interest produces a poor representation of the signal and introduces a lower frequency not present in the original signal.

TABLE F9-5 **Recommended Filter Setting and Sampling Rate for Polysomnography Signals**

	Low Frequency	High Frequency	Sampling Rate (samples/sec) (Minimum/Desired)
EEG	0.3 Hz	35 Hz	200 / 500
EOG	0.3 Hz	35 Hz	200 / 500
EMG	10 Hz	100 Hz	200 / 500
ECG	0.3 Hz	70 Hz	200 / 500
Thermal air flow Chest, abdominal bands	0.1	15 Hz	25 / 100
Snoring	10 Hz	100 Hz	200 / 500
Nasal pressure	0.03 or DC	100 Hz (if snoring has to be visualized)	25 / 100
Oximetry	DC	—	10 / 25
PAP flow	DC	—	25 / 100
Body position	DC	—	1

DC, Direct current; *ECG*, electrocardiography; *EEG*, electroencephalography; *EMG*, electromyography; *EOG*, electrooculography; *Hz*, hertz; *PAP*, positive airway pressure.

In Table F9-5, the sampling rates recommended by the AASM scoring manual[3,4,6] are provided. Some digital PSG systems have the ability to record different signals at different sampling rates. An adequate sampling rate is required for accurate representation of the recorded signal, but other factors to consider include digital resolution and monitor resolution. A/D conversion is characterized by the dynamic range (the range of voltages accepted by the A/D converter) and the resolution.[1] The dynamic range may be expressed as the amplified or unamplified signal range. The resolution depends on the A/D converter as well as the dynamic range. A 12-bit DC converter provides $2^{12} = 4096$ digital values (bits) or a 16-bit converter $= 65,536$ values across the dynamic range. A typical A/D converter might have a dynamic range for the amplified signal of 5 V ($\pm$ 2.5 V). Commonly, a set amplification is applied to all AC signals before A/D conversion (e.g., a gain of 1250). If an amplification of 1250 is assumed, the dynamic range (peak to peak) of an A/D converter with an amplified voltage range of 5 V expressed as the unamplified signal would be approximately 4000 μV (4000 μV $\times 1250 = 5,000,000$ $\mu V = 5.0$ V). If a 12-bit A/D converter is used, this would result in a resolution of 0.97 μV/bit (4000 μV/4096 digital values). Ultimately, the computer program uses only a small portion of the data for the display, as monitor resolution (in pixels per displayed time duration) is usually much less than the sampling rate. A minimum monitor resolution of 1600 $\times$ 1200 pixels is recommended by the *AASM Scoring Manual*. The monitor typically can display only a fraction of the available data, especially when a large time window (e.g., 120 seconds) is displayed. Monitor aliasing may distort the appearance of the signal. Viewing data with a smaller time window (10 seconds per screen) effectively increases monitor sampling rate per displayed second. If 30 seconds is displayed for a monitor with 1600 horizontal pixels, the maximum resolution is 53 samples per second (versus 200 values per second, a typical sampling rate).

LOW-FREQUENCY AND HIGH-FREQUENCY FILTERS AND NOTCH FILTERS

Any signal of interest may be contaminated by unwanted low- or high-frequency signals, including 60 Hz artifact (from nearby AC power lines). Filters attenuate or eliminate these unwanted frequencies. For example, a low filter (high pass filter) attenuates the amplitude of very low frequency signals such as skin galvanic potentials. A high filter (low pass filter) attenuates the amplitude of high-frequency signals. For example, high-frequency muscle activity in the EEG signals is attenuated. A schematic illustration of the effects of low- and high-frequency filters is shown in Figure F9-7. A notch filter (60 Hz) attenuates a narrow band of frequencies to reduce 60 Hz artifact. As noted above *wide band pass filtering by the amplifier occurs before the signal is digitized and stored* (e.g., 0.1 to 100 Hz). Further filtering may be applied before the recorded signals are displayed during acquisition or review *but this filtering does not change the recorded data.* As noted above, default low and high filter settings and information on the notch filter being on or off may be stored for each channel to be displayed.

The amount of signal reduction of a given frequency by an analog or digital filter is given in decibels (dB). The amount of signal reduction in decibels is given by the formula 20 log (voltage-out/voltage-in), where voltage-out and voltage-in are the amplitude of the signal entering and leaving the filter, respectively.

A signal reduction of approximately 30% (voltage-out/voltage-in ratio of approximately 0.7) corresponds to a 3 dB reduction. A 50% reduction in signal corresponds to a 6 dB reduction. The exact ratio is 0.707, but we will use 0.7 for simplicity. Different filter settings (0.3 Hz, 1 Hz, etc.) specify the "cutoff frequency" of a filter, which is the frequency of the signal that is reduced by 3 dB (to 70% of original signal or 30% reduction). Filters are also characterized by the "roll off," that is the slope of the attenuation curve. In Figure F9-8, a 0.3-Hz low

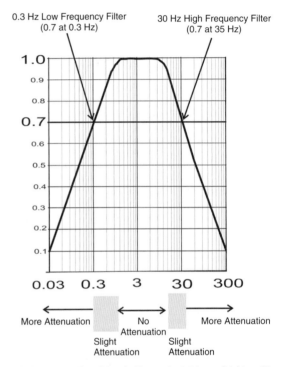

FIGURE F9-8 ■ Combined effects of a 0.3-hertz (Hz) low filter and a 30-Hz high filter. The vertical (y axis) is the amount of attenuation (1.0 = no attenuation, 0.7 means the signal is reduced to 0.7 of the original voltage). The x axis is frequency in hertz using a logarithmic scale. The cutoff frequency for the low and high filters is 0.3 and 30 Hz, respectively (−3 dB or attenuation to approximately 0.7). The American Association of Sleep Medicine (AASM) recommends high filter of 35 Hz, but the behavior is very similar to the 30-Hz high filter illustrated in the figure.

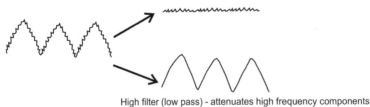

FIGURE F9-7 ■ Schematic effects of low-frequency (high-pass) and high-frequency (low-pass) filters. Signals typically contain both low and high frequency components. Low filters are used to attenuate low-frequency signals, and high filters are used to attenuate the high-frequency signals. The amount of attenuation depends on the filter setting, the signal frequency, and the type of filter (e.g., 3 decibels [dB] or 6 dB).

fitter setting attenuates a 0.3-Hz signal to 70%. Frequencies *lower* than 0.3 Hz are attenuated even more. Signals with a frequency slightly higher than 0.3 Hz are slightly attenuated. Signals with a frequency 5 to 10 times higher are not attenuated at all. In the same figure, a 30-Hz high-frequency (low-pass) filter attenuates a 30-Hz signal to 70% of the original signal. Frequencies *higher* than 30 Hz are attenuated even more. Signals slightly lower than 30 Hz are also attenuated slightly. Signals lower than 30 Hz by a factor of 0.05 to 0.1 are not attenuated. The combination of a low filter and a high filter is called a *band pass filter*. The AASM recommends a high filter of 35 Hz, but the behavior is very similar to the 30-Hz filter, which is shown for simplicity. Using a low filter of 0.3 and high filter of 35 Hz means that frequencies of interest for recording of EEG and EOG of 0.5 Hz to 16 Hz are minimally attenuated. The effects of different low filter settings on slow wave activity is shown in Figure F9-9. Typical low filter settings are 0.1, 0.3, 0.5, 1, 3, 5, 10 Hz. Typical higher filter settings are 12, 15, 35, 50, 70, 100 Hz.

Sometimes, low filter settings are specified as a time constant rather than a cutoff frequency. For a 3-dB filter, the relationship between the time constant and the cutoff frequency is given by:

$$\text{time constant} = 1/(2\pi \times \text{cutoff frequency})$$

For example, a 0.3-Hz (3-dB) low filter has a time constant of approximately 0.53 seconds. The lower the cutoff frequency, the longer is the time constant.

The *AASM Scoring Manual* specifies recommended low and high filter settings. Using a low filter of 0.3 Hz and a high filter of 35 Hz does not attenuate signals of interest except for slight attenuation of signals in the low part of the slow wave activity range (0.5 to 2 Hz). On the other hand, an EMG signal has higher-frequency components, and filtering out more lower-frequency components is desirable, so a low filter of 10 Hz and a high filter of 100 Hz are specified.

VIDEO-AUDIO PSG

Today, most digital systems allow for the simultaneous recording of video and audio signals. Ideally, the video should be synchronized with the recorded EEG and other signals. This will allow the reviewer to see patient movement corresponding exactly to a given time point in the recorded PSG signals. For example, facial twitching can be noted during a particular EEG pattern. Video PSG is an important development and allows the reviewer to confirm the patient position as well as document unusual behavior (e.g., parasomnias) during the night. Video files are often quite large and are usually compressed (e.g., MPEG4). The size of the file will depend on the quality of the video (10 or 25 frames per second). Simultaneous audio is also usually available, and this is very useful for documenting teeth grinding (bruxism), talking during parasomnias, snoring, and other vocal behaviors during the recording.

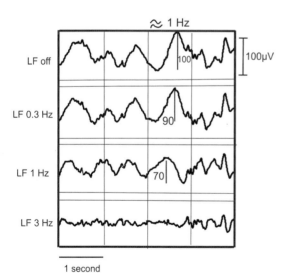

FIGURE F9-9 ■ The effect of different low-frequency filters settings (3 dB filter) on slow wave activity. Note that activity of about 1 hertz (Hz) is decreased to 0.70 by a 1-Hz filter and attenuated significantly more at higher low-filter settings. The further below the cutoff frequency, the more a signal is attenuated. Also, note that the 1-Hz signal is attenuated slightly by the 0.3-Hz filter.

REFERENCES

1. Berry RB: *Fundamentals of sleep medicine*, Philadelphia, 2012, Saunders, pp 13–26.
2. Berry RB: *Sleep medicine pearls*, ed 2, Philadelphia, 2003, Hanley and Belfus, pp 67–69.
3. Iber C, Ancoli-Israel S, Chesson A, Quan SF: for the American Academy of Sleep Medicine: *The AASM manual for scoring of sleep and associated events: rules, terminology and technical specifications*, ed 1, Westchester, IL, 2007, American Academy of Sleep Medicine.
4. Berry RB, Brooks R, Gamaldo CE, et al: for the American Academy of Sleep Medicine: *The AASM manual for the scoring of sleep and associated events: rules, terminology and technical specifications*, Version 2.1, Darien, IL, 2012, American Academy of Sleep Medicine. www.aasmnet.org, Accessed July 3, 2014.
5. Epstein CM: Aliasing in the visual EEG: a potential pitfall of video display technology, *Clin Neurophysiol* 114:1974–1976, 2003.
6. Silber MH, Ancoli-Israel S, Bonnet MH, et al. The Visual scoring of sleep in adults, *J Clin Sleep Med* 15:121–131, 2007.

A Patient with Artifact in Many Channels

QUESTIONS

1. In Figure P15-1, what is the problem electrode?

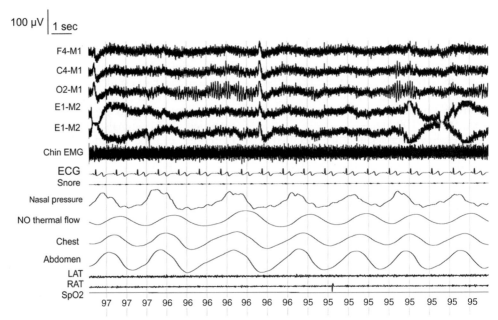

FIGURE P15-1 ■ A 20-second tracing showing a significant artifact in many of the channels. NO thermal flow is the nasal-oral thermal flow signal.

2. In Figure P15-2, a 4-second tracing of a montage showing each electrode as recorded versus the reference electrode (REF) is shown. For each channel, the low frequency filter is 0.1 hertz (Hz0), the high-frequency filter is 70 Hz, and the 60-Hz notch filter is turned off. Which electrode(s) is (are) faulty?

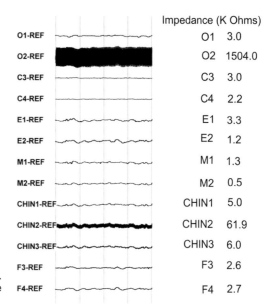

	Impedance (K Ohms)	
O1-REF	O1	3.0
O2-REF	O2	1504.0
C3-REF	C3	3.0
C4-REF	C4	2.2
E1-REF	E1	3.3
E2-REF	E2	1.2
M1-REF	M1	1.3
M2-REF	M2	0.5
CHIN1-REF	CHIN1	5.0
CHIN2-REF	CHIN2	61.9
CHIN3-REF	CHIN3	6.0
F3-REF	F3	2.6
F4-REF	F4	2.7

FIGURE P15-2 ■ A 4-second tracing of a referential montage. The impedance of each electrode is shown. *REF,* Reference electrode.

ANSWERS

1. **Answer:** The reference electrode is the problem.

   Discussion: In referential recording all of the electrodes are recorded versus the reference electrode (REF). That is, F4-REF, M1-REF, and so on are recorded using a differential alternating current (AC) amplifier.[1] Different combinations of referentially recorded electrodes may be displayed by digital subtraction (F4-REF − M1-REF = F4-M1). The position of the REF electrode is not standardized but is often placed at or near Cz (vertex). In Figure P15-1, all the referential derivations display a 60 Hz artifact. This artifact is discussed in more detail in Fundamentals 11. The pattern means that either every referentially recorded electrode is faulty (unlikely) or that the REF electrode is faulty. Note that none of the channels with true bipolar recording (nasal oral thermal air flow, chest, abdomen, right anterior tibial electromyography [EMG], left anterior tibial EMG, or electrocardiography [ECG]) or direct current (DC) recording (nasal pressure, saturation of peripheral oxygen [SpO_2]) are affected. The reference electrode is usually placed near Cz at the vertex. Most digital polysomnography (PSG) systems have a montage that displays each referentially recorded electrode as recorded versus REF (see Figure P15-2). This allows one to determine if an electrode is faulty. For example, if F4-M1 shows a 60 Hz artifact, both F4-REF and M1-REF can be visualized to determine if F4 or M1 is the faulty electrode. If M1 is faulty, other derivations containing M1 should be faulty. Another approach would be to determine if changing to F3-M1 or F4-M2 eliminated the problem.

2. **Answer:** Electrodes O_2 and Chin2 are faulty.

   Discussion: Figure P15-2 displays each electrode recorded versus the REF. This is the actual method by which the activity at individual electrodes is recorded. It is apparent that O_2-REF and Chin2-REF display a 60-Hz artifact (dark band or rope-like tracing). As expected both O_2 and Chin2 have a high impedance. The recommended impedance is 5 kilo ohms but 5 to 10 is acceptable.[2–4] Prior to recording, the impedance of all electrodes should be measured. Many digital PSG systems allow recording of impedance values during actual data acquisition.

CLINICAL PEARLS

1. If all derivations of referentially recorded electrodes are faulty, suspect the reference electrode as the problem. Bipolar and DC channels are not influenced by a faulty REF electrode.

2. The ideal impedance of each electrode is 5 kilo Ohms or less (less than 10 acceptable).

3. Using a display view with each referentially electrode displayed versus REF (as the electrodes are actually recorded) may be useful in quickly identifying problem electrodes. If all the displayed derivations are faulty, this would suggest that the common electrode (REF) was faulty.

REFERENCES

1. Berry RB: *Fundamentals of sleep medicine*, Philadelphia, 2012, Saunders, pp 13–26.
2. Iber C, Ancoli-Israel S, Chesson A, Quan SF, for the American Academy of Sleep Medicine: *The AASM manual for scoring of sleep and associated events: rules, terminology and technical specifications*, ed 1, Westchester, IL, 2007, American Academy of Sleep Medicine.
3. Silber MH, Ancoli-Israel S, Bonnet MH, et al, The visual scoring of sleep in adults, *J Clin Sleep Med* 15:121–131, 2007.
4. Berry RB, Brooks R, Gamaldo CE, et al, for the American Academy of Sleep Medicine: *The AASM manual for the scoring of sleep and associated events: rules, terminology and technical specifications*, Version 2.03, Darien, IL, 2012, American Academy of Sleep Medicine. www.aasmnet.org, Accessed July 3, 2014.

Indications for Polysomnography, Portable Monitoring, and Actigraphy

The American Academy of Sleep Medicine (AASM) practice parameters[1–6] outline the indications for polysomnography (PSG). PSG is the standard test for diagnosis of suspected sleep-related breathing disorders (SRBDs), narcolepsy (when combined with a multiple sleep latency test [MSLT]), positive airway pressure (PAP) titration, evaluation of parasomnias (under certain conditions), determining the efficacy of prior surgical treatment for obstructive sleep apnea, and determining the efficacy of oral appliance (OA) treatment for OSA (PSG while wearing the OA) (Box F10-1). Limited channel sleep testing (LCST) performed unattended in the home may also be used for the diagnosis of obstructive sleep apnea (OSA) and evaluation of surgical and OA treatment of OSA. LCST usually does not record electroencephalography (EEG), electrooculography (EOG), or electromyography (EMG) derivations and therefore cannot determine the amount of sleep recorded. LCST has also been called *Out-of-Center Sleep Testing* (OCST), *home sleep testing* (HST), and portable monitoring (PM). For the remainder of this discussion, the term *OCST* will be used, although unattended LCST may occur in the hospital. Clinical guidelines for the use of OCST have been published outlining recommended indications, procedures, and devices.[7] In general, OCST is acceptable for diagnosis of OSA in patients with high pretest probability of moderate to severe OSA in the absence of certain comorbidities and for determining the adequacy of prior surgery for OSA or effectiveness of current OA treatment for OSA.[2,6–8]

DIAGNOSTIC PSG

PSG is the standard diagnostic study for evaluation of a suspected obstructive or central sleep apnea. A diagnostic study may be repeated if the initial study was negative for sleep apnea and a high clinical index of suspicion for this disorder exists. PSG should be performed preoperatively for planned surgery to treat snoring or suspected OSA. Even if the main goal of surgery is treatment of snoring, evaluation for OSA is important. If unsuspected moderate to severe OSA is present, this may change treatment. A PSG is indicated after surgery for OSA (after surgical healing) to document effectiveness. The practice parameters specify "in moderate to severe OSA," although most clinicians would perform a PSG after surgery for mild OSA as well. A PSG is indicated after adjustment of an OA for OSA (not for primary snoring) to document efficacy. The 2005 AASM practice parameters for PSG recommended a sleep study with the patient using an OA for treatment of moderate to severe OSA to document efficacy.[2] In a subsequent practice parameter on OA treatment of OSA, a PSG to document efficacy was recommended for OSA of all severities.[6] For patients with prior effective surgical treatment (documented by PSG), the PSG may be repeated at a later time if symptoms of sleep apnea return. For a patient using an OA as treatment for OSA, the PSG may also be repeated while the patient wears the OA if the symptoms return. PSG is *not* recommended in patients on continuous positive airway pressure (CPAP) treatment who are doing well. If the patient is being treated on CPAP and is *not* doing well, a repeat PSG study on CPAP is indicated.[2] However, before this expensive procedure, it is essential to document adequate objective adherence and to optimize treatment and the mask interface. PSG is also indicated if a patient on CPAP gains more than 10% of body weight to determine if the pressure is adequate. If a patient on CPAP loses more than 10% of body weight, a diagnostic PSG is indicated to determine whether CPAP is still needed or if a lower level of CPAP will be effective.

BOX F10–1	Indications for Polysomnography (PSG)

PSG INDICATED

Diagnostic PSG

1. Diagnosis of suspected sleep-related breathing disorders (OSA, central sleep apnea).
2. Repeat PSG is indicated if the initial PSG was negative + high clinical suspicion for OSA.
3. Preoperative PSG before planned surgery for snoring or OSA.
4. Evaluation of suspected narcolepsy (in combination with MSLT).
5. Evaluation of suspected periodic limb movement disorder (but *not* restless legs syndrome).
6. Evaluation of suspected **complicated** parasomnia:
   a. Nocturnal behavior possibly caused by seizures
   b. Atypical parasomnia behavior (frequent episodes each night, stereotypical behavior, or behavior unusual for age)
   c. Nocturnal behavior or parasomnia that has resulted in injury to the patient or others (or has the potential to do so)
   d. Presumed parasomnia or nocturnal seizure disorder that does not respond to conventional treatment, or
   e. Legal or forensic implications of nocturnal behavior.

PAP Titration (PSG on PAP)

1. Patients: AHI > 15/hour (hr) with or without symptoms, AHI ≥5/hr with symptoms or comorbidities.
2. Full night of PSG titration.
3. Split:
   • AHI >40 during 2 hours of monitoring in the initial diagnostic portion.
   • AHI 20–40 special clinical circumstances (long apnea or severe desaturation).

   • 3 hours remain for PAP titration.
   • Repeat PSG for PAP titration if inadequate PAP titration portion of study.

Follow-up PSG

1. After surgery for moderate to severe OSA—usually 3–6 months after surgery.
2. After previous surgery for OSA if symptoms return.
3. After adequate adjustment of oral appliance for OSA (all severities).

Repeat PSG (Diagnosis or PAP Titration)

1. After ≥10% weight loss in patient on CPAP (PSG without CPAP) to determine if CPAP still needed.
2. After ≥10% weight gain to determine whether CPAP is adequate.
3. Clinical symptoms return in patient on CPAP (consider MSLT if narcolepsy suspected).
4. Clinical symptoms return after surgery for OSA or on OA treatment for OSA.

PSG NOT INDICATED

1. Routine follow-up of a patient doing well on PAP treatment.
2. Evaluation of asthma or chronic lung disease (unless OSA is suspected).
3. Evaluation of insomnia except under certain circumstances.
4. Evaluation to document diagnosis of depression.
5. Evaluation of uncomplicated parasomnias for which a clinical diagnosis is sufficient.
6. Evaluation of a circadian rhythm sleep disorder.
7. Evaluation of patients with known seizure disorders who have no nocturnal complaints.

Adapted from references 1, 2, and 9.
AHI, Apnea–hypopnea index; *CPAP,* continuous positive airway pressure; *MSLT,* multiple sleep latency test; *OSA,* obstructive sleep apnea; *PAP,* positive airway pressure.

PATIENTS AT HIGH RISK FOR OSA

The 2005 AASM practice parameters for PSG also mentioned a number of circumstances in which OSA is very common.[2] However, PSG is *not* routinely indicated in those circumstances unless a clinical evaluation reveals a *reasonable suspicion* for OSA. The disorders discussed included patients with systolic or diastolic heart failure, recent or past stroke or transient ischemic attack (TIA), coronary artery disease, and tachyarrhythmias or bradyarrhythmias. Most clinicians would also place resistant hypertension or pulmonary hypertension of unknown etiology in this category. The practice parameters do list neuromuscular diseases as a group of disorders in which

PSG is indicated for evaluation of sleep-related symptoms. Routine evaluation of chronic lung disease is not an indication for PSG unless coexistent OSA is suspected. *Nocturnal oximetry* is a useful tool for determining whether nocturnal oxygen desaturation is occurring in a patient with chronic obstructive pulmonary disease (COPD). *A sawtooth pattern is suggestive of sleep apnea.*

PSG TITRATION

A PSG for PAP titration is the standard procedure to select a level of pressure for treatment.[1,2,9] The titration may be performed on a separate night after a diagnostic PSG or during the second part of the night during a split study or partial-night study. A split sleep study is recommended when (1) the diagnostic portion shows an apnea–hypopnea index (AHI) greater than 40 per hour with at least 2 hours of monitoring, (2) an AHI of 20 to 40 is accompanied by special clinical circumstances such as severe desaturation or arrhythmia thought to be caused by OSA, and (3) at least 3 hours remain for the PSG titration.[1,2,9] If the PSG titration does not last at least 3 hours or is not adequate, a repeat PSG titration is indicated. Many sleep centers allow split studies in milder patients especially when mandated by insurance providers.

OCST (UNATTENDED LIMITED CHANNEL SLEEP TESTING)

The devices used for these studies usually do not record EEG and are usually unattended. The Centers for Medicare and Medicaid Services (CMS) uses the nomenclature *home sleep testing* for limited channel sleep studies. In the past, the term *portable monitoring* (PM) was commonly used in the literature. Recently, the nomenclature *out-of-center sleep testing* (OCST, or OOC sleep testing) has been used by the AASM.[8,10]

The traditional classification of monitoring devices for the diagnosis of sleep apnea was originated by Ferber and colleagues (Table F10–1).[11,12] The CMS uses the term home sleep testing (HST) and has a different classification for monitoring (Table F10-2).[13,14] Various types of HST devices were assigned temporary G-codes (still used in some locales). A specific G-code was not assigned to monitoring using peripheral arterial tonometry (PAT). The most recent classification of OCST is one that uses common procedural codes (CPT) as listed in Table F10-3. It is not clear what would qualify as monitoring of sleep (CPT 9580). Presumably limited EEG or EOG monitoring or estimates of sleep using PAT (see below) would qualify. Another classification of OCST devices, termed *SCOPER* (Sleep, Cardiovascular, Oximetry, Position, Effort, and Respiratory), was used in a review of device technology, which was published in an attempt to improve the classification of the wide variety of devices.[14]

The results of OCST is often called the *apnea–hypopnea index*, although the denominator of the metric is monitoring time rather than total sleep time (TST). This metric has also been called the *respiratory event index* (REI) by the AASM and the *respiratory disturbance index* (RDI) by CMS. Since the publication of the 2008 revision of the National Carrier Determination (NCD) 240.4 on CPAP treatment,[13] CMS now allows patients to qualify for PAP

TABLE F10–1	Classification of Sleep Testing			
	Level I: Attended PSG	**Level II: Unattended PSG**	**Level III: Modified Portable Sleep Apnea Testing**	**Level IV: Continuous Single or Dual Bioparameter Recording**
Measures (channels)	Minimum of seven channels including EEG, EOG, chin EMG, ECG, air flow, respiratory effort, oxygen saturation	Minimum of seven channels including EEG, EOG, chin EMG, heart rate or ECG, air flow, respiratory effort, oxygen saturation	Minimum of four, including ventilation (at least two channels of respiratory movement or respiratory movement and air flow), heart rate or ECG, and oxygen saturation	Minimum of one oxygen saturation, flow, or chest movement
Body position	Documented or objectively measured	Possible	Possible	NO
Leg movement	EMG	Optional	Optional	NO
Personnel interventions	Possible	NO	NO	NO

From Littner MR: Portable monitoring in the diagnosis of the obstructive sleep apnea syndrome, *Semin Respir Crit Care Med* 26:56-67, 2005; and Ferber R, Millman R, Coppola M, et al: ASDA standards of practice: portable recording in the assessment of obstructive sleep apnea, *Sleep* 17:378-392, 1994.

ECG, Electrocardiography; *EEG,* electroencephalography; *EMG,* electromyography; *EOG,* electrooculography; *PSG,* polysomnography.

TABLE F10-2 **CMS Classification of Sleep Testing and G Codes**

Code	Type	Setting	Monitoring
N/A	I	In facility attended	
G0398	II	Unattended in or out of a sleep laboratory facility or attended in a sleep laboratory facility	Minimum of seven channels, including EEG, EOG, EMG, ECG/heart rate, oxygen saturation, anterior tibial EMG
G0399	III	Unattended in or out of a sleep laboratory facility or attended in a sleep laboratory facility	Minimum of four channels and must record ventilation, oximetry, and ECG or heart rate
G0400	IV	Unattended in or out of a sleep laboratory facility or attended in a sleep laboratory facility	Minimum of three channels
No code		Unattended in or out of a sleep laboratory facility or attended in a sleep laboratory facility	Minimum of three channels including peripheral arterial tonometry, actigraphy, and oximetry

CMS, Center for Medicare and Medicaid Services; *ECG*, electrocardiography; *EEG*, electroencephalography; *EMG*, electromyography; *EOG*, electrooculography.
G-codes are Healthcare Common Procedure Coding System (HCPCS) codes that are used to identify temporary procedures and professional services. The codes are still used for HST in some locales.

TABLE F10-3 **Common Procedural Terminology Codes for OCST (HST)**

95800	Sleep study, unattended, simultaneous recording; heart rate, oxygen saturation, respiratory analysis (e.g., by air flow or peripheral arterial tone) and sleep time
95801	Sleep study, unattended, simultaneous recording; minimum of heart rate, oxygen saturation and respiratory analysis (e.g., by air flow or peripheral arterial tone)
95806	Sleep study, unattended, simultaneous recording of heart rate, oxygen saturation, respiratory air flow and respiratory effort (e.g., thoracoabdominal movement)

treatment on the basis of an HST, provided certain guidelines are followed. The specific rules vary according to local carrier determinations (LCDs). In general, a physician who is Board-certified or Board-eligible (BC/BE) in sleep medicine or associated with a sleep center accredited by the AASM or the Joint Commission is allowed to interpret the HSTs. The durable medical equipment (DME) providers are not allowed to perform HST on patients who will be provided with PAP equipment. Medicare and many insurance providers also now pay for HST[14] and in fact, some require HST for initial diagnostic testing of OSA unless certain comorbidities are present.

INDICATIONS FOR OCST AND PATIENT SELECTION

OCST is most useful in patients with a high probability of having moderate-to-severe OSA and in those for whom PSG poses special problems. Patients with immobility, with safety issues, or in whom PSG will be delayed and urgent treatment is needed may benefit from OCST. OCST is not indicated for screening asymptomatic populations. In the future, OCST

BOX F10-2 **High-Risk Groups for Obstructive Sleep Apnea in which Polysomnography Should Be Considered**

Congestive heart failure
Coronary artery disease
Prior cerebrovascular accident or transient ischemic attack
Intractable hypertension
Neuromuscular disorder
Nocturnal arrhythmias

may be validated for screening special high-risk populations (Box F10-2). The AASM has published clinical guidelines for portable monitoring and subsequently accreditation standards for OCST. The indications and exclusions for OCST are listed in Box F10-3. The OCST standards specify that acceptable OCST devices must satisfy requirements for CPT codes as listed in Table F10-3 provide an AHI equivalent to that obtained by PSG, and allow review and editing of the raw data. Adequately trained personnel should either place the monitoring equipment on the patients or train them on the application of the sensors. This is essential to

BOX F10-3	Indications for Unattended Portable Monitoring or Out-of-Center Sleep Test

INDICATIONS:

1. Diagnosis of obstructive sleep apnea (OSA) in patients with high probability of having moderate-to-severe OSA (without comorbidities or other sleep disorders).
2. Diagnosis of OSA in patients in whom laboratory polysomnography (PSG) is not possible by virtue of immobility, safety, or critical illness.
3. To document the efficacy of non–positive airway pressure (PAP) treatments for OSA (oral appliances, upper airway surgery, weight loss).

CONDITIONS FOR PM (CGPM):

1. PM must be performed in conjunction with a **comprehensive sleep evaluation** supervised by a board-certified or board-eligible (BC/BE) sleep physician (CPMG).
2. No comorbid medical conditions that may degrade PM accuracy:
   * Severe pulmonary disease
   * Neuromuscular disease
   * Congestive heart failure

3. No clinical suspicion of other sleep disorders (PSG needed for optimal diagnosis and treatment):
   * Central sleep apnea
   * Narcolepsy
   * Periodic limb movement disorder
   * Parasomnias
   * Circadian rhythm sleep disorders

CONDITIONS FOR PM (OCST STANDARDS)

1. Information provided by health care provider must adhere to criteria of high pretest probability of OSA and **limited comorbidities** (as described in the AASM clinical guidelines or practice parameters).

OTHER PATIENT GROUPS NOT OPTIMAL CANDIDATES FOR PM

1. Obesity hypoventilation syndrome
2. Low daytime saturation of peripheral oxygen (SpO_2) or hypoventilation for any cause
3. Patients on high dose potent narcotics
4. Patients on 24-hour supplemental oxygen

From Collop NA, Anderson WM, Boehlecke B, et al: Clinical guidelines for the use of unattended portable monitors in the diagnosis of obstructive sleep apnea in adult patients. Portable Monitoring Task Force of the American Academy of Sleep Medicine, *J Clin Sleep Med* 3:737-747, 2007.
CGPM, Clinical Guidelines for Portable Monitoring; *OCST*, AASM Out-of-Center Sleep Testing Accreditation Standards (now combined with in facility standards, see Reference 8).

avoid a high percentage of technically inadequate studies. If patients place the sensors, up to 30% of studies may be technically inadequate.[15] The PM data must be viewed in the raw form, and if automated scoring is used, it must be edited for accuracy. For quality assurance, standard operating procedures for the PM process must exist. To verify adequate scoring, interrater reliability on scoring of PM studies must be assessed on a routine basis and documented. A physician must look at the raw data (to ensure it is technically adequate and scored correctly) as well as the data summary before making an interpretation. It was recommended that PSG be interpreted by a BC/BE sleep physician or a physician associated with an accredited sleep center. If PM is inadequate technically or if the study results are negative in a patient with a high pretest probability of having OSA, an attended PSG should be performed.

OCST DEVICES

A large number of devices are available. Type III (CPT 95806) devices are the most common and provide a measurement of air flow (nasal pressure, oronasal thermal sensor, or both), respiratory effort (one or two effort belts), and oximetry arterial oxygen saturation by pulse oximetry [SpO_2] and derived heart rate) (Figure F10-1). Many have a position sensor and actigraphy to assist in determining when the patient is awake. Snoring may be derived from the nasal pressure tracing or a separate sensor. The recent SCOPER analysis[10] states that insufficient evidence exists to state that both nasal pressure and thermistor are required to adequately diagnose OSA using OCST devices. Many of the simpler devices use a single air flow sensor.

Unique PM devices that detect respiratory events by recording changes in sympathetic tone (rather than air flow) using PAT are also available (CPT 95801).[16] Devices using this technology, which are worn on the wrist, utilize two finger probes—a PAT probe and an oximetry probe—worn on separate digits of the same hand. The PAT signal is a measure of the blood volume in the digit. When sympathetic tone increases this stimulates alpha receptors in the vasculature of the fingers mediating vasoconstriction. The vasoconstriction reduces finger blood volume and the PAT signal. Because surges in sympathetic tone follow respiratory event termination, the combination of a decrease in PAT signal, a fall in pulse oximetry (SpO_2) followed by an increase in the SpO_2, and an increase in heart

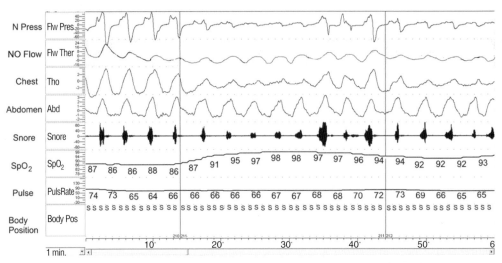

FIGURE F10-1 ■ A 60-second tracing showing an obstructive hypopnea with a type 3 (95806) device (PDX Philips-Respironics). An oronasal thermal sensor (NO flow) as well as nasal pressure (NPres), chest and abdominal respiratory inductance plethysmography bands, snore (snore sensor), oximetry, derived pulse, and body position are shown. (From Berry RB: *Fundamentals of sleep medicine*, Philadelphia, 2012, Saunders, p 201.)

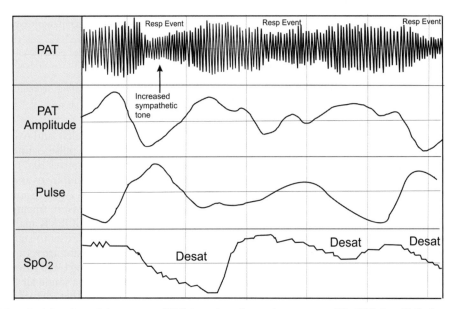

FIGURE F10-2 ■ Peripheral arterial tonometry (PAT) detection of a respiratory event. The PAT signal falls (increased sympathetic tone) associated with an increase then a decrease in pulse and arterial oxygen desaturation. SpO_2, Arterial oxygen saturation by pulse oximetry. (From Berry RB: *Fundamentals of sleep medicine*, Philadelphia, 2012, Saunders.)

rate allows determination of respiratory events (Figure F10-2). Nonrespiratory arousals would not reduce the SpO_2. The device has a built-in actigraphy to help with estimation of an appropriate index time (used to compute an event index). Recently, the combination of actigraphy and the PAT signal has been used to determine estimates of wakefulness, non–rapid eye movement (NREM) sleep, and REM sleep because the sympathetic tone characteristics of these sleep stages differ. If sleep is reported, the device would satisfy CPT 95800. Newer models also have a body position sensor and a snore sensor. The device

cannot be used in patients on alpha blockers (e.g., terazosin) and with patients who are in atrial fibrillation. In Patient 16, practical considerations, including the choice of a PM device and procedure for using OCST devices, are discussed.

ACTIGRAPHY

Actigraphy utilizes a portable device (the actigraph) usually worn on the wrist that records movement over an extended period (Figure F10-3). Sleep-wake patterns are estimated from the pattern of

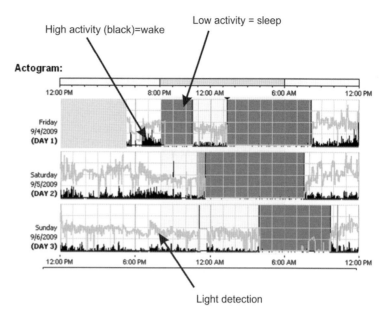

High activity (black)=wake

Low activity = sleep

Actogram:

Light detection

FIGURE F10-3 ■ An example of actigraphy. In this patient, the time of the sleep period was highly variable. On Friday, the patient appears to have fallen asleep for about 2 hours in the early evening following by a period of wake then a major sleep period during the night. (Adapted from Berry RB: *Fundamentals of sleep medicine*, Philadelphia, 2012, Saunders, p 206.)

BOX F10–4	**Indications for Actigraphy**

1. To assess the sleep-wake patterns of normal individuals. (S)
2. To assist in evaluation of suspected circadian rhythm sleep disorders.
   (Guideline):
   - Advanced sleep phase (G)
   - Delayed sleep phase (G)
   - Shift work disorder (O)
   - Free-running circadian rhythm sleep disorder (non-24-hr) (O)
   - Jet lag disorder (G)
3. When PSG is not available, actigraphy provides an estimate of total sleep time in obstructive sleep apnea (OSA). When used with respiratory monitoring, actigraphy may improve the accuracy in assessing severity (AHI). (S)
4. Actigraphy is **indicated** to characterize **circadian rhythm patterns** or sleep disturbance in individuals with **insomnia**, including **insomnia with depression**. (O)
5. Actigraphy is indicated to determine circadian pattern and estimate average daily sleep time in individuals complaining of hypersomnia. (O)
6. Actigraphy is useful in assessing **response to therapy** in:
   - Circadian rhythm sleep disorders
   - Insomnia

S, G, O = Standard, Guideline, Option level of recommendation. Strength of recommendation S>G>0.
Adapted from reference 18.

---

movement. Software is available to estimate TST and wake time from the data. The estimates of TST and wake time are more accurate in normal individuals than in patients with sleep disorders. However, the sleep-wake pattern of actigraph data is extremely valuable in documenting patterns of sleep and wake. This information is useful for evaluation of patients with insomnia and circadian rhythm disorders. AASM practice parameters for the use of actigraphy have been published in 2005 and most recently in 2007 (Box F10-4).[17,18] Actigraphy was *not* recommended for determination of sleep latency or TST in insomnia (although it is often used to estimate these parameters). Actigraphy is indicated for determining the sleep-wake patterns of patients with insomnia and circadian rhythm disorders and for determining the response to therapy in patients with circadian rhythm disorders. Studies of actigraphy have usually compared the results with that of PSG or sleep logs. However, actigraphy does not measure sleep (EEG) or the subjective experience of sleep (sleep logs). The information from actigraphy and sleep logs is complementary.

REFERENCES

1. Standards of Practice Committee Task Force: Practice parameters for the indications of polysomnography and related procedures, *Sleep* 20:406–422, 1997.
2. Kushida CA, Littner MR, Morgenthaler T, Alessi CA: Practice parameters for the indications for polysomnography and related procedures: an update for 2005, *Sleep* 28:499–521, 2005.
3. Littner MR, Kushida C, Wise M, et al: Practice parameters for clinical use of the multiple sleep latency test and the maintenance of wakefulness test, *Sleep* 28:113–121, 2005.

4. Littner M, Kramer M, Kapen S, et al: Practice parameters for using polysomnography to evaluate insomnia: an update, *Sleep* 26:754–760, 2003.

5. Morgenthaler TI, Lee-Chiong T, Alessi C, et al: Practice parameters for the clinical evaluation and treatment of circadian rhythm sleep disorders, *Sleep* 30:1445–1459, 2007.

6. Kushida CA, Morgenthaler T, Littner MR, et al: Practice parameters for the treatment of snoring and obstructive sleep apnea with oral appliances: an update for 2005, *Sleep* 29:240–243, 2006.

7. Collop NA, Anderson WM, Boehlecke B, et al: Clinical guidelines for the use of unattended portable monitors in the diagnosis of obstructive sleep apnea in adult patients. Portable Monitoring Task Force of the American Academy of Sleep Medicine, *J Clin Sleep Med* 3:737–747, 2007.

8. Accreditation Standards (updated 3/14/14) http://www.aasmnet.org/resources/pdf/accreditationstandards.pdf. Accessed April 26, 2014.

9. Kushida CA, Littner MR, Hirshkowitz M, et al: Practice parameters for the use of continuous and bilevel positive airway pressure devices to treat adult patients with sleep-related breathing disorders, *Sleep* 29:375–380, 2006.

10. Collop NA, Tracy SL, Kapur V, et al: Obstructive sleep apnea devices for out-of-center (OOC) testing: technology evaluation, *J Clin Sleep Med* 7(5):531–548, 2011.

11. Ferber R, Millman R, Coppola M, et al: ASDA standards of practice: portable recording in the assessment of obstructive sleep apnea, *Sleep* 17:378–392, 1994.

12. Ferber R, Millman R, Coppola M, et al: ASDA standards of practice: portable recording in the assessment of obstructive sleep apnea, *Sleep* 17:378–392, 1994.

13. Department of Health and Human Services, Center for Medicare and Medicaid Services. Decision memo for continuous positive airway pressure (CPAP) therapy for obstructive sleep apnea (OSA) CAG#0093R, Mar 13, 2008.

14. Centers for Medicare and Medicaid Services: Decision memo for sleep testing for obstructive sleep apnea, CAG-00405N), Aug 5, 2009.

15. Golpe R, Jimenex A, Carpizo R: Home sleep studies in the assessment of sleep apnea/hypopnea syndrome, *Chest* 122:1156–1161, 2002.

16. Ayas NT, Pittman S, MacDonald M, White DP: Assessment of a wrist-worn device in the detection of obstructive sleep apnea, *Sleep Med* 4:435–442, 2003.

17. Littner MR, Kushida DA, Anderson WM, et al: Standards of Practice Committee of the American Academy of Sleep Medicine: Practice parameters for the role of actigraphy in the study of sleep and circadian rhythms: an update for 2002, *Sleep* 26:337–341, 2003.

18. Morgenthaler T, Alessi C, Friedman L, et al: Practice parameters for the use of actigraphy in the assessment of sleep and sleep disorders: an update for 2007, *Sleep* 30:519–529, 2007.

PATIENT 16

Out-of-Center Sleep Testing versus Portable Monitoring

QUESTIONS

1. Which of the four scenarios describes an appropriate patient for out-of-center sleep testing (OCST)?

   A. A 30-year-old man with loud snoring and witnessed apneas. The patient's medical problems include hypertension and diabetes. He denies cataplexy. Physical examination shows a Mallampati 4 upper airway.

   B. A 50-year-old woman has insomnia that is resistant to multiple hypnotics. She does snore and have frequent awakenings. She is taking thyroid replacement medication. Physical examination shows a Mallampati 4 upper airway.

   C. A 60-year-old man has congestive heart failure, atrial fibrillation, and nocturnal dyspnea. He snores loudly but denies daytime sleepiness. Physical examination shows a Mallampati 4 upper airway and pedal edema.

   D. A 50-year-old man with chronic obstructive pulmonary disease (COPD) was noted to have a sawtooth pattern on nocturnal oximetry. He is currently on nocturnal oxygen and has an awake saturation of arterial oxygen (SaO_2) of 92%. Physical examination shows a Mallampati 4 upper airway.

2. What type of respiratory event is shown (Figure P16-1)?

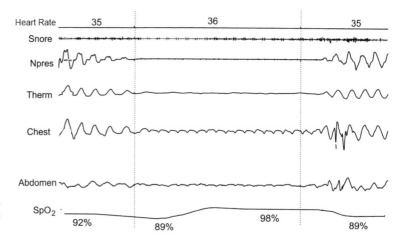

FIGURE P16-1 ■ A 60-second tracing of a respiratory event recorded with limited channels.

3. What is the problem with this set of results from an out of center sleep test (OCST)?

Monitoring Time	6 Hours		
Apnea-hypopnea index (/hr)	5	Desaturations (no.)	180
Obstructive apneas (no.)	10	ODI (no./hr)	20
Mixed apneas (no.)	0	Low SaO$_2$ (%)	88
Central apnea (no.)	0	—	—
Hypopneas (no.)	20	—	—

ODI = oxygen desaturations/hr.

ANSWERS

1. **Answer:** A

Discussion: The most appropriate patient for OCST is one with a moderate to high probability of obstructive sleep apnea (OSA) and no comorbidities that may degrade the accuracy of the study[1]. Patient A has snoring, witnessed apnea, daytime sleepiness and a high Mallampati score. He has no comorbidities that may degrade the accuracy of OCST and is a good candidate for this type of sleep study. Patient B may not be sleeping well, and it is important to know if sufficient sleep and sufficient REM sleep is recorded during the sleep study. Insomnia is usually not an indication for polysomnography (PSG), but when patients do not respond to usual hypnotic or behavioral treatment for insomnia and complain of frequent awakenings, snoring, or both, a PSG is indicated[2]. Patient B also has evidence of a crowded upper airway (a high Mallampati score). Patient C has congestive heart failure and atrial fibrillation. He has a reasonable chance of having central sleep apnea with Cheyne-Stokes breathing (CSB). Although it is possible to recognize CSB from most portable monitoring equipment tracings, he may not respond to continuous positive airway pressure (CPAP) or auto-adjusting PAP (APAP), and thus he will eventually need a PSG for PAP titration. A split sleep study is likely more cost effective[3]. One can also see the ECG signal, rather than a pulse rate. Most portable monitoring equipment records a heart rate derived from the oximeter rather than an ECG signal. Patient D has COPD and likely has sleep apnea as well, given the sawtooth pattern on oximetry. If placed on PAP, he will likely require supplemental oxygen. The clinical guidelines for OCST recommend that patients with significant comorbidities, for example, significant COPD, congestive heart failure, neuromuscular disorders (and/or suspected

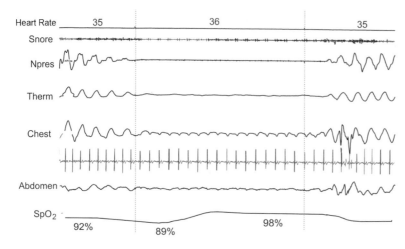

FIGURE P16-2 ■ Electrocardiography frequency was recorded in this limited channel study and allowed easier identification of cardiac pulsations rather than respiratory effort.

hypoventilation), and the need for supplemental oxygen, should be studied with a PSG. If OCST is positive in these patients, they are not good candidates for unattended auto-titration to select an effective pressure for CPAP treatment or for chronic treatment with APAP. Proper selection of patients for alternative PAP titration or treatment is discussed in Patient 54. Diagnostic accuracy is not the only consideration for choosing PSG rather than OCST. How the patient will be further evaluated and treated if the diagnostic study confirms the presence of sleep apnea should be taken into consideration when choosing the diagnostic procedure.

2. **Answer:** Central apnea

   Discussion: What appears to be respiratory efforts in the chest and abdomen channels are, in fact, chest movements from cardiac pulsations in a person with a low heart rate (Figure P16-2). Although one might recognize this from the heart rate tracing showing a low rate, the addition of an ECG provides easily discernible evidence that this is true. This patient actually underwent a limited-channel attended sleep study with the use of routine PSG equipment rather than a PSG because of a shortage of available staff. Most OCST devices do not record electrocardiography (ECG) frequencies, and the tracing would appear as shown in Figure P16-3. An ECG trace is very useful in this patient and shows that the R-R interval is the same as the time interval between "respiratory effort" (e.g., cardiac pulsations). If a patient has atrial fibrillation or frequent premature beats, the oximetry estimate of heart rate may be much lower than the actual heart rate. For example, if someone is in atrial or ventricular bigeminy, only every other beat may provide sufficient signal to the oximetry probe for the oximetry software to detect a heartbeat.

3. **Answer:** The oxygen desaturation index (ODI) is much higher than the AHI.

   Discussion: As hypopneas must be scored solely on the basis of desaturation in most OCST devices (no sleep recorded), the ODI and the AHI should be approximately the same. If some obstructive apneas were not associated with desaturation or if desaturations were noted without obvious air flow changes, the two might differ slightly. However, in Patient C, the ODI and the AHI are very different (Figure P16-3). Review of the actual tracings showed that the nasal pressure signal was faulty for much of the night. The automatic scoring on this device used the nasal pressure signal to detect hypopneas. The technologist should have caught the problem and hand-scored the events by using the changes in chest and abdomen respiratory inductance plethysmography (RIP) signals or in this case the RIPflow (time derivative of the RIPsum = RIPchest + RIPabdomen). Nasal pressure signals on OCST devices may be faulty if the nasal cannula comes out of the nostrils. Most sleep centers use small pieces of tape to stabilize the nasal cannula (applied across the cannula where in crosses the cheek area). When the OCST was rescored, the AHI was 21 per hour (similar to ODI).

   OCST devices with multiple signals (nasal pressure, two RIP belts, and oximetry) provide backup signals if one sensor fails. However, the more sensors the device uses the more difficult for the patient to apply the OCST device.[3] This can increase the technical failure rate. If the patient

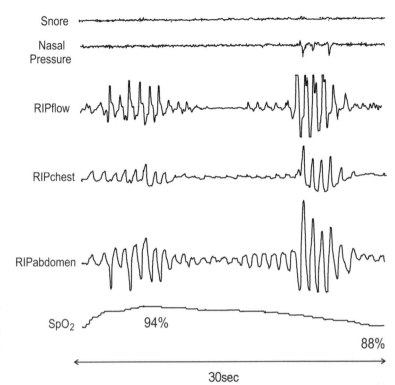

Snore

Nasal Pressure

RIPflow

RIPchest

RIPabdomen

SpO₂   94%

88%

30sec

FIGURE P16-3 ■ Tracing from out-of-center sleep test (OCST) showing the nasal pressure signal is not functioning (nasal cannula may have come out of the nose). The study was rescored using RIP-flow (the time derivative of the RIPsum).

attaches the sensors at home use of a simple device with fewer sensors may be preferable. In designing a OCST program one must consider how the devices will be placed and returned to the sleep center. Some programs with simple devices can simply mail the device to the patient. Others have the patient come to the sleep center for detailed instruction on sensor placement (or placement of sensors by a technologist). The patient must then either return the OCST device in person or by mail.

CLINICAL PEARLS

1. Good candidates for OCST are those patients with a moderate to high probability of having OSA without comorbidities that might degrade the accuracy of PSG or who will need a PSG titration if the diagnostic study is positive (a split study may be more cost effective).

2. PSG enables one to know if sufficient sleep was recorded (and enough REM sleep), to accurately determine if a patient has OSA. One can also observe the ECG rather than heart rate. Using a PSG for diagnosis also provides the option of an immediate PSG PAP titration (if the diagnostic study is positive and the patient qualifies for a split sleep study). Patients with central apneas, hypoventilation, or the need for supplemental oxygen all benefit from a PSG titration rather than unattended auto-titration or treatment with APAP.

3. Heart rate (derived from the oximeter) rather than ECG is recorded by most OCST devices, and one may miss important ECG events or other causes of abnormal heart rate with OCST compared with PSG.

4. When choosing an OCST device consider whether the patient or a technologist will place the sensors. Devices with more channels provide backup signals but are more difficult for the patient to successfully place at home (see reference 3).

REFERENCES

1. Collop NA, Anderson WM, Boehlecke B, et al: Clinical guidelines for the use of unattended portable monitors in the diagnosis of obstructive sleep apnea in adult patients. Portable Monitoring Task Force of the American Academy of Sleep Medicine, *J Clin Sleep Med* 3:737–747, 2007.
2. Kushida CA, Littner MR, Morgenthaler T, Alessi CA: Practice parameters for the indications for polysomnography and related procedures: an update for 2005, *Sleep* 28:499–521, 2005.
3. Purdy S, Berry RB: Portable monitoring. In Mattice C, Brooks R, Lee-Chiong T, editors: *Fundamentals of sleep technology*, 2012, Lippincott-Williams and Wilkins, pp 482–501.

FUNDAMENTALS 11

Artifacts

Artifacts in the electroencephalography (EEG), electrooculography (EOG), and electromyography (EMG) derivations caused by inadequate electrode application, the effects of the environment (warm room), or patient movement with respiration are common in polysomnography.[1-3] It is essential that they be recognized during recording to allow for intervention by the sleep technologist. Postrecording interventions can minimize the effects of most of the artifacts on the ability to accurately stage sleep. For example, the application of backup electrodes allows a change in derivation to one not using a faulty electrode.

Electrode popping is a common artifact that makes the staging of sleep very difficult. It is characterized by a sharp (short duration) high-amplitude deflection secondary to an electrode pulling away from the skin (sudden loss of signal) (Figure F11-1). The popping is usually regular and often corresponds to body movement with each breath. The high amplitude of the artifact may be clipped (not displayed beyond a certain positive and negative amplitude) to avoid overlap into the next channel (Figure F11-2). Electrode popping is usually caused by movement of an electrode from either direct pressure or pulling on the electrode wire associated with body

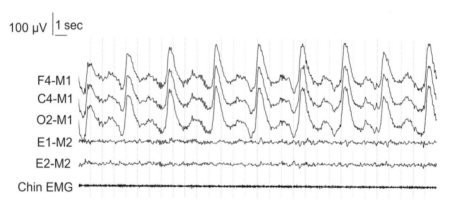

FIGURE F11-1 ■ An example of electrode popping. The faulty electrode was M1. This should be suspected, as this electrode was the only one common to all the affected derivations and none of the unaffected derivations. Derivations F3-M2, C3-M2, and O1-M2 could be used.

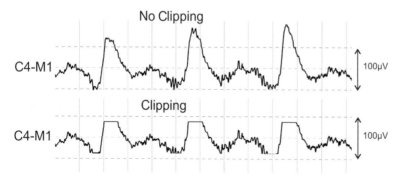

FIGURE F11-2 ■ Popping artifact without and with clipping of waveforms. Clipping prevents the signal from overlapping with the tracing of an adjacent channel. Clipping may usually be turned on or off.

movement during respiration. If the conductive gel between the electrode and the shin dries, this makes the electrodes susceptible to even slight movement. At the time of recording, adding electrode gel, reapplication of the problem electrode, or rerouting the electrode wire may eliminate the problem. After recording, the artifact can frequently be handled by switching to an alternative derivation that does not use the problem electrode. For example, if electrode O2 is the problem, the derivation O1-M2 may be used. In Figure F11-1, M1 is the likely problem electrode, as all derivations that contain electrode are affected and the shape of the deflection is similar in all affected derivations. Note that derivations containing M2 are not affected.

While it is possible that F4,C4, and O2 were all faulty, this is unlikely. In addition, one may temporarily change the F4-M1 to F4-M2, and elimination of the artifact will verify that M1 is the problem. Switching the display to the alternative derivations F3-M2, C3-M2, and O1-M2 eliminated the artifact.

Sixty-cycle artifact in EEG, EOG, or EMG tracings is a common problem in sleep study recording and is recognized on the usual 30-second view by a very dense uniform squared off or "rope like" tracing that does not vary (Figure F11-3). It is caused by contamination of the recorded signal with 60-hertz (Hz) electrical activity from nearby power lines. A 60-Hz artifact may be minimized by correct application of electrodes and proper design of the sleep laboratory. Alternating current (AC)–coupled differential amplifiers record low-voltage EEG and EOG signals by amplifying the difference in voltage between two electrodes while rejecting the common-mode signal consisting of higher-voltage, 60-Hz, background activity. The

background 60-Hz activity is rejected (common signals will cancel) only if the electrode impedances are low and fairly equal. If one electrode is faulty (disconnected or high impedance), then the 60-Hz AC activity will be more prominent. Although most AC amplifiers have 60-Hz notch filters to eliminate 60-Hz activity, these filters may not prevent 60-Hz activity from being prominent when electrode impedances are very different. The ideal impedance of electrodes is below 5 kilo-ohms (acceptable ≤10 kilo-ohms). Electrode impedance should be checked by the sleep technician after electrode application. Routine use of 60-Hz notch filters may make recognition of 60-Hz contamination harder to detect. If the amplitude of the signal from a derivation is **greatly increased** by turning off the 60-Hz notch filter, this is evidence that the 60-Hz artifact is present. It is important to note that EEG and EOG derivations commonly use a high filter of 35 Hz, so much of the 60-Hz activity is filtered out even when the notch filter is off. The effect of adding or removing the notch filter is more prominent in chin or leg EMG derivations that use a high filter of 100 Hz. If the 60-Hz artifact is caused by a single electrode, it should be replaced during recording. In Figure F11-4, three panels of the same signals are shown. When the 60-Hz filter is off, prominent 60-Hz artifact is seen in the chin EMG (left panel). When the 60-Hz notch filter is on, the activity is dramatically reduced (center panel). In the last panel, the 60-Hz filter is off, but the 60-Hz artifact is not present. In this panel, the chin2 EMG electrode has been replaced. This documents that this electrode is faulty. Although changing the chin derivation allows proper sleep staging (in this case stage R), the ideal intervention would have been replacement of the chin2 electrode.

A slow-frequency artifact is characterized by a slowly undulating movement of the baseline of affected channels (Figure F11-5). The artifact often has a high voltage and may mimic slow wave activity (SWA). A slow-frequency artifact is often classified as either sweat artifact or respiratory artifact. A respiratory artifact is characterized by slow undulations in phase with the patient's respiration. The respiratory artifact often has a higher frequency compared with a sweat artifact but may have a similar appearance if the patient's respiratory rate is relative low (8 to 12 breaths per minute). A slow-frequency artifact not synchronous with respiration (e.g., sweat artifact) is believed to be secondary to the effects of perspiration. Sweat (high in sodium chloride) alters the electrode potential, thereby producing an artifact that mimics delta waves and results in overscoring of stage N3. Sweat artifact is usually

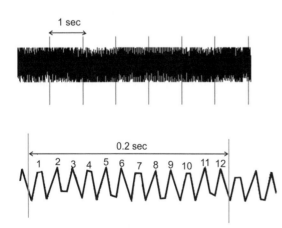

FIGURE F11-3 ■ A 60-Hz artifact as it appears in a 30-second window and blown up to show oscillation (12 × 5 = 60).

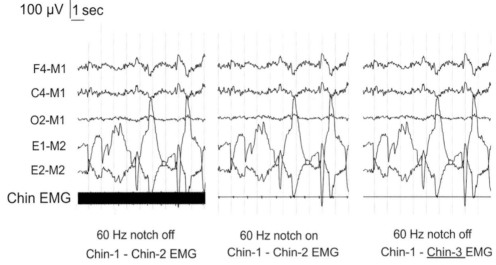

FIGURE F11-4 ■ In the left panel, a 60-hertz (Hz) artifact is noted on chin electromyography (EMG). In the middle panel, the artifact is eliminated by a 60-Hz filter. In the right panel, using a chin EMG derivation that does not use the faulty electrode (chin2 EMG) eliminates the artifact without the need for a 60-Hz notch filter. The recommended high filter for the chin derivations is 100 Hz.

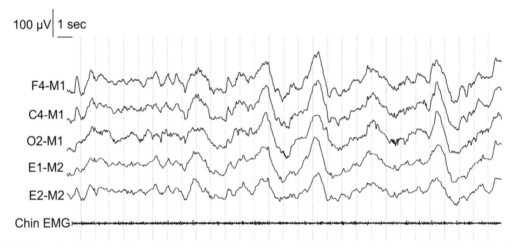

FIGURE F11-5 ■ A slow artifact (sweat artifact). A slow undulation of the signal is seen here in all of the derivations. The undulations were not in phase with respiration. When the room was cooled, the pattern resolved. This artifact makes accurate scoring of stage N3 difficult.

present in all of the EEG or EOG derivations but may be localized if sweat is affecting mainly selected electrodes. For example, if the area between the head and the pillow becomes sweaty, only the mastoid electrode on that side may be affected. The respiratory artifact is caused by pressure on an electrode (or pulling on the electrode) with each respiration. In this case, the artifact is often coming from one or more electrodes on the side on which the patient is lying. For example, if a patient is sleeping in the left lateral position, the M1 electrode is between the patient and the pillow, and movement of the electrode with respirations will affect all derivations containing M1. Of note, both respiratory artifact and sweat artifact may appear in the same individual,[3] and sometimes it is impossible to determine if sweat or respiration is causing the slow-frequency artifact. If a single electrode is the problem, changing derivations to one that does not use the problem electrode may be a solution. If a sweat artifact is the problem, interventions include reducing the room temperature, uncovering the patient, using a fan, or all of these measures. As a last-ditch alternative, the setting of the low-frequency filter may be increased (e.g., from 0.3 to 1 Hz). Unfortunately, this maneuver decreases the amount of SWA that is depicted but still may be preferable to a totally unscorable record. In the patient whose tracing is illustrated in Figure F11-5, the slow-frequency artifact was not synchronous with respiration and involved all derivations. The room temperature was lowered, and the problem resolved.

ECG AND PULSE ARTIFACT

ECG artifact is one of the most common and easily recognizable recording artifacts. It may be identified by sharp deflections in the signals of affected channels corresponding exactly in time to the QRS of the electrocardiography (ECG) tracing. In Figure F11-6, two small dark circles in F4-M1 are placed over two prominent deflections caused by an ECG artifact. Fortunately, the ECG artifact does not interfere a great deal with visual sleep staging, as the artifact does not mimic the usual EEG patterns used for sleep staging. The artifact may be minimized by placing the mastoid electrodes sufficiently high (behind the patient's ear) so that they are over bone instead of neck tissue (fat). Linking the two mastoid electrodes either physically by a jumper cable at the electrode box or using derivations where the reference electrode is an average of M1 and M2 may minimize the ECG artifact. This works because if the ECG voltage

vector is toward one mastoid, it is away from the other. Hence, the ECG component of the two signals tend to cancel each other out

PULSE ARTIFACT

A pulse artifact is similar to an ECG artifact except that rather than electrical interference, the artifact is caused by movement of an electrode resulting from the pulsation of an underlying artery. As the arterial pulse occurs after the QRS complex the timing of the artifact is delayed following each QRS. In Figure F11-7, the ECG (E) and pulse artifacts (P) are shown.

MUSCLE ARTIFACT

Muscle artifact in the EEG and EOG is caused by increased muscle tone in the muscles underlying the EEG and EOG electrodes. Often, this will resolve as the patient relaxes and falls asleep (Figure F11-8).

SNORING OR RESPIRATORY CHIN EMG ARTIFACT

An increase in chin EMG amplitude may sometimes be seen with each inspiration (Figure F11-9). This is especially common during

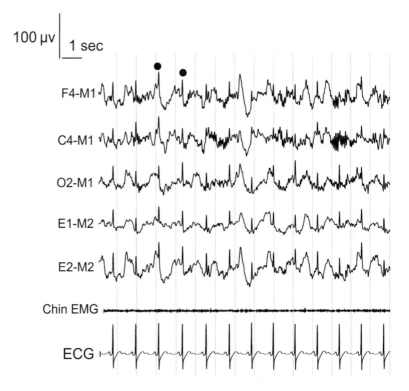

FIGURE F11-6 ■ An electrocardiography (ECG) artifact. The sharp deflections (*dark circles*) are synchronous with deflections in the ECG.

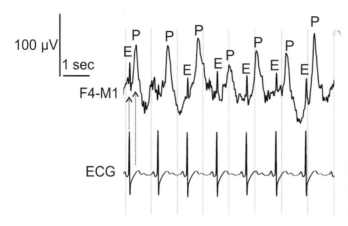

FIGURE F11-7 ■ This figure shows an electrocardiography (ECG) artifact (*E*) concurrent with the R wave and pulse artifact (*P*) following the QRS. While all derivations showed *E*, only the one with F4 showed *P*.

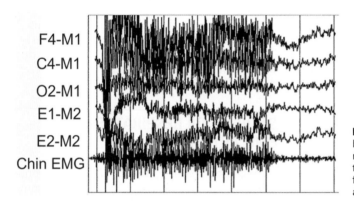

FIGURE F11-8 ■ A muscle artifact seen during biocalibrations when the individual being monitored was asked to grit his teeth and then relax. Turning the 60-hertz (Hz) notch filter on or off had little effect showing the artifact was not caused by the 60-Hz artifact.

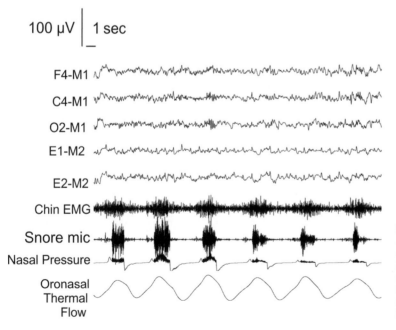

FIGURE 11-9 ■ A snoring artifact is noted on chin electromyography (EMG). Note the evidence of inspiratory snoring in the snore microphone (snore mic) and as high-frequency oscillations in the nasal pressure signal. Inspiration is upward.

snoring or anytime the upper airway is narrowed. The genioglossus (tongue protruder) has increased EMG activity with each inspiration, and the muscle attaches to the mandible in the midline. EMG electrodes below the mandible may pick up the increased inspiratory activity of the genioglossus, especially if the electrodes are near the midline. Another possible cause is simply movement of chin electrode wires with each inspiration. During snoring, high-frequency oscillations are often found superimposed on the slow varying nasal pressure signal (if the high-frequency filter setting is appropriate, e.g., 100 Hz).

CLINICAL PEARLS

1. Electrode popping artifact is characterized by a high-voltage sharp deflection occurring at regular intervals and present in all derivations containing the affected electrode that is pulling away from the skin during movement (usually with each respiration). Drying of the electrode gel may cause electrode popping.

2. A 60-Hz artifact is characterized by a dense ropelike or bandlike artifact. When a 60 Hz artifact is present in a derivation, this usually results from a high-electrode impedance in one of the electrodes. A large increase in amplitude in the signal when the 60-Hz notch filter is turned off (especially prominent when the high-frequency filter is 100 Hz), is evidence that significant 60-Hz contamination is present. The faulty electrode should be replaced or a different derivation used for viewing the signal.

3. A slow-frequency artifact is characterized by a slowly undulating baseline signal and is usually the effect of perspiration on one or more electrodes (sweat artifact) or movement of one or more electrodes with respiration (respiratory artifact). If a sweat artifact is present cooling the patient (reducing room temperature, using a fan, uncovering the patient) may resolve the problem. A slow-frequency artifact makes scoring stage N3 difficult

4. An ECG artifact may be easily recognized as sharp deflections in the affected leads corresponding to the QRS complex in the ECG lead. Proper application of the mastoid electrodes and double referencing (using an average of M1 and M2) may prevent or minimize this artifact.

REFERENCES

1. Berry RB: *Fundamentals of sleep medicine*, Philadelphia, 2012, Saunders, pp 51–56.
2. Berry RB: *Sleep medicine pearls*, ed 2, Philadelphia, 2003, Hanley and Belfus.
3. Siddiqui F, Osuna E, Walters AS, et al: Sweat artifact and respiratory artifact occurring simultaneously in polysomnogram, *Sleep Med* 7(2):197–199, 2006.

Patients with Eye Movements of Interest

QUESTIONS

1. What sleep stage is shown in Figure P17-1? The patient has a history of traumatic brain injury from an explosion.

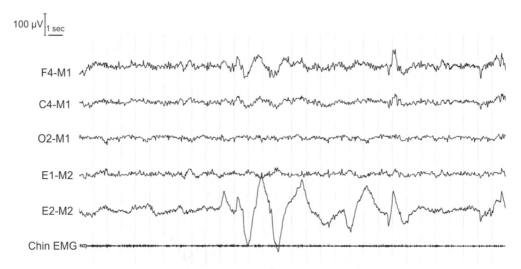

FIGURE P17-1 ■ A 30-second epoch.

2. A patient with snoring and difficulty falling asleep is noted to have the 30-second tracing shown in Figure P17-2 soon after lights-out. What sleep stage is present?

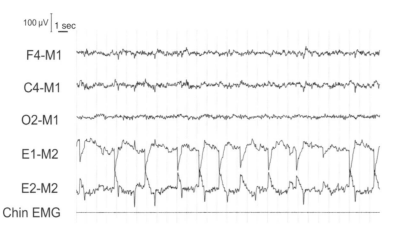

FIGURE P17-2 ■ A 30-second tracing.

3. A 32-year-old female undergoes monitoring for snoring. The patient complained of being too warm, and severe sweat artifact was present in the tracings for the first half of the study. To score the study, the low filter setting for the electroencephalography (EEG) and electrooculography (EOG) derivations were changed from 0.3 Hz to 1 Hz. What is responsible for the abnormality noted in the sleep architecture?

Sleep Architecture:		Total Night		Normal Range
Total recording time	(min)	450		(425–462)
Total sleep time	(min)	431		(394–457)
Sleep efficiency	(%)	98		(90–100)
Sleep latency	(min)	1.0		(0–19)
REM latency	(min)	85		(69–88)
Sleep Stages				
Awake (WASO):	(min)	18.0		(0–26) minutes
			%TST	
Stage N1:	(min)	14.0	3.2	(3–6) (%)
Stage N2:	(min)	295	68.4	(46–62) (%)
Stage N3:	(min)	20.5	4.8	(10–21) (%)
Stage R:	(min)	101	23.4	(21–31) (%)

Hz, Hertz; *REM*, rapid eye movement; *TST*, total sleep time; *WASO*, wakefulness after sleep onset.

ANSWERS

1. **Answer**: Stage R. A prosthetic left eye is present.

   Discussion: Prior to reading a sleep study, the clinician should review the biocalibration tracings to determine if the eye movement derivations are functioning correctly and to detect unusual patterns. In this patient, no deflections in E1-M2 are noted (Figure P17-3). Review of the history and technologist notes documented that the patient had a prosthetic left eye. His left eye had been removed following severe injury from an explosion. The tracing in P17-1 is REM sleep (stage R) and the absence of out-of-phase deflections in the EOG derivations is caused by absence of the left eye. In the biocalibration tracing, the command at B was "Open the eyes." Recall that with eye closure, the globe is turned upward (Bell phenomenon), and with eye lid opening, the globe moves downward. Downward movement away from E2 causes upward deflections in E2-M2 (and F4-M1). At A, the downward deflection in F4-M1 is in parallel to the downward deflection in E2-M2 as the right eye moves toward both E2 and F4 (following the command "Look up"). Also, note the pattern associated with eye blinks.

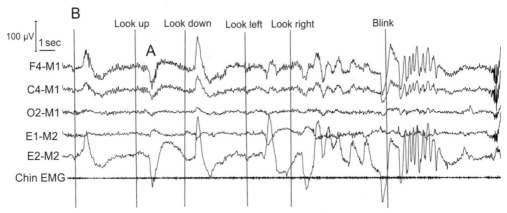

FIGURE P17-3 ■ A biocalibration tracing from the same patient as in Figure P17-1. Lack of deflections in E1-M2 was caused by an absent left eye.

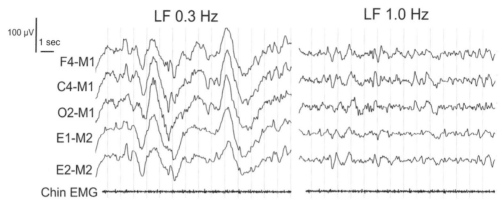

FIGURE P17-4 ■ Two 15-second tracings at different low-filter settings. The low frequency (1 Hz) reduced the slow artifact but also reduced the amplitude of slow waves.

2. **Answer:** Stage W. Reading eye movements are noted.

Discussion: The pattern of eye movements noted in Figure P17-2 is consistent with reading eye movements (see Fundamentals 2). The pattern consists of slow rightward movement, followed by an abrupt shift back to the left to start reading the next line. The patient in question was reading using an e-Reader under the covers. Video monitoring with infra-red illumination revealed a light under the covers. The technologist informed the patient that reading was allowed only before lights-out.

3. **Answer:** A low-filter setting of 1 Hz reduced the amount of stage N3 sleep as the amplitude of slow wave activity (SWA) was attenuated.

Discussion: Use of a low filter of 1 Hz attenuates wave forms with a frequency of 1 Hz to 0.7 of the unfiltered amplitude and further attenuates lower-frequency activity. Frequency of 1 to 2 Hz is attenuated slightly (see Fundamentals 9). Thus, frequency activity in the 0.5- to 2-Hz range is attenuated by a 1 Hz low filter and may not meet the 75-microvolt (μV) peak-to-peak criteria to be scored as SWA. In Figure P17-4, the effect of changing the low filter setting is illustrated in the patient with sweat artifact. If some change in filtering is not performed, it may be nearly impossible to score stage N3 if large-amplitude sweat artifact is present. The ideal intervention is promptly cooling the patient, rather than manipulation of the low-frequency filter. Unfortunately, this was not done during monitoring of the patient in the first part of the night when SWA is most prominent.

Of note, 0.3 Hz is chosen for the routine low filter setting to minimize effects on the EEG signal from unwanted slowly varying voltages (electrogalvanic signals from variations in skin moisture) without significantly reducing slow wave activity. However signals in the low portion of the slow wave activity range (0.5 to 2 Hz) are slightly attenuated.

CLINICAL PEARLS

1. The tracings recorded during biocalibration should be reviewed prior to reading a sleep study. Special attention should be paid to the function of the EOG electrodes (derivations) to note any unusual pattern that might affect sleep staging.

2. Reading eye movements have a characteristic pattern associated with a slow rightward scan of the printed line with a rapid shift leftward to begin reading the new line. When in doubt, review the video to establish that the patient was, indeed, reading.

3. An increase in the low filter setting from 0.3 to 1 Hz will reduce SWA but may be necessary if significant slow artifact is present. A low filter of 0.3 reduces 0.3 Hz activity to 0.7 of the unfiltered amplitude and reduces lower frequency activity even more. Frequencies slightly above 0.3 Hz (0.3 to 1 Hz) are slightly attenuated.

BIBLIOGRAPHY

Berry RB, Brooks R, Gamaldo CE, et al., for the American Academy of Sleep Medicine: *The AASM manual for the scoring of sleep and associated events: rules, terminology and technical specifications*, Version 2.0.3, www.aasmnet.org, Darien, IL, 2014, American Academy of Sleep Medicine.

Iber C, Ancoli-Israel S, Chesson A, Quan SF, for the American Academy of Sleep Medicine: *The AASM manual for scoring of sleep and associated events: rules, terminology and technical specifications*, ed 1, Westchester, IL, 2007, American Academy of Sleep Medicine.

Silber MH, Ancoli-Israel S, Bonnet MH, et al: The visual scoring of sleep in adults, *J Clin Sleep Med* 15:121–131, 2007.

A Patient with Artifacts in the EEG and EOG Derivations

QUESTION

1. What change in the frontal derivation (right panel) was performed to reduce the artifact shown in the left panel (Figure P18-1)?

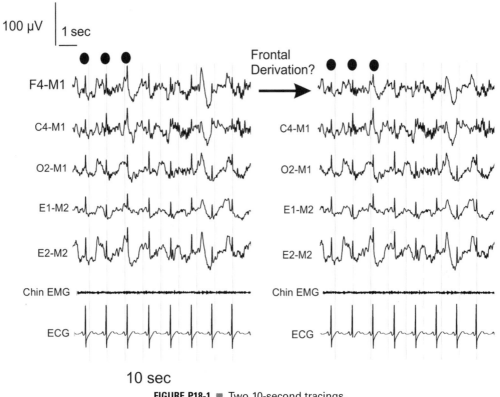

FIGURE P18-1 ■ Two 10-second tracings.

QUESTION

2. What artifact is present in F4-M1 in Figure P18-2? What is the problem electrode? How can you confirm the type of artifact?

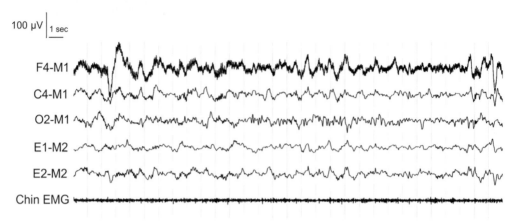

FIGURE P18-2 ■ A 30-second tracing with an artifact in F4-M1.

QUESTION

3. What type of artifact is present in Figure P18-3? The patient is lying on the right ear.

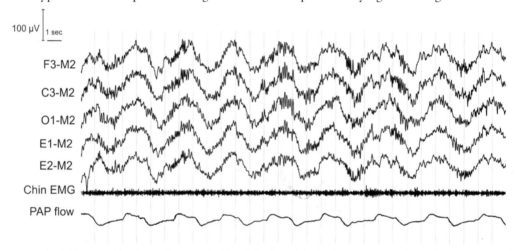

FIGURE P18-3 ■ A 30-second tracing with an artifact in all displayed derivations. Here, positive airway pressure (PAP) flow is the air flow signal for the accurate flow sensor in the PAP device. This tracing is from a PAP titration study.

ANSWERS

1. **Answer:** F4-AVG (M1, M2)

   Discussion: The electrocardiography (ECG) artifact present in the derivation F4-M1 is reduced by using linked or averaged mastoid electrodes F4-AVG (M1, M2). This reduces, but does not eliminate, the ECG artifact spikes (compared with the EEG without linked mastoids (*left panel*) dark circles).[1] ECG artifact is discussed in Fundamentals 11.

2. **Answer:** 60-Hz artifact in F4-M1

   Discussion: The artifact in F4-M1 in Figure P18-2 is a 60-Hz artifact causing a dense bandlike pattern. When the high filter setting was changed from 35 Hz (the recommended high filter) to 70 Hz (Figure P18-4), a dramatic increase in the artifact was noted (60-Hz notch filter off). When a 60-Hz notch filter was applied, this reduced the artifact, confirming that a 60-Hz signal was contaminating F4-M1. This figure illustrates the point that when a high filter setting of 35 Hz is used, turning the 60-Hz filter on or off makes much less difference with respect to a decrease in a 60-Hz artifact.[1] A high filter of 35 Hz significantly attenuates a 60-Hz artifact. Electrode F4 is the problem, as other derivations containing M1 are not involved. The electrode impedance of F4 was 25 kilo-ohms, whereas the impedance of M1 was 5 kilo-ohms. Ideally the electrode impedance

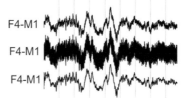

FIGURE P18-4 ■ The effect of different filter settings on the artifact in derivation F4-M1. The 60 Hz notch filter has more effect if the high filter setting is 70 Hz.

should be 5 kilo ohms or less (acceptable <10 kilo ohms). The ideal intervention would be replacement or repair of the electrode F4. During review, one can switch to the derivation F3-M2.

3. **Answer:** Respiratory artifact

   Discussion: Although the artifact in Figure P18-3 looks, at first glance, like sweat artifact affecting all channels, note that the sway is synchronous with respiration (in this case positive airway pressure [PAP] flow). That is, a respiratory artifact is present.[1-3] A respiratory artifact is often secondary to the patient lying on one of the mastoid electrodes, with movement of the electrode associated with breathing. This patient is lying on M2, and all derivations containing M2 are affected. By changing to electroencephalography (EEG) derivations using M1, the artifact is eliminated (Figure P18-5). The artifact persists in the electrooculography (EOG) derivations using M2. In this case, one could substitute M1 for M2 in the EOG derivations during review.[4] A recent revision of the AASM scoring manual states that if electrode M2 is faulty, M1 may be used in the EOG derivations (e.g., E1-M1, E2-M2). Ideally M2 should be repaired or replaced during monitoring.[4] It is possible for sweat and respiratory artifact to coexist. For example, sweat affecting a mastoid electrode between the patient's head and pillow. In this case, cooling the patient may reduce the artifact.[2]

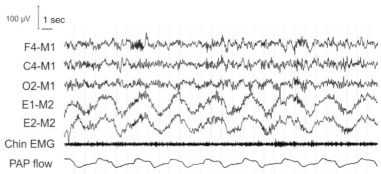

FIGURE P18-5 ■ The epoch in Figure P18-3 is shown with a change in the electroencephalography derivations to those using mastoid electrode M1.

CLINICAL PEARLS

1. Use of an average of M1 and M2 for the reference in the EEG and EOG derivations may help reduce the ECG artifact. Another option is to physically link the electrodes at the jack box.

2. A 60-Hz artifact is characterized by dark, bandlike activity. Because the recommended high filter cutoff frequency for EEG and EOG derivations is 35 Hz, this reduces 60-Hz activity, even if the 60-Hz notch filter is OFF. If the notch filter is ON, one may fail to note 60-Hz contamination, even if it is significant. Unless the electrode impedances are checked during the study, one might fail to note that one of the electrodes is faulty.

3. The pattern of the respiratory artifact appears similar to a sweat artifact, but the undulations are synchronous with breathing. The artifact is usually caused by one of the mastoid electrodes moving with breathing (less commonly from the effect of perspiration on a mastoid electrode). The affected electrode is often between the patient's head and the pillow when the patient is sleeping in the lateral posture. The fact that one of the mastoid electrodes is causing the problem can be easily confirmed if switching to derivations using the other mastoid eliminates the artifact. Of note, what appears to be a respiratory artifact may respond to cooling of the patient if sweat is affecting the performance of the faulty electrode.

REFERENCES

1. Berry RB: *Fundamentals of sleep medicine*, Philadelphia, 2012, Saunders, pp 51–56.
2. Siddiqui F, Osuna E, Walters AS, et al: Sweat artifact and respiratory artifact occurring simultaneously in polysomnogram, *Sleep Med* 7(2):197–199, 2006.
3. Avidan A, Fetterolf J: Artifacts. In Avidan A, Barkoukis TJ, editors: *Review of sleep medicine*, ed 3, Philadelphia, 2012, Saunders, pp 536–608.
4. Berry RB, Brooks R, Gamaldo CE, et al., for the American Academy of Sleep Medicine: *The AASM manual for the scoring of sleep and associated events: rules, terminology and technical specifications*, Version 2.0.3, www.aasmnet.org, Darien, IL, 2014, American Academy of Sleep Medicine.

FUNDAMENTALS 12

Monitoring Respiration

Monitoring of respiration during polysomnography requires, at a minimum, sensors to detect air flow, respiratory effort, and arterial oxygen saturation (Table F12-1). Recording these parameters allows detection of apnea (cessation of air flow), hypopnea (reduction in air flow), arterial oxygen desaturation, as well as classification of apneas as obstructive, mixed, or central (see Fundamentals 13). Additional sensors are used to detect snoring and estimate the partial pressure of arterial carbon dioxide (PCO_2; detection of hypoventilation). Signals derived from respiratory inductive plethysmography thoracoabdominal effort belts may be used to detect apnea and hypopnea. The *American Academy of Sleep Medicine (AASM) Scoring Manual*[1] makes recommendations concerning sensors to be used for respiratory monitoring. The background and

rationale for the recommendations concerning respiratory sensors has also been published.[2] *The convention used in this book is for inspiratory signals to be upward and expiratory signals to be downward.*

AIR FLOW

Oronasal thermal sensors placed in or near the nostrils and extending over the mouth detect either nasal or oral air flow by detecting a change in temperature of the sensor (inhaled air cooler, exhaled air warmer). An oronasal thermal sensor is the recommended sensor to detect apnea. Thermal devices include thermocouples (change in voltage with temperature), thermistors (change in resistance with temperature), or polyvinylidene

TABLE F12-1 Sensor Used to Monitor Air Flow or Tidal Volume

	Physiology	Advantage	Disadvantage
Pneumotachography (PTN)	Pressure drop across linear resistance PTN = Flow × Resistance	Accurate Detects air flow limitation	Requires mask over nose and mouth
Oronasal thermal sensor (Thermistors Thermocouples Polyvinylidene (PVDF) sensors)	Detects change in temperature	Detects both nasal and oral air flow Recommended for scoring apnea	Signal not proportional to flow (except PVDF)
Nasal Pressure (NP)	$NP = K1 \cdot (Flow)^2$ $Flow = K2 \cdot \sqrt{NP}$	Sensitive to decreases in flow Flattening of the waveform detects air flow limitation Recommended for scoring hypopnea	Does not detect oral flow
RIPsum	= RIPchest + RIPabdomen Changes in signal are an estimate of **tidal volume**	Backup if flow sensors at nose or mouth are not functional	Most accurate if respiratory inductance plethysmography (RIP) calibrated Requires thoracoabdominal belts
RIPflow	Time derivative of RIPsum Changes in signal an estimate of air flow	Backup if flow sensors at nose or mouth are not functional	Most accurate if calibrated Requires thoracoabdominal belts

difluoride (PVDF) sensors (change in signal with temperature or pressure). A limitation of thermocouples and thermistors is that the signal is not proportional to the magnitude of air flow. Hence, they are not ideal for detection of hypopneas (reductions in air flow).

A nasal pressure transducer is the recommended sensor to detect hypopnea in clinical diagnostic studies. Although pneumotachography using a mask over the nose and mouth can accurately measure flow by determining the pressure drop across a linear resistance (Equation 1), this method is not practical for clinical studies. Instead, nasal pressure (NP) monitoring uses a nasal cannula placed in the nares and connected to a pressure transducer. NP monitoring determines the pressure drop across the nasal inlet during air flow. However, the resistance is not linear, and flow is proportional to the square root of the nasal pressure signal (Equation 2).[2,3]

Pneumotachograph

Pressure difference = Flow · Resistance

Flow = Pressure difference · (1/Resistance)

(Equation 1)

Nasal pressure

$$NP = K1 \cdot (Flow)^2$$
$$Flow = K2 \cdot \sqrt{NP}$$

(Equation 2)

(K1, K2 are constants)

The NP signal underestimates flow at low flow rates and overestimates flow at higher flow rates (Figure F12-1, *A*). A square root transformation of the NP signal is a more accurate estimate of nasal flow. The apnea + hypopnea index is slightly lower if a square root transformation of the NP signal is used to score respiratory events

compared with the untransformed signal, but the difference is not clinically significant in most patients.[4] Snoring may be detected as a high-frequency oscillation in the NP signal. The shape of the inspiratory NP waveform provides additional information as a flattening of the signal occurs during air flow limitation (high upper airway resistance) (see Figure F12-1, *B*).

A limitation of NP monitoring is that oral flow is not well detected. If the patient is mouth breathing during a hypopnea, the NP tracing may falsely suggest that apnea is present (Figure F12-2). The *AASM Scoring Manual*[1] recommends use of both an oronasal thermal sensor and NP monitoring to monitor air flow during a diagnostic study to accurately detect both apnea and hypopnea (Table F12-2; Figure F12-3). During positive airway pressure (PAP) titration studies, the output of the PAP device (accurate[5] internal sensor) is the recommended sensor. The signal provides an accurate estimate of air flow and shows air flow limitation.[7] The signal is too under-sampled to show snoring. As discussed below, in pediatric patients monitoring exhaled PCO_2 may be used to detect apnea (not a measure of air flow).

ALTERNATIVE SENSORS FOR APNEA AND HYPOPNEA

Alternative sensors for detection of apnea and hypopnea may be used when the recommended sensors are not functioning (Table F12-3). Some of the alternative apnea and hypopnea sensors do not directly measure air flow. Respiratory inductance plethysmography (RIP) is used to monitor respiratory effort (see below).[2,3] Changes in the

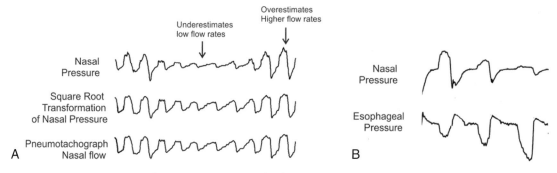

FIGURE F12-1 ■ **A,** The untransformed nasal pressure (NP) is proportional to the square of the flow rate. The signal underestimates flow at low flow rates and overestimates high flow rates. A square root transformation of the NP is an accurate estimate of nasal flow. Inspiration in this figure is upward. **B,** Flattening of the inspiratory waveform of the nasal pressure signal detects air flow limitation and is a sensitive indicator of high upper airway resistance. Here, the deflections in the esophageal pressure are an estimate of the pressure drop across the upper airway. Flattening of the nasal pressure is associated with increased deflections in the esophageal pressure. Inspiration is upward.

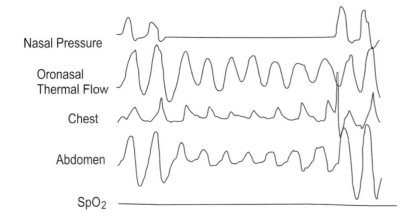

Nasal Pressure

Oronasal
Thermal Flow

Chest

Abdomen

SpO₂

FIGURE F12-2 ■ Hypopnea (reduction in air flow). The nasal pressure signal is flat as the patient is breathing through the mouth during the event. Saturation of peripheral oxygen (SpO_2) is the pulse oximetry signal.

TABLE F12-2	**Recommended Sensors for Detecting Apnea and Hypopnea**	
	Adult	**Pediatric**
Apnea	**Diagnostic:** Oronasal thermal sensor (including PVDF air flow sensor) **PAP titration:** PAP device flow	Same
Hypopnea	**Diagnostic:** Nasal Pressure with or without square root transformation **PAP titration:** PAP device flow	Same

Adapted from References 1 and 2.
PAP, Positive airway pressure; *PVDF,* polyvinylidene.
Note: Diagnostic study: use both oronasal thermal sensor and NP. PAP titration study: use PAP device flow.

TABLE F12-3	**Alternative Sensors for Scoring Respiratory Events (Diagnostic Study)**	
	Adult	**Pediatric**
Apnea	Nasal Pressure RIPsum RIPflow PVDFsum (Acceptable)	Nasal Pressure RIPsum RIPflow End tidal PCO₂ (Acceptable)
Hypopnea	Oronasal thermal sensor RIPsum RIPflow Dual RIP belts PVDFsum (Acceptable)	Oronasal thermal sensor RIPsum RIPflow Dual RIP belts

Adapted from References 1 and 2.
As listed in the *AASM Scoring Manual,* all sensors are "recommended" except for the sensors listed as acceptable.
NP, With or without square root transformation; *PCO₂,* partial pressure of arterial carbon dioxide; *PVDF,* polyvinylidene difluoride; *PVDFsum,* the sum of chest and abdominal PVDF belts; *RIP,* calibrated or uncalibrated; *RIPsum,* sum of thorax and abdominal RIP signals (estimate of tidal volume); *RIPflow,* time derivative of RIPsum (estimate of airflow).

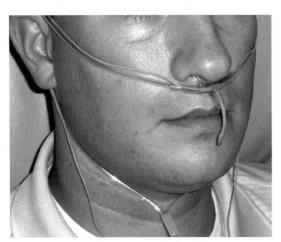

FIGURE F12-3 ■ A patient wearing a nasal cannula and oronasal thermal sensor. The oronasal thermal sensor can detect both nasal and oral air flow. (From Berry RB. Fundamentals of sleep medicine, Philadelphia, 2012, Saunders, p 104.)

sum of chest and abdominal RIP belts (RIPsum) during breathing are a semiquantitative estimate of tidal volume when RIP is calibrated (Figure F12-4). The RIPsum signal has minimal excursions during an apnea (tidal volume = 0) and reduced excursions during hypopnea. The time derivative of the RIPsum is called the *RIPflow* and is an estimate of air flow. If the RIPsum is not available, hypopnea may be detected by a reduction in deflections in both the thoracoabdominal RIP belt excursions. In clinical practice, uncalibrated RIP is commonly used but changes

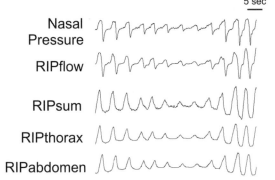

5 sec

Nasal Pressure

RIPflow

RIPsum

RIPthorax

RIPabdomen

FIGURE F12-4 ■ Use of RIPsum and RIPflow. Deflections in the RIPsum estimate tidal volume and deflections in RIPflow are an estimate of air flow. In this patient, RIP-flow and the nasal pressure have a very similar pattern.

in the RIPsum or RIPflow signals compared with baseline breathing may also be used to detect apnea and hypopnea.

The end-tidal PCO_2 signal is listed as an acceptable alternative sensor for apnea detection in pediatric patients in the *AASM Scoring Manual*.[1] A more accurate description of the signal is exhaled PCO_2 (capnography). The side stream method of capnography[6] is most commonly used in polysomnography and consists of gas suctioned via a nasal cannula, with tips located in the nostrils to an external sensor at bedside. During apnea, no CO_2 is exhaled (PCO_2 signal = 0 as room air suctioned). Mouth breathing and

occlusion of the nasal cannula may impair the ability of end-tidal PCO_2 monitoring to detect apnea. A delay in the start of the apnea by PCO_2 monitoring is caused by the time required for exhaled PCO_2 sample to reach the sensor at bedside (Figure F12-5). The value of the capnography signal is usually given as millimeters of mercury (mm Hg).

RESPIRATORY EFFORT

The gold standard sensor to detect respiratory effort is esophageal manometry (Table F12-4 and Figure F12-6). During inspiration, intrathoracic pressure becomes negative, and the change in intrathoracic pressure may be measured using a balloon, transducer-tipped catheter, or a fluid-filled catheter, each with the tip placed in the lower esophagus. Esophageal pressure monitoring may be used to detect an absence of inspiratory effort (e.g., central apnea = absent esophageal pressure excursions), and the magnitude of the esophageal excursions provide an estimate of the magnitude of respiratory effort (greater effort associated with more negative esophageal pressure excursions).

Esophageal manometry is rarely performed in clinical practice. Instead, the monitoring of thoracoabdominal excursions is used to detect the presence of respiratory effort. The magnitude of these excursions may or may not be proportional

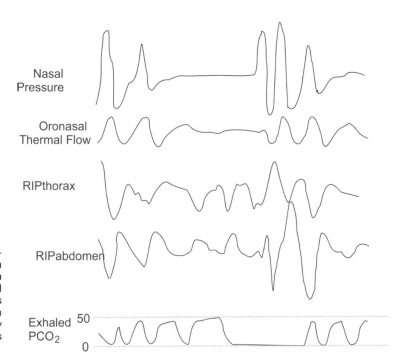

Nasal Pressure

Oronasal Thermal Flow

RIPthorax

RIPabdomen

Exhaled PCO_2 50   0

FIGURE F12-5 ■ Use of exhaled partial pressure of arterial carbon dioxide (PCO_2) to detect apnea (no deflection in oronasal thermal flow signal). When no CO_2 is exhaled the signal = 0, as room air is suctioned. Note the delay in the start of the apnea as detected by PCO_2 = 0.

TABLE F12-4	**Other Sensors Recommended for Sleep Monitoring**	
	Adult	**Pediatric**
Respiratory Effort	Esophageal manometry Dual RIPbelts Dual PVDF belts (acceptable)	Esophageal manometry Dual RIPbelts
Snoring*	Piezoelectric sensor Microphone Nasal pressure transducer	same
Hypoventilation	*Diagnostic study:* End-tidal PCO_2 or Transcutaneous PCO_2 *PAP titration study:* Transcutaneous PCO_2	same

Adapted from Reference 1.
*Use of sensor [recommended], monitoring [optional]
Monitoring of hypoventilation:
Adults: Optional
Pediatrics: Diagnostic study—recommended; PAP titration—optional

to esophageal pressure excursions, yet for routine clinical sleep monitoring, the detection of respiratory effort to differentiate central and obstructive apnea is the major concern. The technology available for respiratory effort belts includes strain gauges, impedance plethysmography, RIP, and belts with piezoelectric or PVDF sensors[2] (see Table F12-4). An advantage of the RIP technology is that inductance of the band and ultimately the signal output depends on the entire cross-sectional area enclosed by the band.[7] Effort belts with piezoelectric or PVDF sensors typically use a single sensor between belt material surrounding the thorax or abdomen. The signal depends on variations in the tension on the sensor which may or may not reflect the magnitude of thoracoabdominal excursions.

As noted above the signal from the dual RIP belts may be calibrated such that excursions in the RIPsum provide a semiquantitative estimate of tidal volume.[2,3]

$$RIPsum = a \cdot RIPchest + b \cdot RIP \text{ abdomen}$$

Here, *a* and *b* are constants determined using a calibration procedure. However, calibration is rarely performed in clinical settings, and in practice, *a* and *b* are chosen as 0.50 so that the excursions of RIPsum, RIPchest, and RIPabdomen channels are of comparable magnitude. RIP bands often show paradoxical movement, that is, one inward (usually up) and one outward during high upper airway resistance (very negative intrathoracic pressure) or when either the chest wall muscles or thoracic cage or the diaphragm are weak.

ARTERIAL OXYGEN SATURATION

Continuous measurement of the partial pressure of arterial oxygen (PaO_2) during sleep studies is not feasible. Instead of PaO_2, the arterial oxygen saturation (SaO_2; (oxygenated hemoglobin × 100/total hemoglobin) is estimated during sleep studies by continuous recording of pulse oximetry (SpO_2), typically with finger or ear probes. In sleep monitoring, *arterial oxygen desaturation* is usually defined as a decrease in the SaO_2 of 3% or 4% or more from baseline. Note that the nadir in SaO_2 commonly follows apnea (hypopnea) termination by approximately 6 to

Air Flow

Esophageal Pressure

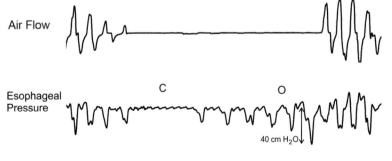

40 cm H_2O

FIGURE F12-6 ■ A mixed apnea is shown (C central portion, O obstructive portion). At **C**, inspiratory effort (the small deflections reflect cardiac pulsations) is lacking. The obstructive part (*O*) is characterized by inspiratory effort that progressively increases until apnea termination.

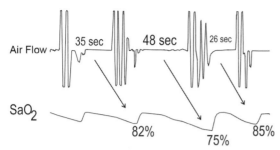

FIGURE F12-7 ■ The nadir in pulse oximetry follow apnea termination. Longer apneas are associated with more severe desaturation. (Reproduced from Berry RB: *Sleep medicine pearls*, ed 2, Philadelphia, 2003, Saunders, p 86.)

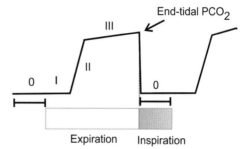

CAPNOGRAPHY - Exhaled CO_2 versus time

Phases of exhaled PCO_2

0 Inspiration (PCO_2=0, inhaled gas)

I Dead space (no CO_2 exhaled)

II Mixture of dead space and alveolar gas

III Alveolar plateau

FIGURE F12-8 ■ Schematic of the exhaled partial pressure of arterial carbon dioxide (PCO_2) values versus time (capnography). The value at end-expiration (end-tidal) is an estimate of the alveolar PCO_2 and therefore the arterial PCO_2. The arterial PCO_2 usually exceeds the end-tidal PCO_2 by about 5 millimeters of mercury (mm Hg; 2 to 7). The arterial to end-tidal PCO_2 difference is larger in patients with lung disease.

8 seconds (longer in severe desaturations) (Figure F12-7). This delay is secondary to circulation time and instrumental delay (the oximeter averages over several[1] cycles before producing a reading). The AASM scoring manual recommends the use of pulse oximetry with a maximum acceptable signal averaging time of 3 seconds or less at a heart rate of 80 beats per minute. Longer averaging times may reduce the ability to detect desaturations.

OTHER RESPIRATORY SENSORS

Snoring is detected as oscillations in the unfiltered nasal pressure signal, piezoelectric sensors placed on the neck to detect vibration, or acoustic sensors (e.g., a microphone) to record sound.[2] The ability of the sensor to detect simulated snoring is typically tested before lights-out.

The gold standard method for documenting hypoventilation is the processing of an arterial sample for determination of the arterial partial pressure of CO_2 ($PaCO_2$). Given the difficulty of drawing an arterial sample during sleep, surrogate estimates are commonly used. The recommended sensors for detection of hypoventilation are end-tidal PCO_2 (diagnostic study) or transcutaneous PCO_2 (diagnostic or PAP titration study). A schematic of the waveform of exhaled PCO_2 is shown in Figure F12-8. The end-tidal PCO_2 is an estimate of the arterial PCO_2. The end-tidal PCO_2 is generally around 5 mm Hg lower than the arterial PCO_2 because of anatomic and physiologic dead space ($PCO_2 = 0$), which dilutes the alveolar PCO_2.[2,6] Higher differences between the end-tidal PCO_2 and the arterial values occur when lung disease is present. To be valid, a plateau should be seen in the exhaled PCO_2 waveform. Capnography may be performed during PAP titration using a nasal cannula under the mask. However, the exhaled sample may be diluted, and hence the *AASM Scoring Manual*[1] does not recommend measurement of end-tidal PCO_2 during PAP titration (although some clinicians find this measurement useful). It is important to remember that the magnitude of signal excursion in the capnography signal depends entirely on the highest value of PCO_2 in the exhaled breath rather than the magnitude of tidal volume or flow. Signal excursions may persist during inspiratory apnea if small expiratory puffs with a high PCO_2 are present.

Measurement of transcutaneous PCO_2 ($TcPCO_2$) depends on the fact that heating of capillaries in the skin causes increased capillary blood flow and makes the skin permeable to the diffusion of CO_2. The CO_2 in the capillaries diffuses through the skin and is measured by an electrode at the skin surface. The measured value is corrected for the fact that heat increases the skin CO_2 production and the measured value exceeds the $PaCO_2$ measured at 37°C. $TcCO2$ electrodes are calibrated with a reference gas.

The accuracy of transcutaneous PCO_2 measurement is not impaired by mask ventilation or mouth breathing.[2,8] However, the signal has a slower response time than the end-tidal PCO_2 signal. After a change in the $PaCO_2$ the transcutaneous value may not reflect the change for 2 or more minutes, depending on the device.

REFERENCES

1. Berry RB, Brooks R, Gamaldo CE, et al: for the American Academy of Sleep Medicine: *The AASM manual for the scoring of sleep and associated events: rules, terminology and technical specifications,* Version 2.1, Darien, IL, 2012, American Academy of Sleep Medicine. www.aasmnet.org, Accessed July 3, 2014.
2. Berry RB, Budhiraja R, Gottlieb DJ, et al: Rules for scoring respiratory events in sleep: update of the 2007 AASM Manual for the Scoring of Sleep and Associated Events, *J Clin Sleep Med* 8(5):597–619, 2012.
3. Farré R, Montserrat JM, Navajas D: Noninvasive monitoring of respiratory mechanics during sleep, *Eur Respir J* 24:1052–1060, 2004.
4. Thurnheer R, Xie X, Bloch KE: Accuracy of nasal cannula pressure recordings for assessment of ventilation during sleep, *Am J Respir Crit Care Med* 146:1914–1919, 2001.
5. Condos R, Norman RG, Krishnasamy I, et al: Flow limitation as a noninvasive assessment of residual upper-airway resistance during continuous positive airway pressure therapy of obstructive sleep apnea, *Am J Respir Crit Care Med* 150:475–480, 1994.
6. Kodali BS: Capnography outside the operating rooms, *Anesthesiology* 118(1):192–201, 2013.
7. Stats BA, Bonekat W, Harris CD, Offord KP: Chest wall motion in sleep apnea, *Am Rev Respir Dis* 130:59–63, 1984.
8. Kirk VG, Batuyong ED, Bohn SG: Transcutaneous carbon dioxide monitoring and capnography during pediatric polysomnography, *Sleep* 29:1601–1608, 2006.

PATIENT 19

Respiratory Monitoring Questions

QUESTIONS

1. Choose the filter settings for B and C in Figure P19-1 that would produce the appearance of the nasal pressure signal. Note the filter settings for A.

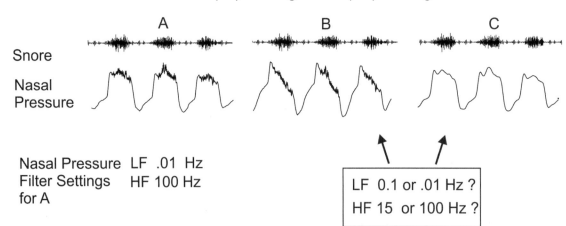

FIGURE P19-1 ■ Snore and nasal pressure tracing displayed with different low frequency (LF) and high frequency (HF) filter settings for filter settings for the nasal pressure signal. Inspiration is upward.

2. What is the most accurate estimate of the patient's arterial PCO_2 (partial pressure of carbon dioxide) shown in Figure P19-2?
   A. 45 mm Hg (millimeters of mercury)
   B. 38 mm Hg
   C. 52 mm Hg
   D. 20 mm Hg

3. A tracing from a sleep study of a 30-year-old patient with an awake saturation of peripheral oxygen (SpO_2) of 94% is shown in Figure P19-3. The patient has neuromuscular weakness. Is hypoventilation present?

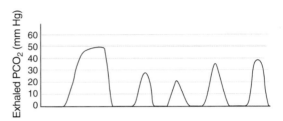

FIGURE P19-2 ■ Exhaled PCO_2 tracing. PCO_2, partial pressure of carbon dioxide.

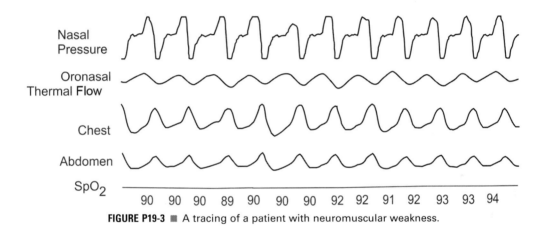

FIGURE P19-3 ■ A tracing of a patient with neuromuscular weakness.

ANSWERS

1. **Answer**: B (LF 0.1, HF 100 Hz), C (LF 0.01, HF 15 Hz)

   Discussion: The nasal pressure signal is proportional to the square of the flow. During air flow limitation, the inspiratory portion of the waveform is flattened. A constant flow during a period in which the driving pressure varies is consistent with air flow limitation (upper airway narrowing). Flattening can be best seen when the nasal pressure signal is recorded and displayed as a DC (direct current) signal. The signal can also be recorded and displayed as an AC (alternating current) signal if the AC amplifier and display low filter (LF) setting is sufficiently low (e.g., 0.01 or 0.03 Hz). If 0.1 Hz is used as the low filter setting, then the flattening is not seen (see Figure P19-1, *B*). If a PSG system uses AC amplifiers with default LF setting of 0.1 Hz, the nasal pressure signal cannot be accurately recorded as an AC signal (even if display LF setting is appropriate). Snoring can be noted in the inspiratory portion of the nasal pressure waveform as rapid oscillations if the high filter setting is 100 Hz (see Figure P19-1, *B*). If the high filter (HF) setting is relatively low (e.g., 15 Hz), the high frequency oscillations are greatly attenuated (see Figure P19-1, *C*). The filter settings for nasal pressure recommended by the *AASM Scoring Manual*[1] are LF = (DC, 0.01, 0.03 Hz) and HF = 100 Hz.

2. **Answer:** C.

Discussion: The arterial PCO_2 is usually 2 to 7 mm Hg higher than the end tidal PCO_2 measured by capnography.[2,3] Alveolar units with a high ventilation–perfusion ratio contribute gas with a low PCO_2 to the exhaled sample (physiologic dead space). This lowers the measured end-tidal PCO_2 relative to the arterial PCO_2. The arterial PCO_2 – end tidal PCO_2 difference is increased if lung disease is present (more ventilation–perfusion mismatch). In the example shown, the answer C is most correct, as it is slightly above the end-tidal value of the first wave form of approximately 49 mm Hg. The other waveforms do not display a plateau and do not provide reliable estimates of the arterial PCO_2. They are likely caused by small breaths (the exhaled sample is a mixture of PCO_2 from the anatomic dead space and alveolar lung units).

   The side-stream method of capnography[2,3] is usually used for sleep monitoring. Exhaled gas is suctioned via a nasal cannula to a sensor at bedside. If no exhalation occurs, room air gas is suction ($PCO_2 = 0$ mm Hg). There is a delay from the time a breath is exhaled until an increase in PCO_2 is noted in the capnography tracing secondary to the time it takes for the exhaled sample to reach the sensor (Figure P19-4). Mouth breathing and occlusion of the sampling nasal cannula with secretions impair the accuracy of end-tidal PCO_2 monitoring. Small breaths result in mixture of dead space and alveolar gas being sampled (rather than a sample from the alveoli), and this results in a low peak PCO_2 value and absence of an alveolar plateau. Why does an alveolar plateau exist? Its presence means that multiple lung units have fairly similar alveolar PCO_2. The more inhomogeneous the PCO_2 from different lung units (ventilation–perfusion mismatch), the steeper is the plateau. As noted in Fundamentals 12, exhaled PCO_2 is listed as an acceptable alternative method for detecting apnea in children in the *AASM Scoring Manual*. Both capnography (end-tidal PCO_2 measurement) and transcutaneous PCO_2 measurement are listed as recommended surrogates of the arterial PCO_2 for detection of hypoventilation in adults and children during a diagnostic test. Note that only transcutaneous PCO_2 is recommended during PAP titration studies. The concern is that the alveolar sample will be diluted by a high flow of gas from the PAP device. However, some sleep centers use a small nasal cannula under the PAP mask to better sample exhaled gas and find this method useful. More research is needed in this area.

3. **Answer:** Hypoventilation cannot be scored without a measure of the arterial PCO_2.

Discussion: The *AASM Scoring Manual*[1] states that hypoventilation during sleep can be scored using a measurement of the arterial PCO_2 (almost never used) or a surrogate measure of the arterial PCO_2. Hypoventilation cannot be scored on the basis of arterial oxygen desaturation without apnea or hypopnea. In this situation, worsening ventilation–perfusion mismatch during sleep may cause hypoxemia in the absence of hypoventilation. During diagnostic testing, the end-tidal PCO_2 or transcutaneous PCO_2 are acceptable surrogates of the arterial PCO_2. During PAP titration, the transcutaneous PCO_2 is recommended. For adults hypoventilation during sleep may be scored if the PCO_2 is >55 mm Hg for ≥ 10 minutes or a ≥ 10 mm Hg increase occurs in PCO_2 from wakefulness to sleep to a value >50 mm g for ≥ 10 minutes (Fundamentals 13). In the patient in Figure P19-3, the awake end-tidal PCO_2 was 43 mm Hg. When the CO_2 channels are added to the displayed montage (Figure P19-5, one can see that the increase in PCO_2

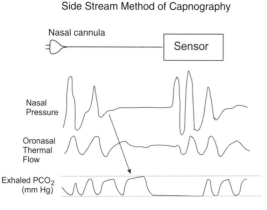

Side Stream Method of Capnography

FIGURE P19-4 ■ The side-stream method of capnography. The capnography tracing is delayed relative to the air flow signals.

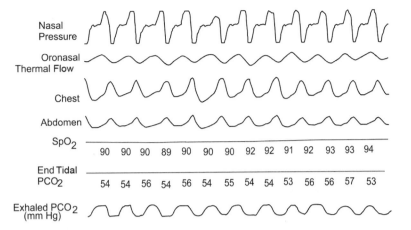

FIGURE P19-5 ■ The same tracing shown in Figure P19-4 with CO_2 channels visible. The end-tidal PCO_2 channel is the maximum PCO_2 value for the last second while the exhaled PCO2 is the capnography waveform. Note the plateaus in CO_2 waveforms. *PCO₂,* partial pressure of carbon dioxide.

is >10 mm Hg above the awake value). In this patient, a PCO_2 of 53 or higher was present for over 100 minutes. Therefore, hypoventilation during sleep was present. Note that an alveolar plateau was present in most but not all breaths (e.g., breaths 1 and 2 but not breath 3).

CLINICAL PEARLS

1. The nasal pressure channel must have appropriate low and high filter settings to properly display the useful information provided by the recording of this signal. Recommended settings are LF = DC or 0.01 to 0.03; and HF = 100 Hz.

2. With rare exceptions, the arterial PCO_2 is approximately 5 mm Hg (2 to 7 mm Hg) above the end-tidal PCO_2 measured with capnography. To be a reliable estimate of the arterial PCO_2, a plateau in the exhaled PCO_2 versus time waveform should be noted. Small breaths may not reflect the true end-tidal PCO_2, as the exhaled gas contains a mixture of dead space ($PCO_2 = 0$) and alveolar gas. Patients with lung disease have a large difference between the arterial PCO_2 and the end-tidal PCO_2 and a steep alveolar plateau.

3. A diagnosis of hypoventilation during sleep requires measurement of the arterial PCO_2 (almost never performed) or an acceptable surrogate of the arterial PCO_2. The presence of arterial oxygen desaturation without apnea or hypopnea is not sufficient to score hypoventilation.

4. The AASM scoring manual recommends end-tidal PCO_2 or transcutaneous PCO_2 for diagnostic studies and transcutaneous PCO_2 for PAP titration studies.

REFERENCES

1. Berry RB, Brooks R, Gamaldo CE, et al for the American Academy of Sleep Medicine: *The AASM manual for the scoring of sleep and associated events: rules, terminology and technical specifications*, Version 2.0.3, www.aasmnet.org, Darien, Illinois, 2014, American Academy of Sleep Medicine.
2. Kodali BS: Capnography outside the operating rooms, *Anesthesiology* 118(1):192–201, 2013.
3. D'Mello J, Butani M: Capnography, *Indian J Anaesthesiol* 46:269–278, 2002.

FUNDAMENTALS 13

Respiratory Event Definitions in Adults

The definitions used to score respiratory events in sleep research and clinical practice have varied considerably over the last 15 years.[1] Variation in definitions makes it difficult to compare the results of different clinical investigations or between different sleep centers. A consensus conference in 1999 published recommendations to attempt to standardize definitions for research (also known as the *Chicago criteria*).[2] In 2001, a clinical practice review committee of the American Academy of Sleep Medicine (AASM) published definitions[3] for hypopnea, and these were subsequently adopted by the Centers for Medicare and Medicaid (CMS). Previously, CMS had only recognized apneas for identification of patients with obstructive sleep apnea. To help standardize sleep monitoring the AASM appointed task forces to make recommendations with regard to monitoring technology and event definitions for analysis of sleep studies, including respiratory event definitions.[4] The 2007 *AASM Scoring Manual*[5] published respiratory event definitions based on a review of the literature and consensus. For adults, two definitions of hypopnea were provided, one was recommended (similar to CMS definition based on flow and arterial oxygen desaturation) and an alternative definition was based on flow, desaturation, and arousal. In 2012, a sleep apnea definitions task force of the AASM made recommendations for updated definitions.[6] The revised rules were published in the *AASM Scoring Manual*[7] and are used in this chapter. The scoring manual is periodically updated and the reader should check for changes. A recent change is that two hypopnea definitions are again provided (one recommended and one acceptable). The acceptable definition is compatible with the CMS hypopnea definition. Alternative sensors are used when the recommended sensor signal is not reliable.

APNEA

The scoring criteria for an apnea are listed in Box F13-1. In adults, the recommended sensor

---

> **BOX F13-1** **Apnea (Adults)**
>
> Score a respiratory event as an apnea when BOTH of the following criteria are met:
> 1. A drop exists in the peak signal excursion by $\geq 90\%$ of baseline using an oronasal thermal sensor (diagnostic study), PAP device flow (titration study) or an alternative apnea sensor (diagnostic study).
> 2. The duration of the $\geq 90\%$ drop in sensor signal is ≥ 10 seconds.

for scoring apnea in the oronasal thermal sensor (diagnostic study) or positive airway pressure (PAP) device flow (titration study). Recommended alternative apnea sensors (diagnostic study) include the nasal pressure, RIPsum, and RIPflow (all recommended). Use of the sum (PVDFsum) from chest and abdominal polyvinylidene difluoride (PVDF) belts is acceptable as an alternative apnea sensor (see Fundamentals 12).

Note that an apnea does not have to be associated with arterial oxygen desaturation. If a portion of a respiratory event that would otherwise meet criteria for a hypopnea meets criteria for apnea, the entire event should be scored as an apnea. The **duration** of the event is from the nadir in flow **preceding** the first breath that is clearly reduced to the **start** of the first breath that approximates baseline breathing (measured based on oronasal thermal signal or alternative apnea sensor). The classification of apneas as obstructive, mixed, or central is shown in Box F13-2.

HYPOPNEA

The definition of hypopnea continues to be controversial.[1,6] Different definitions of hypopnea that have appeared in notable publications are listed in Table F13-1. The major controversy involves whether hypopneas should be scored based on flow and an associated arousal when

BOX F13-2	Classification of Apneas

1. Score an apnea as **obstructive** if it meets apnea criteria and is associated with continued or increased inspiratory effort throughout the entire period of absent air flow.
2. Score an apnea as **central** if it meets apnea criteria and is associated with absent inspiratory effort throughout the entire period of absent air flow.
3. Score an apnea as **mixed** if it meets apnea criteria and is associated with absent inspiratory effort in the initial portion of the event, followed by resumption of inspiratory effort in the second portion of the event.

arterial oxygen desaturation is not significant. Currently the AASM scoring manual provides a recommended and an acceptable hypopnea definition (Box F13-3).

Recommended alternative hypopnea sensors in adults and pediatric patients include oronasal thermal sensor, RIPsum, RIPflow, and dual respiratory inductance plethysmography (RIP). Use of the sum from chest and abdominal polyvinylidene difluoride (PVDF) belts is acceptable as an alternative hypopnea sensor (see Fundamentals 12). Hypopnea duration is measured the same as for apnea except that the nasal pressure tracing is used.

Classification of Hypopneas

Scoring hypopneas as central or obstructive is optional in the *AASM Scoring Manual* (Boxes F13-4 and F13-5). Definitive hypopnea classification would require an accurate measure of air flow and effort (esophageal manometry)[8] (Figure F13-2). As esophageal manometry is rarely used, an increase in upper airway resistance is inferred from snoring, flattening of the nasal pressure waveform, paradoxical movement of chest and abdominal effort bands, or all of these.

TABLE F13-1	Hypopnea Definitions		
	Drop in Flow	**Duration**	**Required Associated Event**
Chicago criteria*	50%	≥10 sec	— —
	Any discernable drop using accurate flow sensor	≥10 sec	≥3% Desaturation or arousal
2007 AASM-A/CMS[†]	≥30%	≥10 sec	≥4% Desaturation
2007 AASM-B[†]	≥50%	≥10 sec	≥3% Desaturation or arousal
AASM recommended[‡]	≥30%	≥10 sec	≥3% Desaturation or arousal
AASM acceptable[‡]	≥30%	≥10 sec	≥4% Desaturation

From CMS Centers for Medicare and Medicaid Services.
*From Reference 2 (obstructive apnea-hypopnea event).
[†]From Reference 5.
[‡]From Reference 7.

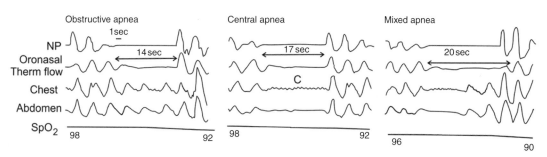

FIGURE F13-1 ■ Obstructive, central, and mixed apneas. The chest respiratory inductance plethysmography (RIP) belt in the central apnea shows small oscillations (*C*) caused by movement of the chest with each heartbeat, but these do not constitute respiratory effort. For apnea, the duration is measured from the nadir in the flow preceding the first breath that is clearly reduced until the start of the first breath that approximates baseline breathing. Here, *flow* refers to oronasal flow with a thermal device, which is used to score apneas; and *NP* refers to nasal pressure which is used to score hypopneas. Inspiration is upward. (Adapted from Berry RB: *Fundamentals of sleep medicine*, Philadelphia, 2012, Saunders, p 124.)

BOX F13-3	Hypopnea Definitions

AASM Recommended

Score a respiratory event as a hypopnea if ALL of the following criteria are met:
1. The peak signal excursions drop by ≥0% of pre-event baseline using nasal pressure (diagnostic study), PAP device flow (titration study), or an alternative hypopnea sensor (diagnostic study).
2. The duration of the ≥30% drop in signal excursion is ≥10 seconds.
3. There is a ≥3% oxygen desaturation from pre-event baseline or the events is associated with an arousal.

AASM Acceptable

Score a respiratory event as a hypopnea if ALL of the following criteria are met:
1. The peak signal excursions drop by ≥30% of pre-event baseline using nasal pressure (diagnostic study), PAP device flow (titration study), or an alternative hypopnea sensor (diagnostic study).
2. The duration of the ≥30% drop in signal excursion is ≥10 seconds.
3. There is a ≥4% oxygen desaturation from pre-event baseline.

Adapted from Berry RB, Brooks R, Gamaldo CE, et al., for the American Academy of Sleep Medicine: *The AASM manual for the scoring of sleep and associated events: rules, terminology and technical specifications*, Version 2.1, www.aasmnet.org, Darien, Illinois, 2014, American Academy of Sleep Medicine.

BOX F13-4	Obstructive Hypopnea

If electing to score obstructive hypopneas, score a hypopnea as **obstructive** if ANY of the following criteria are met (see Figure F13-3):
1. Snoring during the event.
2. Increased inspiratory flattening of the nasal pressure or PAP device flow signal compared with baseline breathing.
3. Associated thoracoabdominal paradox occurs during the event but not during pre-event breathing.

Adapted from Berry RB, Brooks R, Gamaldo CE, et al., for the American Academy of Sleep Medicine: *The AASM manual for the scoring of sleep and associated events: rules, terminology and technical specifications*, Version 2.1, www.aasmnet.org, Darien, Illinois, 2014, American Academy of Sleep Medicine.

Obstructive hypopnea is primarily caused by an increase in upper airway resistance. However, respiratory effort may fall from baseline at the start of obstructive hypopneas (Figure F13-3). Central hypopnea is primarily caused by a drop in inspiratory effort (Figure F13-4). It is also possible to have mixed hypopnea, but this type of event was not defined in the *AASM Scoring Manual*.

BOX F13-5	Central Hypopnea

If electing to score central hypopneas, score a hypopnea as **central** if NONE of the following criteria is met:
1. Snoring during the event.
2. Increased inspiratory flattening of the nasal pressure or PAP device flow signal compared with baseline breathing.
3. Associated thoracoabdominal paradox occurs during the event but not during pre-event breathing.

Adapted from Berry RB, Brooks R, Gamaldo CE, et al., for the American Academy of Sleep Medicine: *The AASM manual for the scoring of sleep and associated events: rules, terminology and technical specifications*, Version 2.1, www.aasmnet.org, Darien, Illinois, 2014, American Academy of Sleep Medicine.

RESPIRATORY EFFORT–RELATED AROUSAL (RERA)

RERAs are respiratory events characterized by increasing respiratory effort leading to an arousal that *do not meet criteria for apnea or hypopnea* (Box F13-6).

If the AASM acceptable definition of hypopnea (drop in flow + ≥4% desaturation) is used, most *RERAs* events (Figure F13-5) do not meet the criteria to be scored as hypopneas because of absence of an associated arterial oxygen desaturation of required severity. If the recommended AASM hypopnea definition is used, very few RERA events occur as RERA events using the acceptable hypopnea definition meet critieria for hypopneas using the recommended definition (Figure F13-6).[9,10] Scoring RERAs when using a hypopnea definition requiring an associated desaturation is believed to be clinically relevant, as the sleep fragmentation associated with respiratory arousals in the absence of arterial oxygen desaturation may be associated with a complaint of daytime sleepiness or fatigue. Some patients have an apnea–hypopnea index (AHI) <5 hour, based on hypopneas requiring an associated desaturation, but will have an AHI + RERA index ≥5/hr. RERA events are sometimes called *upper airway resistance events*.

Use of esophageal manometry is the gold standard for detection of increased respiratory effort. As this is method is uncommonly used, most often RERAs are scored on the basis of flattening of the nasal pressure waveform. If RERAs are compared on the basis of NP (flow-limitation RERAs) versus esophageal manometry, the RERA indices are highly correlated and similar.[11] However, some RERA events are detected only by NP and others only by esophageal manometry.

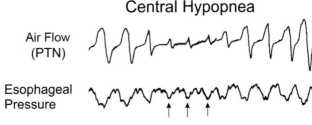

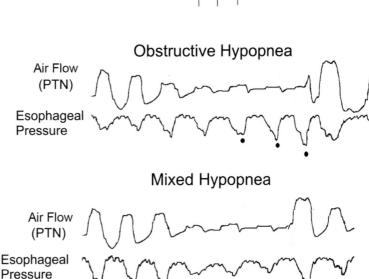

FIGURE F13-2 ■ Hypopneas defined with air flow by pneumotachography and respiratory effort by esophageal manometry. In central hypopneas, the air flow profile remains rounded, and the reduction in flow is proportional to the decrease in effort (*3 arrows*). In obstructive hypopneas, flow falls despite an increase in respiratory effort. Note that the inspiratory air flow is flattened. In mixed hypopneas, *there is* a combination of fall in effort and air flow limitation is present. Inspiration is upward. (Adapted from Berry RB: *Fundamentals of sleep medicine*, Philadelphia, 2012, Saunders, p 129.)

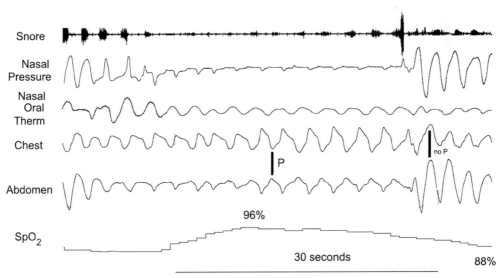

FIGURE F13-3 ■ An example of obstructive hypopnea. Here, chest and abdomen are respiratory inductance plethysmography (RIP) effort belts. Snoring is present. Flattening of the nasal pressure occurs during the event (round shape before and after the hypopnea). During the event, thoracoabdominal paradox (P) exists, whereas after the event, paradox is not present (*no P*). Paradox occurs when high upper airway resistance (very negative intrathoracic pressure) exists or the chest wall is easily collapsed (paralysis of chest wall muscles, structural problems). This event would meet any of the hypopnea criteria listed in Table F3-1. Inspiration is upward. (Reproduced from Berry RB: *Fundamentals of sleep medicine*, Philadelphia, 2012, Saunders, p 130.)

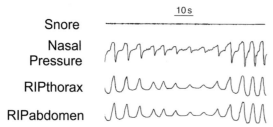

FIGURE F13-4 ■ Central hypopnea. Nasal pressure excursions have a rounded profile, and no evidence of snoring or thoracoabdominal paradox exists. The decrease in nasal pressure is proportional to the decrease in effort belt excursion. Inspiration is upward.

BOX F13-6	**RERA Definition** (*AASM Scoring Manual*)

Scoring respiratory effort-related arousals is **optional** as noted in Parameters to be Reported.

If electing to score respiratory effort–related arousals, score a respiratory event as a respiratory effort–related arousal (RERA) if a sequence of breaths lasting ≥ 10 seconds is characterized by increasing respiratory effort or by flattening of the inspiratory portion of the nasal pressure (diagnostic study) or PAP device flow (titration study) waveform leading to arousal from sleep **when the sequence of breaths does not meet criteria for an apnea or hypopnea.**

HYPOVENTILATION

Hypoventilation during wakefulness is usually defined as a partial pressure of arterial carbon dioxide ($PaCO_2$) >45 mm Hg. During clinical sleep monitoring, continuous monitoring of $PaCO_2$ is not possible. According to the *AASM Scoring Manual*, acceptable surrogates of the $PaCO_2$ include end-tidal PCO_2 (diagnostic study) or transcutaneous PCO_2 (diagnostic or PAP titration). The AASM criteria for hypoventilation are shown in Box F13-7.

CHEYNE-STOKES BREATHING

Cheyne-Stokes breathing (CSB) is a form of periodic breathing, with central apneas or central hypopneas at the nadir of effort and a crescendo–decrescendo pattern of breathing between respiratory events (Box F13-8) (Figure F13-7). CSB is most commonly seen in patients with congestive heart failure (systolic and diastolic) and less commonly following a stroke. The longer the ventilatory phase between central apneas, the longer is the

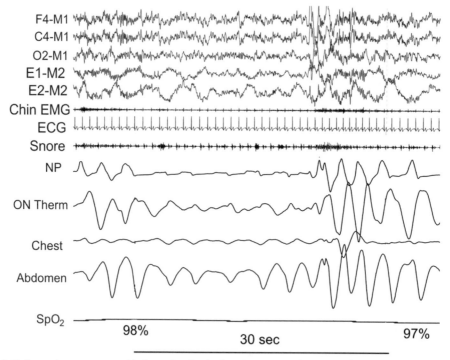

FIGURE F13-5 ■ A respiratory event with flattening in the inspiratory nasal pressure (NP) waveform followed by an arousal but no associated desaturation. This event meets AASM scoring manual recommended hypopnea criteria based on the associated arousal. The event would NOT meet the acceptable hypopnea criteria. If the acceptable hypopnea definition is used, the event meets criteria for a RERA.

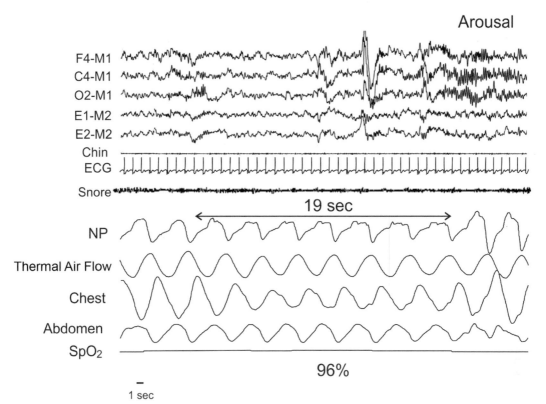

FIGURE F13-6 ■ A respiratory effort–related arousal (RERA) using either the recommended or acceptable hypopnea definition. Neither a 30% drop in nasal pressure signal or arterial oxygen desaturation is noted. Flattening of the nasal pressure (NP) signal exists, with virtually no drop in amplitude of excursions. Note the sudden transition from a flat waveform to a round one at the time of the arousal. (Adapted from Berry RB: *Fundamentals of sleep medicine,* Philadelphia, 2012, Saunders, p 126.)

BOX F13-7	Hypoventilation Definition

Monitoring hypoventilation is **optional**

If electing to score hypoventilation, score hypoventilation during sleep if EITHER of the below occur:
a. There is an increase in the arterial PCO_2 (or surrogate) to a value >55 mm Hg for ≥10 minutes.
b. There is ≥10 mm Hg increase in arterial PCO_2 (or surrogate) during sleep (in comparison to an awake supine value) to a value exceeding 50 mm Hg for ≥10 minutes.

circulation time and the lower is the cardiac output and ejection fraction. Patients with congestive heart failure (CHF) and a normal ejection fraction have a much shorter cycle time than those with systolic dysfunction, but the cycle time is usually >40 seconds. In addition each ventilatory phase in CSB is usually composed of ≥5 breaths.

AHI AND RDI

The AHI is the number of apneas and hypopneas per hour of sleep. The term *respiratory disturbance index* (RDI) is often used as another term for the AHI. However, the *AASM Scoring Manual* recommends that the RDI be used for the sum of the AHI and the RERA index (number of RERAs per hour of sleep). The centers for Medicare and Medicaid uses the term RDI for the number of apneas and hypopneas per hour of monitoring (for limited channel monitoring where sleep is not recorded). Another term, *respiratory event index* (REI), is recommended for use with limited channel monitoring. It is important to carefully determine the definition of RDI when reading publications or sleep study reports as well as the definition used for scoring hypopneas.

$$RDI = AHI + RERA\ index$$

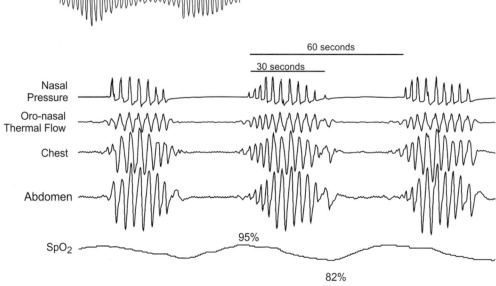

FIGURE F13-7 ■ Cheyne-Stokes breathing. Note the long ventilatory phase and cycle length (60 seconds). This patient had an ejection fraction of 20%. The nadir in the arterial oxygen saturation by pulse oximetry (SpO_2) following an event is very delayed because of the long circulation time. In the upper left hand corner, Cheyne-Stokes breathing with a central hypopnea at the nadir in breathing is illustrated. (Reproduced from Berry RB: *Fundamentals of sleep medicine*, Philadelphia, 2012, Saunders, p 133.)

| BOX F13-8 | **Cheyne-Stokes Breathing** |

Score Cheyne-Stokes breathing if BOTH of the following are met:
a. There are episodes of ≥ 3 consecutive central apneas and/or central hypopneas separated by a crescendo and decrescendo change in breathing amplitude with a cycle length of ≥ 40 seconds.
b. There are ≥ 5 central apneas and/or central hypopneas per hour of sleep associated with the crescendo/decrescendo breathing pattern recorded over ≥ 2 hours of monitoring.
Note 1: Cycle length is the time from the beginning of a central apnea to the end of the next crescendo–decrescendo respiratory phase (start of the next apnea).
Note 2: Central apneas that occur within a run of Cheyne-Stokes breathing should be scored as individual apneas as well.

REFERENCES

1. Redline S, Sander M: Hypopnea, a floating metric: implications for prevalence, morbidity estimates, and case finding, *Sleep* 20:1209–1217, 1997.
2. American Academy of Sleep Medicine Task Force: Sleep-related breathing disorders in adults: recommendations for syndrome definition and measurement techniques in clinical research. The Report of an American Academy of Sleep Medicine Task Force, *Sleep* 22:667–689, 1999.
3. Meoli AL, Casey KR, Clark RW: Clinical Practice Review Committee–AASM: Hypopnea in sleep disordered breathing in adults, *Sleep* 24:469–470, 2001.
4. Redline S, Budhiraja R, Kapur V, et al: The scoring of respiratory events in sleep: reliability and validity, *J Clin Sleep Med* 3:169–200, 2007.
5. Iber C, Ancoli-Israel S, Chesson A, Quan SF, for the American Academy of Sleep Medicine: *The AASM manual for the scoring of sleep and associated events: rules, terminology and technical specifications*, ed 1, Westchester, IL, 2007, American Academy of Sleep Medicine.
6. Berry RB, Budhiraja R, Gottlieb DJ, et al: Rules for scoring respiratory events in sleep: update of the 2007 AASM Manual for the Scoring of Sleep and Associated Events, *J Clin Sleep Med* 8(5):597–619, 2012.
7. Berry RB, Brooks R, Gamaldo CE, et al., for the American Academy of Sleep Medicine: *The AASM manual for the scoring of sleep and associated events: rules, terminology and technical specifications*, Version 2.0.3, www.aasmnet.org, Darien, IL, 2014, American Academy of Sleep Medicine.
8. Berry RB: *Fundamentals of sleep medicine*, Philadelphia, PA, 2012, Saunders.
9. Cracowski C, Pepin JL, Wuyam B, Levy P: Characterization of obstructive nonapneic respiratory events in moderate sleep apnea syndrome, *Am J Respir Crit Care Med* 164:944–948, 2001.
10. Masa JF, Corral J, Teran J, et al: Apneic and obstructive nonapnoeic sleep respiratory events, *Eur Respir J* 34:156–161, 2009.
11. Ayappa I, Norman RG, Krieger AC, et al: Non-invasive detection of respiratory effort–related arousals (RERAs) by a nasal cannula/pressure transducer system, *Sleep* 23:763–771, 2000.

Identifying Respiratory Events

QUESTIONS

1. What type of respiratory event is shown in Figure P20-1?

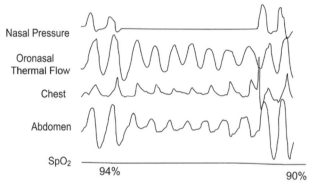

FIGURE P20-1 ■ A respiratory event.

2. What type of event is shown in Figure P20-2?

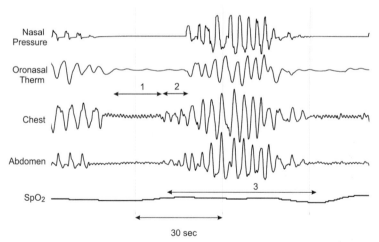

FIGURE P20-2 ■ A respiratory event. Inspiration is upward.

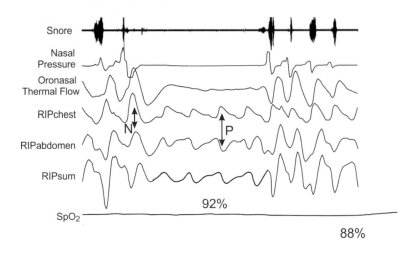

FIGURE P20-3 ■ A respiratory event. The label *N* identifies no thoracoabdominal paradox (signals are slightly out of phase), and *P* signifies paradoxical motion of the chest and abdominal belt signals.

3. In Figure P20-3, why does the oronasal thermal sensor indicate that an apnea is present, whereas the RIPsum suggests that a hypopnea is present?

ANSWERS

1. **Answer**: Hypopnea (obstructive hypopnea)

   Discussion: The *recommended sensor for apnea detection is the oronasal thermal sensor*. In Figure P20-1, the nasal pressure signal appears to show absent air flow (e.g., apnea). However, this pattern may occur with mouth breathing. The oronasal thermal signal shows reduced but not absent flow; therefore, hypopnea is scored on the basis of the drop in the nasal pressure excursions and the presence of an arterial oxygen desaturation. When scoring respiratory events, an orderly approach, focusing first on apnea and then hypopnea, can help avoid incorrectly identifying an event.

   In Figure P20-1, note the paradox in the chest and abdominal belt signals during the event. Before the event, the two signals are slightly out of phase (maximal excursions are not at the same time), but the lack of desynchrony increases during the event to frank paradoxical motion. Paradoxical movement of the chest and abdomen is often noted during obstructive apnea or hypopnea. However, while thoracoabdominal paradox during respiratory events is consistent with upper airway narrowing or closure, this finding is not always present, even if respiratory inductance plethysmography (RIP) is used to detect respiratory effort. The ability to see paradox depends on optimal placement of the effort belts and may differ between different brands of RIP belts, and may be influenced by how negative intrathoracic pressure is during obstructive events (level of respiratory effort). Effort bands should be placed at the point of maximum thoracic and abdominal contractions, respectively. Using calibrated RIP may also improve the ability to see paradox, identify when the chest and abdominal movements are out of phase, or both.

   During normal inspiration, both the chest and the abdomen expand as intrathoracic pressure becomes more negative. Paradoxical motion is characterized by chest compartment expansion and abdominal compartment contracting, or vice versa (Figure P20-4). Paradox in the chest and abdominal band signals occurs during episodes of high upper airway resistance, with chest wall muscle weakness (worse during rapid eye movement [REM] sleep), with diaphragmatic weakness, or with an immature flexible chest wall. During episodes of high upper airway resistance, the intrathoracic pressure swings may become very negative, and this may pull a weak or paralyzed diaphragm upward (abdomen sucked inward). On the other hand, a weak or unstable chest wall the chest may be sucked inward during inspiration while the abdomen expands (contraction of the diaphragm pushes abdominal contents downward). If respiratory inductance bands are calibrated, during an obstructive apnea, the chest and abdominal band excursions are exactly equal but opposite in direction, and the RIPsum (RIPchest + RIPabdomen) is zero. Recall that deflections in RIPsum are estimates of the tidal volume. In apnea tidal volume is zero and in hypopna tidal volume is reduced (Figure P20-5). Use of RIP effort belts may also detect more subtle alterations of chest and abdominal synchrony, as seen when movements are slightly out of phase (peak chest deflection is earlier than peak abdominal belt deflection, or vice versa). Obstructive events may result in out-of-phase motion of the chest and the abdomen, even if paradox is absent.

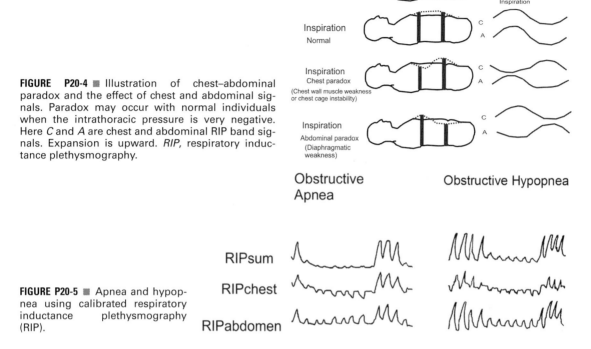

FIGURE P20-4 ■ Illustration of chest–abdominal paradox and the effect of chest and abdominal signals. Paradox may occur with normal individuals when the intrathoracic pressure is very negative. Here *C* and *A* are chest and abdominal RIP band signals. Expansion is upward. *RIP*, respiratory inductance plethysmography.

FIGURE P20-5 ■ Apnea and hypopnea using calibrated respiratory inductance plethysmography (RIP).

2. **Answer:** Mixed apnea. The delay in the saturation nadir following the event is due to a long circulation time.

   Discussion: The tracing in Figure P20-2 shows a mixed apnea with long central (1) and short obstructive (2) portions of the apnea (using oronasal thermal signal to score apnea). When the central portion is much longer than the obstructive portion, the two or three obstructed breaths may be missed and the event incorrectly scored as a central apnea. In typical mixed apnea, the obstructive portion is equal to or longer than the central portion. However, the central portion of mixed apnea may be longer, especially in a patient with underlying Cheyne-Stokes breathing. Note the crescendo–decrescendo pattern of respiration between apneas. The oximetry tracing also provided an important clue that heart failure is present. Note the long delay in the nadir of the saturation of peripheral oxygen (SpO_2) (3), which is 50 seconds following the cessation of apnea. This is caused by a long circulation time.

   In the typical patients with obstructive sleep apnea, who manifest some mixed apneas, the central portion is typically short. The initial central apnea occurs because the PCO_2 is below the apneic threshold and respiratory effort ceases. The low PCO_2 is caused by the preceding increased ventilation following an arousal or preceding respiratory event that "overshoots" blowing the PCO_2 below a level that triggers ventilation during sleep (apneic threshold). This type of mixed apnea usually resolves on positive airway pressure (PAP) treatment. The patient in Figure P20-2 developed Cheyne-Stokes central apnea when place on PAP (upper airway obstruction eliminated) because of the underling central sleep apnea disorder (ventilatory control instability).

3. **Answer:** Use of uncalibrated RIP

   Discussion: The RIPsum (sum of chest and abdominal RIP band signals) may be used as an alternative sensor for scoring apnea and hypopnea when the recommended sensor is not functioning. When using calibrated RIP, the deflections in the RIPsum are an estimate of the tidal volume. When using uncalibrated RIP, the deflections in the RIPsum signal, when compared with baseline breathing, can be used to detect apnea (nearly absent deflections, e.g., tidal volume=0) or hypopnea (reduced tidal volume). With the use of calibrated RIP, during apnea, the chest and abdominal signals cancel each other exactly (see Figure P20-5). With the use of uncalibrated RIP, the signals may not cancel each other exactly. An event believed to be an apnea with the use of an oronasal thermal sensor could be a hypopnea with RIPsum. For this reason, the oronasal thermal sensor is the recommended sensor for scoring apnea. However, if the oronasal thermal sensor is not functioning, the RIPsum may be used to detect apnea. It is possible that some events that are actually apneas will be scored as hypopneas using the RIPsum (if the event in question is associated with an oxygen desaturation or arousal). The RIPflow is the time derivative of the RIPsum signal and is an estimate of air flow (see Fundamentals 12) and may also be used as an apnea alternative sensor.

CLINICAL PEARLS

1. Use the oronasal thermal sensor signal to score apnea. If this signal is not functioning, the nasal pressure, RIPsum, or RIPflow signals may be used. The nasal pressure signal may falsely indicate apnea when mouth breathing is occurring. When using uncalibrated RIP, the RIPsum or RIPflow signal deflections may not be reduced to 90% of baseline during apnea. Misclassification of apnea as a hypopnea, and vice versa, has little clinical significance if the event in question is associated with an arterial oxygen desaturation or an arousal (may be scored as a hypopnea). Apneas and hypopneas are summed to determine the apnea+hypopnea index.

2. Paradoxical movement of the chest and abdomen is often noted during obstructive apnea or hypopnea. However, paradox may not always be seen even when using RIP effort belts. Proper effort belt placement improves the ability to see paradox. In addition, rather than paradox, the two signal deflections may simply be increasingly out of phase during an obstructive event.

3. If the central portion of a mixed apnea is much longer than the obstructive portion, it may be easy to miss the two or three obstructive breaths at the end of the event. This type of mixed apnea is commonly seen in patients who have both obstructive sleep apnea and underlying Cheyne-Stokes central apnea.

4. A delay in the nadir the oximetry tracing following a respiratory event is a clue that a long circulation time may be present (low cardiac output).

BIBLIOGRAPHY

1. Berry RB, Budhiraja R, Gottlieb DJ, et al: Rules for scoring respiratory events in sleep: update of the 2007 AASM Manual for the Scoring of Sleep and Associated Events, *J Clin Sleep Med* 8(5):597–619, 2012.
2. Dempsey JA: Crossing the apnoeic threshold: causes and consequences, *Exp Physiol* 90(1):13–24, 2005.
3. Farré R, Montserrat JM, Navajas D: Noninvasive monitoring of respiratory mechanics during sleep, *Eur Respir J* 24:1052–1060, 2004.
4. Iber C, Davies SF, Chapman RC, Mahowald MM: A possible mechanism for mixed apnea in obstructive sleep apnea, *Chest* 89 (6):800–805, 1986.
5. Staats BA, Bonekat HW, Harris CD, Offord KP: Chest wall motion in sleep apnea, *Am Rev Respir Dis* 130:59–63, 1984.

PATIENT 21

Two Patients with Possible Central Apnea

QUESTIONS

1. A patient with loud snoring was studied with polysomnography (PSG). In Figure P21-1, an apnea was noted. The patient had predominantly obstructive apnea, but this event was scored as a central apnea. Do you agree?

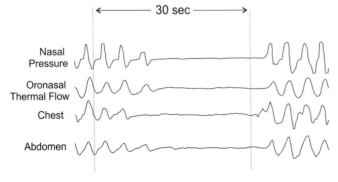

FIGURE P21-1 ■ Is this central or obstructive apnea?

2. Small deflections in the nasal pressure and chest and abdominal belts (respiratory inductance plethysmography [RIP]) were noted (Figure P21-2). Is this a central apnea?

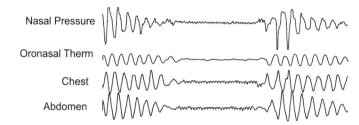

Nasal Pressure
Oronasal Therm
Chest
Abdomen

FIGURE P21-2 ■ Is this a central apnea?

ANSWERS

1. **Answers:** An obstructive apnea is present.

Discussion: The event depicted in Figure P21-1 is actually an obstructive apnea, even though minimal deflection in the chest and abdominal channels are noted. In patients with consecutive apneas, the respiratory effort between events is often composed of very large excursions in the chest wall and abdominal tracings. Often, an auto-scale gain feature is used to keep the chest and abdominal tracings within the channel width (avoiding overlap into adjacent channels). However, the reduction in gain to achieve this purpose may result in very small amplitude deflections in the chest and abdominal effort channels during the respiratory event, suggesting that a central apnea is present. If one increases the gain, it is often possible to determine that persistent effort is occurring (Figure P21-3).

Misclassifying obstructive events as central is more likely if the chest and abdominal effort belts are not tightened snuggly and are not placed in positions of maximum movement during respiration. The optimal position of the effort belts may vary between patients. The most sensitive method of detecting respiratory effort is esophageal manometry. However, this method is rarely used in clinical studies. RIP is the recommended method in adults and children to detect respiratory effort using thoracoabdominal movement (in adults using polyvinylidene fluoride belts is acceptable). However, even when calibrated, RIP may falsely classify events as being central, as it may not detect feeble respiratory effort in up to 9% patients.[1] It should be noted that thoracoabdominal excursions often decrease during obstructive events and may not accurately reflect the level of inspiratory effort (Figure P21-4, *A*). During upper airway narrowing, paradoxical motion of the chest and abdominal effort belts may occur, but this is not invariably present. During obstructive hypopnea, the small deflections in the effort belts simply reflect the fact that modest changes have occurred in chest or abdominal volume because of the small tidal volume. It should be noted that even esophageal pressure deflections often

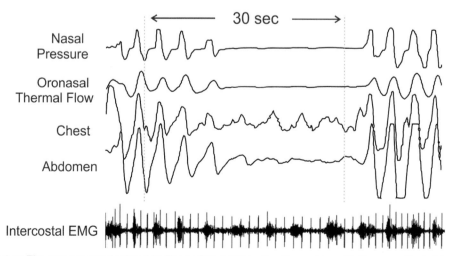

30 sec

Nasal Pressure
Oronasal Thermal Flow
Chest
Abdomen
Intercostal EMG

FIGURE P21-3 ■ The same event depicted in Figure P21-1. When the channel sensitivity was adjusted to maximize chest and abdominal deflections, this resulted in obvious excursions during the apnea (an obstructive apnea). This is confirmed by inspiratory burst in the intercostal electromyography (EMG) channel.

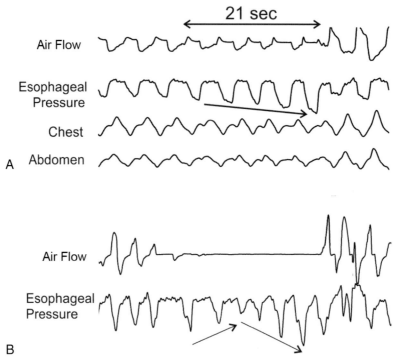

FIGURE P21-4 ■ **Panel A,** There is a fall in chest and abdominal excursions (RIPbands) during an obstructive hypopnea while respiratory effort actually increases (*arrow*). **Panel B,** Respiratory effort during the obstructive apnea falls during the initial portion of the event and then increases until event termination. In both **A** and **B,** inspiration is upward.

decrease during the initial part of obstructive events (see Figure P21-4, *B*) with falling ventilatory drive but then increases until event termination. If ventilatory drive totally ceases in the initial part of an obstructive event, then a mixed apnea occurs. Falling ventilatory drive at the start of obstructive apnea may be caused by hypocapnia (following large breaths following a previous apnea) as well as transition from wakefulness to sleep.

It is possible to record the activity of intercostal muscles (external intercostal is inspiratory) using the same electromyography (EMG) technique as for leg or chin EMG (see Figure P21-3).[2] Usually, two electrodes are placed in the 7th or 8th intercostal space in the right axillary line (right side to minimize electrocardiography [ECG] artifact). In this position, they may also pick up some diaphragmatic activity, as this muscle attaches to the chest wall at that location. As seen in Figure P23-3, definite inspiratory bursts in the intercostal EMG are noted during the apnea confirming that it is obstructive. The current *AASM Scoring Manual*[3] does not list use of intercostal EMG as an acceptable method for monitoring respiratory effort because of the paucity of published studies. However, in some sleep centers, it is used routinely for clinical studies as an adjunct to other methods of monitoring respiratory effort.

2. **Answer:** A central apnea is present with cardioballistic artifact in the chest and abdominal effort tracings.

Discussion: Small deflections in the chest and abdominal effort tracings (see Figure P21-2) may be prominent during central apnea and reflect movement of the chest or abdomen associated with cardiac pulsations. The oscillations do not reflect respiratory effort, and the event in Figure P21-2 is a central apnea. It is often stated that detection of cardiac pulsations in the nasal pressure Figure P21-2 or PAP flow signal is evidence for an open upper airway.[4] Of interest, during central apneas the upper airway may close in up to 20% of central events.[5] However, some studies in animals have demonstrated cardiac associated deflections in the air flow signal, even if the upper airway is closed during central apnea.[6] On the other hand, during obstructive apnea (closed airway and inspiratory effort present), cardiac oscillations in the air flow are almost never seen. Thus, the presence of oscillations suggests that central apnea is present but whether or not this means the upper airway is open remains somewhat controversial.

CLINICAL PEARLS
1. Adjustment of chest and abdominal effort channel sensitivity to increase deflections may be necessary to avoid misclassifying obstructive apneas as central apneas. Even with calibrated RIP belts, some apneas may be misclassified as being central in nature.
2. Small deflections in the chest and abdominal effort channels with spacing approximating the ECG R–R interval are not caused by respiratory effort but reflect movement of the chest and abdomen from cardiac pulsations.
3. Thoracoabdominal excursions tend to decrease during obstructive respiratory events and may not accurately reflect the fact that respiratory effort is high or increasing.
4. If cardiac pulsations are noted in the nasal pressure or PAP flow during an apnea, this suggests that the apnea is central. Some studies suggest that the upper airway is open in such a circumstance (open airway central apnea), but this remains somewhat controversial.
5. Intercostal or diaphragmatic EMG may be used an adjunctive method to document respiratory effort.

REFERENCES

1. Staats BA, Bonekat HW, Harris CD, Offord KP: Chest wall motion in sleep apnea, *Am Rev Respir Dis* 130:59–63, 1984.
2. Stoohs RA, Blum HC, Knaack L, et al: Comparison of pleural pressure and transcutaneous diaphragmatic electromyogram in obstructive sleep apnea syndrome, *Sleep* 28:321–329.
3. Berry RB, Brooks R, Gamaldo CE, et al., for the American Academy of Sleep Medicine: *The AASM manual for the scoring of sleep and associated events: rules, terminology and technical specifications*, Version 2.0.3, www.aasmnet.org, Darien, Illinois, 2014, American Academy of Sleep Medicine.
4. Ayappa I, Norman RG, Rapoport DM: Cardiogenic oscillations on the airflow signal during continuous positive airway pressure as a marker of central apnea, *Chest* 116:660–666, 1999.
5. Badr SM, Toiber F, Skatrud JB, Dempsey J: Pharyngeal narrowing/occlusion during central apnea, *J Appl Physiol* 78:1806–1815, 1995.
6. Morrell MJ, Badr MS, Harms CA, Dempsey JA: The assessment of upper airway patency during apnea using cardiogenic oscillations in the airflow signal, *Sleep* 18(8):651–658, 1995.

PATIENT 22

Why is the Arterial Oxygen Desaturation Severe?

A 50-year-old man with very loud snoring underwent sleep testing. When awake and supine, his arterial oxygen saturation by pulse oximetry (SpO_2) was 94%. A summary of the respiratory events from the sleep study is displayed in Table P22-1. The tracing in Figure P22-1 was done while the patient was in the supine position. His body mass index (BMI) is 35 kilograms per meter squared (kg/m^2).

TABLE P22-1 Summary of Respiratory Events

Totals sleep time (minutes)	360 minutes	Desaturations	260 (no.)
REM sleep (minutes)	90 minutes	Low SpO_2 NREM	80 %
		Low SpO_2 REM	60 %
Obstructive apneas (number [no.])	57	Time ≤88%	60 minutes
Central apneas (no.)	1	—	
Mixed apneas (no.)	2		
Hypopneas (no.)	200		
AHI (no./hour)	43.3		
AHI NREM (no./hour)	34		
AHI REM (no./hour)	70		

AHI, Apnea–hypopnea index; *NREM*, non–rapid eye movement; *REM*, rapid eye movement; *SpO₂*, arterial oxygen saturation by pulse oximetry.

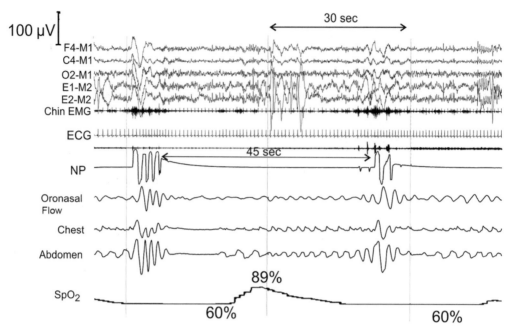

FIGURE P22-1 ■ A tracing showing a mixed apnea while the patient is sleeping **supine**. Oronasal flow is measured by a thermal sensor and the chest and abdomen effort belts use respiratory inductance plethysmography (RIP). The SpO_2 is measured by pulse oximetry. *NP*, Nasal pressure.

QUESTION

1. Name four factors that would explain the severe desaturation noted in the tracing for this patient. What are other factors that could worsen desaturation in other patients?

ANSWER

1. **Answers:** In this patient: Stage R, supine position, obesity, long respiratory event, and only a few breaths between respiratory events. An additional factor in other patients is a low awake SpO_2.

   Discussion: A number of factors may worsen the severity of arterial oxygen desaturation in patients with obstructive sleep apnea (OSA) (Table P22-2).[1-3] Patients with a higher BMI desaturate more severely, and the effect of obesity is accentuated during rapid eye movement (REM) sleep, in the supine position, and in men more than in women.[3] A low baseline SpO_2 (partial pressure of arterial oxygen [PaO_2]) is also a factor. The primary reason is that a given fall in PaO_2 is associated with a greater fall in the SaO_2 the awake SaO_2 is on the steep part of the oxyhemoglobin saturation curve. Long respiratory events with only a few breaths between back-to-back events also worsens the desaturation. The expiratory reserve volume is the difference between the functional residual capacity (end-expiratory lung volume) and the residual volume (lung volume at maximum exhalation). A low FRC means that oxygen stores are lower at the time of the breath-hold.[4] In addition, breathing at low lung volumes causes increased ventilation perfusion mismatch as some airway are closed during tidal volume breathing. Obesity tends to lower the functional residual capacity (FRC; especially compared with the residual volume [RV]). In pulmonary function testing, the most common finding in obesity is a low expiratory reserve volume (ERV) mainly because of a fall in the FRC. A high RV may occur with air trapping caused by chronic lung disease. Patients with both OSA and chronic obstructive pulmonary disease (COPD) tend to have severe desaturation, especially if they have a low awake SpO_2. The supine posture is associated with worse oxygen desaturation in OSA even when the drop in oxygen is adjusted for event duration.[5]

TABLE P22-2 **Factors Worsening Arterial Oxygen Desaturation**

- Higher BMI
  - More effect during REM than during NREM sleep
  - More effect during supine than lateral sleep
  - More effect on men than in women.
- Lower baseline awake supine PaO_2 or SaO_2
- Lower ERV = (FRC – RV).
  - Low FRC—obesity
  - High RV—obstructive airways disease (COPD)
- Longer event duration
- Greater change in V_T (hypopnea)
- Short ventilatory period between apnea
- REM sleep versus NREM sleep (REM events are also longer)
- Supine versus lateral position

BMI, Body mass index; *COPD*, chronic obstructive pulmonary disease; *ERV*, expiratory reserve volume; *FRC*, functional residual capacity; *NREM*, non–rapid eye movement; *PaO₂*, arterial partial pressure of oxygen; *REM*, rapid eye movement; *RV*, residual volume; *SaO₂*, arterial oxygen saturation; *V_T*, tidal volume.

REM sleep has several important consequences in patients with OSA. First, the apnea–hypopnea index (AHI) is usually higher during REM sleep. The respiratory events tend to be longer, and the arterial oxygen desaturation more severe.[6] An exception is when patients have most REM sleep in the lateral position. An interaction occurs between body position and REM sleep as far as the severity of arterial oxygen desaturation.[7] The circumstance most likely to be associated with worsened desaturation is supine REM sleep.

In the current patient, the tracing shows a long mixed apnea during REM sleep; note the REMs in the electrooculography (EOG) channels. Very few breaths occur between respiratory events. The patient is also quite obese and sleeping in the supine position. On the positive side, his awake SpO_2 of 94% was not significantly decreased.

CLINICAL PEARLS

1. Both the AHI and the severity of arterial oxygen desaturation should be considered when the severity of sleep apnea is assessed. A patient may have a high AHI but relatively mild arterial oxygen desaturation. On the other hand, a patient may have only a moderate increase in the AHI but very severe desaturation (often during REM sleep).

2. Factors worsening the severity of desaturation include a low baseline awake SpO_2, obesity, supine posture, REM sleep, long respiratory events with short respiration between events, and a low ERV.

3. REM sleep is usually associated with the highest AHI, the longest respiratory events, and the most severe desaturation.

4. There is an interaction between body position and REM versus NREM sleep. In general AHI-REM-supine> AHI-NREM-supine>AHI-REM-non-supine> AHI-NREM-non-supine. The severity of arterial oxygen desaturation is usually greater in supine REM sleep than nonsupine REM sleep.

REFERENCES

1. Bradley TD, Martinez D, Rutherford R, et al: Physiological determinants of nocturnal arterial oxygenation in patients with obstructive sleep apnea, *J Appl Physiol* 59:1364–1368, 1985.
2. Series F, Cormier Y, La Forge J: Influence of apnea type and sleep stage on nocturnal postapneic desaturation, *Am Rev Respir Dis* 141:1522–1526, 1990.
3. Peppard PE, Ward NR, Morrell MJ: The impact of obesity on oxygen desaturation during sleep disordered breathing, *Am J Respir Crit Care Med* 180:788–793, 2009.
4. Findley LJ, Ries AL, Tisi GM, Wagner PD: Hypoxemia during apnea in normal subjects: mechanisms and impact of lung volume, *J Appl Physiol* 55:1777–1783, 1983.
5. Oksenberg A, Khamaysi I, Silverberg DS, Tarasiuk A: Association of body position with severity of apneic events in patients with severe nonpositional obstructive sleep apnea, *Chest* 118:1018–1024, 2000.
6. Findley LJ, Wihoit SC, Surrat PM: Apnea duration and hypoxemia during REM sleep in patients with obstructive sleep apnea, *Chest* 87:432–436, 1985.
7. Oksenberg A, Arons E, Nasser K, et al: REM-related obstructive sleep apnea: the effect of body position, *J Clin Sleep Med* 6(4):343–348, 2010.

FUNDAMENTALS 14

Respiratory Events in Children

The *American Academy of Sleep Medicine (AASM) Scoring Manual* published definitions for respiratory events in children in 2007.[1] The scoring manual was updated in 2012[2,3] and now is updated once or twice a year. The reader should check the latest version for changes in the rules discussed in this chapter. The pediatric scoring rules differ from adult rules in several important aspects. If an adult is breathing at 12 beats per minute (beats/min), a minimum apnea duration of 10 seconds corresponds to two breaths (5 seconds per breath). As children may breathe at considerably faster rates compared with adults, event duration criteria are based on the duration of two breaths during baseline breathing rather than the absolute duration of 10 seconds. This minimum duration is used for obstructive and mixed apneas and hypopneas. As discussed below, central apneas are scored differently in children than in adults, as central apneas frequency occur after sigh breaths in normal children and likely have no clinical significance unless prolonged or followed by an arousal or arterial oxygen desaturation.

AGES FOR WHICH PEDIATRIC RESPIRATORY SCORING RULES APPLY

Criteria for respiratory events during sleep for infants and children may be used for children under 18 years, and an individual sleep specialist may choose to score children 13 years or older using adult criteria.

Several studies[4,5] suggest that the apnea–hypopnea index (AHI) will be higher in adolescent patients when using pediatric rules compared with the adult rules presented in the 2007 version of the *AASM Scoring Manual*. The adult rules required desaturation to score a hypopnea, whereas the rules for children allowed scoring of hypopneas based on an associated arousal. As the current recommended adult and pediatric hypopnea rules are similar except for the duration of the event, less difference may now exist in the AHI when using adult versus pediatric rules.

PEDIATRIC APNEA RULE[2]

Score a respiratory event as an apnea if it meets ALL of the following criteria:
1. A drop occurs in the peak signal excursion by ≥90% of the pre-event baseline using an oronasal thermal sensor (diagnostic study), positive airway pressure (PAP) device flow (titration study), or an alternative apnea sensor (diagnostic study).
2. The duration of the ≥90% drop lasts at least the minimum duration, as specified by obstructive, mixed, or central apnea duration criteria.
3. The event meets respiratory effort criteria for obstructive, central, or mixed apnea.

Obstructive Apnea Rule[2]

Score a respiratory event as **obstructive apnea** if it meets apnea criteria for at least the duration of two breaths during baseline breathing **AND** is associated with the presence of respiratory effort through the entire period of absent air flow.

In Figure F14-1 a short obstructive apnea is noted lasting only two breaths (two inspiratory efforts). Even though the duration is short, a desaturation is noted.

Mixed Apnea Rule[2]

Score a respiratory event as **mixed apnea** (Figure F14-2) if it meets apnea criteria for at least the duration of two breaths during baseline breathing, is associated with absent respiratory effort during one portion of the event, AND inspiratory effort is present in another portion, *regardless of which portion comes first*.

Central Apnea Rule[2]

Score a respiratory event as **central apnea** (Figure F14-3) if it meets apnea criteria, is associated with absent inspiratory effort through the

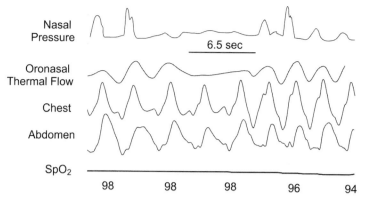

FIGURE F14-1 ■ Obstructive apnea in a 4-year-old child. The oronasal air flow signal shows absent air flow for 6.5 seconds or the duration of two inspiratory efforts. Even though the event is short, a fall in saturation of peripheral oxygen (SpO$_2$) still occurs. The child did not arouse at the end of the event.

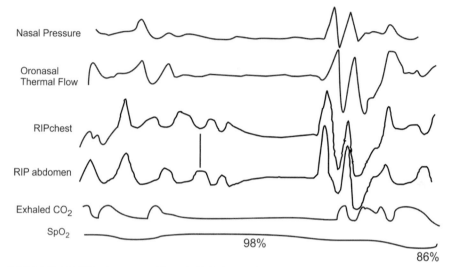

FIGURE F14-2 ■ Mixed apnea with an initial obstructive portion followed by central portion. (Image courtesy of Dr. Carole Marcus.)

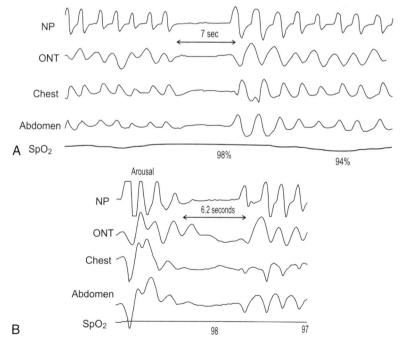

FIGURE F14-3 ■ Two central pauses in breathing. **A,** This event meets criteria for central apnea based on the associated arterial oxygen desaturation. **B,** This central pause in breathing occurs following an arousal and is not followed by either an arousal or arterial oxygen desaturation and is not 20 seconds or more in duration. The event is not scored as a central apnea.

entire duration of the event, AND at least one of the following criteria is met:

1. The event lasts 20 seconds or longer.
2. The event lasts at least the duration of two breaths during baseline breathing and is associated with an arousal or $\geq 3\%$ oxygen desaturation.
3. In infants younger than 1 year of age, the event lasts at least the duration of two breaths during baseline breathing and is associated with a decrease in heart rate to less than 50 beats/min for at least 5 seconds or less than 60 beats/min for 15 seconds.

PEDIATRIC HYPOPNEA RULE[2]

Score a respiratory event as **hypopnea** if it meets ALL of the following criteria:

1. The peak signal excursions drop by $\geq 30\%$ of pre-events baseline using nasal pressure (diagnostic study), PAP device flow (titration study), or an *alternative* hypopnea sensor (diagnostic study).
2. The duration of the $\geq 30\%$ drop in signal excursion lasts for ≥ 2 breaths.
3. Oxygen desaturation is $\geq 3\%$ from pre-event baseline, or the event is associated with an arousal.

The scoring of hypopneas as central or obstructive events is optional as noted in Parameters to be Reported in the *AASM Scoring Manual*.[2]

Obstructive Hypopnea Rule[2]

Score hypopnea as **obstructive** if ANY of the following criteria are met:

1. Snoring during the event.
2. Increased inspiratory flattening of the nasal pressure or PAP device flow signal compared with baseline breathing.
3. Associated thoracoabdominal paradox occurs during the event but not during pre-event breathing.

Central Hypopnea Rule[2]

The *AASM Scoring Manual* states that the scoring hypopneas as central or obstructive events is optional.[2]

Score hypopnea as **central** if NONE of the following criteria is met:

1. Snoring during the event.
2. Increased inspiratory flattening of the nasal pressure or PAP device flow signal compared with baseline breathing.
3. Associated thoracoabdominal paradox occurs during the event but not during pre-event breathing.

PEDIATRIC RERA RULE[2]

Scoring respiratory effort–related arousals (RERAs) is **optional** as noted in parameters to be reported in the *AASM Scoring Manual*.[2]

Score a respiratory event as an RERA if a sequence of breaths last ≥ 2 breaths (or the duration of two breaths during baseline breathing) when the breathing sequence is characterized by increasing respiratory effort, flattening of the inspiratory portion of the nasal pressure (diagnostic study), or PAP device flow (titration study) waveform, snoring, *or an elevation in the end-tidal PCO_2 (partial pressure of carbon dioxide)* leading to arousal from sleep when the sequence of breaths does not meet criteria for apnea or hypopnea.

PEDIATRIC HYPOVENTILATION RULE[2]

Monitoring hypoventilation in children is **recommended** during a diagnostic study and **optional** during a PAP titration study.[2]

Score hypoventilation during sleep when >25% of the total sleep time (TST), as measured by either the arterial PCO_2 or surrogate, is spent with a PCO_2 >50 millimeters of mercury (mm Hg).

Surrogates include end-tidal PCO_2 or transcutaneous PCO_2 during the diagnostic study or transcutaneous PCO_2 during a titration study. This scoring rule is based on data in normal children that shows only 2.2% of children demonstrated end-tidal CO_2 >50 mm Hg for >50% of TST.[6]

PERIODIC BREATHING RULE

Score a respiratory event as **periodic breathing** if ≥ 3 episodes of central apnea last >3 seconds separated by ≤ 20 seconds of normal breathing[2] (Figure F14-4).

Of note, central pauses in breathing that occur within a run of periodic breathing should be scored as individual apneas as well (if they meet criteria for central apnea). Of note, periodic breathing is normal in premature infants and is also noted in variable amounts in full-term infants, with a decrease in frequency during the first year of life. One study showed periodic breathing in 38.6% of normal infants through age 9 months.[7] Normal values for the extent of periodic breathing are not yet established across age groups.

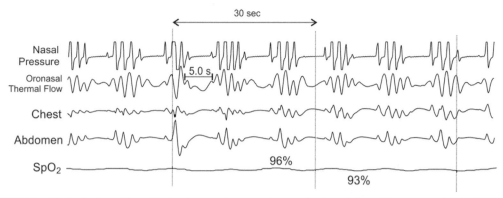

FIGURE F14-4 ■ Periodic breathing. Cycle of central pauses in respiration airflow. The pauses in respiratory are scored as central apneas if they meet the criteria for scoring central apnea follow by respiration less than or equal to 20 seconds in duration.

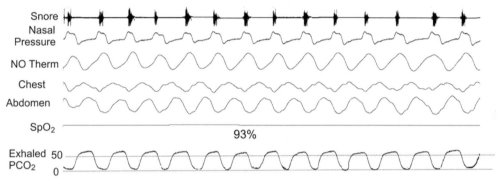

FIGURE F14-5 ■ An example of a pattern of obstructive hypoventilation. In this patient the partial pressure of carbon dioxide (PCO_2) was >50 mm Hg for 40% of the total sleep time.

OBSTRUCTIVE HYPOVENTILATION

In children, episodes of prolonged loud snoring, air flow limitation, or both may occur in association with only mild drops in the saturation of peripheral oxygen (SpO_2). If capnography is performed there is an increase in the end-tidal PCO_2 above that during baseline breathing. The *AASM Scoring Manual* does not provide criteria for the diagnosis of obstructive hypoventilation as a discrete event, but the cumulative increase in PCO_2 may qualify for a diagnosis of hypoventilation.

RESPIRATORY PARAMETERS REPORTED IN PEDIATRIC POLYSOMNOGRAPHY

1. AH = number of apnea + number of hypopneas
2. AHI = number of apneas and hypopneas per hour of sleep: $60 \times AH \div TST$ in minutes

3. AHI during supine and nonsupine sleep
4. AHI non–rapid eye movement (NREM) and AHI REM
5. OD = Number of arterial oxygen desaturations; low SpO_2
6. Oxygen desaturation index (ODI) = (OD X 60)/TST in minutes
7. RERA = number of RERAs, RERA index, RERAs per hour
8. Obstructive AHI (OAHI) = number of obstructive and mixed apneas + hypopneas per hour
9. Maximum end-tidal PCO_2 and time spent with a $P_{ET}CO_2$ >50 mm Hg (absolute time or as %TST)

REFERENCES

1. Iber C, Ancoli-Israel S, Chesson A, et al for the American Academy of Sleep Medicine: *The AASM manual for scoring of sleep and associated events: rules, terminology and technical specifications*, Westchester, Illinois, 2007, American Academy of Sleep Medicine.
2. Berry RB, Brooks R, Gamaldo CE, et al for the American Academy of Sleep Medicine. *The AASM manual for the scoring of sleep and associated events: rules, terminology and technical specifications*, Version 2.0.3, www.aasmnet.org, Darien, Illinois, 2014, American Academy of Sleep Medicine.

3. Berry RB, Budhiraja R, Gottlieb DJ, et al: Rules for scoring respiratory events in sleep: update of the 2007 AASM manual for the scoring of sleep and associated events, *J Clin Sleep Med* 8(5):597–619, 2012.
4. Tapia IE, Karamessinis L, Bandla P, et al: Polysomnographic values in children undergoing puberty: pediatric vs. adult respiratory rules in adolescents, *Sleep* 31:1737–1744, 2008.
5. Accardo JA, Shults J, Leonard MB, et al: Differences in overnight polysomnography scores using the adult and pediatric criteria for respiratory events in adolescents, *Sleep* 33:1333–1339, 2010.
6. Montgomery-Downs HE, O'Brien LM, Gulliver TE, Gozal D: Polysomnographic characteristics in normal preschool and early school-aged children, *Pediatrics* 117:741–753, 2006.
7. Horemuzova E, Katz-Salamon M, Milerad J: Breathing patterns, oxygen and carbon dioxide levels in sleeping healthy infants during the first nine months after birth, *Acta Paediatr* 89(11):1284–1289, 2000.

PATIENT 23

Sickle Disease and an Unexplained Low Arterial Oxygen Saturation

A 12-year-old African American female with known sickle cell disease is monitored for suspected sleep apnea.

- Physical examination: Bilaterally enlarged tonsils
- Laboratory study: hematocrit 26%
- Summary of sleep study results: apnea–hypopnea index (AHI): 14.2 events per hour with 2 obstructive apneas, 2 central apneas, 87 hypopneas, and a minimal arterial oxygen saturation (SaO_2) of 80%

The 30-second tracing shown in Figure P23-1 was typical for non–rapid eye movement (NREM) sleep.

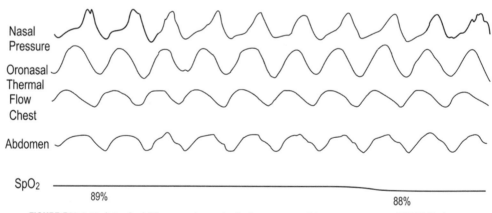

FIGURE P23-1 ■ A typical 30-second epoch during non–rapid eye movement (NREM) sleep.

QUESTION

1. What is the etiology of the low SpO_2 (arterial oxygen saturation by pulse oximetry) during apparently stable breathing?

ANSWER

1. **Answer:** An abnormal oxygen hemoglobin dissociation curve.

   Discussion: The SaO_2 is measured noninvasively during sleep studies by pulse oximetry (SpO_2) to detect arterial oxygen desaturation and hypoxemia. The SaO_2 is usually defined as the amount of oxyhemoglobin (O_2Hb) divided by the sum of the O_2Hb and the deoxygenated or reduced hemoglobin (RHb) (see Equation P23-1).

   $$SaO_2\% = (O_2Hb) \times 100/(O_2Hb + RHb) \qquad \text{(Equation P23-1)}$$

   The relationship between SaO_2 and PaO_2 is given by the oxygen–hemoglobin dissociation curve. The usual position of the curve for hemoglobin A (HbA) and the factors that shift the curve right and left are illustrated in the left panel of Figure P23-2 and Table P23-1. Decreased body temperature, low hydrogen ion concentration (high pH), low 2,3 diphosphoglyceric acid (DPG), and low $PaCO_2$ shift the curve to the left. High body temperature, high hydrogen ion concentration (low pH), increased 2,3 DPG, and high $PaCO_2$ shift the curve to the right.

   The oxygen hemoglobin dissociation curve for sickle hemoglobin (HbS) is shifted to the right, and a higher PaO_2 is present for a given SaO_2. In the current patient, an arterial blood gas was obtained at the end of the study while the patient was awake and breathing room air. The values were a pH of 7.44, a $PaCO_2$ of 37 mm Hg, a PaO_2 of 90 mm Hg, and bicarbonate (HCO_3) of

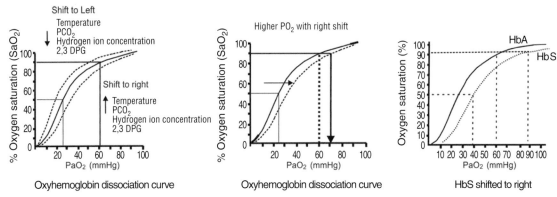

FIGURE P23-2 ■ **Left panel,** The normal oxygen hemoglobin dissociation curve and factors that shift the curve. **Middle panel,** If the curve is shifted to the right the PaO_2 for a given SaO_2 is increased. **Right panel,** The curve for hemoglobin S (HbS) is shifted to the right. The oxygen hemoglobin dissociation curve showing the values for hemoglobin (Hb) A (*solid line*) and a patient with Hb S (*dashed line*). For the patient with Hb S, the P50 is 38 mm Hg, and an SaO_2 value of 92% corresponds to a PO_2 of approximately 90 mm Hg. Adapted from Berry RB: Fundamentals of sleep medicine, p 143.

TABLE P23-1	Approximate PaO₂ Corresponding to SaO₂	
	Hb A	**Hb S**
SaO₂ (%)	PaO₂ (mm Hg)	PaO₂ (mm Hg)
50	27	38
75	40	50
90	60	87

Note: Assuming normal body temperature and pH.

25.3 millimoles per liter (mmol/L). The SpO_2 measurement at same time was 92%. Thus, the PaO_2 during NREM sleep was likely normal in this patient. Of note, patients with sickle cell disease may have some HbA if they have recently been transfused.

Pulse Oximetry

Pulse oximetry provides an estimate of the SaO_2 (SpO_2) by determining the absorption of two wavelengths of light (660 nanometers [nm] [red] and 940 nm [infrared]) by hemoglobin (Hb) in capillary blood. This determines the relative amount of the O_2Hb (oxygenated Hb) and RHb (reduced or deoxygenated Hb). The absorption of radiation at 660 nm is much greater with RHb than with O_2Hb, while O_2Hb absorbs slightly more radiation at 940 nm (Figure P23-3, *A*). The ability of SpO_2 to determine the SaO_2 is based on the empirical observation that the ratio (R) of the absorbance of light at the two wavelengths is related to the SaO_2 (see Figure P23-3, *B*). This relationship (calibration curve) is determined experimentally by determining R at varying SaO_2 for each oximetry performed. To specifically determine the absorbance of arterial blood, the alternating current (AC) (pulse-added absorbance) at each wavelength is divided by the direct current (DC) (background absorbance) to account for the effect of the absorption of the radiation by venous blood and tissue. SpO_2 is accurate down to about 70%. Whereas values below 70% are often reported, it is important to keep in the mind that they probably do not correspond accurately to the actual SaO_2. If carboxyhemoglobin (COHb) is present, this causes the SpO_2 measurement to overestimate HbO_2 as absorption of COHb for 660 nm is similar to O_2Hb. However, the major effect is decreasing the amount of Hb that can bind oxygen. This will be discussed below. If methemoglobin (MetHb) is present, the SpO_2 moves toward 85% (R = 1) as the absorption of the two wavelengths is similar for MetHb.

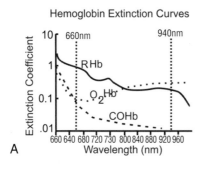
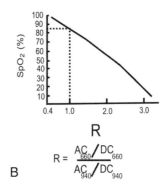

FIGURE P23-3 ■ **A,** Hemoglobin extinction curves for reduced hemoglobin (RHb), oxyhemoglobin (O_2Hb), and carboxyhemoglobin (COHb) at different wavelengths of light. Note that the y-axis is a log scale. **B,** Empirical curve of the ratio of absorption of radiation at wavelengths of 660 and 940 nm. AC = the pulse added absorption; DC = the steady state or background absorbance. Note at R = 1, the arterial oxygen saturation (SpO_2) is 85%. (**A** and **B,** Adapted from Tremper KK, Barker SJ: Pulse oximetry, *Anesthesiology* 70:108-109, 1989.)

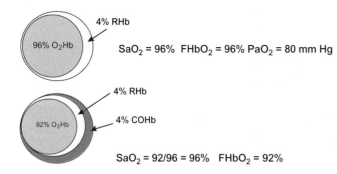

SaO_2 oxyhemoglobin as a fraction of hemoglobin available for binding

$FHbO_2$ oxyhemoglobin as a fraction of total hemoglobin

FIGURE P23-4 ■ Illustration of the difference between the SaO_2 and the FO_2Hb. The PaO_2 is 80 mm Hg and the SaO_2 96%. For simplicity the graph assumes that COHb does not shift the oxygen-hemoglobin association curve. HbCO actually causes a leftward shift of the oxygen hemoglobin dissociation curve (Higher SaO_2 for a given PaO_2, e.g., for $PO_2 = 80$; $SaO_2 = 96.3\%$).

FO$_2$Hb versus SaO$_2$

The majority of the oxygen-carrying capacity of the blood is from oxygen bound to Hb with a small fraction of dissolved oxygen (see Equation P23-2). When fully saturated, a gram of Hb carries about 1.34 milliliters per deciliter (mL/dL) of oxygen (1 dL = 100 mL).

Oxygen content of arterial blood (CaO$_2$ in [mL O$_2$/100 mL])

$$CaO_2 = 1.34 \text{ mL } O_2/g \times [Hb \text{ (g/100 mL)}] \times SaO_2 + 0.003 \text{ } PaO_2, \qquad \text{(Equation P23-2)}$$

where the SaO$_2$ is given as a fraction of one (e.g., 0.95)

However, determining the oxygen-carrying capacity of Hb is complicated by the fact that both COHb and MetHb are forms of circulating Hb that do not bind oxygen but shift the oxyhemoglobin dissociation curve to the left. COHb occurs when carbon monoxide (CO) binds to Hb. Smokers have increased levels of COHb. MetHb occurs when the normal ferrous state (Fe2 +) of the iron moiety in Hb is oxidized to the ferric stage (Fe3 +). Significant methemoglobinemia can occur after exposure to certain medications (dapsone) or in congenital methemoglobinemia but is uncommon in the sleep center. It may cause a low SpO$_2$ reading with a normal PaO$_2$ (arterial blood is brown) (see below). The sum of the concentrations of O$_2$Hb, RHb, COHb, and MetHb equals the total hemoglobin concentration ([Hbtotal]) (see Equation P23-3) and the sum of the fractional concentrations equals 100% (see Equation P23-3).

$$[Hbtotal] = [O_2Hb] + [RHb] + [COHb] + [MetHb] \qquad \text{(Equation P23-3)}$$

where [O$_2$Hb] concentration of oxygenated hemoglobin, similar for RHb, COHb, and MetHb
and
[Hbtotal] = total concentration of hemoglobin
  FO$_2$Hb = fractional concentration of hemoglobin
    = ([O$_2$Hb] × 100)/[Hbtotal]
(with similar definitions for FRHb, FCOHb, and FMetHb)

$$FO_2Hb + FRHb + FCOHb + FMetHb = 100\% \qquad \text{(Equation P23-4)}$$

The SaO$_2$ may be expressed by using fractional concentrations:

$$SaO_2 = FO_2Hb \times 100 \div (100 - FCOHb - FMetHb)$$

For example, if the FO$_2$Hb = 85%, FCOHb = 8%, and FMetHb = 2%, then FRHb = 5%
SaO$_2$ = 85 × 100 /(100 − 8 − 2) = 85 × 100 ÷ 90 = 94%, although FO$_2$Hb = 85%.

The true oxygen carrying capacity of the Hb depends on FO$_2$Hb not SaO$_2$. FO$_2$Hb may be substituted into Equation P23-2 for the SaO$_2$ to calculate the true oxygen carrying capacity of blood. On the other hand, the SaO$_2$ reflects the percentage of the Hb that is available for oxygen binding that is bound to oxygen (oxygenated) at the current PaO$_2$.

Some blood gas laboratories actually measure the PaO$_2$ but determine the SaO$_2$ from a table. Therefore, it is important to know if the SaO$_2$ in an arterial blood gas report was determined by actual measurement of FO$_2$Hb, FCOHb, and FCOMet. **Co-oximetry** accurately determines the concentrations of O$_2$Hb, COHb, and MetHb using four or more wavelengths of light. When reading co-oximetry results, it is important to understand whether or not FHbO$_2$, SaO$_2$, or both are being reported. The SaO$_2$ depends only on the PaO$_2$ and the binding properties of hemoglobin available for binding (e.g., not bound to COHb or MetHb). The presence of COHb shifts the O$_2$Hb saturation curve to the left, but this effect is not large unless the COHb is quite high. Of note, the oxygen-carrying capacity of blood depends on the FO$_2$Hb and Hbtotal. On the other hand, the PaO2 is inferred from the SaO$_2$.

Although COHb affects the typical SpO$_2$ value (2 wave length pulse oximetry measurement of SaO$_2$), the reading is usually similar to the SaO2 but lower than the FO$_2$Hb. For every percentage of COHb above zero, the SaO$_2$ is about 1% higher than the FO$_2$Hb. In the sleep center, the main objective of pulse oximetry is to infer baseline oxygenation and changes in oxygenation caused by respiratory events. In summary, when COHb is present, the SpO$_2$ slightly overestimates the SaO$_2$, and the FO$_2$Hb is lower than the actual SaO$_2$ (Table P23-2). Because of a left shift of the hemoglobin dissociation curve, the PaO$_2$ is slightly lower for a given SaO$_2$. However, at the COHb levels typically seen in the sleep center, this means that a normal SpO$_2$ would correspond to a normal PaO$_2$ even if the FO$_2$Hb is lower than the SpO$_2$ and SaO$_2$.

If a patient has a lower than expected SpO$_2$ while awake in the sleep center, a number of possibilities should be considered (Box P23-1), including true hypoxemia, a faulty oximetry probe,

TABLE P23-2 **Determination of FO$_2$Hb and SaO$_2$ with Co-oximetry in a Patient with an Elevated COHb**

PaO$_2$	62 mm Hg
FO$_2$Hb	86%
FCOHb	5.1%
MetHb	0.1%
SaO$_2$	91% = FO$_2$Hb $\times$ 100 $\div$ (100 − FCOHb − FMetHb) = 86 $\times$ 100 $\div$ (100 − 5.2) = 91%
SpO$_2$ (simultaneous)	92%

BOX P23-1 **Causes of Low SpO$_2$ in the Absence of Obstructive Sleep Apnea**

1. True hypoxemia
   - Residence at high altitude
   - Hypoventilation
   - Ventilation perfusion mismatch
     - Usually with severe obesity or lung disease
   - Shunt (right to left; e.g., congenital heart disease with shunt)
2. Normal PO$_2$ with low SaO$_2$
   - Abnormal hemoglobin (e.g., sickle cell disease)
   - Other factors shifting Hb saturation curve to the right
3. Incorrect SpO$_2$
   - Methemoglobin (SpO$_2$ moves toward 85%)
   - Faulty SpO$_2$ probe
   - Poor perfusion; compression of circulation to digit with probe attached
   - Finger nail polish

poor signal quality because of poor perfusion, and a rightward shift in the O$_2$Hb saturation curve caused by the factors illustrated in Figure P23-1 (including an abnormal Hb). If oximetry issues are ruled out, arterial blood gas measurement is needed to determine whether hypoxemia is, in fact, present (if clinically indicated). In this situation, co-oximetry analysis could also determine whether significant COHb or MetHb is present and determine a true SaO$_2$ and the true fraction of Hb that is oxygenated (FHbO$_2$). A low SaO$_2$ in a patient with a normal PO$_2$ may be caused by an abnormal Hb or other factors that shift the O$_2$Hb dissociation curve to the right.

True causes of hypoxemia in the sleep center include residence at high altitude (low inhaled PO$_2$), ventilation–perfusion mismatch, lung disease, cardiac shunt, and hypoventilation. While hypoxemia caused by residence at high altitude, ventilation–perfusion mismatch or hypoventilation will improve with the addition of supplemental oxygen, minimal improvement with occur with a patient with congenital heart disease and a right-to-left shunt. Hypoventilation may be documented with measurement of end-tidal PCO$_2$ or transcutaneous PCO$_2$.

In the current patient, the presence of an abnormal Hb resulted in a low SaO$_2$ for a normal PaO$_2$. Other causes of a low SaO$_2$ include hypoventilation, ventilation–perfusion mismatch, or shunt (PaO$_2$ low, SaO$_2$ low), technical problems with oximetry (PaO$_2$ normal, SaO$_2$ low).

CLINICAL PEARLS

1. Several causes of a low SpO$_2$ are encountered in the sleep center in a patient with no discrete respiratory events. True hypoxemia may be caused by ventilation–perfusion mismatch (obesity or lung disease), hypoventilation, or a cardiac or pulmonary right-to-left shunt. A normal PO$_2$ associated with a low SpO$_2$ may be caused by an abnormal Hb (rightward shift of the O$_2$Hb saturation curve), and technical problems with oximetry, including a faulty probe or poor perfusion to the digit with the probe attached.

2. Methemoglobinemia (MetHb) causes the SpO$_2$ to approach 85% as MetHb levels increase. Acquired methemoglobinemia (e.g., caused by medications such as dapsone) should be suspected in the setting of cyanosis, low pulse oximetry readings, and chocolate-brown blood on arterial blood gas sampling with normal arterial PaO$_2$ values.

3. The major effect of COHb is to reduce the fraction of the total Hb that available for binding by oxygen. The SpO$_2$ and SaO$_2$ values are usually similar but the FO$_2$Hb is lower.

4. Co-oximetry is needed to accurately determine the SaO$_2$ and FHbO$_2$ when significant MetHb or COHb is present. Co-oximetry uses the absorption of four or more wavelengths of light. Routine pulse oximetry uses only two wavelengths of light.

5. Co-oximetry should be performed when the PaO$_2$ is significantly lower or higher than expected based on the SpO$_2$.

BIBLIOGRAPHY

Barker SJ, Tremper KK: The effects of carbon monoxide inhalation of pulse oximetry and transcutaneous PO_2, *Anesthesiology* 66:677–679, 1987.

Barker SJ, Tremper KK, Hyatt J: Effects of methemoglobin on pulse oximetry and mixed venous oximetry, *Anesthesiology* 7:112–117, 1989.

Roughton FJW, Darling RC: The effect of carbon monoxide on the oxyhemoglobin dissociation curve, *Am J Physiol* 141:17–31, 1944.

Spoon KC, Ramar K: Unexplained hypoxemia, *J Clin Sleep Med* 7(6):679–680, 2011.

Toffaletti J, Zijlstra W: Misconceptions in reporting oxygen saturation, *Anesth Analg* 105:S5–S9, 2007.

Tremper KK, Barker SJ: Pulse oximetry, *Anesthesiology* 70:98–108, 1989.

Wagner MH, Berry RB: A patient with sickle disease and a low baseline sleeping oxygen saturation, *J Clin Sleep Med* 3:313–315, 2007.

PATIENT 24

Central Apnea and Obstructive Hypoventilation in Children

QUESTIONS

1. Figure P24-1 shows a 60-second tracing in a 3-month-old infant. How many of the central pauses in respiration are scored as central apneas?

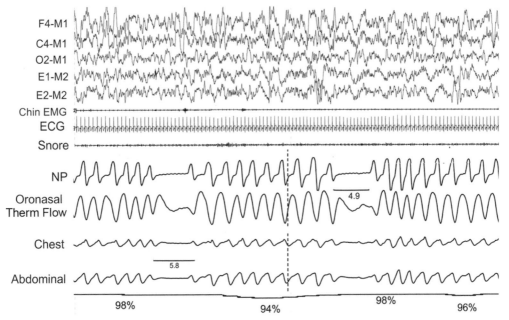

FIGURE P24-1 ■ A 60-second tracing in a 3-month-old infant.

2. Figure P24-2 shows a 30-second tracing in a 4-year-old child. The end-tidal PCO_2 was over 50 mm Hg for 30% of the total sleep time. What type of event is depicted below?

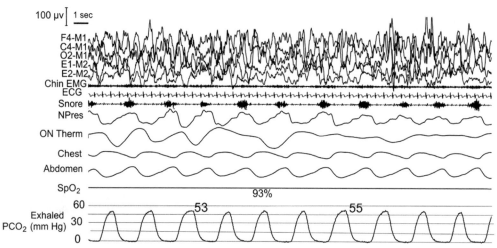

FIGURE P24-2 ■ A 30-second tracing in a 4-year-old child. *Npres*, Nasal pressure; *ON Therm*, oronasal thermal air flow sensor.

ANSWERS

1. **Answer:** The first event is scored as a central apnea.

   Discussion: The rule for scoring central apneas in children and infants is listed below[1]:
   Score a respiratory event as a **central apnea** if it meets apnea criteria, is associated with absent inspiratory effort throughout the entire duration of the event, AND at least one of the following is met:
   a. The event lasts 20 seconds or longer.
   b. The event lasts at least the duration of two breaths during baseline breathing and is associated with an arousal or $\geq 3\%$ oxygen desaturation.
   c. For infants younger than 1 year of age, the event lasts at least the duration of two breaths during baseline breathing and is associated with a decrease in heart rate to less than 50 beats per minute for at least 5 seconds or less than 60 beats per minute for 15 seconds.
   According to this rule, the first but not the second event would be scored as a central apnea. The first event but not the second event is associated with a desaturation $\geq 3\%$. One could question whether a 2% desaturation is also not clinically significant, but that is the current central apnea scoring rule. Note that neither central respiratory pause was associated with arousal.

2. **Answer:** Obstructive hypoventilation

   Discussion: Figure P24-2 depicts a period of increased PCO_2 (by exhaled CO_2) greater than 50 mm Hg. The question informs us that the PCO_2 was above 50 mm Hg for 30% of the total sleep time. Note the snoring and air flow limitation (flattened nasal pressure waveform) without discrete changes in flow consistent with apnea or hypopnea. Also note the mild drop in the SaO_2. In this patient, the awake SaO_2 was 98%. Pediatric patients with obstructive sleep apnea tend to have apneas and hypopneas mainly during REM sleep, whereas long periods of hypoventilation are often present during NREM sleep.[2]
   The PCO_2 was over 50 mg for 30% of total sleep time, therefore hypoventilation is present. The rule for scoring hypoventilation during sleep in pediatric patients is given below.[2,3] Note that this differs from the adult rule and that >50 mm Hg NOT ≥ 50 mm Hg is used as the defining metric.
   Obstructive Hypoventilation[1]:
   Score hypoventilation during sleep when $>25\%$ of the total sleep time as measured by either the arterial PCO_2 or surrogate is spent with a $PCO_2 > 50$ mm Hg.

REFERENCES

1. Berry RB, Brooks R, Gamaldo CE, et al, for the American Academy of Sleep Medicine: *The AASM manual for the scoring of sleep and associated events: rules, terminology and technical specifications, Version 2.0.3.* Darien, IL, 2014, American Academy of Sleep Medicine. www.aasmnet.org.
2. Berry RB, Budhiraja R, Gottlieb DJ, et al: Rules for scoring respiratory events in sleep: update of the 2007 AASM Manual for the Scoring of Sleep and Associated Events, *J Clin Sleep Med* 8(5):597–619, 2012.
3. Montgomery-Downs HE, O'Brien LM, Gulliver TE, Gozal D: Polysomnographic characteristics in normal preschool and early school-aged children, *Pediatrics* 117:741–753, 2006.

Electrocardiography Monitoring During Sleep Studies

Polysomnography (PSG) generally involves recording only one electrocardiographic (ECG) channel, although some PSG systems allow for the monitoring of multiple leads. Historically, ECG recordings used a paper speed of 25 millimeters per second (mm/sec). A 10-second window of digital PSG is equivalent to a paper speed of 30 mm/sec, and thus, visualizing of the ECG channel in a 10-second window mimics the usual appearance of the ECG. Figure F15-1 shows ECG waveforms and useful terminology. The 2007 *AASM Scoring Manual* published criteria for scoring cardiac events during sleep (Box F15-1). A single lead (modified lead II) (see Figure F15-1, *A*) with a low filter setting of 0.3 hertz (Hz), a high filter setting of 70 Hz and a minimum sampling rate of 200 Hz is recommended. The ECG is often recorded as a true bipolar signal using inputs from the two electrodes shown if Figure F15-1. However, multiple ECG electrodes may be recorded in a referential manner, and various combinations may be displayed. If ECG_{neg} and ECG_{pos} denote the two electrodes pictured in Figure F15-1, then the derivation $ECG_{neg} - ECG_{pos}$ provides an upright QRS in the ECG channel.

SINUS RHYTHM DURING SLEEP

In lead II, sinus rhythm is characterized by an upright p-wave, an R-wave, and a T-wave (see Figure F15-1). Normally, a slight speeding of the heart with inspiration and slowing with expiration occur. If the variability in heart rate with respiration is significant, this is often called *sinus arrhythmia* (Figure F15-2). **Sinus tachycardia in sleep** is scored when sustained (>30 seconds) heart rate >90/min is present in adults. In children, heart rates are much faster and must be adjusted according to age. **Sinus bradycardia during sleep** is scored with a sustained heart rate of <40/min in adults and in children 6 years or older.

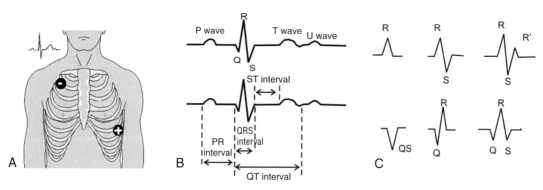

FIGURE F15-1 ■ **Panel A,** AASM modified lead II electrode positions. **Panel B,** Components of electrocardiography (ECG) waveform and interval definitions are illustrated. **Panel C,** Nomenclature of components of QRS. The Q-wave is the initial negative deflection and R-wave the initial positive deflection. Nomenclature of components of the QRS complex are illustrated. (**Panel A,** adapted from Iber C, Chesson A, Ancoli-Israel S, et al: *The scoring of sleep and associated events: rules, terminology and technical specifications,* ed 1, Westchester, IL, 2007, American Academy of Sleep Medicine; **Panels B** and **C,** From Wagner GS [ed]: *Marriott's practical electrocardiography,* ed 9, Philadelphia, 1994, Williams & Wilkins, pp 11-13.)

BOX F15-1	Scoring Electrocardiography Changes during Sleep

- Score **sinus tachycardia** during sleep for a sustained heart rate >90 beats per minute for adults.
- Score **sinus bradycardia** during sleep for a sustained heart rate <40 beats/min for ages 6 years through adulthood.
- Score **asystole** for cardiac pauses >3 seconds for ages 6 years through adulthood.

- Score **wide-complex tachycardia** for a rhythm lasting a minimum of three consecutive beats at a rate >100 beats/min with a QRS duration ≥120 milliseconds (msec; 0.12 seconds [sec]).
- Score **narrow-complex tachycardia** for a rhythm lasting a minimum of three consecutive beats at a rate >100 beats/min with a QRS duration <120 msec (0.12 sec).

Note: Sustained means >30 seconds in duration.

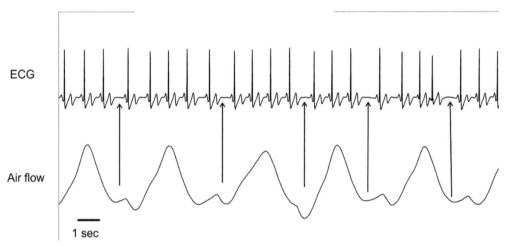

FIGURE F15-2 ■ Sinus arrhythmia. Heart rate slows during exhalation (*arrows*). In this figure, inspiration is upward.

HEART RATE CHANGES IN OBSTRUCTIVE SLEEP APNEA

In normal individuals, heart rate is lower during non–rapid eye movement (NREM) sleep than during wakefulness. This is thought to be caused by parasympathetic predominance during sleep. In patients with obstructive sleep apnea (OSA), the heart rate varies in cycles: slowing with apnea onset; increasing slightly, staying the same, or decreasing during apnea; and increasing in the postapneic period (Figure F15-3). Early studies attributed the slowing of heart rate during apnea to increased vagal tone and hypoxia. The slowing was diminished by atropine and supplemental oxygen. Bonsignore and coworkers found that during apnea, the heart rate could increase, stay the same, or decrease, depending on relative amounts of parasympathetic tone and sympathetic tone. Although the cyclic changes in heart rate are sometimes referred to as *brady-tachycardia*, the

heart rate often remains between 60 and 90 beat per minute (beats/min) in most patients.

BRADYCARDIA AND SINUS PAUSES

The common causes of a slow heart rate during sleep are listed in Box F15-2. A slow heart rate during sleep (sustained heart rate <40 beats/min) may be a normal variant, associated with the effects of medications (e.g., beta-blockers), caused by high parasympathetic tone, or associated with disease of the conduction system (SA node, AV node). The *AASM Scoring Manual* recommends scoring asystole if a sinus pause is >3 seconds for ages 6 years through adulthood (Figure F15-4).

ATRIOVENTRICULAR BLOCK

Examples of atrioventricular (AV) block are displayed in Figure F15-5. First-degree AV

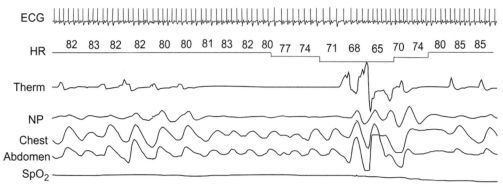

FIGURE F15-3 ■ Heart rate (HR) slows with the onset of apnea and then speeds at apnea termination. This may be visualized by an increase followed by a decrease in the R–R interval. The HR tracing from the oximeter averages over several heart beats, and the change in the HR signal lags behind changes in the R–R interval.

BOX F15-2	Causes of a Slow Heart Rate during Sleep

- Sinus in bradycardia (<40 /min); can be a normal variant
- Sinus node dysfunction
- Sinus pauses

- Atrioventricular block
- Medications
- Increased vagal tone (obstructive sleep apnea)

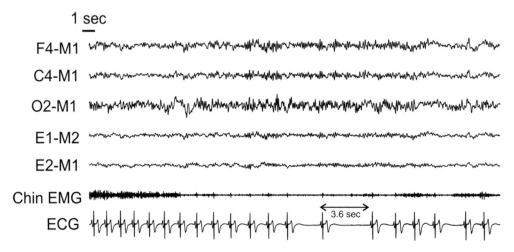

FIGURE F15-4 ■ A sinus pause during a sleep study. The *AASM Scoring Manual* recommends scoring asystole when the sinus pause is >3 seconds.

---

block is defined as a P–R interval >0.2 seconds. Second-degree block, Mobitz I (Wenchkebach), is characterized by a progressive increase in P–R interval followed by a nonconducted p-wave. Second-degree block, Mobitz II, is characterized by a nonconducted p-wave without preceding PR prolongation. Third-degree AV block is characterized by absence of conduction of p-waves. The pacemaker is in the AV node or ventricles. The p-waves and QRS complexes have no fixed relationship.

TACHYCARDIA DURING SLEEP

Common causes of a fast heart rate during sleep are listed in Box F15-3. Sinus tachycardia during sleep is defined as a sustained heart rate over

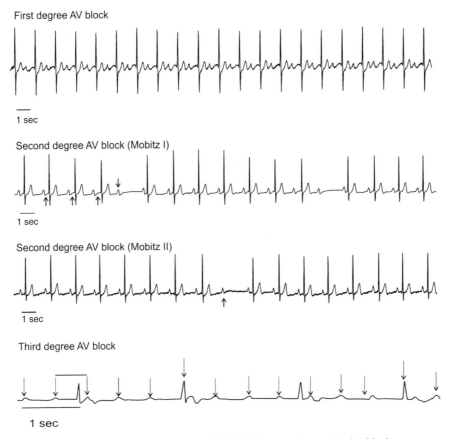

FIGURE F15-5 ■ First-, second-, and third-degree atrioventricular blocks.

BOX F15-3	Common Causes of Tachycardia During Polysomnography

- Sinus tachycardia
- Wide-complex tachycardia
- Narrow-complex tachycardia
- Atrial flutter
- Atrial fibrillation

90 beats/min in adults and in children over 6 years. For narrow-complex (Figure F15-6) and wide-complex (Figure F15-7) tachycardia, **a minimum of three beats** with a **rate >100 per minute** must be present. For narrow-complex tachycardia, the QRS duration is <0.12 seconds, and for wide-complex tachycardia, the QRS duration is >0.12 seconds. Wide-complex tachycardia is usually assumed to be ventricular tachycardia unless proven otherwise (see Figure F15-7). However, supraventricular tachycardia may present with a wide QRS if aberrant AV conduction occurs. Ventricular tachycardia and supraventricular tachycardia with aberrancy cannot be differentiated with a single ECG channel and hence the term *wide-complex tachycardia* is used. Sustained ventricular tachycardia (>30 seconds in duration) or ventricular tachycardia of any duration in a patient in distress is a medical emergency.

Two other common rhythms that may or may not be associated with a ventricular rate over 100 beats/min include atrial flutter and atrial fibrillation (Figure F15-8). Atrial flutter is composed of sawtooth flutter waves (rate 250–300 beats/min) with the R–R intervals being regular or irregular (constant or variable block). At 2/1 block, the ventricular rate is about 150 beats/min and

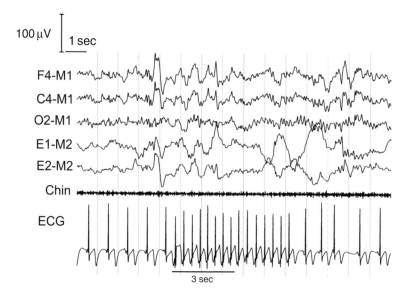

FIGURE F15-6 ■ Narrow-complex tachycardia in a 15-second tracing. Rate of approximately 160 per minute. The rate may be found by counting the number of QRS complexes in 3 seconds (8) and multiplying by 20.

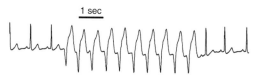

FIGURE F15-7 ■ Wide-complex tachycardia. The rate must be >100 beats per minute with at least three complexes with a QRS duration >0.12 seconds.

maybe mistaken for sinus tachycardia. However, a sinus rhythm of this high a rate is unlikely to be encountered in an individual in a sleep center. Atrial fibrillation is characterized by an irregular–irregular rhythm without p-waves (variable R–R intervals). Both atrial flutter and atrial fibrillation are usually present with a narrow QRS complex but may be a cause of wide-complex tachycardia if aberrant conduction is present.

PREMATURE BEATS

Premature beats (PBs) are usually classified on the basis of the width of the QRS interval, with wide-complex PBs referred to as *premature ventricular contractions* (PVCs) and narrow complex BPs as *supraventricular premature beats* (SVPBs). However, SVPBs may be associated with a wide QRS if aberrant conduction is present. If an ectopic p-wave can be identified before a narrow QRS premature beat, the term *premature atrial contractions* (PACs) is often used. When PBs follow every other sinus beat, bigeminy is said to be present, following every second sinus beat (trigeminy) and every third sinus beat (quadrigeminy) (Figure F15-9). Two successive PVCs are often called a *couplet*. When three successive wide beats with a rate >100 beats/min occurs, the pattern meets the criteria for wide-complex tachycardia.

PACEMAKERS

Pacemakers with a single ventricular pacing lead (in the right ventricle) result in a wide-complex QRS when ventricular pacing occurs (Figure F15-10). A rhythm may convert from a narrow-complex rhythm (normal sinus) to a wide-complex rhythm if the atrial rate falls below a set threshold or if the atrial beat is not conducted. The sudden appearance of a wide-complex rhythm may cause panic in the sleep center. *Therefore, it is important to know if a patient being monitored has a pacemaker.* The fact that paced rhythms are almost always below 90 per minute should be appreciated. A person cannot have wide-complex tachycardia without tachycardia.

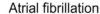

Atrial fibrillation

1 sec

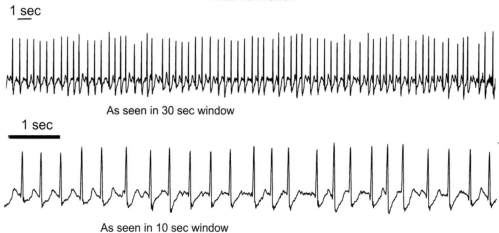

As seen in 30 sec window

1 sec

As seen in 10 sec window

Atrial flutter

1 sec

As seen in 30 sec window

1 sec

As seen in 10 sec window

FIGURE F15-8 ■ Examples of atrial flutter and atrial fibrillation depicted as seen in 30-second and 10-second windows.

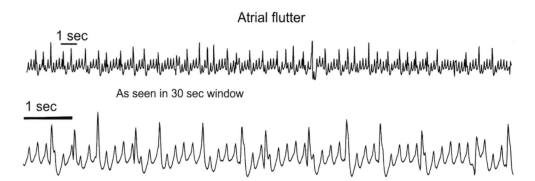

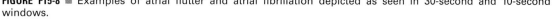

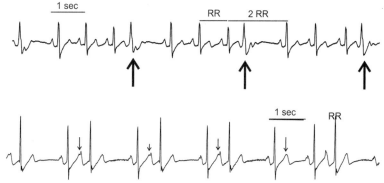

FIGURE F15-9 ■ The top line shows ventricular quadrigeminy, with a wide beat after every 3 sinus beats. The bottom line shows atrial bigeminy from premature atrial contractions. The small arrow shows the ectopic p-wave buried in the preceding T-wave.

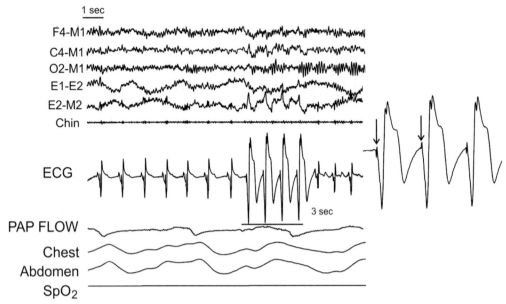

FIGURE 15-10 ■ Sudden appearance of wide-complex QRS. In the blow-up, ventricular pacer spikes can be appreciated. The rate is approximately 80 (4 beats in 3 seconds = 80 beats in 60 seconds). Therefore, this is not wide-complex tachycardia but, rather, ventricular pacing.

BIBLIOGRAPHY

Berry RB, Brooks R, Gamaldo CE, et al., for the American Academy of Sleep Medicine: *The AASM manual for the scoring of sleep and associated events: rules, terminology and technical specifications*, Version 2.03, Darien, IL, 2012, American Academy of Sleep Medicine. www.aasmnet.org, Accessed April 14, 2014.

Caples SM, Rosen CLK, Shen WK, et al: The scoring of cardiac events during sleep, *J Clin Sleep Med* 3:147–154, 2007.

Iber C, Chesson A, Ancoli-Israel S, et al: *The scoring of sleep and associated events: rules, terminology and technical specifications*, ed 1, Westchester, IL, 2007, American Academy of Sleep Medicine.

Wagner GS, editor: *Marriott's practical electrocardiography*, 9 ed, Philadelphia, 1994, Williams & Wilkins.

A Patient with Slowing of Heart Rate During Sleep

Patient A: A 70-second tracing from a patient with loud snoring and witnessed apnea is shown in Figure P25-1.

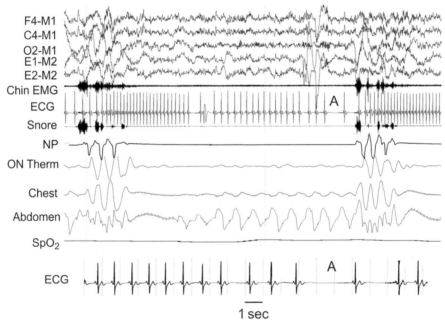

FIGURE P25-1 ■ A 70-second tracing with an enlargement of a portion of the electrocardiogram below.

QUESTION

1. Describe the changes seen on electrocardiography (ECG) at A. NP refers to nasal pressure, and ONTherm refers to the oronasal thermal sensor signal.

ANSWER

1. **Answer:** Bradycardia associated with a mixed obstructive apnea and a 3.2-second sinus pause (asystole).

   Discussion: The *AASM Scoring Manual* recommends **scoring asystole if a sinus pause is >3 seconds in duration for ages 6 years through adult.**[1,2] A review paper providing evidence for cardiac scoring rules quotes normative data in young healthy subjects[2] and shows sinus pauses to be longer in males (range 1.20–2.06 seconds) than in females (1.08–1.92 seconds). In trained athletes, up to 37% had sinus pauses between 2 and 3 seconds. A study of a cohort of 40- to 79-year-old individuals found the longest pause during sleep to be 2 seconds.[3] For this reason, sinus pauses of 3 seconds or longer are scored as asystole.

In normal individuals, the heart rate is lower during NREM sleep than during wakefulness. This is thought to be caused by parasympathetic predominance during sleep.[4] In patients with obstructive sleep apnea (OSA), heart rate varies in cycles: slowing with apnea onset, increasing slightly, staying the same, or decreasing during apnea and increasing dramatically in the postapneic period.[4,5] Early studies emphasized the slowing of heart rate during apnea and attributed this finding to increased vagal tone and hypoxia.[6] The slowing was diminished by atropine and supplemental oxygen. The increased vagal tone during apnea is the result of hypoxic stimulation of the carotid body during absent ventilation. With resumption of respiration, inflation of the lungs decreases vagal tone, and the hypoxic influences on sympathetic tone are unmasked (tachycardia). Later studies of heart rate in sleep apnea[5,7] have not consistently found a reduction in heart rate in the last part of apnea. Bonsignore and coworkers[4] found that heart rate could increase during apnea, stay the same, or decrease depending on relative amounts of parasympathetic and sympathetic tone. One investigation suggested that the individual differences in the effect of apnea on heart rate may be secondary to differences in the response of the carotid body to hypoxia.[7] Although the cyclic changes in heart rate are sometimes referred to as *brady-tachycardia*, the heart rate often remains between 60 and 90 beats per minute (beats/min) in most patients. Recall that in adults, sinus bradycardia during sleep is defined by the *AAMS Scoring Manual* as a sustained heart rate less than 40 per minute.[2]

Guilleminault and colleagues[8] reported on 400 patients with sleep apnea: 48% had some type of arrhythmia; 20% had more than two premature ventricular contractions (PVCs) per min during sleep; 7% had severe bradycardia to less than 30 beats/min; 3% had nonsustained ventricular tachycardia; and 5% and 3% had Mobitz type I and type II second-degree block, respectively. Sinus arrest from 2.5 to 13 seconds was noted in 11%. In a prospective study by Harbison and coworkers, the ECG of 45 patients with recently diagnosed OSA underwent Holter monitoring for 18 hours after diagnosis and again after 2 to 3 days of continuous positive airway pressure (CPAP).[9] Only 8 of the 45 had significant rhythm disturbances, including ventricular tachycardia, atrial fibrillation, supraventricular tachycardia, and second- or third-degree heart block. In 7 of these 8 patients, CPAP resulted in the abolition of rhythm disturbances.

The parasympathetic predominance during apnea in some patients may have little significance except in cases of significant bradycardia or heart block. A study by Becker et al. documented a reversal of atrioventricular conduction block on CPAP treatment.[10] The periods of tachycardia and elevated blood pressure following apnea increase myocardial oxygen demand when hypoxemia coexists, predisposing to ischemia and possibly tachyarrhythmias. In normal individuals, sleep usually is a time of reduced heart rate and reduced ischemia. Patients with OSA may not enjoy the same protection. PVCs are not uncommon in patients with OSA. However, in some patients, the PVC frequency is actually lower during sleep. Shepard and associates[11] found no correlation between the SaO_2 (saturation of arterial oxygen) at desaturation and PVC frequency during sleep unless the SaO_2 was less than 60%.

Heart rate variability has been used as a tool to study the balance of parasympathetic and sympathetic tones in patients with OSA. During wakefulness, these patients show less heart rate variability compared with normal individuals. This is thought to be secondary to an increase in sympathetic tone that is still present during the day. After successful treatment with CPAP, heart rate variability may increase, which suggests a drop in sympathetic activity. Khoo and coworkers[12] found that CPAP treatment of OSA improved vagal heart rate control and that the degree of improvement varied directly with the amount of adherence with CPAP use.

CLINICAL PEARLS

1. A sinus pause of 3 seconds or longer is considered as asystole according to the *AASM Scoring Manual*. Patients with sleep apnea may have increases in vagal tone during respiratory events and increases in sympathetic tone following event termination. The increased vagal tone may worsen heart block or symptomatic bradycardia.

2. Patients with untreated obstructive sleep apnea have a decrease in heart rate variability because of increased sympathetic tone. The increase in sympathetic tone at night may still present during the day in some patients. Adequate CPAP treatment decreases sympathetic tone and increases heart rate variability.

3. The *AASM Scoring Manual*[2] defines sinus bradycardia during sleep (for ages 6 years through adulthood) as a sustained heart rate less than 40 beats/min (sustained means > 30 seconds).

4. The *AASM Scoring Manual*[2] defines sinus tachycardia during sleep as a sustained heart rate greater than 90 beats/min.

REFERENCES

1. Caples SM, Rosen CLK, Shen WK, et al: The scoring of cardiac events during sleep, *J Clin Sleep Med* 3:147–154, 2007.
2. Iber C, Chesson A, Ancoli-Israel S, et al: *The scoring of sleep and associated events: rules, terminology and technical specifications,* ed 1, Westchester, IL, 2007, American Academy of Sleep Medicine.
3. Bjerregaard P: Mean 24 hour heart rate and pauses in healthy subjects 40–79 years of age, *Eur Heart J* 4:44–51, 1983.
4. Bonsignore MR, Romano S, Marrone O, et al: Different heart rate patterns in obstructive sleep apnea during NREM sleep, *Sleep* 20:1167–1174, 1997.
5. Weiss JW, Remsburg S, Garpestad E, et al: Hemodynamic consequences of obstructive sleep apnea, *Sleep* 19:388–397, 1996.
6. Zwillich C, Devlin T, White D, et al: Bradycardia during sleep apnea. Characteristics and mechanisms, *J Clin Invest* 69:1286–1292, 1982.
7. Sato F, Nishimura M, Sinano H, et al: Heart rate during obstructive sleep apnea depends on individual hypoxic chemosensitivity of the carotid body, *Circulation* 96:274–281, 1997.
8. Guilleminault C, Connoly SJ, Winkle RA: Cardiac arrhythmia and conduction disturbances during sleep in 400 patients with sleep apnea syndrome, *Am J Cardiol* 52:490–494, 1983.
9. Harbison J, O'Reilly P, McNicholas WT: Cardiac rhythm disturbances in obstructive sleep apnea syndrome: effects of nasal continuous positive airway pressure therapy, *Chest* 118:591–595, 2000.
10. Becker H, Brandenburg U, Peter JH, et al: Reversal of sinus arrest and atrioventricular conduction block in sleep apnea during nasal continuous positive airway pressure, *Am J Respir Crit Care Med* 151:215–218, 1995.
11. Shepard JW Jr., Garrison MW, Grither DA, et al: Relationship of ventricular ectopy to oxyhemoglobin desaturation in patients with obstructive sleep apnea, *Chest* 88:335–340, 1985.
12. Khoo MC, Belozeroff V, Berry RB, Sassoon CSH: Cardiac autonomic control in obstructive sleep apnea: effects of long term CPAP therapy, *Am J Respir Crit Care Med* 164:807–812, 2001.

Patients with a Sudden Increase in Heart Rate

Patient A: A 50-year-old man was evaluated for snoring and witnessed apnea. He denied daytime sleepiness but did report waking up gasping for air. A tracing of his sleep study is shown in Figure P26-1. The two enlargements show the details of the cardiac rhythm more clearly.

QUESTION

1. What was the change in cardiac rhythm during this respiratory event?

Patient B: A 40-year-old woman was referred by her cardiologist on suspicion of sleep apnea. She had undergone several electrical cardioversions in the past for atrial fibrillation. Figure P26-2 shows a 30 second epoch. The patient started the study in sinus rhythm.

QUESTION

2. What is the rhythm? What would you adjust to better assess the electrocardiography (ECG) changes?

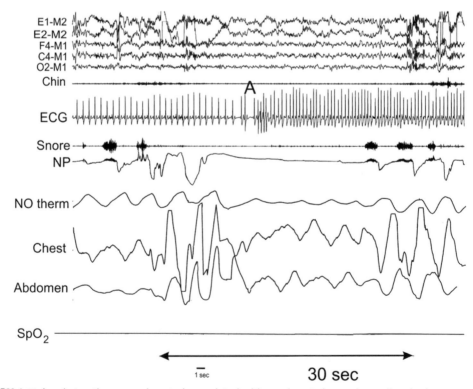

FIGURE P26-1 ■ An obstructive apnea is noted associated with an abrupt change in cardiac rhythm.

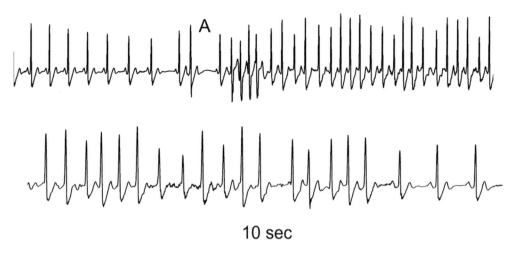

10 sec

FIGURE P26-1—cont'd Two magnified views of the electrocardiogram are shown below the longer tracing.

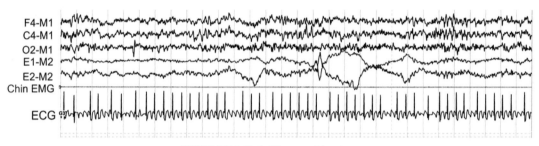

FIGURE P26-2 ■ A 30-second tracing.

ANSWERS

1. **Answer:** The onset of atrial fibrillation with a moderately fast ventricular response

   Discussion: Atrial fibrillation (AF) is the most common cardiac arrhythmia and its prevalence has increased significantly in past three decades.[1-3] Hypertension, thyroid disease, coronary artery disease, cardiomyopathy, and structural heart diseases are conventionally associated with high risk of AF.[2,3] Recently, a high prevalence of obstructive sleep apnea (OSA) has been noted among patients with AF, indicating that OSA might be contributing to initiation and progression of AF.[4,5]

   The relationship between AF and OSA is unclear. Is this an association, or is the presence of OSA a risk factor for developing AF? Gami and colleagues[6] found that the risk of developing AF was more closely associated with obesity and the degree of arterial oxygen desaturation than with the apnea–hypopnea index (AHI). OSA could increase the risk of AF by multiple mechanisms, including high sympathetic tone and negative intrathoracic pressure (stretch of the atrial walls). Certainly, if OSA is associated with significant nocturnal hypoxemia, an increased risk of developing AF does appear to exist. Untreated OSA also appears to worsen arrhythmia control whether by medications,[7] direct current cardioversion,[8] radiofrequency ablation,[9,10] or pulmonary vein isolation.[11] Some studies also suggest that if OSA is present, continuous positive airway pressure (CPAP) treatment may help reduce the risk of recurrence. Kanagala and associates[8] found that patients with untreated OSA had a higher recurrence of AF after cardioversion compared with patients without a diagnosis of sleep apnea. Appropriate treatment with CPAP in OSA was associated with a lower recurrence of AF. Fein et al. found that CPAP reduces the recurrence of AF after radiofrequency ablation.[10]

   Mehra and coworkers[12] evaluated a cohort of older men and found that sleep-disordered breathing was associated with AF and complex ventricular events (CVEs). The prevalence of CVE was associated with OSA and hypoxemia, whereas AF was associated with central sleep apnea (CSA).

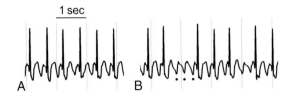

1 sec

A   B

FIGURE P26-3 ■ The electrocardiogram in Figure P26-2 as seen in a 10-second window. At *A*, the rhythm could be mistaken for sinus rhythm at 120 beats per minute. On the left, during a period of increased block, the flutter waves are clearly seen (*small dots*).

An evaluation of the Sleep Heart Health cohort found that although the rate of arrhythmias was low, the relative risk of AF or nonsustained ventricular tachycardia was much higher following respiratory events.[13]

Ryan and coworkers[14] performed a randomized, controlled trial of CPAP in patients with heart failure to determine if the frequency of ventricular premature beats (VPBs) would decrease. The study found that CPAP did reduce their VPB frequency (58% reduction) during sleep. The urinary norepinephrine concentration also decreased. No changes were noted in the control group.

In the current patient, a premature atrial contraction is followed by a pause and then the onset of AF with a heart rate of around 120 beats per minute (beats/min).

The patient remained in AF for the remainder of the night. He was referred to cardiology, and a CPAP titration was ordered.

2. **Answer:** Atrial flutter

Discussion: The R–R interval is irregular, but this is caused by variable block. In atrial flutter, the "flutter wave" frequency is 240 to 350 beats/min but is usually around 300 beats/min and 2 to 1, 3 to 1, and 4 to 1 block results in heart rates for around 150, 75, and 60 beats/min, respectively. A common finding is a heart rate of 150 that is mistaken for "sinus tachycardia." Sometimes, the flutter waves are buried in the preceding T-wave. The flutter waves are best seen by switching to a 10 second window. During periods of greater block, flutter waves more easily visualized. It is helpful to switch to a 10 second window to identify ECG patterns (Figure P26-3). The presence of untreated OSA makes treatment of recurrent atrial flutter more difficult.[15] The current patient was found to have very mild sleep apnea (she declined treatment) and was referred to cardiology for management of her atrial flutter.

CLINICAL PEARLS

1. A high percentage of patients with AF have OSA. The relationship between OSA and AF is still being evaluated. Most data suggest that patients with significant OSA associated with significant hypoxemia are at risk of AF.

2. Studies suggest that untreated OSA decreases control of AF with medications and increases the risk of recurrence after direct cardioversion, radiofrequency catheter ablation, or pulmonary vein isolation. Studies suggest that CPAP may reduce the risk of recurrence in patients with OSA.

3. Atrial flutter may be associated with variable block and an irregular rhythm. Usually, flutter waves may be seen during periods of higher block. Some patients have long periods of 2 to 1 block, and the rhythm is mistaken for sinus tachycardia. A fixed heart rate of 120 to 150 beats/min should always raise the suspicion of atrial flutter.

4. Changing to a 10-second window allows visualization of the electrocardiogram with a similar appearance as noted on routine electrocardiography.

REFERENCES

1. Goyal SK, Sharma A: Atrial fibrillation in obstructive sleep apnea, *World J Cardiol* 5(6):157–163, 2013.
2. Wolf PA, Benjamin EJ, Belanger AJ, et al: Secular trends in the prevalence of atrial fibrillation: the Framingham Study, *Am Heart J* 131:790–795, 1996.
3. Calkins H, Brugada J, Packer DL, et al: HRS/EHRA/ECAS expert consensus statement on catheter and surgical ablation of atrial fibrillation: recommendations for personnel, policy, procedures and follow-up, *Europace* 9:335–379, 2007.

4. Gami AS, Pressman G, Caples SM, et al: Association of atrial fibrillation and obstructive sleep apnea, *Circulation* 110:364–367, 2004.
5. Braga B, Poyares D, Cintra F, et al: Sleep-disordered breathing and chronic atrial fibrillation, *Sleep Med* 10:212–216, 2009.
6. Gami AS, Hodge DO, Herges RM, et al: Obstructive sleep apnea, obesity, and the risk of incident atrial fibrillation, *J Am Coll Cardiol* 49:565–571, 2007.
7. Monahan K, Brewster J, Wang L, et al: Relation of the severity of obstructive sleep apnea in response to anti-arrhythmic drugs in patients with atrial fibrillation or atrial flutter, *Am J Cardiol* 110:369–372, 2012.
8. Kanagala R, Murali NS, Friedman PA, et al: Obstructive sleep apnea and the recurrence of atrial fibrillation, *Circulation* 107:2589–2594, 2003.
9. Naruse Y, Tada H, Satoh M, et al: Concomitant obstructive sleep apnea increases the recurrence of atrial fibrillation following radiofrequency catheter ablation of atrial fibrillation: clinical impact of continuous positive airway pressure therapy, *Heart Rhythm* 10:331–337, 2013.
10. Fein AS, Shvilkin A, Shah D, et al: Treatment of obstructive sleep apnea reduces the risk of atrial fibrillation recurrence after catheter ablation, *J Am Coll Cardiol* 62(4):300–305, 2013.
11. Hoyer FF, Lickfett LM, Mittmann-Braun E, et al: High prevalence of obstructive sleep apnea in patients with resistant paroxysmal atrial fibrillation after pulmonary vein isolation, *J Interv Card Electrophysiol* 29(1):37–41, 2010.
12. Mehra R, Stone KL, Varosy PD, et al: Nocturnal Arrhythmias across a spectrum of obstructive and central sleep-disordered breathing in older men: outcomes of sleep disorders in older men (MrOS sleep) study, *Arch Intern Med* 169:1147–1155, 2009.
13. Monahan K, Storfer-Isser A, Mehra R, et al: Triggering of nocturnal arrhythmias by sleep-disordered breathing events, *J Am Coll Cardiol* 54:1797–1804, 2009.
14. Ryan CM, Usui K, Floras JS, Bradley TD: Effect of continuous positive airway pressure on ventricular ectopy in heart failure patients with obstructive sleep apnea, *Thorax* 60:781–785, 2005.
15. Bazan V, Grau N, Valles E: Obstructive sleep apnea in patients with typical atrial flutter: prevalence and impact on arrhythmia control outcome, *Chest* 143(5):1277–1283, 2013.

FUNDAMENTALS 16

Monitoring Limb and Other Movements During Sleep

The presence and frequency of limb movements (LMs) during sleep is documented by recording the electromyography (EMG) activity of muscles involved in producing the movement.[1-5] The EMG activity of the right and left anterior tibialis muscles is routinely monitored. However, in patients with suspected REM sleep behavior disorder (RBD), arm muscle EMG activity is also often recorded (Figure F16-1). In these patients, abnormal EMG activity in arm as well as leg muscles and chin derivations may be demonstrated. The classic periodic leg movement consists of extension of the big toe, dorsiflexion at the ankle, and sometimes flexion at the knee and hip, similar to the leg movement with the Babinski reflex.

Leg EMG activity is recorded using bipolar alternating current (AC) amplifiers with surface electrodes by using methods similar to those used to record chin EMG activity. The electrodes should have an impedance less than 10 kilo-ohms (less than 5 kohms is preferred). The recommended low and high filter display settings are 10 hertz (Hz) and 100 Hz, respectively.[2,3] Use of a 60-Hz notch filter is not recommended. As discussed below, since voltage amplitude criteria are used to identify significant LMs, *the relaxed leg EMG activity should be less than ± 5 microvolts (μV)*. This requires low electrode impedance. Having the patient move the left

and right legs (wiggle toes) is part of the biocalibration series. Separate EMG electrodes are placed along the long axis of the belly of the anterior tibialis muscle around the middle of the muscle (see Figure F16-1). The *AASM Scoring Manual*[2,3] recommends that the electrodes be placed either 2 to 3 cmH_2O (centimeters of water) apart or one third the length of the anterior tibialis muscle, whichever is shorter. Both legs should be monitored for the presence of leg movements. Using a separate channel (tracing) for each leg is strongly recommended. Combining electrodes from the two legs to give a single recorded channel may suffice in some clinical settings, although it should be recognized that this strategy may reduce the number of detected LMs.

CRITERIA FOR LEG MOVEMENTS AND PERIODIC LIMB MOVEMENTS IN SLEEP

In the following discussion, individual leg (limb) movements are denoted by **LMs**, individual periodic leg movements as **PLMs**, and the polysomnography finding of periodic limb movements in sleep as **PLMS**. Although leg movements were typically monitored, the term **periodic limb**

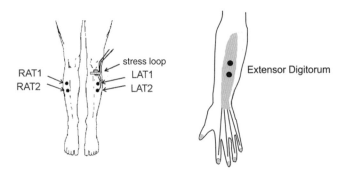

FIGURE F16-1 ■ On the left, placement of electrodes for monitoring right and left anterior tibialis electromyography (EMG) activity (left and right anterior tibialis [RAT, LAT]) is illustrated. On the right, placement of electrodes for monitoring the activity of forearm muscles (extensor digitorum superficialis and Flexor digitorum superficialis) is illustrated. (Reproduced from Berry RB: *Fundamentals of sleep medicine*, Philadelphia, 2012, Saunders.)

BOX F16-1	**Criteria for a Leg Movement**

A significant leg movement (LM) event is defined by the following (see Figure F16-2):
1. **Minimum** duration of a LM event is 0.5 seconds.
2. **Maximum** duration of a LM event is 10 seconds.
3. The **minimum amplitude** of a LM event is an 8 µV increase in electromyography (EMG) voltage above resting EMG.
4. The timing of the **onset of an LM event** is defined as the point at which an 8 µv increase occurs in EMG above resting EMG (see Figure F16-2).
5. The timing of the **ending of an LM event** is defined as the **START** of a period lasting at least 0.5 seconds during which the EMG does not exceed 2 µv above the resting EMG (see Figure F16-2).

Adapted from Berry RB, Brooks R, Gamaldo CE, et al., for the American Academy of Sleep Medicine: *The AASM manual for the scoring of sleep and associated events: rules, terminology and technical specifications*, Version 2.0.3, www.aasmnet.org, Darien, Illinois, 2014, American Academy of Sleep Medicine. Accessed July 3, 2014.

BOX F16-2	**Criteria for a PLM Series**

A periodic limb movement (PLM) series as defined by the AASM Scoring Manual:
1. The minimum number of consecutive leg movement (LM) events to define a PLM series is **4 LMs.**
2. The minimum period length between LMs (*defined as the time between onsets of consecutive LMs*) to include them as part of an PLM series is **5 seconds.**
3. The maximum period length between LMs (*defined as the time between onsets of consecutive LMs*) to include them as part of an PLM series is **90 seconds.**
4. Leg movements on two different legs separated **by less than 5 seconds between movement onsets** are counted as a **single** leg movement.

Adapted from Berry RB, Brooks R, Gamaldo CE, et al., for the American Academy of Sleep Medicine: *The AASM manual for the scoring of sleep and associated events: rules, terminology and technical specifications*, Version 2.0.3, www.aasmnet.org, Darien, Illinois, 2014, American Academy of Sleep Medicine. Accessed July 3, 2014.

Note: The time between two legs movements is measured from **onset to onset**.

Quick summary: At least four consecutive LMs with onset to onset of 5 to 90 seconds should occur to qualify as a PLM series. LMs on different legs are counted as one LM if the onsets are less than 5 seconds apart.

FIGURE F16-2 ■ A schematic illustrating criteria for onset and offset of leg movements. (Adapted from Zucconi M, Ferri R, Allen R, et al: The official World Association of Sleep Medicine [WASM] Standards for Recording and Scoring Periodic Leg Movements in Sleep [PLMS] and Wakefulness [PLMW] developed in collaboration with a task force from the International Restless Legs Syndrome Study Group [IRLSSG], *Sleep Med* 7:175-183, 2006.)

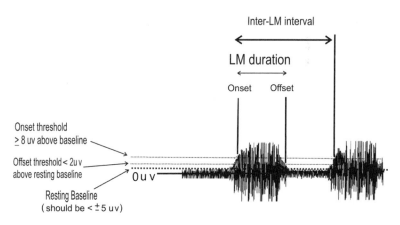

movements is used to be more inclusive. As noted above, the resting anterior tibialis EMG activity should be less than ± 5 µV (Figure F16-2). The *AASM Scoring Manual* criteria for a significant LM and for an LM to be considered a PLM (part of a PLM series) are listed in Boxes F16-1 and F16-2, respectively. LMs on two different legs separated by <5 seconds between movement onsets are counted as a single LM (Figure F16-3).

LEG MOVEMENTS ASSOCIATED WITH RESPIRATORY EVENTS ARE NOT SCORED

An LM should **not** be scored if it occurs during the period between 0.5 seconds preceding and 0.5 seconds following an apnea, hypopnea, or RERA (LMs associated with a respiratory event are not

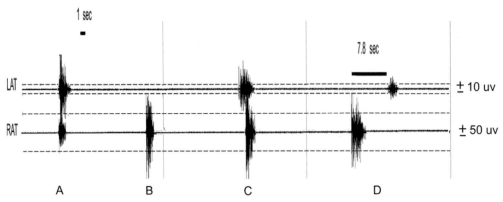

FIGURE F16-3 ■ A 90-second tracing of the left and right anterior tibialis (LAT and RAT) on electromyography is shown. The broken lines in LAT tracing are +10 microvolts (µV)amplitude lines. The dark bars are durations in seconds. According to the scoring rules, a total of five periodic limb movements (PLMs) are shown. Group A has one PLM. Group B has one PLM. Group C has one PLM, as LMs on different legs have an onset separated by less than 5 seconds and are considered a single leg movement. Group D has two PLMs.

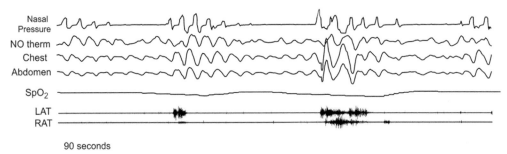

FIGURE F16-4 ■ Leg movements associated with respiratory events are not included in PLM series.

scored). When a respiratory event interrupts a series of LMs, a PLM series may continue after the respiratory event if the time period between the onset of the last LMs preceding the respiratory event and the first LM after the respiratory event is less than 90 seconds.[2,3] It is not uncommon for LMs to be noted at apnea termination, even if an associated cortical arousal is not present. In Figure F16-4, the leg EMG bursts associated with respiratory events are not scored as LMs or PLMs.

ASSOCIATION OF AROUSALS WITH PERIODIC LIMB MOVEMENTS

Leg Movements and Arousals

According to the *AASM Scoring Manual*, an arousal and a limb movement that occur in a PLM series should be considered associated with each other if they occur simultaneously or when there is <0.5 seconds between the end of one event and the onset of the other event regardless of which is first (Figure F16-5).[2,3] This recommendation differs from previous criteria, which required the arousal to follow the onset of the PLM by not more than 3 seconds.

When two PLMs occur with an interval of less than 10 seconds and each is associated with a 3-second arousal, only the first arousal should be scored, although both LMs may be scored. In this scenario, the arousal index and the PLMS arousal index, but not the PLMS index, would be influenced by not scoring the second "arousal." The rationale is that 10 seconds of sleep must precede events scored as an arousal.

PERIODIC LIMB MOVEMENTS IN SLEEP

Of note, the term PLMS implies that PLMs **occur during sleep**. The *AASM Scoring Manual*[2,3] recommends reporting the number of PLMs in sleep and the periodic limb movement index (PLMSI), which is the number of PLMs per hour of sleep. The number of PLMs associated with arousal and the PLMS arousal index (PLMSAI) should also be reported.

PLMS index (PLMSI) = no. of PLMs × 60/TST in min

PLMS arousal index × (PLMSAI) = (no. of PLMs with arousal) × TST in min

where TST = total sleep time

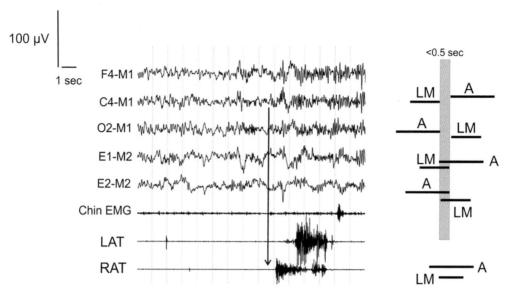

FIGURE F16-5 ■ The two leg movements (LMs) are considered to be one periodic limb movement (PLM). The onset of the LM in the RAT channel is less than 5 seconds before the onset of the LM in the LAT channel. The onset of the LM in the right anterior tibialis (RAT) is less than 0.5 seconds after the onset of the arousal. To the right, a schematic of relationship between LMs considered to be associated with an arousal (A) is shown.

PERIODIC LIMB MOVEMENTS IN WAKEFULNESS

The *AASM Scoring Manual* has not recommended criteria for scoring PLMs during wakefulness (PLMW). The World Association of Sleep Medicine in collaboration with the International Restless Legs Syndrome Study Group (IRLSSG)[5] has published recommendations for scoring PLMW. Of note, frequent PLMW events are highly suggestive of restless leg syndrome.

OTHER LEG MOVEMENT ACTIVITY

The *AASM Scoring Manual* lists criteria for other LM activities, including hypnagogic foot tremor (HFT), alternating leg movement activity (ALMA), and excessive fragmentary myoclonus (EFM) (Figure F16-6).[2–10] These phenomena are not felt to have clinical significance. HFT and ALMA often occur during wakefulness or follow arousals. HFT and ALMA should be not be confused with PLMs (Table F16-1), as the bursts are much closer together (higher frequency). HFT and ALMA are similar, but the EMG bursts alternate between the legs in ALMA. Patients with the REM sleep behavior disorder (RBD) may have phasic EMG activity in the legs also known as *transient muscle activity* (TMA). The pattern is spikier than in PLMs. PLMS may occur during REM sleep, but this occurrence is less common than the occurrence during non-REM (NREM) sleep. PLMs during REM sleep may be seen in patients with narcolepsy and RBD.

EXCESSIVE FRAGMENTARY MYOCLONUS

Fragmentary EMG bursts are common during REM sleep but when seen in NREM may meet criteria for EFM. It most cases, no movements are visible or, if present, are much like the small twitch-like movements of the fingers and toes seen intermittently during REM sleep in normal individuals. To qualify for EFM, the EMG pattern must be noted during at least 20 minutes of NREM sleep (Box F16-3).

BRUXISM

Bruxism (tooth grinding or clenching) may occur during any stage of sleep or at arousal from sleep. The phenomenon is most common in stages N1 and N2 and least common during REM sleep. During sleep, jaw contractions are either tonic (jaw clenching) or phasic (intermittent bursts of activity) and if phasic are termed *rhythmic masticatory muscle activity* (RMMA). Of note, a diagnosis of bruxism consists of more than detection of RMMA; evidence tooth grinding or clenching must be present. Although the *AASM Scoring Manual*[2,3] specifies diagnostic criteria for changes in chin EMG (Box F16-4), rhythmic muscle artifact in the electroencephalography

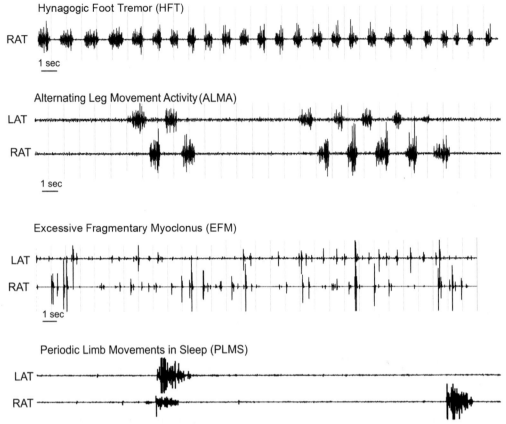

FIGURE F16-6 ■ Patterns of hypnagogic foot tremor, alternating leg movement activity, and excessive myoclonus. A pattern typical of PLMS is also shown for comparison. This is assuming that the two leg movements shown are part of a group of four or more periodic limb movements (PLMs). Note that the nearly simultaneous leg movements in LAT (left anterior tibial) EMG and RAT (right anterior tibial) EMG are considered one leg movement.

TABLE F16-1   Characteristics of HFT and ALMA versus PLMS

	LMs Bursts	Duration	Burst Frequency	Sleep Required
HFT	Minimum of 4 Not Alternating	250-1000 msec	0.3 to 4.0 Hz (.25 to 3.3 seconds between bursts)	No
ALMA	Minimum of 4 Alternating	100-500 msec	0.5 to 3.0 Hz (.33 to 2 seconds between bursts)	No
PLMS	Minimum of 4	0.5 to 10 sec	5 to 90 seconds	Yes

ALMA, Alternating leg movement activity; *HFT,* hypnagogic foot tremor; *Hz,* hertz; *PLMS,* polysomnography finding of periodic limb movement.

BOX F16-3	Scoring Excessive Fragmentary Myoclonus (EFM)

The following rules define EFM:
1. The usual maximum electromyography (EMG) burst duration seen in EFM events is **150 milliseconds (msec).**
2. At least **20 minutes of NREM sleep with FM** must be recorded.
3. At least **5 EMG potentials per minute** must be recorded.

Adapted from references 2 and 3.

(EEG) and electrooculography (EOG) derivations associated with jaw movement or clenching is often more prominent than a rhythmic pattern on chin EMG (see Figure F16-7). Recording of the masseter muscles with EMG versus chin EMG is much more sensitive for detection of rhythmic contractions. Note that the same pattern of bruxism may occur while patients are having a snack or chewing gum (RMMA) during polysomnography (PSG). Audio recording is needed to confirm that the recorded RMMA is, indeed, bruxism (minimum of two episodes of audible tooth grinding or clenching episodes per night).

BOX F16-4	Scoring Bruxism

The following rules define bruxism:
1. Bruxism may consist of brief (phasic) or sustained (tonic) elevations of chin electromyography (EMG) activity that are at least **twice the amplitude of the background EMG.**
2. Brief elevations of chin EMG activity are scored as bruxism if they are **0.25 to 2 seconds in duration** and if **at least three such elevations occur in a regular sequence.**
3. Sustained elevations of chin EMG activity are scored as bruxism, if the **duration is more than 2 seconds.**
4. A period of at least 3 seconds of stable background chin EMG must occur before a new episode of bruxism can be scored.
5. Bruxism can be scored reliably by audio in combination with PSG by a **minimum of 2 audible tooth grinding episodes per night of polysomnography (PSG)** in the absence of epilepsy.

Adapted from Berry RB, Brooks R, Gamaldo CE, et al., for the American Academy of Sleep Medicine: *The AASM manual for the scoring of sleep and associated events: rules, terminology and technical specifications*, Version 2.0.3, www.aasmnet.org, Darien, Illinois, 2014, American Academy of Sleep Medicine. Accessed July 3, 2014.

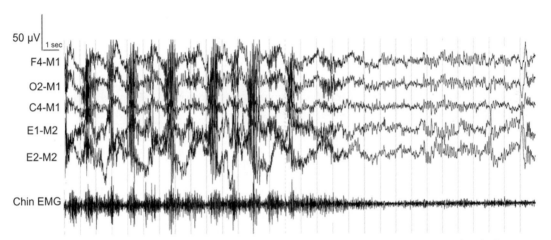

FIGURE F16-7 ■ A pattern of bruxism. Audio monitoring revealed the sound of loud tooth grinding.

RHYTHMIC MOVEMENTS IN SLEEP AND RHYTHMIC MOVEMENT DISORDER

Rhythmic movements during sleep (RMS) are most common in infants and children but may also occur in adults. A diagnosis of rhythmic movement disorder (RMD) implies as associated dysfunction.[11] Here, we will discuss RMS patterns. In Box F16-5, criteria for scoring rhythmic activity during sleep are listed. Observation with video is obviously essential to confirm the diagnosis. In general, the movements are periodic, slower in frequency than in seizure activity, and may involve movement artifact in the EEG, EOG, chin EMG, and leg EMG channels, depending on the type of activity. Typical activity includes head banging and head or body rocking or rolling (see Figure F16-8). Respiratory channels may also be affected. RMS may be seen during wakefulness, sleep, or the transition.

BOX F16-5	Scoring RMs in RMD

The following rules defines the PSG characteristics of RMD:
1. The minimum frequency for scoring RMD is 0.5 Hz.
2. The maximum frequency for scoring RMD is 2.0 Hz.
3. The minimum number of individual movements required to make a cluster of rhythmic movements is four movements.

Adapted from Berry RB, Brooks R, Gamaldo CE, et al., for the American Academy of Sleep Medicine: *The AASM manual for the scoring of sleep and associated events: rules, terminology and technical specifications*, Version 2.0.3, www.aasmnet.org, Darien, Illinois, 2014, American Academy of Sleep Medicine. Accessed July 3, 2014.
HZ, Hertz; *PSG,* polysomnography; *RM,* rhythmic movement; *RMD,* rhythmic movement disorder.

REM SLEEP BEHAVIOR DISORDER

Making a diagnosis of RBD requires PSG evidence of REM sleep without atonia and either video PSG showing dream enacting behavior

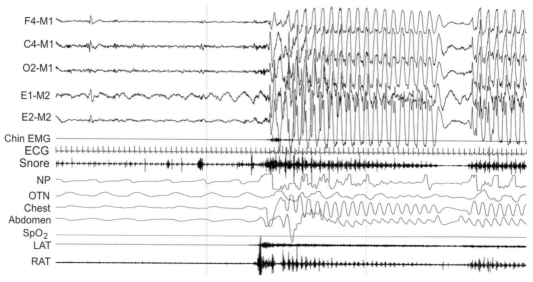

FIGURE F16-8 ■ Body rolling in an adult. This is a 90-second tracing.

BOX F16-6	**Scoring Rules for the Electromyography Activity Associated with the REM Sleep Behavior Disorder Rules**

The polysomnography (PSG) characteristics of rapid eye movement (REM)–related sleep behavior disorder (RBD) are characterized by either or both of the following features:

1. Sustained muscle activity in REM sleep on **chin electromyography (EMG)**
2. Excessive transient muscle activity during REM or **chin or limb EMG**

DEFINITIONS:

Sustained muscle activity in REM sleep is defined as an epoch of REM sleep with at *least 50% of the*

duration of the epoch having a chin EMG amplitude greater than the minimum amplitude in non-NREM sleep.

Excessive transient muscle activity in REM sleep: In a 30-second epoch of REM sleep divided into 10 sequential 3-second mini-epochs, at least 5 (50%) of the mini-epochs contain bursts of transient muscle activity. In RBD, excessive transient muscle activity bursts are 0.1 to 5.0 seconds in duration and at least 4 times as high in amplitude as the background EMG activity.

Adapted from Berry RB, Brooks R, Gamaldo CE, et al., for the American Academy of Sleep Medicine: *The AASM manual for the scoring of sleep and associated events: rules, terminology and technical specifications*, Version 2.0.3, www.aasmnet.org, Darien, Illinois, 2014, American Academy of Sleep Medicine. Accessed July 3, 2014.

or a compatible clinical history of episodes of dream enacting behavior.[11] The scoring rules for identifying EMG activity associated with RBD are listed in Box F16-6. A typical 30-second epoch of REM sleep without atonia is illustrated in Figure F16-9. It may be difficult to differentiate PLMS activity from activity associated with REM sleep without atonia. The complicating factor is that while PLMS is infrequent during REM sleep in most individuals, it is more frequent in patients with narcolepsy and RBD.[12] In addition, patients with narcolepsy often have evidence of RBD. How many epochs of REM sleep without atonia are needed for a diagnosis of RBD? Several methods have been proposed, but no consensus exists.[13–18] In the ICSD-3[11] it is noted that the finding of > 27% of 30 second epochs of stage R with sustained or phasic chin EMG activity or phasic activity in the flexor

digitorum superficialis was highly specific for a diagnosis of RBD. This is based on work by Frauscher et al.[15] One study of the EMG of many different muscles in patients with RBD[18] found that the combination most and found the combination most likely to show activity in REM sleep was the mentalis muscle + anterior tibial muscle + flexor digitorum brevis. However, the combination of the mentalis muscle + anterior tibial muscle + flexor digitorum superficialis (FDS) was almost as good, and the FDS recording had less artifact. The same group chose the latter combination in other studies to determine EMG diagnostic criteria for RBD.[15] In that study, EMG activity in the chin and arms was more specific than activity in the legs for making a diagnosis of RBD. Given this information, monitoring of both arm and leg EMG is recommended in patients with suspected RBD. REM without atonia may be seen

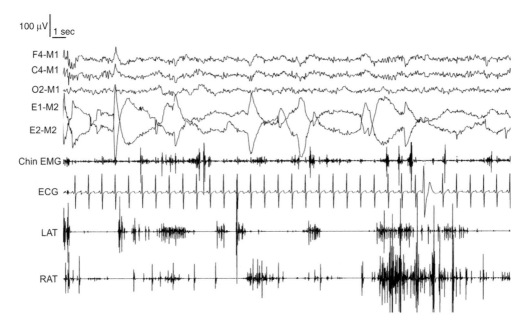

FIGURE F16-9 ■ A 30-second tracing of stage R with transient muscle activity seen in the right anterior tibialis (RAT) and left anterior tibialis (LAT). Both sustained EMG activity and TMA is also seen intermittently in the chin EMG.

in patients taking selective serotonin reuptake inhibitors (SSRIs). Winkelman and James[19] found that tonic submental EMG activity during REM sleep was significantly more common in patients taking antidepressants than in a control group. Trends for more phasic activity also were observed in the anterior tibialis ($p = 0.09$) and submental EMG as well. The study included a relatively small number of individuals; with a larger study, the increased phasic activity in the chin and legs would likely have reached statistical significance.

REFERENCES

1. Coleman RM: Periodic movements in sleep (nocturnal myoclonus) and restless legs syndrome. In Guilleminault C, editor: *Sleeping and waking disorders: indications and techniques*, Boston, 1982, Butterworths, pp 265–295.
2. Iber C, Ancoli-Israel S, Chesson A, Quan SF, for the American Academy of Sleep Medicine: *The AASM manual for the scoring of sleep and associated events: rules, terminology and technical specification*, ed 1, Westchester, IL, 2007, American Academy of Sleep Medicine, pp 41–42.
3. Berry RB, Brooks R, Gamaldo CE, et al., for the American Academy of Sleep Medicine: *The AASM manual for the scoring of sleep and associated events: rules, terminology and technical specifications*, Version 2.0.3, www.aasmnet.org, Darien, Illinois, 2014, American Academy of Sleep Medicine. Accessed July 3, 2014.
4. Walters AS, Lavigne G, Hening W, et al, The scoring of movements in sleep, *J Clin Sleep Med* 3:155–167, 2007.
5. Zucconi M, Ferri R, Allen R, et al: The official World Association of Sleep Medicine (WASM) standards for recording and scoring periodic leg movements in sleep (PLMS) and wakefulness (PLMW) developed in collaboration with a task force from the International Restless Legs Syndrome Study Group (IRLSSG), *Sleep Med* 7:175–183, 2006.
6. Chervin RD, Consens FB, Kutluay E: Alternating leg muscle activation during sleep and arousals: a new sleep-related motor phenomenon? *Mov Disord* 18:551–559, 2003.
7. Vetrugno R, PIazzi G, Provini F, et al: Excessive fragmentary hypnic myoclonus: clinical and neurophysiological findings, *Sleep Med* 3:73–76, 2001.
8. Berry RB: A woman with rhythmic foot movements, *J Clin Sleep Med* 3:749–751, 2007.
9. Constentino FI, Iero I, Lanuzza B, et al: The neurophysiology of the alternating leg muscle activation (ALMA) during study of one patient before and after treatment with pramipexole, *Sleep Med* 7:63–71, 2006.
10. Wichniak A, Tracik F, Geisler P, et al: Rhythmic foot movements while falling asleep, *Mov Disord* 16:1164–1170, 2001.
11. American Academy of Sleep Medicine. International classification of sleep disorders, ed 3, Darien, IL, 2014, American Academy of Sleep Medicine.
12. Fantini ML, Michaud M, Gosselin N, et al: Periodic leg movements in REM sleep behavior disorder and related autonomic and EEG activation, *Neurology* 59 (12):1889–1894, 2002.
13. Consens F, Chervin RD, Koeppe RA, et al: Validation of polysomnographic score for REM sleep behavior disorder, *Sleep* 28:993–997, 2005.
14. Lapierre O, Montplaisir J: Polysomnographic features of REM sleep behavior disorder: development of a scoring method, *Neurology* 42:1371–1374, 1992.
15. Frauscher B, Iranzo A, Gaig C, et al: Normative EMG values during REM sleep for the diagnosis of REM sleep behavior disorder, *Sleep* 35(6):835–847, 2012.
16. Montplaisir J, Gagnon JF, Fantini ML, et al: Polysomnographic diagnosis of idiopathic REM sleep behavior disorder, *Mov Disord* 25(13):2044–2051, 2010.
17. Iranzo A, Frauscher B, Santos H, et al, for the SINBAR (Sleep Innsbruck Barcelona) Group: Usefulness of the SINBAR electromyographic montage to detect the motor and vocal manifestations occurring in REM sleep behavior disorder, *Sleep Med* 12(3):284–288, 2011.
18. Frauscher B, Iranzo A, Högl B, et al: Quantification of EMG activity during REM sleep in multiple muscles in REM sleep behavior disorder, *Sleep* 31:724–731, 2008.
19. Winkelman JW, James L: Serotonergic antidepressants are associated with REM sleep without atonia, *Sleep* 27(2):317–321, 2004.

Identifying Movements During Sleep

QUESTIONS

1. In Figure P27-1, a 180-second tracing during non–rapid eye movement (NREM) sleep is shown. How many periodic limb movements (PLMs; leg movements [LMs] in a PLM series) are present in these 180 seconds? Assume that three PLMs are present in the epochs preceding and following the depicted segment.

2. What pattern of LMs is noted in the 30-second tracing in Figure P27-2?

3. What type of monitoring is needed to diagnose the problem noted in the tracing shown in Figure P27-3?

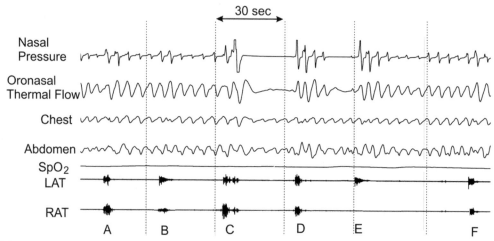

FIGURE P27-1 ■ A 180-second tracing during non–rapid eye movement (NREM) sleep. *LAT*, Left anterior tibial; *RAT*, right anterior tibial. Assume four PLMs are present to the left and another four PLMs are present to the right of the 180 segment.

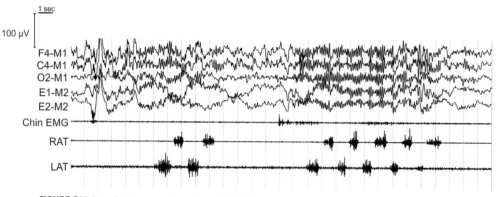

FIGURE P27-2 ■ A 30-second tracing. *LAT*, Left anterior tibial; *RAT*, right anterior tibial.

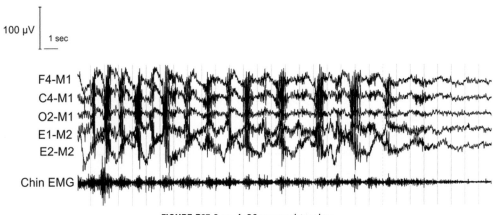

100 μV

1 sec

F4-M1

C4-M1

O2-M1

E1-M2

E2-M2

Chin EMG

FIGURE P27-3 ■ A 30-second tracing.

ANSWERS

1. **Answer:** Three PLMs. The LMs at the end and start of the two apneas (C, D, E) are not counted. The LMs at A, B, and F occur simultaneously on different legs are each considered are one leg movement. This assumes sufficient PLMs are present before and following the depicted segment so that there are at least four contiguous PLMs (minimum of four to define a PLM series).

Discussion: Leg movements occurring from 0.5 seconds before a respiratory event to 0.5 seconds after a respiratory event are not counted as PLMs. These events are thought to be associated with the respiratory events. Note that a PLM series can continue even if interrupted by a respiratory event. For example if a LM occurs 3 seconds after an obstructive apnea it can be considered part of a PLM series before the apnea so long as the time between the last LM preceding the apnea and the LM following the apnea is no more than 30 seconds. In patients with both frequent respiratory events and frequent LMs, it may be difficult to determine what phenomenon is the primary event. (Are LMs associated with respiratory events, or are the changes in respiration due to arousals from LMs?). An increase in respiration may occur, following an arousal associated with LMs and a subsequent fall in respiration on the return to sleep. In Figure P27-4, associated with the LM and arousal, a big breath is followed by smaller breaths followed by another LM and arousal. Are the LMs causing arousal and the appearance of respiratory events because of the large breaths following arousal? The presence of signs of air flow limitation such as flattening of the nasal pressure or snoring prior to the arousal would support the impression that a respiratory arousal caused by high respiratory effort is the primary event with an LM associated with the arousal. However, in patients with both frequent LMs and frequent respiratory events, scoring may be challenging. In one study (Yang et al) of patients with obstructive sleep apnea (OSA), respiratory events associated with LMs were associated with a greater increase in heart rate. It is not known if the LMs are simply a marker for a more significant arousal or if they play a role in the arousal process.

2. **Answer:** Alternating leg movement activity (ALMA)

Discussion: The frequency of ALMA bursts are 0.5 to 3 hertz (Hz) (maximum distance onset to onset is 2 seconds). The minimum distance onset to onset for LMs forming part of a PLM series is 5 seconds. A minimum of four electromyography (EMG) bursts must have occurred to diagnose ALMA. The bursts alternate between the legs. ALMAs often occur during arousal as noted in Figure P27-2.

3. **Answer:** Audio monitoring

Discussion: Bruxism (Box P27-1) (tooth grinding or clenching) may occur during any stage of sleep or be associated with arousal from sleep. It is most common in stages N1 and N2 and least common during rapid eye movement (REM) sleep. During sleep, jaw contractions are either tonic (jaw

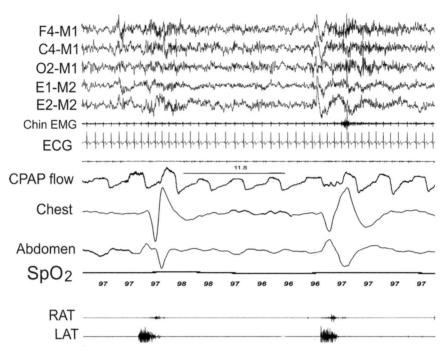

FIGURE P27-4 ■ Is the appearance of a reduction in airflow between leg movements caused by a larger than normal breath following the arousal or due to a reduction in airflow due to upper airway narrowing? Here, the air flow profile following arousal is relatively round. Note the large breath at each arousal.

BOX P27-1	Scoring Bruxism

The following rules define *bruxism*:
1. Bruxism may consist of brief (phasic) or sustained (tonic) elevations of chin electromyography (EMG) activity that are at least **twice the amplitude of the background EMG.**
2. Brief elevations of chin EMG activity are scored as bruxism if they are **0.25 to 2 seconds in duration** and if **at least three such elevations occur in a regular sequence.**
3. Sustained elevations of chin EMG activity are scored as bruxism, if the **duration is more than 2 seconds.**
4. A period of at least 3 seconds of stable background chin EMG must occur before a new episode of bruxism can be scored.
5. Bruxism may be scored reliably by audio in combination with polysomnography PSG by a **minimum of two audible tooth grinding episodes per night of PSG** in the absence of epilepsy.

American Academy of Sleep Medicine: *International classification of sleep disorders*, ed 3, Darien, IL, 2014, American Academy of Sleep Medicine.

---

clenching) or phasic (intermittent bursts of activity) termed rhythmic masticatory muscle activity (RMMA). Of note, a diagnosis of bruxism consists of more than detection of RMMA; audible tooth grinding must be present (see Fundamentals 16). Audio recording is needed to confirm that the recorded RMMA is, indeed, bruxism (minimum of two episodes of audible tooth grinding or clenching episodes per night). The identification of bruxism in the AASM scoring manual is based on the chin EMG. However, in some patients the muscle artifact in the EEG and EOG due to the RMMA may be more prominent than changes in the chin EMG.

TABLE P27-1	**Characteristics of HFT and ALMA versus PLMs**			
	Leg Movement Bursts	**Duration**	**Burst Frequency**	**Sleep Required**
HFT	Minimum of 4 Not alternating	250–1000 milliseconds (msec)	0.3–4.0 Hz (0.25–3.3 seconds between bursts)	No
ALMA	Minimum of 4 Alternating	100–500 msec	0.5–3.0 Hz (0.33–2 seconds between bursts)	No
PLMS	Minimum of 4	0.5–10 seconds	5–90 seconds	Yes

ALMA, Alternating leg movement activity; *HFT*, hypnagogic foot tremor; *PLMS*, periodic limb movement series.

CLINICAL PEARLS

1. LMs during respiratory events are (from 0.5 seconds before to 0.5 seconds after a respiratory event) not counted as PLMs. In some patients with both frequent respiratory events and frequent LMs, it may be difficult to determine the primary event.

2. ALMA EMG bursts have a higher frequency than LMs in a PLM series. The maximum distance between ALMA bursts (onset to onset) is 2 seconds, which is much less than the minimum distance between LM bursts in a PLM series (5 seconds) (Table P27-1).

3. Audio monitoring is needed to confirm a diagnosis of bruxism. A diagnosis of bruxism requires the characteristic electroencephalography (EEG) or electromyography (EMG) pattern of rhythmic masticatory activity as well as at least two audible episodes of clenching or grinding of teeth. The rhythmic activity associated with bruxism may be more prominent in the EEG and electrooculography (EOG) derivations than in the chin EMG is some patients.

BIBLIOGRAPHY

American Academy of Sleep Medicine: *International classification of sleep disorders*, ed 3, Darien, IL, 2014, American Academy of Sleep Medicine.

Berry RB, Brooks R, Gamaldo CE, et al: for the American Academy of Sleep Medicine: *The AASM manual for the scoring of sleep and associated events: rules, terminology and technical specifications*, Version 2.0, Darien, IL, 2012, American Academy of Sleep Medicine. www.aasmnet.org, Accessed?

Stoohs RA, Blum HC, Suh BY, Guilleminault C: Misinterpretation of sleep-breathing disorder by periodic limb movement disorder, *Sleep Breath* 5(3):131–137, 2001.

Walters AS, Lavigne G, Hening W, et al: The scoring of movements in sleep, *J Clin Sleep Med* 3:155–167, 2007.

Yang CK, Jordan AS, White DP, Winkelman JW: Heart rate response to respiratory events with or without leg movements, *Sleep* 29(4):553–556, 2006.

A Child with Repeated Movements During Sleep

A 5-year-old male was evaluated for snoring and daytime behavior problems. His mother also reported that he was observed to have repeated movements during sleep. The child was not taking any medications. A 30-second tracing is shown in Figure P28-1.

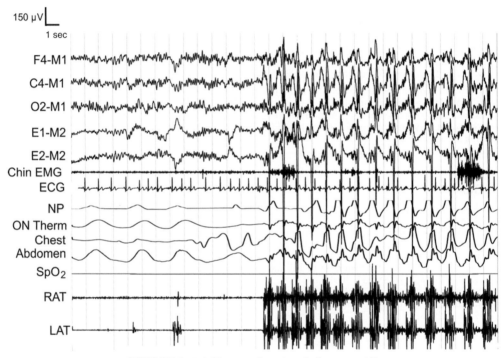

FIGURE P28-1 ■ A 30-second tracing during stage W.

QUESTION

1. What does the 30-second tracing show?

ANSWER

1. **Answer:** Rhythmic movements (RMs) during sleep

   Discussion: The sleep related rhythmic movement disorder (RMD) is characterized by repetitive, stereotypical, and rhythmic motor behaviors (not tremors) that occur predominantly during drowsiness or sleep and involve large muscle groups. The occurrence of significant clinical consequences differentiates RMD from developmentally normal sleep-related movements. Diagnostic criteria for

---

BOX P28-1 | **Sleep Related Rhythmic Movement Disorder: Diagnostic Criteria ICSD-3[1]**

Criterial A to D must be met

A. The patient exhibits repetitive, stereotypical, and rhythmic motor behaviors involving large muscle groups.

B. The movements are predominantly sleep related, occurring near nap or bedtime, or when the individual appears drowsy or asleep.

C. The behaviors result in a significant complaint as manifest by at least one of the following:*

1. Interference with normal sleep
2. Significant impairment in daytime function
3. Self-inflicted bodily injury or likelihood of injury if preventive measures are not taken

D. The rhythmic movements are not better explained by another movement disorder or epilepsy.

---

*When no clinical consequences of the rhythmic movements are present, the rhythmic movements are simply noted, but the term *rhythmic movement disorder* is not used.

---

the sleep-related RMD are listed in Box P28-1. A diagnosis of RMD versus RMs implies clinical consequences (or potential consequences), including evidence of bodily injury or the potential for injury if preventative measures are not applied. A number of types of RMD have been described:

1. Body rocking type: The whole body is rocked while on the hands and knees.
2. Head banging type: The head is forcibly moved, striking an object.
3. Head rolling type: The head is moved laterally, typically while the patient is in a supine position.
4. Other type: Includes body rolling, leg rolling, and leg banging.

Rhythmic humming or inarticulate sounds often accompany the body, head, or limb movements and may be quite loud. Head banging often occurs in the prone position, with repeated lifting of the head or the entire upper torso, and forcible banging of the head back down into the pillow or mattress.

At 9 months of age, 59% of all infants have been reported to exhibit one or more of the following sleep-related RMs: body rocking (43%), head banging (22%), or head rolling (24%). At 18 months, the overall prevalence has been reported to decline to 33% and by 5 years to only 5%. Most pediatric studies have found no gender difference in the prevalence of RMD.[1-3] The disorder can persist into childhood and adulthood. In some studies, an association between RMD and attention deficit disorder was observed. Over 50 cases of RMD have been reported in adolescents and adults, with a male preponderance found in adults.[4,5]

RMs have been reported in association with restless legs syndrome (RLS), obstructive sleep apnea (OSA), narcolepsy,[6] REM sleep behavior disorder (RBD),[5-7] and attention-deficit-hyperactivity disorder (ADHD). RMs may be used as conscious strategy to relieve the urge to move or the uncomfortable sensations associated with RLS. With continuous positive airway pressure (CPAP), obstructive sleep apnea (OSA)–associated RMD often improves.[8-9] Individuals with narcolepsy may initiate RM to terminate episodes of sleep paralysis.[6]

Video-polysomnography (PSG) studies have shown RMs to occur most often in association with stages N1 and N2 sleep. In one study, 46% occurred while the subject was falling asleep (stage W) or during NREM sleep; 30% during both NREM and REM sleep; and 24% only during REM sleep. The exclusively REM-related RMs occur more frequently in adults.

The *AASM Scoring Manual* rules for scoring the PSG features of RMD are listed in Box P28-2. In most patients, electroencephalography (EEG) shows normal activity between episodes of rhythmic behavior (although often obscured by movement artifact). A frequency of 0.5 to 2 Hz corresponds to a duration between movements of 0.5 to 2 seconds.

BOX P28-2 | *AASM Scoring Manual* **Rules for Scoring the Polysomnography Features of Rhythmic Movement Disorder**

1. The following define the polysomnographic characteristics of rhythmic movement disorder:
   a. The minimum frequency for scoring rhythmic movements is 0.5 hertz (Hz).
   b. The maximum frequency for scoring rhythmic movements is 2.0 Hz.
   c. The minimum number of individual movements required to make a cluster of rhythmic movements is four movements.
   d. The minimum amplitude of an individual rhythmic burst is two times the background electromyography (EMG) activity.

Note: Time-synchronized video-polysomnography (PSG), in addition to PSG is needed to make the diagnosis.

Often no treatment is needed for the RMD unless a risk of self-injury or the potential for self-injury exists. In others with violent movements, bed padding may be necessary.

In the present patient, the video showed head banging. In Figure P28-1, the RMs are seen as rhythmic activity in multiple channels—especially prominent in the leg tracings—but also in channels recording respiration. RM artifact is noted in the EEG and electrooculography (EOG) channels. The frequency of RMs in this patient is about 1 hertz (Hz). The chief consequence was parental concern about the child injuring himself. However, no injury had been noted because the banging occurred against a soft mattress. A diagnosis of rhythmic movements but not the rhythmic movement disorder was made. Parental reassurance was given. The PSG showed snoring but no OSA.

REFERENCES

1. American Academy of Sleep Medicine: *International classification of sleep disorder*, ed 3, Darien, IL, 2014, American Academy of Sleep Medicine.
2. Berry RB, Brooks R, Gamaldo CE, et al., for the American Academy of Sleep Medicine: *The AASM manual for the scoring of sleep and associated events: rules, terminology and technical specifications*, Version 2.03, Darien, IL, 2012, American Academy of Sleep Medicine. www.aasmnet.org, Accessed July 3, 2014.
3. Mayer G, Wilde-Frenz J, Kurella B: Sleep related rhythmic movement disorder revisited, *J Sleep Res* 16:110–116, 2007.
4. Stepanova I, Nevsimalova S, Hanusova J: Rhythmic movement disorder in sleep persisting into childhood and adulthood, *Sleep* 28:851–857, 2005.
5. Xu Z, Anderson KN, Shneerson JM: Association of idiopathic rapid eye movement sleep behavior disorder in an adult with persistent, childhood onset rhythmic movement disorder, *J Clin Sleep Med* 5:374–375, 2009.
6. Pizza F, Moghadam KK, Franceschini C, et al: Rhythmic movements and sleep paralysis in narcolepsy with cataplexy: a video-polygraphic study, *Sleep Med* 11:423–425, 2010.
7. Manni R, Terzaghi M: Rhythmic movements in idiopathic REM sleep behavior disorder, *Mov Disord* 22:1797–1800, 2007.
8. Chirakalwasan N, Hassan F, Kaplish N, et al: Near resolution of sleep related rhythmic movement disorder after CPAP for OSA, *Sleep Med* 10:497–500, 2009.
9. Gharagozlou P, Seyffert M, Santos R, Chokroverty S: Rhythmic movement disorder associated with respiratory arousals and improved by CPAP titration in a patient with restless legs syndrome and sleep apnea, *Sleep Med* 10:501–503, 2009.

Subjective and Objective Measures of Sleepiness

Excessive daytime sleepiness (EDS) is defined as sleepiness that occurs in a situation when an individual would usually be expected to be awake and alert. EDS is said to affect at least 5% of the general population. Causes of EDS include sleep deprivation or inadequate sleep, a number of sleep disorders (obstructive sleep apnea [OSA], narcolepsy, idiopathic hypersomnia, periodic limb movement disorder [PLMD]), sleep disturbance from medical conditions, medication side effects, and depression (usually complaints of insomnia as well as hypersomnia). The degree of sleepiness may be assessed by using subjective and objective measures of sleepiness.

SUBJECTIVE MEASURES

Questionnaires such as the Stanford Sleepiness Scale or the Epworth Sleepiness Scale (ESS)[1] are measures of self-rated symptoms of sleepiness. The Stanford Sleepiness Scale (Table F17–1) measures subjective feelings of sleepiness ("fogginess, beginning to lose interest in staying awake"). A score above 3 is considered "sleepy." In contrast, the ESS measures self-rated average sleep propensity (chance of dozing) over eight common situations that almost everyone encounters. The propensity to fall asleep is rated as 0, 1, 2, or 3, where 0 corresponds to "never" and 3 to "a high chance of dozing" (Table F17–2). The maximum score is 24, and normal is assumed to be 10 or less. ESS scores of 16 or greater are associated with severe sleepiness.

The correlation between the ESS and objective measures of sleepiness is low, and in some studies, the two measures were not correlated. The conflicting findings may depend on the methods and the population evaluated. The multiple sleep latency test (MSLT), an objective measure of sleepiness, determines a **mean sleep latency (MSL)** during five naps spread across the daytime hours

TABLE F17–1 Stanford Sleepiness Scale

Degree of Sleepiness	Scale Rating
Feeling active, vital, alert, or wide awake	1
Functioning at high levels, but not at peak; able to concentrate	2
Awake, but relaxed; responsive but not fully alert	3
Somewhat foggy, let down	4
Foggy; losing interest in remaining awake; slowed down	5
Sleepy, woozy, fighting sleep; prefer to lie down	6
No longer fighting sleep, sleep onset soon; having dreamlike thoughts	7
Asleep	X

TABLE F17–2 Epworth Sleepiness Scale

Situation: "Usual Way of Life in Recent Times"	Chance of Dozing Score 0, 1, 2, 3
Sitting and reading	0–3
Watching television	0–3
Sitting, inactive in a public place (e.g., a theater or a meeting)	0–3
As a passenger in a car for an hour without a break	0–3
Lying down to rest in the afternoon when circumstances permit	0–3
Sitting talking to someone	0–3
Sitting quietly after a lunch without alcohol	0–3
In a car, while stopped for a few minutes in the traffic	0–3
Total	0–24 (0–10 = normal)

Adapted from Johns MW: A new method for measuring daytime sleepiness: the Epworth Sleepiness Scale, *Sleep* 14:540-545, 1991.
0 = Would **NEVER** doze
1 = **SLIGHT** chance of dozing
2 = **MODERATE** chance of dozing
3 = **HIGH** chance of dozing

(short latency = greater sleepiness). A higher ESS was correlated with a lower MSL in some[1] but not all studies.[2] The ESS correlates roughly with the severity of obstructive sleep apnea[3] and improves (lower score) after continuous positive airway pressure (CPAP) treatment.[4] Although it is not a perfect metric, the ESS is easy to administer, is a standard part of the evaluation of most sleep patients, and is repeated at each clinic visit for patients on PAP treatment.

OBJECTIVE MEASURES OF SLEEPINESS OR THE ABILITY TO STAY AWAKE

Multiple Sleep Latency Test

The MSLT is used to quantify the degree of daytime sleepiness and to support a diagnosis of narcolepsy.[5–8] The two main MSLT findings are the mean sleep latency (MSL), an objective measure of the tendency to fall asleep and the number of sleep-onset rapid eye movement (REM) periods (SOREMPs). **Sleep latency** is the time from lights-out (LO) to the beginning of the first epoch of any stage of sleep. The shorter the sleep latency, the greater the objective sleepiness. SOREMPs on the MSLT are defined as REM sleep within 15 minutes of **clock time** following sleep onset. Normal individuals are expected to have 0 or 1 SOREMP. The MSLT must be preceded by polysomnography (PSG) during the patient's normal sleep period to document an adequate amount of nocturnal sleep (minimum total sleep time [TST] = 360 minutes) and absence of another sleep disorder that may explain daytime sleepiness and abnormal MSLT findings. Many factors may alter the findings of the MSLT, so considerable clinical judgment is needed to avoid an error in interpretation. A population-based study of the Wisconsin Sleep Cohort found multiple SOREMPs in 13.1% of males and 5.6% of females.[9,10]

Mean Sleep Latency Findings

An MSL of <10 minutes is said to be consistent with excessive sleepiness (<5 minutes severe sleepiness; 5–10 moderate sleepiness; 10–15 mild or borderline sleepiness), but as seen in Table F17-3, up to 30% of normal individuals have an MSL of <8 minutes.[8] Patients with narcolepsy have a very short MSL on average (around 3 minutes), but up to 16% have an MSL >5 minutes. Patients with idiopathic hypersomnia and OSA have moderate sleepiness (MSL in the 6 to 7 min range), but a wide range of values exists in these groups.

TABLE F17-3	MSL Findings on the MSLT
	MSL (min) (mean ± SD)
Normal	10.4 ± 4.3 (four naps) 11.6 ± 5.2 (five naps) 30% MSL <8 min 16% MSL <5 min
Narcolepsy	3.1 ± 2.9 (Diagnostic criteria <8 min) 16% MSL >5 min
Idiopathic hypersomnia	6.2 ± 3.0 (Diagnostic criteria ≤8 min)
Sleep apnea	7.2 ± 6.0 min
Traditional MSL ranges	<5 min = severe sleepiness 5 to <10 = moderate sleepiness >10 to 15 = mild (borderline) sleepiness

Data from Arand D, Bonnet M, Hurwitz T, et al: A review by the MSLT and MWT Task Force of the Standards of Practice Committee of the AASM. The clinical use of the MSLT and MWT, *Sleep* 28:123-144, 2005.
min, Minutes; *MSL,* mean sleep latency; *MSLT,* multiple sleep latency test; *SD,* standard deviation.

MSLT Protocol

The MSLT consists of five naps started every 2 hours, with the first nap started 1.5 to 3 hours after the termination of nocturnal sleep[5–7] (Table F17–4). For a more detailed listing of the protocol, see Reference 7. Although not addressed in the most recent MSLT standard of practice guidelines, prior versions specified that the patient change to daytime attire after awakening from the PSG. Standard frontal, central, occipital, electrooculography (EOG) and chin electromyography (EMG) monitoring is recommended. At the start of the MSLT, the standard instruction is *"Please lie quietly, assume a comfortable position, keep your eyes closed, and try to fall asleep."* Each MSLT nap is terminated if no sleep occurs within 20 minutes of LO (maximum sleep latency is 20 minutes). If sleep occurs, the MSLT continues for another 15 minutes of **clock time** (from sleep onset). If REM sleep occurs within this period, an SOREMP is said to have occurred. Between naps, the individual stays out of bed and is prevented from sleeping. Medications that may affect daytime sleepiness or the propensity for REM sleep are withheld for 2 weeks preceding the study. The individual is instructed to maintain a normal sleep schedule with adequate sleep. Some sleep centers have patients complete a sleep log. The ICSD-3[11] recommends that actigraphy be used to document normal sleep for 1 or 2 weeks prior to the MSLT. A urine drug screen is used in many sleep centers to document absence of medications that may affect the MSLT results.

TABLE F17–4 Comparisons of MSLT and MWT Protocols

	MSLT	MWT (40 min)
Preceding PSG	Required	If clinically indicated
Naps/trials	5	4
Nap/trial times	2-hr intervals starting 1.5–3 hr after PSG ends	2-hr intervals starting 1.5–3 hr after wakeup time
Sleeping posture/ light	Ad lib, supine, lateral	Sitting up in bed with head supported Dim light behind the patient
Test termination	No sleep for 20 min after start of study After 15 min from **onset** of first stage of sleep ("clock time")	No sleep for 40 min after start of study After first epoch of unequivocal sleep (three consecutive epochs of stage N1 or a single epoch of any other stage of sleep)
Sleep latency	First epoch of sleep	First epoch of sleep (15 consecutive sec in a 30-sec epoch)
REM periods	Monitoring for 15 min of clock time after sleep onset to detect SOREMPs	N/A Amount of all stages of sleep specified in report
Additional considerations	Sleep logs "may be obtained" for 1 to 2 wks before MSLT Stop cigarette smoking at least 30 min before nap Abstain from caffeine day of study Stop stimulating activities, including vigorous activity, for at least 15 min before nap	No guidance No guidance No guidance No guidance

Adapted from Johns MW: A new method for measuring daytime sleepiness: the Epworth Sleepiness Scale, *Sleep* 14:540-545, 1991; Littner MR, Kushida C, Wise M, et al: Practice parameters for clinical use of the multiple sleep latency test and the maintenance of wakefulness test, *Sleep* 28:113-121, 2005.

hr, Hour; *min,* minutes; *MSLT,* multiple sleep latency test; *MWT,* maintenance of wakefulness; *N/A,* not applicable; *PSG,* polysomnography; *REM,* rapid eye movement; *SOREMP,* sleep-onset REM sleep period; *wk,* week.

Indications for the MSLT

The indications for the MSLT[7] are listed in Table F17-5. The MSLT is used to support a diagnosis of narcolepsy in a patient with complaints of daytime sleepiness. If the test is not diagnostic, it may be repeated if a high suspicion for narcolepsy exists. The test is not indicated to determine the degree of sleepiness in a patient with sleep apnea (treated or untreated).

Diagnosis of Narcolepsy with the MSLT

The MSLT criteria to support a diagnosis of narcolepsy[9] include a MSL ≤ 8 minutes and ≥ 2 SOREMPs. In the ICSD-3, a SOREMP on the nocturnal PSG may count for one of the two SOREMPs. Other reasons for abnormal MSLT findings such as untreated sleep apnea, prior sleep or REM sleep deprivation or restriction, or recent withdrawal of an REM sleep–suppressing medication should be ruled out. Use of the MSLT in children and adolescents is discussed in Patients 32 and 33.

Interpretation of the MSLT

In normal individuals, the MSL on a five-nap MSLT exceeds that on a four-nap MSLT. MSL

TABLE F17-5 When the MSLT Is and Is NOT Indicated

MSLT Indicated
- Confirmation of suspected narcolepsy (Standard)
- Suspected idiopathic hypersomnia (Option)—to help differentiate idiopathic hypersomnia from narcolepsy

MSLT Not Indicated (Standard)
- Routine evaluation of patients with OSA
- Change in sleepiness in OSA after CPAP treatment
- Evaluation of sleepiness in medical or neurologic conditions (other than narcolepsy)
- Evaluation of sleepiness in insomnia

Repeat MSLT Indicated (Standard)
- Initial MSLT affected by extraneous or unusual conditions
- Appropriate study conditions not present during initial testing
- Ambiguous or uninterpretable findings
- Clinical suspicion of narcolepsy not confirmed by an earlier MSLT

From reference 7.
CPAP, continuous positive airway pressure; *MSLT,* multiple sleep latency test; *OSA,* obstructive sleep apnea.
Level of evidence: standard > guideline > option.

TABLE F17-6   **MSLT Findings in Patients Evaluated for Daytime Sleepiness**

	Narcolepsy with Cataplexy*	Narcolepsy without Cataplexy†	Sleep-Related Breathing Disorder
≥2 SOREMP+MSL <5 min	67%	75%	4%
≥2 SOREMP+MSL <8 min	71%	91%	6%
SOREMP on PSG	33%	24%	1%

Data from Aldrich MS, Chervin RD, Malow BA: Value of the multiple sleep latency test (MSLT) for the diagnosis of narcolepsy, *Sleep* 1997;20:620-629.
MSL, Mean sleep latency; *MSLT*, multiple sleep latency test; *PSG*, polysomnography; *SOREMP*, sleep-onset *REM* sleep period.
*Narcolepsy diagnosed on basis of cataplexy even if MSLT did not meet criteria.
†Diagnosed by repeat MSLT if necessary).

tends to increase with age and is shortest on the third or fourth nap. Of note, generally, a breakfast is provided 1 hour before the first nap and a light lunch between naps 2 and 3. The requirement of ≥2 SOREMPs is much more specific for narcolepsy than a short MSL (30% of normals have a MSL <8 minutes). Causes of a "false-positive MSLT" include untreated sleep apnea (Table F17-6), a habitually delayed sleep period, prior sleep deprivation or restriction, and recent withdrawal of an REM sleep–suppressing medication. A minimum of 360 minutes of sleep should be recorded on the nocturnal PSG for the MSLT results to be considered reliable. If only the first two naps have SOREMPs, one should always consider the possibility that these are caused by a normally delayed awakening time (typical in adolescents). False-negative MSLTs may occur with the concurrent use of REM sleep–suppressing medication and in patients with a diagnosis of narcolepsy based on a history of cataplexy. A large meta-analysis of the MSLT found two or more SOREMPs had a sensitivity of 0.78 and specificity of 0.93 for the diagnosis of narcolepsy.[8] In a study by Aldrich et al. that combined patients with narcolepsy with and without cataplexy, the sensitivity was 0.78. (MSL <8 minutes and 2 or more SOREMPs). In the absence of cataplexy or a low cerebrospinal fluid (CSF) hypocretin level, a diagnosis of narcolepsy depends on the MSLT. Thus, a false-negative MSLT calls for repeat testing when the initial MSLT was negative. The false-negative rate of the MSLT was lower in a recent study requiring that cataplexy be associated with presence of the human leukocyte antigen (HLA) DQB1*602 allele (eliminating false-positive cataplexy). The requirement of both cataplexy and the presence of the HLA DQB1*602 is based on the fact that virtually all patients with hypocretin deficiency and cataplexy are positive for this HLA antigen. In that study, the sensitivity was 92% for identifying patients with narcolepsy and hypocretin

deficiency. In any case, false-negative MSLT results are not rare. Patients with disorders associated with SOREMP on the MSLT may also have a nocturnal SOREMP (on the PSG). In the study of Aldrich et al., a nocturnal SOREMP was present in 33% of those with narcolepsy plus cataplexy and 24% of the time in those with narcolepsy without cataplexy (see Table F17-6). In the study and Andlauer et al.,[12] the finding of a nocturnal SOREMP had a high positive predictive value (PPV) for narcolepsy with hypocretin deficiency but was present in only 50% of the patients.

Diagnosis of Narcolepsy in a Patient with OSA

A low proportion of patients with untreated OSA may have MSLT findings consistent with narcolepsy.[13,14] OSA must be adequately treated before MSLT is performed to avoid a false-positive result. Use of the MSLT to evaluate patients with OSA on CPAP who were still sleepy (to rule out a combination of narcolepsy and OSA) was not addressed in the most current MSLT practice parameters. In prior parameters, it was suggested that the PSG be performed on CPAP to document effective treatment and the MSLT be performed on CPAP.[5,6] In this case, the PAP device flow is often recorded along with derivations to detect sleep. A reasonable period of PAP treatment and objective measures of adherence (over several weeks) should precede the MSLT.

Maintenance of Wakefulness Test

The maintenance of wakefulness (MWT) was designed to test the patient's ability to stay awake.[13] The test differs from MSLT in a number of ways (see Table F17-4). Although the MWT has been used in both the 20-minute and the 40-minute versions,[7,15–17] the longer test was recommended by the American Academy of Sleep Medicine (AASM) practice parameters.

The MWT has been used to assess the effects of sleep disturbance and treatment on the ability of patients to stay awake as reflected by MSL (longer MSL better ability to stay awake).[14,15] The MWT tests characteristics different from those tested by the MSLT. For example, some patients with a short MSL on the MSLT may have a normal sleep latency on the MWT. In research, the MWT is often used to document the effects of treatment from alerting agents.

Specific Indications for the Use of the MWT

The AASM practice parameters for the use of the MWT list specific indications:[7]
1. The MWT 40-minute protocol may be used to assess an individual's ability to remain awake when his or her ability to remain awake constitutes a public or personal safety issue. (Option)
2. The MWT may be indicated in patients with excessive sleepiness to assess response to treatment. (Guideline)

MWT Protocol

The recommended 40-minute MWT protocol is outlined by the AASM practice parameters (see Table F17–4).[7] A four-nap protocol is standard. Note that sleep latency is defined as the time from LO to the start of any epoch of sleep. The requirement of a preceding PSG is left up to the clinician (optional). In contrast to the MSLT, during the MWT, the patient sits upright in bed (head and shoulders comfortably supported), and the instruction before LO is: *"Please sit still and remain awake for as long as possible. Look directly ahead of you, and do not look directly at the light."* Of note, it is essential that the testing individual be observed and not allowed to use extreme measures (hitting self, moving in bed) to maintain alertness.

Each MWT nap lasts a maximum of 40 minutes after LO. The nap is terminated if no sleep has occurred in 40 minutes, if three consecutive epochs of stage N1 are noted, or any single epoch of other stages of sleep are noted. A low-intensity light is present behind the patient's head just out of the visual field (usually a nightlight).

MWT Normative Data

Normative data for the MWT from a systematic review of MWT studies[8] are provided in Table F17-7. Using the 40-minute MWT, 59% of patients were able to stay awake for

TABLE F17-7	Normative Data for the Maintenance of Wakefulness Test (MWT)
MSL (mean ± SD)	30.4 ± 11.2
MSL lower limit (95% confidence interval)	8 min
MSL > 8 min	97.5% of normal individuals
MSL = 40 min (stay awake in all naps)	59% of normal individuals

From Arand D, Bonnet M, Hurwitz T, et al: A review by the MSLT and MWT Task Force of the Standards of Practice Committee of the AASM. The clinical use of the MSLT and MWT, *Sleep* 28:123-144, 2005.
min, Minutes; *MSL*, mean sleep latency; *SD*, standard deviation; *SL*, sleep latency based on the time from lights-out until the first epoch of any stage of sleep.

40 minutes on each nap. The 95% lower confidence level was 8 minutes (97.5% had MSL >8 minutes). Banks et al.[16] studied normal subjects and found that MSL to the first epoch of unequivocal sleep during the 40-minute trial MWT was 36.9 ± 5.4 (standard deviation [SD]) minutes. The lower normal limit, defined as 2 SD below the mean, was therefore 26.1 minutes. In this study, the SD was much lower than in the systematic review.

Conversely, these data do little to set a standard for individuals in whom alertness is essential for personal and public safety. Certainly, staying awake for all trials is an appropriate expectation for individuals requiring the highest level of safety. Therefore, whereas an MSL less than 8 minutes is abnormal, an MSL of 8 to 40 minutes is of uncertain significance. A "normal" MWT finding is no guarantee of what will happen in the work environment. The ability to maintain alertness (different than the ability to maintain wakefulness) may depend on adherence to treatment, prior TST, medication side effects, and circadian factors. A study of patients with OSA during actual 90-minute driving sessions on the road, with a driving instructor intervening if necessary, determined inappropriate line crossing[17] based on video recording. Two groups, one "very sleepy" with an MWT MSL less than 19 minutes and one "sleepy" with an MSL of 20 to 33 minutes, had significantly higher line crossings compared with controls and patients with mild sleepiness (MWT MSL 34–40 minutes). This study suggested that an MSL <33 minutes is consistent with impaired alertness to perform a task such as driving. Of note, the sleep latency on the MWT increases with age similar to the sleep latency on the MSLT.[7]

Relationship between the MSLT and the MWT

Some of the differences in MSLT and MWT protocols are outlined in Table F17-4. When Sangal and associates[18] administered both the MSLT and the MWT to a group of patients with EDS, the correlation between MSL scores on the two tests was significant but low ($r = 0.41$; $p < 0.001$). Several individuals did not fall asleep during the MWT but had some degree of daytime sleepiness as assessed by the MSLT. Table F17-8 illustrates classification of a group of OSA patients according to MSL (low or high) on four-nap MSLT and MWT. The study found that 15% of the patients were sleepy (MSL low) but able to stay awake (MWT high).

TABLE F17-8 Comparison of MSLT and MWT in Sleep Apnea Patients (N = 170)*

Sleep Apnea	MWT MSL Low	MWT MSL High
MSLT MSL high	15%	34%
MSLT MSL low	36%	15%

Data from Sangal RB, Thomas L, Mitler MM: Maintenance of wakefulness test and multiple sleep latency test: measurements of different abilities in patients with sleep disorders, *Chest* 101:898-902, 1992.

MSL, Mean sleep latency; *MSLT*, multiple sleep latency test; *MWT*, maintenance of wakefulness test.

*Cutoff low and high MSLT and MWT based on median values for the studies (7.5-min MSL on the MSLT and 30-min MSL on the MWT).

Note: 15% of patients were in the sleepiest group by MSLT but by MWT were in the group better at maintaining wakefulness.

CLINICAL PEARLS

1. The ESS measures self-rated average sleep propensity (chance of dozing) over eight common situations. The scale ranges from 0 to 24 with 10 or less being considered normal.

2. The MSLT objectively measures the tendency to fall asleep (MSL) and the propensity to have SOREMPs.

3. The MSLT consists of five naps spaced every 2 hours beginning 1.5 to 3 hours after the wake-up time.

4. The MSLT should be preceded by a PSG to detect causes of sleepiness such as sleep apnea and to verify adequate sleep before the MSLT. The MSLT findings are not considered reliable if less than 360 minutes of sleep are recorded.

5. The MSLT diagnostic criteria for narcolepsy include an MSL ≤8 minutes and two or more SOREMPs. A SOREMP occurring on the PSG may be counted as one of the two required SOREMPs. However, a negative MSLT does *not* absolutely rule out narcolepsy, as the sensitivity of the MSLT for diagnosing narcolepsy is about 78% to 92% (depending on the study).

6. The MSLT diagnostic criteria for idiopathic hypersomnia include an MSL ≤8 minutes and 0 to 1 SOREMPs in five naps (and the preceding nocturnal sleep study).

7. In patients with OSA, adequate treatment must precede the MSLT as untreated OSA can result in an abnormal MSLT. Up to 6% of untreated patients with OSA will have a MSLT meeting criteria for narcolepsy.

8. If narcolepsy is suspected in patients with known OSA, the evaluation includes a PSG on CPAP to document good treatment and adequate sleep and a subsequent MSLT on CPAP. This assumes a period of adequate treatment for the OSA before testing.

9. Medications that may affect MSLT sleep latency (stimulants, sedatives) or the number of SOREMPs (REM sleep–suppressing medications) should be withdrawn for 10 days to 2 weeks before testing, if possible.

10. The MWT objectively quantifies a patient's ability to remain awake in a situation predisposing to sleep (dimly lit room, sitting on a bed). The use of four naps of up to 40 minutes in duration is recommended. Each MWT nap is terminated after 40 minutes if no sleep has been recorded, after three consecutive epochs of stage N1, or after a single epoch of any other sleep stage (N2, N3, or R). Sleep latency is defined as the time from lights out until the *first epoch of any stage of sleep*.

REFERENCES

1. Johns MW: A new method for measuring daytime sleepiness: the Epworth Sleepiness Scale, *Sleep* 14:540–545, 1991.
2. Benbadis SR, Mascha E, Perry MC, et al: Association between the Epworth Sleepiness Scale and the multiple sleep latency test in a clinical population, *Ann Intern Med* 130:289–292, 1999.
3. Gottlieb DJ, Whitney CW, Bonekat WH, et al: Relation of sleepiness to respiratory disturbance index, *Am J Respir Crit Care Med* 159:502–507, 1999.
4. Patel SR, White DP, Malhotra A, et al: Continuous positive airway pressure therapy in a diverse population with obstructive sleep apnea, *Arch Intern Med* 163:565–571, 2003.
5. Carskadon MA: Guidelines for the multiple sleep latency test, *Sleep* 9:519–524, 1986.
6. Standards of Practice Committee, American Sleep Disorders Association: The clinical use of the multiple sleep latency test, *Sleep* 15:268–276, 1992.
7. Littner MR, Kushida C, Wise M, et al: Practice parameters for clinical use of the multiple sleep latency test and the maintenance of wakefulness test, *Sleep* 28:113–121, 2005.
8. Arand D, Bonnet M, Hurwitz T, et al: A review by the MSLT and MWT Task Force of the Standards of Practice Committee of the AASM. The clinical use of the MSLT and MWT, *Sleep* 28:123–144, 2005.
9. Singh M, Drake CL, Roth T: The prevalence of multiple sleep-onset REM periods in a population-based sample, *Sleep* 29:890–895, 2006.
10. Mignot E, Lin L, Finn L, et al: Correlates of sleep-onset REM periods during the Multiple Sleep Latency Test in community adults, *Brain* 129:1609–1623, 2006.
11. American Academy of Sleep Medicine: *International classification of sleep disorders*, ed 3, Darien, IL, 2014, American Academy of Sleep Medicine.
12. Andlauer O, Moore H, Jouhier L, et al: Nocturnal rapid eye movement sleep latency for identifying patients with narcolepsy/hypocretin disorder, *JAMA Neurol* 70(7):891–902, 2013.

13. Aldrich MS, Chervin RD, Malow BA: Value of the multiple sleep latency test (MSLT) for the diagnosis of narcolepsy, *Sleep* 20:620–629, 1997.
14. Chervin RD, Aldrich MS: Sleep onset REM periods during multiple sleep latency tests in patients evaluated for sleep apnea, *Am J Respir Crit Care Med* 161:426–431, 2000.
15. Doghramji K, Mitler MM, Sangal RB, et al: A normative study of the maintenance of wakefulness test (MWT), *Electroencephalogr Clin Neurophysiol* 103:554–562, 1997.
16. Banks S, Barnes M, Tarquinio N, et al: The maintenance of wakefulness test in normal healthy subjects, *Sleep* 27(4):799–802, 2004.
17. Philip P, Sagaspe P, Taillard J, et al: Maintenance of wakefulness test, obstructive sleep apnea syndrome and driving risk, *Ann Neurol* 64:410–416, 2008.
18. Sangal RB, Thomas L, Mitler MM: Maintenance of wakefulness test and multiple sleep latency test: measurements of different abilities in patients with sleep disorders, *Chest* 101:898–902, 1992.

PATIENT 29

Two Patients with Questionable MSLT Results

Patient A: You are asked to render a second opinion on the presence or absence of narcolepsy in a 24-year-old woman. Two years ago, the patient had an episode of syncope, but a concern existed about possible cataplexy. The patient underwent polysomnography (PSG) and a multiple sleep latency test (MSLT). The PSG showed adequate sleep (actually total sleep time [TST] was slightly prolonged), and the MSLT showed a sleep latency of 4 minutes with two sleep-onset rapid eye movement periods (SOREMPs). The patient denies cataplexy, and her Epworth sleepiness scale is 6/24 (normal). She does not believe that she has narcolepsy.

QUESTION

1. What questions do you ask patient A to make a decision about the presence or absence of narcolepsy?

Patient B: A 16-year-old male presents for evaluation of daytime sleepiness. He fell asleep while driving, and his car ran off the road. He does not remember being sleepy before the event and reports that he was able to continue driving. The patient denies falling asleep during school, although his mother has received reports otherwise. His grades are excellent. He goes to bed at midnight on weeknights, falls asleep within 10 minutes, and arises, with difficulty, at 6:30 AM. On weekends, he sleeps from 2 AM until noon, with a 10-minute sleep latency. He denies leg restlessness, cataplexy, hypnagogic hallucinations, or sleep paralysis. He consumes two to three caffeinated beverages per day. He has no history of serious illness or trauma. The patient was instructed to increase his sleep time (mainly by going to bed earlier) for at least 2 weeks before sleep testing. The results of the preceding polysomnography and MSLT are shown in Table P29-1 and the sleep diary in Figure P29-1.

TABLE P29-1	**Polysomnography and Multiple Sleep Latency Test Results**		
Lights out: 10:00PM	Lights on: 6:00 AM		
Total Recording time	480 minutes	Stage N1 (%TST)	5%
Total Sleep time			
Sleep Latency			
REM latency			
Wake after Sleep Onset			
Apnea-hypopnea Index			
MSLT			
Mean Sleep Latency	4 minutes		
Sleep Onset REM Periods	2 (naps 1 and 3)		
Drug Screen	Negative		

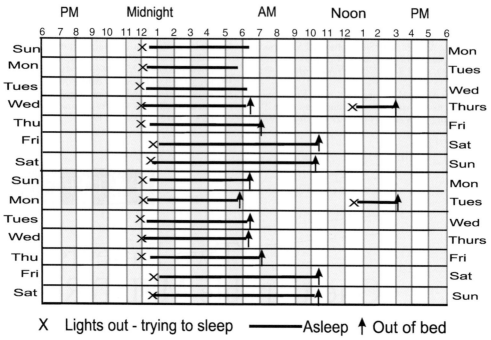

X Lights out - trying to sleep ——Asleep ↑ Out of bed

FIGURE P29-1 ■ Sleep diary (sleep log) for the week before the multiple sleep latency test (MSLT).

QUESTIONS

1. For Patient A, what questions do you ask to make a decision?

2. For Patient B, what is your diagnosis?

ANSWERS

1. **Answer:** Inquire about medications and the quality and amount of sleep prior to the previous MSLT.

   Discussion: The American Academy of Sleep Medicine (AASM) practice parameters for the MSLT state: "Sleep logs may be obtained for 1 week prior to the MSLT to assess sleep-wake schedules." Most sleep centers require that patients complete a sleep diary for at least 7 days prior to testing and regularize their sleep (obtain adequate sleep). Ideally, patients should get at least 7 hours of sleep each night. Sleep restriction may reduce mean sleep latency (MSL) on the MSLT and sometimes result in SOREMPs. If adequate sleep is not obtained prior to the MSLT, this may cause a false-positive result. In addition, the AASM practice parameters state that **MSLT results are "suspect" (unreliable) unless at least 360 minutes of sleep are not recorded on the PSG preceding the MSLT.** When questioned about her sleep before the MSLT, patient A reported that her husband was overseas during the time of her sleep tests and that she was home by herself with a 4-month-old infant. No family member was available to help with child care. She also reported that she had decreased and interrupted sleep prior to the MSLT. Her sister flew in from another state to care for the patient's child while sleep testing was performed. The patient was not on any medications prior to sleep testing. Given the absence of current daytime sleepiness or cataplexy and the history of extremely restricted sleep before prior sleep testing, the second opinion was that the patient did not have narcolepsy and that the MSLT findings were caused by sleep restriction.

2. **Answer:** Behaviorally induced insufficient sleep syndrome (BIISS) and an honest patient.

   Discussion: Although the MSLT results for patient B meet the criteria for the diagnosis of narcolepsy, the sleep diary (see Figure P29-1) reveals that the patient is getting approximately 6 hours of sleep except on weekends. This makes the MSLT findings unreliable. The second fact is that the amount of sleep on PSG preceding the MSLT was <360 minutes, making the results "suspect." The patient reported that he found sleeping in the sleep center very uncomfortable and was "nervous" about the test. The AASM practice parameters state that the "mean sleep latency is influenced by the quantity of prior sleep, sleep fragmentation, clinical sleep disorders such as obstructive sleep apnea, and circadian phase. For these reasons polysomnography must be performed immediately before the MSLT during the patient's usual major sleep period as determined by the sleep clinician. Sleep logs may be obtained for 1 week prior to the MSLT to assess sleep-wake schedules."

This patient was very honest about his sleep (admitting that he did not follow instructions), but others are not so reliable. Bradshaw et al. evaluated a group of 50 patients undergoing an MSLT. They compared self-reported average nightly sleep duration (6.13 ± 1.23 hours), sleep log-recorded average nightly sleep duration (6.99 ± 0.85 hours), and actigraphy-measured average nightly sleep duration (5.56 ± 1.50 hours) for the 2-week period immediately preceding the MSLT. Only actigraphy-measured average nightly sleep duration correlated with the MSL on the MSLT. This study suggests that actigraphy would be valuable in assessing pretesting sleep quality and regularity. Both sleep logs and self-report overestimated the amount of sleep. Janjua et al. reported on a patient who had an abnormal MSLT that normalized over several days of sleep extension. Thus, one night of recovery sleep of adequate duration may not be enough to provide reliable MSLT results. Of interest, after sleep deprivation, on the first night of recovery sleep, stage N3 rebound occurs, but stage R rebound may not occur until the second night of recovery sleep. In the current patient, the relative amount of stage R was increased. A possible explanation is the curtailment of the final hours of sleep by the early rise time for school (relative loss of stage R sleep). In any case, while the study results did not rule out narcolepsy, the results could not be used to reliably make a diagnosis of this disorder. Instead, the patient's parents did not allow him to drive until he clearly obtained at least 7 hours of sleep each night. An earlier bedtime was mandated, and electronic media, including cell phones and tablets, were not permitted in the patient's bedroom after 10 PM. The daytime sleepiness dramatically improved with the additional sleep.

CLINICAL PEARLS

1. At a minimum, the patient should be required to keep a sleep log for at least 7 days (preferably 14) before an MSLT. It is likely that actigraphy is more reliable and may eventually be mandated before the MSLT.

2. When reviewing information about a prior MSLT, it is important to question the patient regarding the quantity and quality of sleep prior to the study and about the medication being taken at the time of the study. These factors may significantly alter the interpretation of the MSLT results.

3. A statement about sleep quantity and timing for the week prior to the PSG/MSLT should be included in the MSLT result interpretation.

4. Sleep restriction of even a modest degree may cause false-positive MSLT results.

5. The AASM practice parameters for the MSLT state: "**The use of the MSLT to support a diagnosis of narcolepsy is suspect if TST on the prior night sleep is less than 6 hours.**" The lights-out time and the lights-on time for PSG preceding the MSLT should be adjusted to allow an adequate amount of sleep (at least 7 hours, if possible). For individuals with a routinely late wake-up time, recording time may need to be extended beyond 6:00 AM.

BIBLIOGRAPHY

Bradshaw DA, Yanagi MA, Pak ES, et al: Nightly sleep duration in the 2-week period preceding multiple sleep latency testing, *J Clin Sleep Med* 3(6):613–619, 2007.

Devoto A, Lucidi F, Violani C, Bertini M: Effects of different sleep reductions on daytime sleepiness, *Sleep* 22(3):336–343, 1999.

Dinges DF, Pack F, Williams K, et al: Cumulative sleepiness, mood disturbance, and psychomotor vigilance performance decrements during a week of sleep restricted to 4-5 hours per night, *Sleep* 20(4):267–277, 1997.

Janjua T, Samp T, Cramer-Bornemann M, et al: Clinical caveat: prior sleep deprivation can affect the MSLT for days, *Sleep Med* 4(1):69–72, 2003.

Littner MR, Kushida C, Wise M, et al., for the Standards of Practice Committee of the American Academy of Sleep Medicine. Practice parameters for clinical use of the multiple sleep latency test and the maintenance of wakefulness test, *Sleep* 28:113–121, 2005.

Marti I, Valko PO, Khatami R, et al: Multiple sleep latency measures in narcolepsy and behaviourally induced insufficient sleep syndrome, *Sleep Med* 10(10):1146–1150, 2009.

Turpen KB, Wagner MA: Dangerous driver, *J Clin Sleep Med* 7(No. 4):408–410, 2011.

Evaluating an MSLT

A 20-year-old male complains of excessive daytime sleepiness for a period of 12 months. No history of cataplexy exists. Polysomnography (PSG) was unremarkable, with a normal amount of sleep and (REM) sleep. No respiratory events were noted. The patient then had a multiple sleep latency test (MSLT) and the results of five naps are show below (Figure P30-1 to P30-5). **Lights out (LO) occurred at the end of the epoch denoted by LO.**

QUESTIONS

1. What is the sleep latency and REM latency of each nap?

2. What is the mean sleep latency (MSL)?

3. Does the MSLT support a diagnosis of narcolepsy?

LO at end of epoch 30					Nap 1				
Epoch	30	31	32	33	34	35	36	37	38	39
Stage	LO	W	W	W	N1	N1	N1	N2	N2	N2
Epoch	40	41	42	43	44	45	46	47	48	49
Stage	N1	N2	N2	R	R	R	R	R	R	W
Epoch	50	51	52	53	54	55	56	57	58	59
Stage	W	W	N1	N1	N2	N2	N2	R	R	R
Epoch	60	61	62	63	64	65	66	67	68	69
Stage	R	R	R	R						

FIGURE P30-1 ■ Nap 1.

LO at end of epoch 70					Nap 2				
Epoch	70	71	72	73	74	75	76	77	78	79
Stage	LO	W	W	W	W	W	W	W	W	W
Epoch	80	81	82	83	124	125	126	127	128	129
Stage	W	W	W	W	W	W	W	W	W	W
Epoch	90	91	92	93	94	95	96	97	98	99
Stage	W	W	W	W	W	W	W	W	W	W
Epoch	100	101	102	103	104	105	106	107	108	109
Stage	W	W	W	W	W	W	W	W	W	W
Epoch	110	111	112	113	114	115	116	117	118	119
Stage	W									

FIGURE P30-2 ■ Nap 2 lights out (LO) is at the end of epoch 70.

LO at end of epoch 110				Nap 3					
Epoch	110	111	112	113	114	115	116	117	118	119
Stage	LO	W	W	N1	N1	N1	N1	N1	N2	W
Epoch	120	121	122	123	124	125	126	127	128	129
Stage	W	N1	N1	N2	N2	N2	N2	N2	N2	N3
Epoch	130	131	132	133	134	135	136	137	138	139
Stage	N2	N3	N3	N3	N3	N3	N3	N3	N3	N3
Epoch	140	141	142	143	144	145	146	147	148	149
Stage	N3	N3	N3							

FIGURE P30-3 ■ Nap 3 lights out (LO) at the end of epoch 110.

LO at end of epoch 150				Nap 4					
Epoch	150	151	152	153	154	155	156	157	158	159
Stage	LO	W	W	W	W	W	R	R	W	N1
Epoch	160	161	162	163	164	165	166	167	168	169
Stage	N1	N2	N2	R	R	W	N1	N2	N2	N2
Epoch	170	171	172	173	174	175	176	177	178	179
Stage	N2	N2	N3	N3	N3	N3	N3	W	N1	N1
Epoch	180	181	182	183	184	185	186	187	188	189
Stage	N2	N2	N3	N3	N3					

FIGURE P30-4 ■ Nap 4 lights out (LO) at the end of epoch 150.

LO at end of epoch 190					Nap 5				
Epoch	190	191	192	193	194	195	196	197	198	199
Stage	LO	W	W	W	W	N1	W	W	W	W
Epoch	200	201	202	203	204	205	206	207	208	209
Stage	N1	N2	N2	N2	N2	N2	N2	W	W	W
Epoch	210	211	212	213	214	215	216	217	218	219
Stage	N1	N1	N1	N2	N2	N2	N2	W	R	R
Epoch	220	221	222	223	224	225	226	227	228	229
Stage	R	R	R	R	R	R	R	R	R	R

FIGURE P30-5 ■ Nap 5 lights out (LO) at the end of epoch 190.

ANSWERS

Answer: For questions for 1 and 2, see Table P30-1.

TABLE P30-1   **MSLT Findings**

Nap	Sleep Latency	REM Latency
Nap 1	1.5 min (3 epochs)	4.5 min (9 epochs)
Nap 2	20 min (40 epochs)	No REM
Nap 3	1 min (2 epochs)	No REM
Nap 4	2.5 min (5 epochs)	0 min (0 epochs)
Nap 5	2.0 min (4 epochs)	11.5 (23 epochs)
	Mean sleep latency = 5.4 min	3 SOREMPs

min, Minutes; *MSL*, mean sleep latency; *REM*, rapid eye movement; *SOREMPs*, sleep-onset REM periods.

3. **Answer:** Yes, the MSL is ≤8 minutes,[1,4] and three sleep-onset REM periods (SOREMPs) are present.

Discussion: In the standard MSLT protocol, naps occur every 2 hours, starting about 1.5 hours after the normal wake-up time. For example, for a wake-up time of 6:30 AM, naps might start at 8:00 AM, 10:00 AM, noon, 2:00 PM and 4:00 PM. Before nap 1, a light breakfast is provided. After the second nap, the individual being tested has a light lunch. Before each nap, the subject is given the chance to use the restroom. Between naps, the individual is out of bed and *observed to ensure that no sleep occurs.*

During each nap following lights-out, the patient is given **20 minutes to fall asleep**. If sleep does not occur (any stage of sleep), the nap is terminated. In this case, the sleep latency is 20 minutes. After sleep onset, each nap study is continued for another **15 minutes of clock time** (not sleep time). This procedure is followed even if stage R occurs soon after sleep onset. In some sleep centers, the MSLT is terminated after four naps when two or more SOREMPs have already been recorded. However, this practice is not recommended. It is possible that the physician reading the study may not agree with the technologist's detection of stage R on some naps.

In nap 1 of the present study, the first epoch of sleep was 34. The sleep latency was three epochs or 1.5 minutes (start of first epoch of monitoring to start of first epoch of sleep). The REM latency sleep was 9 epochs or 4.5 minutes (start of the first epoch of sleep to the start of the first epoch of stage R). Note that the nap continued for 15 minutes (clock time) following the start of the first epoch of sleep. This was done even though many epochs of stage R were recorded. In nap 2, no sleep occurs for 20 minutes, and therefore the sleep latency is 20 minutes. In nap 3, the sleep latency is short (1 minute), but no REM sleep occurs. In nap 4, the sleep latency is 5 epochs or 2.5 minutes. The first epoch of sleep is stage R, so the REM latency = 0 minutes. In nap 5, the sleep latency is 2 minutes (4 epochs), as the first epoch of sleep is epoch 195. The REM latency is 11.5 minutes (23 epochs), as the first epoch of stage R is epoch 218.

CLINICAL PEARLS

1. The REM latency is the time from the start of the first epoch of sleep until the first epoch of stage R.
2. If no sleep occurs within 20 minutes, the MSLT is terminated, and the sleep latency is 20 minutes.
3. The MSLT continues for 15 minutes (30 epochs) of clock time following sleep onset regardless of the occurrence of REM sleep.

BIBLIOGRAPHY

Standards of Practice Committee, American Sleep Disorders Association: The clinical use of the multiple sleep latency test, *Sleep* 15:268–276, 1992.

Littner MR, Kushida C, Wise M, et al: Practice parameters for clinical use of the multiple sleep latency test and the maintenance of wakefulness test, *Sleep* 28:113–121, 2005.

Arand D, Bonnet M, Hurwitz T, et al: A review by the MSLT and MWT Task Force of the Standards of Practice Committee of the AASM. The clinical use of the MSLT and MWT, *Sleep* 28:123–144, 2005.

Scoring an MSLT and an MWT

Patient A: The following are consecutive 30-second epochs during a multiple sleep latency test (MSLT) nap (Figures P31-1 and P31-2). Lights-out is at the **start** of epoch 1. For brevity, only the first four epochs are shown.

Epoch 1

Epoch 2

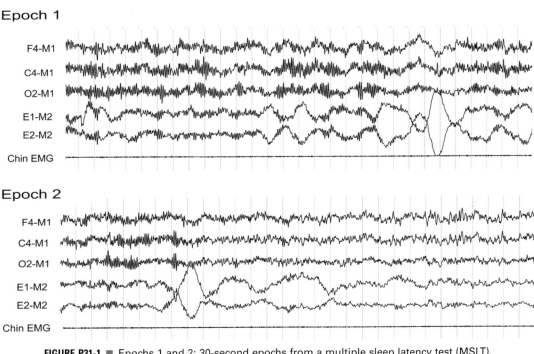

FIGURE P31-1 ■ Epochs 1 and 2: 30-second epochs from a multiple sleep latency test (MSLT).

Epoch 3

Epoch 4

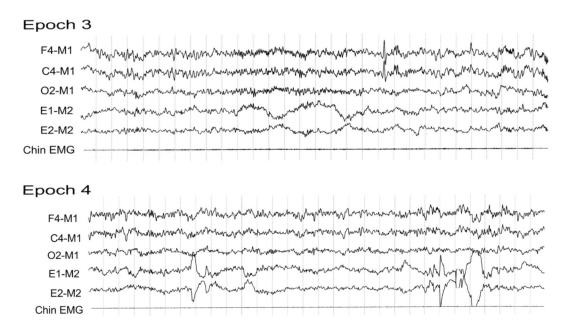

FIGURE P31-2 ■ Epochs 3 and 4: 30-second epochs from a multiple sleep latency test (MSLT).

Patient B: A nap from a maintenance of wakefulness test (MWT) is shown in Figure P31-3.

Patient C: A patient with obstructive sleep apnea (OSA) lost his driver's license when he had an automobile accident believed to have been caused by sleepiness. Since that time, he has been strictly adhering to continuous positive airway pressure (CPAP) treatment. He required the addition of modafinil 400 milligrams (mg) daily to normalize his alertness. He is trying to demonstrate his alertness to the agency determining his eligibility for reinstatement of his driver's license. Polysomnography (PSG) was performed, and it documented a very good treatment outcome and sleep quality with the current level of CPAP. The CPAP information was downloaded, and it again confirmed excellent adherence. An MWT that included 40-minute naps was performed (Table P31-1). The patient took his normal dose of modafinil upon awakening as he does at home.

QUESTIONS

1. What is the sleep latency and rapid eye movement (REM) latency of this nap?

2. What is the sleep latency? Why was the nap stopped after epoch 56?

3. Does the MWT demonstrate sufficient ability to stay awake for the patient to be allowed to drive?

LO at end of epoch 30					Nap 1				
Epoch	30	31	32	33	34	35	36	37	38	39
Stage	LO	W	W	W	W	W	W	W	W	W
Epoch	40	41	42	43	44	45	46	47	48	49
Stage	W	W	W	W	W	W	W	W	W	W
Epoch	50	51	52	53	54	55	56	57	58	59
Stage	W	W	W	W	N1	N1	N1			

FIGURE P31-3 ■ A nap from a maintenance of wakefulness test (MWT).

TABLE P31-1 **MWT Results for Patient C**

Nap	Sleep Latency (min)
Nap 1	34
Nap 2	40
Nap 3	35
Nap 4	40
Mean	37.2

min, Minutes; *MWT*, maintenance of wakefulness test.

ANSWERS

1. **Answer:** Sleep latency 0.5 minutes (30 seconds), REM latency 1 minute

   Discussion: Epoch 1 is stage W, as alpha rhythm is present for the majority of the epoch. Epoch 2 is stage 1, as the alpha rhythm occupies less than 50% of the epoch. Therefore, the sleep latency is 30 seconds (one epoch). Epoch 3 is stage N1. Note slow eye movements and the vertex sharp wave at the end of the epoch. Epoch 4 is stage R (REMs, low chin [EMG] tone). Therefore, the REM latency is 2 epochs or 1 minute. It is important to remember that the REM latency is defined as the time from sleep onset to stage R onset.[1,2]

2. **Answer:** Sleep latency is 23 epochs (11.5 minutes). The MWT is stopped after three consecutive epochs of stage N1 or a single epoch of any other stage of sleep (stages N2, N3, and R).

   Discussion: The MWT differs from the MSLT as summarized in Table P31-2. It is important to understand the differences:

   During the MWT the patient should be observed, and interventions to maintain wakefulness such as hitting or constantly moving are not allowed. No guidance is provided for the patient taking or not taking the usual stimulant medications. The goal of the study would determine whether taking medications was appropriate. If the goal is to determine the objective alertness during the current clinical state, it would seem logical for the patient to mimic the usual circumstances of life (e.g., all regular medications).

3. **Answer:** The MWT provides evidence for the ability to stay awake.

   Discussion: A systematic review of normative data for the 40-minute MWT found that 59% of patients were able to stay awake for 40 minutes on each nap. The 95% lower confidence limit was 8 minutes (97.5% had MSL >8 minutes). The standard deviation (SD) was wide, making it difficult to set a lower limit of normal. Banks et al.[3] studied normal subjects and found a mean sleep latency to the first epoch of unequivocal sleep during the 40-minute trial MWT was 36.9 ± 5.4 (SD) minutes. The lower normal limit, defined as 2 SD below the mean, was therefore 26.1 minutes. In this study, the SD was much lower than in the systematic review. However, these data do little to set a standard for individuals in whom alertness is essential for personal and public safety. Certainly, staying awake for all trials is an appropriate expectation for individuals requiring the highest level of safety (airline pilots). Therefore, whereas an MWT MSL <8 minutes is abnormal, an MSL of 8 to 40 minutes is of uncertain significance. *A "normal" MWT finding is no guarantee of what will happen in the work environment.* The ability to maintain alertness (different from the ability to maintain wakefulness) may depend on adherence to treatment, prior total sleep time (TST), medication side effects, and circadian factors. Of note, the sleep latency on the MWT increases with age, as does the sleep latency on the MSLT.

   Studies using driving simulators have attempted to provide a performance-based test of alertness. A study by George et al.[7] found decreased performance in a group with OSA and a group

TABLE P31-2	**Comparison of MSLT and MWT**	
	MSLT	**MWT**
PSG before test	Required	Optional
Number of naps	5	4 (40-minute version)
Posture	In bed	Sitting in bed with head supported
Light	Dark	Dim light (light source behind the patient—5-watt night light)
Test stopped	After 20 minutes if no sleep After 15 minutes from sleep onset	After 3 consecutive epochs of stage N1 After a single epoch of stages N2, N3, or R
Command	"Please lie quietly, assume a comfortable position, keep your eyes closed, and try to fall asleep."	"Please sit still, and remain awake for as long as possible. Look directly ahead of you, and do not look directly at the light."

Adapted from reference 1.
MSLT, Multiple sleep latency test; *MWT*, maintenance of wakefulness test; *PSG*, polysomnography.

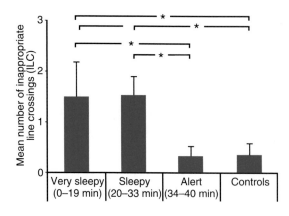

FIGURE P31-4 ■ The mean number of inappropriate line crossings (ILCs) in four groups of patients divided by the maintenance of wakefulness test (MWT) sleep latency. The very sleepy and sleepy groups had significantly more ILCs than the alert and control groups ($p < 0.05$). (From Philip P, Sagaspe P, Taillard J, et al: Maintenance of wakefulness test, obstructive sleep apnea syndrome and driving risk, *Ann Neurol* 64:410-416, 2008.)

with narcolepsy compared to a control group. However, about one half of the participants in the OSA and narcolepsy groups did as well as controls. A study by Phillip et al.[8] tested patients with OSA during actual 90-minute driving sessions on the road, with a driving instructor intervening when necessary (the test car had two steering wheels). Inappropriate line crossing (ILC) was determined by video recording. Results from three groups of patients were compared with results from controls (Figure P31-4). The very sleepy (MWT MSL 0–19 minutes) and sleepy (MWT MSL 20–33 minutes) had significantly higher number of ILCs compared with the controls. The alert patient group (MWT MSLT 34–40 minutes) performed as well as the control group. On the basis of this study, those with an MWT MSL of 34 to 40 minutes could be considered to have normal alertness to function on a task such as driving.

In the current patient, the MSL was 37.2 minutes suggesting that the patient had an ability to stay awake that would be considered normal or near-normal by most studies. His ability to stay awake would be dependent on continued use of CPAP and modafinil as the patient was doing at the time of the study. A letter stating the results of the study was sent to the state agency adjudicating requests for reinstatement of driver's licenses. The patient ultimately received a driver's license and has been accident free for 2 years.

CLINICAL PEARLS

1. Normative data for the MWT suggest a wide range in the normal ability to remain awake. It is difficult to define a "normal" lower limit of normal for the MSL. On the basis of available data, one might say that a lower limit of normal is 26 minutes or that a MSL 34 to 40 minutes represents normal alertness in some studies of driving ability.

2. The MWT differs from the MSLT in several says. Four naps of up to 40 minutes are recommended. Each nap is terminated after three consecutive epochs of stage N1 or one epoch of stages N2,N3, or R. In the MWT, the patient is sits upright in bed, with the head supported. A dim light is positioned behind the patient's head.

3. The MWT sleep latency is the time from lights-out to the first epoch of any stage of sleep.

4. About 59% of normal subjects can maintain wakefulness for all four naps in an MWT.

5. PSG is not required before the MWT but may be useful (as in patient C).

6. No guidance is provided with regard to the use of stimulants or other medications before an MWT. Most clinicians would allow patients to take their usual medications to assess the degree of alertness relevant to their daily functioning.

7. The ability to maintain alertness (different from the ability to maintain wakefulness) depends on adherence to treatment, prior total sleep time (TST), medication side effects, motivation, and circadian factors. A normal MWT is no guarantee that a patient can maintain a required degree of alertness in real life situations.

REFERENCES

1. Littner MR, Kushida C, Wise M, et al: Practice parameters for clinical use of the multiple sleep latency test and the maintenance of wakefulness test, *Sleep* 28:113–121, 2005.
2. Arand D, Bonnet M, Hurwitz T, et al: A review by the MSLT and MWT Task Force of the Standards of Practice Committee of the AASM. The clinical use of the MSLT and MWT, *Sleep* 28:123–144, 2005.

3. Banks S, Barnes M, Tarquinio N, et al: The maintenance of wakefulness test in normal healthy subjects, *Sleep* 27(4):799–802, 2004.
4. Doghramji K, Mitler MM, Sangal RB, et al: A normative study of the maintenance of wakefulness test (MWT), *Electroencephalogr Clin Neurophysiol* 103:554–562, 1997.
5. Poceta JS, Timms RM, Jeong D, et al: Maintenance of wakefulness test in obstructive sleep apnea syndrome, *Chest* 101:893–902, 1992.
6. Marshall NS, Barnes M, Travier N, et al: Continuous positive airway pressure reduced daytime sleepiness in mild to moderate obstructive sleep apnea: a meta-analysis, *Thorax* 61:430–434, 2006.
7. George CFP, Boudreau AC, Smiley A: Comparison of simulated driving performance in narcolepsy and sleep apnea patients, *Sleep* 19:711–717, 1996.
8. Philip P, Sagaspe P, Taillard J, et al: Maintenance of wakefulness test, obstructive sleep apnea syndrome and driving risk, *Ann Neurol* 64:410–416, 2008.

FUNDAMENTALS 18

Sleepiness and Sleep Complaints in Children

Prepubertal pediatric patients are less likely to complain of symptoms of sleepiness compared with adults with sleep disorders or sleep restriction. In disorders such as childhood obstructive sleep apnea (OSA), daytime sleepiness is rarely the most prominent complaint unless sleep apnea is accompanied by sleep restriction. The manifestations of sleepiness may include inattention, learning difficulty, and behavioral problems. The "BEARs" screening tool is a guide for primary physicians[1] but is also useful for sleep physicians. BEARS stands for B = bedtime issues, E = excessive daytime sleepiness, A = awakenings, R = regularity and duration of sleep, S = snoring.

For older children, a modified Epworth Sleepiness Scale (ESS) with the last item "chance of dozing in a car while stopped for a few minutes in traffic" replaced by "doing homework or taking a test." The question about sitting quietly after lunch has "without alcohol" removed. A four-item Pediatric Sleep Questionnaire (PSQ-SS)[2] has also been used (Table F18-1). Parents' answers are obtained, but the physician is encouraged to ask the child for input. In one study, the test distinguished children with sleep-disordered breathing from controls.

Survey results suggest that many parents' knowledge about the sleep needs of their children is limited.[3] In one survey study, 23% of children did not have a consistent bedtime, 25% had a bedtime later than 9 PM, 23% had at least one electronic device in the bedroom, and 56% frequently fell asleep with an adult present. Both positive and negative sleep habits tended to cluster together. Children who had irregular and late bedtimes were more than twice as likely to get insufficient sleep that those with regular and early bedtimes. About 25% of children were getting less than the recommended sleep amount for age, and just 13% of parents believed that their children were getting insufficient sleep.

TABLE F18-1	**Pediatric Sleep Questionnaire**

1. Does your child wake up feeling unrefreshed in the morning?
2. Does your child have a problem with sleepiness during the day?
3. Does your child appears sleepy during the day according to comments of a teacher or other supervisor?
4. Is your child hard to wake up in the morning? Responses are *Yes*, *No*, or *Don't Know*. If at least 2 of the 4 are positive, the child is classified as subjectively sleepy.

From Chervin RD, Hedger KM, Dillon JE, Pituch KJ: Pediatric Sleep Questionnaire (PSQ): validity and reliability of scales for sleep-disordered breathing, snoring, sleepiness, and behavioral problems, *Sleep Med* 1:21-32, 2000.

NORMAL SLEEP DURATION

As shown in Figure F18-1, the average normal sleep duration from age 6 to 10 years is from 11 to 10 hours.[4] Studies of sleep in children before the age of electronic media more accurately represent actual sleep needs. In evaluating daytime sleepiness, it is important for sleep physicians who are not pediatricians to know the usual sleep requirements. The 50th percentile sleep duration for children of 5, 10, and 15 years is approximately 11, 10, and 8.5 hours, respectively. If school wake-up time is at 6:00 AM, 10-year old children should go the bed at 8 PM. It is also important to note that while napping is common in young children, it starts to decrease at age 3 and by age 7 is uncommon (Figure F18-2). The age at which napping ceases is variable. However, a return to napping in a child who previously stopped taking naps or napping at age 7 or later may be a sign of excessive daytime sleepiness.

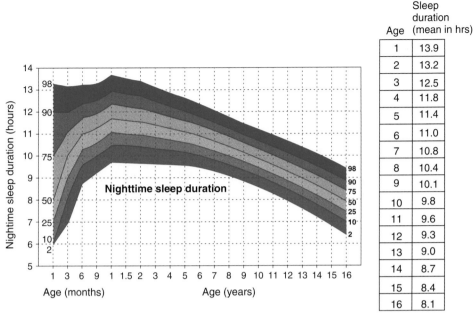

Age	Sleep duration (mean in hrs)
1	13.9
2	13.2
3	12.5
4	11.8
5	11.4
6	11.0
7	10.8
8	10.4
9	10.1
10	9.8
11	9.6
12	9.3
13	9.0
14	8.7
15	8.4
16	8.1

FIGURE F18-1 ■ ?(Redrawn from Iglowstein I, Jenni OG, Molinari L, et al: Sleep duration from infancy to adolescence: reference values and generational trends, *Pediatrics* 111:302-307, 2003.)

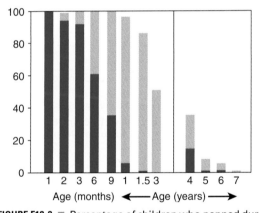

FIGURE F18-2 ■ Percentage of children who napped during the first 7 years after birth. *For 1 month to 3 years:* dark bars represent 2 or more naps per day, and light bars represent only 1 nap per day. *For 4 to 7 years:* dark bars represent napping every day, and light bars represent napping occasionally. (Redrawn from Iglowstein I, Jenni OG, Molinari L, et al: Sleep duration from infancy to adolescence: reference values and generational trends, *Pediatrics* 111:302-307, 2003.)

MSLT IN CHILDREN AND ADOLESCENTS

Much of our information about the multiple sleep latency test (MSLT) results in normal children comes from the work of Caraskadon and coworkers.[5-8] The mean sleep latency (MSL) of prepubertal children was >18 minutes, with many children not falling asleep in any naps (Figure F18-3). The MSL in adolescents is considerably lower. In addition, many adolescents have a delayed sleep phase. The study by Caraskadon et al.[6] found a delay in the timing of the dim light melatonin onset (DLMO). The DLMO is a marker of circadian phase. In the same study, sleep was monitored with actigraphy, and adolescents did *not* to go to bed earlier on school days when the wake-up time was much earlier and had reduced sleep times. In this study *two REM episodes on the MSLT occurred in 16% of participants in 10th grade, and one REM episode occurred in 48%.* When those with REM sleep on one or both morning MSLTs were compared with those without morning REM, significant differences included shorter sleep latency on the first test, less slow wave sleep the night before, and later DLMO phase in those who had morning REM. It was concluded that clinicians should be cautious about interpreting morning REM sleep episodes as abnormal.

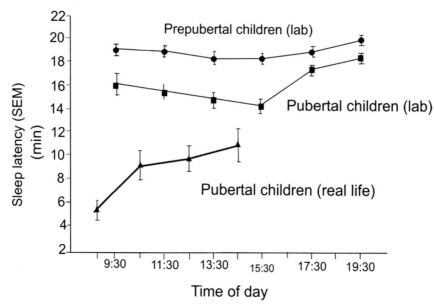

FIGURE F18-3 ■ Sleep latency (on the multiple sleep latency test [MSLT]) profiles in well-slept prepubertal (*circles*; N=22) and pubertal (*squares*; N=25) adolescents under laboratory conditions (data from reference Carskadon et al., 1980) and from pubertal adolescents under real life situations (*triangles*; N=26; data from Carskadon et al., 1998). In the former case, all participants were on a fixed sleep schedule with bedtime at 2200 and rise time at 0800; in the latter case, participants were on a self-selected schedule in which the mean bedtime was 2238 and the mean rise time was 0601. (From Jenni O, Carskadon MA: Sleep behavior and sleep regulation from infancy to adolescence—normative aspects, *Sleep Med Clin* 2: 321-329, 2007; data from Carskadon MA, Harvey K, Duke P, et al: Pubertal changes in daytime sleepiness, *Sleep* 2:453-460, 1980; Carskadon MA, Wolfson AR, Acebo C, et al: Adolescent sleep patterns, circadian timing, and sleepiness at a transition to early school days, *Sleep* 21:871-881, 1998.)

CLINICAL PEARLS

1. The normal sleep duration and sleep need in children is often unappreciated by parents and clinicians. Sleep restriction is a common cause of sleepiness in children.

2. Sleepiness in children may manifest itself as inattentive, impulsive, and aggressive behavior.

3. The 50th percentile sleep duration for children of 5, 10, and 15 years is approximately 11, 10, and 8.5 hours, respectively. Daytime sleepiness may be caused by inadequate time allowed for nocturnal sleep.

4. A return to napping is a sign of daytime sleepiness in a child.

5. Prepubertal children have a long MSL on the MSLT naps (many do not fall asleep in any naps).

6. Adolescents have a shorter sleep latency compared with prepubertal children, a delayed sleep phase, and a tendency for sleep-onset REM periods (SOREMPs) on early MSLT naps.

REFERENCES

1. Owens JA, Dalzell V: Use of the "BEARS" sleep screening tool in a pediatric residents' continuity clinic: a pilot study, *Sleep Med* 6(1):63–69, 2005.
2. Chervin RD, Hedger KM, Dillon JE, Pituch KJ: Pediatric Sleep Questionnaire (PSQ): validity and reliability of scales for sleep-disordered breathing, snoring, sleepiness, and behavioral problems, *Sleep Med* 1:21–32, 2000.
3. Owens JA, Jones C, Nash R: Caregivers' knowledge, behavior, and attitudes regarding healthy sleep in young children, *J Clin Sleep Med* 7(4):345–350, 2011.
4. Iglowstein I, Jenni OG, Molinari L, Largo RH: Sleep duration from infancy to adolescence: reference values and generational trends, *Pediatrics* 111:302–307, 2003.
5. Carskadon MA, Harvey K, Duke P, et al: Pubertal changes in daytime sleepiness, *Sleep* 2:453–460, 1980.
6. Carskadon MA, Wolfson AR, Acebo C, et al: Adolescent sleep patterns, circadian timing, and sleepiness at a transition to early school days, *Sleep* 21:871–881, 1998.
7. Carskadon MA, Dement WC: Multiple sleep latency tests during the constant routine, *Sleep* 15(5):396–399, 1992.
8. Jenni O, Carskadon MA: Sleep behavior and sleep regulation from infancy to adolescence—normative aspects, *Sleep Med Clin* 2:321–329, 2007.

A Teenager with Sleep-Onset REM

An 18-year-old female college student complained of severe daytime sleepiness but no cataplexy. The patient has fallen asleep during morning classes on several occasions. Polysomnography (PSG) followed by a multiple sleep latency test (MSLT) was ordered. The patient brought a sleep diary (Figure P32-1) of her sleep for 1 week before the study. These data, the PSG data, and the MSLT results are shown below (Tables P32-1 and P32-2).

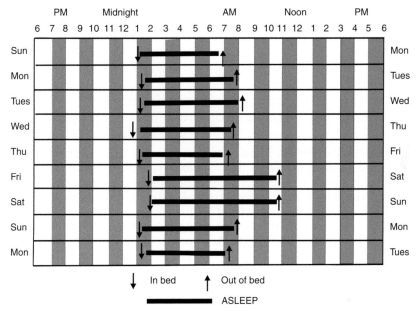

FIGURE P32-1 ■ Sleep log for the week prior to sleep testing.

TABLE P32-1 Polysomnography Results

Lights-Out:		10:00 PM	Lights-On:	06:06 AM	Normal Range
Sleep Architecture					
Total recording time	(min)	486.0			(422–470)
Total sleep time	(min)	450.0			(408–452)
Sleep efficiency	(%)	96.5			(94–98)
Sleep latency	(min)	15.0			(1–15)
REM latency	(min)	70.0			(78–122)
Sleep Stages					
Wakefulness after sleep onset	(min)	10.0			(5–20) min
			(% of TST)		
Stage N1	(min)	9.5	2.1		(2–7)%
Stage N2	(min)	200.5	44.6		(46–58)%
Stage N3	(min)	100.0	22.2		(11–24)%
Stage R	(min)	140.0	31.1		(22–29)%
AHI	0/hour				
PLMS index	4/hour				

AHI, Apnea–hypopnea index; *min*, minutes; *PLMS*, periodic limb movement series.

TABLE P32-2 **MSLT Results**

	Sleep Latency	REM Present
Nap 1	3.0 min	Yes
Nap 2	2.0 min	Yes
Nap 3	10.0 min	No
Nap 4	11.0 min	No
Nap 5	13.0 min	No
Mean	7.8	

min, Minutes; *MSLT*, multiple sleep latency test; *REM*, rapid eye movement.

QUESTION

1. What is your diagnosis?

ANSWER

1. **Answer:** False-positive MSLT because of chronically delayed sleep period and chronic sleep restriction

Discussion: The MSLT shows a reduced mean sleep latency (MSL) and two sleep-onset rapid eye movement (REM) periods (SOREMPs). Taken at face value this suggests that narcolepsy without cataplexy could be present.[1,2] However, a number of features cause concern. First, the amount of REM sleep on PSG is increased, suggestive of prior REM sleep restriction, and the nocturnal sleep latency of 15 minute is longer than expected if the patient has narcolepsy. The sleep diary shows a stable delayed sleep onset time, decreased total sleep time, and much longer sleep on the weekends. These findings and the fact that both SOREMPs were on the first two naps suggest that the results are explained by a chronically delayed sleep period and chronic sleep restriction. Also note that the shortest sleep latencies were noted on the first naps.

Limited normative MSLT data on children and adolescents are available. The majority of what is known on this topic comes from the work of Carskadon and coworkers.[3-6] Table P32-3 shows sleep latency data from children and preadolescents (Tanner stages I-V) as well as from older adolescents.[3,4] Of note, the older adolescents in this study had a sleep period between 10:00 PM and 08:00 AM. The sleep latency of children and preadolescents was significantly **longer** than that of adolescents. In Tanner 1, the MSL was almost as long as the maximum duration of testing if no sleep occurs (20 minutes). **Many children who no longer take daily naps may not sleep during any MSLT nap.** On the basis of the data in Table P32-3, one might conclude that for children up to about age 11 years (prepubertal) an MSL of <12 minutes is abnormal (more than 2 standard deviations [SD] below the mean). In this digital age, many adolescents go to bed later (and wake up earlier on school days), so the data listed in Table P32-3 may not apply to them. With such a compressed week-day sleep period, they would be expected to be even sleepier.

TABLE P32-3 **MSLT Findings in Children and Adolescents**

Stage of Development	Typical Ages	Mean Sleep Latency (minutes)	Standard Deviation
Tanner stage 1	<9 years	19.0	1.8
Tanner stage 2	9–11	18.5	2.1
Tanner stage 3	11–12.5	16.5	2.8
Tanner stage 4	12.5–14	15.5	3.3
Tanner stage 5	14+	16.1	1.5
Older adolescents		15.7	3.5

From References 3 to 6.

In addition to having a shorter sleep latency compared with prepubertal children, adolescents frequently have a delayed circadian phase, with most teenagers having bedtimes between 10:30 to 11:00 PM or later. In one study of the MSLT in 10th graders (26 subjects), **two SOREMPs** were seen in 16% of the participants and **one SOREMP** was noted in 48%.[6] The majority of the SOREMPs were observed in the morning naps. Therefore, one must be cautious about making the diagnosis of narcolepsy in adolescents based on SOREMPs that occur only in the first two naps.

A recent practice parameter publication concerning PSG and MSLT in children stated: "The collective evidence demonstrated that the MSLT is technically feasible and can provide meaningful results in developmentally normal children age 5 years and older."[7] As noted above, normative data indicate that children who are prepubertal or at early pubertal stages would be less likely to fall asleep during an MSLT compared with older adolescents, suggesting that the standard protocol may underestimate their sleepiness. Some researchers have lengthened the naps to 30 minutes in children to detect milder degrees of sleepiness. Others have suggested that an MSL of 12 minutes represents significant sleepiness.[8] However, studies in childhood narcolepsy have found the MSL to be much shorter than 8 minutes (<5 minutes), implying that the standard criteria for the mean sleep latency (≤8 minutes) will permit an accurate diagnosis of narcolepsy in most children.[9] However, one should keep in mind that an MSL from 8 to 12 minutes is consistent with daytime sleepiness in prepubertal children.

In the current patient, detailed questioning revealed that the patient rarely fell asleep in classes in the afternoon or watching TV or doing homework in the evening. A diagnosis of chronic sleep restriction and delayed sleep period rather than narcolepsy was made. The patient was instructed to go to bed earlier and keep a regular sleep schedule. A goal of at least 7 to 8 hours of sleep was recommended. An alternative to an earlier bedtime would be to schedule late morning and afternoon classes. A diagnosis of the delayed sleep phase disorder (see Patient 112) was considered. However, the sleep latency of only 15 minutes on the PSG with a lights out time of 10 PM made this diagnosis unlikely. The delayed sleep period was felt to be behaviorally induced by the desire to pursue electronic social media rather than an intrinsic delay in circadian rhythms. Patients with the delayed sleep phase also have typical onset sleep times of 2 AM or later.

CLINICAL PEARLS

1. A sleep log (diary) or actigraphy for 1 to 2 prior to the MSLT is essential for detection of chronic sleep patterns that may affect MSLT findings.

2. Adolescents and other individuals with a delayed sleep period may have two SOREMPs. Therefore, if the only REM periods occur in the first two naps of the MSLT, the results could be false positive for narcolepsy.

3. Prepubertal children above the age of daily napping have long sleep latencies during the day. For these children, an MSL of 8 to 12 minutes may be considered abnormal. The sleep latency of adolescents is shorter than that of prepubertal children.

4. Many adolescents have a delayed sleep phase and chronically short sleep time during the week because of early school start time.

REFERENCES

1. Littner MR, Kushida C, Wise M, et al: Practice parameters for clinical use of the multiple sleep latency test and the maintenance of wakefulness test, *Sleep* 28:113–121, 2005.
2. Arand D, Bonnet M, Hurwitz T, et al: A review by the MSLT and MWT Task Force of the Standards of Practice Committee of the AASM. The clinical use of the MSLT and MWT, *Sleep* 28:123–144, 2005.
3. Carskadon M: The Second decade. In Gulleminault C, editor: *Sleeping and waking disorders: indications and techniques*, Boston, 1982, Butterworth, pp 99–125.
4. Carskadon MA, Dement WC: Multiple sleep latency tests during the constant routine, *Sleep* 15:396–399, 1992.
5. Carskadon MA, Harvey K, Duke P, et al: Pubertal changes in daytime sleepiness, *Sleep* 2:453–460, 1979.
6. Carskadon MA, Wolfson AR, Acebo C, et al: Adolescent sleep patterns, circadian timing, and sleepiness at a transition to early school days, *Sleep* 21:871–881, 1998.
7. Aurora RN, Lamm CI, Zak RS, et al: Practice parameters for the non-respiratory indications for polysomnography and multiple sleep latency testing for children, *Sleep* 35(11):1467–1473, 2012.
8. Gozal D, Wang M, Pope DW Jr.: Objective sleepiness measures in pediatric obstructive sleep apnea, *Pediatrics* 108:693–697, 2001.
9. Aran A, Einen M, Lin L, et al: Clinical and therapeutic aspects of childhood narcolepsy-cataplexy: a retrospective study of 51 children, *Sleep* 33:1457–1464, 2010.

Sleep in Children

Patient A: The hypnogram of a 3-month-old child is shown in Figure P33-1. As features of stage N1, N2, and N3 were not yet developed, sleep was staged as stage W, stage N, and stage R.

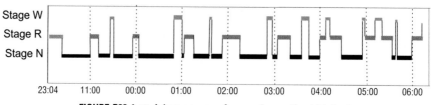

FIGURE P33-1 ▪ A hypnogram from a 3-month-old infant.

Patient B: An 8-year-old child is brought by his parents for snoring and behavior problems. The child's pediatrician is concerned about the possibility of sleep apnea. During the interview, it is determined that at age 5, the child stopped taking daytime naps. However, at age 7, he had resumed napping on the weekends. The parents also admitted that bedtime was often delayed to 9:30 to 10:00 PM. Typical wake-up time for the family was 6 AM to allow the parents to arrive at work on time.

QUESTIONS

1. How much sleep does patient A likely get in 24 hours? Is the amount of night time sleep greater than daytime sleep?

2. Is patient B getting enough sleep? What is the significance of the return of napping behavior?

ANSWERS

1. **Answer:** Patient A (3-month-old) gets about 14 to 16 hours of sleep over a 24-hour period). The hypnogram shows about 7 hours of sleep. So for this infant the amount of nighttime and daytime sleep are each about 50% of the total sleep time in a 24-hour-period.

   Discussion: The sleep of newborn term infants is typically 16 to 18 hours, equally distributed across day and night with sleep episodes of 3 to 4 hours interrupted by feeding.[1–3] By 10 to 12 months of age sleep has consolidated into a major nocturnal period of approximately 8 hours with several long naps during the day (about 14 hours of sleep over a period of 24 hours). However, there is considerable variability. The hypogram in Figure P33-1 shows about 7 hours of sleep.

2. **Answer:** A return to napping in a child who previously had stopped napping is a sign of daytime sleepiness. The estimated sleep need of a 7-year-old child is 10 to 11 hours. The child is sleeping for only 8 to 9 hours.

   Discussion: The recommended sleep time for children varies among different authorities,[1–3] but Table P33-1 shows typical recommendations. In many families, some members arrive home as late as 7 PM, and because of early sleep and work starting time, they often wake up at 6 AM. As both parents work in many families, the children must wake up with the parents to be taken to school or daycare. Electronic media provide distractions for children as they are often taken into the bedroom unless restricted by parents. These factors have resulted in inadequate sleep in many children.

TABLE P33-1	Typical Recommendations for Sleep Duration in Children and Adolescents
Age	**Duration of Sleep**
<1 year	14–16 hours
1–3 years	12–14 hours
3–6 years	10–12 hours
7–12 years	10–11 hours
12–18 years	8–9 hours

In evaluating daytime sleepiness, it is important for sleep physicians who are not pediatricians to know the usual sleep requirements for children. The 50th percentile sleep duration for children of 5, 10, and 15 years is approximately 11, 10, and 8.5 hours, respectively. If school wake-up time is 6:00 AM, 10-year-old children should go the bed between 8 and 9 PM.

CLINICAL PEARLS

1. In infants, entry into sleep via stage R is normal, and the sleep cycle (NREM to REM) is shorter (40–60 minutes) than in adults (70–90 minutes).

2. In evaluation of daytime sleepiness in children, detailed questions about sleep duration is essential. Parents may not understand the sleep requirements for normal children.

3. A return to napping in a child previously nap free is a sign of daytime sleepiness.

4. In evaluating daytime sleepiness, it is important for sleep physicians to know the usual sleep requirements for children. The 50th percentile sleep duration for children of 5, 10, and 15 years is approximately 11, 10, and 8.5 hours, respectively. If school wake-up time is at 6:00 AM, a 10-year-old child should go the bed between 8 and 9 PM.

REFERENCES

1. Kahn A, Dan B, Groswasser J, et al: Normal sleep architecture in infants and children, *J Clin Neurophysiol* 13:184–197, 1996.
2. Seldon S: Polysomnography in infants and children. In Sheldon SH, Ferber R, Kryger MH, editors: *Principles and practice of pediatric sleep medicine*, Philadelphia, 2005, Saunders, pp 49–71.
3. Iglowstein I, Jenni OG, Molinari L, Largo RH: Sleep duration from infancy to adolescence: reference values and generational trends, *Pediatrics* 111:302–307, 2003.

FUNDAMENTALS 19

Diagnosis of Obstructive Sleep Apnea Syndromes in Adults

ADULT OBSTRUCTIVE SLEEP APNEA: DIAGNOSTIC CRITERIA

The apnea–hypopnea index (AHI), defined as the number of apneas and hypopneas per hour of sleep, is the main metric used for the diagnosis of obstructive sleep apnea (OSA).[1,2] Sometimes the respiratory disturbance index (RDI) is also used, but the meaning of this metric has varied between sleep centers. The recent update to the *American Academy of Sleep Medicine (AASM) Scoring Manual*[2] defines the RDI as the number of apneas, hypopneas, and respiratory effort–related arousals (RERAs) per hour of sleep (RDI = AHI + RERA index). The definitions of respiratory events are discussed in Fundamentals 12. *The International Classification of Sleep Disorders*, 3rd edition (ICSD-3), criteria for a diagnosis of the OSA syndrome in adults[3] are displayed in Box F19-1.

Although the ICSD-3 does not use the parameter RDI, the diagnostic criteria for adult OSA are equivalent to an RDI ≥ 15/hour or an RDI ≥ 5 with symptoms or comorbidities. The criteria recognize that patients may have clinically significant disease even if asymptomatic when certain comorbidities are present (hypertension, a mood disorder, cognitive dysfunction, coronary heart disease, stroke, congestive heart failure, atrial fibrillation, or type 2 diabetes mellitus). The word "predominantly" is used because patients may have some central apneas or central hypopneas, but obstructive events predominate.

EVALUATION OF PATIENTS

Recent clinical guidelines for the evaluation, management, and long-term care of OSA in

---

BOX F19-1	ICSD-3 Diagnostic Criteria Obstructive Sleep Apnea: Adults

(A AND B) OR C SATISFY THE CRITERIA

A. The presence of one or more of the following:
 1. The patient complains of sleepiness, nonrestorative sleep, fatigue, or insomnia symptoms.
 2. The patient wakes with breath holding, gasping, or choking.
 3. The bed partner or other observer reports habitual snoring, breathing interruptions, or both during the patient's sleep.
 4. The patient has been diagnosed with hypertension, a mood disorder, cognitive dysfunction, coronary heart disease, stroke, congestive heart failure, atrial fibrillation, or type 2 diabetes mellitus.

B. Polysomnography (PSG) or out-of-center sleep testing (OCST[1]) demonstrates:
 Five or more predominantly obstructive respiratory events (apneas, hypopneas or respiratory effort–related arousals 2 [RERAs]) 3 per hour of sleep during a PSG or per hour of monitoring (OCST[1]).
 OR
C. PSG or OCST[1] demonstrates:
 Fifteen or more predominantly obstructive respiratory events (apneas, hypopneas, or RERAs)[3] per hour of sleep during a PSG or per hour of monitoring (OCST[1]).

Adapted from reference 3.
Notes:
1. OCST may underestimate the true number of obstructive respiratory events per hour because actual sleep is not usually recorded. The term respiratory event index (REI) may be used to denote event frequency based on monitoring time rather than total sleep time.
2. Respiratory effort related arousals cannot be scored using OCST because arousals cannot be identified.
3. Respiratory events defined according the latest version of the *AASM Manual for the Scoring of Sleep and Associated Events.*

TABLE F19-1 **Evaluation of Patients for OSA**

High Risk Patients for OSA	Historical Information	Physical Examination
Obesity (BMI >35)	Snoring?	Increased BMI?
Congestive heart failure	Witnessed apneas or breathing pauses?	Retrognathia?
Atrial fibrillation		Nasal obstruction?
Refractory hypertension	Gasping or choking at night?	Narrow oropharynx?
Type 2 diabetes	Hypertension?	High Mallampati Score?
Nocturnal arrhythmias	Nonrefreshing sleep?	Increased neck circumference?
CVA	Sleepiness? (Epworth Sleepiness Scale)	Evidence of cor pulmonale?
Pulmonary hypertension	Nocturia?	
High-risk driving populations	Morning headaches?	
Preoperative for bariatric surgery	Decreased concentration?	
	Memory loss?	
	Decreased libido?	
	Irritability?	

Modified from Epstein LJ, Kristo D, Strollo PJ, et al: Clinical guideline for the evaluation, management and long-term care of obstructive sleep apnea in adults, *J Clin Sleep Med* 5:263-276, 2009.
BMI, Body mass index; *CVA*, cerebrovascular accident; *OSA*, obstructive sleep apnea.

adults[4] recommended that high-risk populations for OSA be questioned in detail concerning the symptoms of OSA. A number of populations with a high prevalence of OSA have been identified, including patients with refractory hypertension, congestive heart failure, and recent or past cerebrovascular accident or transient ischemic attack (Table F19-1).

OSA SYMPTOMS AND KEY HISTORICAL POINTS

The patient with OSA or bed partner frequently reports excessive daytime sleepiness, loud habitual snoring, gasping choking, witnessed apenas, personality change, morning headache, nocturia, or nonrestorative sleep. The Epworth Sleepiness Scale (ESS) score,[5] a subjective estimate of the propensity to doze off in eight situations, is often (but not invariably) increased. The range of the scale is 0 to 24 with >10 indicating excessive daytime sleepiness (see Fundamentals 17). Only a weak correlation exists between the AHI and either subjective or objective sleepiness. A substantial percentage of patients with OSA do not report daytime sleepiness, and the absence of sleepiness should not discourage further evaluation. However, patients with more severe OSA do have, on average, greater daytime sleepiness.[6] Although men and women with OSA generally report the same symptoms, women may report more insomnia and less witnessed apnea. Women with OSA are also more likely to complain of depression, morning headache, awakenings, and fatigue.[7]

PHYSICAL EXAMINATION

The physical examination of patients with suspected OSA should include measurement of body mass index (BMI) and systemic blood pressure, as well as careful examination of the nose, ears, and oropharynx. Observation of the oropharynx usually reveals a crowded upper airway, and examination of the patient's face in profile may reveal retrognathia. The Mallampati (MP) score of the upper airway was developed to predict the risk of difficult endotracheal intubation (Figure F19-1).[8] The patient's oropharynx is examined with the patient protruding the tongue. The modified Mallampati (MMP) score, also called the *Friedman score*, is performed without the patient protruding the tongue. A high MP or MMP score (3 or 4) is associated with a greater risk of having OSA as well as OSA of greater severity. Measurement of neck circumference and observation of signs of right heart failure may also be informative. A greater neck circumference increases the risk of OSA. A neck size greater than 17 inches in men and 16 inches in women suggests the possibility of OSA.[9,10] However, a normal MP score, a thin neck, or the presence of both does not rule out OSA. It is important to note that retrognathia or a high arched palate (lateral narrowing) may also predispose a person to OSA.

LABORATORY TESTING IN OSA

Laboratory testing in patients with OSA is usually not indicated apart from routine health maintenance unless a particular problem such as hypothyroidism is suspected. In patients with severe

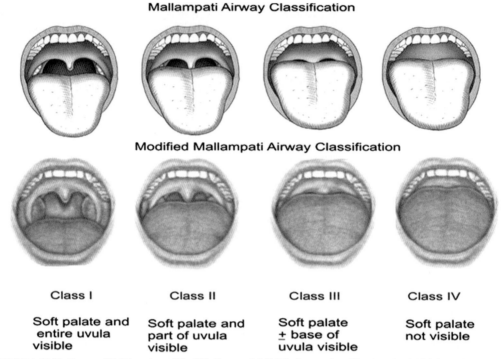

Mallampati Airway Classification

Modified Mallampati Airway Classification

Class I	Class II	Class III	Class IV
Soft palate and entire uvula visible	Soft palate and part of uvula visible	Soft palate ± base of uvula visible	Soft palate not visible

FIGURE F19-1 ■ Mallampati (MP) and modified Mallampati (MMP) airway classification. In the Mallampati maneuver, patients are instructed not to emit sounds but to open the mouth as wide as possible and protrude the tongue as far as possible. In the MMP, the patient is instructed to open the mouth as wide as possible without emitting sounds. (**MP,** Reproduced with permission from Friedman M, Tanyeri H, La Rosa M, et al: Clinical predictors of obstructive sleep apnea, *Laryngoscope* 109:1901-1907, 1999; and **MMP,** Reproduced with permission from Nuckton TJ, Glidden DV, Brownder WS, Claman DM: Physical examination: Mallampati score as an independent predictor of obstructive sleep apnea, *Sleep* 29:903-908, 2006.)

nocturnal hypoxemia, polycythemia (increased hematocrit) may be present. An unexplained elevation in the serum carbon dioxide (CO_2; composed primarily of bicarbonate [HCO_3]) on electrolyte testing is suggestive of chronic compensation for hypercapnia (in the absence of evidence for causes of metabolic alkalosis). Pulmonary function testing, chest radiography, and arterial blood gas testing are indicated in patients with a low awake arterial oxygen saturation (SaO_2) or suspected hypoventilation to evaluate the role of lung disease as a cause of impaired gas exchange and to document hypoventilation.

PREDICTION OF THE PRESENCE OF OSA

A number of clinical indices and questionnaires have been developed to predict the presence of OSA on the basis of symptoms, signs, and measurements. Although they have had some success, they are neither satisfactorily sensitive nor specific enough to be a substitute for objective documentation of the presence of OSA by a sleep study. An adaptation of a prediction rule developed by

Flemons and coworkers[9,10] used an adjusted neck circumference (see Box F19-2) to classify patients on the basis of low, moderate, or high probability. Netzer and colleagues[11] studied the utility of the Berlin Questionnaire (see Box F19-3) to predict whether patients were at high risk or low risk of OSA. The questionnaire consists of three categories: (1) snoring and witnessed apnea, (2) being

BOX F19-2	Prediction of Obstructive Sleep Apnea Based on Adjusted Neck Circumference

Neck circumference (NC) = NC measured in cm
A. If hypertension present, +4
B. If habitual snoring present, +3
C. If gasping or choking present, +3
Adjusted NC = NC + A + B + C
Probability of obstructive sleep apnea (OSA) based on adjusted NC:
<43 cm (17 inches) = low probability
43–48 cm (17–19 inches) = moderate probability
> 48 cm (19 inches) = high probability

From Flemons WW: Obstructive sleep apnea, *N Engl J Med* 347:498-504, 2002.

| BOX F19-3 | Berlin Questionnaire |

Height _____ meter (m) Weight _____ kilogram (kg) Age_____ Male/Female
Please choose the correct response to each question.

Category 1

1. Do you snore?
   a. Yes*
   b. No
   c. Don't know
   If you snore:
2. Your snoring is:
   a. Slightly louder than breathing
   b. As loud as talking
   c. Louder than talking*
   d. Very loud—can be heard in adjacent rooms*
3. How often do you snore?
   a. Nearly every day*
   b. 3–4 times/week (wk)*
   c. 1–2 times/wk
   d. 1–2 times/month (mo)
   e. Never or nearly never
4. Has your snoring ever bothered other people?
   a. Yes*
   b. No
   c. Don't know
5. Has anyone noticed that you quit breathing during your sleep?
   a. Nearly every day*
   b. 3–4 times/wk*
   c. 1–2 times/wk
   d. 1–2 times/mo
   e. Never or nearly never

Category 2

6. How often do you feel tired or fatigued after your sleep?
   a. Nearly every day*
   b. 3–4 times/wk*
   c. 1–2 times/wk
   d. 1–2 times/mo
   e. Never or nearly never
7. During your waking time, do you feel tired, fatigued, or not up to par?
   a. Nearly every day*
   b. 3–4 times/wk*
   c. 1–2 times/wk
   d. 1–2 times/mo
   e. Never or nearly never
8. Have you ever nodded off or fallen asleep while driving a vehicle?
   a. Yes*
   b. No
   If yes:
9. How often does this occur?[†]
   a. Nearly every day
   b. 3–4 times/wk
   c. 1–2 times/wk
   d. 1–2 times/mo

Category 3

10. Do you have high blood pressure?
    a. Yes
    b. No
    c. Don't know

*Items are considered positive.
[†]Item 9 in category 2 should be noted separately but is not involved in determining a positive or negative score.
If two or more items in category 1 are positive, category 1 is positive.
If two or more items in category 2 are positive, category 2 is positive.
Category 3 is positive if the answer to item 10 is positive OR if the BMI is greater than 30 kg/m^2.
Overall Scoring:
High risk of OSA: Two or more categories scored as positive.
Low risk of OSA: Only one or no category scored.

sleepy, tired, or fatigued more than three or four times a week or nodding off while driving a vehicle, and (3) the presence of hypertension or a BMI >30. After questionnaire completion, patients were studied through portable monitoring. The Berlin Questionnaire identified patients with an AHI >5 per hour (hr) (based on assignment to the high-risk group) with a sensitivity of 0.86 and a specificity of 0.77. The STOP-BANG (Snoring, Tired, Observed apnea, (blood) Pressure, Body mass index, Age, Neck circumference, Gender) Questionnaire is a screening tool that has been used for preoperative evaluation to detect sleep

apnea (see Table F19-2). A study of 2467 patients found sensitivities of 84%, 92%, and 100% for AHI cutoffs of >5/hr, >15/hr, and >30/hr.[12]

DIAGNOSTIC TESTING FOR SUSPECTED SLEEP APNEA

Attended PSG is the gold standard to determine whether OSA is present and to classify the severity.[13,14] An entire night of diagnostic monitoring or the initial diagnostic portion of

TABLE F19–2	**STOP-BANG Scoring Model**	
1. **S**noring	Do you snore loudly (loud than talking or loud enough to be heard through closed doors)?	Yes/No
2. **T**ired	Do you often feel tired, fatigued, or sleepy during daytime?	Yes/No
3. **O**bserved Apnea	Has anyone observed you stop breathing during your sleep?	Yes/No
4. Blood **P**ressure	Do you have been or are you being treated for high blood pressure?	Yes/No
5. **B**MI	BMI > 35 kilograms per meters squared (kg/m^2)?	Yes/No
6. **A**ge	Age older than 50 years old?	Yes/No
7. **N**eck Circumference	Neck circumference >40 centimeters (cm)?	Yes/No
8. **G**ender	Male?	Yes/No

High risk of OSA: answering yes to three or more items.
Low risk of OSA: answering yes to less than three items.
BMI, Body mass index.

a split (partial night) study may be used. The second part of a split study is used as a positive airway pressure (PAP) titration. The Center for Medicare and Medicaid Services (CMS) formerly required a minimum of 2 hours of sleep (not monitoring) during the diagnostic portion to qualify a patient for reimbursement of continuous PAP (CPAP) treatment. Currently, if less than 2 hours of sleep is recorded, the number of events to qualify the patient should be the same as if 2 hours of sleep had been recorded.[14] For example, if an AHI of 15/hr or higher qualifies a patient for CPAP (symptoms not required), the total number of apneas and hypopneas must be ≥30. The second part of the night typically has a greater proportion of rapid eye movement (REM) sleep (stage R). Therefore, an entire night of monitoring is usually needed for patients with milder OSA, who frequently have OSA primarily during REM sleep. However, even in more severe patients, the diagnostic portion of a split study may underestimate the severity of the AHI and the degree of arterial oxygen desaturation because relatively little REM sleep is recorded in the first part of the night. In the past, recommended criteria for performing a split study were (1) AHI ≥40/hr or AHI ≥20/hr with severe desaturation, and (2) at least 3 hours remaining for a PAP titration. However, criteria for performing a split study may depend on the patient's insurance and local practice.

The classic PSG findings in patients with OSA are listed in Box F19-4. The degree of abnormality in the sleep architecture varies with severity. Patients with severe OSA usually have a high arousal index, increases in wakefulness after sleep onset (WASO) and stage N1 sleep, and decreases in stage N3 or stage R

sleep. A typical classification of OSA severity based on the AHI (or RDI in some sleep centers) is 5 to <15/hr = mild, 15 to <30 = moderate, and ≥30 = severe OSA. The AHI (RDI) is the most widely used metric for classification of severity, but it is also important to characterize the severity of arterial oxygen desaturation. A widely accepted standard for the characterization of the severity of desaturation does not exist. It is common to present the number of desaturations (usually defined as a drop in the SaO_2 >3 or 4%), the lowest SaO_2, the average SaO_2 at desaturation, and the time below various saturations. For example, a commonly used metric is the time at or below an SaO_2 of 88%.

Because the AHI is often higher in the supine position and during REM sleep[15,16] presentation of the AHI for those conditions in the sleep study report may be useful (Table F19-3). The diagnosis of postural OSA is usually made when the AHIsupine is greater than twice the AHInonsupine (some clinicians also require the AHInonsupine to be normal). REM-associated OSA is usually defined as a normal AHI during NREM sleep associated with an elevated AHI during REM sleep. However, clinicians also use the term to denote patients with a relatively mild AHI in non-REM (NREM) sleep but moderate to severe elevation in AHI during REM sleep. An interaction between body position and sleep stage also is present. The AHI tends to be higher during supine than nonsupine REM sleep. The longest respiratory events and most severe desaturations are usually present during supine REM sleep.[16] It is important to note that in milder OSA patients, the total night AHI may vary, depending on the amounts of supine or REM sleep recorded. Since REM sleep usually

| BOX F19-4 | Polysomnography Findings in Adult Obstructive Sleep Apnea |

EEG Findings

- Increased WASO and stage N1
- Reduced stage N3
- Reduced stage R (REM sleep)
- Increased respiratory arousals

Respiratory Findings

- Snoring
- Obstructive, mixed, and central apneas
- Obstructive hypopneas
- AHI: mild 5 to <15/hr, moderate 15–30/hr, severe >30/hr

- Postural OSA AHI supine >2 × AHI nonsupine
- AHI REM > AHI NREM (common finding)
- Apnea duration REM > NREM
- Arterial Oxygen Desaturation
  - Lowest SaO_2 during REM sleep
  - Longest REM periods in the early morning hours typically associated with the lowest SaO_2

Cardiac

- Cyclic variation in heart rate

AHI, Apnea–hypopnea index; *EEG*, electroencephalogram; *NREM*, non–rapid eye movement; *OSA*, obstructive sleep apnea; *REM*, rapid eye movement; *SaO2*, arterial oxygen saturation; *WASO*, wakefulness after sleep onset.

TABLE F19-3 Typical Presentation of Respiratory Events

	Total	Supine	Nonsupine	NREM	REM
TST	360	60	300	290	70
OA	50	14	10	4	20
MA	5	0	0	0	0
CA	1	1	1	1	1
Hypopnea	40	19	5	20	4
Total events	50	34	16	25	25
AHI	8.3	34	3.2	5.2	21.4

AHI, Apnea–hypopnea index; *CA*, central apnea; *MA*, mixed apnea; *NREM*, non–rapid eye movement sleep; *OA*, obstructive apnea; *REM*, rapid eye movement sleep; *TST*, total sleep time.
Supine 16% of TST; REM 19% of TST.

comprises 20% or less of the total sleep time (TST), large changes in the REM AHI result in relatively small changes in the entire night's AHI. However, for patients with mild OSA, this may change an AHI from "normal" (e.g., 4/hr) to mild OSA (7 to 8/hr). The amount of supine sleep may have a large impact on the entire night's AHI. For the patient whose data are listed in Table F19-3, the AHI would be much higher if more supine sleep was recorded. Some sleep centers also report event duration, which is typically longer in REM sleep than in NREM sleep.

Cyclic variation in heart rate is typically noted during the repeated episodes of obstructive events (see Fundamentals 15). Heart rate slows at the start of the events and increases at event termination. Often, heart rate remains between 60 and 100 beats per minute (beats/min). A standard part of most PSG reports is to present the maximum, minimum, and average heart rates along with notations of abnormalities (premature ventricular contractions, atrial fibrillation, sinus pauses).

OUT-OF-CENTER SLEEP TESTING

The use of out-of-center sleep testing (OCST), also known as *portable monitoring* (PM), *home sleep testing* (HST), *home sleep apnea testing* (HSAT), or *limited-channel sleep testing* (LCST), is discussed in detail in Fundamentals 10. Use of OCST is most appropriate when PSG is difficult to perform because of immobility or safety issues, when a delay in obtaining a PSG occurs because of problems with access or availability and the clinical situation is urgent, when a high probability of OSA exists, when complicated comorbidities are not present, and when coexisting sleep disorders that may benefit from PSG are not present (Table F19-4).[14,15,17,18] Of note, the AHI derived from testing without electroencephalography (EEG) provides a number of events per hour of monitoring time, not TST. The Centers for Medicare and Medicaid define RDI as the number or apneas and hypopneas per hour of monitoring.[14,16] Others have suggested the term *respiratory event index* (REI). The use of monitoring time versus

TABLE F19-4 **Use of OCST versus PSG**	
OCST Acceptable	**PSG needed**
Immobility or safety issues	Low probability of OSA
	Comorbidities present
Delay in obtaining PSG	Central sleep apnea suspected
Moderate to high probability of OSA	Congestive heart failure
	Hypoventilation
	Neuromuscular weakness
Absent comorbidities	Supplemental oxygen
	Potent narcotics
Absent indication for PSG	Parasomnia suspected
	Previous negative OCST with a high clinical suspicion of OSA

OCST, Out-of-center sleep testing; *PSG*, polysomnography.

TST reduces the AHI. For example, if PSG and OCST both identify 100 events, the TST is 6 hours, and the monitoring time is 7 hours, then the AHI PSG $= 100/6$ and the AHI PM $= 100/7$. Therefore, the AHI by OCST will likely be less than that by PSG, even if similar numbers of respiratory events are detected. The possibility of a false-negative OCST should always be considered. This could occur if the patient does not sleep well during the OCST, with the result that monitoring time greatly exceeds TST or if minimal REM sleep was recorded. Most OCST device cannot determine the amount of sleep or REM sleep. If a high index of suspicion for OSA exists but an OCST is negative for OSA, a PSG should be performed.[17,18]

CLINICAL PEARLS

1. A significant proportion of patients diagnosed with OSA do not complain of daytime sleepiness.
2. Women with OSA may have more prominent symptoms of insomnia and fatigue compared with men.
3. A high MP or MMP score for the upper airway is a predictor of OSA.
4. Patients with habitual snoring, witnessed apnea or gasping, hypertension, and a large neck circumference are at increased risk for having OSA.
5. Questionnaires are not sufficiently sensitive or specific to obviate the need for objective testing to determine the presence or absence of OSA.
6. In patients with milder OSA, the amount of supine and REM sleep may determine if the overall AHI is in the normal range or elevated (AHI ≥ 5/hr). For patients with moderate to severe OSA, lack of a normal amount of supine sleep, REM sleep, or both may result in a sleep study AHI that underestimates the true severity of the disorder.
7. The severity of OSA may be underestimated by the AHI and lowest SaO_2 values obtained during the diagnostic portion of a split sleep study.
8. If an OCST is negative in a patient with a moderate to high suspicion of OSA, a PSG is needed to avoid a false-negative result.

REFERENCES

1. Iber C, Ancoli-Israel S, Chesson A, Quan SF: for the American Academy of Sleep Medicine: *The AASM manual for scoring of sleep and associated events: rules, terminology and technical specifications*, 1 ed, Westchester, IL, 2007, American Academy of Sleep Medicine.
2. Berry RB, Brooks R, Gamaldo CE, et al, for the American Academy of Sleep Medicine: *The AASM manual for the scoring of sleep and associated events: rules, terminology and technical specifications*, Version 2.0.3. Darien, IL, 2014, American Academy of Sleep Medicine.
3. American Academy of Sleep Medicine: *International classification of sleep disorders*, ed 3, Darien, IL, 2014, American Academy of Sleep Medicine.
4. Epstein LJ, Kristo D, Strollo PJ, et al: Clinical guideline for the evaluation, management and long-term care of obstructive sleep apnea in adults, *J Clin Sleep Med* 5:263–276, 2009.
5. Johns MW: Daytime sleepiness, snoring, and obstructive sleep apnea. The Epworth Sleepiness Scale, *Chest* 103:30–36, 1993.
6. Gottlieb DJ, Whitney CW, Bonekat WH, et al: Relation of sleepiness to respiratory disturbance index, *Am J Respir Crit Care Med* 159:502–507, 1999.
7. Shepertycky MR, Bano K, Kryger MH: Differences between men and women in the clinical presentation of patients diagnosed with obstructive sleep apnea syndrome, *Sleep* 28:309–314, 2005.
8. Nuckton TJ, Glidden DV, Browder WS, Claman DM: Physical examination: Mallampati score as an independent predictor of obstructive sleep apnea, *Sleep* 29:903–908, 2006.
9. Flemons WW: Obstructive sleep apnea, *N Engl J Med* 347:498–504, 2002.
10. Flemons W, Whitelaw WA, Bryant R, Remmers JE: Likelihood ratios for a sleep apnea clinical prediction rule, *Am J Respir Crit Care Med* 150:1279–1285, 1994.
11. Netzer NC, Stoohs RA, Netzer CM, et al: Using the Berlin questionnaire to identify patients at risk for the sleep apnea syndrome, *Ann Intern Med* 131: 485–491, 1999.
12. Chung F, Yegneswaran B, Liao P, et al: STOP questionnaire: a tool to screen patients for obstructive sleep apnea, *Anesthesiology* 108:812–821, 2008.

13. Kushida CA, Littner MR, Morgenthaler T, et al: Practice parameters for the indications for polysomnography and related procedures. An update for 2005, *Sleep* 28:499–521, 2005.

14. Revision of *NCD240.4 CPAP Therapy for OSA*. Transmittal R96 (recent revision): https://www.cms.gov/transmittals/downloads/R96NCD.pdf. Accessed September 26, 2013.

15. Oksenberg A, Arons E, Nasser K, et al: REM-related obstructive sleep apnea: the effect of body position, *J Clin Sleep Med* 6(4):343–348, 2010.

16. Findley LJ, Wilhoit SC, Suratt PM: Apnea duration and hypoxemia during REM sleep in patients with obstructive sleep apnea, *Chest* 87(4):432–436, 1985.

17. Collop NA, Anderson WM, Boehlecke B, et al: Clinical guidelines for the use of unattended portable monitors in the diagnosis of obstructive sleep apnea in adult patients. Portable Monitoring Task Force of the American Academy of Sleep Medicine, *J Clin Sleep Med* 3:737–747, 2007.

18. American Academy of Sleep Medicine: *Standards for accreditation of out of center sleep testing (OCST) in adult patients*, http://www.aasmnet.org/resources/pdf/OCSTstandards.pdf. Accessed?.

PATIENT 34

A Patient with a Negative Out-of-Center Sleep Test

A 35-year-old man reported that his wife complained that he snored very loudly and that this was a source of major distress for his wife. She did report some witnessed apneas. His primary care physician ordered a home sleep test. The patient had an Epworth sleepiness scale of 12. No history of cataplexy or symptoms of the restless legs syndrome was present.

Physical examination: Saturation of arterial oxygen (SaO_2) 96%; body mass index (BMI) 32; HEENT: Mallampati 4 upper airway; Neck 17 inch in circumference. The physical examination was otherwise normal.

Out-of-center sleep test (OCST): A type 3 study was performed using nasal pressure, chest and abdominal respiratory inductance plethysmography (RIP) effort belts, and oximetry (Figure P34-1). The device also had a body position sensor. Snoring and heart rate signals were derived from the nasal pressure and oximetry, respectively. The overall apnea–hypopnea index (AHI) was 2.8 per hour (hr) (Table P34-1). Intermittent snoring was noted on the raw tracings for most of the night.

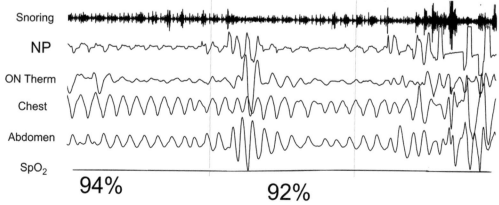

FIGURE P34-1 ■ A 90-second tracing from the home sleep study.

TABLE P34-1 Out-of-Center Sleep Test Results

Monitoring time	420 **min**
Obstructive apneas (#)	8
Mixed apneas (#)	0
Central apneas (#)	2
Hypopneas (#)	10
Apnea–hypopnea index (AHI) (#/hr)	2.8
AHI—supine (#/hr)	2.8
AHI—nonsupine (#/hr)	n/a
%Supine	100%
Oxygen desaturations (#)	20
Minimum saturation of arterial oxygen (SaO_2)	88%
Time $\leq$ 88%	0 **min**
Heart rate—mean bpm	60
Heart rate—maximum bpm	80
Heart rate—minimum bpm	50

AHI, number of events per monitoring time (also known as the REI); *bpm*, beats per minute; #, Number.

QUESTION

1. Do you recommend treatment for snoring or further evaluation?

ANSWER

1. **Answer:** Polysomnography (PSG) should be performed.

   Discussion: A major concern about the use of OCST (also known and *home sleep testing* home sleep apnea testing, or *portable monitoring*) to diagnose obstructive sleep apnea (OSA) is that a false-negative result may be obtained. This patient could be considered to have a high probability of having OSA, on the basis of the history of snoring, witnessed apnea, and a high Mallampati score. He did not have comorbidities that are felt to make OCST less desirable. These include congestive heart failure, neuromuscular weakness, hypoventilation, or significant chronic obstructive pulmonary disease (COPD). Therefore, OCST in this patient is reasonable. However, the test was negative for OSA.

   A number of reasons exist for the AHI by OCST being lower than the AHI of PSG. First, the AHI by OCST is really the number of events per *monitoring time rather than total sleep time* (TST). The Centers for Medicare and Medicaid refers to this metric as the *respiratory disturbance index* (RDI). However, this is poor use of the term, considering it usually refers to the AHI + RERA (respiratory effort–related arousal) index. The term *respiratory event index* (REI) is the recommended alternative. In any case, dividing by a larger number lowers the REI. For example, suppose OCST and PSG both detect 30 events. The TST is 5.5 hours, and the monitoring time is 7 hours. The AHI by PSG is 30/5.5 = 5.5 and by OCST is 30/7 = 4.3/hr. The effect of using monitoring time rather than TST is usually small; however, the poorer the sleep efficiency, the more the REI by OCST will underestimate the AHI. If the OCST sensors do not function well for the entire monitoring period, the total number of events by OCST would also be underestimated. Many OCST devices do have a position sensor, so the amount of *supine monitoring time* may be noted, but the amount of **supine sleep** and the amount of **REM sleep** cannot be determined. Although it can be hypothesized that a patient should sleep better at home, some patients are anxious about pulling out the sensors unknowingly and not having a sleep technologist available to remedy the problem. Therefore, some patients actually may sleep poorly during an OCST. In addition, the use of most OCST devices precludes the scoring of hypopneas based on arousals as electroencephalography (EEG) is not recorded.

   In the current patient, review of the raw tracings revealed snoring and air flow limitation. Frequent episodes of abrupt change from a flat profile to large breaths with a round profile occurred. These changes were likely due to arousals. However, the SaO_2 rarely dropped by more than 1% to 2% following the events. When questioned, the patient reported very poor sleep on the night of the study.

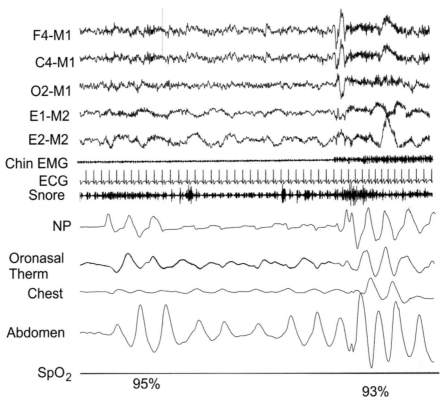

FIGURE P34-2 ■ Obstructive hypopnea scored on the basis of the associated arousal.

When a diagnostic PSG was performed, the AHI was 20/hr according to the AASM recommended hypopnea definition based on desaturation or arousal. His oxygen desaturation index was 10/hr. About 50% of the hypopneas were scored on the basis of an associated arousal (Figure P34-2). Using a hypopnea definition requiring a 4% desaturation, the AHI was 10/hr. When questioned, the patient did report that he did not sleep well during the OCST. The TST in the sleep center was normal.

CLINICAL PEARLS

1. If the OCST is negative but a moderate to high clinical suspicion for OSA exists, PSG should be performed to eliminate the possibility of a false-negative study. This is especially true if the patient reports sleeping much worse than normal while wearing the OCST device.

2. Review of the raw tracings from the OCST and the tabular data are important to verify an adequate technical quality, accurate scoring, and evidence of respiratory events that would likely be scored as hypopneas if the ability of the detect an arousal was provided.

3. OCST devices cannot determine the amount of sleep or rapid eye movement (REM) sleep. If a patient sleeps poorly, one must rely on patient report. Very reduced sleep can cause a false negative study.

BIBLIOGRAPHY

Collop NA, Anderson WM, Boehlecke B, et al: Clinical guidelines for the use of unattended portable monitors in the diagnosis of obstructive sleep apnea in adult patients. Portable Monitoring Task Force of the American Academy of Sleep Medicine, *J Clin Sleep Med* 3:737–747, 2007.

American Academy of Sleep Medicine: Standards for accreditation of out of center sleep testing (OCST) in adult patients. http://www.aasmnet.org/resources/pdf/ OCSTstandards.pdf. Accessed?.

Purdy S, Berry RB: Portable monitoring. In Mattice C, Brooks R, Lee-Chiong T, editors: *Fundamentals of sleep technology*, Philadelphia, 2012, Lippincott-Williams and Wilkins, pp 482–501.

Berry RB, Brooks R, Gamaldo CE, et al., for the American Academy of Sleep Medicine: *The AASM manual for the scoring of sleep and associated events: rules, terminology and technical specifications*, Version 2.0.3. Darien, IL, 2014, American Academy of Sleep Medicine. www.aasmnet.org.

A 30-Year-Old Woman with Unexplained Daytime Sleepiness

A 30-year-old woman is referred by her primary physician for evaluation of daytime sleepiness occurring over a period of at least 2 years. Previous evaluation, including a sleep study, had been unrevealing. The Epworth Sleepiness Scale (ESS) was 16/24 (severe sleepiness). The patient's usual bedtime was 10 PM. She typically fell asleep in 15 minutes or less. Multiple awakenings of unknown etiology occurred. Usually, the patient returned to sleep fairly quickly. The final awakening was at 6:00 AM. The patient did not feel refreshed in the morning. At this time, she was not in a relationship, but during previous relationships, her partners had noted her snoring, especially when she had consumed alcohol. The patient slept only 1 hour longer on the weekends. She denied symptoms of cataplexy (emotionally induced weakness), sleep paralysis, or hypnagogic hallucinations. The patient also denied symptoms of restless legs syndrome or unusual behaviors during sleep. The patient reported that her present job was demanding, but she denied feeling depressed or having less pleasure in life. She had a large group of friends and pursued many hobbies.

Physical examination: Thin, healthy-appearing woman, with a body mass index (BMI) of 26 kilograms per square meter (kg/m^2); HEENT examination showed a Mallampati 2 score of the upper airway, with a high arched palate and mild retrognathia.

Laboratory studies: Vitamin D levels, thyroid function studies, complete blood cell count (CBC), and metabolic panel were all unremarkable.

QUESTION

1. What evaluation do you suggest?

ANSWER

1. **Answer:** After detailed history and examination, polysomnography (PSG) followed by multiple sleep latency test (MSLT), if indicated

Discussion: The evaluation of excessive daytime sleepiness may be straightforward in patients with obvious severe obstructive sleep apnea (OSA) but difficult in many other patients.

The first concern is to characterize sleepiness. It is important to attempt to differentiate between fatigue and sleepiness. Fatigue is more suggestive of depression or a medical condition. One may ask, "Do you feel like you can fall asleep easily while resting in a quiet room?" In Fundamentals 12, the ESS is discussed in detail. In brief, the ESS is a series of eight questions, in which the patient is asked to estimate the propensity to fall asleep (0 never, 1, 2, 3 frequently). The range of scores is 0 to 24. Patients with narcolepsy and idiopathic hypersomnia report, by far, the highest scores. In Table P35-1, typical ESS scores are listed for some of the most common sleep disorders.[1] Usually, an ESS score of 10 or less is considered normal. Note the very high ESS scores in patients with narcolepsy and idiopathic hypersomnia. The ESS may not characterize the degree of sleepiness in every person. Direct questions such as "Do you have problems at work, at school, driving, or doing repetitive work due to sleepiness?" may help detect significant subjective sleepiness. Falling asleep while standing, eating, or sitting on the toilet is a sign of severe sleepiness.

Historical elements of interest are listed in Table P35-2, along with a list of conditions frequently associated with daytime sleepiness. Questions about habitual snoring, witnessed apnea, or cataplexy are among the most helpful. Witnessed apnea, which is the most useful historical element concerning OSA and cataplexy is the only symptom specific for narcolepsy. Weakness triggered by laughter or hearing a joke, maintenance of consciousness during the event, and brief

TABLE P35-1   **Epworth Sleepiness Scale in Different Disorders**

Disorder	ESS Mean (SD)
Normal	5.9 (2.2)
Primary snoring	6.5 (3.0)
Obstructive sleep apnea	11.7 (4.6)
Narcolepsy	17.5 (3.1)
Idiopathic hypersomnia	17.9 (3.1)
Insomnia	2.2 (2.0)
Periodic limb movement disorder	9.2 (4)

From Johns MW: A new method for measuring daytime sleepiness: the Epworth sleepiness scale, *Sleep* 14(6):540-545, 1991.
ESS, Epworth Sleepiness Scale; *SD*, standard deviation.

TABLE P35-2   **Differential Diagnosis and Key Elements and Clues**

Disorder	Historical Elements	Procedures and Clues
Insufficient sleep	Bedtime, sleep latency, awakenings, total sleep duration, sleep on work/school days versus the weekend?	Sleep logs Actigraphy Sleeping much longer on the weekend
Medications	Symptoms started at the time a medication was started or dose increased	Include over the counter medications
Obstructive sleep apnea	Snoring Witnessed apneas: most important predictor Recent weight gain Morning dry mouth	Polysomnography Patients who have minimal falls in the saturation of arterial oxygen (SaO_2) are more challenging
Narcolepsy	Early age of onset (teens to adolescence) Cataplexy: only symptoms specific for disorder Sleep paralysis, hypnogogic hallucinations: these are reported in up to 50% of normal individuals	Severe sleepiness
Idiopathic hypersomnia	Sleep drunkenness Very long sleep time (some patients) Unrefreshing naps	Sleep drunkenness (difficulty waking up)
Hypersomnia caused by medical disorder	Chiari malformation: headaches with exertion Parkinson disease Hypothyroidism	Headaches with exertion Tremor, gait disturbance
Periodic limb movement disorder (PLMD) or restless leg syndrome (RLS)	Symptoms of RLS Bed partner report of leg kicks	RLS rarely presents with a complaint of sleepiness, suspect additional disorders PLMs common in obstructive sleep apnea (OSA), narcolepsy
Depression	Depressed mood Ahedonia: loss of interest and pleasure Feelings of guilt Reduced energy Thoughts about suicide	Depression may be associated with both insomnia and hypersomnia (more common in atypical depression, bipolar depression)

duration (seconds to minutes) are all characteristics of typical cataplexy. Rather than asking patients if they feel depressed, ask instead about the symptoms of depression (lack of pleasure or interest in life). In bipolar depression, a previous episode of mania or hypomania may have occurred. One may ask, "Were you ever hospitalized for a 'nervous breakdown'?". It is useful to ask about any changes in medication, job, or relationships that occurred at the time of the onset of sleepiness. Patients may not connect the relationship between starting a sedating antihistamine, a beta blocker, or pain medications with the onset of sleepiness.

The physical examination should note the BMI (obesity a major risk factor for OSA) and the presence of hypertension (a risk factor for OSA). Examination of the head and neck should be performed to assess for signs of upper airway compromise (high Mallampati score, retrognathia) and neck circumference (>16 inches in women, 17 in men), and neurologic examination should look for tremor and abnormality of gain and muscle tone.

A sleep log and preferably actigraphy should be used to more objectively determine the actual amount of sleep and the pattern of sleep in the patient. Recall is very inaccurate. The history of sleeping much longer on the weekend is suggestive of insufficient sleep. Often a trial of sleep extension is the first intervention to improve daytime sleepiness.

If the above information does not provide a definite explanation for sleepiness, a sleep study may be indicated. If the clinical suspicion of OSA is very high, a diagnostic or split sleep study is indicated. Otherwise, a PSG followed by an MSLT is an approach that will avoid having to repeat the PSG if no sleep apnea is found. If significant sleep apnea is found during PSG, the MSLT can be canceled. Regularizing sleep and getting 7 to 8 hours of sleep per night before PSG or possible MSLT may also be useful as the patient may experience improvement is sleepiness in preparation for the MSLT.

Patients with OSA who do not have significant arterial oxygen desaturations with most events may be a challenge to identify. Guilleminault et al.[2] reported on a group of patients believed to have idiopathic hypersomnia based on sleep studies showing an apnea–hypopnea index (AHI) of <5 per hour (hr) and arousal index >10/hr (arousals from any cause) and an MSLT eliminating the possibility of narcolepsy. Sleep studies in these patients using esophageal pressure monitoring identified respiratory events associated with crescendo increases in inspiratory effort (increased esophageal pressure deflections) followed by arousal. These events did not meet the criteria for either apnea or hypopnea (based on 4% desaturation). The events were called *upper airway resistance* (UAR) *events*. This patient group was noted to exhibit improvement in subjective and objective sleepiness after treatment with modalities usually reserved for patients with sleep apnea. The term *upper airway resistance syndrome* (UARS) was used to identify the condition in these patients. The mean arousal index of the group was 33/hr (range 16–52) and the mean maximally negative esophageal pressure nadir was –37 centimeters of water (cm H_2O). In general, studies have suggested that patients with UARS tend to be thinner than typical patients with OSA and that most but not all complain of snoring. Most sleep clinicians feel that UARS is actually a variant of OSA rather than a distinct syndrome. On the basis of this premise, the 1999 American Academy of Sleep Medicine (AASM) consensus conference defined respiratory effort–related arousals (RERAs) rather than UARS events.[3] An RERA was characterized by increasing respiratory effort (esophageal pressure) lasting 10 seconds or longer that did not meet the criteria for hypopnea. In the *AASM Scoring Manual*,[4,5] RERAs are scored on the basis of flattening of the nasal pressure signal for 10 seconds or longer (or increased effort by esophageal pressure) associated with an arousal when the criteria for a hypopnea were not met (see Fundamentals 13 for hypopnea and RERA definitions). Studies have shown that arousals associated with flattening of the nasal pressure correlated well with those associated with increased esophageal pressure deflections.[7] (Figure P35-1).

The term *respiratory effort–related arousal* has been widely adopted but the UARS is still often used to identify a sleepy patients with an AHI <5/hr (hypopnea based on desaturation) and an increased RERA index. Kristo et al.[6] performed PSG with esophageal pressure monitoring in 527 patients in the military being evaluated for hypersomnia. Using the definition of an AHI <5/hr and RERA index >5/hr, 44 patients were identified as having UARS (8% of the population). The mean ESS was approximately 15,[6] consistent with moderate to severe sleepiness (normal 10 or less). Thus, patients with UARS are not rare (up to one tenth of patients were evaluated for sleepiness) and may have very significant daytime sleepiness.

Using the formula, respiratory disturbance index (RDI) = AHI (hypopnea based on ≥4% desaturation) + RERA index, most patients with UARS with an AHI <5/hr will have an RDI ≥5/hr. That is, they would be diagnosed as having OSA based on the RDI. However, the Centers for Medicare and Medicaid (CMS) does not include RERAs in the metric used to diagnose OSA, and hypopnea must be based entirely on flow and ≥4% desaturation.[8] Using the *AASM Scoring Manual*[5] the *recommended* definition of hypopnea (≥3% desaturation *or* arousal), most previous RERA events are now scored as hypopneas[9-11] and most patients with "UARS" will have an AHI ≥ 5/hr and will be diagnosed as having OSA. It is believed that using a more inclusive definition of hypopnea will identify a wider spectrum of patients who would benefit from treatment. One study of a cohort of thin, sleepy patients who benefited from treatment of OSA, found that using the CMS definition of hypopnea almost 40% of cohort would not be diagnosed with OSA.[12] However, CMS has not accepted the for hypopnea definition recommended by the AASM. The AASM now recognizes the CMS definition of hypopnea as an *acceptable* hypopnea definition.[5]

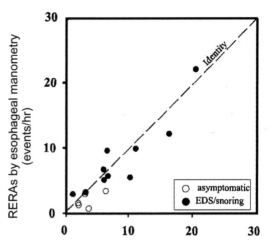

FIGURE P35-1 ■ Flow limitation arousals and respiratory effort–related arousals (RERAs) by esophageal monitoring were highly correlated, although not identical. (From Ayappa I, Norman RG, Krieger AC, et al: Non-invasive detection of respiratory effort–related arousals [RERAs] by a nasal cannula/pressure transducer system, *Sleep* 23:763-771, 2000.)

Flow limitation events with arousal by nasal cannula (events/hr)

TABLE P35-3 **Sleep Study Results**

Total sleep time (minutes)	420		
AASM hypopneas (no)	140	AASM AHI (no/hour)	21.4
CMS hypopneas (no)	10	CMS AHI (no/hour)	2.8
Obstructive apneas (no)	10	Desaturations ($\geq$ 4%) (no)	20
Mixed apneas (no)	0	Desaturations ($\geq$ 3%) (no)	20
Central apneas	0	Low SaO_2%	88%

CMS hypopnea = $\geq$ 30% drop in flow + $\geq$ 4% desaturation (acceptable AASM hypopnea definition).
AASM hypopnea = $\geq$ 30% drop in flow + $\geq$ 3% desaturation *or* an arousal.
AASM, American Academy of Sleep Medicine; *AHI,* apnea–hypopnea index; *CMS,* Centers for Medicare and Medicaid Services; *SaO_2,* arterial oxygen saturation.

In the current patient, a sleep study revealed an elevated AHI of 24.1/hr when the AASM recommended hypopnea definition was used (Table P35-3). Using the CMS hypopnea definition (acceptable AASM hypopnea definition), the AHI was less than 5/hr (although the RDI was equal to the AHI using the AASM recommended hypopnea definition). Most of the hypopneas were associated with 1% or 2% drops in the SaO_2. In the past, this patient would have been diagnosed as having UARS, but currently she would be diagnosed as having moderate OSA. She was treated with an oral appliance, and the AHI dropped to below 7/hr with resolution of her symptoms.

CLINICAL PEARLS

1. Evaluation of a patient for a complaint of daytime sleepiness requires careful history taking and physical examination.

2. The differential diagnosis of daytime sleepiness includes OSA, narcolepsy (with and without cataplexy), idiopathic hypersomnia, insufficient sleep, medications, medical disorders, the periodic limb movement disorder, and depression.

3. In snoring patients without a strong history for OSA, consider ordering a PSG followed by MSLT (if indicated). This approach avoids the need for a repeat PSG if OSA is not documented.

4. Thin patients may be less likely to have significant desaturation following respiratory events. Use of a more inclusive definition of hypopnea will identify a wider spectrum of patients with OSA who will benefit from treatment.

5. The term *respiratory effort–related arousal* is recommended by the AASM rather than the term *upper airway resistance event,* even though the latter terminology is commonly used. Some events scored as a hypopnea on the basis of an associated arousal (desaturation < 3%) using the AASM recommended hypopnea definition will be scored as RERAs if the acceptable AASM hypopnea definition is used.

6. An AHI based on the AASM **recommended** hypopnea definition or the RDI (AHI+RERA index) based on AASM **acceptable** (CMS) hypopnea definition will diagnose most patients with OSA who are symptomatic but exhibit very mild drops in the SaO_2 associated with respiratory events.

REFERENCES

1. Johns MW: A new method for measuring daytime sleepiness: the Epworth sleepiness scale, *Sleep* 14(6):540–545, 1991.
2. Guilleminault C, Stoohs R, Clerk A, et al: A cause of excessive daytime sleepiness. The upper airway resistance syndrome, *Chest* 104(3):781–787, 1993.
3. American Academy of Sleep Medicine Task Force: Sleep-related breathing disorders in adults: recommendations for syndrome definition and measurement techniques in clinical research. The Report of an American Academy of Sleep Medicine Task Force, *Sleep* 22(5):667–89.8, 1999.
4. Iber C, Ancoli-Israel S, Chesson AL Jr., Quan SF: *The AASM manual for the scoring of sleep and associated events: rules, terminology and technical specifications*, Westchester, IL, 2007, American Academy of Sleep Medicine.
5. Berry RB, Brooks R, Gamaldo CE, et al., for the American Academy of Sleep Medicine: *The AASM manual for the scoring of sleep and associated events: rules, terminology and technical specifications*, Version 2.0.3, Darien, IL, 2012, American Academy of Sleep Medicine. www.aasmnet.org, Accessed June 1, 2014.
6. Kristo DA, Lettieri CJ, Andrada T, et al: Silent upper airway resistance syndrome: prevalence in a mixed military population, *Chest* 127(5):1654–1657, 2005.
7. Ayappa I, Norman RG, Krieger AC, et al: Non-invasive detection of respiratory effort–related arousals (RERAs) by a nasal cannula/pressure transducer system, *Sleep* 23:763–771, 2000.
8. Department of Health and Human Services: *Decision memo for continuous positive airway pressure (CPAP) therapy for obstructive sleep apnea (OSA)*. CAG#0093R. March 13, 2008: http://wwwcmshhsgov/mcd/viewdecisionmemoasp?id=204 2008. Accessed?.
9. Masa JF, Corral J, Teran J, et al: Apnoeic and obstructive nonapnoeic sleep respiratory events, *Eur Respir J* 34(1):156–161, 2009.
10. Cracowski C, Pepin JL, Wuyam B, Levy P: Characterization of obstructive nonapneic respiratory events in moderate sleep apnea syndrome, *Am J Respir Crit Care Med* 164:944–948, 2001.
11. American Academy of Sleep Medicine: Rules for scoring respiratory events in sleep: update of the 2007 AASM manual for the scoring of sleep and associated events. Deliberations of the Sleep Apnea Definitions Task Force of the American Academy of Sleep Medicine, *J Clin Sleep Med* 8(5):597–619, 2012.
12. Guilleminault C, Hagen CC, Huynh NT: Comparison of hypopnea definitions in lean patients with known obstructive sleep apnea hypopnea syndrome, *Sleep Breath* 13:341–7.5, 2009.

PATIENT 36

Women with Loud Snoring

Patient A: A 30-year-old woman in the third trimester of her first pregnancy was noted by her husband (a physician) to snore heavily during the night. This occurred although she spent nearly all of the night sleeping in the lateral decubitus position. The patient had gained about 25 pounds during the pregnancy. During regular visits with her obstetrician, all fetal monitoring indicated a healthy pregnancy. No history of snoring prior to the pregnancy was present. Because the patient had been complaining of fatigue and was taking frequent naps, her husband was concerned that she might have obstructive sleep apnea (OSA). He had not heard any pauses in breathing during sleep. The patient denied falling asleep while watching television or reading during the day.

Physical Examination: General: healthy, gravid appearance; HEENT: moderately congested nasal mucosa, edematous palate and uvula; neck: 15-inch circumference; extremities: trace edema.

Patient B: A 60-year-old widow lives by herself, but when vacationing with friends, she was told that she snored loudly. She denied daytime sleepiness but admitted to fatigue. In addition, she reported waking up about four to five times every night. She attributed her fatigue to sleep disturbance. She also admitted to weight gain of about 10 pounds. The patient said she slept about 7 hours nightly and took occasional naps. Her Epworth Sleepiness Scale (ESS) score was 8/24. Her primary care physician wanted to place her on an antidepressant after he was unable to find a reason for her fatigue. She felt that the cause of her sleepiness was the frequent awakenings. The patient presented asking for help with her frequent awakenings and fatigue.

Physical examination: Remarkable for some retrognathia and a Mallampati 4 upper airway. The neck circumference is 14 inches. The body mass index (BMI) is 29 kilograms per square meter (kg/m^2).

QUESTIONS

1. Should a sleep study be performed?

2. Could this patient have sleep apnea?

ANSWERS

1. **Answer:** A sleep study is unnecessary for snoring associated with pregnancy, unless there are clinical indicators to increase the index of suspicion for sleep apnea.

   Discussion: Pregnancy is associated with a number of physiologic changes that affect respiration during wakefulness and sleep. The first trimester is often associated with increased sleepiness and total sleep time (TST) with a decrease in stages 3 and 4 and REM sleep. In the second trimester sleep normalizes.[1-3] In the third trimester, sleep again is commonly disturbed secondary to frequent urination, backache, fetal movement, leg cramps, and heartburn. Restless leg syndrome may appear or become worse during pregnancy. A high level of progesterone (a respiratory stimulant) in the third trimester is associated with a lowering of the arterial partial pressure of carbon dioxide (PCO_2). Growing abdominal girth results in an upward displacement of the diaphragm. In addition, edema develops in the nasal passages and pharynx. These last two changes result in snoring in up to 30% of all pregnant women.

   O'Brien et al.[4] screened 1719 pregnant women and found that 34% reported snoring, with 25% reporting pregnancy-onset snoring. After adjusting for confounders, pregnancy-onset snoring (but not chronic snoring) was independently associated with gestational hypertension (odds ratio [OR] 2.36) and preeclampsia (OR 1.59) but not gestational diabetes. On the basis of this study, pregnancy-onset snoring should increase the concern for the need for additional screening or monitoring. Wilson et al.[5] recruited 380 women in the second trimester of pregnancy from an antenatal clinic. All participants completed the Berlin Questionnaire at recruitment, with a subset of 43 women repeating the questionnaires at the time of polysomnography (PSG) at 37 weeks' gestation. Fifteen of 43 (35%) women were confirmed to have an apnea-hypopnea index (AHI) ≥ 5 per hour (hr). Prediction of AHI $\geq 5/hr$ at 37 weeks, based on the Berlin Questionnaire completed in the second trimester, had a sensitivity of 0.93, specificity of 0.50, positive predictive value (PPV) of 0.50, and negative predictive value (NPV) of 0.93. The main problem was a low PPV due to false positives. This is not surprising, as increased sleepiness, fatigue, and daily snoring are common in pregnancy and all factors addressed in the questionnaire. The authors concluded that traditional screening tools for OSA may not work well in pregnant women. Their analysis identified a high snoring volume, BMI ≥ 32 kg/m^2 and tiredness upon awakening as the strongest independent predictors of sleep-disturbed breathing (SDB) during pregnancy. Facco et al.[6] studied a cohort of pregnant women at high risk for sleep apnea (women with chronic hypertension, pregestational diabetes, obesity, prior history of pre-eclampsia, or a combination of all these factors), who completed a sleep survey composed of the Berlin Questionnaire and the ESS and participated in an overnight sleep evaluation with the Watch-PAT100 (WP100), a wrist-mounted device designed to diagnose sleep apnea, defined as AHI $\geq 5/hr$. Using multivariable statistics, demographic, clinical, and subjective symptoms that were independently associated with sleep apnea were determined and a prediction rule for the presence of sleep apnea was developed. The predictive capacity of this newly developed system was compared with that of the Berlin Questionnaire and the ESS using receiver-operating curve (ROC) statistics. They found that the ESS and the Berlin Questionnaire did not work well in this group. Conversely, a model incorporating frequent snoring, chronic hypertension, age, and BMI performed significantly better. In summary, the best method to screen pregnant patients for OSA remains to be determined. Traditional screening tools may be associated with a significant number of false positive results.

   Studies have shown that a significant percentage of patients developing gestational hypertension or pre-eclampsia have OSA. Pre-eclampsia is characterized by pregnancy-induced hypertension and significant amounts of protein in urine. If left untreated, it may develop into eclampsia and life-threatening seizures during pregnancy. One study[7] suggested that air flow limitation may worsen blood pressure during pregnancy in patients with pre-eclampsia in the absence of overt apnea. A recent investigation[8] found benefit (as assessed by fetal movements) of continuous positive airway pressure (CPAP) in women with snoring and pre-eclampsia. A significant number of patients with gestational hypertension have sleep apnea.[8] The development of gestational hypertension or pre-eclampsia in a snoring patient is an indication for a sleep study.

Home sleep testing, if accurate, might be more acceptable to women in the third trimester compared with PSG. Until recently, the accuracy of home sleep testing compared with PSG has not been studied. O'Brien et al.[8] found that a device based on peripheral arterial tonometry has a high sensitivity and specificity for the diagnosis of OSA in pregnant women. More studies on the use of home sleep testing in pregnant women are needed.

Although snoring is common in pregnant women, overt OSA is believed to be uncommon. However, OSA is likely under diagnosed in pregnancy. Some pregnant patients with OSA continued to have sleep apnea after delivery; thus, pregnancy probably worsened but did not cause sleep apnea in these patients. In summary, indications for sleep monitoring *when snoring is present* during pregnancy (Box P36-1) include witnessed apnea, very loud snoring, gestational hypertension, a previous pregnancy with fetal growth retardation, and severe hypersomnia (especially on awakening) or insomnia. Therapeutic options for sleep apnea are somewhat limited. The safest treatment is nasal CPAP. Close monitoring of both the fetus and the pregnant woman is essential. Some evidence suggests that severe OSA in the mother causes of fetal growth retardation, but this has not been determined conclusively.[11]

BOX P36-1 | Risk Factors for OSA in Pregnancy and Need for Testing in a Snoring Patient

Pregnancy onset snoring	Severe hypersomnia—especially on awakening
Very loud snoring	Prior or current fetal growth retardation
Observed apnea	History of pre-eclampsia
Gestational hypertension or pre-eclampsia	

In the present case, the patient did not have any major risk factor for OSA except for pregnancy-onset snoring. The patient declined a PSG but was willing to undergo a home sleep study. Because of her husband's concerns, a home sleep study was performed, and it showed snoring without sleep apnea.

2. **Answer:** Some differences exist in the presentation of OSA in women compared with men. Given the history of snoring and fatigue, a sleep study is reasonable.

Discussion: Women have many of the same symptoms of OSA as men. However, complaints of insomnia and fatigue tend to be more prominent and snoring and reports of witnessed apnea less prominent. Women with OSA are also more likely to complain of depression, morning headaches, awakenings, and nonrestorative sleep.[12,13] Postmenopausal women are at higher risk for OSA than premenopausal women (about four times more likely to have OSA).[14] The problem of determining the effect of menopause is that postmenopausal women are both older and heavier, both risk factors for OSA. However, postmenopausal women on hormone replacement therapy have a lower risk of OSA, which suggests that hormonal status does play a role.[15] In summary, because OSA complaints in women often center on fatigue and insomnia, the possibility of sleep apnea may be overlooked. If medical causes of fatigue and depression are ruled out, the possibility of occult OSA should be considered. Traditional screening tools for OSA may not work as well in women.

In the current patient, given the history of snoring, frequent awakenings, weight gain, and high Mallampati score, a sleep study was ordered. AHI was 20/hr with mild desaturations. After much hesitation, the patient agreed to try CPAP. After a titration treatment with CPAP of 7 centimeters of water (cm H_2O) was initiated. The patient had difficulty adapting to CPAP, but eventually was adherent to treatment and reported fewer awakenings and improved sleep quality.

CLINICAL PEARLS

1. Snoring is common in pregnancy, especially in the third trimester (at least in 30% of cases).

2. Traditional screening tools for OSA may not work as well in pregnant patients. However, they are better than no screening at all. The major shortcoming is the possibility of false positive results.

3. Observed apnea, very loud snoring, fatigue and sleepiness on awakening, development of gestational hypertension, prior or current fetal growth retardation, and prior pre-eclampsia would all suggest that sleep testing to rule out OSA is indicated in a woman who snores during pregnancy.

4. Given the availability of home sleep testing, it is likely that more pregnant patients will be screened for sleep apnea in the future. However, limited data exist on the accuracy of home sleep testing compared with PSG in pregnant women.

5. If patients with OSA become pregnant, potential harm to the developing fetus is possible if sleep apnea is left untreated. If not already on treatment, these patients warrant a sleep evaluation. Limited data suggest that nasal CPAP is the treatment of choice during pregnancy. Close fetal monitoring is essential.

REFERENCES

1. Facco FL, Kramer J, Ho KH, et al: Sleep disturbances in pregnancy, *Obstet Gynecol* 115:77–83, 2009.
2. Pien GW, Schwab RJ: Sleep disorders during pregnancy, *Sleep* 27:1405–1417, 2004.
3. Ye L, Pien GW, Weaver TE: Gender differences in the clinical manifestation of obstructive sleep apnea, *Sleep Med* 10(10):1075–1084, 2009.
4. O'Brien LM, Bullough AS, Owusu JT, et al: Pregnancy-onset habitual snoring, gestational hypertension, and preeclampsia: prospective cohort study, *Am J Obstet Gynecol* 207(6):487.e1–e9, 2012.
5. Wilson DL, Walker SP, Fung AM, et al: Can we predict sleep-disordered breathing in pregnancy? The clinical utility of symptoms, *J Sleep Res* 22(6):670–678, 2013.
6. Facco FL, Ouyang DW, Zee PC, et al: Development of a pregnancy-specific screening tool for sleep apnea, *J Clin Sleep Med* 8(4):389–394, 2012.
7. Edwards N, Blyton DM, Kirjavainen T, et al: Nasal continuous positive airway pressure reduces sleep induced blood pressure increments in preeclampsia, *Am J Respir Crit Care Med* 162:252–257, 2000.
8. Blyton DM, Skilton MR, Edwards N, et al: Treatment of sleep disordered breathing reverses low fetal activity levels in preeclampsia, *Sleep* 36(1):15–21, 2013.
9. Reid J, Skomro R, Cotton D, et al: Pregnant women with gestational hypertension may have a high frequency of sleep disordered breathing, *Sleep* 34:1033–1038, 2011.
10. O'Brien LM, Bullough AS, Shelgikar AV, et al: Validation of Watch-Pat-200 against polysomnography during pregnancy, *J Clin Sleep Med* 8(3):287–294, 2012.
11. Olivarez SA, Maheshwari B, McCarthy M, et al: Prospective trial on obstructive sleep apnea in pregnancy and fetal heart rate monitoring, *Am J Obstet Gynecol* 202:552.e1–e7, 2010.
12. Shepertycky MR, Bano K, Kryger MH: Differences between men and women in the clinical presentation of patients diagnosed with obstructive sleep apnea syndrome, *Sleep* 28:309–314, 2005.
13. Quintana-Gallego E, Carmona-Bernal C, Capote F, et al: Gender differences in obstructive sleep apnea syndrome: a clinical study of 1166 patients, *Respir Med* 98:984–989, 2004.
14. Young T, Finn L, Austin D, Peterson A: Menopausal status and sleep disordered breathing in the Wisconsin Sleep Cohort Study, *Am J Respir Crit Care Med* 167:1181–1185, 2003.
15. Shahar E, Redline S, Young T, et al: for the Sleep Heart Health Study Research Group: Hormone replacement therapy and sleep disordered breathing, *Am J Respir Crit Care Med* 167:1186–1192, 2003.

FUNDAMENTALS 20

Obstructive Sleep Apnea in Adults: Epidemiology and Variants

EPIDEMIOLOGY OF ADULT OSA

The prevalence of obstructive sleep apnea (OSA) depends on the definition of the respiratory disturbance index (RDI) or apnea–hypopnea index (AHI) criteria, the definition of hypopnea, the method used to detect air flow, and the presence or absence of a requirement that symptoms be present.[1-4] The Wisconsin-based cohort study of state employees younger than 65 years of age found a prevalence of sleep-disordered breathing (SDB) defined as an AHI ≥ 5 per hour (hr) (with hypopneas based on a definition of discernible change in air flow and $\geq 4\%$ desaturation) to be 9% in women and 24% in men.[2] The **OSA syndrome**, defined as the presence of both an increased AHI and self-reported sleepiness, was present in 2% of women and 4% of men. Recent modeling taking into account the obesity epidemic estimated 17% of men and 9% of women age 50-70 years have OSA (AHI $>= 15$/hour).[4] Evidence suggests that a large fraction of patients with OSA remain undiagnosed. It is estimated that in Western countries, up to 5% of the population have undiagnosed OSA syndrome (elevated AHI and symptoms).[3] Some (not all) have found evidence that untreated OSA severity progresses with time.

RISK FACTORS FOR OSA

A number of population-based studies have documented several risk factors for the presence of OSA (Table F20-1).[3] Of these, the most consistent findings have been the presence of obesity and male gender. An association between AHI and obesity has been documented in many studies. Peppard and coworkers[5] found that a 10% increase in weight was associated with a sixfold increase in the risk of developing moderate to severe OSA. Other studies have documented

TABLE F20-1	Risk Factors for Obstructive Sleep Apnea	
Risk Factor	**Evidence**
Obesity—present in roughly 70% of OSA	+++
Male gender	+++
Aging	++
Postmenopausal state	++
Black race	+ (some studies)
Alcohol, smoking, hypothyroidism, acromegaly	±

Adapted from Malhotra A, White DP: Obstructive sleep apnea, *Lancet* 360:237-245, 2002.
OSA, Obstructive sleep apnea, level of evidence +++ >++ > +

a decrease in the AHI with weight loss.[6] The comparative importance of the type of obesity and areas of excess fat (neck versus abdomen) is currently under investigation. Prediction models for OSA have used neck circumference as a predictor.[7] However, one study found neck circumference to correlate best with AHI in women, whereas abdominal girth correlated better with AHI in men.[8] The Wisconsin cohort study by Young et al.[2] found men to have twice the incidence of OSA compared with women. Analysis of the Sleep Heart Health data also showed the risk of OSA in men was greater (odds ratio 1.5).[9] The prevalence of OSA appears to be higher in older adults than in the middle-aged populations. Evidence from the Sleep Heart Health Study shows that SDB prevalence increases from age 40 to around 60 years.[3] After that, the prevalence appears to level off. In older adults, the AHI may be less correlated with excessive sleepiness and increased cardiovascular risk. Although factors such as age and higher body mass index (BMI) complicate the analysis of the effect of the postmenopausal status on the risk for OSA, it appears that postmenopausal women are at increased risk of developing OSA if they are not on hormone replacement treatment.[10,11]

Evidence suggests the possibility that OSA is more common in the African American groups than in white populations. An investigation by Redline and associates[12] found an increase in the risk of OSA to be greater in African Americans than in whites only for those younger than age 25 years. Ip and coworkers[13] found a similar prevalence of OSA in a Chinese population as in whites. The fact that OSA is common in Asian areas where obesity is much less common has led to the hypothesis that craniofacial characteristics of the Asian population might predispose this group to OSA.[14]

In some studies, smoking and alcohol consumption were found to increase the risk of OSA, but the evidence is not considered strong, and no large convincing studies are available. Some, but not all, studies have found an association between hypothyroidism or acromegaly and OSA.

VARIANTS OF SNORING AND OSA

Some of the common variants of snoring and OSA are listed in Box F20-1. Some patients may, in fact, fit into more than one category.

Primary (Simple) Snoring

Snoring may be defined as a vibratory, sonorous noise made during inspiration and, less commonly, expiration. Factors believed to worsen snoring include nasal congestion, the supine posture, and ethanol. Risk factors for snoring include gender (men more than women) and increasing age. Some studies have suggested that up to 60% of men and 40% of women older than age 40 snore to some extent. Snoring is a cardinal symptom of OSA, but not all snorers have OSA. *Simple* or *primary snoring* is defined as the presence of snoring without associated symptoms of insomnia, daytime sleepiness, or sleep disruption. Although the use of polysomnography (PSG) is not necessary unless OSA is suspected, the PSG characteristics of simple snoring would include evidence of snoring on the PSG as detected by audio recording, snore sensor, or vibration in the nasal pressure signal (or technologist report of snoring) *and* the absence of a significant AHI. A recent study by Lee and associates[15] found that *heavy snoring* (defined as the presence of snoring for >50% of the nights) was associated with increased carotid atherosclerosis, independent of other risk factors such as nocturnal hypoxemia and OSA severity. However, to date, other studies have not confirmed this finding. In addition, persons who are heavy snorers are at risk for developing OSA as they age or if significant weight gain occurs. Although not every snorer needs a sleep study, evaluation is recommended if the patient has a moderate to high likelihood of having OSA, is symptomatic, or if a surgical intervention is being considered. PSG is also needed before an oral appliance is made for snoring to rule out significant OSA. If significant sleep apnea is present, this may change the treatment approach.

BOX F20-1	Snoring and OSA Variants
Primary Snoring	AHI <5 per hour (hr), no daytime sleepiness
UARS	Respiratory arousals (RERAs) with few desaturations
	AHI <5/hr when hypopnea definition requires ≥4% desaturation, but RDI ≥5/hr
	AHI ≥5 /hr, using 2012 *AASM Scoring Manual* recommended* definition of hypopnea
Obesity	Obesity BMI >30 kg/m^2
hypoventilation	Daytime PCO_2 >45 mm Hg
syndrome	Hypoventilation not explained by lower airway or parenchymal lung disease or thoracic cage disorder, or neuromuscular disorder
	80% to 90% have OSA, others worsening PCO_2 during sleep
	High morbidity and mortality if not treated
	CO_2 (HCO_3) >27 mEq/L in an obese patient with OSA
	= a clue to evaluate with ABG testing
Overlap	OSA+chronic obstructive pulmonary disease
syndrome	More severe nocturnal desaturation (especially in low awake SaO_2)
	Daytime hypercapnia may be present with only mild reductions in the FEV_1

*Berry RB, Brooks R, Gamaldo CE, et al., for the American Academy of Sleep Medicine: *The AASM manual for the scoring of sleep and associated events: rules, terminology and technical specifications,* Version 2.0.3, www.aasmnet.org, Darien, Illinois, 2014, American Academy of Sleep Medicine.

ABG, Arterial blood gas; *AHI,* apnea–hypopnea sleep index; *FEV₁,* forced expiratory volume in 1 second; *HCO₃,* bicarbonate; *mEq/L,* milliequivalent per liter; *mm Hg,* millimeters of mercury; *OSA,* obstructive sleep apnea; *PCO₂,* partial pressure of carbon dioxide; *RDI,* respiratory disturbance index; *RERA,* respiratory effort–related arousal; *SaO₂,* saturation of arterial oxygen; *UARS,* upper airway resistance syndrome.

Upper Airway Resistance Syndrome

Guilleminault and coworkers[16] identified a group of patients who complained of sleepiness or fatigue but did not have an AHI ≥ 5/hr (thermal devices measured air flow, and hypopneas required desaturation). The group was defined by the presence of a respiratory arousal index >10/hr with esophageal pressure monitoring. The symptoms responded to continuous positive airway pressure (CPAP) or other treatments. The mean arousal index of the group was 33/hr (range 16–52), and the mean maximally negative esophageal pressure nadir was –37 centimeters of water (cm H_2O). Some controversy exists as to whether upper airway resistance syndrome (UARS) is a distinct entity or simply a milder form of OSA.[17] UARS is considered a subtype of OSA in the *International Classification of Sleep Disorders*, Third Edition (ICSD-3).[17] Use of nasal pressure to detect more subtle decreases in air flow as well as air flow limitation (flattening of the inspiratory nasal pressure [NP] waveform) has increased the ability to diagnose patients with milder OSA. If a hypopnea definition requiring a drop in flow + $\geq 4\%$ desaturation is used, most UARS patients with an AHI <5/hour will have an RDI = AHI + respiratory effort–related arousal (RERA) index ≥ 5/hour. Furthermore, if hypopneas are scored on the basis of the *American Academy of Sleep Medicine Scoring Manual* recommended hypopnea definition (requiring either an associated desaturation *or* arousal), most events previously scored as RERAs will be classified as hypopneas.[18,19]

Obesity Hypoventilation Syndrome

Most patients with OSA do not have daytime hypoventilation. Two groups of patients with OSA and hypoventilation include those with obesity hypoventilation syndrome (OHS) and overlap syndrome (a combination of OSA and chronic obstructive pulmonary disease [COPD]). Diagnostic criteria for OHS include obesity (BMI >30 kilograms per meter squared [kg/m^2]), awake (daytime) hypoventilation (partial pressure of carbon dioxide [PCO_2] >45 millimeters of mercury [mm Hg]), and absence of airway or parenchymal lung disease, chest wall disorder (other than obesity), or neuromuscular disorder that explains the hypoventilation.[20] These patients were previously referred to as "Pickwickian." Today, use of this term is discouraged. About 80% to 90% of patients with OHS have OSA as shown by PSG. The other 10% to 20% simply have worsening hypoventilation during sleep without many discrete apneas or hypopneas. The definitive diagnosis of OHS requires arterial blood gas measurement taken while the patient is awake and a PCO_2 of >45 mm Hg. However, arterial blood gas testing is rarely performed on morbidly obese patients with severe OSA unless they have daytime hypoxemia or present with respiratory failure. An elevated serum CO_2 (primarily bicarbonate [HCO_3]) is a very useful indication that a patient with OSA should be tested for hypoventilation. The serum CO_2 is included on routine metabolic or electrolyte laboratory panels. The elevated HCO_3 in OHS patients represents renal compensation for chronic respiratory acidosis (elevated arterial PCO_2). However, an elevated HCO_3 could also be caused by metabolic alkalosis. Mokhlesi and associates[21] found that 20% of 410 patients referred to a sleep center to rule out OSA had OHS. In this study, only 3% of OHS patients had HCO_3 <27 milliequivalents per liter (mEq/L) but only 50% of patients with a HCO_3 of ≥ 27 had OHS. The authors concluded that patients with both OSA and a HCO_3 >27 mEq/L should undergo arterial blood gas testing to determine if hypoventilation is present. Other clues that OHS may be present include a borderline awake SaO_2 (90%–92%) or evidence of significant cor pulmonale. It is important to recognize whether a patient has OHS as well as OSA because this group has a high incidence of complications and increase mortality if not properly treated.[22]

The treatment of OHS includes CPAP or bilevel positive airway pressure (BPAP). Patients with OHS and OSA may respond to CPAP. Those OHS patients without OSA and those with severe hypoventilation are treated with BPAP. Supplemental oxygen may be needed if desaturation persists despite optimized PAP. The awake PCO_2 may improve or normalize if patients with OHS adhere to treatment. The obesity hypoventilation syndrome is discussed in detail in Patient 33.

Overlap Syndrome

Patients with the OSA and COPD may have severe nocturnal oxygen desaturation, awake hypoventilation, or both. An epidemiologic study found that patients with mild COPD have *no* higher incidence of OSA than the general population.[23] However, because both COPD and OSA are common, the combination is common, even if by chance. Of interest, those patients with both airway obstruction and sleep apnea in this study had worsened arterial oxygen desaturation. An early study of a group of patients with OSA and hypoventilation found that the presence of COPD was associated with hypoventilation.[24] Interestingly, patients with COPD alone rarely retain CO_2 until the forced expiratory volume in 1 second (FEV1) is below 1.0 L or 40% of predicted. However, patients with the OSA and mild to moderate COPD may retain CO_2. Patients with overlap syndrome tend to have particularly severe arterial oxygen desaturation at night. They are often assumed to simply have COPD and are treated with nocturnal oxygen alone. This may incompletely reverse the nocturnal hypoxemia and worsen the CO_2 retention during sleep.[25] The long-term outcome of patients with the overlap syndrome may worsen if upper airway obstruction is not addressed.[26] Proper treatment usually requires CPAP or BPAP and supplemental oxygen, if needed. The daytime PCO_2 may improve in some patients with adequate treatment of upper airway obstruction during sleep. Aggressive treatment of the underlying COPD with smoking cessation and bronchodilators may also be helpful in improving gas exchange both during the day and at night. More information about the overlap syndrome is presented in Patient 67.

CLINICAL PEARLS

1. Risk factors for the presence of OSA include obesity, male gender, older age, and postmenopausal status (not on hormonal replacement therapy). Hypothyroidism, acromegaly, cigarettes smoking, and chronic alcohol are also considered risk factors, but the evidence is much less compelling.

2. The two groups of patients with OSA with daytime hypercapnia are those with the OHS and the combination of obstructive airways disease (COPD) and OSA.

3. Approximately 80% of patients with the OHS have OSA. The other 20% have sleep-related worsening of daytime hypercapnia and hypoxemia with relatively few discrete apneas or hypopneas.

4. Patients with OSA and obstructive airway disease (COPD) may have severe arterial oxygen desaturation during sleep and daytime hypercapnia.

REFERENCES

1. American Academy of Sleep Medicine: *ICSD-2 International classification of sleep disorders, diagnostic and coding manual*, ed 2, Westchester, IL, 2005, American Academy of Sleep Medicine.
2. Young T, Palta M, Leder R, et al: The occurrence of sleep-disordered breathing among middle-aged adults, *N Engl J Med* 328:1230–1235, 1993.
3. Young T, Peppard PE, Gottlieb DJ: Epidemiology of obstructive sleep apnea, *Am J Respir Crit Care Med* 165:1217–1239, 2002.
4. Peppard PE, Young T, Barnet JH, et al: Increased prevalence of sleep-disordered breathing in adults, *Am J Epidemiol* 177(9):1006–1014, 2013.
5. Peppard PE, Young T, Palta M, et al: Longitudinal study of moderate weight change and sleep-disordered breathing, *JAMA* 284:3015–3021, 2000.
6. Smith PL, Gold AR, Meyers DA, et al: Weight loss in mildly to moderately obese patients with obstructive sleep apnea, *Ann Intern Med* 103:850–855, 1985.
7. Flemons WW: Obstructive sleep apnea, *N Engl J Med* 347:498–504, 2002.
8. Simpson L, Mukherjee S, Cooper MN, et al: Sex differences in the association of regional fat distribution with the severity of obstructive sleep apnea, *Sleep* 33:467–474, 2010.
9. Young T, Shahar E, Nieto FJ, et al: Predictors of sleep disordered breathing in community dwelling adults: the Sleep Heart Health Study, *Arch Intern Med* 162:893–900, 2002.
10. Young T, Finn L, Austin D, Peterson A: Menopausal status and sleep disordered breathing in the Wisconsin Sleep Cohort Study, *Am J Respir Crit Care Med* 167:1181–1185, 2003.
11. Shahar E, Redline S, Young T, et al: for the Sleep Heart Health Study Research Group: Hormone replacement therapy and sleep disordered breathing, *Am J Respir Crit Care Med* 167:1186–1192, 2003.
12. Redline S, Tishler PV, Hans MG, et al: Racial differences in sleep-disordered breathing in African-Americans and Caucasians, *Am J Respir Crit Care Med* 153:186–192, 1997.
13. Ip M, Lam B, Lauder I, et al: A community study of sleep disordered breathing in middle-aged Chinese men in Hong Kong, *Chest* 119:62–69, 2001.
14. Li KK, Kushida C, Powell NB, et al: Obstructive sleep apnea syndrome: a comparison between Far-East Asian and white men, *Laryngoscope* 110:1689–1693, 2000.
15. Lee SA, Amis TC, Byth K, et al: Heavy snoring as a cause of carotid artery atherosclerosis, *Sleep* 31(9):1207–1213, 2008.
16. Guilleminault C, Stoohs R, Clerk A, et al: A cause of excessive daytime sleepiness: the upper airway resistance syndrome, *Chest* 104:781–787, 1993.
17. American Academy of Sleep Medicine: *International classification of sleep disorders*, ed 3, Darien, IL, 2014, American Academy of Sleep Medicine.
18. Masa JF, Corral J, Teran J, et al: Apnoeic and obstructive nonapnoeic sleep respiratory events, *Eur Respir J* 34:156–161, 2009.
19. Cracowski C, Pépin JL, Wuyam B, Lévy P: Characterization of obstructive nonapneic respiratory events in moderate sleep apnea syndrome, *Am J Respir Crit Care Med* 164:944–948, 2001.
20. Piper AJ, Grunstein RR: Obesity hypoventilation syndrome: mechanisms and management, *Am J Respir Crit Care Med* 183:292–298, 2011.
21. Mokhlesi B, Tulaimat A, Baibussowitsch I, et al: Obesity hypoventilation syndrome: prevalence and predictors in patients with obstructive sleep apnea, *Sleep Breath* 11:117–124, 2007.
22. Nowbar S, Burkart KM, Gonzales R, et al: Obesity-hypoventilation in hospitalized patients: prevalence, effects, and outcome, *Am J Med* 116:1–7, 2004.
23. Sander MH, Newman AB, Haggerty CL, et al: Sleep and sleep disordered breathing in adults with predominantly mild obstructive airway disease, *Am J Respir Crit Care Med* 167:7–14, 2003.
24. Bradley TD, Rutherford R, Lue F, et al: Role of diffuse airway obstruction in the hypercapnia of obstructive sleep apnea, *Am Rev Respir Dis* 134:920–924, 1986.
25. Goldstein RS, Ramcharan V, Bowes G, et al: Effect of supplemental nocturnal oxygen on gas exchange in patients with severe obstructive lung disease, *N Engl J Med* 310:425–429, 1984.
26. Marin JM, Soriano JB, Carrizo SJ, et al: Outcomes in patients with chronic obstructive pulmonary disease and obstructive sleep apnea: the overlap syndrome, *Am J Respir Crit Care Med* 182(3):325–331, 2010.

A 45-Year-Old Man with a Distinct Pattern of Desaturation

A 45-year-old man was evaluated for complaints of heavy snoring for many years and daytime sleepiness (Epworth Sleepiness Scale [ESS] score 12/24) of about a 4-year duration. No history of cataplexy or sleep paralysis was present. The patient did not drink alcohol.

Physical Examination: Height 5 feet 10 inches, weight 180 pounds; HEENT: Mallampati 4, edematous uvula; neck: 15-inch circumference; otherwise normal examination.

A hypnogram of the entire night is shown in Figure P37-1. The PSG results are summarized in Table P37-1.

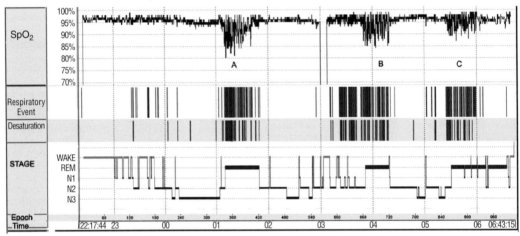

FIGURE P37-1 ■ Hypnogram of Patient 37. All sleep occurred in the supine position. (Adapted from Berry RB: *Fundamentals of sleep medicine*, Philadelphia, 2012, Saunders, p. 194.)

QUESTION

1. Does the overall apnea–hypopnea index (AHI) of 7 per hour (hr) mean this patient has mild obstructive sleep apnea (OSA)? Should he be treated?

ANSWER

1. **Answer:** Rapid eye movement (REM)–related OSA is mild by frequency overall but is severe during REM sleep with severe desaturation during REM sleep.

   Discussion: Some patients have episodes of OSA primarily during REM sleep. Thus, the overall AHI may be low, with low or normal AHI during non-REM (NREM) sleep but moderately to severely increased AHI during REM sleep (see Table P37-1). Other OSA patients will have an elevated AHI during both NREM and REM sleep, with a much higher AHI and more severe desaturation during REM sleep. REM-related OSA is often defined as AHI-REM/AHI-NREM >2 but some also require that the AHI-NREM be <15/hour and the overall AHI ≥5/hr. REM-related OSA is sometimes call REM associated or predominant OSA.

TABLE P37-1	Sleep Study Results			
Total recording time (min)	434.2	Awake (WASO):(min)	20
Total sleep time (min)	389.5	Stage N1 (%TST)	9.8
Sleep efficiency (TST/TIB)	89.6	Stage N2 (%TST)	33.7
Sleep latency (min)	12.5	Stage N3 (%TST)	26.2
REM latency (min)	88.0	Stage REM (%TST)	22.7
Respiratory Events			
AHI (/hr)	7.7	Obstructive apneas (#):	1
AHI NREM (/hr)	1.1	Mixed apneas (#):	0
AHI REM (/hr)	30.0	Central apneas (#):	0
AHI supine (/hr)	8.9	Hypopnea (#):	49
AHI nonsupine(/hr)	0.0		
%TST on back	100		
Oximetry during Sleep			
Minimum SaO_2 NREM (%)	77		
Minimum SaO_2 REM (%)	79		
Desaturations TST (#)	50		
Average SaO_2 at Desat (%)	88.4		
NREM $SaO_2 \leq 88\%$ (min)	4.0		
REM $SaO_2 < 88\%$ (min)	7.6		

AHI, Apnea–hypopnea index; *min*, minutes; *hr*, hour; *NREM*, non–rapid eye movement; *REM*, rapid eye movement; *TIB*, time in bed; *TST*, total sleep time; *SaO₂*, saturation of arterial oxygen; *WASO*, wakefulness after sleep onset.

Despite the common finding of a higher AHI during REM sleep, the reason for this finding is still not clear. It has been assumed that REM sleep, which is associated with muscle hypotonia, should result in a more collapsible upper airway. However, studies of the critical upper airway closing pressure have not confirmed that the airway is more collapsible during REM sleep. It is possible that this method does not accurately represent the physiology of REM sleep. REM sleep is not homogeneous, and upper airway muscle tone is often lowest during bursts of phasic eye movements. In addition, ventilatory drive (esophageal pressure deflections) and upper airway muscle activity often decreases during bursts of phasic eye movements. The frequency of eye movements increases in the later REM periods of the night. Periods of decreased ventilation are also more common and longer during REM sleep in the later part of the night. As in normal individuals, the periods of stage R in OSA patients are longer in the last part of the night and eye movements are more frequent. Thus, it is not surprising that the most severe desaturation usually occurs during the last REM periods of the night. The longest respiratory events usually occur during REM sleep in patients with OSA. In contrast, experimental mask occlusion in normal individuals has shown that subjects arouse more quickly during REM than NREM sleep. The reason for longer events during REM sleep in OSA patients is unknown. In any case, the most severe arterial oxygen desaturation in OSA is during REM sleep.

In the absence of other disorders to explain the excessive daytime sleepiness, many clinicians have empirically treated patients who have REM-related sleep apnea with usual treatments such as nasal continuous positive airway pressure (CPAP). Of note, some patients with REM-related sleep apnea still have some degree of abnormality during NREM sleep with heavy snoring during NREM with or without repetitive respiratory effort–related arousals (RERAs). One study of a group of patients with a low overall AHI (<10/hr) but varying amounts of apnea–hypopnea during REM sleep found that 80% with an AHI-REM >15/hr had a short sleep latency during daytime naps (evidence of excessive sleepiness). Thus, a significantly elevated AHI-REM may justify treatment if the patient is symptomatic (even if the overall AHI is only mildly increased). However, multiple population-based studies have not found evidence of any correlation between the AHI during REM sleep and daytime sleepiness. Of course, even using the entire night AHI, the correlation between the AHI

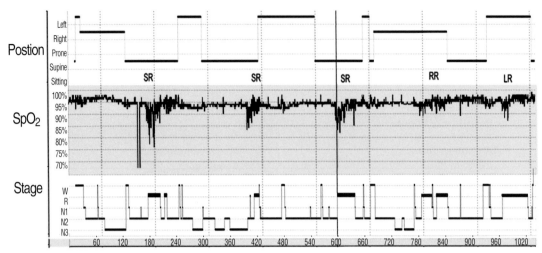

FIGURE P37-2 ■ Interaction between stage R and position. Note more severe desaturation during stage R (rapid eye movement [REM] sleep) in the supine position (supine REM (SR)) compared with that in the left (Left lateral REM (LR)) and right (Right lateral REM (RR)) positions. This patient had REM-associated obstructive sleep apnea (OSA) but the desaturations were worse in the supine position.

and subjective or objective measures of sleepiness in OSA patients is low (around 0.4). Su et al. studied the outcome of PAP treatment in groups with and without REM predominant OSA. REM-predominant OSA was defined as AHI-REM/AHI-NREM >2 and AHI-NREM <15/hr. All functional outcomes improved significantly after PAP therapy in both groups. The groups did not differ in the improvement in outcomes after PAP treatment. The authors concluded that functional outcomes in patients with REM-related OSA improve after treatment with PAP therapy comparable with that observed in patients with OSA not REM related. In an analysis of the MrOS community-based sample of older adult men ≥65 years-old, REM-related OSA was highly prevalent and was associated with objective indices of poorer sleep quality on polysomnography (PSG) but not with subjective measures of daytime sleepiness or quality of life. More outcome studies of REM-related OSA are needed. Until more data are available, treatment of REM-related OSA is recommended if the patient is symptomatic, the AHI during REM sleep is high, or the arterial oxygen desaturation during REM sleep is severe.

Ultimately, in all cases of mild OSA (overall AHI <15/hr), treatment decisions must be based on symptoms, comorbidity, and patient attitudes.

An interaction between REM sleep and posture also exists. The AHI is usually higher during supine than lateral REM sleep. Oksenburg et al. found that the order of AHI severity was: AHI REM supine > AHI NREM supine > AHI REM lateral > AHI NREM lateral.

However, the average length of apneas and hypopneas during REM sleep was similar in the supine and lateral postures. The arterial oxygen desaturation is usually worse in supine REM compared to lateral REM sleep (see Figure P37-2).

In the current patient, the overall AHI was in the mild range but the AHI during REM sleep was severely increased (Table F37-1) and associated with severe arterial oxygen desaturation. Note the pattern of respiratory events and desaturation on the hypnogram (see Table P37-1 and Figure P37-1, *A-C*). Loud snoring was a significant problem for his wife, and he did have symptoms of daytime sleepiness without explanation other than sleep apnea. Long episodes of apnea were noted by the patient's wife, and this concerned her. Long events during REM sleep (up to 50 seconds) were noted during the sleep study. The patient decided to try CPAP and a titration study found that CPAP of 8 centimeters of water (cm H_2O) was effective. Of interest, evidence of significant REM rebound during the CPAP titration was present. The patient was adherent to treatment. His wife noted cessation of snoring, and the patient reported fewer awakenings and a lower ESS score.

CLINICAL PEARLS

1. Some patients with OSA have obstructive apneas and hypopneas primarily during REM sleep (REM related/associated OSA), resulting in a low overall AHI despite frequent events (high AHI) during REM sleep and associated severe arterial oxygen desaturations during REM sleep.

2. The evidence for treatment of OSA present primarily during REM sleep is lacking from population studies looking for a correlation between the REM AHI and daytime sleepiness. However, one outcome study and clinical experience suggest that some patients will benefit from treatment of REM-associated OSA even if the overall AHI is mild.

3. Treatment should be considered in patients with a high AHI or severe desaturations during REM sleep. This is especially true if the patient is symptomatic and the symptoms are attributable to OSA. As with any case of mild OSA, the decision to treat depends on symptoms, the patient's attitude, and comorbidities.

4. An important interaction exists between posture and REM sleep: AHI REM supine > AHI NREM supine > AHI REM lateral > AHI NREM lateral. The worse desaturation is noted during supine REM sleep.

5. The most significant changes in breathing during REM sleep usually occur during the REM periods in the last part of the night when eye movements are most frequent. Often, the most severe desaturation is noted in the final REM periods of the night. An exception is when lateral rather than supine REM sleep is noted in the final REM periods of the night.

BIBLIOGRAPHY

Kass JE, Akers SM, Bartter TC, et al: REM-specific sleep-disordered breathing: a possible cause of excessive daytime sleepiness, *Am J Respir Crit Care Med* 154:167–169, 1996.

Wiegand L, Zwillich CW, Wiegand D, White DP: Changes in upper airway muscle activation and ventilation during phasic REM sleep in normal men, *J Appl Physiol* 71:488–497, 1991.

Penzel T, Moeller M, Becker HF: Effects of sleep position and sleep stage on collapsibility of the upper airways in sleep apnea, *Sleep* 24:90–95, 2001.

Boudewyns A, Punjabi N, Van de Heyning PH, et al: Abbreviated method for assessing upper airway function in obstructive sleep apnea, *Chest* 118:1031–1041, 2000.

Gould GA, Gugger M, Molloy J, et al: Breathing pattern and eye movement density during REM sleep in humans, *Am Rev Respir Dis* 138:874–877, 1988.

Su CS, Liu KT, Panjapornpon K, et al: Functional outcomes in patients with REM-related obstructive sleep apnea treated with positive airway pressure therapy, *J Clin Sleep Med* 8(3):243–247, 2012.

Blackwell T, Yaffe K, Ancoli-Israel S, et al: Osteoporotic Fractures in Men Study Group: Associations between sleep architecture and sleep-disordered breathing and cognition in older community-dwelling men: the Osteoporotic Fractures in Men Sleep Study, *J Am Geriatr Soc* 59(12):2217–2225, 2011.

Khan A, Harrison SL, Kezirian EJ, et al: Osteoporotic Fractures in Men (MrOS) Study Research Group: Obstructive sleep apnea during rapid eye movement sleep, daytime sleepiness, and quality of life in older men in osteoporotic fractures in men (MrOS) sleep study, *J Clin Sleep Med* 9(3):191–198, 2013.

Chami HA, Baldwin CM, Silverman A, et al: Sleepiness, quality of life, and sleep maintenance in REM versus non-REM sleep-disordered breathing, *Am J Respir Crit Care Med* 181(9):997–1002, 2010.

Oksenberg A, Arons E, Nasser K, et al: REM-related obstructive sleep apnea: the effect of body position, *J Clin Sleep Med* 6 (4):343–348, 2010.

Berry RB: Dreaming about an open upper airway, *Sleep* 29(4):429–431, 2006.

Berry RB, Gleeson K: Respiratory arousal from sleep: mechanisms and significance, *Sleep* 20(8):654–675, 1997.

A Patient with Severe Obesity and Hypercapnia

A 30-year-old woman was evaluated for daytime sleepiness and evidence of cor pulmonale. She did report mild snoring and usually slept in a recliner. The patient underwent nocturnal oximetry and was started on supplemental oxygen at night. However, this did not improve her sleepiness.

Physical examination: Morbid obesity

Body mass index (BMI): 45 kg/m^2

HEENT: Mallampati 4; neck—19 inch; chest—decreased breath sounds; cardiovascular— distant heart sounds; leg—3+ edema

Arterial blood gas (ABG) on room air: pH 7.34; arterial partial pressure of carbon dioxide (PCO$_2$) 55; partial pressure of oxygen (PO$_2$) 60 mm Hg.

Saturation of arterial oxygen (SaO$_2$): 92% or room air

Electrolytes: Sodium 140 mEq/L potassium 4.0 mEq/L; chloride 90 mEq/L; carbon dioxide 33 mEq/L

A sleep study was performed while the patient slept in a recliner (patient's request). The patient had severe arterial oxygen desaturation. Apneas and hypopneas were noted mainly during rapid eye movement (REM) sleep. The 30-second tracing in Figure P38-1 was recorded while the patient breathed room air and slept in a recliner. Low-flow oxygen was later added to keep the SaO$_2$ from staying below 85%. After 3 hours of diagnostic monitoring a positive airway pressure (PAP) titration was initiated and end-tidal PCO$_2$ monitoring was changed to transcutaneous PCO$_2$ monitoring.

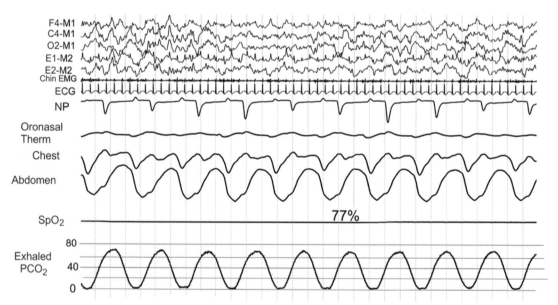

FIGURE P38-1 ■ A 30-second tracing while the patient breathed room air. Supplemental oxygen was later added for the remainder of the diagnostic study.

QUESTION

1. What is your diagnosis?

ANSWER

1. **Answer:** Obesity hypoventilation syndrome (OHS).

   Discussion: The OHS is characterized by obesity and daytime hypercapnia (arterial $PaCO_2$ >45 mm Hg), which cannot be fully attributed to an underlying cardiopulmonary or neurologic disease.[1,2] Hypercapnia worsens during sleep and is often associated with severe arterial oxygen desaturation. Hypoventilation is also usually worse during REM compared with NREM sleep. The majority of patients with OHS have comorbid obstructive sleep apnea (OSA; 80%–90%). In these patients, daytime hypercapnia may improve or even normalize with adequate PAP treatment and sustained adherence to treatment.[3,4] Those patients with OHS but without OSA exhibit sustained or episodic episodes of shallow breathing during sleep associated with worsening hypoventilation and hypoxemia. Patients with the OHS may have few, if any, sleep complaints or may present with considerable sleep disturbance, including reduced sleep efficiency and frequent awakenings. Hypercapnia and hypoxemia may remain unnoticed for quite some time until sudden deterioration with cardiopulmonary arrest or severe decompensation (acute worsening of chronic hypercapnic respiratory failure) develops. Patients with OHS may develop evidence of cor pulmonary and right ventricular hypertrophy. The mortality rate is high if OHS is not diagnosed and treated effectively.

   ## Diagnosis of OHS

   The definitive diagnosis of the OHS requires the presence of obesity (BMI >30 kg/m^2) and an ABG testing while awake, with a PCO_2 of > 45 mm Hg. In addition, the cause of the hypoventilation is not attributed to lung disease, muscle weakness, or a chest wall disorder (other than obesity). An elevated serum CO_2 (primarily bicarbonate [HCO_3]), is a very useful clue that a patient with OSA should be tested for hypoventilation. The serum CO_2 is included on routine metabolic or electrolyte laboratory panels. The elevated HCO_3 in OHS patients represents renal compensation for chronic respiratory acidosis (elevated arterial PCO_2). However, an elevated HCO_3 could also be caused by metabolic alkalosis. Mokhlesi and associates[2] reported that 20% of the 410 patients referred to a sleep center to rule out OSA had OHS. In this study, only 3% of patients with hypercapnia had a HCO_3 level less than 27 milliequivalents per liter (mEq/L) (92% sensitivity), but 50% of patients with HCO_3 of ≥ 27 had hypoventilation. The authors concluded that obese patients with both OSA and a HCO_3 >27 mEq/L should undergo ABG testing. Other clues that OHS may be present include a borderline awake SaO_2 (90%–92%) or evidence of significant cor pulmonale.

   Patients with the OHS are a heterogeneous group. The causes of hypoventilation include nocturnal upper airway obstruction (OSA), decreased respiratory system compliance because of obesity, and intrinsic or acquired abnormalities in ventilatory drive.[4-8] As noted above up to 20% of OHS patients have an AHI <5 per hour (hr) but exhibit both daytime hypercapnia and severe sleep-related hypoventilation and arterial oxygen desaturation. One study characterized patients on the basis of their response to PAP treatment.[8] Some OHS patients were adequately treated with continuous PAP (CPAP) alone. Opening the upper airway with CPAP during sleep restored adequate oxygenation. Others still had persistent oxygen desaturation and hypoventilation despite the absence of apnea or hypopnea. Some with persistent air flow limitation responded to higher levels of CPAP (decreasing the upper airway resistance). Presumably, they could not compensate for a high upper airway resistance even if apnea and hypopnea were not present. Some patients required the addition of supplemental oxygen along with CPAP. Another group of patients required either nasal bilevel PAP (BPAP) or mechanical ventilation with or without oxygen. The group of patients with OHS who manifest hypoventilation without significant OSA are likely to have abnormal ventilatory control or very decreased respiratory system compliance because of extreme obesity. The relative importance of OSA, abnormal ventilatory control, and decreased respiratory system compliance varies among individuals with OHS. Of note, the mortality rate is high among patients with severe OHS who are not treated or do not comply with treatment.[9,10] Nowbar and colleagues[9] studied the outcomes of obese patients admitted to a medical service. Of those who had hypoventilation, the 18-month mortality was 23% compared with 9% in the group with equivalent obesity but no hypoventilation. Of interest, only 6% of the hypoventilation group received treatment for the hypoventilation!

   ## Treatment of OHS

   Piper and coworkers[5] performed a randomized trial that compared CPAP and BPAP for treatment of patients with OHS. Patients with significant residual desaturation (SaO_2 <80%

for >10 minutes) on a level of CPAP that eliminated obstructive events, an acute rise in PCO_2 >10 mm Hg during REM sleep, or an increase in PCO_2 >10 mm Hg in the morning compared with the afternoon were excluded (treated with BPAP). An equivalent reduction in daytime PCO_2 was noted at 3 months in patients randomized to CPAP or BPAP. Adherence to the treatment modalities was also not significantly different. In the BPAP group, the mean inspiratory PAP (IPAP) and expiratory PAP (EPAP) were 16 and 10 cm H_2O, respectively, and the spontaneous mode of BPAP was employed. A few patients in both groups required supplemental oxygen in addition to PAP. OHS patients may require high levels of EPAP to prevent obstructive apnea, and this tends to limit the available range of pressure support unless very high IPAP levels are used. In a study of the effect of NPPV in OHS patients by Berger and colleagues,[6] EPAP values up to 14 cm H_2O and IPAP values up to 25 cm H_2O were needed. The mean IPAP and EPAP values were 18 and 8 cm H_2O, respectively. Patients with OHS may present with acute respiratory failure.[10,11] The treatment of choice is PAP (usually BPAP and oxygen). Severely affected patients may require temporary endotracheal intubation and mechanical ventilation.[11] Tracheostomy may be life saving in patients noncompliant with PAP treatment who have repeated bouts of hypercapnic respiratory failure.

In patients with stable chronic OHS, treatment with PAP may reduce the daytime PCO_2 as well as reduce apnea and hypopnea and nocturnal desaturation. Berthon-Jones and Sullivan[12] showed chronic CPAP treatment of OSA patients with daytime hypoventilation resulted in a leftward shift in the ventilatory response to CO_2 (ventilation plotted versus PCO_2) during the day without a change in slope. The PCO_2 set point is lowered, and ventilation is higher at any given PCO_2. A study by Mokhlesi and associate[3] found that the amount of improvement in the daytime PCO_2 is critically dependent on adherence. Considerable variability existed, but the PCO_2 dropped by about 3 mm Hg for every hour of nightly adherence and reached a plateau with longer than 4.5 hours of use. In summary, the treatment of patients with OHS may require CPAP or BPAP with or without the need for supplemental oxygen. Although CPAP is often sufficient for some patients, most clinicians would use BPAP if the hypoventilation is moderate to severe. Adequate treatment may improve daytime as well as nocturnal gas exchange and prevent apneas and hypopneas.

In the present patient, polysomnography (PSG) during the diagnostic portion of the study revealed only a mild AHI overall (10/hr) but a severely increased AHI during a brief period of REM sleep (40/hr). The patient slept in a recliner, and the AHI may have been higher in the supine position. End-tidal PCO_2 monitoring showed an awake end-tidal PCO_2 of 50 mm Hg that climbed to 70 mm Hg mm Hg during NREM sleep. Values were not obtained during REM sleep because of small tidal volumes making measurements inaccurate. The patient underwent titration with BPAP, and supplemental oxygen was added to keep the SaO_2 over 90%. End-tidal PCO_2 monitoring was changed to transcutaneous PCO_2 monitoring during the PAP titration. On BPAP of 16/8 centimeters of water (cm H_2O) and 3 L/min supplemental oxygen, the AHI was less than 5/hr (including REM sleep), and the SaO_2 remained above 92%. The transcutaneous PCO_2 during sleep was 60 mm Hg on the highest pressures. It was appreciated that if the patient slept in the supine position, much higher pressure would be needed. Ultimately, the patient was treated with BPAP, oxygen, and sleep in a recliner. The average adherence was 6/hr per night. ABG testing 1 month later showed a PCO_2 of 46 mm Hg, and the patient had lost about 25 pounds (mostly edema).

CLINICAL PEARLS

1. The two groups of patients with OSA and daytime hypercapnia are patients with the OHS and the overlap syndrome (OSA+chronic obstructive pulmonary disease [COPD]).

2. A clue that hypoventilation is present in an obese patient with OSA is an elevated CO_2 (HCO_3) on electrolyte testing (>27 mEq/L). ABG testing during wakefulness showing a $PaCO_2$ >45 mm Hg confirms the diagnosis if hypoventilation is not better explained by lung disease, a neuromuscular disorder, or a thoracic cage disorder.

3. About 80% of patients with OHS have OSA. The rest experience hypoventilation during the day with worse hypoventilation at night.

4. Daytime sleepiness may not be present in patients with OHS.

5. Untreated OHS results in a high mortality rate.

6. The treatment of choice for the OHS is CPAP or BPAP. For the group without OSA or for patients with severe hypoventilation, BPAP is recommended. Supplemental oxygen with PAP will be needed for many patients.

7. With adherence to PAP treatment, some patients will have a normalized daytime PCO_2. Patients with normalized daytime PCO_2 on treatment usually have a major component of OSA.

REFERENCES

1. American Academy of Sleep Medicine: *International classification of sleep disorders*, ed 3, Darien, IL, 2013, American Academy of Sleep Medicine.
2. Mokhlesi B, Taulaimat A, Baibussowitsch I, et al: Obesity hypoventilation syndrome: prevalence and predictors in patients with obstructive sleep apnea, *Sleep Breath* 11:117–124, 2007.
3. Mokhlesi B, Tulaimat A, Evans AT, et al: Impact of adherence with positive airway pressure therapy on hypercapnia in obstructive sleep apnea, *J Clin Sleep Med* 2(1):57–62, 2006.
4. Piper AJ, Grunstein RR: Obesity hypoventilation syndrome: mechanisms and management, *Am J Respir Crit Care Med* 183:292–298, 2011.
5. Piper AJ, Wang D, Yee BJ, et al: Randomized trial of CPAP vs bilevel support in the treatment of obesity hypoventilation syndrome without severe nocturnal desaturation, *Thorax* 63:395–401, 2008.
6. Berger KI, Ayappa I, Chatr-Amontri B, et al: Obesity hypoventilation syndrome as a spectrum of respiratory disturbances during sleep, *Chest* 120:1231–1238, 2001.
7. de Llano LA Pérez, Golpe R, Piquer MO, et al: Clinical heterogeneity among patients with obesity hypoventilation syndrome: therapeutic implications, *Respiration* 75:34–39, 2008.
8. Banerjee D, Yee BJ, Piper AJ, et al: Obesity hypoventilation syndrome: hypoxemia during continuous positive airway pressure, *Chest* 131:1678–1684, 2007.
9. Nowbar S, Burkart KM, Gonzales R, et al: Obesity-hypoventilation in hospitalized patients: prevalence, effects, and outcome, *Am J Med* 116:1–7, 2004.
10. Budweiser S, Riedl SG, Jörres RA, et al: Mortality and prognostic factors in patients with obesity-hypoventilation syndrome undergoing noninvasive ventilation, *J Intern Med* 261:375–383, 2007.
11. Shivaram U, Cash ME, Beal A: Nasal continuous positive airway pressure in decompensated hypercapnic respiratory failure as a complication of sleep apnea, *Chest* 104:770–774, 1993.
12. Berthon-Jones M, Sullivan CE: Time course of change in ventilatory response to CO2 with long-term CPAP therapy for obstructive sleep apnea, *Am Rev Respir Dis* 135:144–147, 1987.

FUNDAMENTALS 21

Pediatric Obstructive Sleep Apnea

Significant differences exist in the diagnosis and management of obstructive sleep apnea (OSA) in pediatric patients compared with adults.[1-3] The major differences in the presentation and characteristics of OSA between children and adults are listed in Table F21-1. Although very obese children or those with structural upper airway abnormalities may present with symptoms similar to those in adults, the typical history in childhood OSA is one of inattentiveness, aggressive behavior, and impulsiveness,[1,2] combined with abnormal sleep behaviors observed by the parents. These nocturnal behaviors include snoring, labored breathing, diaphoresis, paradoxical chest movement, or frequent movements during sleep. Less commonly, children may present with failure to thrive. A recent systematic review and associated recommendations for the evaluation and treatment of pediatric OSA is available.[1,2] A summary of the recommendations is listed in Box F21-1.

EPIDEMIOLOGY

The age range of highest prevalence of OSA patients is typically from 4 to 6 years (2 to 8 years, according to some authors) when hypertrophy of the tonsils occurs.[4,5]

A 2008 review of breathing in children concluded that the prevalence of "always snoring" ranged from 1.5% to 6% and "habitual snoring" ranged from 5% to 12%. The prevalence of parent-reported apneic events ranged from

TABLE F21-1	Differences between Children and Adults with Obstructive Sleep Apnea	
	Children	**Adults**
Clinical Findings		
Peak age	Preschool (4–6 years [yr])	50–70 years
Gender ratio	M = F age <13 years M > F if older children included	M > F
Etiology	Adenotonsillar hypertrophy	Obesity or upper airway structure/function
Weight	Failure to thrive to obese, many normal in size	Obese
Excessive daytime sleepiness	Less common	Common
Neurobehavioral	Impulsiveness, aggressiveness, inattention	Impaired vigilance
Polysomnography		
Definition of abnormal	Obstructive apnea index >1/hr OAHI >1.0–1.4	AHI ≥5/hr RDI ≥5/hr (ICSD-3)
Obstruction pattern	Obstructive hypoventilation Apnea during REM sleep	Obstructive apnea/hypopnea Higher AHI in REM sleep
Sleep architecture	Normal	Reduced stage N3 and REM sleep
Sleep stage with OSA	REM (stage R)	REM > NREM
Cortical arousal	Low rates <50% of apneas	High rates 60%–80% of apnea/hypopnea

AHI, Apnea-hypopnea index; *ICSD-3, International Classification of Sleep Disorders*, Third Edition; *NREM*, non–rapid eye movement; *OAHI*, obstructive apnea–hypopnea index; *OSA*, obstructive sleep apnea; *REM*, rapid eye movement.

BOX F21-1	American Association of Pediatrics Recommendations for Evaluation and Treatment of Pediatric Obstructive Sleep Apnea

1. All children/adolescents should be screened for snoring.
2. Polysomnography should be performed in children/adolescents with snoring and symptoms/signs of obstructive sleep apnea syndrome (OSAS); if polysomnography is not available, then alternative diagnostic tests or referral to a specialist for more extensive evaluation may be considered.
3. Adenotonsillectomy is recommended as the first-line treatment of patients with adenotonsillar hypertrophy.
4. High-risk patients should be monitored as inpatients postoperatively.
5. Patients should be re-evaluated postoperatively to determine whether further treatment is required. Objective testing should be performed in patients who are high risk or have persistent symptoms/signs of OSAS after therapy.
6. Continuous positive airway pressure is recommended as treatment if adenotonsillectomy is not performed or if OSAS persists postoperatively.
7. Weight loss is recommended in addition to other therapy in patients who are overweight or obese.
8. Intranasal corticosteroids are an option for children with mild OSAS in whom adenotonsillectomy is contraindicated or for mild postoperative OSAS.

From Marcus CL, Brooks LJ, Draper KA, et al, for the American Academy of Pediatrics: Diagnosis and management of childhood obstructive sleep apnea syndrome, *Pediatrics* 130(3):576-584, 2012.

0.2% to 4%. Using questionnaires filled out by parents, the prevalence of OSA has been estimated to be 4% to 11%. The prevalence by diagnostic studies has been estimated to be 1% to 4% (reported range 0.1%–13%). Evidence suggests that pediatric OSA is more common among children who are heavier. Studies considering younger children (<13 years) have generally found an equal prevalence of OSA in boys and girls. In a majority of studies including older children, a male predominance was found.[4,5] A higher prevalence of pediatric OSA may be found among African Americans compared with whites.

CONSEQUENCES OF CHILDHOOD OSA

Many of the important consequences of untreated pediatric OSA are listed in Box F21-2.[5] They are classified as neurobehavioral, metabolic, and cardiovascular consequences.

Neurobehavioral Consequences

Studies have suggested that both habitual snoring and childhood OSA are associated with behavioral problems, particularly impulsiveness, aggressiveness, and inattentive behaviors.[6] Such behaviors may improve after effective treatment (usually with tonsillectomy and adenoidectomy). Sometimes, a diagnosis of attention-deficit disorder (ADD) is made when a patient, in fact, has OSA. However, one should not assume every child with ADD and hyperactivity (attention-deficit hyperactivity disorder [ADHD]) has OSA. Children with OSA often perform poorly in school and on tests of intelligence, but they improve with treatment. Both hypoxia and sleep fragmentation may cause neurocognitive changes. although some studies suggest that impairment is reversible with treatment, it is still not known if untreated OSA, causes irreversible damage to a component of the central nervous system (CNS).

Although excessive daytime sleepiness is less prominent in childhood OSA compared with

BOX F21-2	Sequelae of Pediatric Obstructive Sleep Apnea

NEUROCOGNITIVE

Decreased quality of life
Aggressive behavior
Poor school performance
Depression
Attention deficit disorder
Hyperactivity
Moodiness

METABOLIC

Elevated C reactive protein
Insulin resistance
Hypercholesterolemia

Elevated transaminases
Decreased insulin-like growth factor
Decreased or altered growth hormone secretion
Increased leptin

CARDIOVASCULAR

Autonomic dysfunction
Systemic hypertension
Absent blood pressure "dipping" during sleep
Left ventricular dysfunction
Pulmonary hypertension
Abnormal heart rate variability
Elevated vascular endothelial growth factor

Adapted from Katz ES, D'Ambrosio CM: Pediatric obstructive sleep apnea syndrome, *Clin Chest Med* 31:221-234, 2010.

OSA in adults, it does occur and may remain unrecognized. Using the multiple sleep latency test (MSLT), daytime sleepiness is thought to occur in between 13% and 40% of patients.[7,8] Daytime sleepiness is often more prominent in obese children with OSA.

Metabolic and Inflammatory Consequences

Untreated pediatric OSA has been associated with a failure to thrive.[5] The possible origin is a reduction in insulin-like growth factor (IGF) associated with decreased secretion of growth hormone. IGF binding protein (IGF-3) correlates with growth hormone secretion and is decreased in some children with OSA. These changes are reversible, and catch-up growth occurs with adequate treatment. Currently, with its epidemic prevalence, obesity is more often noted than failure to thrive. Up to half of childhood OSA patients are obese. Leptin, an adipocyte-secreted hormone, is increased in children with OSA and decreases after treatment.[9,10]

Leukotrienes and their receptors are increased in adenotonsillar tissue and exhaled condensates of children with OSA.[11,12] The combination of nasal inhaled steroid and the leuokotriene inhibitors (montelukast) was found to have benefit in a study of patients with residual sleepiness after tonsillectomy and adenoidectomy.[13] However, long-term success with anti-inflammatory therapy has not been established. Children with OSA may also have elevated serum levels of tumor necrosis factor-alpha (TNF-α), C-reactive protein, interleukin 6 and 8 (IL-6 and IL-8), and interferon-gamma (IFN-γ) levels.[5] These changes may occur independent of obesity.

DIAGNOSIS

The *International Classification of Sleep Disorders*, Third Edition (ICSD-3) diagnostic criteria[14] for pediatric OSA are listed in Box F21-3. Some pediatric sleep centers report not only the AHI but also the obstructive AHI (OAHI = number of obstructive and mixed apneas + hypopneas per hour of sleep) and a central apnea index (CAI). The values of respiratory indices considered diagnostic of pediatric OSA vary, but typically an obstructive apnea index >1/hr or OAHI >1–2/hr is a criterion for diagnosis. The decision to treat is based on symptoms as well as polysomnography (PSG) findings (OAHI). An AHI of 5 to 10/hour is considered moderate and >10/hour severe in children. Most clinicians will treat patients with an AHI of 2 to <5/hour if symptoms are present. A diagnosis of OSA can also be made on the basis of obstructive hypoventilation as defined in Box F21-3 (partial pressure of carbon dioxide [PCO$_2$] >50 millimeters of mercury [mm Hg] for ≥25% of total sleep time [TST]).

PSG IN PEDIATRIC OSA

Most obstructive apnea in pediatric patients occurs during REM sleep (Figure F21-1). However, the most common pattern in pediatric sleep monitoring is "obstructive hypoventilation" (see Fundamentals 14). This pattern consists of long periods of air flow limitation, increased inspiratory effort, increased end-tidal partial pressure of carbon dioxide (P$_{ET}$CO$_2$), and variable amounts of arterial oxygen desaturation. Traditional monitoring using oronasal thermistor flow often demonstrates few changes except for an elevation in P$_{ET}$CO$_2$ and perhaps no or mild drops in the saturation of arterial oxygen

---

BOX F21-3	**Pediatric Obstructive Sleep Apnea: ICSD-3 Diagnostic Criteria (Diagnosis Requires A + B)**

A. The presence of one or more of the following:
   1. Snoring
   2. Labored, paradoxical or obstructed breathing during the child's sleep
   3. Sleepiness, hyperactivity, behavioral problems or learning problems
B. Polysomnography demonstrates one or more of the following:
   1. One or more obstructive or mixed apneas, or hypopneas, per hour of sleep*
   2. A pattern of obstructive hypoventilation, defined as at least 25% of total sleep time with

hypercapnia (PaCO$_2$ >50 mm Hg), arterial oxygen desaturation, or combined hypercapnia and desaturation, in association with one or more of the following: snoring, flattening of the inspiratory nasal pressure waveform, and paradoxical thoracoabdominal motion.
   a. Snoring.
   b. Flattening of the inspiratory nasal pressure waveform.
   c. Paradoxical thoracoabdominal motion.

From American Academy of Sleep Medicine: International classification of sleep disorders, ed 3, Darien, IL, 2014, American Academy of Sleep Medicine.
PaCO$_2$, Partial pressure of arterial carbon dioxide.
*Respiratory events as defined by the latest version of the *AASM Manual for the Scoring of Sleep and Associated Events*.

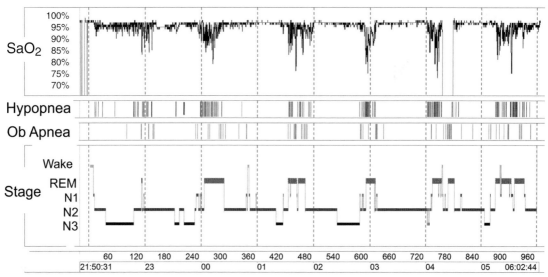

FIGURE F21-1 ▪ Summary of polysomnography in a 4-year-old girl with very loud snoring and disturbed sleep. Note that most of the respiratory events were noted during rapid eye movement (REM) sleep.

(SaO_2). Paradoxical motion of the chest and abdomen may be noted (chest moving inward during inspiration). Nasal pressure monitoring shows air flow limitation (flattening) and reduced but stable flow. This common pattern is the reason the $P_{ET}CO_2$ is an integral part of pediatric sleep studies. The *AASM Scoring Manual*[15] states that sleep-related hypoventilation in children should be scored when >25% of the total sleep time is spent with a PCO_2 >50 mm Hg using transcutaneous carbon dioxide ($TcPCO_2$) monitoring or measurement of $P_{ET}CO_2$.

The sleep architecture of pediatric patients with OSA typically shows a much lower percentage of respiratory events associated with arousals than in adults. The normal sleep architecture is often maintained.

TREATMENT OF PEDIATRIC OSA

Because the majority of pediatric OSA is associated with adenotonsillar hypertrophy, the treatment of choice for most patients in tonsillectomy and adenoidectomy (TNA).[1,2] *However, the severity of OSA does not correlate with tonsillar size.* Other factors such as upper airway structure or obesity affect the impact of tonsillar hypertrophy on breathing during sleep. The epidemic of childhood obesity has tremendous implications for treatments and their outcomes. OSA in obese children is more similar to adult OSA. *However, the current recommendations is for TNA as first line treatment even in obese children if tonsillar hypertrophy is present.* A recent systematic review of TNA treatment of pediatric OSA[2] concluded: "Although the OSA syndrome improved postoperatively, the proportion of patients who had residual OSAS ranged from 13% to 29% in

low-risk populations to 73% when obese children were included and stricter polysomnographic criteria were used. Nevertheless, OSAS may improve after TNA even in obese children, thus supporting surgery as a reasonable initial treatment."[1,2] Certainly, patients with residual symptoms after TNA or those with a pre-treatment OAHI in the moderate to severe range should be restudied. If a significant residual OAHI is present after TNA, possible treatments include weight loss, positive airway pressure (PAP), dental procedures such as rapid maxillary expansion, or medications to reduce adenoidal and tonsillar inflammation.

Medical Treatment of OSA in Pediatric Patients

In obese children, weight management should be instituted even if TNA is planned. Some studies suggest a role for anti-inflammatory medications in the management of adenotonsillar hypertrophy. Such treatments may suffice in patients with mild OSA or when surgery will be delayed or is not possible. As noted above, the combination of nasal inhaled steroid and the leuokotriene inhibitors (montelukast) was found to have benefit in a study of patients with residual sleepiness after tonsillectomy and adenoidectomy.[13]

Tonsillectomy and Adenoidectomy

TNA has been the standard treatment for OSA in pediatric patients for many years (Figure F21-2). Over 400,000 such surgeries are performed per year. It is estimated that PSG is performed in only about 10% of patients undergoing TNA.[18] Studies have shown that history and physical examination are not accurate in

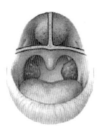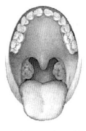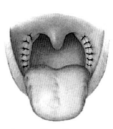

FIGURE F21-2 ■ Tonsillectomy and adenoidectomy. The adenoid and tonsillar tissues are removed and the lateral pharyngeal walls are sutured to prevent collapse. (From Won CHJ, Li KK, Guilleminault C: Surgical treatment of obstructive sleep apnea, *Proc Am Thorac Soc* 5:193-199, 2008.)

predicting the presence or absence of OSA. The size of tonsils is not predictive of OSA. However, the need for routine PSG before TNA for childhood sleep apnea is still debated.[18,19] Recent guidelines published by the American Academy of Pediatrics[2] (see Box F21-1) made the following recommendation: "Polysomnography should be performed in children/adolescents with snoring and symptoms/signs of OSAS." Performing PSG before TNA has a number of advantages: (1) It helps achieve accurate diagnosis and avoid unnecessary surgery; (2) PSG results provide parents with an estimate of chance of surgical success; patients with an elevated AHI may require additional treatment beyond TNA; and (3) PSG and clinical evaluation may reveal factors indicating increased risk for postoperative complications.[20]

Earlier studies found that TNA successfully eliminated OSA in 75% to 100% of patients. Recent prospective studies using postoperative PSG have found lower cure rates (depending on the definition of success).[16,17] A meta-analysis by Brietzke et al.[16] found 82% of patients to be successfully treated for OSA. In the studies analyzed, treatment success varied between studies (AHI <1 to 5/hr). Another meta-analysis of the efficacy of TNA by Friedman and associates[17] found that the percentage of patients with a "cure," defined as an AHI <1/hr, was about 60%. Most patients undergoing TNA do improve, but frequently significant residual OSA persists.

As noted above, TNA is still considered the initial treatment of choice in pediatric patients with OSA and tonsillar hypertrophy,[2] even if obesity is present. Complications from the TNA include bleeding, pain, infection, and weight loss. A list of proposed risk factors for TNA requiring overnight hospitalization or more long-term recovery room monitoring are listed in Box F21-4.[1,2,20] Nasal continuous positive airway pressure (CPAP) may be used to manage postoperative complications in very severely affected individuals. The need for routine postoperative PSG in patients who have undergone TNA (after surgical healing) is also a subject of controversy. The American Academy of Pediatric Guidelines[2] recommends the following: "Patients should be re-evaluated postoperatively to determine whether further treatment is required. Objective testing should be performed in patients who are high risk or have persistent symptoms/signs of OSAS after therapy." High-risk patients would include patients with moderate to severe OSA (AHI of 5–10, or >10/hr, respectively) before surgery as well as those with failure to thrive, craniofacial abnormalities, pulmonary hypertension, or significant obesity. Nasal CPAP and weight loss (if applicable) may be used to treat significant residual OSA after TNA.

Rapid Maxillary Expansion and Distraction Osteogenesis

Rapid maxillary expansion (RME) in conjunction with TNA has been shown to be successful in treating children with OSA and maxillary

---

BOX F21-4	Criteria for Increased Risk of Tonsillectomy and Adenoidectomy

CLINICAL CRITERIA

- Age <3 years
- Craniofacial abnormalities affecting the pharyngeal airway (especially midface hypoplasia or micrognathia or retrognathia)
- Failure to thrive
- Hypotonia
- Obesity
- Neuromuscular disorders

- Cardiac complications of obstructive sleep apnea (OSA) (right ventricular hypertrophy, cor pulmonale)
- Previous upper airway trauma
- Undergoing a uvulopalatopharyngoplasty in addition to tonsillectomy and adenoidectomy (TNA)

POLYSOMNOGRAPHY CRITERIA

- Severe OSA on polysomnography
- Arterial oxygen saturation (SaO_2) nadir less than 70%

Adapted from references 1 and 2.

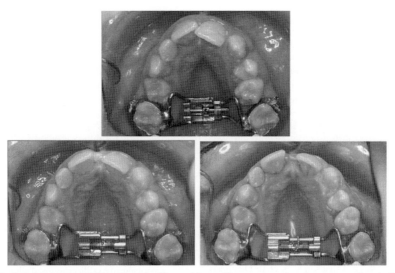

FIGURE F21-3 ■ Occlusal sequence of treatment with rapid maxillary expansion from crowding in the upper central incisors (*top*) to a wide space (*bottom*). Note how the palatal vault has changed. (From Pirelli P, Saponara M, Gulleminault C: Rapid maxillary expansion in children with obstructive sleep apnea syndrome, *Sleep* 27:764, 2004.)

contraction (high arched palate and unilateral or bilateral cross-bite).[21,22,23] RME requires an orthodontic device (Figure F21-3), anchored to two upper molars on each side of the jaw, which applies daily pressure causes each half of the maxilla to grow apart. This technique aims to expand the hard palate laterally, raise the soft palate, and widen the nasal passages. RME needs to occur before cartilage in the suture between left and right maxilla becomes bone (5–16 years of age). *Distraction osteogenesis* is defined as the mechanical induction of new bone between two bony surfaces that are gradually distracted (separated). If RME is not successful or deemed insufficient, mandibular distraction osteogenesis (RMD) is performed surgically.[24] A surgeon uses a saw to create osteotomies in the mandible and then either an internal or an external device is used to expand the bones. Mandibular distraction osteogenesis is often used to treat sleep apnea in patients with severe congenital abnormalities of the mandible (mandibular retrognathia) as in Treacher Collins syndrome or Pierre Robin syndrome.

PAP Treatment in Pediatric Patients

Fundamentals 24 provides guidelines for the titration of PAP in adults and children. Here, a few items of special interest will be discussed. PAP titrations in children require some extra considerations.[25–27] First, split studies are not recommended. If the child without previous mask desensitization undergoes a split-night study, the child maybe frightened, and this will make subsequent CPAP use unlikely. Children are often given masks to play with and wear

during the day before scheduled studies. The child should be desensitized to the mask during the day by wearing it for increasing periods while engaging in a fun activity (e.g., watching a favorite video). This process can takes several weeks and should continue until the child is comfortable with the mask on their face. Pediatric-size masks should be available. Durable medical equipment providers and sleep technologists skilled and willing to provide care for pediatric patients should be part of the team. Studies have shown that structured behavioral interventions help with compliance (graduated exposure, positive reinforcement, dealing with escape and avoidance behavior, and differential reinforcement of distracting activities that allowed the child to wear a mask). As in adults, objective monitoring of adherence is essential to guide treatment in children and adolescents as well. A social support system to educate parents and secure their participation is also essential.

A recent prospective study of PAP adherence in children and adolescents found that adherence is related primarily to family and demographic factors rather than severity of apnea or measures of psychosocial functioning.[28] The authors concluded that further research is needed to determine the relative contributions of maternal education, socioeconomic status, and cultural beliefs to PAP adherence in children, to develop better adherence programs. The involvement of psychologists and social workers skilled at behavioral interventions in children should be an integral part of CPAP programs for children. Recently, a questionnaire has been developed to identify barriers to CPAP use.[29]

CLINICAL PEARLS

1. The presentation of pediatric OSA differs from that in adults. Frequently, behavioral issues and disturbed sleep, rather than daytime sleepiness, prompt evaluation.

2. The treatment of choice of pediatric patients with OSA and tonsillar hypertrophy is TNA, even if obesity is present.

3. Residual sleep apnea is present in a significant proportion of children following TNA. Those with persistent symptoms or risk factors for failure of TNA (obesity, high presurgery AHI, facial abnormalities) should undergo a sleep study after TNA.

4. PAP treatment of children requires special interventions. Split studies are not recommended. Children should have the opportunity to play with and wear masks pre-study until they are comfortable with having the mask on their face. Behavioral techniques such as distracting activities while wearing the mask are useful. Social support to educate parents and secure their active involvement in treatment is essential.

REFERENCES

1. Marcus CL, Brooks LJ, Draper K, et al: Diagnosis and management of childhood obstructive sleep apnea syndrome: clinical practice guideline. American Academy of Pediatrics, *Pediatrics* 130:576–584, 2012.

2. Marcus CL, Brooks LJ, Davidson WS, et al: Diagnosis and management of childhood obstructive sleep apnea syndrome: technical report. American Academy of Pediatrics, *Pediatrics* 130:8714–e755, 2012.

3. Marcus CL: Sleep-disordered breathing in children, *Am J Respir Crit Care Med* 164:16–30, 2001.

4. Lumeng JC, Chervin RD: Epidemiology of pediatric OSA, *Proc Am Thorac Soc* 5:242–252, 2008.

5. Katz ES, D'Ambrosio CM: Pediatric obstructive sleep apnea syndrome, *Clin Chest Med* 31:221–234, 2010.

6. Chervin RD, Archbold KH, Dillon JE, et al: Inattention, hyperactivity, and symptoms of sleep-disordered breathing, *Pediatrics* 109:449–456, 2002.

7. Chervin RD, Weatherly RA, Ruzicka DL, et al: Subjective sleepiness and polysomnography correlates in children scheduled for adenotonsillectomy versus other surgical care, *Sleep* 29(4):495–503, 2006.

8. Gozal D, Kheirandish-Gozal L: Obesity and excessive daytime sleepiness in prepubertal children with obstructive sleep apnea, *Pediatrics* 123:13–18, 2009.

9. Tauman R, Serpero LD, Capdevila OS, et al: Adipokines in children with sleep disordered breathing, *Sleep* 30:443–449, 2007.

10. Nakra N, Bhargava S, Dzuira J, et al: Sleep-disordered breathing in children with metabolic syndrome: the role of leptin and sympathetic nervous system activity and the effect of continuous positive airway pressure, *Pediatrics* 122:e634–e642, 2008.

11. Goldbart AD, Goldman JL, Li RC, et al: Differential expression of cysteinyl leukotriene receptors 1 and 2 in tonsils of children with obstructive sleep apnea syndrome or recurrent infection, *Chest* 12:613–618, 2004.

12. Goldbart AD, Krishna J, Li RC, et al: Inflammatory mediators in exhaled condensate of children with obstructive sleep apnea syndrome, *Chest* 130:143–148, 2006.

13. Kheirandish L, Goldbart AD, Gozal D: Intranasal steroids and oral leukotriene modifier therapy in residual sleep-disordered breathing after tonsillectomy and adenoidectomy in children, *Pediatrics* 117:e61–e66, 2006.

14. American Academy of Sleep Medicine: International classification of sleep disorders, ed 3, Darien, IL, 2014, American Academy of Sleep Medicine.

15. Berry RB, Brooks R, Gamaldo CE, et al., for the American Academy of Sleep Medicine: *The AASM manual for the scoring of sleep and associated events: rules, terminology and technical specifications*, Version 2.0.3, www.aasmnet.org, Darien, IL, 2014, American Academy of Sleep Medicine.

16. Brietzke SE, Gallagher D: The effectiveness of tonsillectomy and adenoidectomy in the treatment of pediatric obstructive sleep apnea/hypopnea syndrome: a meta-analysis, *Otolaryngol Head Neck Surg* 134:979–984, 2006.

17. Friedman M, Wilson M, Chang HW: Updated systematic review of tonsillectomy and adenoidectomy for treatment of pediatric obstructive sleep apnea/hypopnea syndrome, *Otolaryngol Head Neck Surg* 140:800–808, 2009.

18. Hoban TF: Polysomnography should be required both before and after adenotonsillectomy for childhood sleep disordered breathing, *J Clin Sleep Med* 3:675–677, 2007.

19. Friedman N: Polysomnography should not be required before and after adenotonsillectomy for childhood sleep disordered breathing, *J Clin Sleep Med* 3:678–680, 2007.

20. Rosen GM, Muckle RP, Mahowald MW, et al: Postoperative respiratory compromise in children with obstructive sleep apnea syndrome: can it be anticipated? *Pediatrics* 93:784–788, 1994.

21. Cistulli PA, Palmisano RG, Poole MD: Treatment of obstructive sleep apnea syndrome by rapid maxillary expansion, *Sleep* 21:831–835, 1998.

22. Villa MP, Malagola C, Pagani J, et al: Rapid maxillary expansion in children with obstructive sleep apnea syndrome: 12-month follow-up, *Sleep Med* 8:128–134, 2007.

23. Pirelli P, Saponara M, Gulleminault C: Rapid maxillary expansion in children with obstructive sleep apnea syndrome, *Sleep* 27:761–766, 2004.

24. Cohen SR, Simms C, Burstein F: Mandibular distraction osteogenesis in the treatment of upper airway obstruction in children with craniofacial deformities, *Plast Reconstr Surg* 101:312–318, 1998.

25. Marcus CL, Rosen G, Davidson-Ward S, et al: Adherence to and effectiveness of positive airway pressure therapy in children with obstructive sleep apnea, *Pediatrics* 117:e442–e451, 2006.

26. Koontz KL, Slifer KJ, Cataldo MD, Marcus CL: Improving pediatric compliance with positive airway pressure therapy: the impact of behavioral intervention, *Sleep* 26:1010–1015, 2003.

27. Rains JC: Treatment of obstructive sleep apnea in pediatric patients. Behavioral intervention for compliance with nasal continuous positive airway pressure, *Clin Pediatr (Phila)* 34:535–541, 1995.

28. DiFeo N, Meltzer LJ, Beck SE, et al: Predictors of positive airway pressure therapy adherence in children: a prospective study, *J Clin Sleep Med* 8(3):279–286, 2012.

29. Simon SL, Duncan CL, Janicke DM, Wagner MH: Barriers to treatment of paediatric obstructive sleep apnoea: development of the adherence barriers to continuous positive airway pressure (CPAP) questionnaire, *Sleep Med* 13(2):172–177, 2012.

A 5-Year-Old Child with Behavior Problems

A 5-year-old male child had developed behavior problems over the last 6 months. He did not obey his teacher at kindergarten. He often bullied his fellow students and stole their toys. In addition, he seemed hyperactive and was unable to pay attention during class activities. The child's parents reported that he had restless sleep and sometimes snored. A history of daytime sleepiness was not present. The child had been evaluated by his pediatrician who felt that his tonsils were only mildly enlarged. The patient was diagnosed as having the attention deficit/hyperactivity disorder (ADHD) and was being treated with methylphenidate. This resulted in minimal improvement in behavior. The pediatrician ordered a sleep study.

Physical examination: Normal weight and development

HEENT: Mild to moderate tonsillar enlargement

Resting awake saturation of arterial oxygen (SaO_2) 96%, end-tidal partial pressure of carbon dioxide (PCO_2) = 38 mm Hg

The tracing in Figure P39-1 was noted on the sleep study (30-second tracing). The end-tidal PCO_2 tracing is a capnorgram of exhaled PCO_2 versus time. The values of 55 shows a typical end-tidal value in mm Hg.

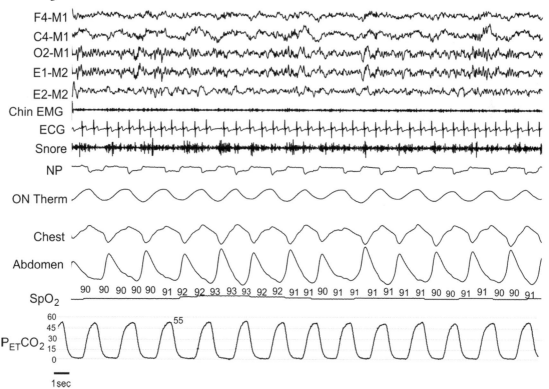

FIGURE P39-1 ■ The awake end-tidal partial pressure of carbon dioxide (PCO_2) was 38 mm Hg. End-tidal PCO_2 is the capnogram (exhaled PCO_2 versus time).

QUESTION

1. What is causing the behavior problems?

ANSWER

1. **Answer:** Obstructive sleep apnea (OSA) syndrome in a child

   Discussion: OSA in children often does not present with complaints of daytime sleepiness. In fact, complaints are often inattentiveness, hyperactivity, and aggressive behavior. A diagnosis of ADHD may have been made in some children who were later found to have OSA. The peak incidence of pediatric OSA is age 4 to 6 years (some studies report 4 to 8 years) when tonsillar hypertrophy is most significant. Although tonsillar enlargement is the etiology in most cases of pediatric OSA, the severity of the disease does not correlate with tonsillar size. The relative size and structure of the other components of the upper airway, as well as upper airway muscle activity, are important for determining the effect of a given degree of tonsillar hypertrophy. Many children with large tonsils have no problems, whereas others with only moderate tonsillar enlargement have severe OSA.

   Many children with sleep-disordered breathing (SDB) will have discrete apneas or hypopneas only during rapid eye movement (REM) sleep. During non-REM (NREM) sleep, often long periods of obstructive hypoventilation occur secondary to high upper airway resistance. When air flow is monitored with thermistors, obstructive hypoventilation may only be detected by a low oxygen saturation or a high end-tidal PCO_2. However, as seen in Figure P39-1, nasal pressure monitoring will often clearly show a severe pattern of air flow limitation.

   In the present case, symptoms of hyperactivity rather than daytime sleepiness were present. The overall apnea–hypopnea index (AHI) was 5 per hour (hr) overall and 30/hr during REM (stage R). The arousal index was 15/hr. The patient displayed long episodes of obstructive hypoventilation (end-tidal $PCO2 > 50$ mm Hg for 40% of total sleep time [TST]). The criteria for scoring hypoventilation in pediatric patients is end-tidal $PCO2 > 50$ mm Hg for $>25\%$ of TST. Note that the thermistor tracing really does not look abnormal. However, the nasal pressure signal clearly shows severe air flow limitation. If nasal pressure was not used, the only clues for hypoventilation would be the low SaO_2, paradoxical motion of the chest and abdomen, and high end-tidal PCO_2. The child was referred for tonsillectomy and adenoidectomy. Within weeks after surgery, his sleep and behaviors were noticeably improved, and the child was weaned off methylphenidate.

CLINICAL PEARLS
1. Children with OSA often present with symptoms of inattentiveness or aggressive behavior rather than excessive daytime sleepiness.
2. The severity of SDB does not correlate with the degree of tonsillar hypertrophy.
3. The peak incidence of pediatric OSA is found in preschoolers (age 4 to 6 years).
4. The predominant pattern of breathing abnormality is often obstructive hypoventilation *without* frequent arousals.
5. Monitoring of end-tidal PCO_2 during polysomnography is essential when studying pediatric patients.

BIBLIOGRAPHY

Marcus CL, Brooks LJ, Draper K, et al: Diagnosis and management of childhood obstructive sleep apnea syndrome: clinical practice guideline. American Academy of Pediatrics, *Pediatrics* 130:576–584, 2012.

Marcus CL, Brooks LJ, Davidson Ward S, et al: Diagnosis and management of childhood obstructive sleep apnea syndrome: technical report. American Academy of Pediatrics, *Pediatrics* 130:e715–755, 2012.

Marcus CL: Sleep-disordered breathing in children, *Am J Respir Crit Care Med* 164:16–30, 2001.

Chervin RD, Archbold KH, Dillon JE, et al: Inattention, hyperactivity, and symptoms of sleep-disordered breathing, *Pediatrics* 109:449–456, 2002.

A Snoring Patient Goes to Surgery

A 55-year-old woman is was scheduled for an elective cholecystectomy. She had a long history of loud snoring but no definite witnessed apnea. Her Epworth Sleepiness Scale (ESS) score was 8/24, and the patient denied fatigue. Her medical problems included obesity, hypertension, and diabetes mellitus.

Physical examination: Obese please female; body mass index (BMI): 34 kg/m^2; HEENT: Mallampati 3 to 4, oropharynx; neck: 16 inches in circumference; cardiovascular: S1/S2 regular; extremities: trace edema.

QUESTIONS

1. How common is obstructive sleep apnea (OSA) in surgical patients?

2. Is the risk of OSA high in this patient (see Table P40-1)?

3. What interventions do you recommend to reduce the risk of perioperative complications in this patient?

TABLE P40-1	STOB-BANG Scoring Model	
1. **S**noring	Do you snore loudly (louder than talking or loud enough to be heard through closed doors)?	Yes / No
2. **T**ired	Do you often feel tired, fatigued, or sleepy during daytime?	Yes / No
3. **O**bserved Apnea	Has anyone observed you stop breathing during your sleep?	Yes / No
4. Blood **P**ressure	Have you been or are you being treated for high blood pressure?	Yes / No
5. **B**MI	BMI >35 kg/m^2?	Yes / No
6. **A**ge	Age older than 50 years?	Yes / No
7. **N**eck Circumference	Neck circumference >40 cm? (15.7 inches)	Yes / No
8. **G**ender	Male?	Yes / No

From Vasu TS, Doghramji K, Cavallazzi R, et al: Obstructive sleep apnea syndrome and postoperative complications: clinical use of the STOP-BANG questionnaire, *Arch Otolaryngol Head Neck Surg* 136:1020-1024, 2010.
BMI, Body mass index.
High risk of OSA: answering yes to three or more items.
Low risk of OSA: answering yes to less than three items.

ANSWERS

1. **Answer:** OSA is very common in surgical patients (20-40%).

2. **Answer:** High risk. On STOP-BANG (1, 4, 6, and 7 are "yes"; 3 or more is a high risk score).

3. **Answer:** Minimize opioids, and provide continuous oximetry monitoring.

   Discussion: In the bariatric surgery population, the prevalence of sleep apnea has been found to be >70%. It is the standard of care for these patients to get a formal sleep evaluation prior to undergoing bariatric surgery. However, patients who are evaluated for general surgery also have a high prevalence of sleep apnea.[1,2] Screening questionnaires such as the Berlin Questionnaire,[3] the STOP-BANG Questionnaire,[4] or the American Society of Anesthesiologists (ASA) checklist are easy to administer preoperatively and have been shown to identify high-risk patients with good sensitivity and specificity. Chung et al.[2] used the Berlin Questionnaire preoperatively and found that 24% of surgical patients were at high risk for sleep apnea. Vasu and coworkers[4] used the STOP-BANG Questionnaire in an elective surgical population and found that 41% of patients were at high risk for sleep apnea, based on the questionnaire. Most patients with sleep apnea are undiagnosed and are therefore unaware of their OSA at the time of the surgery. These patients are at increased risk for perioperative complications. Sedation, anesthesia,[5] and opioids have been shown to cause worsening of sleep apnea in the perioperative period that may lead to an increase in the rate of perioperative complications. Stress for surgery and medications are believed to suppress REM sleep on postoperative nights 1 and 2.[6-8] REM rebound occurs on postoperative nights 3 to 5 and is associated worsening of hypoxemia.[9,10] One study found that postoperative myocardial infarctions occurred in the same time frame as REM rebound and the associated hypoxemia.[11]

It is important to identify OSA in patients preoperatively so that appropriate actions can be taken during perioperative care. A standard protocol for the perioperative management of high-risk patients should be in place to reduce the rate of complications.[12,13] These high-risk patients should also have a formal sleep evaluation for the long-term management of their sleep apnea after discharge from hospital.

A number of interventions have been proposed to reduce the risk of perioperative complications in patients with OSA (Box P40-1). A difficult intubation may be anticipated in a number of patients. Awake extubation in the upright posture is recommended. Using local anesthesia, when possible, minimizing the use of opioids in the postoperative period, and continuous monitoring are among the recommendations.[13] A study by Gali et al.[14] found that decision making combining preoperative screening and detection of problems in the postanesthesia recovery room allowed identification of patients at increased risk for postoperative desaturation events. Often, an overdependence on monitoring of the SaO_2 is seen on medical floors. If a patient is on supplemental oxygen, the partial pressure of arterial carbon dioxide ($PaCO_2$) may be quite high before significant desaturation occurs.[15] If supplemental oxygen is added flow rates should be only as high as needed for SaO_2 in the 94% range. If a patient is known to have OSA, he or she should use his or her CPAP in the postoperative period. In high-risk patients, one might try empirical treatment with automatic positive airway pressure (APAP), assuming that the patients will comply. After hospital discharge, patients should be referred to a sleep specialist or referred for sleep testing by their primary physician.

BOX P40-1	**Perioperative Management of Patients at High Risk of Obstructive Sleep Apnea Syndrome**

PREOPERATIVE EVALUATION

1. History
2. Physical examination
3. Screening questionnaires such as Berlin, ASA, or STOP-BANG to identify high-risk patients
4. Consider a formal sleep evaluation in very high-risk group

INTRAOPERATIVE MANAGEMENT

1. Minimize the surgical stress
2. Reduce the duration of surgery
3. Consider regional or local anesthesia instead of general anesthesia
4. Anticipate difficult intubation
5. Consider awake extubation preferably in semi-upright position

POSTOPERATIVE MANAGEMENT

1. Minimize the use of opioids and sedation after the surgery
2. Consider using acetaminophen, NSAIDs, or regional analgesia for the pain control
3. Continuously monitor oxygenation in the postoperative period
4. Patients with a known diagnosis of sleep apnea should use their CPAP after the surgery
5. Use of auto-CPAP in patients without known sleep apnea could be considered if the clinical suspicion for severe OSA is high.
6. Follow-up at the sleep center for the management of sleep apnea upon discharge from the hospital

From Vasu TS; Grewal R; Doghramji K. Obstructive sleep apnea syndrome and perioperative complications: a systematic review of the literature, *J Clin Sleep Med* 8(2):199-207, 2012.

ASA, American Society of Anesthesiologists; *CPAP*, continuous positive airway pressure; *NSAIDs*, nonsteroidal anti-inflammatory drugs.

CLINICAL PEARLS

1. Although a high prevalence of OSA exists in the surgical population, most patients remain undiagnosed,

2. Screening questionnaires such as the STOP-BANG Questionnaire have a high sensitivity and reasonable specificity
   for detecting patients who are at high risk for OSA.

3. Patients with OSA have an increased risk of perioperative complications.

4. The most severe hypoxemic events occur on the postoperative nights 3 and 5. Rapid eye movement (REM) sleep is suppressed on postoperative nights 1 and 2, and REM rebound is noted on nights 3 to 5. This is one likely mechanism for the delay in the worst hypoxemic events in the postoperative period.

5. Supplemental oxygen impairs the ability of oximetry to detect episodes of hypoventilation.

6. Patients identified as being at high risk for OSA or those with nocturnal desaturations detected in the hospital should have polysomnography after recovery.

REFERENCES

1. Vasu TS, Grewal R, Doghramji K: Obstructive sleep apnea syndrome and perioperative complications: a systematic review of the literature, *J Clin Sleep Med* 8(2):199–207, 2012.
2. Chung F, Ward B, Ho J, et al: Preoperative identification of sleep apnea risk in elective surgical patients, using the Berlin questionnaire, *J Clin Anesth* 19:130–134, 2007.
3. Netzer NC, Stoohs RA, Netzer CM, et al: Using the Berlin Questionnaire to identify patients at risk for the sleep apnea syndrome, *Ann Intern Med* 131:485–491, 1999.
4. Vasu TS, Doghramji K, Cavallazzi R, et al: Obstructive sleep apnea syndrome and postoperative complications: clinical use of the STOP-BANG questionnaire, *Arch Otolaryngol Head Neck Surg* 136:1020–1024, 2010.
5. Eastwood PR, Platt PR, Shepherd K, et al: Collapsibility of the upper airway at different concentrations of propofol anesthesia, *Anesthesiology* 103:470–477, 2005.
6. Knill RL, Moote CA, Skinner MI, et al: Anesthesia with abdominal surgery leads to intense REM sleep during the first postoperative week, *Anesthesiology* 73:52–61, 1990.
7. Rosenberg J: Sleep disturbances after non-cardiac surgery, *Sleep Med Rev* 5:129–137, 2001.
8. Rosenberg-Adamsen S, Skarbye M, et al: Sleep after laparoscopic cholecystectomy, *Br J Anaesth* 77:572–575, 1996.
9. Rosenberg JF, Ullstad TF, Rasmussen J, et al: Time course of postoperative hypoxaemia, *Eur J Surg* 160:137–143, 1994.
10. Rosenberg JF, Wildschiodtz G, Pedersen MH, et al: Late postoperative nocturnal episodic hypoxaemia and associated sleep pattern, *Br J Anaesth* 72:145–150, 1994.
11. Reeder MK, Muir AD, Foex P, et al: Postoperative myocardial ischaemia: temporal association with nocturnal hypoxaemia, *Br J Anaesth* 67:626–631, 1991.
12. Auckley D, Bolden N: Preoperative screening and perioperative care of the patient with sleep-disordered breathing, *Curr Opin Pulm Med* 18(6):588–595, 2012.
13. Joshi GP, Ankichetty SP, Gan TJ, Chung F: Society for Ambulatory Anesthesia consensus statement on preoperative selection of adult patients with obstructive sleep apnea scheduled for ambulatory surgery, *Anesth Analg* 115(5):1060–1068, 2012.
14. Gali B, Whalen FX, Gay PC, et al: Management plan to reduce risks in perioperative care of patients with presumed obstructive sleep apnea syndrome, *J Clin Sleep Med* 3(6):582–588, 2007.
15. Fu ES, Downs JB, Schweiger JW, et al: Supplemental oxygen impairs detection of hypoventilation by pulse oximetry, *Chest* 126(5):1552–1558, 2004.

PATIENT 41

A 50-Year-Old Man with Severe Hypertension

A 50-year-old man with a history of severe hypertension (previous systolic blood pressure 180–190 mm Hg) was admitted to the intensive care unit (ICU) when his physician noted a blood pressure of 230/130 mm Hg in the office. At the time of admission, the patient was being treated with lisinopril and amlodipine for his hypertension, but he had run out of medication. During the first night in the ICU, the patient was noted to have periods of obvious obstructive sleep apnea (OSA) and swings in blood pressure. His blood pressure was monitored on a beat-to-beat basis by using a finger cuff (Penaz method). He adamantly denied symptoms of daytime sleepiness.

Physical examination: Height 5 feet 11 inches, weight 220 pounds; blood pressure 180/95 mm Hg; HEENT: edematous soft palate and uvula, Mallampati 4; neck: 16-inch circumference; chest: clear; cardiac: S4 gallop; extremities: 1+edema.

Laboratory finding: Electrocardiography: Left ventricular hypertrophy

Laboratory finding: Electrocardiography: Left ventricular hypertrophy

In Figure P41-1, air flow and arterial blood pressure were recorded on a two-channel chart during the night in the ICU.

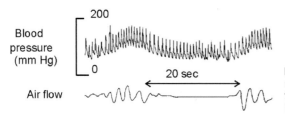

FIGURE P41-1 ■ Noninvasive beat-to-beat blood pressure revealing an increase in blood pressure following apnea termination. (From Berry RB: Sleep medicine pearls, ed 2, Philadelphia, 2003, Saunders, p 191.)

QUESTION

1. Will positive airway pressure treatment of OSA help with blood pressure control?

ANSWER

1. **Answer:** Treatment of OSA will likely improve blood pressure control (especially at night). However, adequate PAP adherence is necessary and the concurrent use of antihypertensive medications will usually be necessary.

   Discussion: Little doubt of an association between OSA and hypertension exists. As seen in most hypertension clinics, a high proportion of patients with hypertension have OSA. The question is whether continuous positive airway pressure (CPAP) and other effective treatments for OSA improve blood pressure control.[1] Results of studies have been conflicting. One problem is variability in CPAP adherence and the diversity of the subjects in the different studies. Another problem is the difficulty of 24-hour blood pressure monitoring (especially during sleep).[2] A recent large meta-analysis of over 1900 patients concluded that the use of PAP in the treatment of OSA results in a modest yet significant reduction in blood pressure, with the greatest effect seen with nocturnal systolic blood pressure.[1]

   Normal persons as well as many patients with hypertension but without sleep apnea have a nocturnal fall in blood pressure. However, 20% to 40% of patients with OSA fail to have the normal nocturnal fall in systemic blood pressure ("nondippers").[3] During obstructive apneas or hypopneas, blood pressure tends to rise slightly and then to rise abruptly at event termination (see Figure P41-1) secondary to arousal from sleep and restoration of breathing associated with sympathetic activation and parasympathetic withdrawal.

   Whether OSA causes daytime (diurnal) as well as nocturnal hypertension is a topic that is still being debated. Animal models of simulated OSA suggest that it can.[4] Several studies have found that OSA is very common in adult populations with hypertension (>30%). This association does not prove causality because patients with hypertension and OSA share common, potentially causative factors such as obesity. Carlson and coworkers[5] found that age, obesity, and sleep apnea were independent and additive risk factors for the presence of hypertension. A prospective study of the Wisconsin cohort found that an increase in the apnea–hypopnea index (AHI) predicted the development of hypertension in the following 4 years (increased incidence) after adjusting for confounding factors such as obesity, age, and smoking.[6] The Sleep Heart Health Study also found a modest increased risk of having hypertension (prevalence) when even mild levels of OSA were present.[7] In contrast to previous findings, a recent analysis of the Sleep Heart Health data found that no relationship existed between the AHI and the risk of incident hypertension (risk of developing hypertension in the next 5 years) when the risk was adjusted for obesity.[8] A trend for a relationship was present when the AHI was >30 per hour (hr). One problem with this analysis is that the population contained relatively few patients with severe OSA. Of note, patients with OSA often have the highest blood pressures in the morning after awakening. Treatment with CPAP can improve early morning blood pressure.[9]

Even if sleep apnea does not cause daytime hypertension, it may well worsen the physiologic impact of the disorder or impair treatment efficacy. For example, Verdecchia and coworkers found that hypertensive patients who failed to have a 10% nocturnal fall in blood pressure had greater left ventricular hypertrophy.[10] Studies have also documented an increase in mortality among nondippers.[11] Studies of populations with resistant hypertension have found a high prevalence of OSA.[12] Therefore, the *possibility of the presence of OSA should be considered in all patients with resistant hypertension.* Two studies have found that CPAP treatment was helpful in patients with resistant hypertension who had OSA.[13,14]

In general, most patients with hypertension with sleep apnea will still continue to require antihypertensive medications when treated with CPAP. However, 24-hour control of blood pressure may improve on CPAP treatment. The current patient was referred for a sleep study which revealed severe OSA. He was started on CPAP, and improvement in blood pressure control in the morning after awakening was noted by the patient. Prior to CPAP, his blood pressure had been at the highest level soon after awakening.

CLINICAL PEARLS

1. Untreated sleep apnea may prevent the normal sleep-associated fall in systemic blood pressure (a cause of non-dipping).

2. The presence of OSA appears to increase the risk of systemic hypertension. However, even if OSA is only an association rather than a cause of hypertension, OSA likely worsens the severity or the consequences of hypertension in many patients.

3. Effective treatment of OSA prevents the cyclic nocturnal increases in blood pressure and may improve daytime blood pressure control, the long-term consequences of hypertension, or both.

4. OSA should be considered in all patients with treatment resistant hypertension. Some studies suggest treatment with CPAP may improve blood pressure control in patients with OSA and resistant hypertension.

REFERENCES

1. Montesi SB, Edwards BA, Malhotra A, Bakker JP: The effect of continuous positive airway pressure treatment on blood pressure: a systematic review and meta-analysis of randomized controlled trials, *J Clin Sleep Med* 8(5):587–596, 2012.
2. Heude E, Bourgin P, Feigel P, et al: Ambulatory monitoring of blood pressure disturbs sleep and raises systolic pressure at night in patients suspected of suffering from sleep-disordered breathing, *Clin Sci (Colch)* 91:4, 1996.
3. Suzuki M, Guilleminault G, Otsuka K, Shimomi T: Blood pressure "dipping" and "non-dipping" in obstructive sleep apnea syndrome patients, *Sleep* 19:382–387, 1996.
4. Brooks D, Horner RL, Kozar LF, et al: Obstructive sleep apnea as a cause of systemic hypertension. Evidence from a canine model, *J Clin Invest* 99:106–109, 1997.
5. Carlson JT, Hedner JA, Ejnell H, Peterson LE: High prevalence of hypertension in sleep apnea patients independent of obesity, *Am J Respir Crit Care Med* 150:72–77, 1994.
6. Peppard PE, Young T, Palta M, Skatrud J: Prospective study of the association between sleep-disordered breathing and hypertension, *N Engl J Med* 342:1378–1384, 2000.
7. Shahar E, Whitney CW, Redline S, et al: Sleep-disordered breathing and cardiovascular disease: cross-sectional results of the Sleep Heart Health Study, *Am J Respir Crit Care Med* 163:19–25, 2001.
8. O'Connor GT, Caffo B, Newman AB, et al: Prospective study of sleep disordered breathing and hypertension, *Am J Respir Crit Care Med* 179:1159–1164, 2009.
9. Becker HF, Jerrentrup A, Ploch T, et al: Effect of nasal continuous positive airway pressure treatment on blood pressure in patients with obstructive sleep apnea, *Circulation* 107:68–73, 2003.
10. Verdecchia P, Schiallica G, Guerrier M, et al: Circadian blood pressure changes and left ventricular hypertrophy in essential hypertension, *Circulation* 81:528–536, 1990.
11. Brotman DJ, Davidson MB, Boumitri M, Vidt DG: Impaired diurnal blood pressure variation and all-cause mortality, *Am J Hypertens* 21:92–97, 2008.
12. Gonzaga CC, Gaddam KK, Ahmed MI, et al: Severity of obstructive sleep apnea is related to aldosterone status in subjects with resistant hypertension, *J Clin Sleep Med* 6:363–368, 2010.
13. Lozano L, Tovar JL, Sampol G, et al: Continuous positive airway pressure treatment in sleep apnea patients with resistant hypertension: a randomized, controlled trial, *J Hypertens* 28:2161–2168, 2010.
14. Dernaika TA, Kinasewitz GT, Tawk MM: Effects of nocturnal continuous positive airway pressure therapy in patients with resistant hypertension and obstructive sleep apnea: effects of nocturnal continuous positive airway pressure therapy in patients with resistant hypertension and obstructive sleep apnea, *J Clin Sleep Med* 5(2):103–107, 2009.

A Patient with Insomnia and Snoring

A 50-year-old man was referred for difficulty falling asleep, frequent awakenings, and nonrestorative sleep. These symptoms had been present for several years. He was particularly distressed when he woke up around 4 AM and could not return to sleep for the remainder of the night. He reported he had been experiencing difficulty sleeping for many years. He took diphenhydramine for sleep, but this made him sleepy during the following day. He denied depression but admitted that he was under stress. He had never been prescribed medications for sleep. Over the last few years, he had gained 10 pounds and was snoring much more loudly. He also noted some increase in nocturia. His only medications were lisinopril and atorvastatin. He rarely drank alcohol. The patient reported an Epworth Sleepiness Scale (ESS) score of 12/24 and admitted to some daytime sleepiness.

Physical examination showed Mallampati 4 upper airway and a 16-inch neck circumference.

A sleep diary showed average sleep latency of 30 to 60 minutes and three to four awakenings per night each about half an hour in duration.

A sleep study was offered, but the patient declined. The patient felt that he could not sleep in the sleep center. However, he would agree to an out-of-center sleep test (OCST). The apnea–hypopnea index (AHI) was 25 per hour, with 175 desaturations to a low saturation of arterial oxygen (SaO_2) of 82%.

A positive airway pressure (PAP) titration in the sleep center was offered to the patient, but he declined that as well.

QUESTION

1. What is your diagnosis? What treatment do you recommend?

ANSWER

1. **Answer:** Comorbid insomnia and obstructive sleep apnea (OSA). The patient was offered a PAP titration in the sleep center and a hypnotic.

   Discussion: As both insomnia and OSA are common problems, it is not surprising that they commonly coexist in an individual. Untreated sleep apnea may cause repeated awakenings, and insomnia may complicate diagnostic sleep studies, the PAP titration, and adherence to PAP treatment. Luyster et al.[1] reviewed the literature of OSA and comorbid insomnia and reported a high prevalence (39%–58%) of insomnia symptoms in patients with OSA, and between 29% and 67% of patients with insomnia have an AHI of >5 per hour (hr). Krakow et al.[2] did a retrospective review of patients failing pharmacotherapy for insomnia. High rates of maladaptive behavior, psychiatric disorders, or OSA (71%) were found. Therefore, OSA is a consideration in patients with insomnia who have failed pharmacotherapy.

   Studies comparing patients with OSA only versus those with OSA plus insomnia[3] suggest that the psychological characteristics of patients with OSA and insomnia are more like those of patients who have only insomnia. It appears that insomnia in patients with OSA is much like the insomnia of those without. Treating the OSA improves insomnia in some patients but often insomnia is unchanged or worse on CPAP. Treatment of both OSA and insomnia is usually needed. For the diagnosis of sleep apnea in a patient with insomnia, patients may be offered a hypnotic for the sleep study. In spite of concerns that hypnotics could worsen sleep apnea, the non-benzodiazepine BZRA hypnotics (zolpidem, eszopiclone) are believed to have a mild impact on sleep apnea (unless hypoventilation is present or the patient is on potent narcotics). Use of a hypnotic in the sleep center is safe, as the patient will be monitored. However, falls in sleep centers in patients taking hypnotics have been reported. A low dose of the hypnotic should be used in older adult patients. It may be prudent to have a family member drive the patient home in the morning after the study. Another approach is to offer a patient a home sleep study with or without a hypnotic. Although this does not follow the American Academy of Sleep Medicine (AASM) guidelines for patients suitable for a home study, this may be all the patient will accept. A retrospective study by Lettieri et al.[4] compared patients undergoing polysomnography (PSG) with and without premedication with zolpidem. Poor-quality polysomnography was defined as sleep time insufficient to allow for diagnosis, incomplete continuous PAP (CPAP) titration with a resulting AHI >10 on the highest level of CPAP achieved, or complete CPAP intolerance. The medicated patients had shorter sleep latency, higher sleep efficiency, and fewer failed studies. The demographics in the two groups (control and hypnotic) were well matched.

Similarly, use of a hypnotic may be considered for PAP titration and PAP treatment—at least in the short term. Some patients have *no* problem sleeping without CPAP but have difficulty falling asleep on CPAP or maintaining sleep. Some clinicians have been hesitant to prescribe hypnotics to patients on CPAP, believing that this may reduce the effectiveness of CPAP. However, a double-blind crossover study by Berry and Patel[5] found that zolpidem, a commonly used hypnotic, did not impair efficacy of a given level of CPAP. It has been hypothesized that using a hypnotic might improve adherence to PAP in some patients. A study by Bradshaw and colleagues[6] using zolpidem did not find an improvement. In contrast, Lettieri and associates[7] found improvement during CPAP titration (sleep quality) and long-term adherence with eszopiclone (a hypnotic with a longer duration of action than zolpidem). It is possible that a longer-acting medication is needed to improve CPAP adherence. Although routine use of a hypnotic cannot currently be recommended for PAP treatment in patients with insomnia, at least temporary use of a hypnotic should be considered if insomnia is a major obstacle to CPAP use. An alternative to the use of hypnotics for long-term PAP treatment in a patient with insomnia is a referral for cognitive behavioral treatment of insomnia (CBT-I). CBT-I could improve the ability of patients with insomnia to sleep on CPAP or assist in the weaning of a hypnotic if the CPAP patient is taking a hypnotic medication.[8,9] Of course, the other option is concurrent CBT-I treatment before or during diagnostic studies or PAP treatment. This approach depends on the patient's attitudes about behavioral treatment and the availability of CBT-I. Clinical guidelines for the treatment of insomnia recommend CBT-I rather than a hypnotic as the treatment of choice for chronic insomnia disorder[9] Fundamentals 38).

In the current patient, OSA was strongly suspected and, indeed, was documented by OCST. The patient accepted a PAP titration with zolpidem 10 milligrams (mg) before the study. If this option had not been accepted an auto-titration at home with or without a hypnotic would have been an option. The patient tolerated CPAP surprisingly well during the PAP titration. He was started on CPAP with zolpidem 10 mg nightly for 2 weeks. The patient's ESS score dropped from 12 to 6, and he reported at most one awakening each night on the combination of zolpidem and CPAP. He attempted to wean off zolpidem (he took 5 mg nightly for 1 week before stopping the medication), but then he could not sleep on CPAP without the medication. He was restarted on zolpidem 10 mg every night at bed time (qhs) and referred for CBT-I with the goal of weaning off the hypnotic. During CBT-I treatment a very slow decrease of 2.5 mg zolpidem every week was attempted. Ultimately, the patient required zolpidem 2.5 mg once or twice weekly.

CLINICAL PEARLS

1. A significant proportion of patients with insomnia have some degree of OSA. A significant percentage of patients with OSA have some degree of insomnia (in some worsened by CPAP).

2. The possibility of coexisting insomnia and OSA should be considered in every patient who complains of insomnia. A history of snoring, breathing pauses, a crowded upper airway, and daytime sleepiness (uncommon in most patients with insomnia) should raise the level of concern. A diagnosis of OSA should also be considered in patients who are refractory to pharmacotherapy for insomnia.

3. Coexisting insomnia may complicate diagnostic and CPAP titration studies as well as CPAP treatment.

4. Use of a hypnotic in the short term for the diagnostic sleep study and PAP titration study and for CPAP initiation is a viable option if no contraindication (e.g., history of drug dependence, ataxia, older adults) exists. Use of a non-benzodiazepine BZRA hypnotic or a sedating antidepressant is an option. A reduced dose should be used in older adults or in hypnotic-naive patients.

5. If a hypnotic is used for a sleep study in a patient not already on medication, extra precautions are indicated. Fall precautions in the sleep center and at home are in order (e.g., assistance to the bathroom). Some sleep centers require that a family member drive the patient home if a hypnotic was taken before a sleep study (especially if the patient is not a chronic hypnotic user).

6. Use of CBT-I along with PAP treatment may also be effective in patients with OSA and insomnia. CBT-I can also be useful in helping patients wean a hypnotic.

7. Some patients who present with insomnia concerns may agree to an OCST even if they refuse PSG. Although not ideal, home testing should detect moderate to severe OSA.

8. Use of a hypnotic may improve CPAP adherence in patients with OSA and insomnia. A safer and effective alternative is concurrent CBT-I (if this treatment is available and acceptable to the patient).

9. In patients with OSA and insomnia, concurrent treatments for both are needed for a good outcome. OSA and insomnia are two separate disorders that have interactions but both need to be separately addressed.

REFERENCES

1. Luyster FS, Buysse DJ, Strollo PJ Jr: Comorbid insomnia and obstructive sleep apnea: challenges for clinical practice and research, *J Clin Sleep Med* 6(2):196–204, 2010.
2. Krakow B, Ulibarri VA, Romero E: Persistent insomnia in chronic hypnotic users presenting to a sleep medical center: a retrospective chart review of 137 consecutive patients, *J Nerv Ment Dis* 198(10):734–741, 2010.
3. Yang CM, Liao YS, Lin CM, et al: Psychological and behavioral factors in patients with comorbid obstructive sleep apnea and insomnia, *J Psychosom Res* 70(4):355–361, 2011.
4. Lettieri CJ, Quast TN, Eliasson AH, Andrada T: Eszopiclone improves overnight polysomnography and continuous positive airway pressure titration: a prospective, randomized, placebo-controlled trial, *Sleep* 31:1310–1316, 2008.
5. Berry RB, Patel PB: Effect of zolpidem on the efficacy of continuous positive airway pressure as treatment for obstructive sleep apnea, *Sleep* 29:1052–1056, 2006.
6. Bradshaw DA, Ruff GA, Murphy DP: An oral hypnotic medication does not improve continuous positive airway pressure compliance in men with obstructive sleep apnea, *Chest* 130:1369–1376, 2006.
7. Lettieri CJ, Eliasson AH, Andrada T, et al: Does zolpidem enhance the yield of polysomnography? *J Clin Sleep Med* 1 (2):129-31.
8. Krakow B, Melendrez D, Lee SA, et al: Refractory insomnia and sleep-disordered breathing: a pilot study, *Sleep Breath* 8:15–29, 2004.
9. Schutte-Rodin S, Broch L, Buysse D, et al: Clinical guideline for the evaluation and management of chronic insomnia in adults, *J Clin Sleep Med* 4(5):487–504, 2008.

PATIENT 43

A Patient with Snoring and Recent Cerebrovascular Accident

A right-handed 65-year-old man had a thrombotic cerebrovascular accident (CVA), which resulted in severe weakness in his left arm and leg. He had a history of hypertension and diabetes mellitus prior to the stroke. He had a long history of mild snoring, but after the CVA, this was noted to worsen. Nocturnal oximetry in the hospital documented desaturations during sleep. You are asked to evaluate the patient about 2 weeks after the CVA.

QUESTIONS

1. Should the patient have a sleep study?

2. If sleep apnea is present is it more likely to be central or obstructive?

3. If sleep apnea is present will positive airway pressure (PAP) treatment improve outcomes?

ANSWERS

1. **Answer:** Yes, some type of sleep study is indicated (preferably polysomnography [PSG]).

2. **Answer:** Obstructive sleep apnea (OSA) is more common.

3. **Answer:** Continuous PAP (CPAP) treatment improved outcomes in some observational studies.

Discussion: A number of studies have shown a high prevalence of sleep-disordered breathing (SDB) in patients soon after a CVA.[1-3] Depending on the study, the prevalence of sleep apnea after a CVA ranges between 50% and 75%. Sleep apnea may precede the occurrence of stroke or appear after the event.[4] Although the predominant form of SDB is OSA, central sleep apnea (CSA) with Cheyne-Stokes breathing (CSB) may also occur.[5] The CSB-CSA is believed to occur early in the post-CVA period and then usually resolves. In contrast, OSA seems to persist after a CVA. However, the temporal relationship between OSA and stroke is not well defined. It is not known whether brain damage from CVA causes sleep apnea or if sleep apnea preceded the stroke. If so, is the presence of sleep apnea an independent risk factor for the development of a CVA? The Sleep Heart Health Study showed an increased risk of having a self-reported CVA (prevalence) if OSA is present.[6] Redline and associates[7] evaluated the Sleep Heart Health data and found an increased risk for incident ischemic stroke in men with mild to moderate OSA. In this study, data were adjusted for a number of confounders that complicated the analysis including obesity. If a causal role for OSA existed in stroke, what are the mechanisms? OSA may predispose to atherosclerosis, hypertension, and early morning hemoconcentration. These factors increase the risk of stroke. During sleep apnea, increases in intracranial pressure (ICP) and decreases in cerebral blood flow occur.[8] An increase in ICP occurs with each apneic event, and the rise tends to be correlated with the length of apnea. The increase in ICP is thought secondary to increases in central venous pressure, systemic pressure, and cerebral vasodilatation from increases in partial pressure of arterial carbon dioxide ($PaCO_2$) during respiratory events. Because cerebral perfusion is proportional to the mean arterial pressure (MAP)–ICP, increases in ICP may reduce perfusion pressure even if MAP also rises. Studies of cerebral blood flow velocity using Doppler monitoring have shown that flow velocity increases in early apnea, and then has approximately a 25% fall below baseline at end apnea.[9]

Some evidence suggests that the presence of OSA in patients who have suffered a CVA is a bad prognostic sign regardless of whether OSA precedes or follows the CVA. Good and coworkers[10] found that the Barthel index (a multifaceted scale measuring mobility and activities of daily living that is used to assess patients after stroke, lower score associated with worse status) was significantly lower in patients with OSA and CVA compared with those with no evidence of OSA after CVA. The presence of OSA was determined at discharge and the Barthel index was lower at 3 and 12 months in the OSA-CVA group. Martinez-Garcia and colleagues[11] found that CPAP treatment reduced the mortality rate after ischemic stroke in patients with concomitant OSA. Other studies[12,13] suggest CPAP treatment may be beneficial in patients with CVA and OSA. However, CPAP adherence tends to be low in patients with a recent CVA. A recent systematic review[14] concluded that existing studies provide sufficient data to establish obstructive SDB as a predictor of all-cause mortality and recurrent vascular events following stroke or TIA. However, the authors concluded that the current data is not sufficiently strong to prove that CPAP treatment will lower the risk of serious adverse outcomes after stroke. This conclusion was based on the fact that a substantial risk of bias was identified in most of the eligible studies concerning CPAP treatment in patients with OSA and a CVA. Additional studies are needed.

The current patient was evaluated with PSG and found to have severe OSA during a split sleep study. CPAP was effective. However, the patient required assistance with placement of the mask. He was started on CPAP during his stay in a rehabilitation facility.

CLINICAL PEARLS

1. A high percentage of patients who have suffered a stroke have some type of sleep apnea.
2. Both OSA and CSA (often with Cheyne-Stokes breathing) may occur. OSA is more common. CSA tends to resolve with time.
3. The presence of OSA increases the risk of incident CVAs.
4. The presence of OSA after CVA is associated with a worse preliminary evidence prognosis.
5. Compliance with CPAP after CVA has been poor, but evidence suggests that treatment may improve prognosis. Further trials are needed.

REFERENCES

1. Barone DA, Krieger AC: Stroke and obstructive sleep apnea: a review, *Curr Atheroscler Rep* 15(7):334, 2013.
2. Culebras A: Sleep, stroke and poststroke, *Neurol Clin* 30(4):1275–1284, 2012.
3. Turkington P, Bamfor J, Wanklyn P, et al: Prevalence and predictors of upper airway obstruction in the first 24 hours after acute stroke, *Stroke* 33:2037–2041, 2002.
4. Para O, Arboix A, Bechichi S, et al: Time course of sleep-related breathing disorders in first-ever stroke or transient ischemic attack, *Am J Respir Crit Care Med* 161:375–380, 2000.
5. Siccoli MM, Valko PO, Hermann DM, Bassetti CL: Central periodic breathing during sleep in patients with acute ischemic stroke—neurogenic and cardiogenic factors, *J Neurol* 255:1687–1692, 2008.
6. Shahar E, Whitney CW, Redline S, et al: Sleep-disordered breathing and cardiovascular disease: cross-sectional results of the Sleep Heart Health Study, *Am J Respir Crit Care Med* 163:19–25, 2001.
7. Redline S, Yenokyan G, Gottlieb DJ, et al: Obstructive sleep apnea-hypopnea and incident stroke: the Sleep Heart Health study, *Am J Respir Crit Care Med* 182:269–277, 2010.
8. Sugita Y, Susami I, Yoshio T, et al: Marked episodic elevation of cerebral spinal fluid pressure during nocturnal sleep in patients with sleep apnea hypersomnia syndrome, *Electroencephalogr Clin Neurophysiol* 60:214–219, 1985.
9. Balfors EM: Impairment of cerebral perfusion during obstructive sleep apneas, *Am J Respir Crit Care Med* 150:1587–1591, 1994.
10. Good DC, Henkle JQ, Gelber D, et al: Sleep disordered breathing and poor functional outcome after stroke, *Stroke* 27:252–259, 1996.
11. Martinez-Garcia MA, Soler-Cataluna JJ, Ejarque-Martinez L, et al: Continuous positive airway pressure treatment reduces mortality in patients with ischemic stroke and obstructive sleep apnea: a five-year follow-up, *Am J Respir Crit Care Med* 180:36–41, 2008.
12. Parra O, Sanchez-Armengol A, Bonnin M, et al: Early treatment of obstructive apnoea and stroke outcome: a randomised controlled trial, *Eur Respir J* 37:1128–1136, 2011.
13. Bravata DM, Concato J, Fried T, et al: Continuous positive airway pressure: evaluation of a novel therapy for patients with acute ischemic stroke, *Sleep* 34:1271–1277, 2011.
14. Birkbak J, Clark AJ, Rod NH: The effect of sleep disordered breathing on the outcome of stroke and transient ischemic attack: a systematic review, *J Clin Sleep Med* 10(1):103–108, 2014.

PATIENT 44

An Patient with Obstructive Sleep Apnea Gets Sleepy While Driving

A 55-year-old man was diagnosed with obstructive sleep apnea (OSA) (apnea–hypopnea index [AHI] 60 per hour [hr]). He had severe sleepiness (Epworth Sleepiness Scale [ESS] score 18/24) before being treated with continuous positive airway pressure (CPAP). The patient currently reports an ESS of 9 (normal). The patient has been using CPAP, although adherence has been inconsistent. He reports sleeping at least 6.5 hours per night. His medications include lisinopril and levothyroxine. He reports that he had previously experienced sleepiness while driving but that this had improved with CPAP. He has never had an automobile accident related to sleepiness (or any accident for over 10 years).

Physical examination: Body mass index (BMI) 35 kg/m^2; HEENT: Mallampati 4; neck 17 inches; Cardiovascular: S1/S2 regular; extremities: no edema.

CPAP Download	
Recent CPAP Adherence Information—Last 30 days	
Days used	25/30
Average use	5 hr 10 minutes
% of nights use >4 hr	80%
Residual AHI	2.1/hr

QUESTION

1. Which of the following are appropriate to tell the patient? (More than one answer may be correct.)
   A. Patients with OSA are at increased risk for an automobile accident.
   B. You are a high-risk driver because of your OSA.
   C. Do not drive if sleepy. Use your CPAP nightly.
   D. Modafinil will decrease your risk of having an accident.

ANSWER

1. **Answer:** A and C are correct.

   Discussion: Sleepiness may account for up to 20% of crashes on monotonous roads, especially highways. OSA is the most common medical disorder that causes excessive daytime sleepiness, increasing the risk for drowsy driving two fold to threefold. The American Thoracic Society (ATS) published an update to the 1994 guidelines concerning recommendations for noncommercial drivers with known or suspected OSA. The recommendations were based on evidence review. A number of conclusions were reached (Box P44-1). Patients with OSA are at two- to threefold higher risk for a motor vehicle accident (MVA) compared with the general population. High-risk individuals with OSA are those who have had an accident or near-accident because of sleepiness. No evidence exists to justify restriction of driving privileges to non–high-risk patients with OSA. Effective treatment with CPAP improves performance on driving simulators, but firm evidence of a reduction in MVAs is lacking. A meta-analysis of nine observational studies by Tregear et al. examining the crash risk of drivers with OSA before and after CPAP found a significant risk reduction following treatment. The study found that daytime sleepiness improves significantly following a single night of treatment, and simulated driving performance improves significantly within 2 to 7 days of CPAP treatment. The authors concluded that CPAP reduces motor vehicle crash risk among drivers with OSA.

   A number of recommendations were made in the ATS clinical guidelines (Table P44-1). High-risk patients with known or suspected OSA should be warned about the potential risk of driving until adequately treated. Most physicians, in fact, would warn high-risk drivers *not* to drive unless treated and document this recommendation in the medical record.

   The topic of commercial drivers and sleep apnea is a different story. It is known that the incidence of OSA in commercial vehicle operators is high. The risk for personal and public injury or death is much greater if these patients have untreated sleep apnea. The Federal Motor Carrier and Safety Administration (FMCSA) oversees authorization of commercial drivers' licenses (CDLs). Drivers must submit to a test by a certified medical examiner (CME) every 2 years. In 1991, guidelines issued by the FMCSA stated that the CME must consider a driver unqualified to drive if suspected or known untreated sleep apnea is present. Until adequately treated, a driver with OSA will not be certified by the CME, and no CDL will be issued. In 1998, a question regarding sleep apnea was added to the CME report. In 2006, the American College of Occupational and Environmental

---

BOX P44-1   Conclusions of ATS Clinical Practice Guideline

1. OSA versus non-OSA is associated with a two- to three times increased overall risk for motor vehicle crashes, but prediction of risk in an individual is imprecise.
2. A high-risk driver is defined as one who has moderate to severe daytime sleepiness and a recent unintended motor vehicle crash or a near-miss attributable to sleepiness, fatigue, or inattention.
3. There is no compelling evidence to restrict driving privileges in patients with sleep apnea if there

has not been a motor vehicle crash or an equivalent event.
4. Treatment of OSA improves performance on driving simulators and might reduce the risk of drowsy driving and drowsy driving crashes.
5. Timely diagnostic evaluation and treatment and education of the patient and family are likely to decrease the prevalence of sleepiness-related crashes in patients with OSA who are high-risk drivers.

TABLE P44-1 Recommendations

All patients being initially evaluated for suspected or confirmed obstructive sleep apnea (OSA)	Question about daytime sleepiness, especially falling asleep unintentionally and inappropriately during daily activities as well as recent motor vehicle accidents or near-misses attributable to sleepiness.
	Patients with these characteristics are deemed high-risk drivers and should be immediately warned about the potential risk of driving until effective therapy is instituted.
	Patient should also be questioned about other factors that may further increase risk such as sleep restriction or alcohol/ or sedatives.
Suspected OSA, high-risk drivers	Evaluation with polysomnography recommended.
	Empiric treatment with continuous positive airway pressure (CPAP) to improve driving risk—not recommended.
Confirmed OSA, high-risk drivers	CPAP treatment recommended, rather than no treatment (strong recommendation, moderate-quality evidence).
Suspected or confirmed OSA, not high risk	Stimulant medications should not be used for the sole purpose of reducing driving risk (weak recommendation, very low–quality evidence).

From Strohl KP, Brown DB, Collop N, et al, ATS Ad Hoc Committee on Sleep Apnea, Sleepiness, and Driving Risk in Noncommercial Drivers: An official American Thoracic Society clinical practice guideline: sleep apnea, sleepiness, and driving risk in noncommercial drivers. An update of a 1994 Statement, *Am J Respir Crit Care Med* 187(11):1259-1266, 2013.

Medicine, the American College of Chest Physicians, and the National Sleep Foundation developed a consensus guideline for triaging commercial drivers with suspected or known sleep apnea. These guidelines were strongly considered by the FMCSA but a recently passed law forbids the FMCSA from issuing regulations that mandate testing of patient at risk for OSA without a formal rule making process. If the CME suspects sleep apnea based on symptoms, testing can still be required. Patients with known OSA are still usually required to provide proof of adherence to treatment. The rationale is to provide a 3-month period, during which lower risk drivers (Table P44-2) with unknown OSA status or nonsleepy drivers with documented mild to moderate OSA can still

TABLE P44-2 Consensus Recommendations for Commercial Drivers

Medically qualified to drive commercial vehicles (CV)	No positive findings on any of the numbered in-service evaluation factors

In-service evaluation recommended (maximum 3 months delay) If driver falls into any one of the five categories	1. Sleep history suggestive of OSA (snoring, EDS, witnessed apnea)
	2. Two or more of the following:
	  BMI > 35 kg/m^2
	  Neck circumference > 17 men > 16 women
	  HTN (new, uncontrolled, unable to control with 2 medications)
	3. ESS > 10
	4. Known OSA, compliance claimed but not documented (must be reviewed within 3 months) If noncompliant, remove from service
	5. AHI > 5 but < 30, no EDS or ESS < 11, no MVAs; no HTN requiring more than 2 medications

Out-of-service immediate evaluation If driver falls into any one of the five categories	1. Observed unexplained sleepiness (asleep in examination or waiting room) or confessed daytime sleepiness 2. MVA related to sleep disturbance (run off the road, at fault, rear end collision)—unless evaluated for sleep disorder in the interim 3. ESS > 16 FOSQ < 18 4. Previously diagnosed sleep disorder (a) noncompliant (CPAP not tolerated); (b) no recent follow-up within recommended time frame; (c) surgical treatment with no follow-up 5. AHI > 30 per hour

Adapted from Hartenbaum N, Collop N, Rosen IM, et al: Sleep apnea and commercial motor vehicle operators: statement from the Joint Task Force of the American College of Chest Physicians, the American College of Occupation and Environmental Medicine, and the National Sleep Foundation, *Chest* 13:902-905, 2006.
AHI, Apnea–hypopnea index; *BMI*, body mass index; *EDS*, excessive daytime sleepiness; *ESS*, Epworth Sleepiness Scale; *FOSQ*, functional outcomes of sleep questionnaire; *HTN*, hypertension; *MVA*, motor vehicle accident; *OSA*, obstructive sleep apnea.

drive while being evaluated and treated, if needed. If OSA is found, it must be treated within 3 months. An in-service examination within no more than 3 months may be performed if the driver meets the criteria in Box P44-1. An out-of-service examination (no driving) is recommended if the patient has known severe untreated sleep apnea, severe sleepiness, or an MVA associated with sleepiness. A driver not falling into any of the three categories is fit to drive if he or she is adherent to treatment (CPAP adherence) and has relief of symptoms. Unfortunately, recently a new law (a product of pressure on Congress from the trucking industry) prevents the FMCSA from issuing a requirement for sleep apnea testing using "guidance" rather than a formal "rule making" process. This will no doubt delay implementation of the consensus recommendations. The FMCSA allows drivers to use modafinil if they are monitored closely by a physician for at least 6 weeks of taking medication (and benefiting). The reader should check for the most current rules of the FMCSA.

The current patient was instructed to continue (and even improve) CPAP adherence and not to drive if sleepy. As he had never had an accident associated with sleepiness, he is not considered a high-risk driver. However, he was informed that an adherence check of his objective use would be ordered in 3 months.

CLINICAL PEARLS

1. Patients with OSA have a two- to threefold risk of having a motor vehicle accident (MVA).
2. Patients with a history of an MVA or near-miss attributable to sleepiness are considered high risk; this group of OSA patients is most likely to have an MVA.
3. During evaluation for suspected OSA or during treatment of known OSA, patients should be questioned about sleepiness while driving and recent accidents caused by sleepiness.
4. High-risk patients with OSA should be warned not to drive if feeling sleepy. Untreated patients should be warned of potential risk until adequately treated. Most physicians warn untreated sleepy patients with OSA not to drive until treated and document this in the medical record.
5. Although CPAP treatment for OSA is recommended, the data that it will definitely reduce the risk of a patient with OSA having an accident do not exist. A large meta-analysis of observational studies found that CPAP does reduce the risk of an MVA in OSA patients.
6. Commercial drivers with known or suspected OSA must be certified by a certified medical examiner before they are issued a commercial drivers license. If they are being treated with CPAP, adherence and benefit must be documented.

BIBLIOGRAPHY

Beran RG, Devereux JA: Road not taken: lessons to be learned from Queen v. Gillett, *Intern Med J* 37:336–339, 2007.
Collop N, Hartenbaum N, Rosen I, Phillips B: Paying attention to at risk commercial vehicle operators, *Chest* 139:637–639, 2006.
Desai AV, Ellis E, Wheatley JR, Grunstein RR: Fatal distraction: a case series of fatal fall-asleep road accidents and their medicolegal outcomes, *Med J Aust* 178:396–399, 2003.
Filtness AJ, Reyner LA, Horne JA: One night's CPAP withdrawal in otherwise compliant OSA patients: marked driving impairment but good awareness of increased sleepiness, *Sleep Breath* 16:865–871, 2012.
Gurtman CG, Broadbear JH, Redman JR: Effects of modafinil on simulator driving and self-assessment of driving following sleep deprivation, *Hum Psychopharmacol* 23:681–692, 2008.
Hartenbaum N, Collop N, Rosen IM, et al: Sleep apnea and commercial motor vehicle operators: statement from the Joint Task Force of the American College of Chest Physicians, the American College of Occupation and Environmental Medicine, and the National Sleep Foundation, *Chest* 13:902–905, 2006.
Kryworuk PW, Nickle SE: Mandatory physician reporting of drivers with medical conditions: legal considerations, *Can J Cardiol* 20:1324–1328, 2004.
Rodenstein D: Sleep apnea: traffic and occupational accidents—individual risks, socioeconomic and legal implications, *Respiration* 78:241–248, 2009.
Strohl KP, Brown DB, Collop N, et al: ATS Ad Hoc Committee on Sleep Apnea, Sleepiness, and Driving Risk in Noncommercial Drivers: An official American Thoracic Society clinical practice guideline: sleep apnea, sleepiness, and driving risk in noncommercial drivers. An update of a 1994 Statement, *Am J Respir Crit Care Med* 187(11):1259–1266, 2013.
Tregear S, Reston J, Schoelles K, Phillips B: Continuous positive airway pressure reduces risk of motor vehicle crash among drivers with obstructive sleep apnea: systematic review and meta-analysis, *Sleep* 33:1373–1380, 2010.
Vakulin A, Baulk SD, Catcheside PG, et al: Driving simulator performance remains impaired in patients with severe OSA after CPAP treatment, *J Clin Sleep Med* 7:246–253, 2011.
Williams SC, Marshall NS, Kennerson M, et al: Modafinil effects during acute continuous positive airway pressure withdrawal: a randomized crossover double-blind placebo-controlled trial, *Am J Respir Crit Care Med* 181:825–831, 2010.
Williams SC, Rogers NL, Marshall NS, et al: The effect of modafinil following acute CPAP withdrawal: a preliminary study, *Sleep Breath* 12:359–364, 2008.

FUNDAMENTALS 22

Obstructive Sleep Apnea: Treatment Overview and Medical Treatments

A number of considerations affect the decision to treat a patient with obstructive sleep apnea (OSA) (Figure F22-1). The first category is the severity of OSA, as based on the apnea-hypopnea index, severity of arterial oxygen desaturation, and association with significant arrhythmias.[1] The second consideration is the presence or absence of symptoms. Symptomatic OSA should always be treated, but the choice of treatment may vary. Symptoms may not correlate with the apnea–hypopnea index (AHI), and the dictum "Treat the patient, not the AHI" should be considered. The third consideration is the impact of OSA on the sleep of the patient's bed partner. Loud snoring and apnea may cause marital discord and impair the sleep of the patient's bed partner.[2] The fourth is the potential increased risk of death or adverse cardiovascular morbidity from untreated OSA. The evidence for increased risk is strongest for severe OSA (AHI >30 per hour [hr]) and in men who are 40 to 70 years of age.[3–5] The evidence is less clear for moderate OSA and for women. However, the presence of certain comorbid conditions such as coronary artery disease, cerebrovascular disease, arrhythmias, or congestive heart failure may increase the risk even for milder degrees of sleep apnea. Given that positive airway pressure (PAP) treatment is safe and effective, treatment of patients with moderate and severe OSA is recommended, even if patients are asymptomatic.

CHOOSING TREATMENT

The choice of treatment modality is based on the severity of OSA as well as patient characteristics and preferences (Table F22-1). Treatment with PAP (Fundamentals 24), surgery (Fundamentals 26) and oral appliances (Fundamentals 27) are discussed in more detail in these chapters. Practice parameters on the use of PAP, oral appliances (OAs), upper airway surgery and medical treatments have been published.[6–9] Although weight loss is included in every category of OSA severity, it is considered an adjunctive measure, as it requires time and weight loss maintenance. For mild asymptomatic OSA, observation may suffice, but patients should be informed that OSA may worsen with weight gain or increasing age. The lateral position may be effective for postural OSA, but long-term studies of effectiveness have yet to be performed. An OA or upper airway surgery (uvulopalatopharyngoplasty [UPPP]) is usually effective for mild OSA. PAP may also be effective in symptomatic patients who are motivated. Many patients with mild OSA will decline surgery, and the absence of

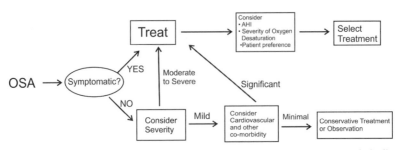

FIGURE F22-1 ■ Algorithm to consider if treatment of obstructive sleep apnea is indicated.

TABLE F22-1	**Treatment of OSA by Severity**			
	Snoring	**Mild OSA**	**Moderate OSA**	**Severe OSA**
AHI		5 TO <15/HOUR	15 TO 30/HOUR	>30/HOUR
Primary Treatment	Observation Treat nasal congestion Lateral positioning	Observation (Asx) Lateral positioning* Oral appliance *or* Upper airway surgery-2	PAP	PAP
Secondary Treatment	Oral appliance *or* Upper airway surgery-1	PAP (if symptomatic and motivated)	Oral appliance *or* Upper Airway Surgery-2	Upper airway surgery-3 *or* Oral appliance
Adjunctive	Weight loss	Weight loss Lateral positioning	Weight loss Lateral positioning	Weight loss Lateral positioning

AHI, Apnea–hypopnea index; *Asx*, asymptomatic; *OSA*; obstructive sleep apnea; *PAP*, positive airway pressure.
*Postural OSA present.
Upper airway surgery 1: Palatal implants, uvulopalatopharyngoplasty (UPPP), laser-assisted uvuloplasty; Upper airway surgery 2: UPPP ± genioglossus advancement, hyoid myotomy (GAHM); Upper airway surgery 3: Maxillomandibular advancement (MMA).

reimbursement of OAs by insurance providers may render this option unacceptable for many patients. For moderate and severe OSA, PAP is the treatment of choice. For moderate OSA, OAs and upper airway surgery are secondary treatments. Both may be effective in selected patients, although success is less reliable than with PAP. However, successful PAP treatment requires adherence. Surgery such as UPPP is listed below OA for moderate OSA treatment, as only about 50% will achieve a significant improvement by AHI, although a higher percentage may have symptomatic improvement. For severe OSA, tracheostomy reliably bypasses upper airway obstruction but is not acceptable to most patients. This procedure is reserved for patients with very severe OSA, who will not adhere to PAP when effective treatment is urgently needed (e.g., recurrent hypercapnic respiratory failure) and the patient is not a candidate for maxillary mandibular advancement. Complex upper airway surgery such as maxillary mandibular advancement may be effective in 80% to 90% of patients. An OA may improve the AHI substantially even in severe OSA, although rarely to <15/hr. In comparing treatment effectiveness, both efficacy and adherence must be considered. If PAP reduces the AHI from 60 to 0/hr but is used only 50% of the night, the average AHI on treatment is 30/hr.

PATIENT EDUCATION BEFORE TREATMENT

Following polysomnography (PSG) or portable monitoring (home sleep testing, limited-channel

sleep testing), the physician ordering the study should discuss the findings and the consequences of untreated sleep apnea with the patient.[1] Factors that may exacerbate OSA, including weight gain, insufficient sleep, medications, and alcohol consumption, should also be addressed. Available treatment options and the pros and cons of each option should be discussed. Although most patients look to the physician for ultimate recommendations, involvement of the patient and spouse in decision making is essential to improve treatment outcomes. Counseling regarding drowsy driving should be provided and documented. Many patients have comorbid conditions such as depression, insomnia, the restless legs syndrome (RLS), or chronic pain that will make compliance with PAP or other treatments more difficult. These problems should be evaluated and treated.

FOLLOW-UP AND OUTCOMES ASSESSMENT

Following treatment initiation, careful follow-up is essential because OSA is a chronic disease. A follow-up sleep study is recommended after upper airway surgery for moderate to severe OSA (most would also recommend for mild OSA) and after final adjustment of an OA as treatment for all severities of OSA.[1,8]

MEDICAL TREATMENT

The American Academy of Sleep Medicine (AASM) has published practice parameters for the medical treatment of OSA (see Table F22-1).[6]

The treatments include weight loss, postural treatment, and modafinil or armodafinil for persistent daytime sleepiness.

Weight Loss

Obesity is a major risk factor for the development of OSA. A body mass index (BMI) of 25 to 29.9 kilograms per square meter (kg/m^2) is considered overweight, >30 is obesity, and >40 is severe obesity. In some studies, approximately 70% of patients with OSA were obese (body weight >120% of predicted). Peppard and colleagues[10] monitored the effects of weight change on AHI. A 10% weight gain predicted an approximate 32% increase in the AHI. A 10% weight loss predicted a 26% reduction in the AHI. A 10% increase in weight was associated with a sixfold increase in the risk of developing moderate to severe OSA. Many studies have documented that weight loss of modest proportions (5%–10% of body weight) may produce significant improvement in sleep apnea[11–13] and decrease upper airway collapsibility.[14] Even patients with mild obesity (110%–115% of ideal body weight) may benefit from weight reduction.

However, the effectiveness of weight loss in reducing the AHI varies among patients. The reason may be that a given amount of weight loss may have more effect on upper body obesity or upper airway anatomy in one individual than in another. Weight loss may also be less effective in reducing the AHI if skeletal abnormalities may play a more prominent role in the pathogenesis of OSA in a given patients. The level of nasal continuous PAP (CPAP) required to maintain upper airway patency may decrease after weight reduction. Lettieri and associates[15] reported a reduction in required CPAP from 11.5 to 8.4 centimeters of water (cm H_2O) after weight loss (BMI dropped from 51 to 32 kg/m^2) in a group of patients undergoing bariatric surgery. However, the magnitude of this effect may vary significantly among patients. Behavioral, surgical, and pharmacologic approaches to weight loss have all been successful in selected groups of patients. The major problem, to date, has been maintenance of weight loss. Techniques have included a low energy diet[12] and life style intervention.[13] Bariatric surgery has been proven to induce weight loss, but many patients have a significant amount of residual sleep apnea.[16] OSA may return even if patients maintain their body weight.[17] The AASM practice parameters for use of medical treatments for OSA recommended that weight loss be combined with a primary treatment for OSA[6] (Box F22-1). This recommendation is based on the fact that weight loss takes time, results vary among patients, and OSA may recur even if initially improved by weight loss. It was stated that bariatric surgery *may* be adjunctive in treatment of OSA in obese patients. This recommendation falls short of the recommendation of bariatric surgery as a primary treatment for OSA given the variable improvement in the AHI. Patients with OSA

BOX F22-1	**American Academy of Sleep Medicine Practice Parameter Recommendations for Medical Treatment of Obstructive Sleep Apnea**

WEIGHT REDUCTION

- Successful dietary weight loss may improve the AHI in obese patients with OSA. (Guideline)
- Dietary weight loss should be combined with primary treatment of OSA. (Option)
- Bariatric surgery may be adjunctive in treatment of OSA in obese patients. (Option)

POSITIONAL THERAPIES

- Positional therapy, consisting of a method that keeps the patient in a nonsupine position, is an effective secondary therapy or can be a supplement to primary therapies for OSA in patients who have a low AHI in the nonsupine versus the supine position. (Guideline)

OXYGEN SUPPLEMENTATION

- Oxygen supplementation is not recommended as a primary treatment for OSA. (Option)

NASAL CORTICOSTEROIDS

- Topical nasal corticosteroids may improve the AHI in patients with OSA and concurrent rhinitis and, thus, may be a useful adjunct to primary therapies for OSA. (Guideline)

MODAFINIL, ARMODAFINIL

- Modafinil is recommended for treatment of residual excessive sleepiness in patients with OSA, who have sleepiness despite effective PAP treatment and who are lacking any other identifiable cause for their sleepiness. (Standard)

OTHER TREATMENTS

- Protriptyline, SSRIs, aminophylline, estrogen preparations with or without progesterone, and short-acting decongestants. These treatments are NOT recommended.

Adapted from Morgenthaler TI, Kapen S, Lee-Chiong T, et al: Practice parameters for the medical therapy of obstructive sleep apnea, *Sleep* 29:1031–1035, 2006.
AHI, Apnea-hypopnea index; *OSA*, obstructive sleep apnea; *PAP*, positive airway pressure; *SSRIs*, selective serotonin reuptake inhibitors.

undergoing bariatric surgery should be given an effective treatment (usually CPAP) in the postoperative period and during weight loss. If a sleep study after significant weight loss documents a "cure," stopping the primary treatment could be considered. If significant OSA persists, a lower level of CPAP may be effective.[15] If CPAP or other treatment for OSA is stopped, patients should be monitored closely for signs and symptoms of recurrence.

Posture and Positional Treatment

Many patients with OSA have a significant worsening of apnea in the supine position.[18-20] Some, but not all, studies have found an increase in upper airway size in the lateral position. Changes in airway shape or size with changes in posture could be caused by an effect of gravity on the tissue surrounding the upper airway or to posterior movement of the tongue in the supine position. Reductions in lung volume in the supine position may also reduce upper airway size. Recent studies suggest that on assuming the supine position, fluid may shift from the lower extremities into the neck and upper airway producing narrowing.[21]

Neill and associates[22] found that elevation of the head by 30 degrees improved airway stability (compared with the supine position) in patients with OSA, as measured by airway occlusion during sleep. In this study, lateral sleep positioning had less of a stabilizing effect compared with elevation of the head. This suggested that sleeping with the head elevated may reduce the AHI more in some patients than sleeping in the lateral position. In the same study, CPAP was also progressively elevated until apneas and hypopneas were abolished. The mean effective pressure was 10.4 cm H_2O in the supine position, 5.3 cm H_2O with the head-elevated position, and 5.5 cm H_2O in the lateral position.

A considerable number of patients with a significant overall AHI have minimal sleep apnea in the lateral position. In fact, many of these patients have chronically favored this position at home. In one study, *approximately 55% of a large group of patients with sleep apnea had positional sleep apnea, defined as an AHI at least two times higher in the supine position than in the nonsupine position.*[18]

Avoiding the supine posture has been proposed as a treatment for sleep apnea. To maintain the lateral posture during sleep, a number of night shirts or straps with foam balls or cushions are available that prevent comfortable supine sleep.[23-26] A cross-over study compared CPAP and postural treatment (foam balls in a backpack) and found that while postural treatment was less effective than CPAP, no difference could be seen in improvement in the Epworth Sleepiness Scale (ESS) or sleep architecture.[24] Permut and colleagues[23] found positional treatment to be as effective as CPAP, as assessed by one night of PSG in a group of patients with mild and positional OSA. McEvoy and associates[25] also found a lower AHI, better oxygen saturation, and better sleep quality in the seated sleeping posture (60 degrees) compared with the supine position. However, a study found poor adherence to the "tennis ball technique."[26] Studies of long-term outcomes with more comfortable positioning devices are needed. Recently, devices with the ability to buzz or vibrate when the patient assumes the supine position have been developed. The buzzing or vibration prompts the patient to change to the lateral posture. These devices also measure adherence and snoring.[27,28] A method to document adherence has been a limitation of positioning devices until recently.

Postural interventions may be used to improve CPAP treatment. An increase in the required CPAP pressure to maintain upper airway patency is commonly required in the supine position compared with the lateral body position.[19,20] Oksenberg and colleagues[19] documented about a 3-cm H_2O difference between the supine and nonsupine postures. As noted previously, Neill and associates[22] noted a significantly less PAP was needed in the lateral position or with the head elevated. In pressure-intolerant patients undergoing CPAP treatment, one approach might be to lower the pressure to one effective in the lateral position and encourage patients to sleep in that position (or use a device to discourage supine sleep), at least during an adaptation period. Nocturnal oximetry at home, observation of the residual AHI recorded on the CPAP device, and a combination of both are methods to document the efficacy of this approach.

Medical Therapies to Improve Nasal Patency

The AASM practice parameters for medical treatments[6] did not recommend the use of short-acting nasal decongestants (see Box F22-1). The major consideration is the development of rhinitis medicamentosa.[29] A study by Kiely and associates,[30] using a placebo-controlled, randomized, cross-over design, found a modest reduction in the AHI in a group of apneic snorers with intranasal fluticasone but no reduction in snoring noise in nonapneic snorers. No improvement was observed in objective sleep quality. Of interest, the improvement in the AHI was correlated with a reduction in the nasal resistance.

A treatment effect is likely only if intranasal steroids improve nasal resistance, and this change may not occur in all patients.

Supplemental Oxygen

Supplemental oxygen may improve nocturnal oxygenation in patients with OSA. In a study by Smith and coworkers,[31] nocturnal supplemental oxygen did not improve objective daytime sleepiness but did improve nocturnal oxygenation in a group of patients with OSA. In general, oxygen does not significantly reduce the AHI or improve daytime sleepiness. Caution is advised in the use of supplemental oxygen in hypercapnic OSA patients because some may develop worsening hypercapnia, especially on high flow rates of oxygen.[32,33] In some studies, acute administration of oxygen caused prolongation of apneas.[34,35] Supplemental oxygen tends to convert central and mixed apneas to obstructive apneas.[36] Loredo and colleagues[37] compared oxygen with CPAP in the treatment of OSA. CPAP improved sleep quality, but supplemental oxygen improved only nocturnal oxygenation. It should also be noted that supplemental oxygen often improves but does not normalize nocturnal oxygen saturation in patients with severe drops in the arterial oxygen saturation.[32] In summary, supplemental nocturnal oxygen is not the treatment of choice for OSA, but individual patients may benefit from this treatment if all other treatment options fail. The AASM practice parameters for medical treatment of OSA state that supplemental oxygen is not indicated for treatment of OSA.[6]

Persistent Daytime Sleepiness on CPAP

A substantial number of patients with OSA continue to have daytime sleepiness despite adequate PAP treatment.[38–44] In such patients, the first steps are to document adequate objective PAP adherence, document effective treatment, and try sleep extension, if indicated. Other causes of persistent daytime sleepiness despite PAP treatment include medications and other sleep disorders (narcolepsy, periodic limb movement disorder, idiopathic hypersomnia, depression). Other sleep disorders should be ruled out, if clinically indicated. Of note, although some might assume 6 hours of nightly CPAP adherence to be "good adherence," in patients with continued daytime sleepiness, the first step would be an attempt at sleep extension to 7 hours. This includes using CPAP during naps. Another option would be an empirically small increase in CPAP pressure. Adequacy of pressure should also be documented because a surprisingly high percentage of patients remain inadequately treated.[45] Many of the current PAP devices give an estimate of the residual AHI. However, the estimated AHI is not always accurate. Finally, a repeat PAP titration may be considered if any suspicion exists that the current level of CPAP is not effective. In addition, other factors such as mouth leak or mask leak could be present that are causing repeated arousals.

Modafinil, Armodafinil, and Stimulants

If daytime sleepiness persists on optimized CPAP treatment and no identifiable additional sleep disorder or cause of sleepiness exists, treatment with an alerting agent (modafinil [Provigil] or armodafinil [Nuvigil]) is indicated.[6] These medications have been shown to improve daytime alertness (subjective and objective) in randomized, placebo-controlled studies in OSA patients with residual sleepiness despite adequate PAP treatment.[38–44,46] The dosing and side effects of these medications are discussed in detail in the chapter on narcolepsy (Fundamentals 33). During treatment with modafinil in patients with OSA, it is essential to document continued adequate adherence to PAP treatment. In one study evaluating the addition of modafinil to CPAP treatment, poorer CPAP use was noted with patients taking modafinil compared with placebo.[39] Patients with OSA who are adherent to PAP treatment are sometimes not able to use CPAP for various reasons (e.g., upper respiratory tract infection). A study by Williams and coworkers[43] documented that use of modafinil did help the patients to function in this circumstance.

Unfortunately, the addition of modafinil has minimal or modest benefits in a significant number of OSA patients who are still sleepy on PAP treatment. Kingshott and colleagues[39] found no improvement in the ESS or the multiple sleep latency test (MSLT) with modafinil but did find an improvement in sleep latency in the maintenance of wakefulness test (MWT). Although stimulants (methylphenidate, dextroamphetamine) are not approved for treatment of persistent sleepiness in OSA by the U.S. Food and Drug Administration (FDA) or the AASM practice parameters, individual patients with persistent daytime sleepiness despite adequate PAP treatment may respond better to stimulants than to modafinil. If clinically indicated, the possibility of coexistent narcolepsy should be ruled out.

Treatment with stimulants in addition to PAP could be tried as "off-label treatment" if patients continue to have disabling sleepiness despite other measures. They should be educated about the side effects and risks involved with these medications. These medications are discussed in detail in Patient 92.

REFERENCES

1. Epstein LJ, Kristo D, Strollo PJ Jr. et al: Adult obstructive sleep apnea task force of the American Academy of Sleep Medicine: clinical guideline for the evaluation, management and long-term care of obstructive sleep apnea in adults, *J Clin Sleep Med* 5:263–276, 2009.
2. Beninati W, Harris CD, Herold DL, Shepard JW Jr: The effect of snoring and obstructive sleep apnea on the sleep quality of bed partners, *Mayo Clin Proc* 74:955–958, 1999.
3. Punjabi NM, Caffo BS, Goodwin JL, et al: Sleep-disordered breathing and mortality: a prospective cohort study, *PLoS Med* 6:e1000132, 2009.
4. Marin JM, Carrizo S, Vicente E, Agusti AGN: Long-term cardiovascular outcomes in men with obstructive sleep apnea-hypopnea with or without treatment with continuous positive airway pressure: an observational study, *Lancet* 365:1046–1053, 2005.
5. Lavie P, Herer P, Lavie L: Mortality risk factors in sleep apnoea: a matched case-control study, *J Sleep Res* 16:128–134, 2007.
6. Morgenthaler TI, Kapen S, Lee-Chiong T, et al: Practice parameters for the medical therapy of obstructive sleep apnea, *Sleep* 29:1031–1035, 2006.
7. Aurora RN, Casey KR, Kristo D, et al: Practice parameters for the surgical modifications of the upper airway for obstructive sleep apnea in adults, *Sleep* 33:1408–1413, 2010.
8. Kushida CA, Morgenthaler TI, Littner MR, et al: American Academy of Sleep Medicine practice parameters for the treatment of snoring and obstructive sleep apnea with oral appliances: an update for 2005, *Sleep* 29:240–243, 2006.
9. Kushida CA, Littner MR, Hirshkowitz M, et al: American Academy of Sleep Medicine Practice parameters for the use of continuous and bilevel positive airway pressure devices to treat adult patients with sleep-related breathing disorders, *Sleep* 29:375–380, 2006.
10. Peppard PE, Young T, Palta M, et al: Longitudinal study of moderate weight change and sleep disordered breathing, *JAMA* 284:3015–3021, 2000.
11. Smith PL, Gold AR, Meyers DA, et al: Weight loss in mildly to moderately obese patients with obstructive sleep apnea, *Ann Intern Med* 103:850–855, 1985.
12. Johansson K, Neovius M, Lagerros YT, et al: Effect of a very low energy diet on moderate and severe sleep apnea in obese men: a randomised controlled trial, *Br Med J* 339:b4609, 2009.
13. Tuomilehto HPI, Seppa JM, Partine MM, et al: Lifestyle intervention with weight reduction first-line treatment in mild obstructive sleep apnea, *Am J Respir Crit Care Med* 179:320–327, 2009.
14. Schwartz AR, Gold AR, Schubert N, et al: Effect of weight loss on upper airway collapsibility in obstructive sleep apnea, *Am Rev Respir Dis* 144:494–498, 1991.
15. Lettieri CJ, Eliasson AH, Greenburg DL: Persistence of obstructive sleep apnea after surgical weight loss, *J Clin Sleep Med* 4:333–338, 2008.
16. Greenburg DL, Lettieri CJ, Eliasson AH: Effects of surgical weight loss on measures of obstructive sleep apnea: a meta-analysis, *Am J Med* 122:535–542, 2009.
17. Pillar G, Peled R, Lavie P: Recurrence of sleep apnea without concomitant weight increase 7.5 years after weight reduction surgery, *Chest* 106:1702–1704, 1994.
18. Oksenberg A, Silverberg DS, Arons E, Radwan H: Positional vs nonpositional obstructive sleep apnea patients, *Chest* 112:629–639, 1997.
19. Oksenberg A, Silverberg DS, Arons E, et al: The sleep supine position has a major effect on optimal nasal CPAP, *Chest* 116:1000–1006, 1999.
20. Pevernagie DA, Shepard JW Jr: Relations between sleep stage, posture and effective nasal CPAP levels in OSA, *Sleep* 15:162–167, 1992.
21. Redolfi S, Yumino D, Ruttanaumpawan P, et al: Relationship between overnight rostral fluid shift and obstructive sleep apnea in nonobese men, *Am J Respir Crit Care Med* 179(3):241–246, 2009.
22. Neill AM, Angus SM, Sajkov D, McEvoy RD: Effects of sleep posture on upper airway stability in patients with obstructive sleep apnea, *Am J Respir Crit Care Med* 155:199–204, 1997.
23. Permut I, Diaz-Abad M, Eissam C, et al: Comparison of positional therapy to CPAP in patients with positional obstructive sleep apnea, *J Clin Sleep Med* 6:238–243, 2010.
24. Jokic R, Klimaszewski A, Crossley M, et al: Positional treatment vs continuous positive airway pressure in patients with positional obstructive sleep apnea syndrome, *Chest* 115:771–781, 1999.
25. McEvoy RD, Sharp DJ, Thornton AT: The effects of posture on obstructive sleep apnea, *Am Rev Respir Dis* 133:662–666, 1986.
26. Bignold JJ, Deans-Costi G, Goldsworthy MR, et al: Poor long-term patient compliance with the tennis ball technique for treating positional obstructive sleep apnea, *J Clin Sleep Med* 5:428–430, 2009.
27. Ravesloot MJ, van Maanen JP, Dun L, de Vries N: The undervalued potential of positional therapy in position-dependent snoring and obstructive sleep apnea-a review of the literature, *Sleep Breath* 17(1):39–49, 2013.
28. Bignold JJ, Mercer JD, Antic NA, et al: Accurate position monitoring and improved supine-dependent obstructive sleep apnea with a new position recording and supine avoidance device, *J Clin Sleep Med* 7(4):376–383, 2011.
29. Doshi J: Rhinitis medicamentosa: what an otolaryngologist needs to know, *Eur Arch Otorhinolaryngol* 266:623–625, 2009.
30. Kiely JL, Nolan P, McNicholas WT: Intranasal corticosteroid therapy for obstructive sleep apnea in patients with co-existing rhinitis, *Thorax* 59:35–55, 2004.
31. Smith PL, Haponik EF, Bleecker ER: The effects of oxygen in patients with sleep apnea, *Am Rev Respir Dis* 130:958–963, 1984.
32. Alford NJ, Fletcher EC, Nickeson D: Acute oxygen in patients with sleep apnea and COPD, *Chest* 89:30–38, 1986.
33. Fletcher E, Munafo DA: Role of nocturnal oxygen therapy in obstructive sleep apnea. Should it be used? *Chest* 98:1497–1504, 1990.
34. Martin RJ, Sander MH, Gray BA, Pennock BE: Acute and long term ventilatory effects in adult sleep apnea, *Am Rev Respir Dis* 125:175–180, 1982.
35. Gold AR, Schwartz AR, Bleecker ER, Smith PL: The effect of chronic nocturnal oxygen administration upon sleep apnea, *Am Rev Respir Dis* 134:925–929, 1986.
36. Gold AR, Bleecker ER, Smith PL: A shift from central and mixed sleep apnea to obstructive sleep apnea resulting from low flow oxygen, *Am Rev Respir Dis* 132:220–223, 1985.
37. Loredo JS, Ancoli-Israel S, Kim E, et al: Effect of continuous positive airway pressure versus supplemental oxygen on sleep quality in obstructive sleep apnea: a placebo-CPAP-controlled study, *Sleep* 29:564–571, 2006.

38. Pack AI, Black JE, Schwartz JR, Matheson JK: Modafinil as adjunct therapy for daytime sleepiness in obstructive sleep apnea, *Am J Respir Crit Care Med* 164:1675–1681, 2001.

39. Kingshott RN, Vennelle M, Coleman EL, et al: Randomized, double-blind, placebo-controlled crossover trial of modafinil in the treatment of residual excessive daytime sleepiness in the sleep apnea/hypopnea syndrome, *Am J Respir Crit Care Med* 163:918–923, 2001.

40. Dinges DF, Weaver TE: Effects of modafinil on sustained attention performance and quality of life in OSA patients with residual sleepiness while being treated with nCPAP, *Sleep Med* 4:393–402, 2003.

41. Black JE, Hirshkowitz M: Modafinil for treatment of residual excessive sleepiness in nasal continuous positive airway pressure–treated obstructive sleep apnea/hypopnea syndrome, *Sleep* 28:464–471, 2005.

42. Weaver TE, Chasens ER, Arora S: Modafinil improves functional outcomes in patients with residual excessive sleepiness associated with CPAP treatment, *J Clin Sleep Med* 5:499–505, 2009.

43. Williams SC, Marshall NS, Kennerson M, et al: Modafinil effects during acute continuous positive airway pressure withdrawal: a randomized crossover double-blind placebo-controlled trial, *Am J Respir Crit Care Med* 181:825–831, 2010.

44. Krystal AD, Harsh JR, Yang RR, et al: A double-blind, placebo-controlled study of armodafinil for excessive sleepiness in patients with treated obstructive sleep apnea and comorbid depression, *J Clin Psychiatry* 71:32–40, 2010.

45. Pittman SD, Pillar G, Berry RB, et al: Follow-up assessment of CPAP efficacy in patients with obstructive sleep apnea using an ambulatory device based on peripheral arterial tonometry, *Sleep Breath* 10:123–131, 2006.

46. Roth T, Rippon GA, Arora S: Armodafinil improves wakefulness and long-term episodic memory in nCPAP-adherent patients with excessive sleepiness associated with obstructive sleep apnea, *Sleep Breath* 12:53–62, 2008.

PATIENT 45

Patient with OSA and Weight Loss

Patient A: A 30-year-old man with sleep apnea and weight loss—height 5 feet 10 inches weight 230 pounds (lb), body mass index (BMI) 34 kilograms per square meters (kg/m^2)—was diagnosed as having severe obstructive sleep apnea (OSA) (apnea–hypopnea index [AHI] 60 per hour [hr]). He underwent a continuous positive airway pressure (CPAP) titration, and on CPAP of 12 centimeters of water (cm H$_2$O), the AHI was 5/hr. Following CPAP treatment, he had a rapid resolution of symptoms. However, he found CPAP unacceptable for his social life and began a dietary weight loss program. After 6 months, he weighed 200 lb and stopped using his CPAP. He reported that he did not snore and that his symptoms of sleepiness had not returned. He underwent repeat polysomnography (PSG) (Table P45-1).

TABLE P45-1	**Effect of Weight Loss**		
	Baseline	**CPAP Titration**	**Repeat PSG after Weight Loss**
Weight lbs	230	230	200
CPAP (cm H$_2$O)	None	12	None
AHI no./hr	70	5	5
AHIsupine #/hr	50	n/a (no supine sleep)	25
AHInonsupine #/hr	45	5	0

AHI, Apnea–hypopnea index; *CPAP*, continuous positive airway pressure; *hr*, hour; *n/a*, not applicable; no sleep in this position recorded; *PSG*, polysomnography.

QUESTIONS

1. What treatment option do you recommend for Patient A?

Patient B: A 40-year-old woman with severe obesity with a BMI of 45 kg/m^2 underwent bariatric surgery, and the BMI fell to 31 kig/m^2 over 6 months. Before surgery she had a split sleep study with an AHI of 45/hr and a low arterial oxygen saturation of 75% in the diagnostic portion and 5/hr on CPAP of 12 cm H$_2$O. The patient did not report daytime sleepiness (Epworth Sleepiness Scale [ESS] of 8). The patient's surgeon would not perform bariatric surgery unless she was compliant with treatment. She started CPAP treatment, although she did not like this therapy. Following weight loss, the patient stopped using CPAP and felt well without snoring or sleepiness.

2. What evaluation do you recommend for Patient B?

Patient C: A 35-year-old woman had resolution of sleep apnea following bariatric surgery. The patient noted a reduction in the body mass index from 38 to 31 kg/m^2 with an associated drop in the AHI from 28 to 8/hr. She used CPAP of 10 cm H$_2$O prior to weight loss. The patient did well for about 1 year after stopping CPAP treatment but over the last 6 months had noted return of symptoms of daytime sleepiness and reported only mild snoring. She had been able to maintain her body weight. Recently, she had noted a significant increase in pedal edema. About 6 months ago, a diuretic used for hypertension treatment had been discontinued.

Physical examination showed obesity and Mallampati 3 upper airway; leg examination showed evidence of venous insufficiency and 3+pedal edema.

3. What do you recommend for Patient C?

ANSWERS

1. **Answer (for Patient A):** Continued weight loss and sleep in the lateral position

Discussion: The American Academy of Sleep Medicine (AASM) practice parameters[1] for use of medical treatments for OSA recommend that weight loss be combined with a primary treatment for OSA. This recommendation is based on the fact that weight loss takes time, results vary among patients, and OSA may recur even if initially improved by weight loss. Both dietary and surgical means of weight loss have been shown to reduce the AHI.[2,3] A sleep study documenting resolution of OSA by weight loss is needed before the primary treatment for OSA can be discontinued. Weight loss maintenance and follow-up are needed as OSA may return even if weight loss is maintained.[4] Patients with mild-to-moderate OSA may have postural sleep apnea. This is usually defined as AHIsupine >2 ×AHInonsupine. Some clinicians also require that the AHI-nonsupine be <5/hour. In the current patient, his AHIsupine was much higher. Because he spent minimal time in the supine position, his overall AHI was near normal.

2. **Answer (for Patient B):** Diagnostic PSG

Discussion: Bariatric surgery is commonly performed as a treatment for morbid obesity. Studies of patients with OSA undergoing bariatric surgery report that OSA rarely completely resolves and that the AHI remains in the moderate to severe range in the majority of patients. Greenburg and coworkers[5] performed a meta-analysis of bariatric surgery and the effects on OSA in morbidly obese patients. Twelve studies including 342 patients were analyzed. The mean BMI was reduced by 17.9 kg/m^2 (baseline 55.3 kg/m^2), and the AHI was reduced from 54.7 to 15.8/hr. The authors concluded that bariatric surgery does result in both dramatic weight loss and improvement of the AHI, but not always to normal levels. Many patients will still likely require treatment of OSA (CPAP and others). In another series of 24 consecutive patients undergoing bariatric surgery, only 4% were cured of OSA. Bariatric surgery may be considered as an adjunctive treatment for OSA. The most common bariatric operation is a Roux-en-Y procedure, although other surgery such as laparoscopic gastric banding may be tried for less obese patients. The mortality of the Roux-en-Y procedure is less than 2%. In the AASM practice parameters for medical treatment of OSA, it is stated that bariatric surgery "may" be an adjunctive treatment for OSA in obese patients. This recommendation falls short of recommendation of bariatric surgery as a primary treatment for OSA treatment given the variable improvement in the AHI. Patients with OSA undergoing bariatric surgery should be provided an effective treatment (usually CPAP) in the postoperative period and during weight loss. If a sleep study after significant weight loss documents a "cure," stopping primary treatment could be considered. If CPAP or other treatment for OSA is stopped, patients should be monitored closely for signs and symptoms of recurrence. In general, CPAP adherence in patients following bariatric surgery is poor and a majority of patients report resolution of snoring despite objective findings that both snoring and OSA are still present after weight loss. If CPAP is needed, the level of positive pressure may be lower after weight loss. Lettieri and associates[6] reported a reduction in required CPAP from 11.5 to 8.4 cm H_2O after weight loss (BMI dropped from 51 to 32 kg/m^2) in a group of patients undergoing bariatric surgery. However, the magnitude of this effect may vary significantly among patients. If a patient continues to use CPAP while losing weight, a sleep study off CPAP is needed to determine if continued CPAP is needed. Young et al[7] found the AHI to be lower after two nights of CPAP withdrawal compared with pretreatment values in a group of OSA patients who did not lose weight. The biggest difference was in severe cases. Some residual effects of CPAP are present soon after withdrawal in individual patients. This carryover effect should be considered before CPAP is discontinued based on a sleep study showing minimal OSA on the first night off CPAP. In Patient B, a diagnostic PSG revealed persistent moderate snoring, an AHI of 15/hr, and moderate snoring. However, the patient declined treatment for the persistent sleep apnea.

3. **Answer (for Patient C):** Diagnostic PSG (followed by PAP PSG titration if indicated)

Discussion: A return of significant sleep apnea has been reported in patients who have previously had resolution following weight loss **_even if weight loss is maintained._** Pillar and colleagues[4] reported on a patient that had recurrence of OSA after previous weight loss without concomitant weight gain. Sampol and associates[8] monitored 24 patients "cured" by weight loss for a mean of 94 months. Six of the 13 patients who maintained weight loss had recurrence of OSA (AHI = 40.5/hr). This illustrates the need for continued clinical follow-up. The etiology of this phenomenon is not understood. It is possible that a return of snoring caused a return of upper airway edema. Studies have suggested that a redistribution of fluid during the supine posture at night may result in worsening sleep apnea.[9] Thus, even if the BMI was unchanged in this patient, it is possible that the lean body mass was lower and amount of body water higher. In study by Redolfi and associates,[10] patients with OSA and venous insufficiency who wore compression stockings during the day showed attenuation of the AHI at night. Compression stockings were thought to minimize redistribution of fluid at night. Other factors such as the effect of sedatives or ethanol could be considered. In Patient C, a sleep study revealed an AHI of 20/hr. A subsequent CPAP titration study showed that a pressure of 7 cm H_2O was effective (lower than her pre–weight loss pressure). Although the cause of worsening OSA in the patient is unknown, the historical association of a return of OSA with appearance of significant pedal edema (and stopping a diuretic medication) is of interest in this patient.

CLINICAL PEARLS

1. Weight loss may result in significant improvement in OSA and is considered an adjunctive treatment for OSA. It is not recommended as a primary treatment except in mild and asymptomatic cases. Weight loss may take time and must be maintained.

2. Improvement in OSA may occur following weight loss induced by both dietary and surgical treatments. Weight loss may improve the AHI, even if obesity is mild.

3. Bariatric surgery may result in significant decreases in the AHI, but often at least moderate OSA may persist. A sleep study is needed to document resolution of OSA before termination of CPAP treatment can be recommended.

4. OSA may return after previous resolution following weight loss, even if weight loss is maintained. If symptoms return, evaluation is needed.

5. A resolution of symptoms and snoring by patient report is not sufficient evidence that OSA has resolved following weight loss. A sleep study is needed.

6. If CPAP is still needed after weight loss, the required pressure may be lower. If clinically indicated, a repeat CPAP titration study could be considered.

REFERENCES

1. Morgenthaler TI, Kapen S, Lee-Chiong T, et al: Practice parameters for the medical therapy of obstructive sleep apnea, *Sleep* 29:1031–1035, 2006.
2. Johansson K, Neovius M, Lagerros YT, et al: Effect of a very low energy diet on moderate and severe sleep apnea in obese men: a randomised controlled trial, *Br Med J* 339:b4609, 2009.
3. Tuomilehto HPI, Seppa JM, Partine MM, et al: Lifestyle intervention with weight reduction first-line treatment in mild obstructive sleep apnea, *Am J Respir Crit Care Med* 179:320–327, 2009.
4. Pillar G, Peled R, Lavie P: Recurrence of sleep apnea without concomitant weight increase 7.5 years after weight reduction surgery, *Chest* 106(6):1702–1704, 1994.
5. Greenburg DL, Lettieri CJ, Eliasson AH: Effects of surgical weight loss on measures of obstructive sleep apnea: a meta-analysis, *Am J Med* 122(6):535–542, 2009.
6. Lettieri CJ, Eliasson AH, Greenburg DL: Persistence of obstructive sleep apnea after surgical weight loss, *J Clin Sleep Med* 4 (4):333–338, 2008.
7. Young LR, Taxin ZH, Norman RG, et al: Response to CPAP withdrawal in patients with mild versus severe obstructive sleep apnea/hypopnea syndrome, *Sleep* 36(3):405–412, 2013.
8. Sampol G, Sagales MT, Marti S, et al: Long-term efficacy of dietary weight loss in sleep apnea/hypopnea syndrome, *Eur Respir J* J12:1156–1159, 1998.
9. White LH, Bradley TD: Role of nocturnal rostral fluid shift in the pathogenesis of obstructive and central sleep apnoea, *J Physiol* 591(Pt 5):1179–1193, 2013.
10. Redolfi S, Arnulf I, Pottier M, et al: Attenuation of obstructive sleep apnea by compression stockings in subjects with venous insufficiency, *Am J Respir Crit Care Med* 184(9):1062–1066, 2011.

PATIENT 46

Postural OSA

A 60-year-old woman was evaluated for loud snoring and mild daytime sleepiness that had persisted for about 1 year. Over that year, she had gained about 10 pounds. The results of a diagnostic polysomnography (PSG) are shown in the table below. Treatment options, including continuous positive airway pressure (CPAP), an oral appliance (OA), and upper airway surgery, were discussed with the patient. Weight loss was also recommended. The patient found all the treatment options other than weight loss unacceptable.

Total sleep time (TST)	380 minutes	% TST supine	70
Rapid eye movement (REM) sleep	70 minutes	% TST nonsupine	30
Apnea–hypopnea index (AHI)	17.3	AHI supine (#/hr)	23
OA (#)	32	AHI nonsupine (#/hr)	4
CA (#)	3	AHI non-REM (NREM) (#/hr)	15.6
MA (#)	0	AHI REM (#/hr)	25
Hypopnea (#)	75		

(#), Number; *TST*, total sleep time; *OA*, obstructive apnea; *CA*, central apnea; *MA*, mixed apnea; *REM*, rapid eye movement sleep.

QUESTION

1. What treatment do you recommend?

ANSWER

1. **Answer:** Position (postural) treatment

Discussion: A considerable number of patients with a significant overall AHI have minimal sleep apnea in the lateral position. In fact, many of these patients have chronically favored this sleeping position at home. Others have slept with the head elevated in a recliner or on a wedge. In one study,[1] approximately 55% of a large group of patients with sleep apnea had positional sleep apnea, defined as an AHI at least two times higher in the supine position than in the nonsupine position. Postural obstructive sleep apnea (OSA) is generally defined as an AHIsupine >2 ×AHInon-supine. Other clinicians also require the AHInonsupine to be less than 5 per hour (hr). Because the amount of supine sleep can dramatically affect the overall AHI in some patients, *the amount of supine sleep should always be noted when interpreting a sleep study or comparing the results of different sleep studies.*

Avoiding the supine posture has been proposed as a treatment for sleep apnea.[2] To maintain the lateral posture during sleep, a number of night shirts or straps with foam balls or cushions are available that prevent comfortable supine sleep (Figure P46-1). Jokic and coworkers[3] performed a randomized cross-over trial of position therapy and CPAP in a group of patients with positional OSA. The positional device consisted of a backpack with a foam ball (10 × 5.5 inches). Positional treatment was slightly less effective than CPAP, but no difference in improvement in the Epworth Sleepiness Scale (ESS), sleep architecture, or subjective sleep quality was observed. No long-term studies of positional therapy have been performed. Permut and colleagues[4] found positional treatment (see Figure P46-1) to be as effective as CPAP as assessed by one night of PSG in a group of patients with mild and positional OSA. McEvoy and associates[5] also found a lower AHI, better oxygen saturation, and better sleep quality in the seated sleeping posture (60 degrees) compared with the supine position. Skinner and coworkers[6] studied the effect of a shoulder-head elevation pillow in mild to moderate OSA. In 7 of 14 patients, the AHI dropped to less than 10/hr. In contrast with CPAP, the AHI was less than 5/hr in all patients. Thus, positional treatment might be effective therapy in a number of patients with positional OSA. However, a study found poor adherence to the "tennis ball technique.[7]" Recently, some new devices[8] that vibrate when the patient is in the supine position have been studied. This vibration reminds the patient to move to the lateral position. The devices can also track adherence and time in each body position. Studies of *long-term* outcomes with more comfortable positioning devices that can monitor adherence are needed.

Postural treatment may also be combined with CPAP with the goal of lowering the required level of CPAP. An increase in the required CPAP pressure to maintain upper airway patency is commonly required in the supine position compared with the lateral body position.[9,10] Oksenberg and leagues[10] documented about a 3-cm H_2O (centimeters of water) pressure difference between supine and nonsupine postures. Neill and associates[2] noted that significantly less PAP (about 4 to 5 cm H_2O less) was needed in the lateral position or with the head elevated. In pressure-intolerant patients undergoing CPAP treatment, one approach might be to lower the pressure to one effective in the lateral position and encourage patients to sleep in that position (or use a device to discourage supine sleep), at least during an adaptation period. Nocturnal oximetry at home, observation of the residual AHI recorded on the CPAP device, or both are methods to document the efficacy of this approach.

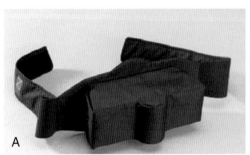
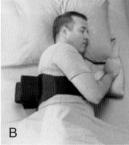

FIGURE P46-1 ■ **A** and **B,** A lateral positioning device. The ZZsoma Positional Sleeper. (From Permut I, Diaz-Abad M, Eissam C, et al: Comparison of positional therapy to CPAP in patients with positional obstructive sleep apnea, *J Clin Sleep Med* 6:238-243, 2010.

CLINICAL PEARLS

1. Postural OSA is common especially in patients with mild-to-moderate OSA.

2. Position (postural) therapy has proven to be effective in short-term studies in patients with postural OSA. Comfortable devices that can record use and time in each body position are needed.

3. Sleep in the lateral position or with the head elevated may reduce the required level of CPAP by 3 to 5 cm H_2O. Postural treatment may be used as an adjunct to CPAP therapy.

4. When comparing the AHI values between studies, the percentage of supine sleep should always be noted.

REFERENCES

1. Oksenberg A, Silverberg DS, Arons E, Radwan H: Positional vs nonpositional obstructive sleep apnea patients, *Chest* 112:629–639, 1997.
2. Neill AM, Angus SM, Sajkov D, McEvoy RD: Effects of sleep posture on upper airway stability in patients with obstructive sleep apnea, *Am J Respir Crit Care Med* 155:199–204, 1997.
3. Jokic R, Klimaszewski A, Crossley M, et al: Positional treatment vs continuous positive airway pressure in patients with positional obstructive sleep apnea syndrome, *Chest* 115:771–781, 1999.
4. Permut I, Diaz-Abad M, Eissam C, et al: Comparison of positional therapy to CPAP in patients with positional obstructive sleep apnea, *J Clin Sleep Med* 6:238–243, 2010.
5. McEvoy RD, Sharp DJ, Thornton AT: The effects of posture on obstructive sleep apnea, *Am Rev Respir Dis* 133:662–666, 1986.
6. Skinner MA, Kingshott RN, Jones DR, et al: Elevated posture for the management of obstructive sleep apnea, *Sleep Breath* 8:193–200, 2004.
7. Bignold JJ, Deans-Costi G, Goldsworthy MR, et al: Poor long-term patient compliance with the tennis ball technique for treating positional obstructive sleep apnea, *J Clin Sleep Med* 5:428–430, 2009.
8. Bignold JJ, Mercer JD, Antic NA, et al: Accurate position monitoring and improved supine-dependent obstructive sleep apnea with a new position recording and supine avoidance device, *J Clin Sleep Med* 7(4):376–383, 2011.
9. Pevernagie DA, Shepard JW Jr.: Relations between sleep stage, posture and effective nasal CPAP levels in OSA, *Sleep* 15:162–167, 1992.
10. Oksenberg A, Silverberg DS, Arons E, et al: The sleep supine position has a major effect on optimal nasal CPAP, *Chest* 116:1000–1006, 1999.

FUNDAMENTALS 23

PAP Modes and Treatment

Positive airway pressure (PAP) is the treatment of choice for patients with moderate to severe obstructive sleep apnea (OSA) and is also effective in patients with "mild" OSA, who are symptomatic and motivated to use the treatment.[1-5] PAP is very effective often lowering the apnea–hypopnea index (AHI) to ≤5/hour (hr). However, some patients do not accept PAP treatment. Inadequate adherence and duration of nightly use are major problems with PAP treatment.[6] Refer to the Fundamentals 25 on adherence. In the current chapter, basic PAP modes will be discussed. More advanced PAP modes (bilevel PAP [BPAP] spontaneously timed [ST], assured pressure support, and adaptive servoventilation) are discussed in Fundamentals 30.

MODES OF PAP

A number of basic modes of delivering PAP exist (Table F23-1). The algorithms used to vary pressure in the more complex devices are undergoing constant change, and the reader should consult the most recent device manual for clinicians from the manufacturer. Continuous positive airway pressure (CPAP) delivers a predetermined constant pressure during both inspiration and exhalation (Figure F23-1). Bilevel positive airway pressure (BPAP) delivers separately adjustable higher inspiratory PAP (IPAP) and lower expiratory PAP (EPAP).[7] In the spontaneous (S) mode, the patient determines the respiratory rate and cycles the device between IPAP and EPAP. In unselected patients, BPAP treatment does not result in higher rates of adherence than CPAP.[8] A Cochrane database analysis of six studies and 285 participants found no significant difference in usage with BPAP compared with CPAP.[9] However, some patients failing CPAP because of pressure intolerance will tolerate BPAP.[10-12] This is especially true of patients having difficulty exhaling or who have complaints of bloating. Some patients with

TABLE F23-1 Basic Modes of Positive Airway Pressure Devices

PAP Mode	Method	Use
CPAP	Continuous pressure during inhalation and exhalation	OSA Some patients with central apnea
BPAP (S mode)	IPAP inspiratory PAP EPAP expiratory PAP PS (pressure support) = IPAP-EPAP	Pressure intolerance OHS, COPD Bloating, mouth leak
Flexible PAP Expiratory pressure relief (Cflex, EPR)	Pressure falls in early exhalation Returns to set pressure at end-exhalation	Pressure intolerance
APAP autotitrating, autoadjusting PAP (autoCPAP)	Titrates between maximum and minimum pressure limits to prevent apnea, hypopnea, airway vibration	PAP treatment without titration Auto-titration (determine optimal CPAP) Pressure intolerance
Auto-BPAP	Titrates IPAP and EPAP between EPAPmin and IPAPmax—algorithms vary	BPAP treatment without titration Pressure intolerance

APAP, Autoadjusting (auto-titrating positive airway pressure); *BPAP*, bilevel positive airway pressure; *COPD*, chronic obstructive pulmonary disease; *CPAP*, continuous positive airway pressure; *EPAP*, expiratory positive airway pressure; *EPR*, expiratory pressure relief; *IPAP*, inspiratory positive airway pressure; *OHS*, obesity hypoventilation syndrome; *OSA*, obstructive sleep apnea; *PAP*, positive airway pressure; *PS*, pressure support; *S mode*, spontaneous mode.

FIGURE F23-1 ■ Modes of positive airway pressure (PAP). On the left, continuous PAP (CPAP) provides a near-constant pressure during inspiration (I) and exhalation (E). In the middle, bilevel PAP (BPAP) provides separately adjustable pressure in inspiration (IPAP) and expiration (EPAP). On the right is an example of expiratory pressure relief, where the pressure drops in early exhalation but returns to the level of CPAP at end exhalation. (From Berry RB: *Fundamentals of sleep medicine*, Philadelphia, 2012, Saunders, pp 315.)

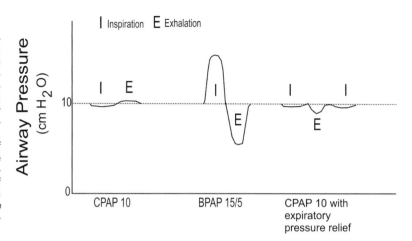

chronic obstructive pulmonary disease (COPD) may tolerate BPAP better than CPAP.[11,12] However, it should be noted that many patients may tolerate high levels of CPAP quite well and that CPAP may be more effective at maintaining an open upper airway (e.g., CPAP of 18 better than BPAP of 20/16). BPAP delivers pressure support (PS = IPAP−EPAP) that is useful for augmenting ventilation in patients with OSA and concomitant hypoventilation. Patients with OSA and hypoventilation include those with the obesity hypoventilation syndrome (OHS) and the "overlap syndrome" (OSA+COPD). Some patients with OHS or overlap syndrome may be adequately treated with CPAP alone.[13,14] However, other patients in this group require BPAP, especially if significant hypoventilation is present. Usually, BPAP without a backup rate is sufficient. Patients with OHS or overlap syndrome may also require the addition of supplemental oxygen to PAP.

Auto-titrating PAP (APAP), also known as auto-adjusting PAP (auto-CPAP) devices vary the delivered pressure between upper and lower pressure limits to eliminate apnea, hypopnea, snoring, and air flow limitation.[15–17] If no events are noted, the pressure is lowered gradually until events recur, at which time the pressure increases again. That is, the device is constantly searching for the lowest effective pressure in any circumstance. The highest pressure is usually needed during supine rapid eye movement (REM) sleep. The devices may be used for unattended auto-titration to find an optimal pressure level for chronic CPAP treatment. The 90th or 95th percentile pressure (pressure exceeded only 10% or 5% of the time) after several days of treatment is usually selected as the treatment pressure.[18] APAP devices may also be used for chronic treatment without the need for polysomnography

(PSG) titration and have the advantage of delivering the lowest effective pressure in any circumstance.[15–17] When APAP was developed, it was hypothesized that this might improve adherence to PAP. For unselected patients, no clinically significant improvement in usage occurs with APAP compared with CPAP (but APAP treatment is no worse).[9,19] A recent large meta-analysis of 30 studies and 1136 participants[9] found a statistically significant differences in machine usage of 0.21 hour (12 minutes) only in studies with a cross-over design. This is not a clinically significant difference. However, individual patients may tolerate APAP better than CPAP.

The *average* pressure using an APAP device is typically only 2 to 3 centimeters of water (cm H_2O) lower than the fixed pressure that would be effective during the entire night but may be up to 6 cm H_2O lower.[20] Of note, *different brands of APAP devices may respond very differently to changes in air flow*.[21] High air leak (mask or mouth leak), which simulates physiologic events, and the inability to differentiate between central and obstructive apnea by these devices may result in errors in APAP titration.[22] PAP devices monitor pressure and flow and have no method of determining whether inspiratory effort is present during an apnea. In the past, some auto-titration algorithms would not titrate above 10 cm H_2O unless snoring and air flow limitation were present. Other algorithms would not continue to increase pressure if this did not reduce apnea (nonresponsive apnea). New technology used by Philips-Respironics attempts to differentiate "clear airway apneas" versus obstructive airway apneas by delivering a small pressure pulse (1 to 2 cm H_2O) after approximately 6 seconds of a reduction in air flow (see Patient 54). If the pressure pulse does produce an increase in flow, this is compatible with a "clear" (open) airway.

If the pressure pulse does not increase flow, the airway is assumed to be closed (obstructed). The APAP device does not increase pressure for "clear airway" apneas. Note that a closed airway may occur with some central apneas.[23] The devices do not monitor respiratory effort and therefore classify central apneas with a closed airway as obstructive apneas. Res Med uses a forced oscillation technique to determine if the upper airway is open or closed (see Patient 51). The use of APAP devices for auto-titration is discussed in more detail Fundamentals 24. When using APAP for chronic treatment either wide (e.g., 6 to 18 cm H_2O) pressure limits or narrow limits of 2 or 3 cm H_2O above and below the 90th or 95th percentile pressure may be used. For example, if a 90% pressure is 10 cm H_2O, the range would be 8 to 12 cm H_2O.

Pressure-intolerant patients may favor the first approach, but if the device does not titrate up fast enough when events occur after changes in body position or sleep stage (e.g., transition to REM sleep), then a narrower pressure limit approach may work better.

AUTO-BPAP

Auto-BPAP devices adjust the delivered IPAP and EPAP to maintain an open airway. The device of Philips-Respironics varies both IPAP and EPAP between pressure limits (EPAPmin, IPAPmax) and the minimum and maximum pressure support may be set (PSmin and PSmax) (Figure F23-2). Typical values for PSmin and PSmax are 4 and 6 cm H_2O. The Auto-BPAP device by Res Med varies the EPAP using a fixed pressure support that can be set by the clinician. Auto-BPAP is useful for BPAP treatment without the need for a titration or in extremely pressure-intolerant patients, for example, a patient with pressure intolerance who requires high pressure.[10,24,25] Of interest, in one

group of patients with poor initial response to CPAP, an aggressive approach to improving adherence (attention to mask interface and humidification issues) was as successful as switching patients to auto-BPAP.[10]

PAP AND SUPPLEMENTAL OXYGEN

The addition of supplemental oxygen to PAP treatment is sometimes necessary. This is discussed in more detail in Fundamentals 24. Nocturnal oximetry on patients using PAP at home is often useful in patients with borderline arterial oxygen saturation by oximetry (SpO_2) during a PAP titration. Oximetry may also reveal that the current treatment pressure is inadequate (sawtooth pattern). It is important to note that the effective fraction of inspired oxygen varies with both the supplemental oxygen flow rate bled into the PAP circuit and the total machine flow. Increase in total flow with higher pressures and higher leak will dilute the supplemental oxygen flow and decrease the effective fraction of inspired oxygen (FiO_2). Sometimes, correcting the leak will improve the effective FiO_2 without the need to increase the supplemental oxygen flow rate.

COMFORT MEASURES
Flexible PAP

Two manufacturers of PAP devices have developed flexible PAP in an attempt to improve patient comfort and adherence. Some PAP devices manufactured by Philips-Respironics provide several comfort options (Cflex, Cflex+, and Aflex) (Figure F23-3).[26,27] ResMed devices offer expiratory pressure relief (EPR). However, convincing data that any of these options improve adherence in unselected patients are

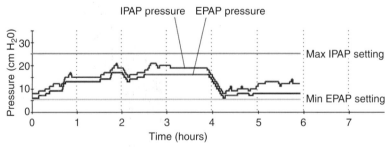

FIGURE F23-2 ■ An overnight pressure-versus-time tracing is shown for a patient using auto-bilevel positive airway pressure (auto-BPAP) with a minimum expiratory positive airway pressure (EPAP) of 6 centimeters of water (cm H_2O) and a maximum inspiratory airway pressure (IPAP) of 25 cm H_2O. The 90% IPAP and EPAP pressures were 19.2 cm H_2O and 16.2 cm H_2O, respectively. The average IPAP and EPAP values were 14.6 cm H_2O and 11.8 cm H_2O, respectively. (From Kakkar RK, Berry RB: Positive airway pressure treatment for obstructive sleep apnea, *Chest* 132:1057-1072, 2007.)

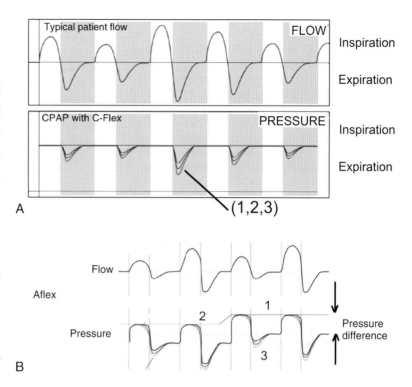

FIGURE F23-3 ■ A, Cflex: The pressure drops at the start of exhalation (the amount depends on expiratory flow and the Cflex setting, 1, 2, or 3) but returns to the set continuous positive airway pressure (CPAP) pressure at end-exhalation. **B,** Aflex. (1) The inspiratory pressure auto-adjusts per auto-adjusting positive airway pressure (APAP); (2) smoothing of transition from inspiration to exhalation; (3) expiratory pressure relief similar to Cflex. The end-expiratory pressure is 2 cm H_2O below the inspiratory pressure (pressure difference = 2 cm H_2O). (From Kushida CA, Berry RB, Blau A et al: Positive airway pressure initiation: a randomized controlled trial to assess the impact of therapy mode and titration process on efficacy, adherence, and outcomes, *Sleep* 34[8]:1083-1092, 2011.)

lacking. In Cflex, expiratory pressure drops at the start of exhalation but returns to the set CPAP at end exhalation. The amount of drop (Cflex 1, 2, 3) is determined by a proprietary algorithm. In general, a greater pressure drop is present for greater flow during exhalation. Cflex is available on APAP devices as well as CPAP. Cflex + adds a smoothing of the transition from inhalation to exhalation. Aflex is a form of APAP that provides a 2 cm H_2O lower end-expiratory pressure than the inspiratory pressure (in addition to the features of Cflex+). The inspiratory pressure is titrated as per usual APAP algorithm (Figure F23-3). For both BPAP and auto-BPAP devices made by Philips-Respironics, a form of expiratory pressure relief is available (Biflex). The technology provides a smoothing of transition from IPAP to EPAP as well as expiratory pressure relief during the EPAP cycle (Biflex 1, 2, 3). ResMed devices provide expiratory pressure relief (EPR) and drop the pressure during the start of exhalation pressure by 1, 2, or 3 cm H_2O (EPR 1,2,3). EPR may be used full time or only during the ramp period. EPR is not available with ResMed APAP devices.

An initial study found that flexible PAP improved adherence by about half an hour using a cross-over design.[27] A number of subsequent studies in patients on CPAP,[26,28–32] APAP,[33] or Aflex[26] have not found an increase in adherence. These modes may still be useful for individual patients who find CPAP difficulty to tolerate (e.g., pressure intolerance). Conversely, some patients actually prefer CPAP to flexible PAP. A recent randomized trial compared CPAP, APAP for 2 weeks followed by CPAP, and APAP with Aflex. No significant difference was observed in adherence or effectiveness.[26]

Ramp

Most PAP devices, with the exception of certain APAP devices, allow the patient to trigger the ramp option. In the ramp option, the pressure starts at a preset level—usually a low level of CPAP—and then slowly increases to the treatment pressure (CPAP) over the set ramp time. Some APAP devices have a "settling time" at a low pressure before the device starts auto-adjusting while others have an adjustable ramp (if the lower pressure APAP limit is above 4 cm H_2O). The ramp option is appealing to patients and may be used during middle of the night awakenings to help the person return to sleep. However, no study has shown that the ramp option increases adherence.

Humidification

Today, most PAP devices come with the option of an integrated heated humidification system. They may be used in the cool humidity (CH) mode, if desired. Heated humidity (HH) permits deliver a greater level of moisture than CH and may be especially useful in patients with mouth leak or nasal congestion. Mouth leak may cause a dramatic fall in relative humidity[34] and a loss of humidity from the upper airway or CPAP system, thus drying the nasal or oral mucosa (Figure F23-4). Drying of the nasal mucosa increases nasal resistance and this is minimized by use of HH.[35,36] The level of humidity (amount of heat applied to the water in the humidifier chamber) can be adjusted by the patient to meet variable needs. An occasional patient will prefer CH (heat turned off) or no humidity at all. Adequate cleaning of the humidifier chamber and hoses does require extra patient effort. One study suggested that use of humidity is associated with an increase in risk of infectious complications[37] that can be reduced with use of a filter.[38] An occasional patient with recurrent sinus infections seems to do better without humidification—but the etiology of this improvement is unclear.

Studies determining whether HH improves either acceptance of CPAP (after titration) or long-term adherence to CPAP treatment have found conflicting results. Massie and associates[39] studied patients who received either HH or CH for 3 weeks (random order), a 2-week washout period of no humidity, and 3 weeks of the alternative humidity. Patients on HH had about half an hour greater objective adherence than those on no humidity. However, several other studies have not found an improvement in adherence[40-44] with the use of HH for PAP treatment. Other investigations could not document a benefit from the "prophylactic" use of HH for titration. A criticism of these studies is that patients with baseline nasal congestion or dryness were not targeted. It seems reasonable to use humidity in patients with complaints of nasal congestion or mouth breathing at baseline. Certainly, in some patients, use of HH is crucial, and in others, it may improve satisfaction. Rain-out in the tubing and the mask is a significant problem for some patients. Lowering the CPAP unit to a level below the bed (water flows back into humidifier chamber by gravity), reducing the humidity setting, or using a tube insulator may help. New technology recently available adjusts the humidifier setting based on room temperature and relative humidity. Heated tubes are now available to prevent rain out in the tube, allowing more aggressive humidification of the air. However, it is not clear that this technology will improve adherence. In the AASM practice parameters for PAP treatment, use of HH is recommended to improve CPAP utilization.[3]

INTERFACES

When CPAP devices became commercially available, the first interfaces were nasal masks. Today, a large and ever increasing types of interfaces are available.[45-48] However, it is still be difficult to obtain a good mask fit in many patients. Nasal pillow masks (Figure F23-5) are often better tolerated compared with traditional nasal masks by patients with claustrophobia and are useful in patients with mustaches or edentulous patients who have no dental support for the upper lip.[48] The masks obviate the need for obtaining a seal on the nasal bridge and may be helpful if patients complain of air leaking into their eyes. It is essential to use a size of pillow large enough to provide a good seal. A wide variety of nasal masks with gel or air cushion interfaces are available. Recently, some "mini" masks that only cover the lower part of the nose have become available. For patients who have severe nasal congestion or open their mouths during PAP treatment, oronasal (full face

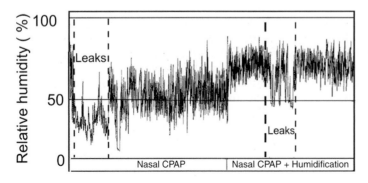

FIGURE F23-4 ■ This tracing shows a fall in the relative humidity at the nasal mask during mouth leaks (leak detected by an oral thermistor). Heated humidification minimized but did not eliminate the fall in relative humidity. *CPAP*, Continuous positive airway pressure. (From Martins de Araujo MT, Vieira SB, Vasquez EC, Fleury B: Heated humidification or face mask to prevent upper airway dryness during continuous positive airway pressure therapy, *Chest* 117:142-147, 2000.)

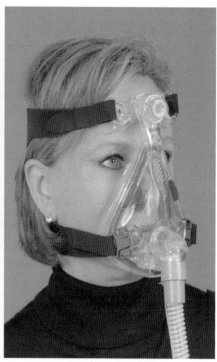
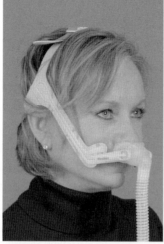
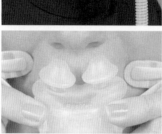

FIGURE F23-5 ■ Positive airway pressure (PAP) interface options. *Left,* A nasal pillows mask (Swift LT for her by ResMed). *Right,* A full face mask (Mirage Quattro by ResMed). (Images used with permission. EPR, ResMed, Swift and Quattro are trademarks of ResMed Limited and are registered in the U.S. Patent and Trademark Office.)

masks)[45,46] and oral interfaces[47] are available. Oronasal masks (see Figure F23-5) have to seal over a large area, and this makes finding a good fit very difficult in some patients. In edentulous patients, oronasal masks may also compress soft tissues. Patients tend to over-tighten masks, and this may cause damage to the nasal bridge or actually impair the ability of the mask to seal. Often, a trial of several masks is needed to find one that patients can use comfortably. This is one situation in which trying several different types of masks in the sleep center before the titration can be very useful. *When the patient is trying on a new mask, it is essential to test the mask fit with the patient's treatment pressure to determine if the seal is adequate.* Adequate care and replacement of masks are also essential to maximize their ability to seal. If the patient gets up to use the bathroom during the night, we encourage disconnection of the hose from the mask rather than taking off the mask. Masks that are removed in the middle of the night often are not replaced. Of note, for unselected patients, the type of interface does not seem to affect adherence.[48] However, finding the right interface for individual patients is very important.

REFERENCES

1. Sullivan CE, Issa FG, Berthon-Jones M, et al: Reversal of obstructive sleep apnoea by continuous positive airway pressure applied through the nares, *Lancet* 1:862–865, 1981.
2. Gay P, Weaver T, Loube D, et al: Evaluation of positive airway pressure treatment for sleep related breathing disorders in adults, *Sleep* 29:381–401, 2006.
3. Kushida CA, Littner MR, Hirshkowitz M, et al: Practice parameters for the use of continuous and bilevel positive airway pressure devices to treat adult patients with sleep related breathing disorders, *Sleep* 29:375–380, 2006.
4. Loube DI, Gay PC, Strohl KP, et al: Indications for positive airway pressure treatment of adult sleep apnea patients. A consensus statement, *Chest* 115:863–866, 1999.
5. Kakkar RK, Berry RB: Positive airway pressure treatment for obstructive sleep apnea, *Chest* 132:1057–1072, 2007.
6. Weaver TE, Grunstein RR: Adherence to continuous positive airway pressure therapy: the challenge to effective treatment, *Proc Am Thorac Soc* 5:173–178, 2008.
7. Sanders MH, Kern N: Obstructive sleep apnea treated by independently adjusted inspiratory and expiratory positive airway pressures via nasal mask, *Chest* 98:317–324, 1990.
8. Reeves-Hoché MK, Hudgel DW, Meck R, et al: Continuous versus bilevel positive airway pressure for obstructive sleep apnea, *Am J Respir Crit Care Med* 151:443–449, 1995.
9. Smith I, Lasserson TJ: Pressure modification for improving usage of continuous positive airway pressure machines in adults with obstructive sleep apnoea, Update

of Cochrane Database Syst Rev 4:CD003531, 2004, *Cochrane Database Syst Rev* 4:CD003531, 2009.

10. Ballard RD, Gay PC, Strollo PJ: Interventions to improve compliance in sleep apnea patients previously non-compliant with continuous positive airway pressure, *J Clin Sleep Med* 3:706–712, 2007.

11. Schafer H, Ewig S, Hasper E, et al: Failure of CPAP therapy in obstructive sleep apnea syndrome: predictive factors and treatment with bilevel positive airway pressure, *Respir Med* 92:208–215, 1998.

12. Schwartz SW, Rosas J, Iannacone MR, et al: Correlates of a prescription for Bilevel positive airway pressure for treatment of obstructive sleep apnea among veterans, *J Clin Sleep Med* 9(4):327–335, 2013.

13. Berger KI, Ayappa I, Chatr-Amontri B, et al: Obesity hypoventilation syndrome as a spectrum of respiratory disturbances during sleep, *Chest* 120:1231–1238, 2001.

14. Piper AJ, Wang D, Yee BJ, et al: Randomized trial of CPAP vs bilevel support in the treatment of obesity hypoventilation syndrome without severe nocturnal desaturation, *Thorax* 63:395–401, 2008.

15. Berry RB, Parish JM, Hartse KM: The use of auto-titrating continuous positive airway pressure for treatment of adult obstructive sleep apnea. An American Academy of Sleep Medicine Review, *Sleep* 25:148–173, 2002.

16. Littner M, Hirshkowitz M, Davila D, et al: Practice parameters for the use of auto-titrating continuous positive airway pressure devices for titrating pressures and treating adult patients with obstructive sleep apnea syndrome. An American Academy of Sleep Medicine report, *Sleep* 25:143–147, 2002.

17. Morgenthaler TI, Aurora RN, Brown T, et al: for the Standards of Practice Committee of the AASM: Practice parameters for the use of autotitrating continuous positive airway pressure devices for titrating pressures and treating adult patients with obstructive sleep apnea syndrome: an update for 2007, *Sleep* 31:141–147, 2008.

18. Masa JF, Jimenez A, Duran J, et al: Alternative methods of titrating continuous positive airway pressure, *Am J Respir Crit Care Med* 170:1218–1224, 2004.

19. Ayas NT, Patel SR, Malhotra A, et al: Auto-titrating versus standard continuous positive airway pressure for the treatment of obstructive sleep apnea: results of a meta-analysis, *Sleep* 27:249–253, 2004.

20. Randerath WJ, Schraeder O, Galetke W, et al: Autoadjusting CPAP therapy based on impedance efficacy, compliance and acceptance, *Am J Respir Crit Care Med* 163:652–657, 2001.

21. Farre R, Montserrat JM, Rigau J, et al: Response of automatic continuous positive airway pressure devices to different sleep breathing patterns: a bench study, *Am J Respir Crit Care Med* 166:469–473, 2002.

22. Coller D, Stanley D, Parthasarathy S: Effect of air leak on the performance of auto-PAP devices: a bench study, *Sleep Breath* 9:167–175, 2005.

23. Badr MS, Toiber F, Skatrud JB, et al: Pharyngeal narrowing/occlusion during central apnea, *J Appl Physiol* 78:1806–1815, 1995.

24. Gentina T, Fortin F, Douay B, et al: Auto bi-level with pressure relief during exhalation as a rescue therapy for optimally treated obstructive sleep apnoea patients with poor compliance to continuous positive airways pressure therapy—a pilot study, *Sleep Breath* 15(1):21–27, 2011.

25. Powell ED, Gay PC, Ojile JM, et al: A pilot study assessing adherence to auto-bilevel following a poor initial encounter with CPAP, *J Clin Sleep Med* 8(1):43–47, 2012.

26. Kushida CA, Berry RB, Blau A: Positive airway pressure initiation: a randomized controlled trial to assess the impact of therapy mode and titration process on efficacy, adherence, and outcomes, *Sleep* 34(8):1083–1092, 2011.

27. Aloia MS, Stanchina M, Arnedt JT, et al: Treatment adherence and outcomes in flexible vs standard continuous positive airway pressure therapy, *Chest* 172:2085–2093, 2005.

28. Bakker J, Campbell A, Neill A: Randomized controlled trial comparing flexible and continuous positive airway pressure delivery: effects on compliance, objective and subjective sleepiness and vigilance, *Sleep* 33:523–529, 2010.

29. Dolan DC, Okonkwo R, Gfullner F, et al: Longitudinal comparison study of pressure relief (C-Flex) vs. CPAP in OSA patients, *Sleep Breath* 13:73–77, 2009.

30. Marshall NS, Neill AM, Campbell AJ: Randomised trial of compliance with flexible (C-Flex) and standard continuous positive airway pressure for severe obstructive sleep apnea, *Sleep Breath* 12:393–396, 2008.

31. Pépin JL, Muir JF, Gentina T, et al: Pressure reduction during exhalation in sleep apnea patients treated by continuous positive airway pressure, *Chest* 136:490–497, 2009.

32. Nilius G, Happel A, Domanski U, Ruhle KH: Pressure-relief continuous positive airway pressure vs constant continuous positive airway pressure: a comparison of efficacy and compliance, *Chest* 130:1018–1024, 2006.

33. Mulgrew AT, Cheema R, Fleetham J, et al: Efficacy and patient satisfaction with autoadjusting CPAP with variable expiratory pressure vs standard CPAP: a two-night randomized crossover trial, *Sleep Breath* 11:31–37, 2007.

34. Martins de Araujo MT, Vieira SB, et al: Heated humidification or face mask to prevent upper airway dryness during continuous positive airway pressure therapy, *Chest* 117:142–147, 2000.

35. Hayes MJ, McGregor FB, Roberts DN, et al: Continuous positive airway pressure with a mouth leak: effect on nasal mucosal blood flow and nasal geometry, *Thorax* 50:1179–1182, 1995.

36. Richards GN, Cistulli PA, Ungar RG, et al: Mouth leak with nasal continuous positive airway pressure increases nasal airway resistance, *Am J Respir Crit Care Med* 154:182–186, 1996.

37. Sanner BM, Fluerenbrock N, Kleiber-Imbeck A, et al: Effect of continuous positive airway pressure therapy on infectious complications in patients with obstructive sleep apnea syndrome, *Respiration* 68(5):483–487, 2001.

38. Ortolano GA, Schaffer J, McAlister MB, et al: Filters reduce the risk of bacterial transmission from contaminated heated humidifiers used with CPAP for obstructive sleep apnea, *J Clin Sleep Med* 3:700–705, 2007.

39. Massie CA, Hart RW, Peralez K, Richards GN: Effects of humidification on nasal symptoms and compliance in sleep apnea patients using continuous positive airway pressure, *Chest* 116:403–408, 1999.

40. Ryan S, Doherty LS, Nolan GM, et al: Effects of heated humidification and topical steroids on compliance, nasal symptoms, and quality of life in patients with obstructive sleep apnea syndrome using nasal continuous positive airway pressure, *J Clin Sleep Med* 5:422–427, 2009.

41. Worsnop CJ, Miseski S, Rochford PD: The routine use of humidification with nasal continuous positive airway pressure, *Intern Med J* 40:650–656, 2009.

42. Nilius G, Domanski U, Franke KJ, Ruhle KH: Impact of a controlled heated breathing tube humidifier on sleep quality during CPAP therapy in a cool sleeping environment, *Eur Respir J* 31:830–836, 2008.

43. Duong M, Jayaram L, Camfferman D, et al: Use of heated humidification during nasal CPAP titration in obstructive sleep apnoea syndrome, *Eur Respir J* 26:679–685, 2005.

44. Mador MJ, Krauza M, Pervez A, et al: Effect of heated humidification on compliance and quality of life in

patients with sleep apnea using nasal continuous positive airway pressure, *Chest* 28:2151–2158, 2005.

45. Prosise GL, Berry RB: Oral-nasal continuous positive airway pressure as a treatment for obstructive sleep apnea, *Chest* 106:180–186, 1994.

46. Sanders MH, Kern NB, Stiller RA, Strollo PJ Jr. et al: CPAP therapy via oronasal mask for obstructive sleep apnea, *Chest* 106:774–779, 1994.

47. Anderson FE, Kingshott RN, Taylor DR, et al: A randomized crossover efficacy trial of oral CPAP (Oracle) compared with nasal CPAP in the management of obstructive sleep apnea, *Sleep* 26:721–726, 2003.

48. Massie CA, Hart RW: Clinical outcomes related to interface type in patients with obstructive sleep apnea/hypopnea syndrome who are using continuous positive airway pressure, *Chest* 123:1112–1118, 2003.

PATIENT 47

Unable to Tolerate Nasal CPAP Because of "Too Much Pressure"

A 30-year-old man with severe obstructive sleep apnea (OSA) stopped using nasal continuous positive airway pressure (CPAP) because the prescribed pressure of 14 centimeters of water (cm H_2O was "too high." When the ramp option was used, he was able to fall asleep on his side, but he woke up later and was unable to tolerate CPAP at the prescription pressure. He also felt that the beginning pressure when the ramp option was activated was "not enough pressure" when he tried to fall asleep on his back. A summary of his original CPAP titration (selected pressure levels) is shown in Table P47-1. The column for 0 pressure is the diagnostic portion of the study. When the patient changed from the left lateral position to the supine position, a CPAP level of 10 cm H_2O was no longer adequate, and it was increased to 11 cm H_2O. At this pressure, few events occurred until the patient entered rapid eye movement (REM) sleep. The CPAP level was increased to 14 cm H_2O to maintain airway patency during supine REM sleep (see Table P47-1).

TABLE P47-1   Sleep Study—CPAP Titration

Pressure (cm H_2O)	0	10.0	10.0	11.0	14
Body position	Left	Left	Supine	Supine	Supine
REM (minutes)	0	0	0	10	30
AHI (events/hour)	55	5	50	15	5
AHI, NREM (#/hr)	55	5	30	5	0
AHI, REM (#/hr)	n/a	n/a	n/a	40	5

AHI, Apnea–hypopnea index; *cm H_2O*, centimeters of water; *CPAP*, continuous positive airway pressure; *n/a*, not applicable; *NREM*, non–rapid eye movement; *REM*, rapid eye movement.

QUESTION

1. What measures could make PAP treatment acceptable to this patient?

ANSWER

1. **Answer:** Auto-adjusting PAP (APAP), bilevel PAP (BPAP), lower CPAP with adjunctive measures (Box P47-1).

BOX P47-1	Interventions for Pressure Intolerance
• Ramp • Flexible PAP • Auto-CPAP (autoadjusting PAP, APAP) • BPAP	• Auto-BPAP • Lower level of CPAP with adjunctive measures (side sleep position, elevation of head) • Temporary reduction in pressure

BPAP, Bilevel positive airway pressure; *CPAP*, continuous positive airway pressure.

Discussion: Studies of PAP adherence have *not* found that higher pressure is associated with lower adherence.[1] However, in individual patients, pressure intolerance may be a major impediment to good adherence. *In other patients, high pressure makes obtaining a good mask seal more difficult or is associated with mouth leak (using a nasal mask).* Several approaches are available when patients have difficulty tolerating the prescribed CPAP. The ramp mode on CPAP units allows a slow increase in airway pressure from a low setting (around 4 cm H_2O) to the prescribed pressure so that the patient can fall asleep at lower pressures. The ramp period (time to reach set pressure) is adjustable on most units. If the patient awakens during the night, the ramp mode can be reinitiated. Two important points concerning ramp: (1) The mask seal must be tested at the final (prescribed) pressure before the ramp is initiated. If this is not done, mask leaks may appear as the pressure increases. (2) A low initial pressure is a problem for some patients. These patients may have trouble falling asleep because of difficulty breathing through the system even when awake. Most CPAP units allow an increase of the initial pressure in the ramp mode (e.g., from 4 to 8 cm H_2O). If not, a short ramp period may be better tolerated than a long one. However, no study has demonstrated that the ramp option really improves acceptance or adherence to CPAP therapy. It may help individual patients.

Flexible PAP (expiratory pressure relief [EPR], Cflex, flexible pressure) was developed to improve tolerance to CPAP (Figure P47-1).[2] Pressure is allowed to drop below the treatment pressure during the start of exhalation but is returned to the treatment pressure at end-exhalation. Different manufacturers have variants of flexible pressure. In Cflex (levels 1, 2, 3, Philips-Respironics), the amount the pressure falls depends on expiratory flow and the setting (1,2,3) using a proprietary algorithm. In EPR (levels 1,2,3, Res Med), the peak fall in pressure is 1, 2, or 3 cm H_2O as specified. EPR may be used full time or only during the ramp period. Aflex (Philips Respironics) is another variant of flexible pressure in which pressure during exhalation is 2 cm H_2O below the inspiratory pressure (see Figure P47-1). A recent large randomized trial by Kushida et al found no advantage for Aflex or APAP compared with CPAP.[2] However, individual patients might find flexible PAP more acceptable.

In unselected patients, BPAP does not improve adherence compared with CPAP.[3] However, a change from CPAP to BPAP may be an effective intervention for pressure intolerance, especially if a patient reports difficulty exhaling, has chronic obstructive pulmonary disease (COPD), bloating, or expiratory muscle weakness.[4] In some sleep centers, during PAP titration, CPAP is automatically changed to BPAP for pressures over 15 cm H_2O. However, many patients actually tolerate high levels of CPAP, and in some, CPAP is more effective. That is, BPAP of 20/16 cm H_2O may not be as effective as CPAP of 18 cm H_2O.

APAP devices attempt to provide the lowest effective pressure in any circumstance. These units apply a variety of detection methods—searching for apnea, hypopnea (air flow), airway vibration (snoring), and inspiratory air flow flattening (an indicator of airway narrowing). The machines

FIGURE P47-1 ■ **A,** Cflex, The pressure drops during exhalation (the amount depends on flow and the setting 1, 2, 3). **B,** Aflex: (1) The inspiratory positive airway pressure is adjusted per auto-adjusting positive airway pressure (APAP); (2) smoothing of transition from inspiration to exhalation; (3) expiratory pressure relief similar to Cflex. The end-expiratory pressure is 2 centimeters of water (cm H2O) below the inspiratory pressure (2 cm H2O pressure difference). (**A,** From Mulgrew AT, Cheema R, Fleetham J, et al: Efficacy and patient satisfaction with autoadjusting CPAP with variable expiratory pressure vs standard CPAP: a two-night randomized crossover trial, *Sleep Breath* 11:31-37, 2007; **B,** From Kushida CA, Berry RB, Blau A, et al: Positive airway pressure initiation: a randomized controlled trial to assess the impact of therapy mode and titration process on efficacy, adherence, and outcomes, *Sleep* 34[8]:1083-1092, 2011.)

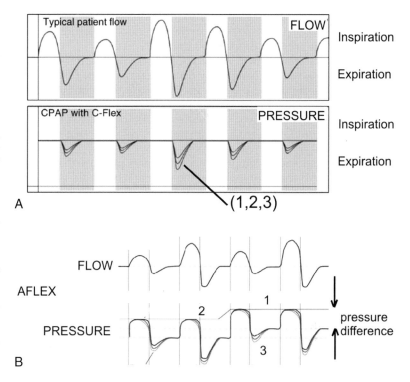

use different algorithms to determine how much the pressure should be increased and how fast. When no events are detected, the units slowly lower the level of pressure. The APAP device changes pressure between the lower and upper pressure limit set by the clinician. The continuous titration of pressures up and down may lower the nightly mean pressure required to maintain airway patency compared with a fixed level of CPAP. For example, while sleeping in the lateral decubitus position, a pressure level of 5 cm H_2O might be adequate while a supine pressure of 10 cm H_2O is required. However, two meta-analyses of published studies comparing adherence with APAP versus CPAP did not find a clinically significant advantage for APAP.[5,6] Individual patients may tolerate APAP better than CPAP.[7] Of note, the difference between the mean nightly pressure on APAP and the fixed CPAP pressure was small in some of the studies comparing APAP and CPAP. One might expect APAP to have the biggest advantage in those patients have considerable variability in the pressure needed during the night (effects of posture and sleep stage). However, this has not been clearly demonstrated.[8] APAP devices also allow for selection of an optimal level of CPAP (auto-titration) or provide the option of chronic treatment with APAP (obviating the need for CPAP titration. The physician may alter the minimum and maximum pressure limits of APAP to adapt to the situation). This may be useful, as some patients may develop episodes of mouth or mask leak causing transient large increases in pressure and arousal. Other patients with require a relatively elevated lower pressure limit to feel comfortable. Pressure levels at each time are stored in memory, and the 90% or 95% pressure (pressure exceeded only 10% or 5% of time) is used to select a fixed CPAP pressure when APAP is used for auto-titration to select an appropriate CPAP level. Some clinicians use APAP for treatment with a tight pressure range, for example, 10 to 14 cm H_2O if the 90% pressure is 12 cm H_2O. Others use a larger pressure gradient (8 to 18 cm H_2O etc.).

Auto-BPAP devices are also now available and are an option for a patient needing BPAP when the optimal treatment pressure is unknown or in extremely pressure intolerant individuals who require relatively high pressure to maintain an open airway.[9,10] In one study, patients with poor tolerance to CPAP were "salvaged" by auto-BPAP, although aggressive intervention in a control group was also effective.[10]

Adjunctive therapy also may decrease the level of pressure required to maintain airway patency. Weight loss may minimize the tendency of the upper airway to collapse. The simultaneous use of an oral appliance may sometimes improve the efficacy of a given level of CPAP. Aggressive treatment of nasal resistance (congestion) also may potentially reduce the required mask pressure. The pressure level at the mask is lower than the inspiratory pressure level in the oropharynx or hypopharynx because of a pressure drop across the nose.

In general, the highest levels of CPAP are needed during supine REM sleep.[11,12] Studies have shown that postural change may decrease the level of CPAP required to keep the airway open.[11] Sleeping in the lateral position may decrease the required pressure in some patients. However, assuming the lateral posture may be ineffective in very obese patients. Moreover, it is difficult to constrain patients to sleep on their sides. Alternatively, a study by Neill et al[13] found that modest head elevation (30%) reduced the pressure required to maintain upper airway patency by almost 5 cm H_2O.

A final approach is simply to accept a lower pressure than the optimal pressure determined during the CPAP trial. For example, the present patient did well at 10 cm H_2O in the supine position until he entered REM sleep. He may be better served by using nasal CPAP at a lower-than-optimal pressure than by stopping therapy altogether. With time, patients tend to adapt to higher pressure. In the current patient, treatment with 11 cm H_2O might be expected to result in an apnea–hypopnea index (AHI) of 5/hr in non-REM (NREM) sleep and 40/hr in REM sleep. Therefore, the overall AHI is likely to be around 16/hr (assuming 20% REM sleep). In many other treatments (surgery, oral appliance) for OSA, an AHI of 15/hr in a patient with a value of 55/hr at baseline would be considered a fairly good response. Accepting less-than-perfect treatment results is especially important for patients with severe OSA, in whom the only effective alternatives are tracheostomy or extensive upper airway surgery (not always available). Overtime, many patients adapt to CPAP and may accept a slow increase in pressure to the one maintaining an open airway in all circumstances. Also, many patients do sleep in the lateral position for much of the night, lowering the needed pressure. *It may also be useful to review the sleep study used to determine a patient's treatment pressure.* Often, pressure is increased too rapidly, and a lower pressure than the final one documented to be effective may be reasonably effective. In fact, in some centers, a trial at reduction in pressure (downward titration) is part of the titration protocol.

In the current case, the patient required much lower pressure during NREM sleep in the lateral sleeping position than during REM in the supine position. He was treated with an APAP device with a minimum pressure of 7 cm H_2O and a maximum pressure of 15 cm H_2O. Figure P47-2 shows pressure information transferred from the device's memory for one night. The wide variation in pressure and the fact that the average pressure (around 10 cm H_2O) is much lower than the peak pressure are apparent. If a single pressure for the entire night were used, a pressure of 14 to 15 cm H_2O would be necessary. The upper pressure limit on APAP was set on the basis of the maximum pressure used during the CPAP titration. A lower pressure limit of 4 to 5 cm H_2O could have been used. However, the patient reported that he found a starting pressure of 4 cm H_2O to be too low. On APAP treatment, the patient was able to tolerate positive pressure. The machine determined that the AHI was less than 10/hr on most nights.

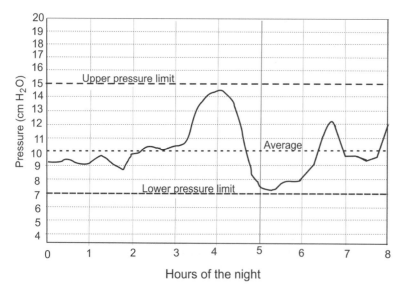

FIGURE   P47-2 ■ Auto-adjusting positive airway pressure (APAP) varies during the night. The average pressure is below a single pressure that would be effective for the entire night (for example CPAP of 14 cm H_2O). From Berry RB: Sleep medicine pearls, ed 2, Philadelphia, 2002, Saunders, p 153.

CLINICAL PEARLS

1. Higher treatment pressure is *not* associated with lower adherence in unselected patients. However, pressure intolerance is a major issue in some patients. Some problems such as mask or mouth leak may improve with a slightly lower pressure.

2. In unselected patients, no pressure mode has been proven to significantly improve adherence.

3. Flexible PAP, APAP, and BPAP are treatment alternatives in patients unable to use nasal positive pressure at the optimal pressure because of pressure intolerance. Individual patients may tolerate these pressure modes better compared with CPAP.

4. Adjunctive measures such as postural changes and weight loss may improve the efficacy of a given level of CPAP (allowing a lower treatment pressure).

5. Many patients are better served by using a less-than-optimal CPAP pressure rather than no effective therapy at all. With chronic treatment, higher levels of CPAP may eventually be accepted by many patients. Postural interventions such as lateral sleep may allow a lower treatment pressure.

6. Review of a prior titration may reveal that higher than necessary pressure was used and thus excessive pressure was prescribed.

REFERENCES

1. Weaver TE, Grunstein RR: Adherence to continuous positive airway pressure therapy: the challenge to effective treatment, *Proc Am Thorac Soc* 5:173–178, 2008.
2. Kushida CA, Berry RB, Blau A, et al: Positive airway pressure initiation: a randomized controlled trial to assess the impact of therapy mode and titration process on efficacy, adherence, and outcomes, *Sleep* 34(8):1083–1092, 2011.
3. Reeves-Hoché MK, Hudgel DW, Meck R, et al: Continuous versus bilevel positive airway pressure for obstructive sleep apnea, *Am J Respir Crit Care Med* 151:443–449, 1995.
4. Schwartz SW, Rosas J, Iannacone MR, et al: Correlates of a prescription for Bilevel positive airway pressure for treatment of obstructive sleep apnea among veterans, *J Clin Sleep Med* 9(4):327–352, 2013.
5. Ayas NT, Patel SR, Malhotra A, et al: Auto-titrating versus standard continuous positive airway pressure for the treatment of obstructive sleep apnea: results of a meta-analysis, *Sleep* 27:249–253, 2004.
6. Smith I, Lasserson TJ: Pressure modification for improving usage of continuous positive airway pressure machines in adults with obstructive sleep apnoea, Update of Cochrane Database Syst Rev 4:CD003531, 2004, *Cochrane Database Syst Rev* 4: CD003531, 2009.
7. Fleetham J, et al: Efficacy and patient satisfaction with autoadjusting CPAP with variable expiratory pressure vs standard CPAP: a two-night randomized crossover trial, *Sleep Breath* 11:31–37, 2007.
8. Series F, Marc I: Importance of sleep stage and body position dependence of sleep apnea in determining benefits to auto-CPAP therapy, *Eur Respir J* 18:170–175, 2001.
9. Gentina T, Fortin F, Douay B, et al: Auto bi-level with pressure relief during exhalation as a rescue therapy for optimally treated obstructive sleep apnoea patients with poor compliance to continuous positive airways pressure therapy–a pilot study, *Sleep Breath* 15(1):21–27, 2011.
10. Ballard RD, Gay PC, Strollo PJ: Interventions to improve compliance in sleep apnea patients previously non-compliant with continuous positive airway pressure, *J Clin Sleep Med* 3(7):706–712, 2007.
11. Oksenberg A, Silverberg DS, Arons E, et al: The sleep supine position has a major effect on optimal nasal CPAP, *Chest* 116:1000–1006, 1999.
12. Pevernagie DA, Shepard JW Jr.: Relations between sleep stage, posture and effective nasal CPAP levels in OSA, *Sleep* 15:162–167, 1992.
13. Neill AM, Angus S, Sajovo D, McEvoy RD: Effects of sleep posture on upper airway stability in patients with obstructive sleep apnea, *Am J Respir Crit Care Med* 155:199–204, 1997.

FUNDAMENTALS 24

PAP Titration and Auto-Titration

Polysomnography (PSG) is the standard method for positive airway pressure (PAP) titration (determination of the optimal pressure) and is usually accomplished either as the second part of a split-night study or during an entire night after a previous diagnostic study. The American Academy of Sleep Medicine (AASM) has published practice parameters for the use of PSG and clinical guidelines for the titration of continuous positive airway pressure (CPAP) and bilevel positive airway pressure (BPAP), as well as titration for noninvasive positive pressure ventilation in the sleep center.[1-3] The practice parameters provide guidance about when a split study is acceptable.[1] A split study is recommended only if the apnea–hypopnea index (AHI) is >40 per hour (hr) (or 20/hr with severe desaturation or arrhythmia) and 2 hours of monitoring have occurred. In addition, at least an additional 3 hours of monitoring time must be available for the PAP titration. If adequate titration is not obtained, repeat PSG titration is indicated. Of note, these recommendations for a split study are based on limited data, and some sleep centers have more lenient criteria for the use of a split study. Sometimes, the use of a split study is mandated by reimbursement issues. The Centers for Medicare and Medicaid Services (CMS) guidelines[4] for qualifying a patient for PAP have been revised to state that if <2 hours of sleep were recorded, the minimum number of apneas and hypopneas must equal the number that would have been required if 2 hours of sleep had been recorded. For example, to meet a cutoff of an AHI of 15/hr, a total of 30 apneas and hypopneas must be recorded.

GENERAL TITRATION CONSIDERATIONS

Before PAP titration, the patient should be educated about obstructive sleep apnea (OSA), PAP treatment, and the PAP titration process.[3,5] They should be given mask interface options. They should try on one or more interfaces while breathing on low pressure (continuous PAP [CPAP] practice). If a split study has been ordered, these events should take place before any diagnostic monitoring begins. A number of interfaces should be available (nasal, oronasal, oral, pillows). Heated humidity should be available as well as a source of supplemental oxygen.

PEDIATRIC CONSIDERATIONS

PAP titrations in children require some extra considerations. Children are often given a mask to play with and try on during the day for at least a week before the scheduled study. The child should be desensitized to the mask during the day by wearing it for increasing periods while engaging in a fun activity (e.g., watching a favorite video). Split-night studies are not recommended for children. If the child without previous mask desensitization undergoes a split-night study, this may frighten the child, and this will make subsequent CPAP use unlikely. Pediatric-size masks should be available. Durable medical equipment providers and sleep technologists skilled and willing to provide care for pediatric age patients should be utilized.[6,7] Studies have shown that structured behavioral interventions help with compliance including graduated exposure, positive reinforcement, dealing with escape and avoidance behavior, and differential reinforcement of distracting activities that allowed the child to wear a mask successfully. For example, rewarding the behavior of watching a video while wearing a mask.

MONITORING DURING POSITIVE PRESSURE TITRATION

Positive pressure devices used in the sleep disorders center provide several analog or digital outputs that can be recorded including the PAP flow, leak, pressure, and tidal volume (Table F24-1). The total flow delivered by the machine is measured by an accurate flow sensor in the PAP device. The total flow is then divided by the device into two components (see Figure F24-1). The

TABLE F24-1	**Monitoring during Positive Airway Pressure or Noninvasive Positive Pressure Ventilation Titration**	
Parameter	**Sensor**	**Reason**
Air flow	Positive airway pressure (PAP) device output (accurate internal flow sensor)	Detection of apnea, hypopnea, and respiratory effort–related arousals (RERAs)
Leak	Leak estimate by PAP or noninvasive positive pressure ventilation (NPPV) device from accurate flow measurement	Intentional + unintentional leak
Snoring	Piezoelectric sensor or microphone	Detection of snoring
Pressure	External pressure transducer or PAP device signal (internal pressure sensor)	Documentation of amount and pattern of pressure delivery
Chest and abdominal movement	Respiratory inductance plethysmography	Differentiating central and obstructive events, detection of paradox

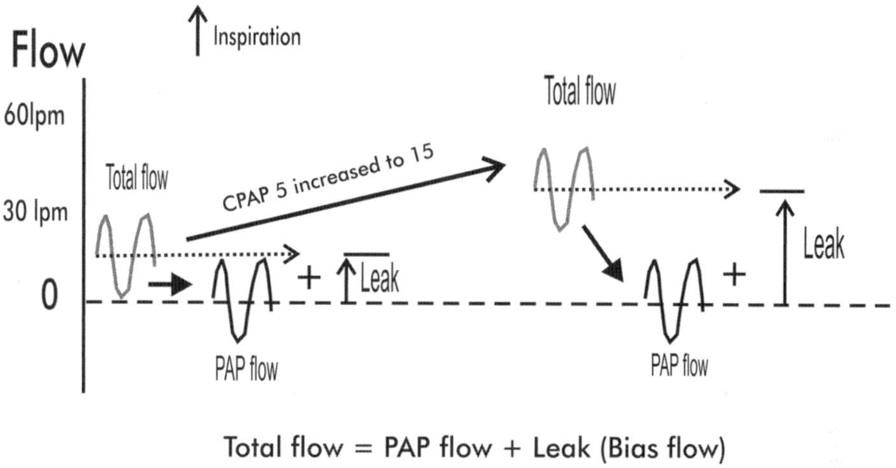

Total flow = PAP flow + Leak (Bias flow)

FIGURE F24-1 ■ When continuous positive airway pressure (CPAP) is increased from 5 to 15 centimeters of water (cm H_2O), the total flow and leak increase. Total flow is partitioned by the device into two components: PAP flow and leak.

PAP flow is sometimes called *PAP device flow*, *PAP flow*, *CPAP flow*, or *Cflow*.

$$\text{Total flow} = \text{PAP flow} + \text{Leak (bias flow)}$$

$$\text{(Equation 1)}$$

$$\text{Leak} = \text{intentional leak}$$
$$\text{(mask non-rebreathing orifices)}$$
$$+ \text{unintentional leak (mask and/or mouth)}$$

$$\text{(Equation 2)}$$

The PAP flow varies with inspiration and expiration while the leak is the constant background (bias) flow. The leak is the sum of the intentional leak and the unintentional leak (mask leak, mouth leak, or both). The intentional leak is the air escaping from the system through small orifices in the mask to prevent rebreathing (washes out carbon dioxide [CO_2]). The amount of intentional leak depends on the mask type and increases with higher delivered pressure

(Figure F24-2). As pressure increases, the leak also increases because the intentional mask leak increases. Recall that PAP devices are leak tolerant, that is, they maintain pressure by increasing the flow. If the leak increases, the device will increase total flow to compensate. The leak signal from some PAP devices represents only the unintentional leak. These devices compute an estimated intentional leak from the pressure and mask type (specified by the technologist) and then subtract this from the total leak. The PAP flow is used to score respiratory events.

The PAP flow signal provides not only an estimate of the magnitude of flow but also information from the inspiratory flow contour. High upper airway resistance is manifested by a flattened inspiratory waveform.[8] The normal shape is a round one. The tracing in Figure F24-3 shows that the PAP flow signal is flat at a pressure of 7 centimeters of water (cm H_2O) and snoring is noted. These findings suggest that

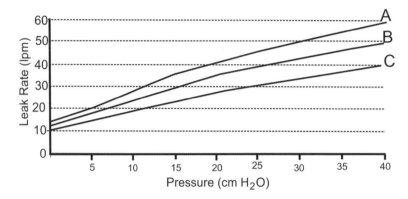

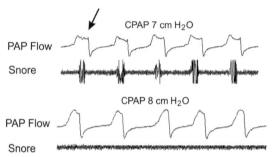

FIGURE F24-3 ■ At continuous positive airway pressure (CPAP) of 7 centimeters of water (cm H_2O), the PAP flow inspiratory waveform is flattened and snoring is noted. At CPAP of 8 cm H_2O, the waveform is round and snoring has been eliminated. (Adapted from Berry RB: *Fundamentals of sleep medicine*, Philadelphia, 2012, Saunders, pp 328.)

significant upper airway narrowing is still present. An increase in CPAP to 8 cm H_2O results in a round signal shape and elimination of snoring. PAP flow signals are usually either filtered or insufficiently sampled to show snoring. Snoring can be detected by a snoring sensor placed on the neck or from pressure vibrations in mask pressure. Sleep center PAP units also provide a "machine pressure" signal that can be recorded. This is the pressure at the machine outlet and may differ slightly from the set pressure (value entered by technologist). The actual mask pressure is slightly lower during inhalation and slightly higher during exhalation. The mask pressure may be significantly lower than the pressure at the device outlet if a large pressure drop occurs across the hose (because of high flow). Mask pressure can also be directly measured by connecting the mask to a pressure transducer. Actual mask pressure can then be recorded.

Recording of the leak signal is useful for the physician reviewing the PAP titration. The trend in the leak is more useful than the absolute number. If the patient has not moved and leak suddenly increases, this is a clue that mouth leak

may be occurring (assuming the patient is wearing a nasal mask). Sometimes, an *increase in leak* may occur with the *onset of rapid eye movement (REM) sleep.* Relaxation in the facial musculature may sometime produce mask or mouth leaks. Observation using video (zooming in) may show an open mouth or fluttering of the lips during mouth leak. *If the flow signal becomes truncated during expiration, this means that part or all of flow during exhalation is not sensed by the machine flow sensor (no flow returning to the hose/device system)* consistent with an expiratory leak from either the mask or the mouth. If the patient is wearing a nasal mask (which has not moved), the sudden appearance of truncated expiratory flow (often associated with vibration in the snoring sensor during exhalation) is suggestive of expiratory mouth leak (Figure F24-4). The technician does not necessarily have to intervene unless mouth leak is arousing the patient or preventing PAP from maintaining a patent airway. If mouth leak is a problem, either using a chin strap or an oronasal mask[9,10] or lowering the pressure could be considered.

Positive pressure titrations may switch from CPAP to bilevel PAP (BPAP) if the patient is pressure intolerant or the arterial oxygen saturation remains low in the absence of discrete respiratory events. BPAP not only eliminates upper airway obstruction but delivers pressure support (PS = IPAP–EPAP). The pressure support can be adjusted to augment tidal volume. Typically, the IPAP—EPAP difference is 4 cm H_2O. This may be increased to treat hypopnea, low tidal volume, or persistent hypoxemia from presumed hypoventilation. For example, patients with obesity hypoventilation syndrome (OHS) may require BPAP for persistent hypoxemia or periods of low tidal volume (Figure F24-5). If the IPAP–EPAP difference is adjusted to augment tidal volume, display and recording of the tidal volume signal from the PAP device may also be very useful (Figure F24-6). The PAP device

FIGURE F24-4 ■ The patient was wearing a nasal mask. No body movement occurred from epoch 600 to 602. Continuous positive airway pressure (CPAP) was increased, and the PAP flow showed a rounder inspiratory waveform. However, the expiratory flow was truncated *(dotted line shows expected shape)*, and an expiratory vibration was detected. When the video was zoomed, the lips were seen to be fluttering during exhalation.

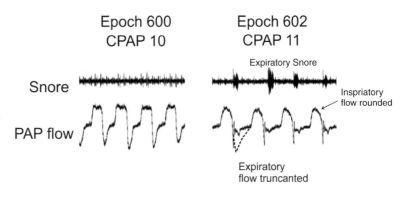

Epoch 600
CPAP 10

Epoch 602
CPAP 11

Expiratory Snore

Snore

PAP flow

Inspriatory
flow rounded

Expiratory
flow truncanted

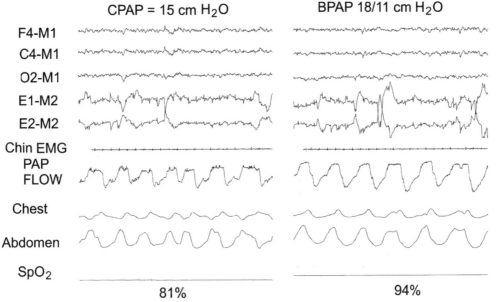

CPAP = 15 cm H$_2$O   BPAP 18/11 cm H$_2$O

F4-M1
C4-M1
O2-M1
E1-M2
E2-M2
Chin EMG
PAP FLOW
Chest
Abdomen
SpO$_2$

81%   94%

FIGURE F24-5 ■ A patient on continuous positive airway pressure (CPAP) of 15 centimeters of water (cm H$_2$O) has persistent hypoxemia during rapid eye movement (REM) sleep, even though discrete respiratory events are absent. One option is to add supplemental oxygen. Another option is to try an increase in CPAP. However, in this patient treatment was changed to bilevel PAP (BPAP), which resulted in an increase in tidal volume and resolution of hypoxemia.

FIGURE F24-6 ■ Although the peak flow on the four breaths (A, B, C, D) was similar the tidal volume varied considerably because of differences in inspiratory time. The units of flow are L/min and tidal volume (mL), respectively. Recording the tidal volume may be useful in patients undergoing positive airway pressure (PAP) titration for nocturnal hypoventilation.

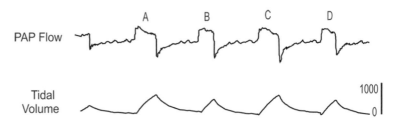

A   B   C   D

PAP Flow

Tidal
Volume

1000

0

provides the tidal volume signal by integration of the flow. Tidal volume depends both on flow and inspiratory time. Therefore, monitoring the flow signal alone may not provide an accurate estimate of ventilation. A detailed discussion of titration for noninvasive positive pressure ventilation is presented in Fundamentals 30. If arterial oxygen desaturation remains low in the absence of discrete events, the addition of supplemental oxygen is another option.

TITRATION PROTOCOL

The recommended PAP titration protocol for adults and children is shown in Tables F24-2 and F24-3.[3] CPAP is usually started at 4 to 5 cm H_2O and then increased for obstructive apneas, hypopneas, respiratory effort–related arousals (RERAs), and snoring. Usually, as pressure is increased, apneas → hypopneas → RERAs → snoring resolve in that order.[11] CPAP is increased in adults after two obstructive apneas, three hypopneas, or five RERAs and no more often than every 5 minutes. When titrating BPAP, starting pressures of 8/4 cm H_2O are typically used. *Both IPAP and EPAP are increased together for obstructive apnea.* For obstructive hypopneas, RERAs, and snoring, the IPAP alone is increased. The clinical guidelines suggest that the IPAP–EPAP difference should be at least 4 cm H_2O but no greater than 10 cm H_2O. Note that during noninvasive positive pressure ventilation (NPPV) titration (see Fundamentals 30), a wider IPAP–EPAP difference is used to augment tidal volume. *Higher PAP is needed for the supine position and during REM sleep.*[12–14] For this reason, an effective pressure during supine REM sleep should be determined, if possible, during the titration.[3] Note that the recommended maximum CPAP and number of events triggering pressure changes are lower in children.

If the patient awakens and complains of excessive pressure, the pressure should be lowered. If this does not work, a switch from CPAP to BPAP or use of flexible PAP may be tried. When switching from CPAP to BPAP, one approach is to use IPAP 2 cm H_2O higher than CPAP and EPAP 2 cm H_2O lower than CPAP. Thus, a change from CPAP of 16, one would use BPAP 18/14 cm H_2O. Another approach is to use IPAP = CPAP and EPAP = IPAP − 4 cm H_2O and titrate pressure upward, if needed. Of note, in pressure-intolerant patients, sleep in the lateral position or with the head elevated may be tried to reduce the required level of pressure.[14] If mouth leak is a problem, a chin strap may be tried, followed by an oronasal mask. In patients with allergic rhinitis or nasal congestion, use of heated humidity (HH) from the start of the study is suggested. Although studies have not shown a benefit from using "prophylactic" HH in all patients, many sleep centers find this to be very useful. Once the nose is congested, this problem is not easily reversed. If excessive mask leak occurs, a readjustment of the mask, change in mask size, or change in mask type is indicated. Overtightening of the mask straps is strongly discouraged. It also is worth mentioning that some patients with severe upper airway narrowing may tolerate a *higher initial pressure* (8–10 cm H_2O) better than the usual lower starting pressure. This is also true of patients already using CPAP at home. If the patient is not able to fall asleep on PAP, the patient should be asked what is bothering him or her. The AASM guidelines also suggest that downward pressure titration could be tried during the study. With any doubt that the pressure was raised too rapidly, a lowering of pressure should be tried. It is also important not to increase pressure for "central hypopneas" that occur following arousal. Sudden increases in mouth or mask leak may mimic respiratory events (see Patient 50). If increases in pressure do not eliminate respiratory events, the technologist should consider the effect of the leak.

TABLE F24-2	**Continuous Positive Airway Pressure Titration Guidelines**	
	Adults and Children >12 Years	**Children <12 Years**
Beginning/minimum pressure (cm H_2O)	4	4
Maximum pressure (cm H_2O)	20	15
Increase CPAP in at least 1 cm H_2O increments no more frequently than every 5 minutes	Increase pressure for ≥2 obstructive apneas ≥3 hypopneas ≥5 RERAs ≥3 minutes of loud or unambiguous snoring	Increase pressure for ≥1 obstructive apnea ≥1 hypopnea ≥3 RERAs ≥1 minutes of loud or unambiguous snoring
Switch to BPAP	Intolerant to CPAP Events still present on CPAP of 15 cm H_2O (option)	

From Kushida CA, Chediak A, Berry RB, et al, for the Positive Airway Pressure Titration Task Force, American Academy of Sleep Medicine: Clinical guidelines for the manual titration of positive airway pressure in patients with obstructive sleep apnea, *J Clin Sleep Med* 4:157-171, 2008.
BPAP, Bilevel positive airway pressure; *cm H_2O*, centimeters of water; *CPAP*, continuous positive airway pressure; *RERAs*, respiratory effort–related arousals.

TABLE F24-3	Bilevel Positive Airway Pressure Titration Guidelines	
	Adults	**Children <12 Years**
Beginning pressure (cm H_2O) IPAP/EPAP	8/4	8/4
Maximum IPAP (cm H_2O)	30	20
Minimum PS (cm H_2O)	4	4
Maximum PS (cm H_2O)	10	10
Increase **both IPAP and EPAP** in at least 1 cm H_2O increments no more frequently than every 5 min	$\geq$3 obstructive apneas	$\geq$1 obstructive apnea
Increase **IPAP** in at least 1 cm H_2O increments no more frequently than every 5 minutes	Increase for $\geq$3 hypopneas $\geq$5 RERAs $\geq$3 minutes loud or unambiguous snoring (may increase)	Increased for $\geq$1 hypopnea $\geq$3 RERAs $\geq$1 minute of loud or unambiguous snoring (may increase)

From Kushida CA, Chediak A, Berry RB, et al, for the Positive Airway Pressure Titration Task Force, American Academy of Sleep Medicine: Clinical guidelines for the manual titration of positive airway pressure in patients with obstructive sleep apnea, *J Clin Sleep Med* 4:157-171, 2008.
cm H_2O, Centimeters of water; *EPAP*, expiratory positive airway pressure; *IPAP*, inspiratory positive airway pressure; *PS*, pressure support = IPAP − EPAP; *RERAs*, respiratory effort–related arousals.

TREATMENT EMERGENT CENTRAL APNEAS

During titration for OSA, central apneas may appear. In most patients, these are hypocapnic central apneas following arousal or are caused by instability in breathing. It is important to note if the apneas are of the Cheyne-Stokes type. A common mistake is to change to BPAP. However, *BPAP without a backup rate can make central apneas worse*. Three choices—wait, pressure down, pressure up—are possible. Often, if the patient reaches stage N3 or stable N2, the central apneas will resolve (wait). If the central apneas followed respiratory arousals from RERAs, an increase in pressure (up) can be tried. If the arousal was caused by a leak, intervention for the leak should be performed. Some patients will respond to a drop in pressure (down). In any case, a relentless increase in pressure should be prevented. The best solution is to simply find a pressure that will eliminate upper airway obstruction. Treatment of emergent central apneas is discussed in Patient 72.

PAP AND SUPPLEMENTAL OXYGEN

The addition of supplemental oxygen to PAP treatment is sometimes needed for patients who exhibit persistent oxygen desaturation after PAP is optimized (elimination of apnea and hypopnea). Persistent hypoxemia in these conditions may be caused by hypoventilation or ventilation–perfusion mismatch (often resulting from chronic lung disease). In some studies of titrations in patients with OHS, a substantial number of patients required the addition of supplemental oxygen. If, while awake and supine, the patient has a saturation of arterial oxygen (SaO_2) of 88% or lower or is already on supplemental oxygen to maintain an acceptable awake SaO_2, the addition of supplemental oxygen will definitely be needed. Recall that the arterial partial pressure of oxygen (PaO_2) falls on the order of 5 to 10 mm Hg during sleep even in normal subjects. Before adding supplemental oxygen, adjusting of the PAP pressure settings may be tried to prevent the need for this additional treatment. If the patient is requiring high oxygen flows, optimizing PAP may allow reduction in the required oxygen flow rate. First, an increase in CPAP may be tried to eliminate unrecognized high upper airway resistance. If this is not successful or not tolerated, CPAP may be changed to BPAP. If optimizing PAP does not relieve hypoxemia, the addition of oxygen is indicated at 1 to 2 liters per minute (L/min) with upward titration to reach a goal of a SaO2 > 90% to 92%. If the patient is on oxygen when awake, higher oxygen flows will usually be needed on PAP. The PAP flow dilutes the supplemental oxygen added to the system and reduces the effective fraction of inspiratory oxygen (fraction of inspired oxygen [FiO_2]) (Figure F24-7).[15,16] Note that increases in flow resulting from pressure increases or increases in mask or mouth leak will further dilute the added oxygen.

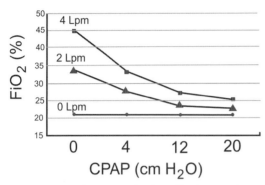

FIGURE F24-7 ■ Reduction in the effective fraction of inspired oxygen (FiO$_2$) for a given supplemental oxygen flow into the positive airway pressure (PAP) system with increasing continuous positive airway pressure (CPAP). This is caused by higher flow on the higher pressures. The effective FiO$_2$ may be further increased by higher mask or mouth leak (higher total flow). (Figure plotted from data in Yoder EA, Klann K, Strohl KP: Inspired oxygen concentrations during positive pressure therapy, *Sleep Breath* 8:1-5, 2004. Adapted from Berry RB: *Fundamentals of sleep medicine*, Philadelphia, 2012, Saunders, p 333.)

ALTERNATIVE METHODS OF STARTING PAP TREATMENT

A number of alternative options are available for starting PAP without using PSG titration after a diagnosis of OSA has been made (PSG or out-of-center sleep test [OCST], e.g., portable monitoring). The titration alternatives may also be used in patients who are unwilling or unable to have standard PSG titration. The alternatives are listed in Box F24-1 and include treating the patient with an APAP device (titration not needed), performing auto-titration at home for several days to a week (at least 3 days optimum) to determine an effective level of CPAP, and starting PAP treatment based on a prediction equation[17] with subsequent adjustment based on symptoms, machine readings, or oximetry.[18–27] Equations to predict the optimal CPAP level have been developed. These may provide an empiric treatment level or a reasonable starting point for PAP titration.[17] Most PAP devices

BOX F24-1	Methods for Starting Positive Airway Pressure

1. PSG titration → CPAP treatment
2. Autotitration → CPAP treatment
3. APAP treatment
4. CPAP treatment with empirical pressure; then adjustments based on symptoms, oximetry, or machine-residual AHI

AHI, Apnea-hypopnea index; *APAP*, auto-adjusting positive airway pressure; *CPAP*, continuous positive airway pressure; *PSG*, polysomnography.

provide an estimate of the residual AHI.[18] Some devices also separate apneas into clear airway apneas and obstructive apneas. Desia and coworkers[18] recently compared the PAP device residual AHI with PSG and found that using a PAP AHI of 8/hr had a sensitivity and specificity of 0.94 and 0.90, respectively, for detecting a PSG AHI greater than 10/hr. Another study found that a low residual AHI by device event detection usually means adequate treatment while a high value (AHI > 10/hr) had only a moderate positive predictive value (false positives).[19] This was caused by device detection of events not associated with arterial oxygen desaturation. A number of studies have validated the approach of a diagnosis by OCST followed by APAP titration at home and CPAP treatment.[21–28] The adherence was either equal or better compared with traditional PSG. These studies often *excluded a significant number of patients* and had a structured system with good follow-up. The results may not apply when careful patient selection, education, and follow-up are not available.

PATIENT SELECTION FOR ALTERNATIVE TITRATIONS

Patients with a number of conditions are not suitable for APAP titration or treatment.[28] These include patients who require, or are likely to require, supplemental oxygen (low baseline SaO$_2$), patients with known or suspected hypoventilation, patients likely to have central apneas (narcotics, congestive heart failure), and patients who may require very high pressures (may need BPAP). Patients with severe pressure intolerance or moderate to severe chronic obstructive pulmonary disease (COPD) who may require BPAP should also undergo PSG titration, if possible. If clinical circumstances mandate the use of APAP titration or APAP treatment, performing oximetry on the final treatment level is essential to rule out persistent desaturation. Auto-BPAP devices may also be used in patients likely to require high pressure. However, high pressure usually results in mask interface issues, so the ability of a sleep technologist to help with mask adjustment is often crucial.

TECHNIQUE OF AUTO-TITRATION

The patient is educated about OSA and PAP treatment and has mask fitting and instructions on use of an APAP device. It is often useful for the patient to take a brief practice nap during which she or he applies the interface, activates the APAP device, and "naps" for about 15 or

20 minutes. This allows identification of interface problems and allows for adjustment or change of interface. The patient then sleeps on the APAP device at home for several nights. Usually, the lower and upper pressure limits of the device are set at 4 and 20 cm H_2O. In large patients likely to require high CPAP, a lower limit of 6 or 8 cm H_2O may be more comfortable. For the pressure-intolerant patient, a lower upper limit of pressure may be chosen. A telephone hotline should be available for interventions similar to that for PAP treatment. The device is then returned and the information transferred to a computer. The quality of the auto-titration may be noted, including the amount of use (adherence), residual AHI, and amount of leak. Typically, either the 95th percentile pressure or the 90th percentile pressure (depending on device) is chosen for chronic PAP treatment. If the APAP titration is suboptimal because of poor adherence, high leak, or high residual AHI, another attempt at auto-titration may be made using a different mask, heated humidity, or other interventions. Alternatively, the patient may be referred for PSG titration. Three examples of typical APAP titrations are shown in Table F24-4). The case of Patient A is ideal, with good adherence, low leak, a 90th percentile pressure well within pressure limits, and a good residual AHI. He could be prescribed CPAP of 12 cm H_2O. The case of Patient B is an example of poor titration. Adherence was poor, and the leak was very high. The patient complained of having a dry mouth despite using a

high humidity setting. He was changed from a nasal mask to a full face mask, and the study was repeated. Patient C showed good adherence, but the residual AHI was very high. Better history taking revealed that he was taking methadone, and central apneas were suspected. He was referred for PSG titration.

REFERENCES

1. Kushida CA, Littner MR, Hirshkowitz M, et al: Practice parameters for the use of continuous and bilevel positive airway pressure devices to treat adult patients with sleep related breathing disorders, *Sleep* 29:375–380, 2006.
2. Kakkar RK, Berry RB: Positive airway pressure treatment for obstructive sleep apnea, *Chest* 132:1057–1072, 2007.
3. Kushida CA, Chediak A, Berry RB, et al: for the Positive Airway Pressure Titration Task Force, American Academy of Sleep Medicine: Clinical guidelines for the manual titration of positive airway pressure in patients with obstructive sleep apnea, *J Clin Sleep Med* 4:157–171, 2008.
4. Department of Health and Human Services Centers for Medicare and Medicaid Services: *National coverage determination (NCD) for continuous positive airway pressure (CPAP) therapy for obstructive sleep apnea (OSA) (240.4)*, http://www.cms.gov/medicare-coverage-database/details/ncd-details.aspx?NCDId=226&ncdver=3&bc=AgAAgAAAAAAA&, Assessed May 23, 2014.
5. Berry RB, Chediak A, Brown LK, et al: for the NPPV Titration Task Force of the American Academy of Sleep Medicine: Best clinical practices for the sleep center adjustment of noninvasive positive pressure ventilation (NPPV) in stable chronic alveolar hypoventilation syndromes, *J Clin Sleep Med* 6(5):491–509, 2010.
6. Koontz KL, Slifer KJ, Cataldo MD, et al: Improving pediatric compliance with positive airway pressure therapy: the impact of behavioral intervention, *SLEEP* 26(8):1010–1015, 2003.
7. Capdevila OS, Kheirandish-Gozal L, Dayat E, Gozal D: Pediatric obstructive sleep apnea, *Proc Am Thorac Soc* 5:274–282, 2008.
8. Condos R, Norman RG, Krishnasamy I, et al: Flow limitation as a noninvasive assessment of residual upper-airway resistance during continuous positive airway pressure therapy of obstructive sleep apnea, *Am J Respir Crit Care Med* 150:475–480, 1994.
9. Prosise GL, Berry RB: Oral-nasal continuous positive airway pressure as a treatment for obstructive sleep apnea, *Chest* 106:180–186, 1994.
10. Sanders MH, Kern NB, Stiller RA, et al: CPAP therapy via oronasal mask for obstructive sleep apnea, *Chest* 106:774–779, 1994.
11. Montserrat JM, Ballester E, Olivi H, et al: Time-course of stepwise CPAP titration. Behavior of respiratory and neurological variables, *Am J Respir Crit Care Med* 152:1854–1859, 1995.
12. Oksenberg A, Silverberg DS, Arons E, et al: The sleep supine position has a major effect on optimal nasal CPAP, *Chest* 116:1000–1006, 1999.
13. Pevernagie DA, Shepard JW Jr: Relations between sleep stage, posture and effective nasal CPAP levels in OSA, *Sleep* 15:162–167, 1992.
14. Neill AM, Angus SM, Sajkov D, McEvoy RD: Effects of sleep posture on upper airway stability in patients with obstructive sleep apnea, *Am J Respir Crit Care Med* 155:199–204, 1997.
15. Yoder EA, Klann K, Strohl KP: Inspired oxygen concentrations during positive pressure therapy, *Sleep Breath* 8:1–5, 2004.

TABLE F24-4	**Examples of Auto-Adjusting Positive Airway Pressure Titration**		
	Patient A	**Patient B**	**Patient C**
Min pressure limit	4	4	4
Max pressure limit	20	20	20
Days used	14/14	3/6	11/12
Average use	6:31	2:02	5:05
90th percentile pressure	11.8	9.5	12.0
Average pressure	9.2	8	8.0
AHI	4.0	3	15
Large leak*	5 min	1 hr	12 min

Pressure in cm H_2O; AHI events/hour, large leak in L/min.
AHI, Apnea–hypopnea index; *cm H_2O*, centimeters of water; *hr*, hour; *min*, minute; 6:31= 6 hrs and 31 min.
*Large leak defined as twice the expected leak from an average mask at the given treatment pressure.

16. Schwartz AR, Kacmarek RM, Hess DR: Factors affecting oxygen delivery with bilevel positive airway pressure, *Respir Care* 49:270–275, 2004.

17. Oliver Z, Hoffstein V: Predicting effective continuous positive airway pressure, *Chest* 117:1061–1064, 2000.

18. Desai H, Patel A, Patel P, et al: Accuracy of auto-titration CPAP to estimate the residual apnea-hypopnea index in patients with obstructive sleep apnea on treatment with auto-titration CPAP, *Sleep Breath* 13:383–390, 2009.

19. Berry RB, Kushida CA, Kryger MH, et al: Respiratory event detection by a positive airway pressure device, *Sleep* 35(3):361–367, 2012.

20. Fitzpatrick MF, Alloway CED, Wakeford TM, et al: Can patients with obstructive sleep apnea titrate their own continuous positive airway pressure? *Am J Respir Crit Care Med* 167:716–722, 2003.

21. Masa JF, Jimenez A, Duran J, et al: Alternative methods of titrating continuous positive airway pressure, *Am J Respir Crit Care Med* 170:1218–1224, 2004.

22. Mulgrew AT, Fox N, Ayas NT, Ryan CF: Diagnosis and initial management of obstructive sleep apnea without polysomnography: a randomized validation study, *Ann Intern Med* 146:157–166, 2007.

23. Berry RB, Hill G, Thompson L, McLaurin V: Portable monitoring and autotitration versus polysomnography for the diagnosis and treatment of sleep apnea, *Sleep* 31:1423–1431, 2008.

24. Antic NA, Buchan C, Esterman A, et al: A randomized controlled trial of nurse-led care for symptomatic moderate-severe obstructive sleep apnea, *Am J Respir Crit Care Med* 179:501–508, 2009.

25. Kuna ST, Gurubhagavatula I, Maislin G, et al: Noninferiority of functional outcome in ambulatory management of obstructive sleep apnea sleep apnea, *Am J Respir Crit Care Med* 183(9):1238–1244, 2011.

26. Skomro RP, Gjevre J, Reid J, et al: Outcomes of home-based diagnosis and treatment of obstructive sleep apnea, *Chest* 138(2):257–263, 2010.

27. Rosen CL, Auckley D, Benca R, et al: A multisite randomized trial of portable sleep studies and positive airway pressure autotitration versus laboratory-based polysomnography for the diagnosis and treatment of obstructive sleep apnea: the HomePAP study, *Sleep* 35(6):757–767, 2012.

28. Morgenthaler TI, Aurora RN, Brown T, et al: for the Standards of Practice Committee of the AASM; American Academy of Sleep Medicine: Practice parameters for the use of autotitrating continuous positive airway pressure devices for titrating pressures and treating adult patients with obstructive sleep apnea syndrome: an update for 2007. An American Academy of Sleep Medicine report, *Sleep* 31(1):141–147, 2008.

Questions About PAP Titration

Patient A: A 30-second tracing is shown in Figure P48-1.

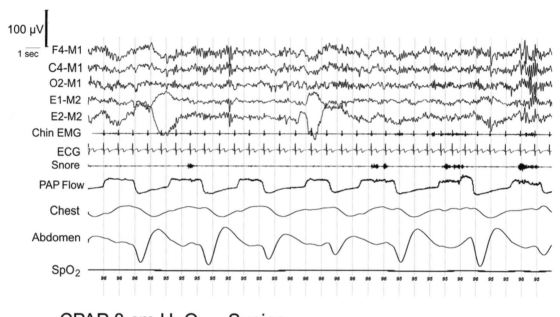

CPAP 8 cm H$_2$O   Supine

FIGURE P48-1 ■ Inspiration is upward. The pattern noted above was present for 3 minutes.

Question A: For patient A, what intervention do you suggest? Does the tracing illustrate the situation likely to require the highest CPAP?

Patient B: A tracing taken from bilevel positive airway pressure (BPAP) titration is shown in Figure P48-2. The patient is on BPAP of 12/8 centimeters of water (cm H$_2$O).

FIGURE P48-2 ■ A patient during bilevel positive airway pressure (BPAP) titration. The patient is on BPAP of 12/8 cm H$_2$O. (Figure adapted from Sanders MH, Kern N: Obstructive sleep apnea treated by independently adjusted inspiratory and expiratory positive airway pressures via nasal mask, *Chest* 98:317-324, 1990.)

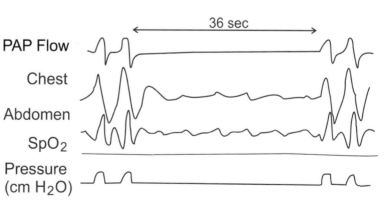

Question B: For patient B, what do you recommend to eliminate the event shown in Figure P48-2?

A. BPAP 13/8
B. BPAP 14/7
C. BPAP 13/9
D. BPAP 12/9

Patient C: A patient with obstructive sleep apnea (OSA) and severe chronic obstructive pulmonary disease (COPD) using supplemental oxygen at 2 L/min for 24 hours a day undergoes a undergoes continuous PAP (CPAP) titration for severe OSA. Tracings on two different levels of CPAP are shown in Figure P48-3. Both tracings are from non–rapid eye movement (NREM) sleep in the supine position.

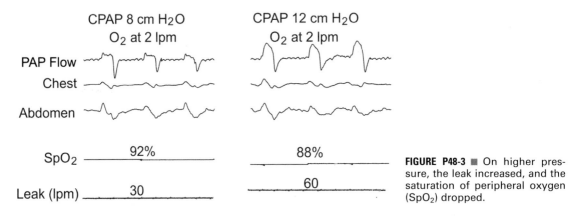

FIGURE P48-3 ■ On higher pressure, the leak increased, and the saturation of peripheral oxygen (SpO₂) dropped.

Question C: For patient C, what is the cause of a lower saturation of peripheral oxygen (SpO_2) on a higher CPAP?

ANSWERS

A. **Answer:** Increase CPAP pressure. Yes, supine REM sleep is the situation usually requiring the highest pressure.

Discussion: The PAP flow provides both magnitude and waveform information. If the inspiratory waveform is flattened, it suggests that high upper airway resistance is still present. If snoring is also present, it is further evidence of a need for higher pressure. In the tracing in Figure P48-1, inspiratory flattening is present, with a long inspiratory time and evidence of snoring. Fine oscillation can be seen in the inspiratory part of the PAP signal—this is not always noted, as the PAP flow signal is too undersampled to reliably show fine detail. Another finding suggesting high upper airway resistance is the paradoxical movement of the chest and abdomen tracings. Although some level of air flow limitation may be accepted if pressure is high or the patient is pressure intolerant, significant air flow limitation warrants an increase in CPAP. At the very edge of the tracing in Figure P48-1, evidence of the start of an arousal can be seen. The highest level of CPAP is usually needed for supine REM sleep. In Patient A, CPAP was increased to 10 cm H_2O with abolition of snoring and air flow limitation. The inspiratory waveform changed from flat to round.

    Recall that as CPAP is sequentially increased, obstructive apnea → hypopnea → snoring → air flow limitation are sequentially eliminated.

B. **Answer:** BPAP 13/9 cm H_2O

Discussion: The event pictured is an obstructive apnea. The AASM *Clinical Guidelines for Titration of Positive Airway Pressure* recommend that for obstructive apnea both the inspiratory PAP (IPAP) and expiratory PAP (EPAP) both be increased (see Fundamentals 24). This maintains the chosen pressure support. An increase in the EPAP as well as IPAP is needed to eliminate obstructive apnea. For obstructive hypopnea, snoring, or respiratory effort–related arousals (RERAs), the IPAP is increased. Any of the answers that increased the EPAP may work, but when using BPAP as treatment for OSA, an IPAP–EPAP difference of *at least* 4 cm H_2O should be used (otherwise why not use CPAP?). The smallest size of the upper airway is typically at end expiration. Sufficient EPAP must be applied to keep the upper airway open at that time. The titration guidelines are summarized in Table P48-1.

TABLE P48-1 Bilevel Positive Airway Pressure Titration Guidelines

	Adults	Children <12 Years
Beginning pressure (cm H$_2$O) IPAP/EPAP	8/4	8/4
Maximum IPAP (cm H$_2$O)	30	20
Minimum PS (cm H$_2$O)	4	4
Maximum PS (cm H$_2$O)	10	10
Increase **both** IPAP **and** EPAP in at least 1 cm H$_2$O increments no more frequently than every 5 minutes	$\geq$3 obstructive apneas	One obstructive apnea
Increase IPAP in at least 1 cm H$_2$O increments no more frequently than every 5 minutes	$\geq$3 hypopneas $\geq$5 RERAs $\geq$3 minutes loud or unambiguous snoring	$\geq$1 hypopneas $\geq$3 RERAs $\geq$1 minute of loud or unambiguous snoring (may increase)

Modified from Kushida CA, Chediak A, Berry RB, et al, for the Positive Airway Pressure Titration Task Force, American Academy of Sleep Medicine: Clinical guidelines for the manual titration of positive airway pressure in patients with obstructive sleep apnea, *J Clin Sleep Med* 4:157-171, 2008.

PS, Pressure support = IPAP – EPAP; *cm H$_2$O*, Centimeters of water; *EPAP*, expiratory positive airway pressure; *IPAP*, inspiratory positive airway pressure; *RERAs*, respiratory effort–related arousals.

C. **Answer:** Higher flow as evidenced by the increased leak is diluting the added flow of supplemental oxygen.

Discussion: The effective inspired oxygen concentration (fraction of inspired oxygen [FiO$_2$]) when supplemental oxygen is added to the PAP circuit depends on both the liter flow of supplemental oxygen **and the PAP flow**. Increases in pressure always increase total flow as the intentional leak increases. If mask leak increases (as it often does) the increase in flow may be fairly large. This may lower the effective FiO$_2$ and result in a lower arterial oxygen saturation (SaO$_2$), even if respiratory events are not present. In the current patient, the increase in pressure did eliminate evidence of air flow limitation (inspiratory waveform changed from flat to round). However, the SaO$_2$ decreased. The supplemental oxygen flow was increased to 3 L/min and the SaO$_2$ rose to 93% for the remainder of the titration. It is important to note that sometimes simply improving the mask seal (lower leak) will increase the FiO$_2$ by reducing the amount of device flow. With lower leak, less device flow is needed to provide the same pressure.

CLINICAL PEARLS

1. Flattening of the PAP device flow inspiratory waveform identifies high upper airway resistance. If persistent snoring and RERAs are present, an increase a pressure is indicated. Some clinicians would recommend an increase in pressure if significant air flow limitation is present even in the absence of snoring or RERAs. If the pressure is low and the patient is not pressure intolerant, an increase in pressure is indicated. If the pressure is high or the patient is pressure intolerant, accepting some degree of air flow limitation may be prudent.

2. When titrating BPAP it is recommended that both IPAP and EPAP be increased together as an intervention for obstructive apnea.

3. Either an increase in pressure (intentional leak) or an increase in mask or mouth leak (unintentional leak) increases the total flow delivered by the PAP device and may dilute the flow of supplemental oxygen lowering the effective fraction of inspired oxygen.

BIBLIOGRAPHY

Sanders MH, Kern N: Obstructive sleep apnea treated by independently adjusted inspiratory and expiratory positive airway pressures via nasal mask, *Chest* 98:317–324, 1990.

Oksenberg A, Silverberg DS, Arons E, et al: The sleep supine position has a major effect on optimal nasal CPAP, *Chest* 116:1000–1006, 1999.

Pevernagie DA, Shepard JW Jr.: Relations between sleep stage, posture and effective nasal CPAP levels in OSA, *Sleep* 15:162–167, 1992.

Condos R, Norman RG, Krishnasamy I, et al: Flow limitation as a noninvasive assessment of residual upper-airway resistance during continuous positive airway pressure therapy of obstructive sleep apnea, *Am J Respir Crit Care Med* 150:475–480, 1994.

Kushida CA, Chediak A, Berry RB, et al: for the Positive Airway Pressure Titration Task Force, American Academy of Sleep Medicine: Clinical guidelines for the manual titration of positive airway pressure in patients with obstructive sleep apnea, *J Clin Sleep Med* 4:157–171, 2008.

Yoder EA, Klann K, Strohl KP: Inspired oxygen concentrations during positive pressure therapy, *Sleep Breath* 8:1–5, 2004.

Schwartz AR, Kacmarek RM, Hess DR: Factors affecting oxygen delivery with bilevel positive airway pressure, *Respir Care* 49:270–275, 2004.

PAP Titration Questions

Patient A: A patient with obstructive sleep apnea (OSA) undergoes an attended positive airway pressure (PAP) titration. Table P49-1 shows the the continuous PAP (CPAP) treatment results. Assume that all sleep occurred in the supine position.

TABLE P49-1	**Positive Airway Pressure Treatment**							
CPAP	**TST**	**REM Sleep**	**AHI**	**AHI REM**	**OSA**	**MA**	**CA**	**H**
(CM H$_2$O)	MIN	MIN	/HR	/HR	NO.	NO.	NO.	NO.
7	30	0	20	0	10	0	0	0
8	30	10	10	30	0	0	0	5
9	30	20	4	6	0	0	0	2
10	30	10	10	0	0	0	5	0
11	30	10	20	0	0	0	10	0

AHI, Apnea–hypopnea index; *CA*, central apnea; *cm H$_2$O*, centimeters of water; *CPAP*, continuous positive airway pressure; *H*, hypopnea; *hr*, hour; *MA*, mixed apnea; *min*, minutes; *No.*, number; *OSA*, obstructive sleep apnea; *REM*, rapid eye movement.

Question A: What pressure do you recommend?
A. 7 cm H$_2$O
B. 8 cm H$_2$O
C. 9 cm H$_2$O
D. 10 cm H$_2$O
E. 11 cm H$_2$O

Patient B: A patient with severe OSA is undergoing a PAP titration. A 60-second tracing is shown in Figure P49-1 with the patient on CPAP of 13 cm H$_2$O.

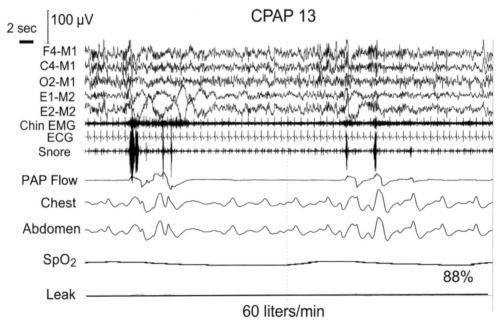

FIGURE P49-1 ■ A 60-second tracing on continuous positive airway pressure (CPAP) of 13 centimeters of water (cm H$_2$O) using a full-face (oronasal) mask.

Question B: What intervention is needed?
A. Increase CPAP to 14 cm H_2O
B. Increase CPAP to 15 cm H_2O
C. Adjust mask
D. Change to BPAP 16/12 cm H_2O

ANSWERS

A. **Answer:** C. CPAP of 9 cm H_2O

Discussion: On CPAP of 9 cm H_2O, the AHI = 4/hr and supine REM sleep was recorded. Higher pressure was associated with central apneas. The optimal pressure is one that effectively reduces respiratory events during supine REM sleep. This circumstance usually requires the highest pressure. Ideally, the arterial oxygen saturation by oximetry (SpO_2) at the treatment pressure should be adequate and consolidated sleep without repeated arousals should be present. The ideal titration is not always attained. If the patient has little REM sleep until the end of the night, minimal time may be available to find an effective pressure. *One should avoid the tendency to simply recommend the highest pressure used during the titration.* Higher-than-needed pressure may have been used. On the other hand, if significant air flow limitation and snoring were present on the highest pressure, slightly higher pressure is probably indicated. Another point to remember is that the "optimal" pressure is one the patient will use consistently. It is better to have an AHI of 10/hr for 7 hours than an AHI of 5/hr for 2 hours and 50/hr for the remaining 5 hours (CPAP not used the last 5 hours). The amount of pressure patients tolerate varies tremendously. The patient estimate of pressure is in the "nose of the beholder." In some patients, as PAP is increased, central apnea is noted to appear. This circumstance may occur before an effective pressure is reached for obstructive events. Treatment emergent central apnea is discussed in Fundamentals 29 and Patient 72. In many patients, a pressure lower than one associated with central apnea is effective at eliminating the majority of respiratory events (even during supine REM sleep). In the current patient, CPAP of 9 cm H_2O was effective during supine REM sleep. Higher pressures were associated with central apneas.

B. **Answer:** Adjust the mask.

Discussion: When mask leak is very high further adjustment (increases) in machine pressure may not result in an increase in mask pressure or effectively treat residual obstructive events. In fact, even higher leak will likely occur. Some leak may be tolerated if it does not arouse the patient or prevent the ability to maintain upper airway patency. However, if leak is high (>50 liters per minute [L/min], total leak), the first intervention is an adjustment of the mask. Adjust the straps or the mask position, change to a different size mask, or change the type of mask. As noted in Fundamentals 24, total leak increases as pressure is increased, and the amount depends on the mask type. Higher pressure causes higher leak through the nonrebreathing (exhalation) orifices use to washout the exhaled carbon dioxide (CO_2) (intentional leak). However, leak over 50 L/min (total leak) is considered high for most mask types at pressures below 20 cm H_2O (Figure P49-2).

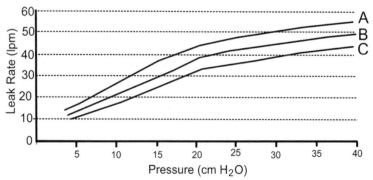

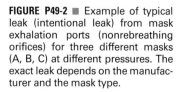

FIGURE P49-2 ■ Example of typical leak (intentional leak) from mask exhalation ports (nonrebreathing orifices) for three different masks (A, B, C) at different pressures. The exact leak depends on the manufacturer and the mask type.

However, often a change in leak is more informative that the absolute value. In PAP devices that output the unintentional leak, a leak over 25 L/min would be considered high. If mouth leak is present and has not responded to a chin strap, a change to an oronasal mask may be tried. High leak may also be associated with severe dryness and nasal congestion and may require an increase in humidity. In assessing PAP titration, it is not enough to simply look at the treatment table. The table does not include information on leak or allow the clinician to determine if an increase in pressure was truly indicated. In the current patient, obstructive apnea is noted, and the leak is high. On CPAP of 10 cm H_2O, the leak had been 30 L/min. A change to a different brand of mask for a better fit resulted in a decrease in leak to 40 L/min, and CPAP of 14 cm H_2O eliminated respiratory events.

CLINICAL PEARLS

1. In choosing an effective treatment pressure from a PAP treatment table, it is important to note more than the AHI. One must note if supine sleep or REM sleep was recorded. If the AHI is elevated, the nature of the residual events should be noted (e.g., central apneas).
2. In choosing an effective treatment pressure, there is no substitute for looking at the sleep tracings. Review of the titration tracings may reveal very high leak or an inappropriate increase in pressure.
3. Although PAP devices are leak tolerant, when very high leak occurs, an increase in machine pressure may not translate into an increase in mask pressure.
4. Recording the PAP device leak can be very useful to the sleep technologist and clinician reading PAP titrations studies.

BIBLIOGRAPHY

Kushida CA, Chediak A, Berry RB, et al: for the Positive Airway Pressure Titration Task Force, American Academy of Sleep Medicine: Clinical guidelines for the manual titration of positive airway pressure in patients with obstructive sleep apnea, *J Clin Sleep Med* 4:157–171, 2008.

Berry RB: Positive airway pressure treatment. In *Fundamentals of sleep medicine*, Philadelphia, 2012, Saunders.

Oksenberg A, Silverberg DS, Arons E, et al: The sleep supine position has a major effect on optimal nasal CPAP, *Chest* 116:1000–1006, 1999.

Pevernagie DA, Shepard JW Jr.: Relations between sleep stage, posture and effective nasal CPAP levels in OSA, *Sleep* 15:162–167, 1992.

A 50-Year-Old Man with Problems During a CPAP Titration

A 50-year-old man with complaints of snoring and excessive daytime sleepiness underwent continuous positive airway pressure (CPAP) titration after an initial diagnostic portion showed an apnea–hypopnea index (AHI) of 30 per hour (hr). The patient initially seemed to do well on 7 centimeters of water (cm H_2O). However, on higher pressures, the AHI was higher. The next morning, he complained of a dry mouth.

Sleep study: Data at selected pressures are shown below. Hypopneas were defined as a 30% reduction in PAP flow associated with an arousal or $\geq 3\%$ desaturation (Table P50-1).

TABLE P50-1 CPAP TITRATION TABLE			
Pressure (cm H_2O)	7	9	11
Monitoring time (minutes)	60	40	40
TST (minutes)	50	30	20
REM (minutes)	30	0	0
Body position	Supine	Supine	Supine
AHI (#/hr)	4.8	24	36
Obstructive apneas (#)	0	0	0
Mixed apneas (#)	0	0	0
Central apneas (#)	2	3	0
Hypopneas (#)	2	16	10
Desaturations (#)	0	2	1
Minimum SaO_2 %	94%	91%	90%
Respiratory arousal index (#/hr)	5	30	30

REM, Rapid eye movement; *SaO₂*, saturation of arterial oxygen; *TST*, total sleep time.

A tracing on CPAP of 9 cm H_2O is shown in Figure P50-1.

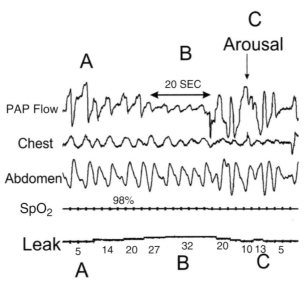

FIGURE P50-1 ■ A 90-second tracing on CPAP of 9 centimeters of water (cm H_2O) is shown. Of note, the leak on 7 cm H_2O was between 10 to 15 liters per minute. The patient is wearing a nasal mask.

QUESTION

1. Why do more events occur at pressures higher than 7 cm H_2O?

ANSWER

1. **Answer:** Overtitration and increased mouth leak on pressures higher than 7 cm H_2O

   Discussion: CPAP treatment tables such as the Table P50-1 are sometimes useful for choosing an appropriate pressure for treatment. However, they do not tell the entire story. It is not uncommon for the AHI to temporarily increase on a given level of CPAP after changes in body position or sleep stage. Higher pressure is almost always needed in the supine position and may also be required after transitions from non-REM (NREM) to REM sleep. Another possibility is an increase in central events. Therefore, one must look not simply at the AHI but at the composition of events. Two other reasons that the AHI might increase at higher pressures are patient intolerance (arousals) and mask or mouth leaks. Arousals may result in what appear to be central apneas or hypopneas on return to sleep. That is, higher flow after arousal with return to lower flow with sleep onset. High mask or mouth leak may also compromise the ability of pressure to maintain airway pressure. The mask pressure is usually only slightly lower than the device pressure (pressure drop across the resistance of the tubing during inspiratory flow). CPAP devices are designed to compensate for leak by increasing flow. High leaks are associated with high flow resulting in a greater pressure drop across the tubing. Therefore, the actual mask pressure may be significantly lower than the pressure at the device during periods of high leak (pressure drop across the resistance of the tube connecting machine and mask).

   Most positive pressure devices used in the sleep laboratory provide several analog or digital outputs that can be recorded. PAP flow is an estimate of flow and is derived from the total flow the machine delivers minus an estimate of the bias flow or leak. The leak signal is also available to be recorded. All CPAP mask interfaces have small orifices for controlled leak that washes out carbon dioxide (CO_2) and prevents rebreathing. This intentional leak increases with the amount of pressure and varies between masks. The total leak is the intentional leak plus the unintentional leak (see Fundamentals 24). The unintentional leak is caused by mask or mouth leak (in the case of a nasal mask). Of note, some PAP devices output a signal based on the total leak and others output a signal based on the unintentional leak (estimate of intentional leak subtracted from total leak).

   Leak information is very useful for a number of reasons. First, a high leak may mean a poor mask seal. If the mask pressure is significantly lower than the machine pressure, this may compromise the ability of pressure to maintain airway patency. High mask leaks may also cause arousal (noise or leaks into the eyes). In a patient wearing a nasal interface, high leak may mean that a significant mouth leak is present. The leak magnitude does not reveal the source of the leak. However, the pattern of leak may be very suggestive. A leak that fluctuates without any evidence of patient movement or increase in pressure in a patient wearing a nasal mask suggests a mouth leak. Sometimes, the low light camera (video recording) will allow the sleep technologist to actually visualize an open mouth or a fluttering of the lips. The PAP flow sensor detects flow via the tubing to the nasal mask. If some portion of the ventilation is via the mouth, this will not register as flow. Periods of nasal and mouth breathing on CPAP may simulate a hypopnea (Figure P50-1). Sometimes no desaturation is associated with such an event. Alternatively, mouth leak may actually compromise the ability to keep the airway open and result in a true hypopnea with an associated desaturation. Patients often arouse during mouth leak. Commonly, *the leak dramatically decreases after arousal when the patient wakes up and closes the mouth.* As noted in Fundamentals 24, truncation of the expiratory flow may also be a clue that mouth leak is present in a patient wearing a nasal mask.

   Of interest, leak may sometimes increase on transition from NREM to REM sleep. With relaxation of the facial muscles (muscle hyptonia during REM) the mouth may open with resulting mouth leak (nasal mask) or leak from the bottom of an oronasal mask. A chin strap under the full-face mask could be necessary in extreme cases to prevent "jaw drop." In Figure P50-2, an increase in total leak is noted on transition to REM sleep. No change in pressure or patient movement was noted.

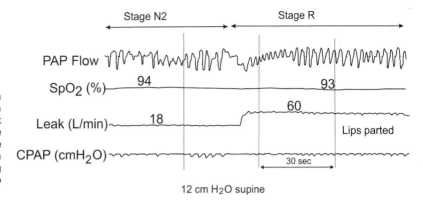

FIGURE P50-2 ■ A change in total leak on transition from non–rapid eye movement (NREM) to REM sleep (stage R). In this case, the increase in leak is caused by mouth leak. The patient was wearing a nasal mask. The video revealed slightly parted lips.

In the current patient, the CPAP was increased from 7 to 9 cm H_2O because of some questionable events during a brief episode of REM sleep. On 7 cm H_2O, the leak had been low and constant at 10 to 15 liters. per minute (L/min) and the AHI was low even during supine REM sleep. On 9 cm H_2O, the leak was higher and fluctuated. Many events like the one pictured at B in Figure P50-1 occurred. Many of the "hypopneas" were associated with arousal followed by a drop in leak. The definition of *hypopnea* used here does not require a desaturation and is based on the associated arousal. In the sample tracing, note the change in flow and leak from A to B. Flow decreases, and leak increases. Leak falls back to a low value after the arousal (C). At arousal, the patient woke up and closed the mouth. Note also that the shape of the flow is round during the "event." This actually is the appearance of a central hypopnea (round inspiratory profile). What should have been done during the titration? The CPAP could have been reduced back to 7 cm H_2O. Alternatively, a chin strap or full face mask could have been applied. The sleep technologist did apply a chin strap and started the patient on heated humidity (HH). HH may help reduce the tendency for mouth leak in patients with nasal congestion. Unfortunately, the pressure was also increased to 11 cm H_2O. This only worsened the situation. Although the patient had an uncomfortable night in the sleep laboratory ("they blasted my mouth open"), he was willing to try CPAP. He was subsequently treated with 7 cm H_2O, a nasal mask, and HH and had near-complete resolution of symptoms.

CLINICAL PEARLS

1. When the AHI worsens with higher positive airway pressure, always consider the possibility than an increase in mouth or mask leak is causing the problem.
2. Recording leak information can be very useful for both the reviewer and the sleep technologist.
3. A fluctuating pattern of leak without change in body position in a patient wearing a nasal mask suggests that mouth leak may be present. At arousal, leak may decrease with mouth closure.
4. Mouth dryness is an important clue that mouth leak could be occurring in a patient using a nasal mask. This is especially true if minimal leak occurred on the same mask and pressure when the patient was awake.
5. Periods of breathing through the nose and mouth may simulate a hypopnea in a patient wearing a nasal mask.
6. With the onset of REM sleep, facial muscles relax, and mask leak (including an oronasal mask) or mouth leak may worsen.

BIBLIOGRAPHY

Berry RB: Medical therapy. In Johnson JT, Gluckman JL, Sanders MH, editors: *Obstructive sleep apnea*, London, U.K., 2002, Martin Dunniz, pp 89–118.

Kushida CA, Chediak A, Berry RB, et al: for the Positive Airway Pressure Titration Task Force, American Academy of Sleep Medicine: Clinical guidelines for the manual titration of positive airway pressure in patients with obstructive sleep apnea, *J Clin Sleep Med* 4:157–171, 2008.

Berry RB: Positive airway pressure treatment. In *Fundamentals of sleep medicine*, Philadelphia, 2012, Saunders.

FUNDAMENTALS 25

PAP Adherence

ADHERENCE—DEFINITIONS AND MEASUREMENT

The major challenge of PAP treatment is to ensure that patient adherence to treatment is adequate.[1,2] Despite the excellent efficacy of PAP devices for reducing the apnea–hypopnea index (AHI), the actual effectiveness may be much lower. For example, if continuous positive airway pressure (CPAP) reduces the AHI from 40 to 5 per hour (hr) but is only used 50% of the night, the mean AHI has only been reduced to 25/hr. The pattern of PAP use is established early and objective adherence (not patient report) is essential to guide treatment. PAP devices can record both blower hours and time at pressure (actual use). Detailed daily information may show important patterns. For example, consistent mask removal at 5 AM. The data obtained from PAP devices often also include useful information on leak as well as an estimate of the residual AHI. Today, PAP machines have both internal memory and removal memory (smart cards, SD cards, flash drives). The removable media can store extensive information on adherence and patterns of use. The recorded device information may be assessed by direct machine interrogation (internal memory) or transferring of information on removable media to a computer. Modems when attached to a PAP device can send information to a central location via telephone lines or wireless technology. The physician or durable medical equipment company (DME) can assess the information from a central server. Information about patient adherence is provided during the critical first weeks of use without requiring the patient to come to clinic or a DME office.

Adherence rates are defined in many ways. Most devices compute the percentage of days used, the average use all days (averaging in 0 hours for days not used), average nightly use (days used), and the percentage of nights used greater than 4 hours. An early paper reporting measurement of objective adherence by Kribbs and coworkers[3] defined regular users as those who used CPAP at least 4 hr/day on at least 70% of nights. In their study, only 46% of patients met this criterion.

PAP ADHERENCE IN LARGE STUDIES

A tremendous variability has existed in the reported rates of PAP adherence. This is attributed to a number of factors, including different populations (moderate to severe OSA versus all patients), different definitions of adherence, different length of follow-up, and different algorithms of initiating PAP treatment and following patients. One of the largest studies of long-term adherence with nasal CPAP reported only 68% of patients were still using CPAP at 5 years.[4] Pepin et al found 79% of patients using CPAP for >4 hours on 70% of nights at 3 months.[5] Sin and coworkers monitored patients with an AHI >20/hr and found >85% were using the device >3.5 hours per night at 6 months. Kohler et al found that 81% of patients were using CPAP at 5 years.[6]

FACTORS INFLUENCING ADHERENCE AND IMPORTANCE OF EARLY ADHERENCE

Factors associated with good versus poor PAP adherence are listed in Table F25-1. However, in general, the factors identified to date explain relatively little of the large variance in CPAP acceptance and adherence.[2,4–7] The level of pressure or pressure mode of treatment (CPAP versus APAP versus BPAP) does not seem to be important[8,9] in unselected patients. Finding an acceptable interface is often the biggest challenge in getting patients to adhere to PAP treatment. However, no evidence exists for the superiority of any type of interface.[10] A high amount of mask leak was associated with poor

TABLE F25-1 **Factors Associated with Good or Poor Adherence**

Good Adherence	Poor Adherence	No Effect
Pretreatment daytime sleepiness	Spouse referral	Level of pressure
Subjective benefit	High nasal resistance	Mask type
High apnea–hypopnea index (AHI) (some studies)	High mask leak	Mode of pressure
High oxygen desaturation index	Poor early adherence	
Good early adherence	Adverse effect on sexual intimacy	
	Race (blacks)	
	Lower socioeconomic group	

adherence in one study,[11] as was a high nasal resistance.[12] A recent study found that the adverse effects of CPAP on sexual intimacy may be a major problem for some patients.[13] If a bed partner reacts negatively to CPAP this may have a negative effect on adherence. Conversely, a major motivation for seeking treatment may be the spouse's complaints about snoring. Unfortunately, spouse referral was associated with poor adherence in one study.[14] The patient must be convinced that CPAP treatment is needed for his or her health as well as the concerns of the bedmate. Involving the spouse in the treatment process has been a part of many PAP programs. If the spouse understands the health risks they may encourage better CPAP use.

In some, but not all, studies, patients with a higher AHI or worse arterial oxygen desaturation[15] showed better adherence. In general, if patients note a symptomatic improvement, this is positive reinforcement for CPAP use. Although early studies found an improvement in adherence with heated humidification,[16] later studies have not confirmed this finding.[17] Heated humidification is likely to have the most benefit in patients with symptoms of nasal congestion and dryness. Although a great deal of effort is spent in intervening for side effects, the presence or absence of side effects does not seem to be a major determinant of PAP use.[2,7] However, in one study, an aggressive approach of intervention for side effects salvaged a significant proportion of patients with initial poor adherence.[18]

Whether CPAP treatment follows a split night (diagnostic or PAP titration) or separate diagnostic and PAP titration studies does not seem to affect PAP adherence. Some studies have suggested that poorer socioeconomic group or race (blacks) is associated with poor adherence.

Early adherence is a good predictor of long-term PAP use. In a study of 32 patients monitored for 9 weeks, the nightly duration of use differed between compliant and noncompliant patients by the fourth night of use.[19] Budhiraja and colleagues[20] found that long-term adherence to CPAP may be predicted as early as 3 days after CPAP initiation.

HOW MUCH ADHERENCE IS ENOUGH?

Weaver and associates[21] studied patients before and after 3 months of therapy and correlated objective adherence with improvement in functioning. Thresholds of the duration of nightly PAP use above which significant improvement was noted were identified for the Epworth Sleepiness Scale (ESS) (≈ 4 hr), multiple sleep latency test (≈ 6 hr), and quality of life (assessed by Functional Outcomes of Sleep Questionnaire) (≈ 7.5 hrs). Thus, as usage increases, subjective sleepiness, then objective sleepiness, then last, quality of life measures improve. The necessary amount of PAP usage depends on which outcome is being evaluated. The current Centers for Medicare and Medicaid (CMS) guidelines state that devices will be reimbursed after 12 weeks only if objective adherence for a period of at least 1 month shows >4 hours use per night for 70% or more of nights and the treating physician documents in a face-to-face meeting that the patient is benefiting from PAP treatment.[22] For most patients, this is not enough PAP use for optimal benefit. Campos-Rodriguez and coworkers followed a historical cohort of 871 patients with obstructive sleep apnea (OSA) for a mean of 48 months.[23] Five-year cumulative survival was highest in the group of patients who used PAP therapy more than 6 hours per night on average (96.4% survival) compared with patients who used PAP from one to 6 hours per night (91.3% survival) and patients who used PAP less than 1 hour per night (85.5%). The same group conducted a prospective cohort study of 55 patients with hypertension.[24] Patients with average use >5.3 hr/day and hypertension at entry to the study had a drop in mean arterial blood pressure of about 4 mm Hg.

INTERVENTIONS TO IMPROVE ADHERENCE

The literature on this subject is somewhat difficult to interpret as most programs use a number of interventions to try to improve adherence[2] (Table F25-2). It is difficult to know whether a given individual component is helpful. Although education about OSA and PAP treatment is recommended, one meta-analysis found no evidence that education alone improves adherence.[25] Comprehensive programs of education (patient and bed partner), early contact, and simple interventions such as a CPAP help line have improved adherence in some studies.[14] Cognitive behavioral interventions have shown promise for improving PAP adherence.[26,27] Timely interventions for side effects and discomforts would also seem reasonable, although not proved to improve adherence.

INTERVENTIONS FOR SIDE EFFECTS

Although for unselected patients a greater number of side effects does not correlate with lower adherence, individual patients may have a large improvement in adherence with an aggressive approach to handling problems[18] (see Table F25-2). Finding a comfortable and well-fitting mask interface is one of the biggest challenges in PAP treatment. Proper sizing and mask adjustment are essential and should be checked at every visit to the physician

---

TABLE F25-2 Interventions for Common PAP Treatment Side Effects

Positive Pressure Side Effects	Interventions
Mask Side Effects	
Air leaks Conjunctivitis Discomfort Noise	Proper mask fitting Proper mask application (education) Different brand or type of mask
Skin breakdown (especially on nasal bridge)	Avoid overtightening—intervene as above for leaks Alternate between different mask types Nasal prongs or pillows—eliminate trauma to nasal bridge Tape or gel barrier for skin protection
Mouth leaks Mouth dryness	Treat nasal congestion, if present (see below) Chin strap Heated humidity Full-face (oronasal) mask Consider BPAP, flexible PAP, lower pressure, APAP
Mask claustrophobia	Nasal pillows/prongs interface Desensitization
Unintentional mask removal	Low pressure alarm Consider increase in pressure Interventions if high leak noted
Nasal Symptoms	
Congestion/obstruction	Nasal steroid and/or antihistamine inhaler Antihistamines (if allergic component) Nighttime topical decongestants (oxymetazoline) as a last resort Nasal saline Humidification (heated) Full face (oronasal) mask - eliminating mouth leak may reduce dryness
Epistaxis Pain	Nasal saline Humidification (heated)
Rhinitis/rhinorrhea	Nasal ipratropium bromide
Other Problems	
Pressure intolerance	Ramp Flexible PAP BPAP APAP Lower prescription pressure temporarily—accept higher AHI Lower pressure + adjunctive measures (elevated head of bed, side sleeping position, weight loss)
Aerophagia or bloating	BPAP, flexible PAP, reduce pressure

AHI, Apnea–hypopnea index; *APAP*, autoadjusting positive airway pressure; *BPAP*, bilevel positive airway pressure; *PAP*, positive airway pressure.

or respiratory therapist providing PAP support. If necessary, a different mask type could be tried. Obtaining a replacement interface or mask cushion on a regular basis is essential. For mouth leaks, the addition of a chin strap, higher humidity, or a full-face mask is an option. Sometimes, a leak will respond to slight lowering of pressure or switch from CPAP to bilevel PAP (BPAP) if all else fails. Nasal pillows may help deal with claustrophobia. Patients with severe claustrophobia may respond to formal desensitization therapy with a psychologist. Unintentional mask removal may indicate a leak or inadequate pressure.

Nasal congestion may be a significant issue. This problem may be addressed with nasal steroids, antihistamines (oral and topical), increased humidity, or reduced mask leak (tends to remove humidity from the system). Studies have demonstrated that loss of *humidity via a leak can dramatically increase nasal resistance.*[28] If a patient reports worsening nasal congestion as the night progresses, suspect leak as the problem. If mouth leak is occurring, a chin strap or oronasal mask may be used. *Some patients are able to tolerate leak if the amount of humidification is increased.*

Bloating may respond to lowering of pressure or switch to auto-PAP (APAP) or BPAP. Rhinitis or rhinorrhea may respond to nasal ipratropium bromide. For pressure intolerance, use of a lower pressure, the addition of flexible CPAP, a change to APAP or BPAP, and education about using the ramp are all options. More information about heated humidity and interventions for pressure intolerance is presented in Patients 47 and 52.

The ability of patients to easily communicate PAP problems to providers is essential. Computer programs by PAP manufactures allow patients to view their adherence and communicate problems. A CPAP hotline or weekly walk-in clinics for PAP problems may be helpful. Recently telemedicine is being used to improve PAP adherence. The use of wireless modems allow the provider the ability to view daily adherence, leak, and residual AHI as well as to change pressure settings from a remote location.

HYPNOTICS, ALCOHOL, AND CPAP

Patients with both insomnia and OSA pose a difficult problem. In addition, some patients who normally have no problems with insomnia will have problems falling asleep or staying asleep on CPAP. Some clinicians have been hesitant to prescribe hypnotics believing that this may reduce the effectiveness of CPAP. One study found that zolpidem, a commonly used hypnotic, did not impair efficacy of a given level of CPAP.[30] It has been hypothesized that using a hypnotic might improve adherence to PAP in some patients. A study by Bradshaw and colleagues[31] using zolpidem did not find an improvement. In contrast, Lettieri and associates[32,33] found improvement during CPAP titration (sleep quality) and long-term adherence with eszopiclone (a hypnotic with a longer duration of action than zolpidem). It is possible that a longer-acting medication is needed to improve CPAP adherence. Although routine use of a hypnotic cannot currently be recommended, at least temporary use of a hypnotic should be considered if insomnia is a major obstacle to CPAP use. Cognitive behavioral treatment of insomnia is another option.

PAP ADHERENCE IN PEDIATRIC PATIENTS

Special interventions are needed to improve acceptance of PAP treatment and adherence in pediatric patients.[34–36] Behavioral techniques such as desensitization (allowing children to play with and wear masks for a week or more before a sleep study), a system of rewards for good adherence, and a team approach using social workers and psychologists are helpful. Education of parents both to the importance of treatment as well as providing parents some techniques for encouraging adherence is essential. Use of a durable medical equipment company with experience dealing with children is also very important.

CLINICAL PEARLS

1. Objective monitoring of adherence is essential for successful PAP treatment.
2. Objective monitoring should be performed early and at continuous intervals.
3. Documenting adequate objective adherence is the first step to evaluate persistent sleepiness despite PAP treatment.
4. While the presence and number of PAP side effects does not predict poor adherence, studies have shown that aggressive intervention for side effects can salvage patients with poor adherence.
5. In patients with poor adherence try to determine if the problem is motivation, adverse spousal reaction to PAP treatment, mask issues, dryness, or pressure issues. Target interventions to what side effects that patient feels are an obstacle to good adherence.

REFERENCES

1. Kakkar RK, Berry RB: Positive airway pressure treatment for obstructive sleep apnea, *Chest* 132:1057–1072, 2007.
2. Weaver TE, Grunstein RR: Adherence to continuous positive airway pressure therapy: the challenge to effective treatment, *Proc Am Thorac Soc* 5:173–178, 2008.
3. Kribbs NB, Pack AI, Kline LR, et al: Objective measurement of patterns of nasal CPAP use by patients with obstructive sleep apnea, *Am Rev Respir Dis* 147:887–895, 1993.
4. McArdle N, Devereux G, Heidarnejad H, et al: Long-term use of CPAP therapy for sleep apnea/hypopnea syndrome, *Am J Respir Crit Care Med* 159:1108–1114, 1999.
5. Pépin JL, Krieger J, Rodenstein D, et al: Effective compliance during the first 3 months of continuous positive airway pressure. A European prospective study of 121 patients, *Am J Respir Crit Care Med* 160:1124–1129, 1999.
6. Sin DD, Mayers I, Man GC, Pawluk L: Long-term compliance rates to continuous positive airway pressure in obstructive sleep apnea: a population-based study, *Chest* 121:430–435, 2002.
7. Engleman HM, Wild MR: Improving CPAP use by patients with the sleep apnoea/hypopnoea syndrome (SAHS), *Sleep Med Rev* 7:81–99, 2003.
8. Smith I, Lasserson TJ: Pressure modification for improving usage of continuous positive airway pressure machines in adults with obstructive sleep apnoea, Update of Cochrane Database Syst Rev 4:CD003531, 2004, *Cochrane Database Syst Rev* 4:CD003531, 2009.
9. Reeves-Hoché MK, Hudgel DW, Meck R, et al: Continuous versus bilevel positive airway pressure for obstructive sleep apnea, *Am J Respir Crit Care Med* 151:443–449, 1995.
10. Massie CA, Hart RW: Clinical outcomes related to interface type in patients with obstructive sleep apnea/hypopnea syndrome who are using continuous positive airway pressure, *Chest* 123:1112–1118, 2003.
11. Valentin A, Subramanian S, Quan SF, et al: Air leak is associated with poor adherence to autoPAP therapy, *Sleep* 34(6):801–806, 2011.
12. Sugiura T, Noda A, Nakata S, et al: Influence of nasal resistance on initial acceptance of continuous positive airway pressure in treatment for obstructive sleep apnea syndrome, *Respiration* 74:56–60, 2007.
13. Ye L, Pack AI, Maislin G, et al: Predictors of continuous positive airway pressure use during the first week of treatment, *J Sleep Res* 21(4):419–426, 2012.
14. Hoy CJ, Vennelle M, Kingshott RN, et al: Can intensive support improve continuous positive airway pressure use in patients with the sleep apnea/hypopnea syndrome? *Am J Respir Crit Care Med* 159:1096–1100, 1999.
15. Kohler M, Smith D, Tippett V, Stradling JR: Predictors of long-term compliance with continuous positive airway pressure, *Thorax* 65:829–32.1, 2010.
16. Massie CA, Hart RW: Clinical outcomes related to interface type in patients with obstructive sleep apnea/hypopnea syndrome who are using continuous positive airway pressure, *Chest* 123:1112–1118, 2003.
17. Ryan S, Doherty LS, Nolan GM, et al: Effects of heated humidification and topical steroids on compliance, nasal symptoms, and quality of life in patients with obstructive sleep apnea syndrome using nasal continuous positive airway pressure, *J Clin Sleep Med* 5:422–427, 2009.
18. Ballard RD, Gay PC, Strollo PJ: Interventions to improve compliance in sleep apnea patients previously non-compliant with continuous positive airway pressure, *J Clin Sleep Med* 3:706–712, 2007.
19. Weaver TE, Kribbs NB, Pack AI, et al: Night-to-night variability in CPAP use over the first three months of treatment, *Sleep* 20:278–283, 1997.
20. Budhiraja R, Parthasarathy S, Drake CL, et al: Early CPAP use identified subsequent adherence to CPAP therapy, *Sleep* 30:320–324, 2007.
21. Weaver TE, Maislin G, Dinges DF, et al: Relationship between hours of CPAP use and achieving normal levels of sleepiness and daily functioning, *Sleep* 30:711–719, 2007.
22. Department of Health and Human Services Centers for Medicare and Medicaid Services: National Coverage Determination (NCD) for Continuous Positive Airway Pressure (CPAP) Therapy For Obstructive Sleep Apnea (OSA) (240.4)
23. Campos-Rodriguez F, Pena-Grinan N, Reyes-Nunez N, et al: Mortality in obstructive sleep apnea-hypopnea patients treated with positive airway pressure, *Chest* 128:624–633, 2005.
24. Campos-Rodriguez F, Perez-Ronchel J, Grilo-Reina A, et al: Long-term effect of continuous positive airway pressure on BP in patients with hypertension and sleep apnea, *Chest* 132:1847–1852, 2007.
25. Smith I, Nadig V, Lasserson TJ: Educational, supportive and behavioural interventions to improve usage of continuous positive airway pressure machines for adults with obstructive sleep apnoea, *Cochrane Database Syst Rev* 2, 2009 CD007736.
26. Richard D, Bartlett DJ, Wong K, et al: Increased adherence to CPAP with a group cognitive behavioral treatment intervention: a randomized trial, *Sleep* 30:635–640, 2007.
27. Aloia MS, Smith K, Arnedt JT, et al: Brief behavioral therapies reduce early positive airway pressure discontinuation rates in sleep apnea syndrome: preliminary findings, *Behav Sleep Med* 5:89–104, 2007.
28. Richards GN, Cistulli PA, Ungar RG, et al: Mouth leak with nasal continuous positive airway pressure increases nasal airway resistance, *Am J Respir Crit Care Med* 154:182–186, 1996.
29. Fox N, Hirsch-Allen AJ, Goodfellow E, et al: The impact of a telemedicine monitoring system on positive airway pressure adherence in patients with obstructive sleep apnea: a randomized controlled trial, *Sleep* 35(4):477–481, 2012.
30. Berry RB, Patel PB: Effect of zolpidem on the efficacy of continuous positive airway pressure as treatment for obstructive sleep apnea, *Sleep* 29:1052–1056, 2006.
31. Bradshaw DA, Ruff GA, Murphy DP: An oral hypnotic medication does not improve continuous positive airway pressure compliance in men with obstructive sleep apnea, *Chest* 130:1369–1376, 2006.
32. Lettieri CJ, Shah AA, Holley AB, et al: CPAP promotion and prognosis—the Army Sleep Apnea Program Trial. Effects of a short course of eszopiclone on continuous positive airway pressure adherence: a randomized trial, *Ann Intern Med* 151:696–702, 2009.
33. Lettieri CJ, Quast TN, Eliasson AH, Andrada T: Eszopiclone improves overnight polysomnography and continuous positive airway pressure titration: a prospective, randomized, placebo-controlled trial, *Sleep* 31:1310–1316, 2008.
34. Rains JC: Treatment of obstructive sleep apnea in pediatric patients. Behavioral intervention for compliance with nasal continuous positive airway pressure, *Clin Pediatr (Phila)* 34:535–541, 1995.
35. Marcus CL, Rosen G, Davidson-Ward S, et al: Adherence to and effectiveness of positive airway pressure therapy in children with obstructive sleep apnea, *Pediatrics* 117:e442–e451, 2006.
36. Koontz KL, Slifer KJ, Cataldo MD, Marcus CL: Improving pediatric compliance with positive airway pressure therapy: the impact of behavioral intervention, *Sleep* 26:1010–1015, 2003.

A Patient with a High Residual AHI on PAP

A 30-year-old man was evaluated by his primary care physician for suspected obstructive sleep apnea (OSA). His insurance company mandated that he have a home sleep test (out-of-center sleep testing [OCST]). The test showed an apnea–hypopnea index (AHI) of 25 per hour (hr) with 40 obstructive apneas, 10 central apneas, and 100 hypopneas. The patient was placed on an auto-adjusting positive airway pressure (APAP) device (pressure range 6 to 16 centimeters of water [cm H$_2$O]) for 2 weeks. The goal was to use auto-titration to pick an effective level of continuous positive airway pressure (CPAP) (Table P51-1).

TABLE P51-1 **APAP Download**	
Days used 14/14 days	
Average use all days	5 hours 10 minutes
Average use days used	5 hours 10 minutes
% of nights >4 hours	90%
Time in large leak	2 minutes
AHI	20/ hour
Apnea index	15/ hour
Hypopnea index	5/ hour
90% pressure	9 cm H$_2$O

AHI, Apnea–hypopnea index; *APAP*, auto-adjusting positive airway pressure; *cm H$_2$O*, centimeters of water.

QUESTION

1. What additional information would be helpful? What do you recommend?

ANSWER

1. **Answer**: Information on the type of residual events: Were they central apneas? Does something in the clinical history suggest that the patient may develop central apneas?

   Discussion: Today, most PAP devices have the ability to provide information about residual respiratory events. The question the clinician must ask is: How accurate are these estimates? It must be kept in mind that the automatic event detection is based entirely on the flow signal (including magnitude, vibration, and flattening of the inspiratory waveform). The device does not know if arterial oxygen desaturation is occurring, if the patient is actually attempting to breathe (no information on respiratory effort), or even if the patient is asleep. The diagnostic algorithms are similar to the ones used in auto-adjusting PAP (APAP) devices to detect apnea, hypopnea, air flow limitation, or respiratory effort–related arousals (RERAs). The exact definitions of detected events vary among devices. In APAP devices, the event detection information is used to make decision about whether changes in pressure are needed. The same event detection algorithms are available on CPAP devices with the ability to estimate the residual AHI, but these devices do not use the information to change pressure.

The clinical utility of the device detected residual AHI has been assessed by several studies with somewhat variable results. As might be guessed, the results depend on the population studied and the definition of hypopnea. In these studies, patients were monitored in the sleep center, and the AHI by device detection and by polysomnography (PSG) were compared. Desai and coworkers[4] compared the AHI by APAP (RemStar AutoPAP, Philips-Respironics) versus manually scored PSG. A device cutoff AHI of 8 events/hr predicted a PSG AHI >10 events/hr with a sensitivity of 0.94 and a specificity of 0.90. The PSG criteria for hypopnea in this study included a decrease in air flow with either a ≥4% decrease in the arterial oxygen saturation or an arousal. Berry et al[3] compared PSG and PAP device event detection (REMstar Auto M-Series, Philips-Respironics, Murrysville, PA), but the required PSG hypopneas to have an associated 4% arterial oxygen desaturation and arousals were not considered. The positive predictive value was 0.67 and negative predictive value was 0.92. The high negative predictive value means that if the device AHI is <10/hr, the PSG AHI is almost always less than 10/hr (good treatment). If the device AHI was >10/hr, then the PSG AHI was >10/hr about 70% of the time. The reason for the false positives was that the device detected "hypopneas" based on air flow that were not associated with desaturation on the PSG (hypopnea not scored). Ultimately, the accuracy of event detection by device depends on the PSG definition of hypopnea and the population studied. In any case, the limitations of the residual AHI estimate must be understood. It is important to remember that a device AHI is the number of events per machine treatment time not total sleep time.

If the PAP device residual events are high and the patient *is not doing well*, intervention is indicated. One might try an empiric increase in pressure (or an increase in the low pressure limit on an APAP device) or order a PSG titration. If the patient *is doing well* clinically, one approach would be to perform oximetry at home on the APAP (or CPAP) to determine if the residual events are associated with significant arterial oxygen desaturation. APAP PSG titration study is also an option, even if the patient is responding clinically. A good clinical response to the current PAP treatment is reassuring, but studies have found that a surprisingly high fraction of patients have high residual AHI levels on their current treatment.

In the past, APAP devices had methods of dealing with possible central apneas that differed between manufacturers. In one case, pressure would not increase above a certain level without coexistence of snoring and air flow limitation. In other devices, if a sequential increase in pressure did not lower the number of residual events, the events were classified as nonresponsive, and further pressure increases were not made by the device. In evaluating the significance of residual events, it is useful to remember the time course of PAP titration. *As PAP is increased the following respiratory events type are sequentially eliminated:*

Obstructive apneas → obstructive hypopneas → snoring/RERAs → air flow limitation

Therefore, if the *residual AHI shows many more apneas than hypopneas, this finding suggests that the apneas are central in nature* (obstructive apneas usually eliminated before hypopneas). Recent PAP devices have the ability to detect "clear airway apneas" and obstructive airway apneas. The terminology "clear airway" is used rather than central apnea because some central apneas may be associated with a closed upper airway. The devices cannot assess respiratory effort so that some "obstructive airway apneas" may actually be central in nature. PAP units by Philips-Respironics identify clear airway apnea by producing a small pressure pulse and determining if associated flow is present. If flow is present, the airway is clear. If no change occurs in flow, the airway is closed (obstructive) (Figure P51-1). The pulse occurs after a period of no (or minimal) air flow; the exact duration is proprietary information but is usually on the order of 6 seconds. If air flow resumes before 10 seconds, the event would *not* be classified as an apnea. PAP devices by Res Med use the forced oscillation technique—a low pressure oscillation with a frequency of 4 hertz (Hz) is superimposed on the current treatment pressure. If oscillations are also detected in the flow signal, the airway is "clear" (open). When a clear airway apnea is detected, APAP devices do not increase pressure.

In the present case, given the fact that the apnea index was greater than the hypopnea index, central apneas were suspected. It was also determined that the patient was taking long-acting morphine for pain. These medications may be associated with central apneas. PSG titration was ordered to determine the nature of the residual AHI and find a level of pressure (or type of PAP) that would effectively reduce the respiratory events. As approval for the PSG was delayed, the patient was given an APAP device that could detect clear airway apneas. After use for 7 days, the report noted in

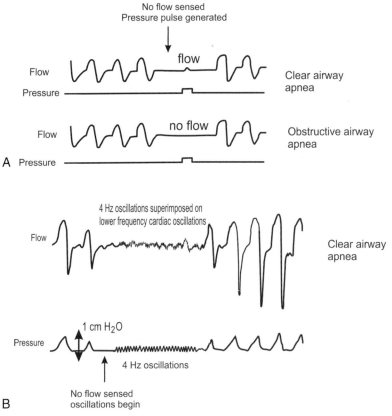

FIGURE P51-1 ■ **A,** Use of a pressure pulse to determine if the airway is open or closed. Recall that closed airways may still be central apneas. **B,** With use of the forced oscillation technique, oscillation in the pressure signal begins once absent air flow is noted. If the airway is not closed, the oscillations will be present in the flow signal.

TABLE P51-2	Results of APAP at Home for 1 Week (Device with Ability to Detect Clear Airway Apneas)
Days used 7/7 days	
Average use all days	5 hours 30 minutes
Average use days used	5 hours 30 minutes
% of nights >4 hours	90%
Time in large leak	2 minutes
AHI (no/hr)	23/hour
Clear airway apnea index (no/hr)	18/hour
Obstructive apnea index (no/hr)	2/hour
Hypopnea index	3/hour
90% pressure (cm H$_2$O)	9.1 cm H$_2$O

AHI, Apnea–hypopnea index.

Table P51-2 was made available. This confirmed the suspicion that most of the residual events were central apneas. Given the evidence from the findings, approval was obtained for PSG titration. The patient was started on CPAP but had many central apneas on treatment. The PAP mode was changed to adaptive-servo-ventilation (see Fundamentals 30), and the AHI was reduced to 7/hr (Table P51-2).

CLINICAL PEARLS

1. The residual AHI information obtained from PAP devices may be helpful but has limitations. If the results do not fit the clinical picture, further evaluation may be needed. In general, if the device AHI is low, treatment is likely effective. If the device AHI is high, this could be a falsely elevated AHI. The residual AHI must be evaluated in the context of the patient's response to treatment. If the patient is doing well, a mild increase in the AHI may not require intervention. If the patient is not doing well, some study to evaluate the effectiveness of PAP treatment is needed.

2. When the device AHI is elevated it is important to look at the nature of the residual events. If the apnea index is greater than the hypopnea index, central apneas should be suspected.

3. PAP devices can now determine if apneas are clear airway apneas or obstructed airway apneas. It is important to remember that devices *cannot assess respiratory effort* and that some of the closed (obstructive) airway apneas could be central apneas.

4. If the patient is not responding to treatment and the AHI is high, PSG titration should be considered. If the patient is hesitant to undergo another study, oximetry on PAP (to determine if oxygen desaturations are occurring on treatment) may be performed or an empiric increase in pressure attempted (if the residual events are not clear airway apneas).

BIBLIOGRAPHY

Pittman SD, Pillar G, Berry RB, et al: Follow-up assessment of CPAP efficacy in patients with obstructive sleep apnea using an ambulatory device based on peripheral arterial tonometry, *Sleep Breath* 10:123–131, 2006.

Baltzan MA, Kassissia I, Elkholi O, et al: Prevalence of persistent sleep apnea in patients treated with continuous positive airway pressure, *Sleep* 29:557–563, 2006.

Berry RB, Kushida CA, Kryger MH, et al: Respiratory event detection by a positive airway pressure device, *Sleep* 35(3):361–367, 2012.

Desai H, Patel A, Patel P, et al: Accuracy of auto-titration CPAP to estimate the residual Apnea-Hypopnea Index in patients with obstructive sleep apnea on treatment with auto-titrating CPAP, *Sleep Breath* 13:383–390, 2009.

Ueno K, Kasai T, Brewer G, et al: Evaluation of the apnea-hypopnea index determined by the S8 auto-CPAP, a continuous positive airway pressure device, in patients with obstructive sleep apnea-hypopnea syndrome, *J Clin Sleep Med* 6:146–151, 2010.

Badr MS, Toiber F, Skatrud JB, et al: Pharyngeal narrowing/occlusion during central apnea, *J Appl Physiol* 78:1806–1815, 1995.

PATIENT 52

Intervention for PAP Problems

Patient A: A 50-year-old man was diagnosed with severe obstructive sleep apnea (OSA) and had been using continuous positive airway pressure (CPAP) of 12 centimeters of water (cm H₂O). A download showed only fair adherence with use >4 hours on about 50% of nights. The residual apnea–hypopnea index (AHI) was 4 per hour (hr). The patient reported that his major problem was bloating and gas.

Question 1: What do you recommend for Patient A?

Patient B: A 40-year-old woman is being treated for moderate OSA. She was using a nasal mask but is unable to use CPAP of 12 cm H₂O for more than 2 to 3 hours per night because of severe dryness. An increase in the humidifier setting from 1 to 4 did not provide much improvement. She notes that nearly all the water in the humidifier chamber was used each night. On CPAP download, the time in large leak was one hour.

Question 2: What do you recommend for Patient B?

ANSWERS

1. **Answer (Patient A):** Switch to bilevel PAP (BPAP) or auto-adjusting PAP (APAP) or lower the CPAP pressure.

   Discussion: Bloating is a significant problem for some patients using CPAP. A number of interventions can be tried. A change from CPAP to BPAP is one intervention. This lowers the pressure during exhalation and may decrease bloating. BPAP may be started with a pressure support of 4 and average pressure equal to the current level of CPAP (BPAP 12/8 instead of CPAP of 10 cm H_2O). The downside is that BPAP devices are considerably more expensive that CPAP devices. Another option is use of APAP. These devices deliver the lowest effective pressure in any circumstance and the mean pressure may be much lower than the level of CPAP needed to maintain an open airway in all circumstances. Use of flexible PAP with a reduction in expiratory pressure during most of exhalation is another approach that may work in some patients. Finally, simply reducing treatment pressure may be effective intervention for bloating if a lower pressure does not result in an unacceptable increase in the AHI. In Patient A, CPAP of 12 cm H_2O was changed to BPAP of 14/10 cm H_2O, with almost complete resolution of bloating symptoms. The average nightly use increased to 6 hours, and the residual AHI remained below 5/hr.

2. **Answer (Patient B):** Mask intervention to reduce leak and adjustment of humidification.

   Discussion (Patient B): When a patient on PAP treatment complains of severe dryness the potential interventions listed in Table P52-1 should considered. If heated humidification is not already being used this should be added. If humidification is being used, an increase in the humidifier setting is the next intervention. If this has not improved dryness, the function of the humidifier should be checked. If the humidifier uses minimal water even on a high setting, malfunction of the humidifier may be an explanation for dryness. The amount of water used by a humidifier depends on the humidifier setting and the flow across the water chamber. PAP devices deliver higher flow in an attempt to compensate for leak.

   Total leak = intentional leak (nonbreathing) + Unintentional leak (mask and/or mouth)

   Recall that the intentional mask leak is higher at higher pressure and a high unintentional leak (mask or mouth) may dramatically increase the total flow. If a high leak and a high humidifier setting are present, most of the water in the humidifier chamber should be used each night. If this is not

TABLE P52-1	**Interventions for Complaints of Severe Dryness or Humidification Problems**
Problem	**Intervention**
High leak - High large leak on download - Humidifier using most of water in chamber - Bed partner report - Suspect mouth leak if good nasal mask fit	Change mask (different size or type) Intervene for mouth leak (try chin strap or full-face mask) Consider lower pressure, APAP or BPAP to reduce mouth or mask leak
Humidifier	Is it working—using water? Is setting optimized? Consider use of a heated tube if rain-out is a limiting the amount of humidification
Mouth breathing	Treat nasal congestion Adequate humidification Chin strap or full face mask
Excessive moisture in mask or tubing (rain-out)	Tube insulator Increased room temperature PAP device below level of bed Reduce humidity setting Heated tube

APAP, Auto-adjusting positive airway pressure; *BPAP*, bilevel positive airway pressure.

the case, the humidifier may not be working. At high humidity settings, moisture may condense in the tubing or mask (rain out). Use of a tube insulator, avoiding an excessively low room temperature, and positioning the CPAP device below the level of the bed (condensed fluid drains into chamber by gravity) may reduce the excessive water in the tube and mask. Currently, some CPAP devices monitor room temperature (and relative humidity) and adjust humidifier heat to limit rain-out. Unfortunately, this may also limit the amount of humidity delivered to the mask. Recently, use of heated tubing has allowed the delivery of high levels of moisture without rain-out. However, with the use of heated tubing, the amount of water in the humidifier chamber may be the limiting factor unless the chamber if refilled during the night.

If humidification has been optimized, the next consideration is to try to reduce leak. High leak removes humidity from the upper airway and may overcome the nose's ability to humidify the inhaled air. If the machine download shows considerable time with a large leak, this requires intervention. Even if the time in "large leak" is low, moderate leak may still occur for most of the night. Large leak for a given pressure is typically defined as two times the expected leak with an average mask at that treatment pressure. Mask refit, education about proper mask placement, and adjustment are the first steps to reduce leak. Regarding mask refit and adjustment, the best approach in clinic is to have the patient in the supine position with the mask placed by the patient at the treatment pressure. *Unless masks are tested under pressure the ability to seal cannot really be assessed.* Sometimes, a fit seem good, but a trial under pressure reveals unacceptable leak. Many patients overtighten masks to try to compensate for a poor fit or poor adjustment of the straps. An apparently great fit may actually seal poorly under pressure. *If dryness and leak have developed only in the last few months*, it may be a sign that the mask needs to be replaced (mask cushion has deteriorated).

If a nasal mask is being used, the possibility of mouth leak could be considered. In Figure P52-1, periods of mouth leak caused drops in the mask's relative humidity. If the nasal mask fits well and is not reported to leak during the night by the patient, this makes mouth leak a real possibility. The bed partner may report observing mouth leak or the intermittent sound of high flow. An empiric trial of a chin strap or a change to a full-face mask are two interventions for mouth leak. On the other hand, some patients with high leak with an oronasal mask will have less leak on the combination of a nasal mask and chin strap. Another intervention for leak is a small decrease in treatment pressure or a change to APAP. A study by Hukins that average leak decreased when patients were switched from CPAP to APAP. This is not surprising as leak increases with pressure. Using APAP, the average pressure is lower than the single level of CPAP required for airway patency in all body positions and sleep stages.

Sometimes, high leak is noted in a patient already using an oronasal (full-face mask). Oronasal masks are difficult to fit, as they require the mask to seal over a large area. In addition, the mandible may move during sleep, causing an interruption in seal. If the patient reports no mask leak at sleep onset, then the possibility of a shift in mask position during sleep or the effect of facial muscle relaxation and jaw droop during sleep are considerations. Some oronasal masks have a ridge to prevent jaw drop. As a last resort, use of a chin strap under the full-face mask may be tried. Another option mentioned previously is a change from a full-face mask to a nasal mask and chin strap. Finally, some patients have difficult-to-fit faces, and in that case, use of a lower treatment pressure will have to be accepted. If a drop in CPAP of only a few centimeters of water makes the mask much easier to seal, a trial of the lower pressure as treatment is a reasonable option.

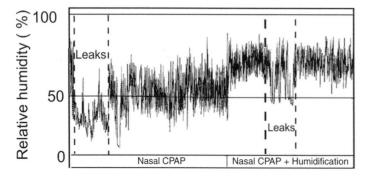

FIGURE P52-1 ■ This tracing shows a fall in the relative humidity at the nasal mask during mouth leaks (leak detected by an oral thermistor). Heated humidification minimized but did not eliminate the fall in relative humidity. *CPAP,* Continuous positive airway pressure. (From Martins de Araujo MT, Vieira SB, Vasquez EC, Fleury B: Heated humidification or face mask to prevent upper airway dryness during continuous positive airway pressure therapy, *Chest* 117:142-147, 2000.)

Although intervention for a complaint of dryness may make a huge difference in the adherence of a given patient, the use of heated humidity has not been demonstrated to improve PAP adherence in unselected patients Humidification may be expected to be most important in patients with nasal congestion and a tendency toward mouth breathing. An early study by Massie et al found that heated humidity modestly improved adherence, but subsequent studies have not found a consistent effect (unselected patients).

CLINICAL PEARLS

1. If significant bloating or gas is a complaint of a patient using CPAP, switching to BPAP or APAP or lowering the level of may improve symptoms of bloating.

2. A complaint of dryness typically means that flow through the system has overwhelmed the humidification mechanisms of the nose or removed humidity from the upper airway–PAP system (e.g., mask leak or mouth leak when using a nasal mask).

3. Heated humidity allows delivery of increased moisture compared with passive humidity, and the setting may be adjusted for comfort.

4. Optimization of humidification includes adjustment of the humidity setting and interventions to reduce rain out and mask or mouth leak.

5. Even if the time of "large leak" on download is modest, complaints of dryness may improve with a reduction in leak (change mask; change mask type; add chin strap; switch from a nasal mask to an oronasal mask, or vice-versa).

BIBLIOGRAPHY

Duong M, Jayaram L, Camfferman D, et al: Use of heated humidification during nasal CPAP titration in obstructive sleep apnoea syndrome, *Eur Respir J* 26:679–685, 2005.

Hukins C: Comparative study of autotitrating and fixed-pressure CPAP in the home: a randomized, single-blind crossover trial, *Sleep* 27(8):1512–1517, 2004.

Martins de Araujo MT, Vieira SB, Vasquez EC, Fleury B: Heated humidification or face mask to prevent upper airway dryness during continuous positive airway pressure therapy, *Chest* 117:142–147, 2000.

Massie CA, Hart RW, Peralez K, Richards GN: Effects of humidification on nasal symptoms and compliance in sleep apnea patients using continuous positive airway pressure, *Chest* 116:403–408, 1999.

Nilius G, Domanski U, Franke KJ, Ruhle KH: Impact of a controlled heated breathing tube humidifier on sleep quality during CPAP therapy in a cool sleeping environment, *Eur Respir J* 31:830–836, 2008.

Ryan S, Doherty LS, Nolan GM, et al: Effects of heated humidification and topical steroids on compliance, nasal symptoms, and quality of life in patients with obstructive sleep apnea syndrome using nasal continuous positive airway pressure, *J Clin Sleep Med* 5:422–427, 2009.

Worsnop CJ, Miseski S, Rochford PD: The routine use of humidification with nasal continuous positive airway pressure, *Intern Med J* 40:650–656, 2009.

Nasal Congestion and Oronasal Masks

Patient A: A 55-year-old man was diagnosed as having severe obstructive sleep apnea (OSA) (apnea–hypopnea index [AHI] = 55 per hour [hr]). After continuous positive airway pressure (CPAP) titration, treatment with nasal CPAP was initiated. Unfortunately, the patient developed severe nasal congestion and was able to use CPAP for only a few hours each night. He had a long history of mild nasal congestion that worsened during the spring. He was treated with a nonsedating oral antihistamine and nasal steroid medications without much improvement. He reported waking up several hours after starting nasal CPAP and being unable to breathe through his nose. A very dry mouth usually was noted at that time. He was started on heated humidity with partial improvement in symptoms. A summary of the CPAP download is shown in Table P53-1.

TABLE P53-1	Positive Airway Pressure Download (Before Intervention)
Average humidity setting	3 (out of 5)
Average use (hours)	3 hours 30 minutes
Average large leak	2 hours
Apnea–hypopnea index (AHI)	4/hour

Question 1: What further therapy would you consider for Patient A?

Patient B: A 70-year-old woman underwent PAP titration after a diagnosis of moderate OSA was made. The titration was started with a nasal mask but leak became very high when pressure was increased to 9 centimeters of water (cm H_2O). Video monitoring revealed a partially open mouth. Heated humidity was added but the problem persisted. A chin strap was tried but was unsuccessful at reducing leak. The patient was changed to a full-face (oronasal) mask. This did reduce the leak, but intermittent leak was still a problem. The patient was titrated to 12 cm H_2O, but the AHI remained slightly above 10/hr.

Question 2: What intervention do you recommend for Patient B? Should a full-face mask (oronasal mask) be used?

Patient C: A 45-year-old man with a modest body mass index (BMI) of 30 kilograms per square meter (kg/m^2) and neck circumference of 15.5 inches was diagnosed as having very severe OSA. He arrived at the sleep center for titration. He was tried on both nasal pillows and traditional nasal masks but complained of inability the breath through his nose. He could not tolerate a nasal mask but was able to use a full face (oronasal) mask. The titration was performed with the full face mask. The optimal pressure appeared to be 16 cm H_2O.

Question 3: What are the challenges of using a full-face (oronasal) mask in Patient C?

ANSWERS

1. **Answer (Patient A):** Optimization of heated humidification, aggressive treatment of nasal congestion, and use an oronasal (full face mask) if necessary.

Discussion (Patient A): Nasal symptoms are common in patients with OSA before treatment, and nasal obstruction itself may be a contributing factor in the development of sleep-disordered breathing (SDB). After starting treatment with nasal CPAP, many patients report new or increased nasal symptoms. Of patients using nasal CPAP, 30% to 50% experience nasal congestion, dry nose and throat, sore throat, and even bleeding from the nose. These side effects may dramatically reduce adherence and may result in cessation of therapy.

It is unclear how nasal CPAP increases or causes nasal symptoms. In some patients, the necessity of nasal respiration draws attention to de novo nasal symptoms. In others, airway pressure on the nasal mucosa induces rhinorrhea by reflex mechanisms. Patients with rhinorrhea may respond to nasal inhalation of an anticholinergic medication (ipratropium bromide). However, in most patients, nasal congestion, rather than rhinorrhea, is the major problem. The etiology of worsening nasal congestion on CPAP is not known with certainty but may be related to mucosal drying. Cold, dry air appears to induce release of mediators from mast cells. Some degree of mouth breathing may initiate a unidirectional air leak (out the mouth), and the loss of moisture from the system overwhelms the capacity of the nasal mucosa to humidify inspired air. Further drying of the nasal mucosa results in more nasal congestion and higher nasal resistance (Figure P53-1), which, in turn, promotes more mouth breathing. Thus, a vicious cycle develops. In many patients, adequate humidification can break this cycle. Richard et al measured nasal resistance in a group of normal individuals before and after breathing on CPAP. CPAP induced little change in nasal resistance. The study subjects then used CPAP with a mouth leak. Nasal resistance increased tremendously (Figure P53-1). The rise in nasal resistance was blunted by application of heated humidity.

If *nasal congestion increases overnight* in a patient using CPAP, drying and mouth or mask leak should be suspected. If mouth leak is suspected and the patient is using a nasal mask, the humidity setting could be increased (may compensate for mild degree of leak). If underlying nasal congestion is present, use of nasal corticosteroids, inhaled antihistamines (astelin), or an oral antihistamine could be tried. Some patients may benefit from a nasal pillow mask, which tends to reduce nasal resistance across the nasal inlet. In patients with inferior turbinate hypertrophy, referral to Otorhinolaryngology for turbinate reduction with radiofrequency ablation could be considered.

Patient A was using a nasal mask but the download showed a large amount of time in large leak (see Table P53-1). He denied leaks from the nasal mask. His wife confirmed that he had air escaping from his mouth and "bubbling." The humidifier setting was increased, and a chin strap was added. The patient was started on nasal steroids. The patient's symptoms improved dramatically. Although a repeat download showed that large leak was still present for 30 minutes on average, the degree of nasal congestion was tolerable and he was able to use CPAP for the entire night.

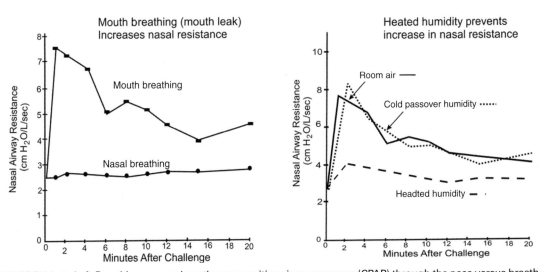

FIGURE P53-1 ▪ *Left,* Breathing on nasal continuous positive airway pressure (CPAP) through the nose versus breathing through the open mouth. Mouth breathing dramatically increases nasal resistance. *Right,* The mouth breathing challenge does not increase resistance if using heated humidity (delivers sufficient moisture to prevent mucosal drying). Passover (cool) humidity was not effective. (From Richard GL, Cistulli PA, Ugar G, et al: Mouth leak with nasal continuous positive airway pressure increases nasal airway resistance, *Am J Respir Crit Care Med* 154:182-186, 1996.)

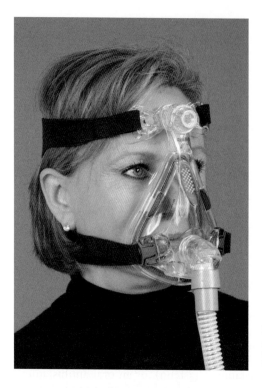

FIGURE P53-2 ■ Example of an oronasal (full face) mask. (Image used with permission. EPR, ResMed, Swift and Quattro are trademarks of ResMed Limited and are registered in the U.S. Patent and Trademark Office.)

2. **Answer:** An oronasal mask could be used, but other options should also be considered.

Discussion: Oronasal masks (Figure P53-2) are useful for patients with severe nasal congestion (unable to breathe via a nasal mask) or mouth leak. If a full-face mask is used during the titration, many patients are automatically started on this type of interface for chronic treatment. However, many patients find sleeping with the oronasal mask to be uncomfortable, and obtaining a good seal with low leak is often difficult. Given the variety of shapes of facial structures and the challenge of beards, finding a good seal is often challenging. In patients with lower dentures, little support for the mask exists in the chin area unless the patients sleep with their dentures on. Sleeping with dentures in place may be needed to obtain a good mask seal. If multiple attempts at finding a suitable full-face mask fail or the patient cannot tolerate the mask because of leak or dryness, other options could be considered. One option is the use of a nasal mask and chin strap. Although widely used, chin straps have not been well studied, and the design is variable. Many are flimsy and ineffective. However, they do work in some patients. Finally as a last resort, use of a lower pressure could be considered—not because of pressure intolerance but to control leak. With a full-face mask in place, pressure may be lowered and the mask adjusted until a combination is effective. Lower pressure or a change to bilevel PAP (BPAP) might also be considered in a patient using a chin strap, as oral venting is often expiratory. In Patient B, review of the study showed a reasonable AHI of 6/hr on CPAP of 8 cm H_2O in the supine position. Lower pressure was effective in the lateral position. Review of the tracings confirmed a large increase in leak with a nasal mask in place on pressures of 9 cm H_2O and above. The patient refused to use an oronasal mask ("that big thing") and was started on a nasal mask, chin strap, an increased humidifier setting, and CPAP of 8 cm H_2O. A download 2 weeks later showed a residual AHI of 5/hr, and the patient was adherent to treatment.

3. **Answer:** Mask seal may be more difficult, adherence was lower in some studies, and higher pressure may be needed compared to one effective using a nasal mask.

Discussion: Oronasal mask (see Figure P53-2) provide a useful interface alternative, but they have issues. As discussed in Patient B, obtaining a good seal with an oronasal mask may be difficult, as a good seal must be obtained over a large area of the face. Patients frequently prefer sleeping with a smaller interface and even experience claustrophobia with a full-face mask. Several studies were been unable to find evidence that use of an oronasal mask worsened adherence. However, other studies, including an analysis of a large French cohort (Borel et al) found use of an oronasal mask was associated with lower adherence. A higher pressure may be needed with an oronasal compared to a nasal interface. This may be caused by posterior displacement of the mandible during use of the oronasal mask, which moves the tongue to a more posterior position. When facial muscles relax with sleep, the tension in the oronasal mask straps tends to pull the mandible backward and downward narrowing the upper airway.

Patient C had severe nasal congestion at the start of the titration. The availability of an oronasal mask saved the titration. However, over the long term, an effort was made to change to a nasal mask. His nasal congestion was treated with nasal steroids and antihistamines. He found sleeping with the oronasal mask difficult once he was less sleepy (after several weeks of treatment). He was tried on a nasal pillow mask and chin strap with heated humidity. He found tolerating CPAP of 16 cm H_2O more difficult with the pillow mask and pressure was dropped to CPAP of 14 cm H_2O. Machine download after a month showed good adherence and an AHI of 3/hr.

CLINICAL PEARLS

1. Nasal symptoms are a major cause of adherence problems with nasal CPAP therapy.

2. Mouth leaks may further increase nasal resistance by setting up a unidirectional flow out the mouth (leak) and drying the nasal mucosa.

3. Oronasal masks may be very useful for PAP treatment of patients with severe nasal congestion or those with mouth leak. However, these masks have some issues.

4. Some studies have found equivalence in treatment effectiveness with oronasal and nasal interfaces, whereas others have found lower adherence and a need for high pressure with oronasal masks.

5. Oronasal mask may increase upper airway resistance because of the mandible being pulled down and back (tension from head straps) when facial muscles relax during sleep. This may especially true in patients lacking mandibular dentition or who overtighten the mask.

6. Although a full face mask (oronasal) mask may salvage a titration in a given patient with severe nasal congestion, this does not mean the a full face mask must always be used by the patient for chronic CPAP treatment.

7. A nasal mask and chin strap, aggressive medical treatment of nasal congestion, and use of adequate heated humidity may be an alternative to the use of full face (oronasal) mask.

BIBLIOGRAPHY

Richard GL, Cistulli PA, Ugar G, et al: Mouth leak with nasal continuous positive airway pressure increases nasal airway resistance, *Am J Respir Crit Care Med* 154:182–186, 1996.

Prosise GL, Berry RB: Oral-nasal continuous positive airway pressure as a treatment for obstructive sleep apnea, *Chest* 106:180–186, 1994.

Sanders MH, Kern NB, Stiller RA, et al: CPAP therapy via oronasal mask for obstructive sleep apnea, *Chest* 106:774–779, 1994.

Borel JC, Gakwaya S, Masse JF, et al: Impact of CPAP interface and mandibular advancement device on upper airway mechanical properties assessed with phrenic nerve stimulation in sleep apnea patients, *Respir Physiol Neurobiol* 183:170–176, 2012.

Teo M, Amis T, Lee S, et al: Equivalence of nasal and oronasal masks during initial CPAP titration for obstructive sleep apnea syndrome, *Sleep* 34:951–955, 2011.

Bakker JP, Neill AM, Campbell AJ: Nasal versus oronasal continuous positive airway pressure masks for obstructive sleep apnea: a pilot investigation of pressure requirement, residual disease, and leak, *Sleep Breath* 16:709–716, 2012.

Ebben MR, Oyegbile T, Pollak CP: The efficacy of three different mask styles on a PAP titration night, *Sleep Med* 13:645–649, 2012.

Mortimore IL, Whittle AT, Douglas NJ: Comparison of nose and face mask CPAP therapy for sleep apnoea, *Thorax* 53(4):290–292, 1998.

Borel JC, Tamisier R, Dias-Domingos S, et al: for the Scientific Council of The Sleep Registry of the French Federation of Pneumology (OSFP): Type of mask may impact on continuous positive airway pressure adherence in apneic patients, *PLoS One* 8(5):e64382, 2013.

Davis SS, Eccles R: Nasal congestion: mechanisms, measurement and medications. Core information for the clinician, *Clin Otolaryngol Allied Sci* 29(6):659–666, 2004.

Auto-Titration

Patient A: A 50-year-old man underwent an out-of-center sleep test (OCST) and was diagnosed as having severe obstructive sleep apnea (OSA) (apnea–hypopnea index [AHI] 60 per hour [hr]). His insurance provider denied preapproval for a polysomnography (PSG) positive airway pressure titration. He underwent auto-titration at home for 2 weeks, and the results are listed in Table P54-1.

TABLE P54-1 Auto-Adjusting Positive Airway Pressure Titration Results for Patients A and B

	Patient A	Patient B
Minimum pressure limit (cm H_2O)	4	4.0
Maximum pressure limit (cm H_2O)	20	14.0
Days used	14/14	3/6
Average use	6 hours 31 minutes	2 hours 2 minutes
90th percentile pressure (cm H_2O)	11.8	14.0
Average pressure (cm H_2O)	9.2	8
AHI	4.0	13.6
Large leak	5 minutes	1 hours 30 minutes

Large leak is defined as leak >2 times the average leak of interfaces at a given pressure.
AHI, Apnea–hypopnea index; *cm H2O*, centimeters of water.

Question 1: What level of CPAP do you recommend for Patient A?

Patient B: A 30-year-old man was diagnosed with severe OSA during PSG. Positive airway pressure (PAP) titration was attempted, but the patient could not tolerate continuous PAP (CPAP). He declined to return for PSG titration. He was very pressure intolerant, according to the technologist's notes. Auto-titration was performed with a relatively low upper pressure limit (see Table P54-1).

Question 2: What is the next step for Patient B?

ANSWERS

1. **Answer (Patient A):** CPAP of 12 centimeters of water (cm H_2O) based on the 90th percentile pressure

   Discussion: After a diagnosis of OSA has been made by PSG or an out of center sleep test (OCST), a number of options for starting PAP therapy without a PSG titration are available.[1–9] (Box P54-1). These options are especially relevant if the diagnosis of OSA is based on an OCST and if PSG is not readily available for financial or scheduling reasons. Titration alternatives may also be used for patients who are unwilling or unable to have a standard PSG PAP titration. The alternatives for starting CPAP in a patient with OSA include treating the patient with an APAP device (titration not needed), performing auto-titration at home for several days to a week (at least 3 days optimum) with subsequent CPAP treatment based on the results, and starting PAP treatment based on a prediction equation with subsequent adjustment based on symptoms, machine readings, and nocturnal oximetry. Equations to predict the optimal CPAP level have been developed.[2–4]

   How effective is the approach of using unattended auto-titrating PAP devices to determine an effective level of CPAP? Studies have shown that with proper patient selection, education, and follow-up, the outcomes resemble those of PSG PAP titration.[2,5–9] However, *most studies excluded a significant number of patients*, and a well-structured systematic approach with good patient education was used. Key elements of successful auto-titration are noted in Box P54-2.

BOX P54-1	Alternative Methods of Starting Positive Airway Pressure

- PSG titration → CPAP treatment
- Autotitration → CPAP treatment
- APAP treatment

- CPAP treatment with empirical pressure then adjustments based on symptoms, bedmate observations, oximetry, or machine-residual AHI

AHI, Apnea-hypopnea index; *APAP*, auto-adjusting positive airway pressure; *CPAP*, continuous positive airway pressure; *PSG*, polysomnography.

BOX P54-2	Technique of Auto-Titration

| Patient selection (exclusions) | • Use polysomnography (PSG) titration rather than auto-adjusting positive airway pressure (APAP) titraton if:
  • Daytime supplemental oxygen
  • Hypoventilation
  • Severe hypoxemia
  • Neuromuscular weakness
  • Congestive heart failure
  • Moderate to severe chronic obstructive pulmonary disease (COPD)
  • Central apnea likely (narcotics, noted on diagnostic study) | Education

Auto-titration | • Education about obstructive sleep apnea (OSA) and PAP treatment
• Mask fitting
• Practice nap
• Duration—three nights to 1 or 2 weeks
• Is auto-titration adequate?
  • Adequate adherence
  • Absence of excessive leak
  • Residual apnea–hypopnea index (AHI) <10 per hour
• Select 90th or 95th percentile pressure for CPAP treatment |

Patient Selection for APAP Titration or APAP Chronic Treatment: Patients with a number of conditions are not suitable for APAP titration or treatment and should undergo PSG titration, if possible (see Box P54-2). These include patients who require or are likely to require supplemental oxygen (low baseline saturation of arterial oxygen [SaO_2]), patients with hypoventilation, patients who have central apneas on the diagnostic study or those likely who may have treatment emergent central apneas (narcotics, congestive heart failure), and patients who may require very high pressures. Many patients with moderate to severe lung disease often require both PAP and supplemental oxygen and should undergo PSG titration, if possible. If an auto-titration is performed on patients with very severe arterial oxygen desaturation, nocturnal oximetry on CPAP or auto-adjusting PAP (APAP) is advised to determine if supplemental oxygen is needed in addition to PAP.

Technique of Auto-Titration: The patient is educated about OSA and PAP treatment and has mask fitting and instructions on use of an APAP device. It is often useful for the patient to take a brief practice nap during which she or he applies the interface, activates the APAP device, and "naps" for about 15 or 20 minutes. This allows identification of interface problems and allows for adjustment or change of interface. The patient then sleeps on the APAP device at home for several nights. Usually, the pressure limits of the device are set from 4 to 20 cm H_2O. Patients with a high body mass index (BMI) or large neck circumference are likely to require high CPAP and a starting with pressure of 4 cm H_2O may be uncomfortable (insufficient to fall asleep). In this situation, a higher low pressure limit is chosen (8–10 cm H_2O). For the pressure-intolerant patient, using an upper limit of pressure lower than 20 cm H_2O may also improve adherence during the auto-titration. A telephone hotline should be available for interventions similar to one used for chronic PAP treatment. The APAP device is then returned and the information transferred to a computer. The quality of the auto-titration is noted, including the amount of use (adherence), the residual AHI, and amount of leak. Typically, either the 95th percentile pressure or the 90th percentile pressure (depending on device) is chosen for chronic PAP treatment. If the APAP titration is suboptimal because of poor adherence, high leak, or high residual AHI, another attempt may be made using a different mask, heated humidity, or other interventions. Alternatively, the patient may be referred immediately for PSG PAP titration. This option is recommended for patients with very poor adherence to APAP. If two attempts at APAP titration are unsuccessful, the patient should definitely be referred for PSG titration. In Patient A, the auto-titration was ideal (Table P54-1) with good adherence, low leak, a 90th percentile pressure well within the pressure limits, and a good residual AHI. On the basis of this information, CPAP of 12 cm H_2O was used for chronic treatment.

2. **Answer (for Patient B):** A repeat APAP titration or PSG PAP titration

Discussion: The results for Patient B (see Table P54-1) show a high leak, low adherence, a high residual AHI, and *a 90th percentile pressure at the upper pressure limit*. On the basis of this information, either a repeat auto-titration (different mask, settings) or PSG PAP titration is needed.

High leak is associated with poor auto-titrations and ultimately poor adherence to CPAP.[10,11] In general, APAP devices do not function very well when the leak is high. Valentin et al[11] found that, the adherence during auto-titration was predictive of the adherence on subsequent CPAP treatment. Patient B is an example of a poor auto-titration with high leak, poor adherence, and a high residual AHI. The patient complained of being dry despite using a high humidity setting. He reported that his nasal mask was not leaking. This information raised the possibility of a mouth leak with loss of humidity. The patient could be changed from a nasal to a full-face mask or a chin strap added to the nasal mask and the auto-titration repeated. Poor adherence during an APAP titration identifies a patient as high risk for CPAP failure.

The 90th percentile pressure of the APAP titration for patient B is at the upper pressure limit (see Table P54-1, Patient B), and the residual AHI was higher than desired. When the 90th percentile pressure is at the upper pressure limit, it means that the device is constrained from further increases in pressure that could be needed. Although not included in Table P54-1, the AHI in this patient was not caused by an elevated clear airway apnea index. Figure P54-1 shows the titration information from a single night. Note that pressure is constrained by the upper pressure limit (A). The event flags displayed below the pressure tracings show that frequent obstructive apneas (OA) are present. This suggests that high pressure and a higher upper pressure limit are needed in this patient. On the other hand, using higher pressure would not be useful unless the high leak was addressed. While the high residual AHI is a concern, the poor adherence identifies a patient as risk for CPAP treatment failure.

In view of pressure intolerance, low adherence, high leak, and a high residual AHI (suggesting the need for high pressure), the patient was referred for a PSG titration. He ultimately needed bilevel PAP (BPAP) for pressure intolerance, and several full-face mask changes during the titration were needed to find an acceptable interface.

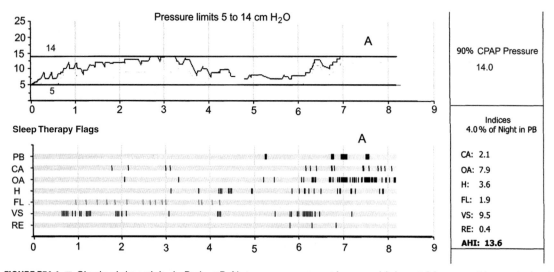

FIGURE P54-1 ■ Single night activity in Patient B. Note pressure cannot increase higher at A because it is constrained by the upper pressure limit. At A on the lower graph (sleep therapy flags are detected events), many obstructive apneas (OAs) were noted. Note that relatively few clear airway (CAs) were noted.

CLINICAL PEARLS

1. Auto-titration (followed by CPAP treatment) or chronic APAP treatment are methods of starting PAP treatment without the need for PSG PAP titration.

2. Proper patient selection is needed for auto-titration and APAP treatment. Patients with known or suspected hypoventilation, a low awake or sleeping baseline SaO_2 (likely need for supplemental oxygen), severe lung disease, central apneas, taking potent narcotics, and congestive heart failure (possibility of Cheyne-Stokes breathing) would benefit from PSG titration rather that auto-titration or APAP treatment. Interventions for central apnea, BPAP intervention for hypoventilation, or the addition of supplemental oxygen could be required.

3. High leak is associated with impaired function of APAP devices and associated with poor adherence during the APAP titration and subsequent CPAP treatment.

4. If the 90th percentile pressure (or 95th percentile pressure) is constrained by the upper pressure limit and the AHI remains elevated, either increase the upper pressure limit or intervene for high mask leak if present.

5. PSG titration should be strongly considered if patients using CPAP at a level determined by auto-titration or those on APAP treatment are not clinically responding to current treatment. This assumes that obvious problems with adherence have been addressed and efforts to optimize mask fit and leak have not resulted in clinical improvement.

REFERENCES

1. Morgenthaler TI, Aurora RN, Brown T, et al: Standards of Practice Committee of the AASM: Practice parameters for the use of autotitrating continuous positive airway pressure devices for titrating pressures and treating adult patients with obstructive sleep apnea syndrome: an update for 2007, *Sleep* 31:141–147, 2008.
2. Masa JF, Jimenez A, Duran J, et al: Alternative methods of titrating continuous positive airway pressure, *Am J Respir Crit Care Med* 170:1218–1224, 2004.
3. Oliver Z, Hoffstein V: Predicting effective continuous positive airway pressure, *Chest* 117:1061–1064, 2000.
4. Fitzpatrick MF, Alloway CED, Wakeford TM, et al: Can patients with obstructive sleep apnea titrate their own continuous positive airway pressure? *Am J Respir Crit Care Med* 167:716–722, 2003.
5. Mulgrew AT, Fox N, Ayas NT, Ryan CF: Diagnosis and initial management of obstructive sleep apnea without polysomnography: a randomized validation study, *Ann Intern Med* 146:157–166, 2007.
6. Berry RB, Hill G, Thompson L, McLaurin V: Portable monitoring and autotitration versus polysomnography for the diagnosis and treatment of sleep apnea, *Sleep* 31:1423–1431, 2008.
7. Antic NA, Buchan C, Esterman A, et al: A randomized controlled trial of nurse-led care for symptomatic moderate-severe obstructive sleep apnea, *Am J Respir Crit Care Med* 179:501–508, 2009.
8. Kuna ST, Gurubhagavatula I, Maislin G, et al: Noninferiority of functional outcome in ambulatory management of obstructive sleep apnea, *Am J Respir Crit Care Med* 183(9):1238–1244, 2011.
9. Rosen CL, Auckley D, Benca R, et al: A multisite randomized trial of portable sleep studies and positive airway pressure autotitration versus laboratory-based polysomnography for the diagnosis and treatment of obstructive sleep apnea: the home PAP study, *Sleep* 35(6):757–767, 2012.
10. Coller D, Stanley D, Parthasarathy S: Effect of air leak on the performance of auto-PAP devices: a bench study, *Sleep Breath* 9(4):167–175, 2005.
11. Valentin A, Subramanian S, Quan SF, et al: Air leak is associated with poor adherence to auto-PAP therapy, *Sleep* 34(6):801–806, 2011.

A Man with OSA Still Sleepy on Nasal CPAP

A 55-year-old man with obstructive sleep apnea (OSA) complained that his continuous positive airway pressure (CPAP) treatment was not working, even though he used it every night. He was started on nasal CPAP at 12 centimeters of water (cm H_2O) based on a split-night study. His wife denied that the patient was snoring on positive pressure ("unless he took it off during the night"). The patient denied problems with mask leaks or dry mouth. He did admit to sometimes removing the mask when he got up during the night to urinate. His Epworth Sleepiness Scale (ESS) score was 20 before CPAP and 14 after CPAP treatment. He reported sleeping 7 hours per night. No history of cataplexy, hypnogogic hallucinations, or symptoms of the restless leg syndrome existed. Results of machine information download are shown in Table P55-1, and 1-month usage information for the patient is shown in Figure P55-1.

TABLE P55-1	CPAP Information		
Days used	28/30	% of nights >4 hours use	90%
Average daily use (all days)	4 hours 10 minutes	AHI	6.5/hour
Average use (days used)	4 hours 20 minutes	Time in large leak	10 minutes

AHI, Apnea–hypopnea index; *CPAP*, continuous positive airway pressure.

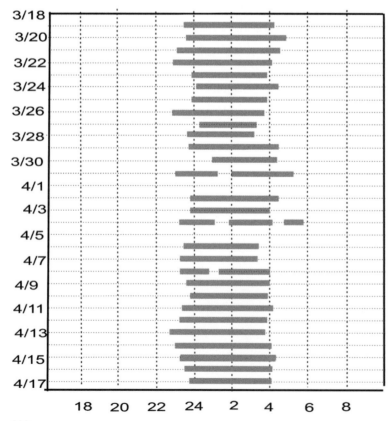

FIGURE P55-1 ■ One month of adherence information in graphical format.

QUESTION

1. Why is the patient still sleepy? Should another CPAP titration be performed?

ANSWER

1. **Answer:** Inadequate CPAP adherence, early removal of mask; optimize adherence before ordering another PAP titration.

   Discussion: A number of possibilities need to be considered when a patient reports persistent sleepiness on PAP (Box P55-1). Although a repeat CPAP titration may be indicated, many other interventions should be attempted before ordering this expensive test.

   The first step in evaluation of complaints of persistent sleepiness on CPAP is obtaining objective adherence information. Objective adherence should be obtained early (1 or 2 weeks, or sooner, after starting CPAP), at regular intervals during the first 6 months of treatment and at every clinic visit. Today, most insurance providers require a face-to-face patient visit after at least 1 month of CPAP use but within the first 3 months to document patient benefit and adequate adherence (usually defined as use >4 hours on ≥70% of nights). The pattern of use may also be instructive. For example, some patients have nights when no CPAP is used at all. Others discontinue CPAP use early in the morning. An important point to remember is that most patients need 7.5 hours of sleep to be well rested. In Figure P55-2, the benefits of CPAP treatment may be seen to improve with greater duration of use. *Although as little as 4 hours of use will often improve subjective sleepiness, most patients require greater use for normalization of sleepiness.* In many patients, the first intervention is educating them about the need to use PAP all night and to obtain an adequate amount of sleep. A typical story is removal of mask for a 4- to 5-AM bathroom trip. Patients should be instructed to leave the mask in place and simply disconnect the hose from the mask. They should also be reminded that the worst desaturation occurs during rapid eye movement (REM) sleep in the early morning hours. Education helps convince the patient to use the mask longer each night.

BOX P55-1	Differential of Persistent Sleepiness on CPAP

1. Inadequate CPAP treatment
   - Inadequate adherence (for optimal rest—7 hours of sleep on PAP)
   - Inadequate pressure
   - Mask leak, mouth leak, or both arousing patient
2. Disturbance of sleep from other factors (leak, pain)
3. Another sleep disorder—narcolepsy, insufficient sleep syndrome, RLS, PLMD
4. Depression or mood disorder
5. Chronic pain syndromes
6. Medical conditions/medications disturbing sleep
7. Entity "Residual sleepiness of OSA"

CPAP, Continuous positive airway pressure; *OSA,* obstructive sleep apnea; *PLMD,* periodic limb movement disorder; *RLS,* restless leg syndrome.

FIGURE P55-2 ■ Note the values are a percentage of normal values rather than the raw values. The Epworth Sleepiness Scale (ESS) is a higher percentage of normal as the amount of continuous positive airway pressure (CPAP) increases. *FOSQ,* Functional outcomes of sleep questionnaire (higher score better qualify of life); *MSLT,* multiple sleep latency test (measures objective sleepiness [mean sleep latency increases with treatment]). (From Weaver TE, Maislin G, Dinges DF, et al: Relationship between hours of CPAP use and achieving normal levels of sleepiness and daily functioning, *Sleep* 30:711-719, 2007.)

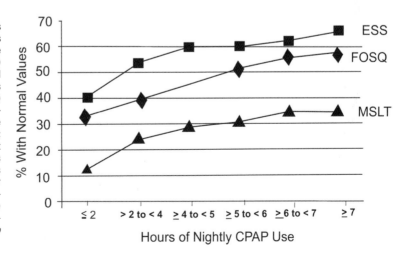

TABLE P55-2 Useful Questions at CPAP Follow-Up		
Questions to ask	**Possible Problems**	**Interventions**
Average nightly use	Overestimation of usage	Objective adherence
Snoring on CPAP	Inadequate pressure Weight gain High leak	Increase pressure (unless high leak) Weight loss Reduce leak
Mask discomfort	Incorrect mask size Old mask (cushion deterioration) Wrong mask type Incorrect application	Change mask size Replace mask regularly Change mask type Educate about mask application
Air blowing out of the mouth	Mouth leak	Chin strap Full-face (oronasal) mask Heated humidity
Mask leak causing noise, arousals, eye irritation	Poor mask fit or application	Refit mask or change mask; educate
Dry mouth	Mouth leak Mask leak Nasal congestion No humidification used Humidity setting too low	Intervene for mask or mouth leak Treat nasal congestion Add heated humidity Increase humidity setting Check humidifier function (if not using water)
Pulling mask off unconsciously during the night	Mask or mouth Leak Mask discomfort Inadequate pressure	Mask off alarm Improve mask seal and comfort Consider increase in pressure Consider PAP titration study

CPAP, Continuous positive airway pressure.

Many devices provide information on the residual apnea–hypopnea index (AHI), amount of snoring and amount of leak. However, the residual AHI is not always accurate and is most helpful if low (high predictive value for good treatment). If the AHI is high the result is accurate about 60% to 80% of the time. One option would be to perform oximetry at home on the current CPAP. A persistent sawtooth pattern documents inadequate treatment. If the amount of leak is high, simply improving the seal of the mask interface may normalize the AHI. In general, a slight increase in the residual AHI would not be expected to have a significant impact on alertness. However, inexperienced clinicians *may to be more concerned about a residual AHI of 10/hr than the need for the patient to use CPAP for much more than 4 hours.*

In Table P55-2, useful questions for the patient and bedmate are listed. Questioning the bedmate about snoring, mask and mouth leaks may be very instructive. Snoring on CPAP is a simple way to detect the need for slightly higher pressure. On the other hand, if the leak is high, improvement in mask fit or adjustment of the mask is essential before increasing pressure. If mouth leak is suspected (nasal mask), the addition of a chin strap or switch to a full face mask could be considered. *When trying new masks, it is essential to pressurize them in the office to immediately detect a poor fit or poor adjustment.* The other issue is that mask should be changed on a regular basis. The cushions on old masks may lose their ability to seal if the material deteriorates. Patients often overtighten their masks in an attempt to compensate for poor mask fit or seal. Different mask type or sizes should be tried, if necessary.

In discussing adherence issues with patients, it is important to emphasize that many patients who ultimately do well with CPAP have difficult periods of adaptation. Reminding patients of the long-term benefits and being supportive may establish a good relationship. In this regard, having the patient join OSA support groups may help. Patients who hear success stories from other patients may be more likely to persist during the adaptation period.

If inadequate CPAP treatment is eliminated as a cause for persistent sleepiness, other sleep disorders and medical disorders must be considered. Patients with OSA may have narcolepsy (ask about cataplexy), periodic limb movement disorder, depression, and chronic pain syndromes. Medications are also a cause of daytime sleepiness. It is important to recall that insufficient sleep is the most common cause of daytime sleepiness. Although CPAP adherence of 6 hours per night is considered "good adherence," many patients will benefit from more sleep (using CPAP). Another potential problem is the 1-hour afternoon nap without using CPAP.

If all else fails, repeat titration may be ordered. To maximize benefit, the sleep study order should include definite instructions, including the patient's current pressure and mask. If narcolepsy is suspected, polysomnography (PSG) on CPAP and multiple sleep latency test (MSLT) to follow while the patient uses CPAP could be considered. However, a group of patients with OSA but without another sleep disorder do appear to have persistent daytime sleepiness despite adequate CPAP adherence and treatment (Hypersomnia due to Medical Condition, see Fundamentals 34). No more specific diagnostic category exists for these patients.

A diagnosis of hypersomnia caused by a medical disorder could be considered. Modafinil (racemic) and armodafinil (R-enatiomer of modafinil) are approved by the U.S. Food and Drug Administration (FDA) for persistent sleepiness in patients who have OSA despite treatment. If modafinil is started, it is important to monitor the patients to ensure that PAP adherence does not decrease. Modafinil does not prevent nocturnal hypoxemia and the impact of OSA on blood pressure and cardiovascular morbidity. An occasional patient will not respond to modafinil, and the off-label use of a traditional stimulant (dextroamphetamine, methyphenidate) could be considered. The use of modafinil is discussed in sections on narcolepsy.

In the present case, the adherence pattern shows that CPAP was used on nearly all nights but that *the duration of use was not optimal.* CPAP was removed around 4 AM nearly every night. Although the residual AHI was slightly above 5/hr, this would have a minor effect on the restorative nature of sleep. The patient's wife reported that no snoring or apnea was noted. When confronted with objective data, the patient admitted that he rarely replaced the CPAP when he got up to urinate at night. Putting the mask and headgear back on seemed too difficult at 4 AM. The patient was instructed to keep his mask on and simply disconnect the hose at the mask. He also admitted that by 4 AM his mask was uncomfortable. A different brand of mask was prescribed. The patient was educated about the severity of oxygen desaturation during REM sleep in the last hour or two of the night. On a return visit in 4 weeks, the average night compliance had increased to 6.5 hours and the ESS score was now 12/24. On a subsequent visit after another 3 months, the average nightly adherence was 7.5 hours and the ESS score was 9/24 (normal).

CLINICAL PEARLS

1. Objective adherence information is essential to optimize PAP treatment and should be a part of every follow-up visit. Objective adherence information should be obtained within the first week of treatment and at regular intervals.

2. Questioning the bedmate about the presence of snoring, apnea, mask leak, or mouth leak can be helpful.

3. Although the minimum PAP usage acceptable for most insurance providers to continue to pay for CPAP treatment is 4 hours per night on 70% or more of nights, this is much too little sleep on CPAP for many patients to have a full resolution of symptoms.

4. Attention should be paid to a pattern of early removal of CPAP (4 AM bathroom trip) and education provided to the patient about the importance of using PAP for the entire night.

5. The device residual AHI information is helpful but is not always accurate. If the result does not fit the clinical picture, the accuracy should be questioned. A low AHI is highly predictive of good treatment efficacy, but an elevated AHI is not always correct. If leak is elevated, it should be optimized. If the AHI is elevated a slightly higher pressure could be tried (assuming leak optimized first). Oximetry could be performed at home of CPAP. The definitive study is PSG titration, but the technologist should be informed of the current pressure to avoid wasting time on pressures that are much too low to be effective.

6. If the combination of high leak and high AHI is present, the first intervention is correction of leak, although an increase in pressure may also be needed.

7. If narcolepsy is suspected, a PSG using CPAP followed by an MSLT using CPAP should be ordered. It is important that medications affecting REM sleep be discontinued before the study (ideally 2 weeks before the study). (see patient 89).

8. If residual sleepiness is present in a patient with OSA after treatment is optimized, the addition of an alerting agent may be effective (modafinil, armodafinil). Adherence should be monitored closely, as some patients tend to use CPAP less once an alerting agent is started.

BIBLIOGRAPHY

Kakkar RK, Berry RB: Positive airway pressure treatment for obstructive sleep apnea, *Chest* 132:1057–1072, 2007.

Budhiraja R, Parthasarathy S, Drake CL, et al: Early CPAP use identified subsequent adherence to CPAP therapy, *Sleep* 30:320–324, 2007.

Weaver TE, Maislin G, Dinges DF, et al: Relationship between hours of CPAP use and achieving normal levels of sleepiness and daily functioning, *Sleep* 30:711–719, 2007.

Berry RB, Kushida CA, Kryger MH, et al: Respiratory event detection by a positive airway pressure device, *Sleep* 35(3):361–367, 2012.

Valentin A, Subramanian S, Quan SF, et al: Air leak is associated with poor adherence to autoPAP therapy, *Sleep* 34(6):801–806, 2011.

Pack AI, Black JE, Schwartz JR, Matheson JK: Modafinil as adjunct therapy for daytime sleepiness in obstructive sleep apnea, *Am J Respir Crit Care Med* 164(9):1675–1681, 2001.

Schwartz JR, Khan A, McCall WV, et al: Tolerability and efficacy of armodafinil in naïve patients with excessive sleepiness associated with obstructive sleep apnea, shift work disorder, or narcolepsy: a 12-month, open-label, flexible-dose study with an extension period, *J Clin Sleep Med* 6(5):450–457, 2010.

PATIENT 56

A Retired Nurse with Nocturia and Snoring

Discussion: A retired 65-year-old female nurse had a long history of snoring. However, her major complaint was three to four nocturnal awakenings to urinate. It often required 30 minutes to an hour to return to sleep. She did not take diuretics after noon and restricted her fluid and salt intake without improvement in nocturia. The patient also eliminated beverages containing caffeine. Her primary care doctor evaluated her and found no evidence of urinary tract infection or glycosuria. The patient's medications included lisinopril and levothyroxine. The patient lived by herself, so no observer could comment of the presence of apnea. The patient reported feeling tired and groggy in the morning as well as mild daytime sleepiness (Epworth Sleepiness Scale [ESS] score of 12). She attributed these symptoms to the nocturia. Her first statement to the sleep physician interviewing her was that she "knew all about CPAP and did not want it."

Physical examination: Body mass index (BMI) 31 kilograms per square meter (kg/m^2); HEENT Mallampati 3; neck 16 inches; chest clear to auscultation; cardiovascular: regular rhythm, no murmurs; extremities: no edema

QUESTION

1. Is a sleep study indicated? Could the nocturia be caused by untreated sleep apnea?

ANSWER

1. **Answer:** Polysomnography (PSG) is indicated, given the unexplained awakenings and nocturia.

   Discussion: The presentation of obstructive sleep apnea (OSA) in older adults appears to differ from that in younger individuals.[1,2] A study by Endeshaw[2] of community-dwelling patients age >62 years found that traditional risk factors such as snoring, BMI, and neck circumference were not significantly associated with OSA. An apnea–hypopnea index (AHI) of 15 or more per hour (hr) was independently associated with not feeling well rested in the morning, a higher ESS score, and greater frequency of nocturia.

Snoring may be less reported in older adults because of decreased hearing acuity in the bed partner or the fact that the bed partner may also have OSA. Postmenopausal women have four times the risk of developing OSA compared with premenopausal women. Available information suggests that the presence of untreated sleep apnea increases the risk of cognitive decline in older women.[3] Treating OSA in patients with dementia with continuous positive airway pressure (CPAP) may improve outcomes.[4] Therefore, identification and treatment of OSA in older adults is important both for quality of life issues as well as maintenance of intellectual function. Studies also suggest that adherence to PAP is no worse in older adult patients.[5]

It has been a common clinical observation that many patients with OSA who start CPAP treatment report fewer awakenings to urinate. Hajduk and coworkers[6] found a high incidence of pathologic nocturia (PN; defined as ≥2 urination events per night) in OSA patients. The percentage of PN was 47.8% and age, arousal index, AHI, and measures of oxygenation were predictors of the presence of PN. Some of the reported effects of CPAP treatment could be attributed to better sleep. However, studies have shown reduced sodium excretion in patients with OSA treated with CPAP. Krieger and colleagues[7] found that patients with OSA had greater urinary flows and great urinary sodium excretion compared with controls. Nasal CPAP resulted in a reduction in urinary flow and sodium and chloride excretion. Fitzgerald and coworkers[8] found that CPAP decreased nocturia in OSA patients. A second study by Krieger et al found evidence of increased guanosine 3'5'-cyclic monophosphate excretion in untreated patients with OSA, which reflects atrial natriuretic peptide (ANP) release.[9] The authors hypothesized that atrial stretch during sleep apnea induced release of ANP, which caused increased sodium excretion. Umlauf and associates[10] also found increased nocturia and elevated urinary ANP, when the AHI was greater than or equal to 15/hr. However, not all studies have found an increase in ANP in patients with OSA and nocturia.[11] Other studies[12] suggest that high nocturnal blood pressure may cause a higher glomerular renal filtrate (GRF) and naturesis.[11] Gjørup et al[12] concluded that the higher fractional excretion of sodium in untreated OSA is likely attributable to pressure natriuresis. The correlation between mean arginine vasopression (AVP) levels and blood pressure suggested to the authors that AVP may be part of the pathogenetic mechanism underlying hypertension in these patients. In summary, the mechanism of nocturnal natriuresis and nocturia in untreated OSA has not been firmly established. However, convincing evidence suggests that treatment with CPAP reduces the nocturnal natriuresis and nocturia.

The present patient agreed to a diagnostic sleep study only after much discussion. The study showed an AHI of 60/hr, with 50% of events being obstructive apneas and 50% hypopneas. The arterial oxygen desaturation was frequent but mild. The results surprised the patient, who reluctantly agreed to proceed with CPAP titration. The most convincing argument was information that nocturia might decrease. During the night in the sleep center, only one awakening to urinate was noted, and the patients slept well on CPAP. The patient reported that she sleeps very well on CPAP at home with zero or one episode of nocturia per night. She is now enthusiastic about CPAP treatment.

CLINICAL PEARLS

1. The presentation of OSA in older adults is different. Patients are less likely to be obese or complain of snoring. Older patients with OSA are more likely to complain of not feeling well rested in the morning and nocturia.

2. Nocturia in older men is frequently assumed to be caused by benign prostatic hyperplasia (BPH), diuretics, or bladder dysfunction, so the clue that OSA could be present is often missed.

3. Nocturia is frequently present in patients with OSA and often improves following effective CPAP treatment.

4. The etiology of OSA associated nocturia is not known with certainty. Studies have consistently shown a nocturnal natriuresis in untreated OSA but have not agreed on the mechanism. Increased ANP or higher nocturnal blood pressure (increased GFR) may be possible causes.

5. CPAP adherence is not worse in older adults.

6. Nocturnal hypoxemia, untreated OSA, or a combination of both is a risk factor for the development of cognitive impairment in older adults.

7. Preliminary evidence suggests that CPAP treatment in patients with dementia and OSA may improve outcomes.

REFERENCES

1. Russell T, Duntley S: Sleep disordered breathing in the elderly, *Am J Med* 124(12):1123–1126, 2011.
2. Endeshaw Y: Clinical characteristics of obstructive sleep apnea in community-dwelling older adults, *J Am Geriatr Soc* 54 (11):1740–1744, 2006.

3. Yaffe K, Laffan AM, Harrison SL, et al: Sleep-disordered breathing, hypoxia, and risk of mild cognitive impairment and dementia in older women, *JAMA* 306(6):613–619, 2011.
4. Cooke JR, Ayalon L, Palmer BW, et al: Sustained use of CPAP slows deterioration of cognition, sleep, and mood in patients with Alzheimer's disease and obstructive sleep apnea: a preliminary study, *J Clin Sleep Med* 5(4):305–309, 2009, 2011.
5. Parish JM, Lyng PJ, Wisbey J: Compliance with CPAP in elderly patients with OSA, *Sleep Med* 1(3):209–214, 2000.
6. Hajduk IA, Strollo PJ, Jasani RR, et al: Prevalence and predictors of nocturia in obstructive sleep apnea hypopnea syndrome—a retrospective study, *Sleep* 26:61–64, 2003.
7. Krieger J, Imbs JL, Schmidt M, Kurtz D: Renal function in patients with obstructive sleep apnea. Effects of nasal continuous positive airway pressure, *Arch Intern Med* 148:1337–1340, 1988.
8. Fitzgerald MP, Mulligan M, Parthasarathy S: Nocturic frequency is related to severity of obstructive sleep apnea, improves with continuous positive airways treatment, *Am J Obstet Gynecol* 194:1399–1403, 2006.
9. Krieger J, Schmidt M, Sforza E, et al: Urinary excretion of guanosine 3′:5′-cyclic monophosphate during sleep in obstructive sleep apnea patients with and without nasal continuous positive airway pressure, *Clin Sci (Lond)* 76:31–37, 1989.
10. Umlauf MG, Chasens ER, Greevy RA, et al: Obstructive sleep apnea, nocturia and polyuria in older adults, *Sleep* 27:139–144, 2004.
11. Rodenstein DO, D'Odemont JP, Pieters T, Aubert-Tulkens G: Diurnal and nocturnal diuresis and natriuresis in obstructive sleep apnea. Effects of nasal continuous positive airway pressure therapy, *Am Rev Respir Dis* 145(6):1367–1371, 1992.
12. Gjørup PH, Sadauskiene L, Wessels J, et al: Increased nocturnal sodium excretion in obstructive sleep apnoea. Relation to nocturnal change in diastolic blood pressure, *Scand J Clin Lab Invest* 68(1):11–21, 2008.

PATIENT 57

A Patient with Claustrophobia

A 50-year-old man had mild obstructive sleep apnea (OSA) (apnea–hypopnea index [AHI] = 10 per hour [hr] and minimum saturation of arterial oxygen [SaO_2] = 90%) on a previous partial-night sleep study. Use of a split-night study was mandated because of insurance issues. During the continuous positive airway pressure (CPAP) titration portion of the study, the patient slept very little and could not tolerate CPAP because of claustrophobia. Because daytime sleepiness was severe (Epworth Sleepiness Scale [ESS] = 16) and sleep apnea mild the patient's primary physician ordered polysomnography (PSG) followed by a multiple sleep latency test (MSLT) to rule out narcolepsy. No cataplexy was reported. However, severe OSA was noted on PSG (AHI 40/hr, with frequent mild to moderate arterial oxygen desaturations). The MSLT was cancelled.

QUESTIONS

1. Why was the severity of OSA underestimated by the first study?

2. What treatment alternatives do you offer to this patient?

ANSWERS

Answer 1: The diagnostic portion of a split-sleep study may underestimate OSA severity.

Answer 2: Treatment alternatives include use of a nasal pillow mask, densensitization to masks and CPAP treatment, and nasal expiratory PAP (EPAP).

> **Discussion:** In the current patient, review of the split-night study showed no supine or rapid eye movement (REM) sleep in the diagnostic portion of the study. This is not uncommon, and when judging the severity of OSA, it is useful to know if the AHI was derived on the basis of the diagnostic portion of a split-sleep study or a diagnostic study with limited REM or supine sleep.

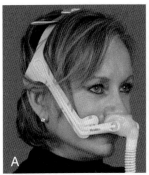
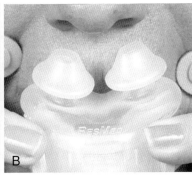
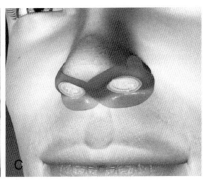

FIGURE P57-1 ■ **A** and **B,** A nasal pillows mask (Swift LT, ResMed, Poway, CA). **C,** Nasal EPAP device. Single-use valves are inserted into each nostril and sealed with adhesive. (**A** and **B,** From Berry RB: *Fundamentals of sleep medicine,* Philadelphia, 2012, Saunders, p 322, from Berry RB, Kryger MH, Massie CA: A novel nasal expiratory positive airway pressure (EPAP) device for the treatment of obstructive sleep apnea: a randomized controlled trial, *Sleep* 34[4]:479-485, 2011.)

Patients who do not tolerate PAP via traditional nasal masks or full-face masks may tolerate titration or treatment with a nasal pillows mask. These masks provide a seal through the use of cone shaped pillows that insert into each nostril (Figure P57-1, *A* and *B*). Pressure causes the pillow material to expand slightly and creates a seal. A variety of these masks are available, and the major issue is finding the correct size of pillow mask for each patient. Finding a mask with the proper pillow shape and angle of entry into the nostrils may require trying several brands of masks. Using too small a pillow size causes leak unless the mask is overtightened, and this may cause nasal pain with prolonged use, even if tolerated briefly. Some patients also do not like head straps, and for such patients, masks that fit around the ears are available. Nasal pillow masks are especially useful in patients with mustaches and for edentulous patients who have no dental support to resist the mask pressure on the upper lip. Some patients have difficult-to-seal nasal bridges or have problems with air leak into the eyes. These patients may do well with a nasal pillows mask. A water-based gel may be used to avoid irritation of the entry area into the nose caused by the pillow. In our experience, *when patients are switched from a traditional nasal mask to a pillows mask, they often complain that the pressure feels much higher.* The pressure drop across the nasal inlet is eliminated. A slightly lower pressure may be needed when changing to a nasal pillow mask.

If severe claustrophobia is present, even the use of a nasal pillows mask may not be tolerated. In this case, desensitization, with or without the assistance of a behavioral specialist such as a psychologist, may be tried. In general, the techniques involve slowly introducing the object that causes distress, for example, wearing a mask while watching television during the day for progressive periods. Very low CPAP pressure could be used or the mask adjusted to minimize rebreathing. Densensitization may be used with or without relaxation treatment or the addition of an anxiolytic medication. An example is to construct a behavioral hierarchy which, in increasing order of perceived difficulty, consists of the following five "steps": (1) wearing the CPAP nasal pillow mask at home for 1 hour each day while awake; (2) attaching the mask to the CPAP apparatus, switching the unit to the "on" position and practicing breathing through the mask for 1 hour while watching television, reading, or performing some other sedentary activity; (3) using CPAP during 1-hour, scheduled naps at home; (4) using CPAP during initial 3 to 4 hours of nocturnal sleep, and (5) using CPAP through an entire night's sleep. When the patient reports performing one step for 5 consecutive days without anxiety, he or she is encouraged to move to the next, more difficult step. For more details see the article by Edinger and Radtke.

Nasal EPAP

One-way valves inserted into each nostril and sealed with band-aid adhesive provide PAP during exhalation (nasal EPAP) (Provent, Theravent, Inc.) (see Figure P57-1, *C*). Inspiration is without resistance, but exhalation meets a resistance, and back pressure is generated. The mechanism of action is unknown but likely includes an increase in end-expiratory lung volume, an increase upper airway size by pneumatic effect, or a slight increase in partial pressure of carbon dioxide (PCO_2) (stabilizes breathing). About 50% to 60% of patients have *a 50% decrease in the AHI or a reduction in the AHI to less than 10/hr.* Patients with OSA severity of all degrees may respond. The treatment AHI is not reliably as low as CPAP but may be acceptable to patients not tolerating CPAP for multiple reasons, including claustrophobia. *Because nasal EPAP is not effective in all patients, a sleep study with the device in place must be ordered to document adequate OSA treatment.* Customized nasal cannulas are available and may be attached to the nasal EPAP valves to enable recording nasal pressure.

Some patients doing well on CPAP treatment may use nasal EPAP for convenience while traveling. Side effects are minimal, and the main obstacle to use is difficulty falling asleep with the device in place. It takes several nights to adapt to nasal EPAP. Patients are instructed to breathe in through the nose and out through the mouth until they fall asleep. Thirty-day starter packs use graded increases in resistance to improve adaptation. The devices are single-use items. Patients cannot have severe nasal obstruction or an allergy to the band-aid adhesive. A lower resistance device for preventing snoring is sold without a prescription. Mouth leak causes a drop in pressure, and if intermittent mouth leak is a problem, a chin strap could be used. Postural treatment may also be added to improve effectiveness.

CLINICAL PEARLS

1. The severity of OSA may be underestimated by the diagnostic portion of split-night (partial-night) studies.
2. Problems with the mask interface are the most frequent side effects of PAP treatment.
3. The clinician must be persistent in trying different sizes, types, and brands of interfaces until an adequate one is found (trial and error).
4. Claustrophobia may be approached by using nasal pillow–type interfaces and desensitization.
5. Nasal EPAP provides a treatment option for patients unable to tolerate PAP. Adaptation to the device takes several nights. A sleep study while the patient wears the device must ordered to document efficacy. Nasal EPAP is effective in about 50% of patients across all AHI severities.

BIBLIOGRAPHY

Massie CA, Hart RW: Clinical outcomes related to interface type in patients with obstructive sleep apnea/hypopnea syndrome who are using continuous positive airway pressure, *Chest* 123:1112–1118, 2003.

Ryan S, Garvey JF, Swan V, et al: Nasal pillows as an alternative interface in patients with obstructive sleep apnoea syndrome initiating continuous positive airway pressure therapy, *J Sleep Res* 20(2):367–373, 2011.

Berry RB, Kryger MH, Massie CA: A novel nasal expiratory positive airway pressure (EPAP) device for the treatment of obstructive sleep apnea: a randomized controlled trial, *Sleep* 34(4):479–485, 2011.

Kryger MH, Berry RB, Massie CA: Long-term use of a nasal expiratory positive airway pressure (EPAP) device as a treatment for obstructive sleep apnea (OSA), *J Clin Sleep Med* 7(5):449–453, 2011.

Means MK, Edinger JD: Graded exposure therapy for addressing claustrophobic reactions to continuous positive airway pressure: a case series report, *Behav Sleep Med* 5(2):105–116, 2007.

Edinger JD, Radtke RA: Use of in vivo desensitization to treat a patient's claustrophobic response to nasal CPAP, *Sleep* 16(7):678–680, 1993.

Chasens ER, Pack AI, Maislin G, et al: Claustrophobia and adherence to CPAP treatment, *West J Nurs Res* 27(3):307–321, 2005.

An Obese 12-Year-Old with Sleep Apnea and Enlarged Tonsils

A 12-year-old boy (body mass index [BMI]% = 99)* underwent evaluation for complaints of snoring, restlessness, inattention, and declining school performance. The patient had no other medial problems. Physical examination showed enlarged tonsils and obesity. The patient underwent a sleep study, which demonstrated severe obstructive sleep apnea (OSA) (Table P58-1).

TABLE P58-1 Sleep Study Results	
TST (min)	393.5
AHI total (#/hr)	20.1
AHI NREM (#/hr)	15.2
AHI REM (#/hr)	39.0
OA (#)	38
CA (#)	4
MA (#)	0
Hypopneas (#)	90
Low SpO_2 NREM	82%
Low SpO_2 REM	82%
$ETCO_2$	Peak 62 torr

AHI, Apnea–hypopnea index; *CA*, central apnea; *MA*, mixed apnea; *ETCO2*, end-tidal carbon dioxide; *OA*, obstructive apnea; *min*, minutes; *NREM*, non–rapid eye movement; *REM*, rapid eye movement; *SpO2*, saturation of peripheral oxygen; *TST*, total sleep time.

QUESTION

1. What treatment do you recommend?
   A. Continuous positive airway pressure (CPAP)
   B. Tonsillectomy and adenoidectomy (TNA)
   C. Weight loss
   D. Intranasal steroids, montelukast, or both

ANSWER

1. **Answer:** (B) Tonsillectomy and Adenoidectomy (TNA)

   Discussion: TNA is the treatment of choice for pediatric patients with adeno-tonsillar hypertrophy diagnosed with significant OSA, even if they are obese and the OSA is severe. Recall that in pediatric patients ages 4 to 8 years, an AHI of 5-10 is considered moderate and >10/hr is severe. The rationale for TNA as the initial treatment is that most patients receive some benefit from TNA, and compliance

*BMI% ≥85 to <95% = overweight; ≥95% obese; ≥99% high risk. BMI% is the BMI value based on a population. For example 85 BMI% means a BMI above or at 85% of the population for a given age and gender.

to PAP, even with the best support system, is around 50%. It is acknowledged that significant residual OSA is still present in at least one third of patients following treatment with TNA. Predictors of residual OSA following TNA are listed in Box P58-1. The absolute and relative contraindications for TNA are listed in Box P58-2. Risk factors for perioperative complications associated with TNA are listed in Box P58-3. Those with risk factors for complications should have surgery performed in the hospital with careful monitoring after surgery. Polysomnography (PSG) should be performed after surgical healing if residual symptoms of sleep apnea are present or if the patient is at high risk for significant residual apnea–hypopnea index [AHI]. If mild OSA is still present after TNA, use of nasal steroids or montelukast (Singulair) may be tried. Montelukast is a selective and orally active leukotriene receptor antagonist that inhibits the cysteinyl leukotriene CysLT1 receptor. Adeno-tonsillar tissue contains an abundance of these receptors. Studies have shown benefit either with or without previous TNA. Weight loss is recommended for obese children with OSA, but significant weight loss is often difficult to obtain and maintain.

The current patient was obese with a severely elevated AHI. He underwent TNA in the hospital but did well. A PSG after 3 months showed an AHI of 5/hour but symptoms had dramatically improved.

BOX P58-1	Risk Factors for Persistent OSA after TNA

1. High presurgery AHI (> 10/hour)   3. Craniofacial abnormalities
2. Obesity   4. Neuromuscular disease

From Marcus CL, Brooks LJ, Draper KA, et al, for the American Academy of Pediatrics: Diagnosis and management of childhood obstructive sleep apnea syndrome, *Pediatrics* 130(3):e714-e755, 2012; Marcus CL, Brooks LJ, Draper KA, et al, for the American Academy of Pediatrics: Diagnosis and management of childhood obstructive sleep apnea syndrome (Technical Report), *Pediatrics* 130(3):576-584, 2012.
AHI, Apnea–hypopnea index; *OSA*, obstructive sleep apnea; *TNA*, tonsillectomy and adenoidectomy.

BOX P58-2	Contraindications for Adeno-Tonsillectomy

ABSOLUTE CONTRAINDICATIONS	RELATIVE CONTRAINDICATIONS
No adeno-tonsillar tissue (tissue has previously been surgically removed)	Very small tonsils or adenoids Morbid obesity and small tonsils or adenoid Bleeding disorder refractory to treatment Submucous cleft palate Other medical conditions making patient medically unstable for surgery

---

BOX P58-3	Risk Factors for Perioperative Complications from TNA

Severe OSAS on polysomnography* Cardiac complications of OSAS Failure to thrive Obesity	Craniofacial anomalies Neuromuscular disorders Current respiratory infection

---

From Marcus CL, Brooks LJ, Draper KA, et al, for the American Academy of Pediatrics: Diagnosis and management of childhood obstructive sleep apnea syndrome, *Pediatrics* 130(3):e714-e755, 2012.
OSAS, Obstructive sleep apnea syndrome; *TNA*, tonsillectomy and adenoidectomy.
*Note: It is difficult to provide exact polysomnographic criteria for severity because these criteria will vary depending on the age of the child; additional comorbidities such as obesity, asthma, or cardiac complications of OSAS and other polysomnographic criteria that have not been evaluated in the literature such as the level of hypercapnia.

CLINICAL PEARLS

1. In pediatric patients with enlarged tonsillar tissue, TNA is recommended as the initial treatment for OSA, even if the AHI is severely increased and obesity is present. Most patients with adeno-tonsillar hypertrophy will receive benefit.

2. Repeat PSG after TNA is needed in patients who are still symptomatic or in those at high risk for a significant residual AHI after TNA.

3. Nasal steroids and oral montelukast are treatment options for persistent mild OSA after TNA.

4. CPAP is used for moderate to severe residual OSA following TNA.

5. Weight loss is always recommended for obese children with OSA, but it takes time and is often difficult to maintain.

BIBLIOGRAPHY

Marcus CL, Brooks LJ, Draper KA, et al: for the American Academy of Pediatrics: Diagnosis and management of childhood obstructive sleep apnea syndrome, *Pediatrics* 130(3):e714–e755, 2012.

Marcus CL, Brooks LJ, Draper KA, et al: for the American Academy of Pediatrics: Diagnosis and management of childhood obstructive sleep apnea syndrome (Technical Report), *Pediatrics* 130(3):576–584, 2012.

Kheirandish L, Goldbart AD, Gozal D: Intranasal steroids and oral leukotriene modifier therapy in residual sleep-disordered breathing after tonsillectomy and adenoidectomy in children, *Pediatrics* 117(1):e61–e66, 2006.

Goldbart AD, Goldman JL, Veling MC, Gozal D: Leukotriene modifier therapy for mild sleep-disordered breathing in children, *Am J Respir Crit Care Med* 172(3):364–370, 2005.

Tapia IE, Marcus CL: Newer treatment modalities for pediatric obstructive sleep apnea, *Paediatr Respir Rev* 14(3):199–203, 2013.

PATIENT 59

Persistent OSA after TNA

A 10-year-old boy (body mass index percentage [BMI%] = 103*) was evaluated for symptoms of snoring, restlessness, obesity, behavioral issues, and declining school performance. He underwent a sleep study which demonstrated severe OSA, and the sleep study results are listed in Table P59-1. He was seen for follow-up 3 months after surgery, and his family reported that his snoring and restlessness at night had improved but not resolved entirely. He continued to have problems with behavior and school performance.

TABLE P59-1 Sleep Study Results Before and After TNA

	Prior to TNA	After TNA
TST (min)	393.5	466.5
AHI total (#/hr)	31.6	9.7
AHI NREM (#/hr)	29.8	6.7
AHI REM (#/hr)	39.0	15.0
OA (#)	38	2
CA (#)	4	9
Hypopneas (#)	165	64
Low SpO$_2$ NREM	82%	94%
Low SpO$_2$ REM	82%	88%
ETCO$_2$	Peak 62 torr	Peak 53 torr

AHI, Apnea–hypopnea index; *CA*, central apnea; *ETCO$_2$*, end-tidal carbon dioxide; *OA*, obstructive apnea; *min*, minutes; *NREM*, non–rapid eye movement; *REM*, rapid eye movement; *SpO$_2$*, saturation of peripheral oxygen; *TNA*, tonsillectomy and adenoidectomy; *TST*, total sleep time.
No mixed apneas were recorded

---

*BMI% ≥85 to <95% = overweight; ≥95% obese; ≥99% high risk. BMI% is the BMI value based on a population. For example 85 BMI% means a BMI above or at 85% of the population for a given age and gender.

QUESTION

1. Is further treatment warranted for this boy? If so, what are the options for additional treatment?

ANSWER

1. **Answer:** Yes, further treatment is indicated. Consider continuous positive airway pressure (CPAP).

   Discussion: On his initial sleep study, this boy was found to have severe obstructive sleep apnea (OSA), with both nocturnal and daytime symptoms. The initial treatment of choice for most children with OSA and adeno-tonsillar hypertrophy is tonsillectomy and adenoidectomy (TNA). Children with severe OSA seen on their initial study, residual symptoms, or both should be reevaluated after TNA to determine evidence of residual OSA. The patient's family reported an improvement but lack of complete resolution of his symptoms and ongoing behavioral and academic issues. His post-TNA study demonstrated improvement in his OSA but residual moderate obstruction with residual hypoxemia and hypercarbia. This patient should have additional treatment for his residual OSA because of his abnormal apnea–hypopnea index (AHI) and significant ongoing symptoms. Note that in children, severity by the AHI is very different from that in adults. Most clinicians consider a normal AHI to be <1, an AHI of 1 to 4/hr (mild OSA), an AHI of 5 to 10 (moderate OSA), and >10/hour (severe OSA). Many pediatricians obstructive AHI (OAHDI, does not include central apnea) to determine severity.

   Options for treatment in patients with residual AHI after TNA include PAP, weight loss, and use of montelukast or nasal steroids, which may be combined. The rational for the use of montelukast or nasal steroids is that often some adenoidal or tonsillar tissue remains. Montelukast is a leukotriene inhibitor that may reduce tonsillar tissue. Although most normal children will have a significant resolution of their OSA symptoms, recent reports show 60% of children may have residual OSA and obese children are more likely to have incomplete resolution of their OSA after TNA. Weight loss is always a goal for patients with obesity. However, weight loss is difficult to accomplish and may take an extended period. Additional therapy should be offered to improve this child's sleep and give him a better chance of improving his daytime symptoms. PAP treatment may be accomplished in children, but the approach is different from that for adults. Children should be desensitized gradually to the CPAP mask to improve their acceptance of PAP in the short term and the long term. Split-night studies should not be attempted unless the child has had a previous positive experience with CPAP. If the laboratory staff attempts to "make" the child wear CPAP, it may result in frightening the patient and decreasing the likelihood that the child will be able to use PAP in the long run. The child should take the mask home and gradually increase the time wearing the mask while engaging in a fun activity (e.g., watching a favorite movie or video). The technologists should be experienced, patient, and willing to work with children. Positive reinforcement should be used ("catch them doing something good") to encourage the patient during PAP titration. Objective assessment should be obtained in children as in adults to determine actual PAP use, leak, and residual AHI. Patients should be monitored closely to resolve problems with PAP initiation promptly. Children will require reevaluation of their PAP needs more frequently compared with adults, as children continue to grow and develop. Behavioral specialists play a key role in helping children and their families overcome barriers to the use of CPAP.

   An additional option for treating residual OSA after TNA is treatment with montelukast with or without nasal steroids. Recent studies have shown improvement in residual OSA after TNA with montelukast and nasal steroids. Additional studies have shown improvement in OSA with montelukast treatment without prior TNA.

   Rapid maxillary expansion (RME) is an orthodontic procedure that increases the width of the maxilla, reduces nasal resistance and may be helpful in patients with a maxillary transverse deficiency or "cross-bite." Clinically, a maxillary transverse deficiency is suspected when the upper jaw is too narrow for upper teeth to occlude properly with mandibular teeth. Several studies have demonstrated the effectiveness of RME in children with OSA syndrome (OSAS). However, further research is needed to determine the best approach to children with both adeno-tonsillar hypertrophy and maxillary transverse deficiency.

Given current patient's symptoms, CPAP treatment was offered. His family was very involved and supportive. The patient took a mask home to practice for several weeks. He gradually increased his time wearing the mask. PAP titration was performed, and CPAP of 7 centimeters of water (cm H_2O) effectively reduced the respiratory events. After the patient was started on CPAP, his behavior improved considerably, according to his parents. He also started a structured weight loss program.

CLINICAL PEARLS

1. Following TNA, pediatric patients with OSA should be evaluated for residual symptoms and if present should be restudied to determine if significant OSA is still present.

2. Although hard and fast rules do not exist, generally an AHI >5 or the presence of symptoms would warrant initiation of additional treatment after TNA.

3. Treatments for residual OSA following TNA include weight loss, intranasal steroids, and leukotriene inhibitors (e.g., montelukast), and PAP.

4. PAP treatment in children requires a period of adaptation to the mask and family involvement. A multidisciplinary team, including pediatric sleep specialists, psychologists, respiratory therapists, and nurses skilled in dealing with children, should be utilized.

BIBLIOGRAPHY

Marcus CL, Brooks LJ, Draper KA, et al: for the American Academy of Pediatrics: Diagnosis and management of childhood obstructive sleep apnea syndrome, *Pediatrics* 130(3):e714–e755, 2012.

Marcus CL, Brooks LJ, Draper KA, et al: for the American Academy of Pediatrics: Diagnosis and management of childhood obstructive sleep apnea syndrome (Technical Report), *Pediatrics* 130(3):576–584, 2012.

Kheirandish L, Goldbart AD, Gozal D: Intranasal steroids and oral leukotriene modifier therapy in residual sleep-disordered breathing after tonsillectomy and adenoidectomy in children, *Pediatrics* 117(1):e61–e66, 2006.

Goldbart AD, Goldman JL, Veling MC, Gozal D: Leukotriene modifier therapy for mild sleep-disordered breathing in children, *Am J Respir Crit Care Med* 172(3):364–370, 2005.

Pirelli P, Saponara M, Guilleminault C: Rapid maxillary expansion in children with obstructive sleep apnea syndrome, *Sleep* 27:761–766, 2004.

Villa MP, Malagola C, Pagani J, et al: Rapid maxillary expansion in children with obstructive sleep apnea syndrome: 12-month follow-up, *Sleep Med* 8:128–134, 2007.

Villa MP, Rizzoli A, Miano S, Malagola C: Efficacy of rapid maxillary expansion in children with obstructive sleep apnea syndrome: 36 months of follow-up, *Sleep Breath* 15:179–184, 2011.

PATIENT 60

CPAP Treatment in a Child

A 12-year-old boy (body mass index percentage [BMI%] = 104*) underwent tonsillectomy and adenoidectomy (TNA) after a sleep study documented severe obstructive sleep apnea (OSA) (apnea–hypopnea index [AHI] 30 per hour). After surgery, he continued to have significant daytime sleepiness and was doing poorly in school. A weight loss program was begun but was not successful. Nasal steroids and montelukast treatment had been tried with minimal improvement in symptoms. Polysomnography (PSG) was performed after TNA (Table P60-1).

TABLE P60-1	Sleep Study
	After TNA
TST	440.5 min
AHI total	12.0
AHI NREM	7.0
AHI REM	18.0
OA	2
CA	9
Hypopneas	64
Low SpO$_2$ NREM	92%
Low SpO$_2$ REM	84%
ETCO$_2$	Peak 53 torr

AHI, Apnea–hypopnea index; *CA*, central apnea; *ETCO$_2$*, end-tidal carbon dioxide; *OA*, obstructive apnea; *min*, minutes; *NREM*, non–rapid eye movement; *REM*, rapid eye movement; *SpO$_2$*, saturation of peripheral oxygen; *TNA*, tonsillectomy and adenoidectomy; *TST*, total sleep time.

QUESTION

1. What treatment do you recommend?

ANSWER

1. **Answer:** Continuous positive airway pressure (CPAP) treatment.

   Discussion: TNA is usually the first treatment of choice for OSA in children with adeno-tonsillar hypertrophy unless special attributes such as hypoventilation or craniofacial abnormalities are present. In these special populations, tracheostomy with volume ventilation is reserved for the most severe cases. Given the presence of the epidemic of childhood obesity and the fact that a significant proportion of patients have an elevated residual AHI following TNA, the use of CPAP in children will likely increase in the future. Fundamentals 24 provides guidelines for the titration of PAP in adults and children. Here, a few items of special interest will be discussed. PAP titrations in children require some extra considerations (Box P60-1). First, split-night studies are *not* recommended. If the child without previous mask desensitization undergoes

*BMI% ≥85 to <95% = overweight; % ≥95% obese; ≥99% high risk.

BOX P60-1	PAP Indications and Considerations in Children

INDICATIONS FOR PAP IN CHILDREN

- Poor surgical candidates for TNA
- Preparation for surgery in high-risk patients
- Significant residual OSA after TNA
- Hypoventilation

SPECIAL PAP CONSIDERATIONS IN CHILDREN

- No split studies
- Desensitization to mask
- Team comprising a social worker and a psychologist to prepare the child and the family
- DME company and sleep laboratory experienced in dealing with children
- Behavior modification to encourage good adherence
- Reward for good adherence

a split-night study, the child may be frightened, and this will make subsequent CPAP use unlikely. Children are often given masks to play with and try on during the day for a week before scheduled studies. The child should be desensitized to the mask during the day by wearing it for increasing periods while engaging in a fun activity (e.g., watching a favorite video). Pediatric-size masks should be made available. Durable medical equipment providers and sleep technologists who are skilled and willing to provide care for pediatric age patients should be utilized. Studies have shown that structured behavioral interventions help with compliance (graduated exposure, positive reinforcement, dealing with escape and avoidance behavior, praising, and distracting activities that allow the child to wear a mask). As in adults, objective monitoring of adherence is essential to guide treatment. The same is true in children and adolescents.

A study by Marcus et al of CPAP use by children (published in 2006) studied a total of 29 patients. Approximately one third of children dropped out before 6 months. Of the 21 children for whom 6-month adherence data could be downloaded, the mean nightly use was 5.3 ± 2.5 (standard deviation [SD]) hours. Parental assessment of PAP use considerably overestimated actual use. PAP was highly effective, with a reduction in the AHI from 27 ± 32 to 3 ± 5/hour, and an improvement in arterial oxygen saturation nadir from $77 \pm 17\%$ to $89 \pm 6\%$. Results were similar for children who received CPAP versus bilevel PAP (BPAP). Children also had a subjective improvement in daytime sleepiness.

A recent prospective study of PAP adherence in children and adolescents by DiFeo and coworkers found that adherence is related primarily to family and demographic factors rather than to severity of apnea or measures of psychosocial functioning. The authors concluded that further research was needed to determine the relative contributions of maternal education, socioeconomic status and cultural beliefs to PAP adherence in children to develop better adherence programs. Simon et al developed a questionnaire to assess barriers to PAP treatment in children. The involvement of psychologists and social workers skilled at behavioral interventions in children should be an integral part of CPAP programs for children. Recently, a questionnaire has been developed to identify barriers to CPAP use.

In the current patient, the decision was made to proceed with PAP treatment. The patient had the opportunity to try on masks in the clinic with low pressure. An incentive program was planned with the boy's parents. The boy specifically loved watching wrestling on TV. CPAP titration was successful, and the patient was started on CPAP of 8 centimeters of water (cm H_2O) using a nasal mask.

CLINICAL PEARLS

1. Successful PAP treatment requires desensitization to masks in young children.
2. Split-night studies are not recommended.
3. Involvement of parents is crucial.
4. A team approach with social workers, psychologists, and nutritionists is important.
5. PAP treatment is a viable alternative when significant residual OSA persists after TNA.

BIBLIOGRAPHY

Marcus CL, Brooks LJ, Draper K, et al: Diagnosis and management of childhood obstructive sleep apnea syndrome: clinical practice guideline, American Academy of Pediatrics, *Pediatrics* 130:576–584, 2012.

Marcus CL, Brooks LJ, Davidson-Ward S, et al: Diagnosis and management of childhood obstructive sleep apnea syndrome: technical report. American Academy of Pediatrics, *Pediatrics* 130:e714–e755, 2012.

Marcus CL: Sleep-disordered breathing in children, *Am J Respir Crit Care Med* 164:16–30, 2001.

Marcus CL, Beck SE, Traylor J, et al: Randomized, double-blind clinical trial of two different modes of positive airway pressure therapy on adherence and efficacy in children, *J Clin Sleep Med* 8(1):37–42, 2012.

Marcus CL, Rosen G, Davidson-Ward S, et al: Adherence to and effectiveness of positive airway pressure therapy in children with obstructive sleep apnea, *Pediatrics* 117:e442–e451, 2006.

Koontz KL, Slifer KJ, Cataldo MD, Marcus CL: Improving pediatric compliance with positive airway pressure therapy: the impact of behavioral intervention, *Sleep* 26:1010–1015, 2003.

Rains JC: Treatment of obstructive sleep apnea in pediatric patients. Behavioral intervention for compliance with nasal continuous positive airway pressure, *Clin Pediatr (Phila)* 34:535–541, 1995.

DiFeo N, Meltzer LJ, Beck SE, et al: Predictors of positive airway pressure therapy adherence in children: a prospective study, *J Clin Sleep Med* 8(3):279–286, 2012.

Simon SL, Duncan CL, Janicke DM, Wagner MH: Barriers to treatment of paediatric obstructive sleep apnoea: development of the adherence barriers to continuous positive airway pressure (CPAP) questionnaire, *Sleep Med* 13(2):172–177, 2012.

PATIENT 61

A 20-Year-Old Female with Daytime Sleepiness Since Childhood

A 20-year-old female with Prader-Willi syndrome (PWS) and moderately impaired cognitive function (mental retardation) was evaluated for persistent heavy snoring and leg edema. The patient had a long history of obstructive sleep apnea (OSA). Her condition deteriorated after she had a 2-month visit with her parents and a 30-pound weight gain. Before the vacation, she was cared for at an institution specializing in children and young adults with special needs and had been doing well on nasal continuous positive airway pressure (CPAP) of 12 centimeters of water (cm H_2O).

Physical examination: Height 60 inches, weight 210 pounds; very obese, cooperative female

HEENT: Up-sloping palpebral fissures, crowded oropharynx and dependent palate

Neck: 17 inches in circumference

Extremities: 2+ pitting edema, short calves

Neurologic: Oriented to person and place but not date; able to answer simple questions

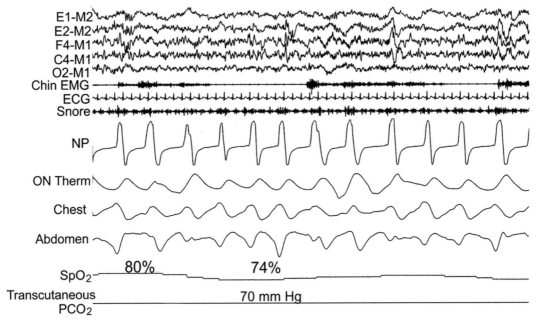

FIGURE P61-1 ■ A 30-second tracing while breathing room air. *NP*, Nasal pressure, *ON Therm*, oronasal thermal sensor.

Figure P61-1 shows the tracing obtained at stage 2 sleep during an initial diagnostic portion off positive pressure ($TcPCO_2$ = transcutaneous partial pressure of carbon dioxide). Later in the study, frank obstructive apneas were noted. The awake $TcPCO_2$ was 50 mm Hg.

QUESTION

1. Why is the saturation of arterial oxygen (SaO_2) so low (74%–80%) and the transcutaneous PCO_2 so high (70 mm Hg) when no discrete breathing events are noted?

ANSWER

1. **Answer:** Hypoventilation associated with PWS.

   Discussion: PWS is characterized by hypothalamic obesity, hyperphagia, hypogonadism, mental retardation, hypotonia (muscle weakness) and behavioral and sleep disorders. The prevalence of this disorder is 1 per 10,000 to 25,000 live births. The syndrome is associated with failure of expression of genes on the long arm of the paternally derived chromosome 15. A deletion of the long arm of this chromosome occurs in approximately 50% to 70% of the patients. Patients with PWS have a characteristic habitus, including short stature, up-sloping palpebral fissures, and short arms and legs. They have abnormal growth hormone secretion. Some exhibit compulsive behaviors. Daytime sleepiness may be an intrinsic manifestation of the disease, although in some patients, it is worsened by sleep-disordered breathing (SDB). Some patients have daytime sleepiness, narcolepsy caused by a medical condition, or hypersomnia resulting from a medical condition (no OSA present, narcolepsy criteria not met).

   One important characteristic of patients with this syndrome is an insatiable appetite leading to massive obesity. In evaluating alterations in ventilatory control, it has been difficult to separate intrinsic problems from those associated with severe obesity. However, the hypoxic ventilatory response was found to be absent or reduced in patients with PWS with or without obesity. This is believed to be secondary to peripheral chemoreceptor dysfunction, although central processing of chemoreceptor information may be involved as well. The hypercapnic ventilatory responses appear to be decreased mainly in obese patients. The arousal response to hypoxia during sleep is virtually absent, and the arousal response to hypercapnia is impaired. Obese patients with PWS may have severe forms of OSA syndrome with severe hypoxia and hypercapnia during sleep. They may also have daytime hypercapnia. Patients demonstrating hypoventilation may require noninvasive ventilation (bilevel PAP [BPAP]).

Treatment of OSA in these patients usually consists of weight loss and some form of PAP therapy or upper airway surgery. Weight reduction often results in considerable improvement in these patients. As patients with PWS have special needs and mental retardation, weight loss is usually only possible in a very structured environment. Special group homes experienced in caring for persons with PWS have had success with weight loss. PAP treatment usually consists of nasal CPAP or BPAP. Very severe cases may require nocturnal ventilatory support via tracheostomy at least until weight loss has been achieved. Growth hormone replacement has been shown to improve muscle strength, decrease body fat, and improve ventilatory control in these patients.

In the present case, the tracing shows what appears to be relatively normal air flow. However, SaO_2 is very low and TcPCO2 high. In fact, the awake PCO_2 is also high. This patient has daytime hypoventilation that worsens during sleep. Later, during the short diagnostic portion of the sleep study, discrete obstructive hypopneas and apneas were noted with even more severe arterial oxygen desaturation. The patient required a combination of bilevel pressure of 16/10 cm H_2O and supplemental oxygen at 2 liters per minute to prevent nocturnal desaturation. After 2 months of treatment and an intensive weight loss program (30-pound weight loss) the daytime $TcPCO_2$ returned to normal, and nocturnal oxygen was no longer needed (demonstrated by nocturnal oximetry). The patient continued treatment on bilevel pressure of 16/10 cm H_2O, although lower levels might have sufficed.

CLINICAL PEARLS

1. PWS is associated with severe obesity, OSA, and abnormal ventilatory control.
2. The ventilatory response to hypercapnia and daytime CO_2 retention (if present) may normalize with weight loss and treatment of OSA.
3. Most patients have an abnormality in chromosome 15.
4. Food restriction (weight control) is an essential component of treatment.
5. Obese patients with PWS and OSA often have very severe desaturations and hypercapnia during sleep.
6. Patients with PWS may have daytime sleepiness caused by narcolepsy due to medical condition, OSA, or PWS (hypersomnia caused by a medical condition).

BIBLIOGRAPHY

Arens R, Gozal D, Omlin KJ, et al: Hypoxic and hypercapnic ventilatory responses in Prader-Willi Syndrome, *J Appl Physiol* 77:231–236, 1994.

Lindgren AC, Hellstron LG, Ritzen EM, Milerad J: Growth hormone treatment increased CO2 response, ventilation and central inspiratory drive in children with Prader-Willi syndrome, *Eur J Pediatr* 158:936–940, 1999.

Manni R, Politini L, Nobili L, et al: Hypersomnia in the Prader-Willi syndrome: clinic-electrophysiological features and underling factors, *Clin Neurophysiol* 112:800–805, 2001.

Yee BJ, Buchanan PR, Mahadev S, et al: Assessment of sleep and breathing in adults with Prader-Willi syndrome: a case control series, *J Clin Sleep Med* 3(7):713–718, 2007.

Nixon GM, Brouillette RT: Sleep and breathing in Prader-Willi syndrome, *Pediatr Pulmonol* 34(3):209–217, 2002.

Meyer SL, Splaingard M, Repaske DR, et al: Outcomes of adenotonsillectomy in patients with Prader-Willi syndrome, *Arch Otolaryngol Head Neck Surg* 138(11):1047–1051, 2012.

Surgical Treatment for Obstructive Sleep Apnea

SURGICAL TREATMENTS FOR OBSTRUCTIVE SLEEP APNEA

A number of surgical procedures are available to treat adults with obstructive sleep apnea (OSA).[1-3] The major options are listed in Table F26-1. Each of the major procedures is discussed briefly below. Surgery for nasal obstruction is considered adjunctive treatment, laser-assisted uvuloplasty (LAUP) and palatal implants are recommended mainly for the treatment of snoring. The use of tonsillectomy and adenoidectomy (TNA) to treat pediatric OSA is discussed in Fundamentals 21.

INDICATIONS FOR SURGICAL TREATMENT

An update of the American Academy of Sleep Medicine (AASM) practice parameters for surgical treatment of OSA was published in 2010 (Table F26-2).[1,2] The practice parameters state that the presence and severity of OSA must be determined before initiating surgical therapy. The patient should be advised about the success of surgical procedures and side effects as well as the success rate of alternative treatments. The practice parameters state that positive airway pressure (PAP) should first be offered to patients with severe OSA, and either PAP or an oral appliance (OA) for patients with moderate OSA. Patients requiring the stepped procedure approach should be informed that multiple surgical procedures may be needed.

EVALUATION FOR POSSIBLE SURGICAL TREATMENT

The AASM practice parameters for surgical treatment of OSA mandate that all patients scheduled for surgery to correct snoring or OSA should undergo polysomonography (PSG) for diagnosis and to assess severity.[1,2] Additional evaluation of patients with snoring or OSA for possible upper airway surgery includes fiberoptic examination of the nose, pharynx, and hypopharynx to evaluate the anatomy for abnormalities and location of narrowing or obstruction. During fiberoptic pharyngoscopy, the patient performs the Müller maneuver (inspiration with the nose occluded). This maneuver is performed to help identify the most prominent site of collapse (retropalatal or retroglossal or hypopharyngeal area).[4] A limitation of this technique, which is typically performed during wakefulness and often in an upright posture, is that the results may not correspond to what happens during supine sleep. Lateral cephalometric radiography is also standard and helps visualize bony

TABLE F26-1	Surgical Options for Treatment of Adult Obstructive Sleep Apnea
Procedure	**Target Area**
• Uvulopalatopharyngoplasty (UPPP)	Retropalatal
• Genioglossus advancement (GA)	Retroglossal
• Hyoid advancement (HA)	Retroglossal
• Maxillomandibular advancement (MMA)	Retroglossal>retropalatal
• Temperature-controlled radiofrequency (RF) and robotic tongue base reduction	Retroglossal

TABLE F26-2	**Summary of AASM Surgical Treatment of OSA Practice Parameter Recommendations**

Procedure	Indications or Conditions
Tracheostomy	Other options do not exist or have failed Clinical urgency (e.g., repeated bouts of hypercapnic respiratory failure)
MMA	Severe OSA Unwilling or unable to tolerate PAP OA considered and undesirable or ineffective
UPPP	Snoring, mild OSA Moderate OSA—only after offering PAP treatment and oral appliances
Palatal implants	"may be effective in some patients with mild OSA" Indicated for OSA treatment *IF* patients cannot tolerate or adhere to PAP therapy and OA treatment is considered and found ineffective and undesirable
GA or HA	No specific recommendations Used for patients with hypopharyngeal narrowing
Multilevel or Stepwise surgery	Upper airway narrowing at multiple sites Patients have failed UPPP as sole treatment

From Caples SM, Rowley JA, Prinsell JR, et al: Surgical modifications of the upper airway for obstructive sleep apnea in adults: a systematic review and meta-analysis, *Sleep* 33:1396-1407, 2010.
AASM, American Academy of Sleep Medicine; *GA*, Genioglossus advancement; *HA*, hyoid advancement; *MMA*, mandibular maxillary advancement; *OA*, oral appliance; *OSA*, obstructive sleep apnea; *PAP*, positive airway pressure; *UPPP*, uvulopharyngopalatoplasty.

abnormalities and the posterior airspace. On cephalometry, patients with OSA tend to have long soft palates, small posterior airspaces (<10 millimeters [mm] behind the tongue), mandibular deficiency, and a low hyoid (long distance from the mandibular plane to the hyoid).

TRACHEOSOTOMY

This procedure bypasses all obstructions and is almost always effective at preventing upper airway obstruction.[5,6] The main use of tracheostomy is for patients who have life-threatening OSA (often obesity hypoventilation syndrome [OHS] with recurrent hypercapnic respiratory failure) and are poorly adherent to PAP treatment. It is also used as a temporary measure while patients recover from other upper airway surgery. The most recent AASM practice parameters state that tracheostomy has been found to be an effective single intervention.[2] However, this "operation should be considered only when other options do not exist, have failed, are refused, or when this operation is deemed necessary by clinical urgency." A number of potential adverse effects of tracheostomy for OSA exist.[5,6] Tracheostomy is discussed in more detail in Patient 62.

SURGERY FOR NASAL OBSTRUCTION

Nasal obstruction may lead to mouth breathing during sleep. This causes rotation of the mandible and retrodisplacement of the tongue base back into the pharynx. The major areas of focus include the nasal valve or alar cartilage area, septum, and turbinates (mostly inferior turbinates). Radiofrequency ablation (RFA) of turbinate hypertrophy may improve nasal continuous PAP (CPAP) adherence in selected patients.[7] Long-term studies are needed to better define the indications for this procedure. A randomized, controlled trial of nasal surgery (versus placebo surgery) found that surgery resulted in improvement in the amount of nasal breathing during sleep (less mouth breathing) but minimal effects on the apnea–hypopnea index (AHI). The surgeries included resection of the deviated nasal septum and submucous resection of the inferior turbinates.[8] Thus, although nasal surgery may improve the quality of life for some patients, it is considered an adjunctive rather than a primary treatment for OSA.

PALATAL IMPLANTS

The Pillar procedure involves insertion of Teflon strips into the palate and may be done in the office or outpatient surgery center. The purpose of the strips is to induce fibrosis which stiffens the palate (reduced snoring). The success is variable and sometimes additional strip insertion is needed.[9] Although the evidence that palatal implant surgery is effective in patients with OSA is very marginal, recent practice parameters state: "Palatal implants may be effective in some patients with mild OSA who cannot tolerate or are unwilling to adhere to PAP therapy, or in whom oral appliances have been considered and found ineffective or undesirable (Option)."[2]

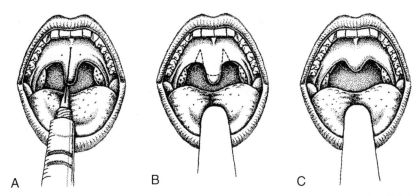

FIGURE F26-1 ■ Laser uvulopalatoplasty. **A,** Local anesthetic is injected. **B,** The carbon dioxide (CO_2) laser is used to excise vertical trenches of the soft palate on either aspect of the uvula up to the muscular sling, and 30% to 90% of the uvula is excised or vaporized. **C,** The postoperative result necessitates 4 to 5 weeks for complete healing and scarring to produce traction forces to improve airway patency. (**A-C,** From Li KK, Powell NB, Riley RW: Surgical management of OSA. In Lee-Chiong TL, Sateia MJ, Carskadon MA [eds]: *Sleep medicine,* Philadelphia, 2002, Hanley & Belfus, p 439, reproduced with permission.)

LASER-ASSISTED UVULOPLASTY

Laser-assisted palatoplasty or uvuloplasty (LAP or LAUP) was introduced as a treatment for snoring.[9] In this procedure, only a small portion of the uvula or soft palate is removed (Figure F26-1). Usually, two trenches are cut on either side of the uvula. Sometimes the end of the uvula is also removed. With time and scarring, the palate stiffens and elevates. This procedure may be done on an outpatient basis with the use of local anesthesia. It is generally considered a treatment for snoring but has been used for very mild sleep apnea when suitable upper airway anatomy exists. The long-term efficacy of LAP remains to be established. The 2010 AASM practice parameters for surgical treatment of OSA[2] state "LAUP is NOT routinely recommended as a treatment for obstructive sleep apnea syndrome (Standard)."

RADIOFREQUENCY ABLATION (ALSO KNOWN AS RADIOFREQUENCY VOLUMETRIC TISSUE REDUCTION [RFVTR])

RFA has been used in the upper airway usually with temperature control of the probe tip. A probe is inserted in the area of interest and tissue is heated to create cellular damage. With time the tissue shrinks. RFA has been used for treatment of the soft palate, base of the tongue, and treatment at multiple levels.[10] Somnoplasty (a variant of RFA) is a method of palatoplasty for treatment of snoring, appears to be well tolerated (possibly less pain), but is not more effective than the traditional uvulopalatopharyngoplasty (UPPP). It may be performed as an outpatient procedure. Repeated treatments may be needed. The same technique may be used for turbinate reduction. Several other procedures that utilize cautery or injection of sclerotic agents to stiffen the palate have also been used.[9] The 2010 AASM practice parameters for surgical treatment of OSA state: "RFA can be considered as a treatment in patients with mild to moderate OSA who cannot tolerate or who are unwilling to adhere to PAP, or in whom oral appliances have been considered and have been found ineffective or undesirable (Option)."

UVULOPALATOPHARYNGOPLASTY

UPPP is an operation that removes residual tonsillar tissue, the uvula, a portion of the soft palate, and redundant tissue from the pharyngeal area (Figure F26-2).[11-13] Its disadvantages include the need for general anesthesia and considerable postoperative pain. The most frequent complication is velopharyngeal insufficiency, which is manifested as some degree of nasal reflux when drinking fluids. This usually resolves within a month following surgery. Other potential complications include voice change, postoperative bleeding, nasopharyngeal stenosis (secondary to scarring), or a persistent globus sensation. However, the major problem with UPPP is less-than-perfect efficacy as a treatment for OSA.[1,14] UPPP does not address airway narrowing behind the tongue or in the hypopharynx; therefore, it is not universally effective in preventing sleep apnea. UPPP is generally reasonably effective in decreasing the incidence or

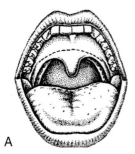
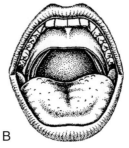
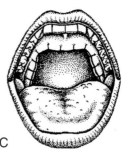

FIGURE F26-2 ■ Technique of uvulopalatopharyngoplasty. **A,** Redundant soft palate and tonsillar pillar mucosa are outlined. **B,** Tonsils, tonsil pillar mucosa, and posterior soft palate are excised. **C,** Mucosal flaps of the lateral pharyngeal wall and nasal palatal muscle are advanced to the anterior pillar and or mucosa of the soft palate. (**A-C,** From Li KK, Powell NB, Riley RW: Surgical management of OSA. In Lee-Chiong TL, Sateia MJ, Carskadon MA [eds]: *Sleep medicine*, Philadelphia, 2002, Hanley & Belfus, p 439, reproduced with permission.)

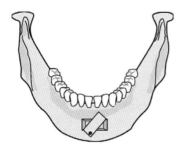
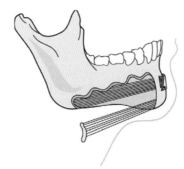

FIGURE F26-3 ■ Technique of genioglossus advancement. A rectangular window of symphyseal bone consisting of the geniotubercle is advanced anteriorly, rotated to allow body overlap, and immobilized with a titanium screw. *Left,* Anterior view. *Right,* Lateral view. (From Li KK: Hypoglossal airway surgery, *Otolaryngol Clin North Am* 40:845-853, 2007.)

loudness of snoring (vibration of the soft palate). In general, 40% to 50% of all patients undergoing UPPP have about a 50% decrease in their AHI, to less than 20 per hour (hr), or about a 30% chance of a postoperative AHI dropping below 10/hr.[1,14] The results will, of course, depend on the presurgery AHI and the locations of upper airway obstruction. Frequently, the number of apneas decreases, and the number of hypopneas increases after UPPP. Recent practice parameters for surgical treatment of OSA state: "UPPP as a sole procedure, with or without tonsillectomy, does not reliably normalize the AHI when treating moderate to severe OSA. Therefore, patients with severe OSA should initially be offered positive airway pressure therapy, while those with moderate OSA should initially be offered either PAP therapy or oral appliances (Option)."[2] More information is provided about UPPP in Patient 63.

UVULOPALATAL FLAP

This surgery is a modification of the UPPP and, instead of removing the uvula and soft palate, the uvula is retracted and tucked superiorly under the soft palate. The pharyngeal pillars are sutured back, and the tonsils are removed in this procedure as well. The advantages are less postoperative pain and perhaps less nasopharyngeal reflux. The results are similar to UPPP. The procedure cannot be done if the palate is very long or bulky.[3]

GENIOGLOSSUS ADVANCEMENT OR HYOID ADVANCEMENT

In genioglossus advancement (GA)[15] (Figure F26-3), the attachment of the genioglossus at the genoid tubercle of the mandible is advanced by making a limited rectangular mandibular osteotomy to include the genial tubercle (site of attachment of genioglossus and geniohyoid on the mandible).[15] The rectangular piece of bone with muscular attachments is advanced and rotated to prevent retraction of the piece of bone back into the mandible. A screw is then placed for stabilization.

When initially introduced, the second component of the surgery, hyoid advancement (HA) (Figure F26-4) was called *hyoid myotomy with suspension.* The original surgery consisted of release of the hyoid from its inferior muscular

FIGURE F26-4 ■ Technique of hyoid advancement (HA). The hyoid bone is isolated, the inferior body is dissected cleanly, and the majority of the suprahyoid musculature remains intact. The hyoid is advanced over the thyroid lamina and immobilized with sutures placed through the superior aspect of the thyroid cartilage. *Left,* Anterior view. *Right,* Lateral view. (From Li KK: Hypoglossal airway surgery, *Otolaryngol Clin North Am* 40:845-853, 2007.)

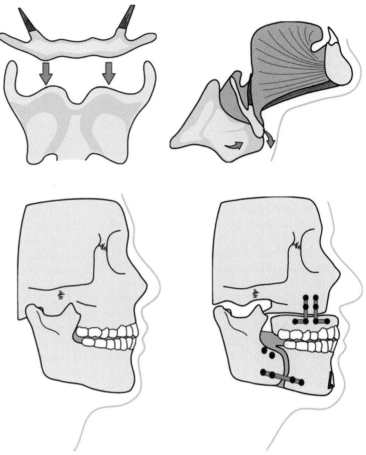

FIGURE F26-5 ■ Technique of maxillomandibular advancement *(lateral view).* The procedure includes a Le Fort I maxillary osteotomy with rigid plate fixation and a bilateral sagittal split mandibular osteotomy with bicortical screw fixation. The advancement is at least 10 millimeters (mm). (From Li KK: Hypoglossal airway surgery, *Otolaryngol Clin North Am* 40:845-853, 2007.)

attachments and suspension from the anterior mandible with suture or ligament. Today, the hyoid is often attached to the superior border of the thyroid cartilage. Some surgeons perform only GA at the first surgery, and HA performed only if needed at a subsequent operation. GA +HA does not require any change in dental occlusion. Complications of GA+HA include transient anesthesia of the lower anterior teeth (all) and, rarely, tooth injury. Indications for GA+HA include a small posterior airspace as shown by lateral cephalometry (<10 mm), an increased mandible-to-thyroid distance (>20 mm) as shown by cephalometry, mandibular deficiency, tongue base prominence on nasopharyngoscopy, or macroglossia.[15]

The recent AASM practice parameters for surgical treatment of OSA[2] did not provide a specific statement about the GA or HA procedure. The practice parameters state: "Multilevel or stepwise surgery (MLS), as a combined procedure or stepwise operations, is acceptable in patients with narrowing of multiple sites in the upper airway, particularly if they have failed UPPP as a sole treatment (Option)."[2]

MAXILLOMANDIBULAR ADVANCEMENT

Maxillomandibular advancement (MMA) is the most complex upper airway surgery, but excluding tracheostomy, this procedure has the best record of success as a treatment for OSA (Figure F26-5). The maxilla and the mandible are advanced together, and both upper and lower teeth are moved to maintain adequate occlusion.[1,3,15,16] The procedure increases the retrolingual and, to a lesser extent, the retropalatal segments of the upper airway. The maxilla is moved by a Le Fort I osteotomy and the mandible by a sagittal split osteotomy. MMA enlarges the pharyngeal and hypopharyngeal areas by moving the skeletal framework and tensions the suprahyoid and velopharyngeal musculature. Although patients with retrognathia may be especially good candidates, this procedure is not limited to patients who have this problem.

In some institutions, MMA is performed only after UPPP and GA+HA. However, for patients with severe OSA, mandibular deficiency, or both,

MMA may also be offered as the initial surgery. If the palate is long, doing UPPP at the same time as MMA is also an option. Numbness of the chin and cheek areas is an expected complication that resolves in 6 to 12 months in most patients. The response rates from MMA vary from 50% to 80% or higher, depending on the definition of surgical success. Li and coworkers[16] reported 95% "cure" rate defined as an AHI <20/hr and at least a 50% reduction. In a group of 36 of 40 patients who were responders, the AHI dropped from 69.6/hr preoperatively to 7.7/hr postoperatively. A recent meta-analysis found MMA to reduce the AHI to less than 20/hr in 80% to 90%.[14] This procedure is usually offered only at large tertiary hospitals by experienced maxillofacial surgeons. The recent AASM practice parameters for surgical treatment of OSA state: "MMA is indicated for surgical treatment of severe OSA in patients who cannot tolerate or are unwilling to adhere to positive airway pressure therapy, or in whom oral appliances, which are often more appropriate in mild and moderate OSA patients, have been considered and found ineffective or undesirable (Option)."[2] The reason for the grade "Option" rather than a higher grade "Guideline" is that the published studies were considered to be of "low quality of evidence" because they were small and not controlled. Other than tracheostomy, the procedure is most likely to significantly improve the AHI in patients with severe OSA, although the AHI is often not normalized.

TONGUE PROCEDURES

In an attempt to avoid surgery involving the mandible or the maxilla, procedures directed at the tongue have also been developed. Tongue base reduction surgery aims to increase the retroglossal airway by removing tongue tissue. Surgical resection, laser resection, and temperature-controlled radiofrequency (TCRF) tongue base reduction have all been tried with varying degrees of success.[17–19] Recently, the use of robotic surgery has allowed better access to the tongue. Postoperative bleeding, odynophagia, tongue abscess, swallowing difficulty, and alterations in speech are potential side effects of surgical tongue procedures.

TONGUE BASE SUSPENSION SUTURE

A suspension suture is looped from the anchor screw on the inner surface of the mandible to the base of the tongue. The suture is tensioned, bringing the tongue forward. The procedure may be performed in less than half an hour and has few side effects (infection, injury to tooth roots, and detachment of screw). The success

rates are variable.[3] The procedure is often performed with UPPP or another procedure.

OVERALL SURGICAL APPROACH

The overall surgical approach depends on OSA severity, upper airway anatomy, prior treatment failures, and patient preference. Obstruction may be classified as types 1 to 3 based on the predominant level of upper airway obstruction.[18] A type 1 obstruction is at the retropalatal area. Type 3 obstruction is at the hypopharyngeal area (behind the tongue or lower), and type 2 is a combined obstruction (palate+hypopharynx). Type 1 patients are considered favorable candidates for palatal procedures (UPPP). Type 3 patients are candidates for procedures addressing the retroglossal space (GA, with or without hyoid advancement). Type 2 patients are candidates for UPPP +GA+HA, UPPP+ tongue base reduction, or MMA. A systematic stepped surgical approach such as the one used at Stanford has been advocated (Figure F26-6).[18] Postoperative PSG is performed in 6 months, and patients with treatment failures may then be offered MMA (if not previously performed). Because an occasional patient with type 2 obstruction will improve with UPPP, in some centers, a retrolingual procedure is added only after UPPP fails. In other centers, patients with severe OSA, severe mandibular deficiency, or very small posterior airspaces are offered *MMA with or without UPPP as the first procedure*. Some patients also want to avoid multiple procedures, and this more aggressive approach may be more acceptable to them.

SUCCESS RATES OF UPPER AIRWAY SURGERY

A recent meta-analysis and synthesis of evidence for success in upper airway surgery was reported by Elshaug and colleagues[14] (Table F26-3). A traditional metric of success has been a 50% reduction in the AHI, 20/hr or less, or both. These authors suggested a more rigorous approach with reduction less than 10 or 5/hr being the goal of success.[14] Phase I surgery included palatal surgery without or without other procedures such as GA or GA+HA. Phase II surgery was MMA with or without additional procedures. Of course, the percentage of procedures deemed successful will depend on the initial severity of the problem. Although surgical results are less than ideal, neither is PAP therapy. For example, a patient with an AHI of 60/hour who uses CPAP for 50% of the night (assume AHI = 0/hour) has an average AHI for the entire night of approximately 30/hour.

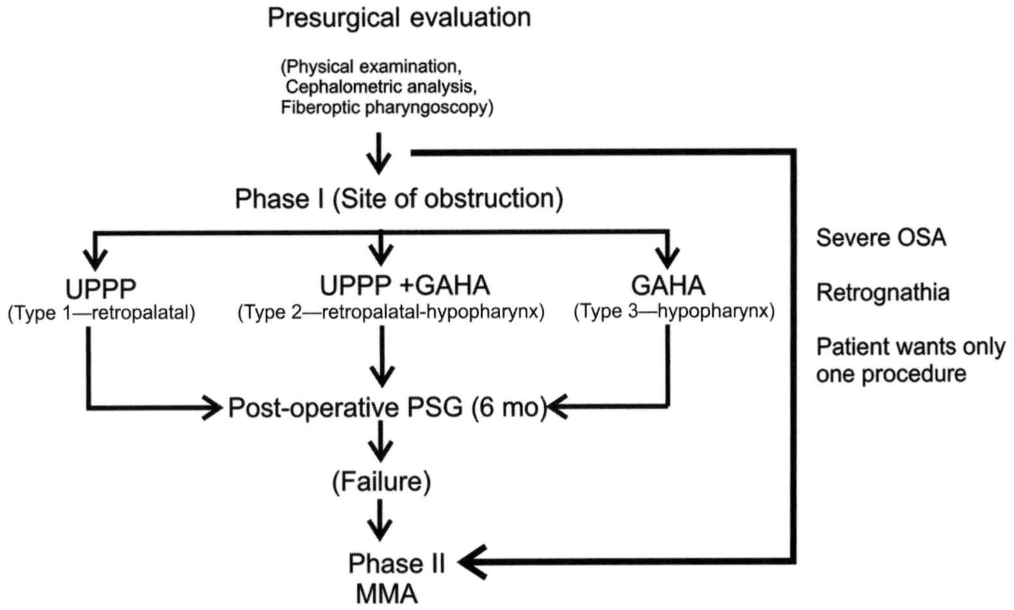

FIGURE F26-6 ■ Stepped surgical approach to treatment of obstructive sleep apnea (OSA) based on the site of upper airway obstruction. *GA+HA*, Genioglossal advancement+hyoid advancement; *MMA*, maxillomandibular advancement; *PSG*, polysomnography; *UPPP*, uvulopalatopharyngoplasty. (Adapted from Li KK, Powell NB, Riley RW: Surgical management of obstructive sleep apnea. In Lee-Chiong TL, Sateia MJ, Caraskadon MA [eds]: *Sleep medicine*, Philadelphia, 2002, Hanley & Belfus, pp 435-446.)

TABLE F26-3 Meta-Analysis Results for Upper Airway Surgery (% Success Rates)

Criteria	50% Reduction in AHI to ≤20/hr	AHI <10/hr	AHI <5/hr
Phase I*	55%	31.5%	13%
Phase II†	86%	45 %	43%

From Elshaug AG, Moss JR, Southcott A, et al: Redefining success in airway surgery for obstructive sleep apnea: a meta-analysis and synthesis of the evidence, *Sleep* 30:461-467, 2007.
AHI, Apnea–hypopnea index; *GA*, genioglossus advancement; *HA*, hyoid advancement; *MMA*, maxillomandibular advancement; *UPPP*, uvulopalatopharyngoplasty.
*Phase I (UPPP, GA, HA, or combination).
†Phase II (MMA).

CLINICAL PEARLS

1. The presence and severity of OSA must be determined before initiating any type of surgical treatment (including treatment for "presumed snoring").

2. Before undergoing surgery patients should be advised of potential success rates and complications as well as treatment alternatives.

3. Tracheostomy is the only surgery uniformly effective for severe OSA, although some series suggest that MMA may approach a 80% to 90% success rate, depending on how surgical success is defined.

4. MMA is indicated for initial treatment of severe OSA in patients who cannot tolerate or are unwilling to adhere to PAP therapy and in whom OAs have been considered and found ineffective or undesirable.

5. UPPP does not reliably normalize the AHI in patients with moderate to severe OSA. Patients with severe OSA should be offered PAP treatment. Patients with moderate OSA should initially be offered PAP therapy or an OA.

REFERENCES

1. Caples SM, Rowley JA, Prinsell JR, et al: Surgical modifications of the upper airway for obstructive sleep apnea in adults: a systematic review and meta-analysis, *Sleep* 33:1396–1407, 2010.

2. Aurora RN, Casey KR, Kristo D, et al: Practice parameters for the surgical modifications of the upper airway for obstructive sleep apnea in adults, *Sleep* 33:1408–1413, 2010.

3. Won CHJ, Li KK, Guilleminault C: Surgical treatment of obstructive sleep apnea, *Proc Am Thorac Soc* 5:193–199, 2008.

4. Sher AE, Thorpy MJ, Spielman AJ, et al: Predictive values of Müller maneuver in selection of patients for uvulopalatopharyngoplasty, *Laryngoscope* 95:1483–1487, 1985.
5. Guilleminault C, Simmons B, Motta J, et al: Obstructive sleep apnea syndrome and tracheostomy, *Arch Intern Med* 141:985–988, 1981.
6. Conway WA, Victor L, Magilligan DJ, et al: Adverse effects of tracheostomy for sleep apnea, *JAMA* 246:347–350, 1981.
7. Powell NB, Zonato AI, Weaver EM, et al: Radiofrequency treatment of turbinate hypertrophy in subjects using continuous positive airway pressure: a randomized, double-blind, placebo-controlled clinical pilot trial, *Laryngoscope* 111:1783–1790, 2001.
8. Koutsourelakis I, Georgoulopoulos G, Perraki E, et al: Randomized trial of nasal surgery for fixed nasal obstruction in obstructive sleep apnea, *Eur Respir J* 31:110–117, 2008.
9. Friedman M, Schalch P: Surgery of the palate and oropharynx, *Otolaryngol Clin North Am* 40:829–843, 2007.
10. Powell NB, Riley RW, Troell RJ, et al: Radiofrequency volumetric tissue reduction of the palate in subjects with sleep-disordered breathing, *Chest* 113:1163–1174, 1998.
11. Fujita S, Conway W, Zorick F, Roth T: Surgical correction of anatomic abnormalities in obstructive sleep apnea. Uvulopalatopharyngoplasty, *Otolaryngol Head Neck Surg* 89:923–934, 1981.
12. Larsson LH, Carlsson-Norlander B, Svanborg E: Four year follow-up after uvulopalatopharyngoplasty in 50 unselected patients with obstructive sleep apnea syndrome, *Laryngoscope* 104:1362–1368, 1994.
13. Fairbanks DNF: Uvulopalatopharyngoplasty complications and avoidance strategies, *Otolaryngol Head Neck Surg* 102:239–245, 1990.
14. Elshaug AG, Moss JR, Southcott A, et al: Redefining success in airway surgery for obstructive sleep apnea: a meta-analysis and synthesis of the evidence, *Sleep* 30:461–467, 2007.
15. Li KK: Hypoglossal airway surgery, *Otolaryngol Clin North Am* 40:845–853, 2007.
16. Li KK, Powell NB, Riley RW, et al: Long term results of maxillomandibular advancement surgery, *Sleep Breath* 3:137–139, 2000.
17. Li K, Powell NB, Riley RW, Guilleminault C: Temperature controlled radiofrequency tongue base reduction for sleep disordered breathing: long term outcomes, *Otolaryngol Head Neck Surg* 127:230–234, 2002.
18. Powell NB: Contemporary surgery for obstructive sleep apnea, *Clin Exp Otolaryngol* 2:107–114, 2009.
19. Friedman M, Hamilton C, Samuelson CG, et al: Transoral robotic glossectomy for the treatment of obstructive sleep apnea-hypopnea syndrome, *Otolaryngol Head Neck Surg* 146(5):854–862, 2012.

PATIENT 62

A Man with Severe OSA and Limited Treatment Options

A 55-year-old man was referred for severe daytime sleepiness of at least a 3-year duration (Epworth Sleepiness Scale [ESS] score of 22/24 – severe). He had been previously evaluated and found to have severe obstructive sleep apnea (OSA). At that time, he was started on nasal continuous positive airway pressure (CPAP), but he could not tolerate this treatment. The patient subsequently underwent uvulopalatopharyngoplasty (UPPP) with limited improvement in his symptoms. He was unable to lose weight but did discontinue drinking alcohol. He was treated with an oral device but found this very uncomfortable despite many adjustments. He fell asleep at work and was passed over for promotion.

Physical examination: Height 5 feet 8 inches; weight 220 pounds; HEENT: large tongue, well-healed palatal defect, mild retrognathia; neck: short, 18-inch circumference; chest: clear; cardiac: distant heart sounds; extremities: 3+ pedal edema; neurologic: patient asleep in the waiting room.

Sleep study (post-UPPP): Apnea–hypopnea index (AHI) 40 per hour (hr), no position dependence; type of events: mixed or obstructive apnea 50%, central apnea 5%, hypopnea 45%; arterial oxygen saturation: 400 desaturations to a low of 60%.

QUESTION

1. What treatment do you recommend?

ANSWER

1. **Answer:** Maxillomandibular advancement (MMA)

Discussion: Patients with severe sleep apnea who do not tolerate nasal CPAP pose a difficult problem for the sleep physician. UPPP may be tried, but it has only a 40% to 50% chance of reducing the AHI by 50%.[1-4] Thus, many patients with severe OSA will continue to have an AHI >20/hr after UPPP. For this reason, today UPPP is rarely offered to patients with severe OSA. Weight loss may be prescribed, but this treatment takes time, and successful maintenance of weight loss is rare. Some patients with severe OSA will respond to treatment with an oral appliance. However, for many patients with severe OSA, effective treatment options beyond nasal CPAP are limited to tracheostomy[5,6] or upper airway surgery more complex than UPPP.[7] In this patient, MMA is the most likely acceptable surgery to result in effective treatment. Tracheostomy would be effective but is unacceptable to most patients. Another approach in this patient might be genioglossus advancement (GA) and hyoid advancement (HA), but given the severity of the OSA and the retrognathia, most physicians would recommend the MMA procedure (if available). If MMA was not acceptable, tongue base reduction surgery may be considered.

Tracheostomy is a highly effective treatment for OSA.[5] However, it is cosmetically unacceptable to most patients. The indications for tracheosotomy in one large series included (1) disabling sleepiness with severe consequences, (2) cardiac arrhythmias with sleep apnea, (3) cor pulmonale, (4) AHI >40/hr, (5) frequent very severe desaturations and (6) no improvement after other therapy. Today, this treatment is usually reserved for patients with the obesity hypoventilation syndrome (OHS) and recurrent hypercapnic respiratory failure and who are not adherent to CPAP or bilevel PAP (BPAP) therapy. Tracheostomy may also be used for perioperative airway protection in selected patients undergoing upper airway surgery. Tracheostomy has significant complications in patients with OSA.[6] Postoperative complications include stomal infection or granulation tissue, accidental decannulation, obstruction of the tube when the patient's head is turned or hyperextended, recurrent purulent bronchitis, and psychosocial difficulties (depression). Noncuffed, size 6 French tubes usually suffice. A longer-than-usual tracheostomy tube may be needed for very obese patients with thick necks. The end of the tracheostomy tube typically is plugged during the day and, because of its small size, air flows around it between the lungs and the upper airway. During sleep, the tracheostomy tube is unplugged to bypass the upper airway obstruction. However, it must not be forgotten that very obese patients may still occlude the tracheostomy opening with "triple chins."

MMA is a treatment alternative for patients who have failed UPPP with or without GA and HA.[1-4,7,8] See Fundamentals 26 for an illustration and a description of the procedure. Some surgeons would recommend MMA as the first surgical procedure in a patient with severe OSA who has retrognathia or in whom multiple surgeries are not acceptable. When MMA is performed as the initial surgery, UPPP may also be performed if the palate is elongated. Indications for MMA are listed in Box P62-1. MMA is also called *maxillomandibular osteotomy and advancement* (MMOA). For patients with retroglossal upper airway obstruction tongue base reduction surgery is another option if an enlarged tongue base is causing obstruction.[9-11]

The American Academy of Sleep Medicine (AASM) practice parameters for surgical treatment of OSA[2] state: "MMA is indicated for surgical treatment of severe OSA in patients who cannot tolerate or are unwilling to adhere to positive airway pressure therapy, or in whom oral appliances, which are often more appropriate in mild and moderate OSA patients, have been considered and found ineffective or undesirable (Option)." The reason for the grade "Option" rather than the higher grade "Guideline" is that the published studies were considered "low quality of evidence" because they were small and not controlled. Other than tracheostomy, MMA is most likely to significantly improve the AHI in patients with severe OSA, although the AHI is often not normalized.

BOX P62-1	**Indications for Maxillomandibular Advancement**

- First surgical option:
  - Severe obstructive sleep apnea (OSA; especially with minimally redundant palate)
  - Retrognathia or facial skeletal deficiency
  - Morbid obesity
  - Adequate health to undergo surgery
- Second surgical option:
  - Failed previous surgical procedures (oral appliance [OA] unacceptable or likely ineffective, intolerant of positive airway pressure [PAP])

The MMA procedure increases the retrolingual and, to a small extent, the retropalatal segments of the upper airway. Numbness of the chin and cheek areas is an expected complication that resolves in 6 to 12 months in most patients.

Response rates up to 90% have been published—depending on the definition of surgical success. Li and coworkers[8] reported 95% "cure" rate defined as an AHI <20/hr and at least a 50% AHI reduction. In a group of 36 of 40 patients who were responders, the AHI dropped from 69.6/hr preoperatively to 7.7/hr postoperatively. A recent meta-analysis found MMA to reduce the AHI to less than 20/hr in 80% to 90% but to less than 10/hour in only 43%.[4] This procedure is usually offered only at large tertiary hospitals by experienced maxillofacial surgeons.

The present patient had persistent, disabling daytime sleepiness and moderate-to-severe oxygen desaturations after UPPP. When presented with the options of tracheostomy or more complex upper airway surgery, he chose the latter. He was evaluated with cephalometric radiography and fiberoptic pharyngoscopy and found to have a very small posterior airspace and evidence of mandibular deficiency.

The options of trying GA + HA first or proceeding directly to MMA were discussed with the patient. The patient already had a UPPP and only wanted one additional surgery. He subsequently underwent a MMA procedure. A sleep study performed 6 months after surgery revealed an AHI of 10/hr overall with minimal drops in the saturation of arterial oxygen (SaO_2). The patient's ESS score was reduced to 12 (mildly increased sleepiness). His performance at work improved, and he was quite satisfied with treatment.

CLINICAL PEARLS

1. The most reliable treatment for severe OSA in patients refusing or not tolerating PAP treatment is tracheostomy. This is rarely indicated except in patients with recurrent hypercapnic respiratory failure (or other severe manifestations of OSA) who are intolerant of PAP. Tracheostomy has a number of side effects as well as being cosmetically unacceptable to most patients.

2. Unless upper airway obstruction is localized to the retropalatal area, UPPP alone is usually ineffective in severe OSA. For this reason a UPPP is generally not indicated for treatment of severe OSA.

3. GA or GA + HA may increase the effectiveness of UPPP by preventing obstruction in the retroglossal hypopharyngeal region. The procedures may be effective if obstruction is present only in the retroglossal/hypopharyngeal areas.

4. MMA is an extensive procedure that is available only in specialized centers, but it is the surgery most likely to be effective in patients with severe OSA (excluding tracheostomy). MMA is often recommended as the initial surgery in patients with severe OSA and retrognathia. It may also be used in patients who have failed UPPP or UPPP + GA + HA.

REFERENCES

1. Caples SM, Rowley JA, Prinsell JR, et al: Surgical modifications of the upper airway for obstructive sleep apnea in adults: a systematic review and meta-analysis, *Sleep* 33:1396–1407, 2010.
2. Aurora RN, Casey KR, Kristo D, et al: Practice parameters for the surgical modifications of the upper airway for obstructive sleep apnea in adults, *Sleep* 33:1408–1413, 2010.
3. Won CHJ, Li KK, Guilleminault C: Surgical treatment of obstructive sleep apnea, *Proc Am Thorac Soc* 5:193–199, 2008.
4. Elshaug AG, Moss JR, Southcott A, et al: Redefining success in airway surgery for obstructive sleep apnea: a meta-analysis and synthesis of the evidence, *Sleep* 30:461–467, 2007.
5. Guilleminault C, Simmons B, Motta J, et al: Obstructive sleep apnea syndrome and tracheostomy, *Arch Intern Med* 141:985–988, 1981.
6. Conway WA, Victor L, Magilligan DJ, et al: Adverse effects of tracheostomy for sleep apnea, *JAMA* 246:347–350, 1981.
7. Li KK: Hypoglossal airway surgery, *Otolaryngol Clin North Am* 40:845–853, 2007.
8. Li KK, Powell NB, Riley RW, et al: Long term results of maxillomandibular advancement surgery, *Sleep Breath* 3:137–139, 2000.
9. Li K, Powell NB, Riley RW, Guilleminault C: Temperature controlled radiofrequency tongue base reduction for sleep disordered breathing: long term outcomes, *Otolaryngol Head Neck Surg* 127:230–234, 2002.
10. Friedman M, Hamilton C, Samuelson CG, et al: Transoral robotic glossectomy for the treatment of obstructive sleep apnea-hypopnea syndrome, *Otolaryngol Head Neck Surg* 146(5):854–862, 2012.
11. Powell NB: Contemporary surgery for obstructive sleep apnea, *Clin Exp Otolaryngol* 2:107–114, 2009.

Upper Airway Surgery in Two Patients

Patient A: A 30-year-old woman complained of fatigue and mild daytime sleepiness of 2-year duration. Her general internist was unable to find an explanation for her fatigue. The patient's husband reported that she snored heavily, especially in the supine position. She had gained 20 pounds over the last 2 years. Polysomnography (PSG) found the patient to have moderate obstructive sleep apnea (OSA) (apnea–hypopnea index [AHI] 20 per hour [hr]). Continuous positive airway pressure (CPAP) titration found CPAP of 8 centimeters of water (cm H_2O) to be very effective, but the patient declined this treatment.

Physical examination: Height 5 feet 3 inches; weight 177 pounds; body mass index (BMI) 31; HEENT: dependent palate, long edematous uvula, tongue normal, prominent pharyngeal tonsils, Mallampati score 3; neck: 14-inch circumference; chest: clear; cardiac: normal; extremities: trace edema.

Fiberoptic upper airway: examination: mainly retropalatal narrowing

Question 1: What treatment options do you suggest for Patient A?

Patient B: A 54-year-old female underwent a sleep study, which showed severe OSA by frequency (AHI 35.1/hr) but moderate desaturation (low saturation of arterial oxygen [SaO_2] 80%) during the diagnostic portion of a split-night sleep study. She tried CPAP but could not tolerate the treatment because of nasal congestion and dislike for masks of any type on her face.

Physical examination: BMI 31; HEENT: nose bilateral inferior turbinate hypertrophy; Mallampati score 4 with dependent palate

Fiberoptic upper airway examination: Bilateral inferior turbinate hypertrophy; prominent tongue base and both retrolingual and retroglossal obstruction during the Müller maneuver.

Question 2: What do you recommend for Patient B?

ANSWER

1. **Answer for Patient A:** Uvulopalatopharyngoplasty (UPPP) or an oral appliance (OA) as alternatives to nasal CPAP

   Discussion: UPPP is an operation that removes residual tonsillar tissue, the uvula, a portion of the soft palate, and redundant tissue from the pharyngeal area (see Fundamentals 26 for an illustration). Its disadvantages include the need for general anesthesia and postoperative discomfort. The most frequent complication is velopharyngeal insufficiency, which is manifested as some degree of nasal reflux when drinking fluids. This usually resolves within a month of surgery. Other potential complications include voice change, postoperative bleeding, and nasopharyngeal stenosis (secondary to scarring) (Box P63-1). A few cases of severe postsurgical bleeding or upper airway obstruction requiring reintubation have been reported. Significant apnea and desaturation may occur during the recovery period in patients with severe OSA. These problems often can be managed with nasal CPAP. Patients with moderate to severe OSA preoperatively should be monitored closely in the post-surgical period. UPPP is rarely performed for severe OSA unless the obstruction is felt to be localized to the palatal area.

   The major problem with UPPP is less-than-perfect efficacy as a treatment for OSA. UPPP does not address airway narrowing behind the tongue or in the hypopharynx; therefore, it is not universally effective in treating sleep apnea. It is more effective in decreasing the incidence or loudness of

---

BOX P63-1	**Complications from Uvulopalatopharyngoplasty**

IMMEDIATE

Pain—may be severe
Velopharyngeal incompetence (fluid out the nose during swallowing)
Voice change
Globus sensation—"mucus in the back of the throat"
Worsening of apnea in the postoperative period

DELAYED

Return of snoring
Worsening of obstructive sleep apnea
Nasopharyngeal stenosis
Increased probability of mouth leak during continuous positive airway pressure treatment

---

snoring (vibration of the soft palate). In general, 40% to 50% of all patients undergoing UPPP have about a 50% decrease in their AHI to <20/hr. Frequently, the number of apneas decreases, and the number of hypopneas increases. Boot et al. found that the effectiveness of UPPP may decrease with time. This is especially likely if weight gain occurs. Thus, patients treated with UPPP should be restudied if symptoms or signs of sleep apnea return. Dickel et al. found worsening of their condition after UPPP in a few patients. It should also be remembered that a split-night sleep study may underestimate the severity of OSA. Sometimes, patients undergo a split-night sleep study only to later decline or not tolerate CPAP. The severity of the OSA may be underestimated by the diagnostic portion of a split-night sleep study.

Several methods have been studied to determine if good responders to UPPP can be identified preoperatively. These methods include cephalometric radiography, computed tomography (CT), magnetic resonance imaging (MRI), fluoroscopy, fiberoptic endoscopy of the upper airway during Müeller maneuvers (precipitating airway collapse), and upper airway pressure monitoring during sleep. In some of these procedures, the patient is upright, and in most the patient is awake; therefore, it is not surprising that predictions of what happens during sleep are less than perfect. Patients with obstruction only in the palatal area are the most likely to respond to UPPP. However, no method can predict with certainty which patients will benefit from this surgery.

UPPP is considered less effective than nasal CPAP because it is less likely to eliminate apnea and normalize sleep. However, when nasal CPAP is refused or not tolerated, UPPP may be a treatment alternative—especially in mild-to-moderate apnea. With disease of this severity, the chances of obtaining a postoperative AHI <15/hr are reasonable. If UPPP fails, the option of again trying nasal CPAP is always available. However, a study by Mortimore et al. suggested that when nasal CPAP is used after UPPP, air leak via the mouth may be more likely. Even if CPAP is more effective than UPPP, if CPAP is not used for the entire night, the average AHI over the entire night on CPAP treatment may be >15/hour.

Patient A had moderate OSA, and she refused a trial of nasal CPAP. An OA is an effective option in mild to moderate OSA. However, when the patient performed a Müller maneuver, nasopharyngoscopy revealed collapse mainly in the retropalatal area; thus, the patient was considered a reasonable candidate for UPPP. In addition, her health insurance would not cover the costs of an OA. She underwent UPPP without complications except for postoperative pain. A PSG performed 3 months months after UPPP showed an AHI of 8/hr, with an arousal index of 10/hr. The patient reported a great improvement in symptoms. Attempts at weight loss have been unsuccessful.

2. **Answer for Patient B:** Treatment options include MMA or UPPP + other surgical options to address hypopharyngeal narrowing (genioglossus advancement (GA) and hyoid advancement (HA), or, tongue base reduction)

Discussion: In patients with severe OSA, MMA is the procedure most likely to achieve success (excluding tracheostomy). However, not all patients are willing to undergo MMA. If obstruction in the hypopharynx is contributing to sleep apnea, other procedures including GA (with or without HA) or tongue base surgery are surgical options (see figures in Fundamentals 26). Many techniques have been used for tongue base reduction, including temperature-controlled radiofrequency ablation and traditional resection. Side effects of tongue reduction have included voice change, difficulty swallowing, temporary pain, and a single report of a tongue abscess. Li et al studied the effect of radiofrequency ablation for tongue reduction and showed the AHI improved from 39.6/hr to 17.9/hr. However, long-term follow-up showed relapse (AHI = 28.7/hr) without major weight gain. Recently, the use of robotic surgery has been used and allows better visualization of the tongue area. The utility of tongue base surgery remains to be defined but may be an option for some patients.

TABLE P63-1   Before and After Upper Airway Surgery in Patient B

Parameter	Presurgery (Diagnostic Portion)	Postsurgery
Total sleep time (min)	116.5	480.5
Rapid eye movement (REM) (min)	15	92
% supine	59.7%	28.9
Apnea–hypopnea index (AHI) (no/hr)	36.0	6.7
AHI non-REM (NREM) (no/hr)	24.8	0.3
AHI REM (no/hr)	108	33.9
Obstructive apnea (no)	4	37
Central apnea (no)	0	0
Mixed apnea (no)	0	0
Hypopnea (no)	66	17
Desaturation (no)	46	50
Low saturation of arterial oxygen (SaO_2)	84%	82%

Patient B had an inferior turbinate reduction, UPPP, and a robotic partial glossectomy and lingual tonsillectomy during a single surgery. She reported excellent improvement in her symptoms. Table P63-1 shows results before and after the procedure. Although the overall AHI was reduced to near normal levels significant sleep apnea was still present during rapid eye movement (REM) sleep. Of note, the overall AHI during the treatment portion of the split study was 0.7/hr.

CLINICAL PEARLS

1. UPPP has roughly a 40% to 50% chance of reducing the AHI by 50%, to less than 20/hr.
2. Patients with obstruction only in the retropalatal area are more likely to respond to UPPP.
3. As subjective improvement exceeds objective response, repeat PSG several months after UPPP is needed to document efficacy.
4. An experienced surgeon and careful monitoring during the postoperative period are essential to reduce immediate complications of UPPP.
5. A significant number of initial responders to UPPP may relapse, especially if weight gain occurs. Patients should be restudied if signs or symptoms of sleep apnea return.
6. GA with or without HA may be used in combination with UPPP in patients with narrowing in both the retropalatal and retroglossal areas. Another option is UPPP with tongue base reduction surgery. For patients with severe OSA and obstruction in both the retropalatal and retroglossal areas, MMA is an effective option.

BIBLIOGRAPHY

Aurora RN, Casey KR, Kristo D, et al: Practice parameters for the surgical modifications of the upper airway for obstructive sleep apnea in adults, *Sleep* 33:1408–1413, 2010.

Boot H, van Wegen R, Poublon RM, et al: Long-term results of uvulopalatopharyngoplasty for obstructive sleep apnea syndrome, *Laryngoscope* 110(3 Pt 1):469–475, 2000.

Elshaug AG, Moss JR, Southcott A, et al: Redefining success in airway surgery for obstructive sleep apnea: a meta-analysis and synthesis of the evidence, *Sleep* 30:461–467, 2007.

Fairbanks DNF: Uvulopalatopharyngoplasty complications and avoidance strategies, *Otolaryngol Head Neck Surg* 102:239–245, 1990.

Fernández-Julián E, Muñoz N, Achiques MT, et al: Randomized study comparing two tongue base surgeries for moderate to severe obstructive sleep apnea syndrome, *Otolaryngol Head Neck Surg* 140(6):917–923, 2009.

Friedman M, Hamilton C, Samuelson CG, et al: Transoral robotic glossectomy for the treatment of obstructive sleep apnea–hypopnea syndrome, *Otolaryngol Head Neck Surg* 146(5):854–862, 2012.

Hudgel DW, Harasick T, Katz RL, et al: Uvulopalatopharyngoplasty in obstructive apnea: value of preoperative localization of site of upper airway narrowing during sleep, *Am Rev Respir Dis* 143:942–946, 1991.

Larsson LH, Carlsson-Norlander B, Svanborg E: Four year follow-up after uvulopalatopharyngoplasty in 50 unselected patients with obstructive sleep apnea syndrome, *Laryngoscope* 104:1362–1368, 1994.

Launois SH, Feroah TR, Campbell WN, et al: Site of pharyngeal narrowing predicts outcome of surgery for obstructive sleep apnea, *Am Rev Respir Dis* 147(1):182–189, 1993.

Li K, Powell NB, Riley RW, Guilleminault C: Temperature controlled radiofrequency tongue base reduction for sleep disordered breathing: long term outcomes, *Otolaryngol Head Neck Surg* 127:230–234, 2002.

Li KK: Hypoglossal airway surgery, *Otolaryngol Clin North Am* 40:845–853, 2007.

Mortimore IL, Bradley PA, Murray JA, et al: Uvulopalatopharyngoplasty may compromise nasal CPAP therapy in sleep apnea syndrome, *Am J Respir Crit Care Med* 54(6Pt1):1759–1762, 1996.

Sasse SA, Mahutte CK, Dickel M, Berry RB: The characteristics of five patients with obstructive sleep apnea whose apnea–hypopnea index deteriorated after uvulopalatopharyngoplasty, *Sleep Breath* 6(2):77–83, 2002.

FUNDAMENTALS 27

Oral Appliance Treatment for Obstructive Sleep Apnea

ORAL APPLIANCES

An oral appliance (OA) may be defined as a device inserted into the mouth for treatment of snoring or obstructive sleep apnea (OSA).[1–3] The two main types are devices moving the tongue forward [4–6] (tongue-retaining device [TRD]/tongue stabilizing device [TSD] [Figure F27-1]) and the mandibular repositioning appliances (MRAs) (Figure F27-2). The TSD/TRDs hold the tongue in a forward position by retaining the tongue in a suction bulb. The MRAs are attached to the dental arches and provide variable degrees of bite opening and mandibular advancement. The MRAs are also called *mandibular advancing devices* (MADs) or *mandibular repositioning devices* (MRDs).

INDICATIONS FOR ORAL APPLIANCES

Practice parameters for use of OAs in the treatment of OSA were published in 2006.[2] Since that time, OAs have improved but the basics remain the same (Box F27-1). OAs are indicated for treatment of snoring and mild and moderate OSA. Positive airway pressure (PAP) is the treatment of choice for moderate OSA, but if the patient cannot tolerate or adhere to PAP treatment, an OA is a viable option. The American Academy of Sleep Medicine (AASM) practice parameters for upper airway surgery suggested that OAs be considered before uvulopalatopharyngoplasty (UPPP) for moderate OSA (although some patients will prefer surgery). For severe OSA, the treatment of choice is PAP, the second being complex upper airway surgery, and last an OA. OAs may substantially reduce the AHI in severe OSA but rarely to normal levels. OAs could be used in patients who have failed UPPP, in combination with PAP, or both. *Patients with postural OSA may be more likely to respond to OAs.*[7]

EVALUATION OF THE PATIENT

Each candidate for an OA should be examined by a qualified dentist to determine whether an OA is feasible and safe from a dental standpoint (Box F27-2). The dental examination should focus on the temporomandibular joint (TMJ), evidence or history of bruxism, quality of dental occlusion, the presence of significant periodontal disease, overall dental health, and protrusive

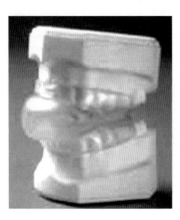
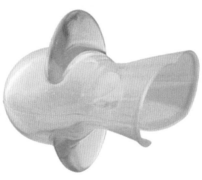

FIGURE F27-1 ■ *Left,* Tongue retaining device (TRD). *Right,* Tongue stabilizing device (TSD). The TRD is fabricated for each patient whereas the TSD comes in three standard sizes (small, medium, large). From Berry RB: Fundamentals of sleep medicine, Philadelphia, 2012, Saunders, p 350.

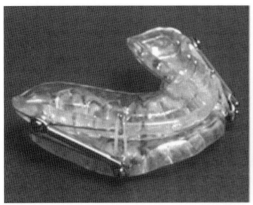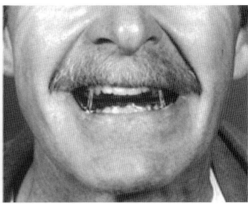

HERBST APPLIANCE

FIGURE F27-2 ■ A Herbst appliance. The side arms allow adjustment of the amount of mandibular protrusion. From Berry RB: Sleep medicine pearls, ed 2, Philadelphia, 2003, Saunders, p 175.

BOX F27-1	Oral Appliance Treatment Guidelines

1. *Initial diagnosis:* Presence or absence of OSA must be determined before OA treatment for snoring or OSA.
2. *Appliance fitting:* OA treatment should be managed by dental practitioners with training in sleep medicine and sleep-related breathing disorders.
3. Cephalometry is not always needed, but if used, qualified professionals should perform and evaluate.
4. Primary snoring—Goal of OA is to reduce snoring to a subjectively acceptable level.
5. OSA—Goals of treatment are resolution of clinical signs and symptoms of OSA, normalization of AHI, and oxyhemoglobin saturation.
6. OAs are indicated for treatment of primary snoring in patients who do not respond to or are not appropriate candidates for weight loss or sleep position change.
7. OA treatment is indicated for mild to moderate OSA.
   a. OA is not as efficacious as CPAP but is preferred by some patients.
   b. OA is indicated with CPAP failures.
   c. OA treatment is indicated when there is failure of weight loss or side sleep position treatments.
8. OAs are not indicated for initial treatment of severe OSA. Upper airway surgery may also supersede use of OA in patients for whom surgery is predicted to be highly effective.

Adapted from Kushida CA, Morgenthaler TI, Littner MR, et al: American Academy of Sleep Medicine. Practice parameters for the treatment of snoring and obstructive sleep apnea with oral appliances: an update for 2005, *Sleep* 29:240-243, 2006.
AHI, Apnea–hypopnea index; *CPAP,* continuous positive airway pressure; *OA,* oral appliance; *OSA,* obstructive sleep apnea.

ability. Cephalometry or dental radiography may be indicated.[8] The patient's occlusion type should be noted. Three classes (types) of skeletal occlusions are illustrated in Figure F27-3. Overbite refers to the vertical overlap between upper and lower incisors and overjet to the horizontal distance between the posterior surface of the upper incisors and the anterior surface of the lower incisors. The expectation may be that patients with mandibular deficiency (retrognathia) would benefit the most from an OA, but the amount of improvement is somewhat unpredictable. Patients with occlusion mainly in the retroglossal area rather than in the retropalatal area might be expected to improve the most with an MRA. However, in one study, some patients with upper airway occlusion mainly in the velopharynx also improved with MRA treatment.[9]

EXCLUSIONS AND CONTRAINDICATIONS

Patients must have a minimal of 6 to 10 healthy teeth in each arch.[1,3] Edentulous patients may be treated with a TRD/TSD. Treatment with dental implants may permit future MRA treatment in patients with insufficient dentition at the time of evaluation. Patients must be able to open the jaw adequately for OA insertion and must have the ability to voluntarily protrude the mandible. Moderate to severe TMJ disease or inadequate protrusive ability are contraindications. Mild TMJ dysfunction may actually improve with the jaw positioned anteriorly during sleep. Moderate to severe bruxism is a contraindication in most cases. Bruxism during sleep may damage some types of OAs. However, bruxism in some patients improves with adequate treatment of

OSA. An experienced dental practitioner should evaluate patients with bruxism for suitability for an OA. A history of bruxism may also alter the choice of the type of OA used.

DEVICES

MRAs come in monobloc (boil and bite) fixed configurations or custom-fitted appliances that can be adjusted to change the amount of mandibular protrusion (advancement). The ideal device has coverage of both arches, provides posterior stabilization, and is adjustable (protrusion may

BOX F27-2	Dental Evaluation for OSA and Device Adjustment

Pre OA evaluation	1. PSG or OCST in all patients (even if only snoring expected)
	2. Dental evaluation
	  • Condition of teeth and gums (minimum 6 teeth in each arch)
	  • Edentulous patients may use TSD
	  • Type of occlusion
	  • TMJ (moderate to severe problems a contraindication)
	  • Bruxism (moderate to severe contraindication)
	  • Ability to open mouth and protrude mandible

Titration	3. Progressive adjustment (protrusion) based on symptoms, bed partner report of snoring, OCST, or PSG 4. During PSG some devices may be titrated

OCST, Out-of-center sleep testing; *OSA*, obstructive sleep apnea; *PSG*, polysomnography; *TMJ*, temporomandibular joint; *TSD*, tongue-stabilizing device.

be changed). A recent study compared a custom-made and thermoplastic OA for the treatment of mild OSA. The custom-made device was more effective.[10] However, custom-made devices are typically much more expensive. OAs are now viewed by the U.S. Food and Drug Administration (FDA) as class 2 medical devices and, as such, must adhere to more detailed standards with special controls.[11] For a list of commonly available devices, the reader is referred to Reference 3 listed at the end of the chapter.

TITRATION OR ADJUSTMENT OF ORAL APPLIANCES

After OAs are fabricated, they are usually adjusted for fit and comfort by the dentist taking care of the patient. Patients are then instructed to slowly increase mandibular protrusion until symptoms improve (cessation of snoring and improvement in sleep quality) or until either the maximum protrusion is reached or further advances are not tolerated. In one study, patients were studied during polysomnography (PSG) and a remotely controlled mandibular appliance was advanced until respiratory events were controlled or until further advances were not tolerated.[12] The results of the PSG OA titration were highly predictive of the effectiveness of chronic OA treatment with a permanent device. In another study, patients were allowed to adjust their devices at home.[13] They subsequently had a PSG wearing the OA and if persistent events were noted, further adjustment during the PSG was performed by protocol (increased protrusion in 1-mm increments). Of the patients completing the protocol, 55% were successfully treated (apnea–hypopnea index [AHI] <10 per hour [hr]) after home titration. However, a total of 64.9% of patients were successfully treated overall with an additional 9.9%

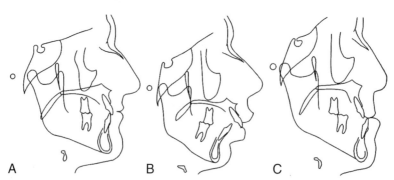

FIGURE F27-3 ■ Lateral cephalometric views of three distinct skeletal occlusions. **A,** A skeletal Class I occlusion. A nearly ideal skeletal and dental balance is present. **B,** A skeletal Class II malocclusion (overjet, or retrognathia). Mandibular deficiency is present. Note the everted lower lip and distance between the upper and the lower incisors. **C,** A skeletal Class III occlusion with mandibular hyperplasia and maxillary hypoplasia (or prognathia). The upper incisor is behind the lower incisor. (**A-C,** From Conely RS: Orthodontic considerations related to sleep disordered breathing, *Sleep Med Clin* 5:71-89, 2009.)

successfully treated after OA adjustment during the PSG (55% + 9.9% total responders). Thus some patients will likely need further adjustments either during or after PSG documenting the efficacy of OA treatment.

ADHERENCE TO ORAL APPLIANCE TREATMENT

Studies of adherence to OA treatment have almost always relied on patient report. Objective monitoring of OA adherence is not possible using small embedded temperature sensing data loggers.[3] This technology will enhance clinical practice and research OA adherence rates tend to decrease with the duration of use.[1,3,14,15] Clark et al reported a 51% of patients were still using an OA at the 3-year follow-up. Of interest, 40% reported some change in occlusion. Another study reported 62% adherence at the 4-year of follow-up.[16] In a questionnaire study of patients with OAs, 5 years after starting treatment, 64% of respondents were using the OA. Of these, 93% were using the OA more than 4 nights per week. In those stopping OA treatment, the causes were discomfort (44%), little or no effect (34%), and the patient changing to CPAP treatment (23%).[17] In cross-over studies of continuous PAP (CPAP), adherence to OA was equal to or better than to CPAP.[18-20]

EFFECTIVENESS COMPARED WITH OTHER TREATMENTS

A number of studies comparing OSA and CPAP[1,3] have shown that OAs are not as effective as CPAP but are effective in a significant proportion of patients (19%–67%) (Table F27-1).[1] In some studies, a significant proportion of patients preferred the OA to CPAP. In a typical study, the baseline AHI was around 30/hr and the AHI was reduced to less than 5/hr on CPAP, and 10 to 15 per hour on an OA (Figure F27-4).

SIDE EFFECTS AND COMPLICATIONS

Commonly side effects of OAs include TMJ pain, myofascial pain, tooth pain, excessive salivation, TMJ sounds, dry mouth, gum irritation, and occlusal changes for several hours after removing the OA in the morning.[1,20,21] These phenomena were observed in a wide range of frequencies from 6% to 86% of patients.[1,3] Patients undergoing TRD and TSD treatments may report a sore tongue or difficulty with the device slipping off during

TABLE F27-1	Range of Effectiveness of Oral Appliance Treatment of Obstructive Sleep Apnea*	
	Mild to Moderate OSA	**Severe OSA**
OA success	57%-81%	14%-61%

From Ferguson KA, Cartwright R, Rogers R, et al: Oral appliances for snoring and obstructive sleep apnea: a review, *Sleep* 29:244-262, 2006.
AHI, Apnea-hypopnea index; *OA*, oral appliance; *OSA*, obstructive sleep apnea.
*Success is defined as a reduction of the AHI to <10/hr.

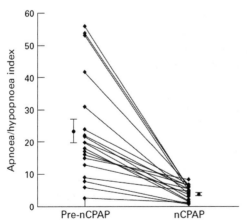
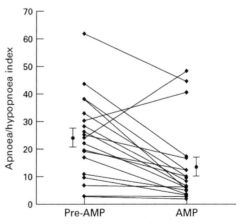

FIGURE F27-4 ■ The apnea–hypopnea index (AHI) as determined by home monitoring before and after treatment with nasal continuous positive airway pressure (nCPAP; *left*) and an anterior mandibular positioner (AMP; *right*). The AHI was significantly reduced (*p* <0.05) by both devices, although the posttreatment AHI was lower with nCPAP. (From Ferguson KA, Ono T, Lowe AA, et al: A short-term controlled trial of an adjustable oral appliance for the treatment of mild to moderate obstructive sleep apnoea, *Thorax* 52:362-368.)

the night. Several studies found long-term changes in dental occlusion but the results vary between studies[1,16,20,21]. The dental changes were usually mild, sometimes beneficial (reduction in overjet), and were often not noticed by the patients.[21] A study by Rose et al[22] found changes in the anteroposterior position of the molars and the inclination of upper and lower incisors changed with MRA treatment (mean follow-up of 30 months).

COMBINATIONS OF ORAL APPLIANCE WITH OTHER TREATMENTS

Use of an OA in patients with persistent sleep apnea after UPPP was reported by Millman and coworkers[23] in 18 patients. The post UPPP AHI was 37.2/hr, and the arterial oxygen saturation (SaO_2) nadir was 84%. With OA treatment, the AHI fell to 15.3/hr, and the SaO_2 nadir was 87.9%. With the addition of a Herbst device, 10 of the patients had a fall in the AHI to less than 10/hr. OAs may be used with CPAP, and some oral devices are specially designed to work with CPAP.

FOLLOW-UP

The practice parameters do not mandate repeat sleep testing for OA treatment of snoring (Box F27-3). For all severities of OSA, repeat sleep testing with the patient wearing the OA is indicated to document effectiveness.[2,24] Unattended out-of-center sleep testing (OCST) or PSG are acceptable methods. During PSG, some devices may be titrated by using a protocol determined by the treating dentist and sleep physician. Follow-up visits with the dentist who fabricated the OA are also indicated every 6 months and then yearly. This is to ensure that side effects are not significant and that the amount of protrusion is optimized. Follow-up with the clinician directing sleep apnea treatment is also indicated to ensure that OSA symptoms are controlled and do not recur. If symptoms return on OA treatment, repeat sleep testing with OA in place is indicated.

BOX F27-3 **Follow-Up after Oral Appliance Treatment**

1. Follow-up sleep testing is not indicated after OA treatment of primary snoring.
2. Follow-up sleep testing with OA in place *IS* indicated after OA treatment of OSA after final adjustments of fit have been performed. Testing is indicated for all OSA severities.
3. PSG or OCST can be used to document OA efficacy.
4. Follow-up visits with dental specialist until optimal fit and efficacy are shown.
5. Follow-up dental visits every 6 months for first year, and annually thereafter.
6. Regular visits with clinician supervising treatment of OSA.
7. Repeat sleep study with OA in place if signs or symptoms of OSA worsen or recur.

OA, Oral appliance; *OCST*, out of center sleep test; *OSA*, obstructive sleep apnea; *PM*, portable monitoring; *PSG*, polysomnography.

CLINICAL PEARLS

1. The presence or absence of OSA must be determined before OA treatment for snoring or suspected OSA. It is important to determine whether OSA or snoring is being treated. If OSA is present, the severity has implications for treatment selection and the probability of success with OA.
2. The OA should be fitted by a qualified dental professional.
3. OAs are indicated for primary snoring and mild to moderate OSA. Patients with moderate OSA should be offered CPAP. If CPAP is not acceptable, OA treatment or surgery are options.
4. CPAP, rather than OA, should be the first treatment for severe OSA. If CPAP is not accepted, upper airway surgery or an OA should be considered.
5. PSG or OCST (with the patient wearing the OA) is needed to document the effectiveness of OA after adjustment.
6. Titration of OAs is possible with PSG (some devices) and may improve the efficacy.
7. Follow-up of OA treatment should include both dental follow-up to address OA side effects and any changes in dentition or occlusion and physician follow-up to assess if symptoms of OSA are well controlled and to verify continued adherence to treatment.
8. A significant number of patients stop using the oral appliance within 3 years (40 to 50%), and some change occurs in occlusion in up to 40%, although the dental changes are usually not significant.

REFERENCES

1. Ferguson KA, Cartwright R, Rogers R, et al: Oral appliances for snoring and obstructive sleep apnea: a review, *Sleep* 29:244–262, 2006.
2. Kushida CA, Morgenthaler TI, Littner MR, et al: American Academy of Sleep Medicine: Practice parameters for the treatment of snoring and obstructive sleep apnea with oral appliances: an update for 2005, *Sleep* 29:240–243, 2006.
3. Sutherland K, Vanderveken OM, Tsuda H, et al: Oral appliance treatment for obstructive sleep apnea: an update, *J Clin Sleep Med* 10(2):215–227, 2014.
4. Lazard DS, Blumen M, Lévy P, et al: The tongue-retaining device: efficacy and side effects in obstructive sleep apnea syndrome, *J Clin Sleep Med* 5:431–438, 2009.
5. Dort L, Brant R: A randomized, controlled, crossover study of a noncustomized tongue retaining device for sleep disordered breathing, *Sleep Breath* 12:369–373, 2008.
6. Deane SA, Cistulli PA, Ng AT, et al: Comparison of mandibular advancement splint and tongue stabilizing device in obstructive sleep apnea: a randomized controlled trial, *Sleep* 32:648–653, 2009.
7. Chung JW, Enciso R, Levendowski DJ, et al: Treatment outcomes of mandibular advancement devices in positional and nonpositional OSA patients, *Oral Surg Oral Med Oral Pathol Oral Radiol Endod* 109:724–731, 2010.
8. Conely RS: Orthodontic considerations related to sleep disordered breathing, *Sleep Med Clin* 5:71–89, 2009.
9. Henke KG, Fratnz DE, Kuna ST: An oral mandibular advancement device for obstructive sleep apnea, *Am J Respir Crit Care Med* 161:420–425, 2000.
10. Vanderveken OM, Devolder A, Marklund M, et al: Comparison of a custom-made and a thermoplastic oral appliance for the treatment of mild sleep apnea, *Am J Respir Crit Care Med* 178:197–202, 2008.
11. Center for Devices and Radiologic Health, U.S. Food and Drug Administration: Class II special controls guidance document: intraoral devices for snoring and/or obstructive sleep apnea: guidance for industry, *FDA Bulletin*.
12. Tsai WH, Vazquez J, Oshima T, et al: Remotely controlled mandibular positioner predicts efficacy of an oral appliance in sleep apnea, *Am J Respir Crit Care Med* 170:366–370, 2004.
13. Krishnan V, Collop N, Scherr S: An evaluation of a titration strategy for prescription of an oral appliance for obstructive sleep apnea, *Chest* 133:1135–1141, 2008.
14. Clark GT, Sohn JW, Hong CN: Treating obstructive sleep apnea and snoring: assessment of an anterior mandibular positioning device, *J Am Dent Assoc* 131(6):765–771, 2000.
15. Clark GT, Blumenfeld I, Yoffe N, et al: A crossover study comparing the efficacy of continuous positive airway pressure with anterior mandibular positioning devices on patients with obstructive sleep apnea, *Chest* 109:1477–1483, 1996.
16. Walker-Engström ML, Tegelberg Å, Wilhelmsson B, Ringqvist I: 4-year follow-up of treatment with dental appliance or uvulopalatopharyngoplasty in patients with obstructive sleep apnea: a randomized study, *Chest* 121:739–746, 2002.
17. de Almeida FR, Lowe AA, Tsuiki S, et al: Long-term compliance and side effects of oral appliances used for the treatment of snoring and obstructive sleep apnea syndrome, *J Clin Sleep Med* 1:143–152, 2005.
18. Ferguson KA, Ono T, Lowe AA, et al: A randomized crossover study of an oral appliance vs nasal-continuous positive airway pressure in the treatment of mild-moderate obstructive sleep apnea, *Chest* 109:1269–1275, 1996.
19. Clark GT, Blumenfeld I, Yoffe N, et al: A crossover study comparing the efficacy of continuous positive airway pressure with anterior mandibular positioning devices on patients with obstructive sleep apnea, *Chest* 109:1477–1483, 1996.
20. Engleman HM, McDonald JP, Graham D, et al: Randomized crossover trial of two treatments for sleep apnea/hypopnea syndrome: continuous positive airway pressure and mandibular repositioning splint, *Am J Respir Crit Care Med* 166:855–859, 2002.
21. Robertson CJ: Dental and skeletal changes associated with long-term mandibular advancement, *Sleep* 24(5):531–537, 2001.
22. Rose E, Statts R, Virchow C, Jonas IE: Occlusal and skeletal effects of an oral appliance in treatment of obstructive sleep apnea, *Chest* 122:871–877, 2002.
23. Millman RP, Rosenberg CL, Carlisle CC, et al: The efficacy of oral appliances in the treatment of persistent sleep apnea after uvulopalatopharyngoplasty, *Chest* 113:992–996, 1998.
24. Collop NA, McDowell W, Boehlecke B, et al: Clinical guidelines for the use of unattended portable monitors in the diagnosis of obstructive sleep apnea in adult patients, *J Clin Sleep Med* 3:737–747, 2007.

A 40-Year-Old Man with Sleep Apnea Unable to Accept CPAP Treatment

A 40-year-old man was evaluated for complaints of loud snoring and daytime sleepiness (Epworth Sleepiness Scale [ES] score of 12). Although he was able to function fairly well, he sometimes fell asleep during important business meetings. His work required him to travel frequently. The patient had read extensively about sleep apnea and wanted to avoid nasal continuous positive airway pressure (CPAP), if possible. He was recently divorced and feared that use of this device would impair his social life. In addition, he wanted to avoid surgery, if possible.

Physical examination: Height 5 feet 10 inches; weight 220 pounds; blood pressure: normal; HEENT: slight retrognathia, palate edematous but otherwise normal, Mallampati 4; neck: 16-inch circumference; cardiac: normal; extremities: no edema

Sleep study: See Table P64-1.

TABLE P64-1	**Sleep Study Results**		
AHI (#/hr)	25	AHIsupine (#/hr)	40
AHI NREM (#/hr)	15	AHInonsupine (#/hr)	15
AHI REM (#/hr)	30	Low SpO$_2$ (%)	89%

AHI, Apnea–hypopnea index; *NREM*, non–rapid eye movement; *REM*, rapid eye movement; *SpO$_2$*, arterial oxygen saturation by pulse oximetry; #, number.

QUESTION

1. What treatment options would you consider for this patient?

ANSWER

1. **Answer:** An oral appliance (OA)

   Discussion: OAs may be an effective treatment in patients with snoring or mild-to-moderate obstructive sleep apnea (OSA). Some patients with severe apnea also will respond. The importance of OAs for treatment of OSA is highlighted by the establishment of the American Academy of Dental Sleep Medicine. OAs work either by retaining the tongue in a forward position (tongue-retaining device) or by moving the mandible forward (thereby indirectly moving the tongue) a so-called mandibular advancing device (MAD). Because the great majority of OAs used are MADs, the term OA is used in the following discussion to refers to this type appliance.

   An evaluation is recommended for all patients for whom the use of an OA is planned, even if only snoring is believed to be present. The finding of more severe OSA than anticipated may change treatment plans. Patients must have a dental evaluation to determine if they are good candidates for an OA. To be effective, OAs require an appliance fitting by a trained dentist to obtain the dental impression and bite registration. The device is then fabricated in a dental laboratory. A few devices composed of thermolabile material may be molded to the patient's teeth in the office ("boil and bite"). However, even with simpler MADs, the involvement of a dentist is recommended because if the mandible is moved too far forward or too rapidly, temporomandibular joint (TMJ) problems may occur. With careful fitting of oral appliances, TMJ problems can be avoided. However, these devices generally are not recommended for patients with pre-existing moderate to severe TMJ problems.

Oral devices frequently induce excess salivation, at least initially, as well as some mild discomfort in the morning. Thus, adherence to treatment is a problem with oral devices as with nasal CPAP. Studies in which both nasal CPAP and OAs were effective have revealed that many patients prefer treatment with an OA. The patient is started on a conservative amount of mandibular advancement, and this is usually increased slowly over several weeks until the desired result is obtained (no snoring etc.). Once the device has been optimally adjusted, a sleep study of some type (polysomnography [PSG] or out-of-center sleep testing [OCST]) is recommended for all severities of OSA to ensure effectiveness. It is also possible to perform further adjustment of the OA in the sleep center during an attended sleep study. This requires a protocol and training of sleep technologists on how to advance the mandible. The efficacy of OAs may improve using OA titration during a PSG. One problem with OA treatment is that it is often difficult to predict the degree of improvement in a given patient. The findings of a study by Chung et al. *suggested demonstration of postural OSA (AHIsupine >2 ×AHInonsupine) was associated with a better response from an oral appliance.*

The patient should be monitored by a dentist to ensure that TMJ or signficant occlusion problems do not develop. Some evidence suggests that after 3 to 5 years of use, OAs may induce some mild shift in the dentition. The patient should also be monitored by a physician to ensure that symptoms of OSA do not reappear.

In the present case, nasal CPAP would be effective, but it was not acceptable to the patient. The other suitable treatment options included uvulopalatopharyngoplasty (UPPP) and other types of upper airway surgery, or OAs. The patient did have a significant postural component to his sleep apnea, which predicted a good result from OA treatment. Respecting the patient's wish to avoid surgery, if possible, he was referred to a dentist experienced in fabricating and adjusting OAs. An impression of the patient's teeth was made, a bite registration was taken, and a dental laboratory prepared a Herbst device (see Fundamentals 27). This device allows forward movement of the jaw (Figure P64-1). It was attached to the teeth on both the maxilla and the mandible and was unlikely to fall out during the night. A sleep study after the OAs was adjusted showed a residual AHI of 10/hour. Although the AHI was not as low as might be possible with CPAP, the patient noted complete resolution of his daytime sleepiness and his ESS score fell from 12 to 8.

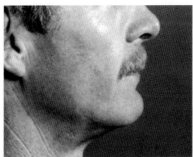 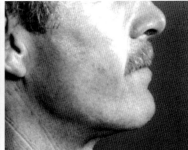

FIGURE P64-1 ■ A lateral view of the patient without and with the Herbst appliance in place. Note that the patient has mild retrognathia, but when the device is worn, the mandible is protruded. Adapted from Berry RB. Fundamentals of Sleep Medicine Pearls pg 350.

Before   Herbst appliance

CLINICAL PEARLS

1. An OA may be effective treatment in mild-to-moderate OSA.

2. Some patients with severe OSA will also have a good response to an OA.

3. Patients with significant TMJ problems are poor candidates for OAs.

4. Involvement of a dentist is crucial in preventing dental complications of OAs.

5. A sleep study (PSG or OCST) after the patient has stabilized on an OA is recommended for patients with mild to severe OSA.

6. An OA should not be used for "presumed snoring" without a sleep study to rule out OSA. If OSA is present this may change treatment plans and follow-up.

BIBLIOGRAPHY

Bailey DR, Hoekema A: Oral appliance therapy in sleep medicine, *Sleep Med Clin* 5:91–98, 2010.

Chung JW, Enciso R, Levendowski DJ, et al: Treatment outcomes of mandibular advancement devices in positional and non-positional OSA patients, *Oral Surg Oral Med Oral Pathol Oral Radiol Endod* 109:724–731, 2010.

Ferguson KA, Cartwright R, Rogers R, et al: Oral appliances for snoring and obstructive sleep apnea: a review, *Sleep* 29:244–262, 2006.

Henke KG, Fratnz DE, Kuna ST: An oral mandibular advancement device for obstructive sleep apnea, *Am J Respir Crit Care Med* 161:420–425, 2000.

Krishnan V, Collop N, Scherr S: An evaluation of a titration strategy for prescription of an oral appliance for obstructive sleep apnea, *Chest* 133:1135–1141, 2008.

Kushida CA, Morgenthaler TI, Littner MR, et al: American Academy of Sleep Medicine: Practice parameters for the treatment of snoring and obstructive sleep apnea with oral appliances: an update for 2005, *Sleep* 29:240–243, 2006.

Vanderveken OM, Devolder A, Marklund M, et al: Comparison of a custom-made and a thermoplastic oral appliance for the treatment of mild sleep apnea, *Am J Respir Crit Care Med* 178:197–202, 2008.

PATIENT 65

A 45-Year-Old Woman Experiencing Daytime Sleepiness After UPPP

A 45-year-old woman with significant daytime sleepiness and fatigue was diagnosed with severe sleep apnea (apnea–hypopnea index [AHI] 36.9 per hour [hr]) (Table P65-1). She underwent continuous positive airway pressure (CPAP) titration but did not tolerate this treatment. After several treatment options were discussed (including an oral appliance [OA]), the patient decided to undergo uvulopalato-pharyngoplasty (UPPP). Surgery was performed, and the patient initially noted improvement in snoring and daytime sleepiness. A sleep study was ordered for 3 months after surgery but was never completed. At 6 months after UPPP, the patient began to have a return of her symptoms of daytime sleepiness and fatigue. The patient admitted that she had gained about 15 pounds since surgery. A repeat sleep study was ordered (see Table P65-1).

Physical examination: Blood pressure 160/90; pulse 88; respirations 16; HEENT: well-healed UPPP palatal defect, moderate-size tongue; chest: clear; cardiac: normal; extremities: no edema

TABLE P65-1 Sleep Study Results		
	Diagnostic	**6 Months After Uvulopalatopharyngoplasty**
Total sleep time (min)	390	400
Rapid eye movement (min)	60	80
Apnea–hypopnea index (AHI) (no/hr)	36.9	16.5
AHI non–rapid eye movement (NREM) (no/hr)	33.9	14
AHI REM (no/hr)	53	30
Obstructive apnea (no)	89	10
Mixed apnea (no)	0	0
Central apnea (no)	0	0
Hypopnea (no)	150	100
Desaturations (no)	239	130
Low saturation of arterial oxygen (%)	80	88

no, Number; *no/hr*, number per hour of sleep.

QUESTION

1. What treatment would you recommend for this patient?

ANSWER

1. **Answer**: An OA and weight loss for persistent obstructive sleep apnea (OSA) after UPPP

   Discussion: UPPP is a treatment option for patients with mild OSA and for moderate OSA if they do not tolerate or accept CPAP. In the American Academy of Sleep Medicine (AASM) practice parameters for surgical treatment of OSA, it is stated that "UPPP as a single surgical procedure, with or without tonsillectomy, does not reliably normalize the AHI when treating moderate to severe OSA". Therefore, patients with severe OSA should initially be offered PAP therapy, and those with moderate OSA should initially be offered either PAP therapy or an OA. However, the benefit of an OA in a given patient is also variable and not all patients have an AHI less than 10/hr on OA treatment. Some patients would rather have a surgical procedure given the need to wear an OA each night for benefit. As illustrated in Patient 63, some patients have a good response to UPPP. The current patient with moderate OSA chose to undergo UPPP as treatment for OSA.

   A significant proportion of patients will experience inadequate improvement after UPPP. Another common scenerio is initial improvement after UPPP with subsequent redevelopment of symptoms (especially with weight gain). Rarely, OSA may worsen after UPPP, possibly secondary to scar tissue at the site.

   What options are available for patients who require additional treatment after UPPP? One option is to ask the patient to lose weight. Weight loss of just 10% to 20% of body weight may dramatically reduce the AHI in some patients. Certainly, weight gain should be avoided in any patient undergoing UPPP. Because weight loss is difficult (and often slow) to achieve and maintain, it should not be relied upon as the sole treatment for OSA except in the mildest cases. In patients with postural OSA after UPPP, use of postural treatment could be considered. A third option is CPAP treatment. This should prove effective. Unfortunately, many patients undergo UPPP because they are unwilling to undergo CPAP. However, some will reconsider this decision and submit to nasal CPAP titration. A study by Montimore et al. study found that mouth leaks are more common on nasal CPAP following UPPP. However, this is not invariably present and may be addressed by a chin strap or full-face mask. Heated humidity may help patients tolerate a mouth leak. A fourth alternative is to proceed to more advanced surgical treatment. A fifth option is to try an OA as treatment for residual OSA. The rationale for trying an OA in UPPP failures is that the UPPP should have decreased obstruction at the retropalatal area and the OA should reduce obstruction behind the tongue and in the hypopharynx. A study by Millman and coworkers has reported success with OA treatment of patients with significant residual OSA after UPPP. Even if the site of obstruction after UPPP is still retropalatal, OA may still be effective. Henke and coworkers found that an OA was effective in some patients with predominantly retropalatal obstruction. The mechanism of this action is not known.

   In the present patient, a sleep study 6 months after UPPP showed persistent, significant sleep apnea, although it had improved from the initial surgery. Of note, before surgery, the patient had been offered more complex upper airway surgery but declined these options. In the table, note that apneas composed a smaller fraction of the respiratory events after UPPP. The patient again declined nasal CPAP treatment and was referred to a dentist. An OA was constructed (mandibular advancement device). With the use of this device, the patient's symptoms improved. A repeat sleep study with the device in place showed an overall AHI of 5/hr. The symptoms of daytime sleepiness improved. She was referred to a dietician and started a structured weight-loss program. In retrospect, it is possible that an OA without UPPP would have been effective. However, it is also possible that both treatments contributed to the desired outcome.

CLINICAL PEARLS

1. Patients who undergo UPPP should be monitored closely. In some patients, symptoms of OSA return after an initial improvement.
2. Nasal CPAP treatment may be more difficult in patients with a previous UPPP because of an increased tendency for mouth leaks.
3. OAs may be a satisfactory treatment for some patients in whom UPPP failed.
4. A sleep study should be ordered to document efficacy of OA treatment for all severities of OSA.

BIBLIOGRAPHY

Aurora RN, Casey KR, Kristo D, et al: Practice parameters for the surgical modifications of the upper airway for obstructive sleep apnea in adults, *Sleep* 33:1408–1413, 2010.

Ferguson KA, Cartwright R, Rogers R, et al: Oral appliances for snoring and obstructive sleep apnea: a review, *Sleep* 29:244–262, 2006.

Henke KG, Frantz DE, Kuna ST: An oral elastic mandibular advancement device for obstructive sleep apnea, *Am J Respir Crit Care Med* 161:420–425, 2000.

Kushida CA, Morgenthaler TI, Littner MR, et al: American Academy of Sleep Medicine: Practice parameters for the treatment of snoring and obstructive sleep apnea with oral appliances: an update for 2005, *Sleep* 29:240–243, 2006.

Millman RP, Rosenberg CL, Carlisle CC, et al: The efficacy of oral appliances in the treatment of persistent sleep apnea after uvulopalatopharyngoplasty, *Chest* 113:992–996, 1998.

Mortimore IL, Bradley PA, Murray JAM, et al: Uvulopalatopharyngoplasty may compromise nasal CPAP therapy in sleep apnea syndromes, *Am J Respir Care Med* 154:1759–1762, 1995.

Sutherland K, Vanderveken OM, Tsuda H, et al: Oral appliance treatment for obstructive sleep apnea: an update, *J Clin Sleep Med* 10(2):215–227, 2014.

Asthma and COPD

OBSTRUCTIVE VENTILATORY DYSFUNCTION

Obstructive ventilatory dysfunction (OVD) describes a pattern of pulmonary dysfunction characterized by spirometry (exhaled volume versus time) showing a reduced forced expiratory volume in 1 second (FEV_1) to forced vital capacity (FVC) ratio (e.g., reduced FEV_1/FVC) and usually a reduced FEV_1 (Figure F28-1). Patients with very mild OVD may have a normal FEV_1 but a reduced FEV_1/FVC ratio. For convenience, the lower limits of normal for FEV_1 and FVC are assumed to be 80% of predicted and the lower limit of normal for the FEV_1/FVC is assumed to be 0.70. Use of a slightly higher value of the FEV_1/FVC for the lower limit of normal is appropriate in younger patients. For example, using 90% of predicted as the lower limit of normal for the FEV_1/FVC ratio may be more sensitive for identification of OVD.

Patients with OVD have normal or increased residual volume (RV), function residual capacity (FRC), and total lung capacity (TLC) (Figure F28-2). The first lung volume to be affected is RV. Most patients with OVD have elevated RV because of air trapping from small

airway narrowing and closure. With more severe disease, the FRC and then the TLC may also be increased (hyperinflation). However, the relative increase in RV is greater than any increase in FRC or TLC. In moderate to severe OVD, the increase in RV is large enough (compared with any increase in TLC) to cause a reduction in FVC (Figure F28-2). The increase in FRC and TLC is caused by loss of lung elastic recoil (emphysema) or airway disease (asthma). *A significant acute response to inhaled bronchodilator is defined by a ≥ 12% increase in FEV1 or FVC with a minimum of 200 milliliters (mL) absolute increase.* Lack of an acute bronchodilator response does not rule out a benefit from chronic bronchodilator therapy. Patients with emphysema have disease of the terminal bronchioles and alveoli with a decrease in the surface for gas exchange. This results in a decreased diffusing capacity for carbon dioxide. In this test, the patient inspires a mixture of carbon monoxide (CO) and helium from RV to TLC and breath-holds for 10 seconds before exhaling. The amount of CO transferred is determined by measuring the carbon monoxide (CO) concentration in the exhaled sample (discarding the initial portion of the sample from the dead space). The units of the DLCO are milliliters per minute per millimeters of mercury (mL/min/mm Hg).

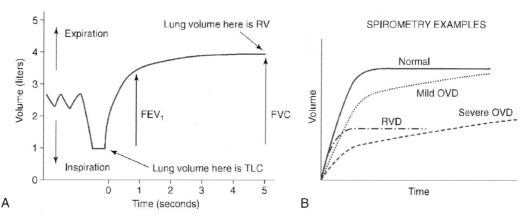

FIGURE F28-1 ■ *Left,* Spirometric parameters are defined including the FEV_1 (the volume exhaled in 1 second) and the FVC (forced vital capacity). *Right,* Patterns as shown in normal individuals and patients with mild and severe OVD. RVD is restrictive ventilatory dysfunction, which is characterized by a reduced FVC but normal FEV_1/FVC ratio.

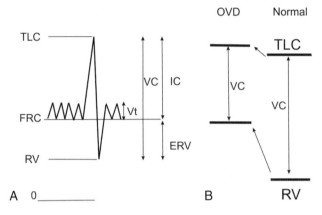

FIGURE F28-2 ■ **A,** Lung volume nomenclature and definition. Total lung capacity (TLC) is lung volume at maximal inhalation. Functional residual capacity (FRC) is the end expiratory lung volume. Residual volume (RV) is the lung volume at maximal exhalation. The vital capacity (VC) is the difference between TLC and RV. The inspiratory capacity (IC) is the difference between TLC and FRC. The expiratory reserve volume (ERV) is the difference between the FRC and the RV. **B,** In obstructive ventilatory dysfunction (OVD), absolute lung volumes are normal or increased. However, VC may be decreased because of an increase in RV exceeding the increase in TLC.

TABLE F28-1	**Spectrum of Obstructive Ventilatory Dysfunction**			
	Diagnosis	**Diffusing Capacity**	**Bronchodilator Response**	**Air Trapping and Hyperinflation**
Asthma	Reversible air flow obstruction (physiologic diagnosis)	Normal	Yes >12% often (15%-25%)	Sometimes (high RV)
Chronic bronchitis	Productive sputum for ≥3 months for more than 2 consecutive years (clinical diagnosis)	Normal	Sometimes 10%–15%	Air trapping (high RV)
Emphysema	Destruction of gas exchanging units and enlargement of terminal airspaces (pathologic diagnosis) + disease of small airways	Decreased	Rarely	Yes high (RV, FRC) or high (RV, FRC, TLC)
Mixed chronic bronchitis and emphysema (COPD)	Combination	Decreased	None or (10%-15%)	Yes

COPD, Chronic obstructive pulmonary disease; *FRC,* functional residual capacity; *RV,* residual volume; *TLC,* total lung capacity.

The common OVD disorders are listed in Table F28-1. These include asthma (bronchospasm = reversible airway obstruction), chronic bronchitis (productive cough or sputum production usually with OVD), and emphysema (destruction of alveoli and increased size of the terminal airspaces). Patients often have a mixture of these manifestations and are said to have chronic obstructive pulmonary disease (COPD). Patients with asthma may have normal pulmonary function between exacerbations that may occur after upper respiratory tract infections, exposure to allergens, or exercise. They typically demonstrate a large improvement in the FEV_1 or FVC after inhaled bronchodilator. Patients with asthma also have bronchial hyperresponsiveness to methacholine challenge (>20% fall in FEV_1 after inhaling low concentrations), allergen challenge, or exercise challenge (>15% fall in FEV_1 after exercise). A diagnosis of asthma may be made in a patient with normal pulmonary function by demonstration of bronchial hyperresponsiveness. Some patients with asthma have persistent air flow obstruction and require inhaled or even oral corticosteroids for improvement. Patients with severe asthma may have hyperinflation and even hypercapnic respiratory failure. Patients with COPD and predominantly chronic bronchitis typically have recurrent exacerbations and tend to have lower partial pressure of arterial oxygen (PaO_2) values earlier in the disease course. Some may develop hypercapnia and cor pulmonale (blue bloaters). Other patients with OVD predominantly have emphysema with severe hyperinflation (caused by loss of lung elastic recoil) and relative preservation of PaO_2 levels until late in the disease course. They present with dyspnea and, because of the relatively spared PaO_2, are called *pink puffers*. In general, an FEV_1 less than 30% to 40% of predicted or 1 liter

(L) for a normal-sized individual indicates very severe disease. Daytime hypercapnia is usually associated with an FEV_1 of 30% to 40% of predicted or less. Patients with the overlap syndrome (COPD+obstructive sleep apnea [OSA]) may develop hypercapnia with higher FEV_1 values. The GOLD criteria for severity COPD are listed in Table F28-2. The severity criteria are based on the *post-bronchodilator FEV_1* as a percentage of predicted, mild $FEV_1 > 80\%$ predicted, moderate FEV_1 50% to 80% of predicted, severe FEV_1 30% to 50% of predicted, and very severe $FEV_1 < 30\%$ of predicted (or 50% with chronic respiratory failure).

NOCTURNAL DESATURATION IN COPD (NONAPNEIC)

Many patients with COPD have significant hypercapnia and hypoxemia at night. Of the patients with COPD, 10% to 15% may also have concomitant OSA that worsens nocturnal gas exchange (overlap syndrome). The typical patterns of *nocturnal oxygen desaturation (NOD)* in a patient with COPD and COPD and OSA are shown in Figure F28-3. The baseline sleeping arterial oxygen saturation (SaO_2) falls 2% to 4% from the awake baseline with minor fluctuations during non–rapid eye movement (NREM) sleep until much larger drops are noted

TABLE F28-2 Gold Criteria for Chronic Obstructive Pulmonary Disease Severity from Lung Function Testing

Stage	Description	Findings (Based on Post-Bronchodilator FEV_1)		Symptoms
0	At risk	Normal Spirometry		Risk factors and chronic symptoms
I	Mild	FEV_1:FVC $\leq$70%	FEV_1 at least 80% of predicted value	May have symptoms
II	Moderate	FEV_1:FVC $\leq$70%	FEV_1 50% to <80% of predicted value	May have chronic symptoms
III	Severe	FEV_1:FVC $\leq$70%	FEV_1 30% to <50% of predicted value	May have chronic symptoms
IV	Very severe	FEV_1:FVC $\leq$70%	$FEV_1 < 30\%$ of predicted value or $FEV_1 < 50\%$ of predicted value + chronic respiratory failure	Respiratory failure: $PaO_2 < 60$ mm Hg with or without $PaCO_2 > 50$ mm Hg while breathing room air at sea levels

From Rabe KF, Hurd S, Anzueto A, et al: Global Initiative for Chronic Obstructive Lung Disease. Global strategy for the diagnosis, management, and prevention of chronic obstructive pulmonary disease: GOLD executive summary, *Am J Respir Crit Care Med* 176:532-555, 2007.
FEV_1, Post-bronchodilator forced expiratory volume in 1 second; *FVC,* forced vital capacity; *PaO_2,* partial pressure of arterial oxygen, *$PaCO_2$,* partial pressure of arterial carbon dioxide.

FIGURE F28-3 ■ **A,** Schematic of typical oximetry in a patient with moderate chronic obstructive pulmonary disease (COPD) and nocturnal oxygen desaturation (NOD). The arterial oxygen saturation by pulse oximetry (SpO_2) falls from a normal or low awake SpO_2 by 2 to 4% to a low baseline SpO_2 during NREM sleep with more significant drops occurring during REM sleep. The lowest desaturation is usually in the early morning hours. **B,** Overlap syndrome—a sawtooth pattern is superimposed on the COPD pattern of nocturnal oxygen desaturation.

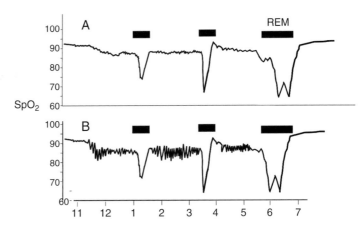

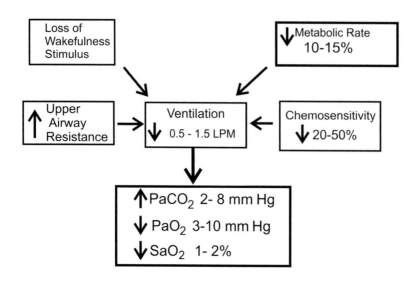

FIGURE F28-4 ■ Normal changes in gas exchange during sleep. *PaCO$_2$,* Arterial partial pressure of carbon dioxide; *PaO$_2$,* arterial partial pressure of oxygen; *SaO$_2$,* arterial oxygen saturation. (Adapted from Mohsenin V: Sleep in chronic obstructive pulmonary disease, *Semin Respir Crit Care Med* 26:109-115, 2005.)

BOX F28-1	Major Mechanisms of Nocturnal Oxygen Desaturation in Chronic Obstructive Pulmonary Disease

- Low awake SaO$_2$—starting on the steep portion of the oxygen–hemoglobin dissociation curve (larger fall in SaO$_2$ for a given fall in PO$_2$)
- Hypoventilation— decreased alveolar ventilation
  - Decreased chemosensitivity (REM < NREM < Wakefulness)
  - Reliance on accessory respiratory muscles and loss of this assistance during REM atonia
  - Increased upper airway resistance

- Drop in alveolar ventilaton > minute ventilation (high dead space and low tidal volume)
- Ventilation-perfusion mismatching (drop in PaO$_2$ exceeds the increase in PaCO$_2$)
  - High closing volume and decreases in FRC— especially during REM-associated hypopnea
- Coexisting sleep apnea (12%–15%)—especially blue bloaters

FRC, Functional residual capacity; *PaCO$_2$,* partial pressure of arterial carbon dioxide; *PaO$_2$,* partial pressure of arterial oxygen; *NREM,* non–rapid eye movement; *REM,* rapid eye movement; SaO2, saturation of arterial oxygen.

during REM sleep (stage R). In contrast, a typical oximetry of a patient with the overlap syndrome shows a low baseline sleeping SaO$_2$ and a saw-tooth pattern consistent with repeated discrete events. Oxygen desaturation is also worse during REM sleep.

During sleep, in normal individuals, the PCO$_2$ increases from 2 to 8 mm Hg and PO$_2$ decreases slightly (Figure F28-4). The causes of nocturnal oxygen desaturation in patients with COPD are listed in Box F28-1. In patients with COPD and awake hypoxemia, the SaO$_2$ levels fall from wakefulness to NREM sleep because even the normal fall in PaO$_2$ with sleep onset (3 to 10 mm Hg) is associated with a greater decrease in SaO$_2$ because of the initial position on the steep part of the oxyhemoglobin dissociation curve (Figure F28-5). The etiology of the significant drops in SaO$_2$ during REM sleep is still being debated. The fall in PO$_2$ usually is greater than the increase in PCO$_2$. Even in normal individuals, ventilation during REM sleep is

irregular, with periods of decreased tidal volume often associated with bursts of REMs. During REM sleep, skeletal muscle hypotonia reduces the contribution from accessory respiratory muscles, and respiration depends on the diaphragm. Periods of inhibition of diaphragmatic activity occur during REM sleep (phasic). Although tidal volume falls in normal individuals, it is associated with minimal changes in the SaO$_2$. In contrast, in patients with COPD, more profound drops in the SaO$_2$ occur during REM sleep compared to NREM sleep. Episodes of desaturation during REM sleep in patients with COPD are characterized by long periods of irregular breathing and reduced tidal volume (Figure F28-6). In contrast to obstructive hypopnea in patients with OSA, the onset and termination of these nonapneic periods of REM desaturation are less well defined. In patients with COPD, the diaphragm is at a mechanical disadvantage because of hyperinflation. The mechanical impairment in diaphragmatic function, coupled with skeletal

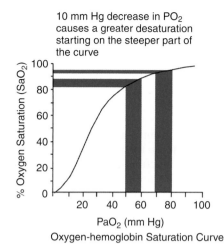

10 mm Hg decrease in PO$_2$ causes a greater desaturation starting on the steeper part of the curve

Oxygen-hemoglobin Saturation Curve

FIGURE F28-5 ■ A fall in partial pressure of arterial oxygen (PaO$_2$) of 10 millimeters of mercury (mm Hg) is associated with a much greater drop in saturation of peripheral oxygen (SaO$_2$) because of the initial position on the steep portion of the oxyhemoglobin dissociation curve. In this example a normal PaO$_2$ is assumed to be 80 mm Hg and a PO$_2$ of 60 mm Hg is consistent with mild hypoxemia. (From Berry RB: Fundamentals of sleep medicine, Philadelphia, 2012, Saunders, p 413.)

muscle hypotonia and periods of diaphragmatic inhibition during REM sleep, results in more significant falls in tidal volume that in normal individuals. The reduced tidal volume in combination with the higher physiologic dead space results in hypoventilation. Patients with lung disease have a high closing volume (volume at which airway closure becomes significant). During periods of breathing with small tidal volumes (breathing a lower lung volume below the closing volume), ventilation–perfusion mismatch worsens, as some lung units are poorly ventilated. Of note, some studies also suggest that the end expiratory lung volume (FRC) may fall during hypoponeic breathing episodes during REM sleep (Figure F28-6).

TIME OF NIGHT AND CIRCADIAN VARIATION IN LUNG FUNCTION

REM episodes in the early morning have greatest REM density and the greatest variation in ventilation even in normal individuals. These REM

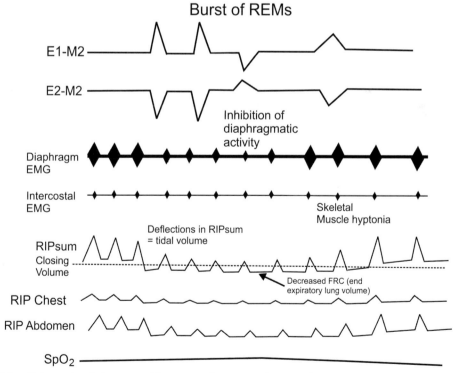

FIGURE F28-6 ■ Schematic of changes with nonapneic oxygen desaturation during phasic rapid eye movement (REM) sleep in a patient with chronic obstructive pulmonary disease (COPD). The chest and abdomen respiratory inductance plethysmography signals are acquired in direct-current mode so that a fall in the expiratory RIPsum documents a reduction in end-expiratory lung volume. Note that the functional residual capacity (FRC) may be normal between events. The deflections in the RIPsum are estimates of tidal volume. Reduced intercostal electromyography (EMG) activity is characteristic of skeletal muscle hypotonia during REM sleep. During phasic bursts of REM, diaphragmatic EMG output is also reduced. Note that while deflections in both the chest and abdominal bands decrease during hypopneic breathing, the chest is more severely affected. During the hypopneic episode breathing occurs below the closing volume increasing ventilation perfusion abnormality. In this schematic inspiration is upward.

periods also are typically longer. There is a circadian increase in lower airway resistance in the early morning hours even in normal persons. In patients with COPD there is an exaggeration of this effect. Due to these REM sleep and circadian factors the lowest FEV_1 and worse oxygen desaturation are often noted in the early morning hours in patients with COPD.

SLEEP QUALITY IN COPD

Sleep quality is impaired with reductions in total sleep time, stage N3 sleep, and REM sleep. In contrast, the wakefulness after sleep onset (WASO) and stage N1 sleep are increased as is the total arousal index. Patients often complain of insomnia but may also complain of daytime sleepiness if OSA is also present. Sleep disturbance does not seem to be greater in COPD patients who have nocturnal oxygen desaturation. It is likely that other factors such as cough, nocturnal dyspnea, and medication side effects

have greater effect than transient hypoxemia on sleep quality. In many COPD patients, the NOD is <15 minutes and confined to the last few REM periods of the night.

ASTHMA

Patients with asthma and those with COPD experience a larger than normal 24-hour variation in lung function with the highest flow rates in the afternoon and lowest flow rates at 4 AM.

The easiest way to diagnose severe nocturnal worsening of asthma is to have the patient record peak flow measurements at bedtime and upon awakening. Although a widely accepted criterion does not exist, a fall in the peak flow of >15% (evening to awakening) supports the diagnosis of nocturnal asthma. The peak expiratory flow rate (PEFR) is the highest flow during forced exhalation and can be measures at home with an inexpensive flow-meter.

CLINICAL PEARLS

1. Patients with COPD may experience nocturnal oxygen desaturation (NOD) without discrete apneas and hypopneas.

2. In COPD, NOD is worse during REM sleep. Hypopneic breathing during REM sleep is characterized by long periods of irregular but reduced tidal volume.

3. A sawtooth pattern on nocturnal oximetry in a patient with COPD suggests the possibility of coexisting sleep apnea (overlap syndrome).

4. If the awake SaO_2 is low, even the normal fall in PO_2 with sleep will result in greater desaturation (drop in SaO_2) because of the initial position on the steep portion of the oxyhemoglobin dissociation curve.

5. Mechanisms of NOD in patients with COPD include a low baseline SaO_2, hypoventilation during phasic REM sleep characterized by low tidal volume, and increased in ventilation–perfusion mismatch during periods of reduced tidal volume.

BIBLIOGRAPHY

American Thoracic Society: Lung function testing: selection of reference values and interpretative strategies, *Am Rev Respir Dis* 144:1202–1218, 1991.

Atanasov ST, Calhoun WJ: The relationship between sleep and asthma, *Sleep Med Clin* 2:9–18, 2007.

Becker HF, Piper AJ, Flynn WE, et al: Breathing during sleep in patients with nocturnal desaturation, *Am J Respir Crit Care Med* 159:112–118, 1999.

Catterall JR, Calverley PMA, MacNee W, et al: Mechanism of transient nocturnal hypoxemia in hypoxic chronic bronchitis and emphysema, *J Appl Physiol* 59:1698–1703, 1985.

Collop N: Sleep and sleep disorders in chronic obstructive pulmonary disease, *Respiration* 80:78–86, 2010.

Crapo RO: Pulmonary function testing, *N Engl J Med* 331:25, 1994.

Douglas NJ, Flenley DC: Breathing during sleep in patients with obstructive lung disease, *Am Rev Respir Dis* 141:1055–1070, 1990.

Fletcher EC, Gray BA, Levin DC: Nonapneic mechanisms of arterial oxygen desaturation during rapid-eye-movement sleep, *J Appl Physiol* 54:632–639, 1983.

Fletcher EC, Miller J, Divine GW, et al: Nocturnal oxyhemoglobin desaturation in COPD patients with arterial oxygen tensions above 60 mm Hg, *Chest* 92:604–608, 1987.

Gould GA, Gugger M, Molloy J, et al: Breathing pattern and eye movement density during REM sleep in humans, *Am Rev Respir Dis* 138:874–877, 1988.

Hudgel DW, Martin RJ, Capehart M, et al: Contribution of hypoventilation to sleep oxygen desaturation in chronic obstructive pulmonary disease, *J Appl Physiol* 55:669–677, 1983.

Kim V, Benditt JO, Wise RA, Sharafkhaneh A: Oxygen therapy in chronic obstructive pulmonary disease, *Proc Am Thorac Soc* 5:513–518, 2008.

Martin RJ, Cicutto LC, Ballard RD: Factors related to the nocturnal worsening of asthma, *Am Rev Respir Dis* 141:33–38, 1990.

Mohsenin V: Sleep in chronic obstructive pulmonary disease, *Semin Respir Crit Care Med* 26:109–115, 2005.

Nocturnal Oxygen Therapy Trial Group: Continuous or nocturnal oxygen therapy in hypoxemic chronic obstructive lung disease, *Ann Intern Med* 93:391–398, 1980.

Rabe KF, Hurd S, Anzueto A, et al: Global Initiative for Chronic Obstructive Lung Disease: Global strategy for the diagnosis, management, and prevention of chronic obstructive pulmonary disease: GOLD executive summary, *Am J Respir Crit Care Med* 176:532–555, 2007.

Sutherland ER: Nocturnal asthma, *J Allergy Clin Immunol* 116:1179–1186, 2005.

35-Year-Old Woman with Asthma and Poor Sleep at Night

A 35-year-old woman had been treated for moderate-to-severe asthma since age 15. Her medications included *fluticasone/salmeterol (100/50) 1 puff two times daily*. During several severe exacerbations, the patient was treated with oral prednisone and had gained about 15 pounds over the last 2 years. Over the last year, the patient had reported frequent awakenings with shortness of breath. In the morning, she usually felt sleepy and somewhat wheezy. The patient's roommate reported that the patient snored loudly, gasping for air during the night.

Physical examination: Height 5 feet 2 inches; weight 130 pounds; general: slightly "Cushingoid" appearance; HEENT: Mallampati 4, with edematous uvula and palate, neck: 15-inch circumference; chest: bilateral expiratory wheezes; cardiac: normal; extremities: no edema

Laboratory findings: Spirometry (3 PM): forced expiratory volume in 1 second (FEV_1) of 1.8 liters (L) (63% of predicted); forced vital capacity (FVC) of 3.0 L (90% of predicted), FEV_1/FVC of 0.60. Table P66-1 shows peak flow measurement at bedtime and in the morning. The patient reported 4 to 5 awakenings with dyspnea each night.

TABLE P66-1 Peak Expiratory Flow Rate (PEFR) Diary (L/min)	
	Peak Flow
Day 1 10 PM	300
Day 2 6 AM	200
Day 2 10 PM	325
Day 3 6 AM	225
Day 3 10 PM	350
Day 4 6 AM	200

Predicted peak flow for this patient is 430 liters per minute (L/min).

QUESTION

1. What is your diagnosis? What other evaluation do you suggest?

ANSWERS

1. **Answers:** Nocturnal asthma (large diurnal variation in air flow). Consider a sleep study to rule out obstructive sleep apnea (OSA).

Discussion: Nocturnal worsening of asthma symptoms and sleep disturbance are significant problems for patients with asthma (Box P66-1). In one study, up to 40% experienced symptoms every night. A normal circadian variation exists in airway function, with the highest air flow in the late afternoon (4 PM) and the lowest in the early morning (4 AM). This normal variation is exaggerated in patients with obstructive airway diseases. The FEV_1 or peak flow may fall as much as 20% to 40% in the morning hours ("morning dippers"). The largest study of the prevalence of nocturnal asthma

BOX P66-1	Manifestations of Nocturnal Asthma

- Morning drop in (FEV$_1$) >15%
- Increased circadian variation in airflow (FEV$_1$)
- Decreased response to BD during early AM
- Increased bronchial hyperresponsiveness
- Nocturnal awakenings with cough/dyspnea

FEV$_1$, Forced expiratory volume in 1 sec; *BD*, bronchodilator.

(NA), reported by Turner-Warwick in 1988, surveyed 7729 people with asthma. The study revealed that 74% woke up at least once each week with asthma symptoms and 65% woke up with symptoms at least 3 times per week. Among those who considered their asthma "mild," 26% woke up every night with symptoms of asthma. A more severe overnight drop in lung function is also associated with greater airway hyperresponsiveness, increased airway inflammation, and a decreased response to inhaled bronchodilators. The etiology of this variation in airway function is multifactorial and includes circadian changes in the amounts of circulating steroids and, possibly, inflammatory mediators in the lungs, as well as variations in cholinergic tone (increased during sleep). Sleep appears to have an adverse effect on asthma, independent of other circadian factors. The easiest way to diagnose severe nocturnal worsening of asthma is to have the patient record peak flow measurements at bedtime and upon awakening. *Nocturnal asthma is usually defined as a morning drop in the FEV$_1$ or peak expiratory flow >15%.* Peak expiratory flow meters may be prescribed to patients who can then routinely monitor their lung function at home. The price varies from about $20 to $30, depending on the quantity purchased.

Treatment of patients with nocturnal asthma should begin with inhaled corticosteroids. This medication has been shown to reduce the circadian fluctuation in airway tone. Patients with continued nocturnal symptoms despite an adequate dose of inhaled corticosteroids may then be treated with the addition of a long-acting inhaled beta-agonist bronchodilator or sustained action oral theophylline. Long-acting inhaled beta-agonists (salmeterol and formoterol) are probably the most popular long-acting bronchodilators for asthma. These drugs are effective treatment for nocturnal asthma and potentially might cause less systemic stimulation and sleep disruption compared with theophylline. Studies comparing salmeterol and theophylline have found salmeterol to either be better or equivalent to theophylline. However, theophylline has been proven effective despite the stimulatory effects of the medication. In dosing theophylline, the goal should be to obtain the highest levels during the time of greatest air flow obstruction (at night and early morning). The downside of theophylline is the need to carefully monitor serum levels to avoid toxicity. Although patients with asthma generally have a greater response to beta-agonists than to anticholinergic medications, vagal tone is increased at night. Studies have shown an improvement in nocturnal peak flow after ipratropium bromide (anticholinergic). A higher bedtime dose (4 puffs) may be needed for a more prolonged duration of action. The sustained action inhaled anticholinergic medication (tiotropium) may also help the symptoms of nocturnal asthma in some patients.

Patients with asthma may have other sleep disorders. If OSA is present, adequate treatment may improve the control of asthma as well as symptoms of daytime sleepiness (see Chan et al.). The reasons that OSA may worsen asthma are unknown at present. Treatment of nocturnal gastroesophageal reflux has also been tried to improve nocturnal asthma. A large study of a proton pump inhibitor (PPI) by Mastronarde et al. found no benefit, but individual patients may benefit from a trial of PPI before the evening meal.

In the current case, spirometry reveals obstructive ventilatory dysfunction (reduced FEV$_1$/FVC ratio) with a mild reduction in the FEV$_1$. The peak flow diary confirmed severe morning dipping with morning peak flow showing about a 30% decline. An increase in the dose of fluticasone or the addition of theophylline or tiotropium was discussed with the patient. An increase in fluticasone/salmeterol to 250/50 micrograms (mcg) twice daily was initiated. Given the history of snoring and daytime sleepiness, a sleep study was ordered, and it revealed an apnea–hypopnea index (AHI) of 30/hr during the diagnostic portion of a split-night sleep study. CPAP of 7 centimeters of water (cm H$_2$O) was found to be effective. Treatment with CPAP was started and resulted in improvement in both the daytime sleepiness and asthma. Morning peak flow rates improved to 275 to 300 liters per minute (L/min). The inhaled fluticasone/salmeterol dose was reduced back to 100/50 mcg, and improved control of nocturnal asthma persisted.

CLINICAL PEARLS

1. A diagnosis of nocturnal worsening of asthma and the degree of diurnal variation in air flow can most easily be documented by peak flow measurements at bedtime and on awakening. A drop in morning air flow of >15% documents nocturnal asthma.

2. Nocturnal asthma may cause severe sleep disturbance and poor sleep quality.

3. When OSA is present in patients with asthma, adequate treatment of OSA may improve the asthma.

4. The first-line treatment for nocturnal asthma is inhaled corticosteroids.

5. The addition of a long-acting bronchodilator is indicated in patients with nocturnal asthma who do not respond to inhaled steroids (or if the required dose of inhaled steroids is higher than desired).

6. Long-acting inhaled beta-agonists taken at bedtime have been shown to improve morning flow rates as well as, if not better than, theophylline and may improve perceptions of sleep quality more compared with theophylline in some patients.

7. If theophylline is used, dosing should be such that the highest levels are during the night or the early morning hours.

BIBLIOGRAPHY

Chan CS, Woolcock AJ, Sullivan CE: Nocturnal asthma: role of snoring and obstructive sleep apnea, *Am Rev Respir Dis* 137:1502–1504, 1988.

Fagnano M, Bayer AL, Isensee CA, et al: Nocturnal asthma symptoms and poor sleep quality among urban school children with asthma, *Acad Pediatr* 11(6):493–499, 2011.

Greenberg H, Cohen RI: Nocturnal asthma, *Curr Opin Pulm Med* 18(1):57–62, 2012.

Holimon TD, Chafin CC, Self TH: Nocturnal asthma uncontrolled by inhaled corticosteroids: theophylline or long-acting beta2 agonists? *Drugs* 61(3):391–418, 2001.

Karpel JP, Busse WW, Noonan MJ, et al: Effects of mometasone furoate given once daily in the evening on lung function and symptom control in persistent asthma, *Ann Pharmacother* 39(12):1977–1983, 2005.

Kerstjens HA, Engel M, Dahl R: Tiotropium in asthma poorly controlled with standard combination therapy, *Ann Pharmacother* 39(12):1977–1983, 2005.

Kraft M, Wenzel SE, Bettinger CM, et al: The effect of salmeterol on nocturnal symptoms, airway function, and inflammation in asthma, *Chest* 111:1249–1254, 1997.

Lafond C, Series F, Lemiere C: Impact of CPAP on asthmatic patients with obstructive sleep apnoea, *Eur Respir J* 29:307–311, 2007.

Mastronarde JG, Anthonisen NR, Castro M, et al: Efficacy of esomeprazole for treatment of poorly controlled asthma, *N Engl J Med* 360(15):1487–1499, 2009.

Selby C, Engleman HM, Fitzpatrick MF, et al: Inhaled salmeterol or oral theophylline in nocturnal asthma? *Am J Respir Crit Care Med* 155:104–108, 1997.

Turner-Warwick M: Epidemiology of nocturnal asthma, *Am J Med* 85:6–8, 1988.

Weersink EJM, Douma RR, Postma DS, et al: Fluticasone propionate, salmeterol xinafoate, and their combination in the treatment of nocturnal asthma, *Am J Respir Crit Care Med* 155:1241–1246, 1997.

Weigand L, Mende CN, Zaidel G, et al: Salmeterol vs Theophylline. Sleep and efficacy outcomes in patients with nocturnal asthma, *Chest* 115:1525–1532, 1999.

PATIENT 67

A 55-Year-Old Man with Chronic Obstructive Pulmonary Disease and Snoring

A 55-year-old man was being treated for moderate to severe chronic obstructive pulmonary disease (COPD) and documented nocturnal oxygen desaturation. Treatment included bronchodilators and nocturnal oxygen therapy at 2 liters per minute (L/min). Despite this treatment, he had severe, persistent pedal edema and carbon dioxide (CO_2) retention. Large doses of diuretics had not improved the pedal edema. His wife reported that he snored and fell asleep in front of the television during the day. The patient attributed this to poor sleep at night.

Physical examination: Height 5 feet 9 inches; weight 200 pounds; blood pressure 150/90 mm Hg; pulse 88; HEENT: edematous uvula, dependent palate (Mallampati 4); neck: 17-inch circumference; chest: bilateral wheezes; cardiac: distant heart sounds; extremities: 3+ pedal edema

Laboratory findings: Spirometry: forced expiratory volume in 1 second (FEV_1) 1.7 L (46% of predicted); forced vital capacity (FVC) 3.0 L (64% of predicted) **FEV1/FVC = 0.57**; arterial blood gas (ABG): pH 7.36, **partial pressure of CO_2 (PCO2) 50 mm Hg**, partial pressure of oxygen (PO_2) 63 mm Hg on room air

Chest radiography: large pulmonary arteries, no pulmonary edema

Nocturnal oximetry: Figure P67-1 is a trace of a portion of a nocturnal recording of arterial oxygen saturation (SaO_2) while that patient breathed room air (study to qualify the patient for nocturnal oxygen).

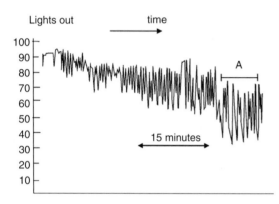

FIGURE P67-1 ■ A portion of overnight oximetry in the patient while he breathed room air. The more severe drops at A are likely associated with REM sleep.

QUESTION

1. Would complete polysomnography (PSG) be useful? What disorder is present?

ANSWER

1. **Answer:** A sleep study is indicated in this patient with the overlap syndrome (OLS).

Discussion: This patient fits the classic description of the "blue bloater" variant of COPD characterized by, hypercapnia plus cor pulmonale. It has been appreciated that many such patients also have obstructive sleep apnea (OSA). Such patients are said to have OLS (COPD + OSA).[1-3] One study found that OSA is no more frequent in patients with COPD than in the general population.[4] That is, the prevalence of OSA in patients with COPD is the same as the general population. Thus, patients do have an overlap of two separate conditions. However, because both conditions are common, the combination is also fairly common. Recognition that a patient with COPD may have OSA (or that a patient with OSA also has COPD) has important implications in terms of morbidity and treatment. A low baseline PO_2 (SaO_2), ventilation–perfusion mismatch secondary to COPD, or a combination of both results in more significant oxygen desaturation during apnea. Thus, patients with OSA + COPD tend to have more severe arterial oxygen desaturation and cor pulmonale. They also may have daytime hypercapnia (even if the FEV_1 is only moderately reduced).

Most patients with OSA do not have daytime CO_2 retention. Those that do usually have a component of COPD or the obesity hypoventilation syndrome OHS.[5] Patients with hypercapnic COPD usually have an $FEV_1 < 1$ L, or 40% predicted. Patients with OLS may retain CO_2 with more moderate degrees of air flow obstruction. Resta et al[6] retrospectively reviewed consecutive patients referred for evaluation of OSA or COPD and divided them into groups of COPD only, OLS, and OSA only (Table P67-1). The OLS group had higher partial pressure of arterial CO_2

TABLE P67-1 **Characteristics of COPD, OLS, and OSA-Only Groups**

	COPD Group (n = 32)	OLS Group (n = 29)	OSA-Only Group (n = 152)
Age (years)	60.1 (10.4)	57.2 (9.5)	48.9 (12.9)
Weight (kilograms [kg])	87.6 (17.5)	**102.2 (20.6)**	106.8 (28.8)
BMI (kg/m²)	31 (7)	36 (6)	39 (10)
FVC (% predicted)	60 (19)	72 (17)	87 (20)
FEV₁ (% predicted)	47 (16)	63 (16)	89 (20)
FEV₁/FVC (%)	59 (9)	67 (5)	87 (9)
PaO₂ (mm Hg)	69 (10.4)	70 (11)	79 (12)
PCO₂ (mm Hg)	40 (5)	45 (5)	39 (4)
AHI (events/h)	6 (5)	40 (20)	42 (23)
%Time SpO₂ − 90%	16 (28)	48 (28)	30 (28)

AHI, Apnea–hypopnea index; *BMI*, body mass index; *COPD*, chronic obstructive pulmonary disease; *FEV₁*, forced expiratory volume in 1 second; *FVC*, forced vital capacity; *OLS*, overlap syndrome; *OSA*, obstructive sleep apnea; *PaO₂*, partial pressure of arterial oxygen; *SpO₂*, saturation of peripheral oxygen.
Data are means (standard deviation [SD]), OLS = OSA + COPD.

($PaCO_2$) than the COPD group, although air flow limitation was milder (FEV_1 higher). The OLS group had a similar apnea–hypopnea index (AHI) as the OSA-only group but higher PCO_2. The OLS group had more severe desaturation than either of the two groups. Table P67-1 illustrates two points. First comparing OLS and OSA only, the OLS group had a higher PCO_2 and worse oxygenation although the AHI was similar. Second comparing the OLS and COPD group, the OLS patients had a higher PCO_2 although the FEV_1 was higher (milder lung disease) in the OLS group compared to the COPD group.

The etiology of the daytime hypercapnia in the OLS is unclear, but OSA may predispose to nocturnal CO_2 retention and blunting of ventilatory drive. In clinical practice, patients with a combination of COPD, OSA, and severe obesity are seen to have significant hypoventilation. It is difficult to know how to label them because they likely have components of both OHS and OLS.

The amount of CO_2 retention in patients with OLS does not necessarily correlate with the AHI. One study comparing OLS patients with or without hypercapnia found no difference in the FEV_1 and AHI between the two groups.[7] The hypercapnic group was heavier and had a history of heavy ethanol use. The authors hypothesized that the patients with hypercapnia had depressed respiratory drives possibly secondary to the effects of alcohol. Effective treatment of OSA in patients with OLS may result in a reduction of daytime PCO_2. Nocturnal CO_2 retention secondary to apnea probably contributes to the development of daytime hypercapnia in patients with OLS.

What are the treatment implications of this combination of diseases (COPD + OSA)? The most obvious implication is that *both diseases need to be well treated for optimal results*. Thus, the awake and sleeping gas exchange of the patient with OSA and COPD may improve when smoking cessation and bronchodilator therapy are added to the treatment of OSA in patients with OLS. On the other hand, adequate treatment of OSA in patients with OLS requires PAP with supplemental oxygen, if needed. PAP treatment should be added, even if the patient is currently on nocturnal supplemental oxygen if significant OSA exists. Treatment of patients with OLS with supplemental oxygen alone may result in significant increases in nocturnal $PaCO_2$, and many not adequately normalize nocturnal oxygen saturation. Alford and colleagues[8] administered 4 L/min supplemental oxygen to 20 men with both OSA and COPD. Although nocturnal oxygenation improved, the duration of obstructive events increased from 25.7 seconds to 31.4 seconds, resulting in an end-apneic PCO_2 increase from 52.8 mm Hg to 62.3 mm Hg, with corresponding decreases in pH. Goldstein et al.[9] performed oximetry and transcutaneous PCO_2 monitoring in groups with hypercapnic COPD alone and hypercapnic OLS during sleep. The effect of the addition of supplemental oxygen was noted. In the COPD-only group, a mild increase in PCO was noted with the addition of supplemental oxygen. In the OLS group, a large increase in PCO_2 was noted with the addition of supplemental oxygen. In Figure P67-2, nocturnal oximetry and transcutaneous PCO_2 tracing are shown for a patient with the hypercapnic OLS and severe hypoxemia. The top tracing on room

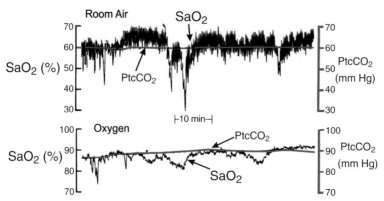

FIGURE P67-2 ■ A patient with obstructive sleep apnea (OSA) and chronic obstructive pulmonary disease (COPD). *Top,* A saw-tooth pattern in the arterial oxygen saturation (SaO_2) is noted while the patient breathes room air. The transcutaneous partial pressure of carbon dioxide ($TcPCO_2$) is approximately 60 mm Hg. *Bottom,* The patient is breathing oxygen. The SaO_2 is improved but the $TcPCO_2$ has increased dramatically up to just below 90 mm Hg. (From Goldstein RS, Ramcharan V, Bowes G, et al: Effect of supplemental nocturnal oxygen on gas exchange in patients with severe obstructive lung disease, *N Engl J Med* 310:425-429, 1984.)

air, shows very severe arterial oxygen desaturation and a sawtooth pattern in the SaO_2 tracing. Note that the transcutaneous PCO_2 is 60 mm Hg. A sawtooth pattern in the nocturnal oximetry tracing is a clue that OSA as well as COPD is present. On the bottom, the patient is on supplemental oxygen, and although the SaO_2 is much improved, the transcutaneous partial pressure of carbon dioxide ($TcPCO_2$) has climbed from approximately 60 mm Hg (top tracing) to approximately 90 mm Hg. This is an example of how supplemental oxygen in patients with OLS and significant hypercapnia may worsen nocturnal hypercapnia.[9] In addition, the SaO_2 is not completely normalized. Fletcher and associates[10] monitored patients with chronic lung disease and OSA, including a group treated with oxygen but no effective treatment for sleep apnea. They found that patients who did not have adequate treatment for OSA had no improvement in their pulmonary hemodynamics, whereas those who had effective treatment of OSA also had improved pulmonary hemodynamics. One should recall the hypoxemia and acidosis results in pulmonary arterial vasoconstriction and pulmonary hypertension. This may result in cor pulmonale. An observational study by Machado et al. of patients with OSA and hypoxemic COPD receiving long-term oxygen therapy (LTOT) found that those who accepted continuous positive airway pressure (CPAP) in addition to oxygen and adhered to treatment had a better survival than those who did not.[11] Another study by Marin and coworkers[12] of patients with OLS found an increased risk of death and hospitalization caused by COPD exacerbations. CPAP treatment was associated with improved survival and decreased hospitalizations.

The optimal treatment of patients with OLS includes treatment of their COPD and treatment of their OSA with CPAP or bilevel positive airway pressure (BPAP) with supplemental oxygen, if needed. If significant CO_2 retention is present, most clinicians would use BPAP. Some patients with COPD have difficulty exhaling on CPAP and may be more adherent to treatment with BPAP compared with CPAP.[13] Patients with OSA and COPD and a low awake PO_2 (and SaO_2) value will likely need both oxygen and PAP to prevent nocturnal oxygen desaturation. When the upper airway obstruction of hypercapnic patients with OLS is adequately treated, the daytime PCO_2 frequently improves.

When should a sleep study be ordered in a patient with known COPD? The major indication is a suspicion of sleep apnea (snoring, daytime sleepiness). *If nocturnal oximetry shows a sawtooth pattern, it means that repeated discrete respiratory events are present and is highly suggestive of some type of sleep apnea.* Another indication for PSG is lack of improvement in cor pulmonale in spite of nocturnal oxygen use. If resources are limited, a simple overnight pulse oximetry test may show the sawtooth pattern suggestive of sleep apnea. However, this approach may be more costly in the long run if PSG for definitive diagnosis and PAP titration are required based on the oximetry results.

In the present patient, oximetry showed the sawtooth pattern of desaturation consistent with OSA (see Figure P67-1). The worsening of the SaO_2 at A is probably secondary to an episode of rapid eye movement (REM) sleep. Note the low baseline SaO_2 and the persistence of decreased SaO_2 after each event. The patient underwent PSG while using his supplemental oxygen. The oxygen flow rate was decreased to provide a baseline sleeping SaO_2 of 92%. At this flow rate, supplemental oxygen did not prevent desaturations caused by apnea and hypopnea (allowing diagnosis of OSA). An AHI of 50/hr was documented in the first 2 hours of the study. Nasal CPAP was titrated but was changed to BPAP because of pressure intolerance. Apnea and hypopnea were abolished at 16/10 centimeters of water (cm H_2O). Addition of oxygen at 3 L/min to BPAP was needed to maintain SaO_2 above 92%. Treatment with a combination of nasal BPAP and oxygen was started, and the patient's daytime sleepiness and pedal edema improved. After 1 month of nasal BPAP and oxygen, the daytime PCO_2 had decreased to 45 mm Hg.

CLINICAL PEARLS

1. A sawtooth pattern on the nocturnal oximetry tracing (SaO_2 versus time) in a patient with COPD suggests that sleep apnea is also present (usually OSA). A definitive diagnosis requires PSG.

2. If a patient with COPD and only mild to moderate air flow obstruction has daytime CO_2 retention, the presence of OLS should be suspected.

3. In OLS, adequate treatment of both COPD and OSA is required.

4. Supplemental oxygen therapy of nocturnal desaturation **alone** is not optimal treatment for most patients with COPD and significant OSA.

5. PAP (CPAP or BPAP) plus oxygen (if needed) is the most effective therapy for patients with COPD and significant OSA. Treatment of the COPD should include by smoking cessation and bronchodilator therapy.

6. Even in patients with COPD and OSA but without hypercapnia, supplemental oxygen may be needed with CPAP (or BPAP) at night.

7. Observational studies suggest that PAP treatment of patients with OLS (compared with nocturnal oxygen alone) have improved survival.

REFERENCES

1. Owens RL, Malhotra A: Overlap syndrome, *Respir Care* 55(10):1333–1346, 2010.
2. Weitzenblum E, Chaouat A, Kessler R, Canuet M: Overlap syndrome. Obstructive sleep apnea syndrome in patients with chronic obstructive pulmonary disease, *Proc Am Thorac Soc* 5:237–241, 2008.
3. McNicholas WT: Chronic obstructive pulmonary disease and obstructive sleep apnea: overlaps in pathophysiology, systemic inflammation, and cardiovascular disease, *Am J Respir Crit Care Med* 180(8):692–700, 2009.
4. Sanders MH, Newman AB, Haggerty CL, et al: Sleep and sleep disordered breathing in adults with predominantly mild obstructive airway disease, *Am J Respir Crit Care Med* 167:7–14, 2003.
5. Bradley TD, Rutherford R, Lue F, et al: Role of diffuse airway obstruction in the hypercapnia of obstructive sleep apnea, *Am Rev Respir Dis* 134:920–924, 1986.
6. Resta O, Foschino Barbaro MP, Brindicci C, et al: Hypercapnia in overlap syndrome: possible determinant factors, *Sleep Breath* 6(1):11–18, 2002.
7. Chan CS, Grunstein RR, Bye PTP, et al: Obstructive sleep apnea with chronic airflow limitation: comparison of hypercapnic and eucapnic patients, *Am Rev Respir Dis* 140:1274–1278, 1989.
8. Alford NJ, Fletcher EC, Nickeson D: Acute oxygen in patients with sleep apnea and COPD, *Chest* 89(1):30–38, 1986.
9. Goldstein RS, Ramcharan V, Bowes G, et al: Effect of supplemental nocturnal oxygen on gas exchange in patients with severe obstructive lung disease, *N Engl J Med* 310:425–429, 1984.
10. Fletcher EC, Schaaf JW, Miller J, Fletcher JG: Long-term cardiopulmonary sequelae in patients with sleep apnea and chronic lung disease, *Am Rev Respir Dis* 135:525–533, 1987.
11. Machado MCL, Vollmer WM, Togeiro SM, et al: CPAP and survival in moderate to severe obstructive sleep apnea syndrome and hypoxemic COPD, *Eur Respir J* 35:132–137, 2010.
12. Marin JM, Soriano JB, Carrizo SJ, et al: Outcomes in patients with chronic obstructive pulmonary disease and obstructive sleep apnea, *Am J Respir Crit Care Med* 182:325–331, 2010.
13. Sampol G, Sagalés MT, Roca A, et al: Nasal continuous positive airway pressure with supplemental oxygen in coexistent sleep apnea-hypopnea syndrome and severe chronic obstructive pulmonary disease, *Eur Respir J* 9:111–116, 1996.

A 55-Year-Old Man with COPD and Nocturnal Desaturation

A 55-year-old man with a long history of heavy smoking and chronic obstructive pulmonary disease (COPD) was referred for evaluation. He had failed to qualify for **daytime** home oxygen therapy on a recent examination (partial pressure of arterial oxygen [PaO_2] = 62 mm Hg). The patient had bouts of mild pedal edema during courses of steroid therapy for exacerbations of COPD. These bouts responded to diuretics. A history of only mild snoring was present, and the patient denied daytime sleepiness. Nocturnal oximetry was ordered to determine if nocturnal desaturation might explain the presence of cor pulmonale.

Physical examination: body mass index (BMI) 29 kilograms per square millimeter (kg/m^2); HEENT: edentulous, Mallampati 2; neck: 15½-inch circumference; chest: decreased breath sounds; cardiac: no murmurs or gallops; extremities: 1+ pedal edema

Pulmonary function testing: forced expiratory volume in 1 second (FEV$_1$) 1.1 liters (L) (29% of predicted); forced vital capacity (FVC) 2.5 L (52% of predicted); FEV1/FVC = 0.44; diffusing capacity 30% of predicted

Arterial blood gas on room air: pH 7.43; partial pressure of carbon dioxide (PCO$_2$) 38 mm Hg; partial pressure of oxygen (PO$_2$) 62 mm Hg; HCO$_3$ 25 millimoles per liter (mmol/L), breathing room air)

Chest radiography: possible mild enlargement of the pulmonary arteries

Nocturnal oximetry: (Figure P68-1): shows a tracing from nocturnal oximetry while the patient breated room air.

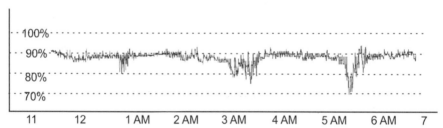

FIGURE P68-1 ■ Nocturnal oximetry breathing room air. The saturation of arterial oxygen (SaO$_2$) was less than 88% for 5 hours. The awake SaO$_2$ was 92%.

QUESTIONS

1. What is causing the nocturnal arterial oxygen desaturation? What treatment should be offered to the patient?

ANSWER

1. **Answer:** COPD with nocturnal oxygen desaturation (NOD). Treatment with nocturnal oxygen.

   Discussion: Patients with COPD may have NOD during sleep for several reasons. First, the normal sleep-associated 8 to 10 mm Hg fall in PO$_2$ has much greater significance if the baseline presleep PO_2 value is on the steep part of the oxyhemoglobin saturation curve (PO_2 50–60 mm Hg). At this range of baseline PO_2, a normal fall in PO_2 during non–rapid eye movement (NREM) sleep results in significant arterial oxygen desaturation (see Fundamentals 28. figure 28-5). Second, periods of sleep apnea of varying significance may occur during NREM and REM sleep (see Patient 67 for COPD+OSA). Third, nonapneic arterial oxygen desaturation may occur during REM sleep. The REM-associated oxygen desaturation may be abrupt and severe. Often, REM-associated oxygen desaturation is associated with hypopneic periods that are not well defined and consist of small and variable tidal volumes over a period as long as several minutes. The REM-associated desaturations are believed to be secondary to hypoventilation during periods of small tidal volume as well as to an increase in ventilation–perfusion (V/Q) mismatch. The PO_2 drop is greater than the PCO_2 increase. Thus, both hypoventilation and ventilation–perfusion mismatch cause hypoxemia. During REM sleep, the diaphragm is the only active muscle of inspiration (REM-associated skeletal muscle hypotonia). In patients with COPD, diaphragmatic function often is compromised secondary to hyperinflation. In addition, neural drive to the diaphragm may fall during bursts of eye movements in REM sleep, producing hypopnea (or central apnea). The increase in V/Q mismatch is believed to be secondary to a decrease in functional residual capacity (end expiratory lung volume) during these REM-related hypopneic episodes. Breathing at low lung volumes with low tidal volumes increases the closing of small airways resulting in a decrease in ventilation compared with perfusion. Because of lung disease, airway closure occurs at higher lung volumes than in normal individuals.

Patients with COPD may have NOD without having sleep apnea even if their daytime PO_2 is ≥60 mm Hg. As expected, the REM-associated desaturations occur every 90 to 120 minutes during the night. The most severe and longest periods of desaturation typically occur in the early morning hours when REM periods are longer and the REM density (number of eye movements per minute) is greater. In contrast, the pattern of arterial oxygen desaturation on an all-night plot in patients with COPD+OSA shows a sawtooth pattern consistent with repetitive, discrete episodes of desaturation (Figure P68-2). In general, patients with COPD with lower saturation of arterial oxygen (SaO_2) and higher PCO_2 during wakefulness are more likely to have significant nocturnal desaturation. However, considerable individual variation exists, and the degree of nocturnal oxygen desaturation cannot be reliably predicted. A study by Fletcher et al. published in 1987 found that 21% of a group of patients with COPD and daytime PO_2 > 60 mm Hg showed some desaturation during sleep, although most of the desaturations were during REM sleep and often brief.

Long-term oxygen therapy (LTOT) has been proven to benefit patients with COPD and a daytime PO_2 ≤ 55% (SaO_2 ≤ 88%) or 55 to 60 mm Hg (SaO_2 ≤ 89%) with evidence of right heart failure or cor pulmonale on electrocardiography (ECG). Such patients qualify for 24-hour oxygen therapy. In addition, patients with ≥ 5 minutes with SaO_2 of ≤ 88% during sleep (nocturnal oximetry) qualify for nocturnal oxygen treatment, according to the Centers of Medicare and Medicaid Services (CMS) and most insurance providers. Slightly less severe nocturnal desaturation may qualify a patient, with certain stipulations. However, no evidence suggests that providing supplemental oxygen improves either survival or sleep quality in patients with desaturation *only* at night (during sleep). Most physicians would offer patients this treatment if they qualify—especially if long periods are spent with SaO_2 less than 88% or if they have evidence of cor pulmonale.

In the original Nocturnal Oxygen Treatment Trial, 21% of the patients screened no longer met the criteria when they were placed on intensive bronchodilator therapy. Some patients with minimal acute improvement in the FEV_1 and FVC after inhaled bronchodilator have steady

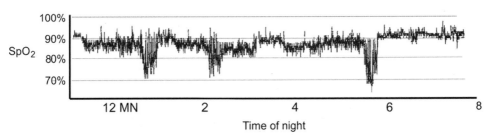

FIGURE P68-2 ■ Nocturnal oximetry is a patient with both chronic obstructive pulmonary disease (COPD) and obstructive sleep apnea (OSA). In this patient, a sleep study found an apnea–hypopnea index (AHI) of 60 per hour.

improvement in oxygenation when treated with smoking cessation and bronchodilator therapy. Therefore, treatment with smoking cessation and bronchodilator therapy is indicated to help improve nocturnal oxygenation. Martin and colleagues studied the effect of ipratropium inhaled four times a day in 36 patients with moderate to severe COPD ($FEV_1 < 65\%$ of predicted). After 4 weeks, nocturnal oxygen saturation improved, subjective sleep quality was better, and total REM time increased. In another triotropium (a long acting anti-cholinergic bronchodilator) also improved nocturnal oxygen saturation, although sleep quality was not affected. Long-acting beta-agonists show similar benefits. Of interest a small short term study by Sposato et al found oral steroids to improve the nocturnal SaO_2 and sleep duration in a group of COPD patients with a daytime $PO_2 > 60$ mm Hg. However, given steroid side effects and limited evidence, steroid treatment for NOD is not recommended. Patients with COPD are often treated with inhaled steroids, but a benefit regarding sleep quality has not been proven. Many patients with COPD complain of sleep disturbance because of cough or shortness of breath. The worst lung function in normal individuals and patients with COPD occur in the early morning hours (as in patients with asthma). To provide adequate treatment and improve nocturnal symptoms throughout the night and in the early morning hours, long-acting bronchodilators (e.g., long-acting beta-agonist or anticholinergic medications) are recommended. Many patients with COPD complain of poor sleep even if treated with bronchodilators. Some studies suggest that benzodiazepine receptor agonists can be used safely (if the patient does not exhibit daytime hypoventilation). Ramelteon (melatonin receptor agonist) and sedating antidepressants are often used instead of benzodiazepine receptor agonists. However, no data exist to support the efficacy of these hypnotics in this situation. Studies of ramelteon in COPD patients have documented safety.

In the present patient, the nocturnal oximetry showed a fall in SaO_2 to below 88% for long periods with further episodes of steep desaturation, likely associated with REM sleep. However, a prominent sawtooth pattern was not present. Contrast the oximetry with one from a patient with the overlap syndrome (see Figure P68-2). A complete sleep study was performed because of the history of loud snoring (despite the fact that the oximetry was not suggestive of sleep apnea). The dramatic falls in SaO_2 were associated with hypopneic breathing during REM sleep (Figure P68-3). The apnea–hypopnea index (AHI) was only 7 per hour. The patient was treated with long-acting bronchodilators and nocturnal oxygen at 2 liters per minute (L/min). Repeat oximetry on this treatment showed resolution of significant desaturation. The patient still complained of poor sleep. He was started on trazodone 50 milligrams (mg) every night, and this seemed to improve his sleep duration.

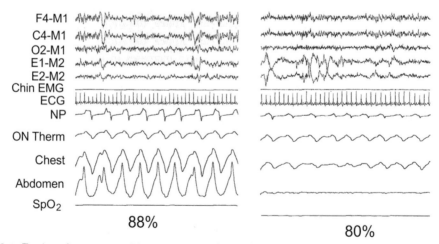

FIGURE P68-3 ■ Tracings from non–rapid eye movement (NREM) sleep on the left panel and REM sleep on the right pane the patient in the supine position. REM sleep was associated with a reduction in tidal volume and nonapneic arterial oxygen desaturation. During REM sleep, the chest wall muscles are hypotonic. Note the minimal deflections in the chest tracings. NP nasal pressure, ON Therm oronasal thermal sensor, chest and abdomen by respiratory inductance plethysmography. (From Berry RB, Harding SM: Sleep and medical disorders, *Med Clin North Am* 88:679-703, 2004.)

CLINICAL PEARLS

1. The usual pattern of nocturnal desaturation caused by COPD is a fall in baseline SaO_2 during NREM sleep with more dramatic falls occurring during episodes of REM sleep. If a pronounced sawtooth pattern is present in the SaO_2 tracing, it suggests that substantial sleep apnea is present.

2. REM-associated desaturation in patients with COPD usually is secondary to periods of hypopneic breathing (low and irregular tidal volumes) and ventilation–perfusion mismatch rather than apnea.

3. The clinical suspicion of sleep apnea is the main indication for ordering a sleep study in patients with COPD. Oximetry is sufficient to evaluate a patient for possible nocturnal oxygen desaturation. If a prominent sawtooth pattern is noted this suggests evaluation for sleep apnea is indicated.

4. The treatment of NOD caused by COPD is supplemental nocturnal oxygen. Studies have proven a benefit for 24-hour supplemental oxygen in patients with an awake $PO_2 \leq 55\%$ ($SaO_2 \leq 88\%$). However, the benefit of oxygen therapy in patients who have *hypoxemia only during sleep* has not been proven.

5. In patients with COPD not qualifying for 24-hour oxygen treatment, nocturnal oximetry may be ordered (especially if cor pulmonale is present) and may document sufficient nocturnal desaturation to qualify the patient for nocturnal oxygen.

6. Smoking cessation and long-acting bronchodilators may improve both oxygenation and night-time symptoms of cough and dyspnea. However, sleep quality often remains poor.

7. Benzodiazepine receptor agonists may be used as hypnotics in patients with COPD with caution if the patients are stable without chronic hypoventilation. However, other sleep disorders (depression, occult sleep apnea) should be addressed. Many clinicians feel more comfortable with use of a sedating antidepressant (eg trazodone) but the evidence for effectiveness is lacking.

BIBLIOGRAPHY

Becker HF, Piper AJ, Flynn WE, et al: Breathing during sleep in patients with nocturnal desaturation, *Am J Respir Crit Care Med* 159:112–118, 1999.

Cannaughton JJ, Catterall JR, Elton RA: Do sleep studies contribute to the management of patients with severe chronic obstructive pulmonary disease? *Am Rev Respir Dis* 138:341–344, 1988.

Catterall JR, Calverley PMA, MacNee W, et al: Mechanism of transient nocturnal hypoxemia in hypoxic chronic bronchitis and emphysema, *J Appl Physiol* 59:1698–1703, 1985.

Douglas NJ, Flenley DC: Breathing during sleep in patients with obstructive lung disease, *Am Rev Respir Dis* 141:1055–1069, 1990.

Fletcher EC, Gray BA, Levin DC: Nonapneic mechanisms of arterial oxygen desaturation during rapid-eye-movement sleep, *J Appl Physiol* 54:632–639, 1983.

Fletcher EC, Luckett RA, Goodnight-White S, et al: A double-blind trial of nocturnal supplemental oxygen for sleep desaturation in patients with chronic obstructive pulmonary disease and a daytime PO_2 above 60 mmHg, *Am Rev Respir Dis* 145:1070–1076, 1992.

Fletcher EC, Miller J, Divine GW, et al: Nocturnal oxyhemoglobin desaturation in COPD patients with arterial oxygen tensions above 60 mm Hg, *Chest* 92(4):604–608, 1987.

Girault C, Muir JF, Mihaltan F, et al: Effects of repeated administration of zolpidem on sleep, diurnal and nocturnal respiratory function, vigilance, and physical performance in patients with COPD, *Chest* 110:1203–1211, 1996.

Hudgel DW, Martin RJ, Capehart M, et al: Contribution of hypoventilation to sleep oxygen desaturation in chronic obstructive pulmonary disease, *J Appl Physiol* 55:669–677, 1983.

Kim V, Benditt JO, Wise RA, Sharafkhaneh A: Oxygen therapy in chronic obstructive pulmonary disease [review], *Proc Am Thorac Soc* 5:513–518, 2008.

Kryger M, Wang-Weigand S, Zhang J, Roth T: Effect of ramelteon, a selective MT(1)/MT (2)-receptor agonist, on respiration during sleep in mild to moderate COPD, *Sleep Breath* 12:243–250, 2008.

Martin RJ, Bartelson BL, Smith P, et al: Effect of ipratropium bromide treatment on oxygen saturation and sleep quality in COPD, *Chest* 115:1338–1345, 1999.

McNicholas WT, Calverly PMA, Edward JC: Long-acting inhaled anticholinergic therapy improves sleeping oxygen saturation in COPD, *Eur Respir J* 23:825–831, 2004.

Nocturnal oxygen Therapy Trial Group: Continuous or nocturnal oxygen therapy in hypoxemic chronic obstructive lung disease, *Ann Intern Med* 93:391–398, 1980.

Roth T: Hypnotic use for insomnia management in chronic obstructive pulmonary disease, *Sleep Med* 10:19–25, 2009.

Ryan S, Doherty LS, Rock C, et al: Effects of salmeterol on sleeping oxygen saturation in chronic obstructive pulmonary disease, *Respiration* 79:475–481, 2010.

Scharf SM, Maimon N, Simon-Tuval T, Bernhard-Scharf BJ, Reuveni H, Tarasiuk A: Sleep quality predicts quality of life in chronic obstructive pulmonary disease, *Int J Chron Obstruct Pulmon Dis* 6:1–12, 2010.

Sposato B, Mariotta S, Palmiero G, et al: Oral corticosteroids can improve nocturnal isolated hypoxemia in stable COPD patients with diurnal $PaO_2 < 60$ mmHg, *Eur Rev Med Pharmacol Sci* 11(6):365–372, 2007.

Stege G, Heijdra YF, van den Elshout FJ, et al: Temazepam 10 mg does not affect breathing and gas exchange in patients with severe normocapnic COPD, *Respir Med* 104:518–524, 2010.

Steens RD, Pouliot Z, Millar TW, et al: Effects of zolpidem and triazolam on sleep and respiration in mild to moderate chronic obstructive pulmonary disease, *Sleep* 16:318–326, 1993.

A Patient with Snoring and Heart Failure

A 50-year-old man was admitted with decompensated heart failure. At the time of admission, he was on a carvedilol, lisinopril, and spironolactone. Previous studies had documented that he had an ejection fraction of 30%. He was believed to have ischemic cardiomyopathy. An acute myocardial infarction was ruled out. He reported snoring but no daytime sleepiness. The patient had episodes of awakening sometimes with shortness of breath. His New York Heart Association Functional Classification is III (marked limitation caused by symptoms).

Physical examination: body mass index (BMI) 32 kilograms per square meter (kg/m^2); HEENT: Mallampati 4; chest: a few rales bilaterally; cardiovascular: regular rhythm with a systolic heart murmur; extremities: 3+ pedal edema

Electrocardiography: atrial fibrillation

Chest radiography: pulmonary edema, cardiomegaly

QUESTION

1. Should this patient be evaluated for sleep apnea?

ANSWER

1. **Answer:** Polysomnography (PSG) is indicated. At the very least, an out-of-center sleep testing (OCST) should be performed. The patient has risk factors for both obstructive sleep apnea (OSA) and central sleep apnea (CSA).

   Discussion: Studies have suggested that sleep-disordered breathing (SDB) is very common in patients with congestive heart failure (CHF). OSA and/or CSA is present in at least 60% to 70% of stable patients with significant CHF (systolic or diastolic) (Table P69-1). Javaheri and colleagues found occult SDB in 45% of a group with stable heart failure and an ejection fraction less than 45%, and CSA was common in the affected individuals. MacDonald and associates studied a group of patients in stable CHF with maximal modern medical management and found 61% to have some form of SDB (31% central apnea and 30% OSA). Oldenburg and coworkers published an observational study of 700 patients with heart failure showed sleep apnea was present in 76% of the patients, including 40% with CSA and 36% with OSA. Studies have also found a high percentage of sleep apnea in patients admitted with decompensated heart failure.

TABLE P69-1	Prevalence of Sleep Apnea			
Author	Patients	% Sleep Apnea	% OSA	% CSA
Javaheri	Stable	45		
MacDonald	Stable	61	30	31
Oldenberg	Stable	76	36	40
Mared	Decompensated	70	3.6	66
Kayat	Decompensated	75	57	18

CSA, Central sleep apnea; *OSA*, obstructive sleep apnea; % sleep apnea = % OSA + % CSA.

Javaheri et al analyzed retrospectively analyzed data concerning Medicare beneficiaries (30,719 patients) with newly diagnosed heart failure and determined that sleep apnea was underdiagnosed. Patients who were tested, diagnosed, and treated for sleep apnea with positive airway pressure (PAP) therapy, supplemental oxygen, or both, had a better 2-year overall survival compared with patients who were tested and diagnosed with sleep apnea but not treated.

Defining what percent of events qualified patients for CSA versus OSA has varied between studies. Indeed, the percentage of central events may vary overnight or from night to night. In some patients, more central events are seen in the second half of the night. During the night, fluid redistributes into the lungs (higher wedge pressure). Pulmonary congestion stimulates J receptors, and this increases ventilatory drive and lowers the arterial partial pressure of carbon dioxide (PCO_2) (increasing the tendency for CSA). Of interest, studies have shown CSA with Cheyne-Stokes breathing (CSB) may occur in diastolic heart failure, but the CSB in these patients has a shorter cycle time than in patients with systolic failure. The presence of CSA-CSB in a patient with CHF is associated with a worse prognosis (Figure P69-1).

As the prevalence of either OSA, CSA-CSB, or both is high in patients with significant systolic or diastolic heart failure, *it should not be assumed that complaints of disturbed nocturnal sleep are simply secondary to heart failure*. A study by Sin and colleagues published in 1999 retrospectively evaluated a group of patients with significant left ventricular failure referred to the sleep laboratory and found that risk factors for OSA included an increased BMI for men and increased age for women. Risk factors for CSA included atrial fibrillation, male gender, age > 60, and hypocapnia. In patients with CHF and OSA, negative intrathoracic pressure, hypoxemia, and increased sympathetic tone are associated with the apneas are believed to negatively affect ventricular function. With regard to CHF and CSA a higher wedge pressure has been associated with lower PCO_2 (Lorenzi-filho et al.) and a higher central AHI (Solin and coworkers). The factors determining the relative amounts of OSA and CSA are illustrated in Figure P69-2.

Treatment of CHF and OSA: Treatment of OSA with continuous PAP (CPAP) in patients with CHF has been found to improve the ejection fraction and symptoms in a number of studies. This appears to occur because of a reduction in sympathetic tone and a decrease in ventricular afterload. However, not all studies have shown a significant benefit. Does CPAP treatment of OSA in a patient with CHF improve outcome? Wang et al published results of a retrospective cohort study of patients with CHF. Those patients with sleep apnea who were diagnosed and treated had a better 2-year survival than those in whom sleep apnea was diagnosed but not treated (adjusted for age, gender, comorbidities). However, to date, no prospective controlled study has confirmed a reduction in mortality with CPAP treatment in patients with CHF + OSA.

Treatment of CHF and CSB-CSA: The first step in treatment is to optimize medical treatment of CHF. In patients with CSA-CSB treatment with CPAP may improve the ejection fraction and markers of increased sympathetic tone. A large trial randomized trial (CANPAP) did not document an improvement in mortality with CPAP compared to standard care. Only 50% of patients

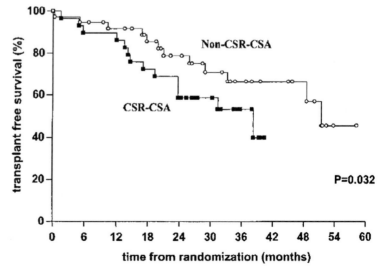

FIGURE P69-1 ■ Transplant-free survival in patients with congestive heart failure with Cheyne-Stokes respiration (CSR) and central sleep apnea (CSR-CSA) was significantly worse than in those with CHF who did not have CSR-CSA. (From Sin DD, Logan AG, Fitzgerald FS, et al: Effects of continuous positive airway pressure on cardiovascular outcomes in heart failure patients with and without Cheyne-Stokes respiration, *Circulation* 02(1):61-66, 2000.

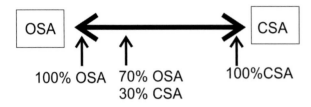

The relative amounts of OSA and CSA vary between patients and within the same patient during a single night

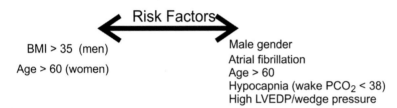

OSA ⟷ CSA

100% OSA 70% OSA 100%CSA
30% CSA

Risk Factors ⟷

BMI > 35 (men)
Age > 60 (women)

Male gender
Atrial fibrillation
Age > 60
Hypocapnia (wake PCO_2 < 38)
High LVEDP/wedge pressure

FIGURE P69-2 ■ Factors associated with obstructive sleep apnea (OSA) versus central sleep apnea (CSA) in patients with congestive heart failure. *LVEDP*, Left ventricular end-diastolic pressure. Data from Sin DD, Fitzgerald F, Parker JD, et al: Risk factors for central and obstructive sleep apnea in 450 men and women with congestive heart failure, *Am J Respir Crit Care Med* 160:64, 1999.)

had an improved AHI with CPAP (AHI <15 per hour [hr]). In the group of responders, improvements in ejection fraction were seen. The titration of CPAP in this study differed from the approach in patients with OSA. CPAP was increased to around 10 to 12 centimeters of water (cm H_2O) as tolerated (and sufficiently high to eliminate obstructive events). This level of pressure had been shown effective in several previous studies. However, it may take time for patients with CHF to adapt to CPAP, and lower pressure was used in some patients. Adaptive servoventilation (ASV) was developed to stabilize breathing in CSB and may reduce both OSA and CSA. It is generally well tolerated and often reduces the AHI to less than 10/hr. ASV is discussed in Fundamentals 30. Short-term studies have shown an improvement in ejection fraction with ASV, but no study has documented an increase in survival. Large studies of ASV in patients with CHF are underway. Other treatment options for CSA-CSB in heart failure patients are discussed in Patient 73.

The current patient underwent a sleep study, which showed both OSA and CSA of the Cheyne-Stokes type. CPAP was tried but did not reduce the central apneas. The patient returned for another titration study, and ASV effectively eliminated both obstructive and central events.

CLINICAL PEARLS

1. Sleep apnea (both OSA and CSA-CSB) is common in patients with systolic or diastolic heart failure, either stable or decompensated. The presence of CSA-CSB is associated with a worse prognosis. Patients with CSA-CSB and diastolic heart failure have shorter cycle lengths compared with those with CSA-CSB and systolic heart failure.

2. Sleep apnea is often unrecognized:
   - Patients are often not sleepy.
   - Nocturnal disturbed sleep and symptoms are often attributed to CHF.
   - Sleep studies are delayed.

3. The relative amount of OSA and CSA in patients with CHF depends on the population being studied and the definitions of OSA and CSA. The proportion of CSA in a given patient is often higher in the second part of the night (possibly because of worse pulmonary congestion, higher wedge pressure) and may vary between nights in the same patient.

4. The treatment of patients with CHF+**OSA** is PAP (e.g., CPAP). Short-term studies have found that CPAP improves cardiac function. Limited data suggest that long-term PAP treatment of OSA in CHF (observational studies) may improve survival.

5. The best treatment for patients with CHF + **CSA-CSB** is not known. The first intervention is optimization of medical treatment of CHF. Most clinicians would treat patients with ASV (unless CPAP was effective during the initial titration study). Short-term studies have shown improvement in ejection fraction and markers of sympathetic activity. However, no study has proven a survival advantage with ASV treatment.

BIBLIOGRAPHY

Arzt M, Floras JS, Logan AG, et al: Suppression of central sleep apnea by continuous positive airway pressure and transplant-free survival in heart failure: a post hoc analysis of the Canadian Continuous Positive Airway Pressure for Patients with Central Sleep Apnea and Heart Failure Trial (CANPAP), *Circulation* 115:3173–3180, 2007.

Bitter T, Faber L, Hering D, et al: Sleep-disordered breathing in heart failure with normal left ventricular ejection fraction, *Eur J Heart Fail* 11:602–608, 2009.

Bradley TD, Logan AG, Kimoff RJ, et al: CANPAP Investigators: Continuous positive airway pressure for central sleep apnea and heart failure, *N Engl J Med* 353:2025–2033, 2005.

Javaheri S, Caref EB, Chen E, et al: Sleep apnea testing and outcomes in a large cohort of Medicare beneficiaries with newly diagnosed heart failure, *Am J Respir Crit Care Med* 183(4):539–546, 2011.

Javaheri S, Parker TJ, Wexler L, et al: Occult sleep-disordered breathing in stable congestion heart failure, *Ann Intern Med* 122:487–492, 1995.

Kaneko Y, Floras JS, Usui K, et al: Cardiovascular effects of continuous positive airway pressure in patients with heart failure and obstructive sleep apnea, *N Engl J Med* 348:1233–1241, 2003.

Khayat RN, Jarjoura D, Patt B, et al: In-hospital testing for sleep disordered breathing in hospitalized patients with decompensated heart failure-report of prevalence and patient characteristics, *J Card Fail* 15(9):739–746, 2009.

Lorenzi-Filho G, Azevedo ER, Parker JD, et al: Relationship of carbon dioxide tension in arterial blood to pulmonary wedge pressure in heart failure, *Eur Respir J* 19(1):37–40, 2002.

MacDonald M, Fang J, Pittman SD, et al: The current prevalence of sleep disordered breathing in congestive heart failure patients treated with beta-blockers, *J Clin Sleep Med* 4:38–42, 2008.

Mared L, Cline C, Erhardt L, et al: Cheyne-Stokes respiration in patients hospitalised for heart failure, *Respir Res* 5:14, 2004.

Oldenburg O, Lamp B, Faber L, et al: Sleep-disordered breathing in patients with symptomatic heart failure: a contemporary study of prevalence in and characteristics of 700 patients, *Eur J Heart Fail* 9:251–257, 2007.

Oldenburg O, Schmidt A, Lamp B, et al: Adaptive servoventilation improves cardiac function in patients with chronic heart failure and Cheyne-Stokes respiration, *Eur J Heart Fail* 10:581–586, 2008.

Pepperell JC, Maskell NA, Jones DR, et al: A randomized controlled trial of adaptive ventilation for Cheyne-Stokes breathing in heart failure, *Am J Respir Crit Care Med* 168:1109–1114, 2008.

Sin D, Fitzgerald F, Parker J: Risk factors for central and obstructive sleep apnea in 450 men and women with congestive heart failure, *Am J Respir Crit Care Med* 160:1101–1106, 1999.

Sin DD, Logan AG, Fitzgerald FS, et al: Effects of continuous positive airway pressure on cardiovascular outcomes in heart failure patients with and without Cheyne-Stokes respiration, *Circulation* 102:61–66, 2000.

Solin P, Bergin P, Richardson M, et al: Influence of pulmonary capillary wedge pressure on central apnea in heart failure, *Circulation* 99(12):1574–1579, 1999.

Teschler H, Döhring J, Wang YM, Berthon-Jones M: Adaptive pressure support servoventilation: a novel treatment for Cheyne-Stokes respiration in heart failure, *Am J Respir Crit Care Med* 164:614–619, 2001.

Tkacova R, Niroumand M, Lorenzi-Filho G, Bradley TD: Overnight shift from obstructive to central apneas in patients with heart failure: role of PCO_2 and circulatory delay, *Circulation* 103:238–243, 2001.

Wang H, Parker JD, Newton GE, et al: Influence of obstructive sleep apnea on mortality in patients with heart failure, *J Am Coll Cardiol* 49(15):1625–1631, 2007.

FUNDAMENTALS 29

Central Sleep Apnea and Sleep-Related Hypoventilation Disorders

This chapter provides an overview of central sleep apnea (CSA) and sleep-related hypoventilation disorders. The *International Classification of Sleep Disorders*, Third Edition (ICSD-3), provides diagnostic criteria for the disorders listed in Box F29-1 and refers to the *American Academy of Sleep Medicine (AASM) Scoring Manual* for definitions of respiratory disorders. Scoring rules for central apneas, *Cheyne-Stokes breathing (CSB)*, and hypoventilaton in adults and children have been discussed in previous chapters (see Fundamentals 13 and 14). CSA and hypoventilation disorders are considered together here, as some patients have both CSA and hypoventilation. The obesity hypoventilation syndrome (OHS) is discussed along with obstructive sleep apnea (OSA) in Fundamentals 19 and 20. *It should be noted that many patients have a combination of obstructive and central apneas and may, in fact, qualify for both diagnoses.*

CENTRAL SLEEP APNEA SYNDROMES

To understand the pathophysiology of CSA, CSA and hypoventilation syndromes it is useful to divide the disorders into hypocapnic and normocapnic–hypercapnic groups. Patients with primary CSA, CSA with CSB (CSA-CSB), CSA due to high-altitude periodic breathing, and treatment-emergent CSA (TE-CSA) disorders exhibit CSA sleep because the arterial partial pressure of carbon dioxide ($PaCO_2$) during sleep transiently falls below the apneic threshold (AT) (Table F29-1). The AT is the value of $PaCO_2$, below which respiration is not triggered during sleep. For most individuals, the apneic threshold is within 1 or 2 millimeters of mercury (mm Hg) of the awake $PaCO_2$. Most normal individuals increase the $PaCO_2$ from 2 to 8 mm Hg during sleep. Patients with hypocapnic CSA have a

---

BOX F29-1	Central Sleep Apnea and Sleep-Related Hypoventilation Disorders—ICSD-3

CENTRAL SLEEP APNEA DISORDERS

1. Primary Central Sleep Apnea
2. Central Sleep Apnea with Cheyne-Stokes Breathing
3. Central sleep apnea Due to High Altitude Periodic Breathing high-altitude periodic breathing
4. Treatment-Emergent Central Sleep Apnea
5. Central sleep apnea Due to Medication or Substance
6. Central sleep apnea due to a Medical Disorder without Cheyne-Stokes Breathing without Cheyne-Stokes breathing
7. Primary Central Sleep Apnea of Infancy
8. Primary Central Sleep Apnea of Prematurity

SLEEP-RELATED HYPOVENTILATION DISORDERS

1. Obesity Hypoventilation Syndrome
2. Congenital Central Alveolar Hypoventilaton
3. Late-Onset Central Hypoventilation with Hypothalamic Dysfunction
4. Idiopathic Central Alveolar Hypoventilation (sleep-related nonobstructive alveolar central hypoventilation, idiopathic)
5. Sleep-related hypoventilation Due to Medication or Substance
6. Sleep-related hypoventilation Due to Medical Disorder

SLEEP-RELATED HYPOXEMIA DISORDER

1. Sleep-related hypoxemia

TABLE F29-1 **Hypocapnic CSA Disorders and Common Characteristics**

Disorders	Characteristics of Disorders
1. Primary CSA 2. CSA with CSB 3. CSA caused by high-altitude periodic breathing 4. Treatment-emergent CSA	1. Central apnea when the sleeping $PaCO_2$ drops below the hypocapnic AT 2. High ventilatory drive 3. Small difference between AT and sleeping $PaCO_2$ 4. Unstable sleep, frequent arousals 5. Long circulation time in CSA-CSB due to CHF 6. Central AHI NREM > REM sleep 7. No awake or sleeping hypoventilation

AHI, Apnea–hypopnea index; *AT*, apneic threshold; *CSA*, central apnea; *CSB*, Cheyne-Stokes breathing; *NREM*, non–rapid eye movement; *PaCO₂*, partial pressure of arterial carbon dioxide; *REM*, rapid eye movement.

TABLE F29-2 **Normocapnic-Hypercapnic CSA or Hypoventilation Syndromes**

Awake PaCO₂	Normal or Increased	
Sleeping $PaCO_2$	• Increased in sleep-related Hypoventilation disorders (awake hypoventilation may or may not be present) • In OHS, by definition, awake hypoventilation is present • Normal or increased in normocapic CSA disorders	
Pathophysiology*	• Abnormal ventilatory control caused by structural (tumor, infarct) or functional dysfunction of ventilatory control centers • Drug or substance suppressing ventilation • Immature ventilatory control centers	• Disorders of structures innervating respiratory muscles, myopathy, disorders of the neuromuscular junction • Chest wall disorders • Pulmonary disorders (airways, parenchyma, pulmonary vasculature)
Disorders	**CSA Syndromes:** • CSA, not CSB caused by medical or neurological condition • CSA due to drug or substance • Primary CSA of infancy • Primary CSA of prematurity	**Sleep-Related Hypoventilation Disorders:** • Idiopathic central alveolar hypoventilation • Congenital central hypoventilation syndrome • Late-onset central hypoventilation with hypothalamic abnormalities • Sleep-related hypoventilation caused by drug or substance • Sleep-related hypoventilation caused by medical or neurologic condition

CSA, Central sleep apnea; *CSB*, Cheyne-Stokes breathing; *OHS*, obesity hypoventilation syndrome; *PaCO₂*, partial pressure of arterial carbon dioxide.
*For pathophysiology: left column associated with CSA or sleep-related hypoventilation, right column associated with sleep-related hypoventilation.

---

smaller difference between the sleeping $PaCO_2$ and the AT. Patients with hypocapnic CSA have normal or decreased awake $PaCO_2$, and sleep-related hypoventilation is not present. The small difference between the sleeping $PaCO_2$ and the AT is due to high ventilatory drive rather than a low $PaCO_2$ (see Manisty et al. 2006).

The normocapnic–hypercapnic CSA or sleep-related hypoventilation group includes those disorders with a normal or increased awake $PaCO_2$ and either CSA, sleep-related hypoventilation, or both CSA and sleep-related hypoventilation (Table F29-2; Figure F29-1). CSA occurs because of abnormal ventilatory control associated with a congenital dysfunction, medication, or a functional or structural abnormality of the ventilatory control centers (tumor, infarct). Patients with

CSA without CSB caused by a neurologic disorder are classified here, but the pathophysiology of the disorder presumably caused by damage to the ventilatory control centers has not been well characterized. Sleep-related hypoventilation may occur because of chest wall disorders, obesity, damage to the neural pathways supplying innervation to the respiratory muscles, disorders of the neuromuscular junction, or myopathies. Sleep-related hypoventilation may also occur in patients with lung disease (parenchymal, airway, or pulmonary vasculature). Hypoventilation during wakefulness may also be present in patients with sleep-related hypoventilation. If hypoventilation is present during wakefulness it invariably worsens during sleep. The obesity hypoventilation syndrome is the only sleep-related breathing

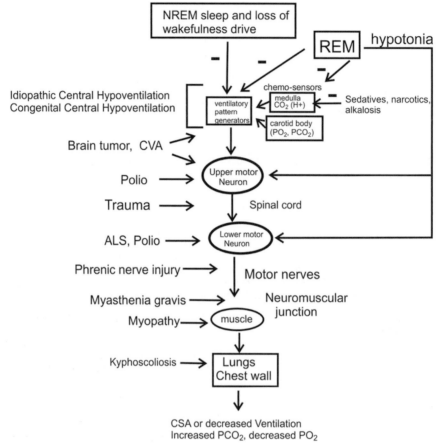

FIGURE F29-1 ■ Mechanisms of normocapnic or hypercapnic central sleep apnea, sleep-related hypoventilation, or both. (Adapted from Berry RB: *Fundamentals of sleep* medicine, Philadelphia, 2012, Saunders, p 393.)

disorder that has a diagnostic criteria requiring hypoventilation during wake.

Primary Central Sleep Apnea

Primary central sleep apnea (idiopathic CSA) is an uncommon disorder (5% of patients with sleep apnea) of unknown etiology (idiopathic) characterized by recurrent central apneas. Symptoms include complaints of snoring, frequent awakenings, sleepiness, or insomnia. These patients tend to be thinner than patients with OSA and are more likely to complain of insomnia. The awake $PaCO_2$ is normal or low (less than 40 mm Hg). Patients with a known medical or neurologic disorder that is believed to cause central apneas are classified elsewhere. Sleep studies in patients with primary CSA typically reveal isolated central apneas or runs of central apneas (a form of periodic breathing). A run of central apneas may follow arousal from a nonrespiratory stimulus. Five or more central apneas or central hypopneas per hour of sleep are

required, and more than 50% of respiratory events must be central. CSB is not present. No evidence of daytime or nocturnal hypoventilation exists. The central apneas occur during stages N1 and N2 and are uncommon during stage N3 and REM sleep. Diagnostic criteria for primary CSA are summarized in Table F29-3 and discussed in detail in Patient 70.

CSA with Cheyne-Stokes Breathing (CSA-CSB)

CSA-CSB is characterized by recurrent central apneas or central hypopneas alternating with a respiratory phase exhibiting a crescendo–decrescendo pattern of flow (or tidal volume). The longer cycle length (>40 seconds and typically 45 to 60 seconds) and the crescendo–decrescendo pattern of breathing distinguishes CSB from other CSA types (Figure F29-2). Central apnea or central hypopnea and the pattern of

TABLE F29-3	**Summary of Diagnostic Criteria for Some of the Major CSA Syndromes**		
Disorder	**Symptoms**	**PSG findings**	**Other Criteria**
Primary central sleep apnea	+ Symptoms	1. CAHI ≥ 5 per hour (hr) 2. Number of CA + CH >50% of the total A + H	Absence of CSB No evidence of daytime or nocturnal hypoventilation
CSA with CSB	+ Symptoms OR atrial fibrillation or flutter, congestive heart failure, or a neurologic disorder	1. CAHI ≥ 5 per hour (hr) 2. Number of CA + CH >50% of the total A + H 3. 1 and 2 occur during either a diagnostic PSG or PAP titration PSG	CA or CH meet criteria for CSB
Treatment emergent CSA	+ Symptoms	Diagnostic study - predominantly obstructive events, AHI ≥ 5/hr PAP titration study-after obstructive events have resolved shows CAHI ≥ 5/hr and >50% of events are central apneas or central hypopneas	CSA not better explained by another CSA disorder (e.g., no CSB, no opioids)
CSA due to drug or substance	+Symptoms	1. CAHI ≥ 5 per hour (hr) 2. Number of CA + CH >50% of the total A + H 3. 1 and 2 occur during either a diagnostic PSG or PAP titration PSG	Absence of CSB • Believed to be caused by opioid or respiratory depressant • Sleep-related hypoventilation may be present
CSA due to medical disorder without CSB	+Symptoms	1. CAHI 5 per hour (hr) 2. Number of CA + CH >50% of the total A + H	Absence of CSB • Believe to be cause by medical or neurological condition • *not* caused by drug or substance • Sleep-related hypoventilation may be present

CA, Central apnea; *CH*, central hypopnea; *CAHI*, central apnea + central hypopnea index; *CSB*, Cheyne-Stokes breathing, as defined in the *AASM Scoring Manual*; *PSG*, polysomnography.
+ Symptoms = presence of sleepiness, insomnia, awakening SOB, snoring, witnessed *A*, apnea; *H*, hypopnea.

breathing must meet the *AASM Scoring Manual* criteria. The vast majority of patients with CSA-CSB have either systolic or diastolic heart failure. Patients may manifest CSA-CSB following a cerebrovascular accident (CVA) or associated with other neurologic disorders. Of note, idiopathic CSA-CSB may also occur. Patients with CSA-CSB have normal or low daytime PaCO$_2$. The ICSD-3 diagnostic criteria for CSA-CSB (see Table F29-3 and Patient 73) require that either symptoms or a comorbid condition must be present (atrial fibrillation, congestive heart failure, neurologic disorder). Symptoms of CSA-CSB include excessive daytime sleepiness, insomnia, or nocturnal dyspnea. If neither symptoms nor comorbid conditions are present, CSA-CSB is simply considered a PSG finding. Five or more central apneas or central hypopneas per hour of sleep with CSB

morphology must be present during either a diagnostic PSG or PAP titration PSG. More than 50% of respiratory events must be central (central apneas or central hypopneas) and meet criteria for CSB during either a diagnostic PSG or PAP titration PSG. Many patients with heart failure have a mixture of obstructive, mixed, and central apneas. In some patients, more central apneas are noted in the later part of the night or when the patient is placed on PAP. A diagnosis of CSA-CSB does not exclude a diagnosis of OSA. In patients with CSA-CSB, arousal from sleep tends to occur at the zenith of respiratory effort (Figure F29-2) between contiguous central apneas or hypopneas, rather than at apnea termination (as in primary CSA). The longer cycle length of CSA-CSB events compared with those in primary CSA is caused by a *long ventilatory phase* (usually five or more breaths) between the apneas or hypopneas.

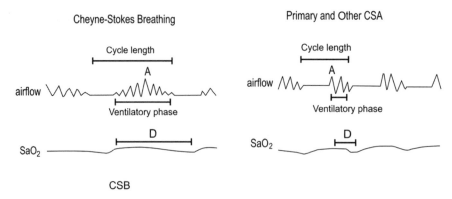

FIGURE F29-2 ■ Difference between central apnea (CSA) with Cheyne-Stokes breathing (CSB) versus CSA with other types of central apnea. *For simplicity, respiratory effort is not shown, but all apneas are assumed to be central.* (Adapted from Berry RB: *Fundamentals of sleep medicine*, Philadelphia, 2012, Saunders, p 384.)

BOX F29-2	Central Sleep Apnea Caused by High Altitude Periodic Breathing—ICSD-3 Diagnostic Criteria (Criterial A-D must be met)

A. Recent ascent to high altitude*
B. The presence of one or more of the following:
   1. Sleepiness
   2. Difficulty initiating or maintaining sleep, frequent awakenings, or nonrestorative sleep
   3. Awakening with shortness of breath or morning headache
   4. Witnessed Apnea

C. The symptoms are clinically attributable to high altitude periodic breathing or polysomnography, if performed, demonstrates recurrent central apneas or hypopneas primarily during non–rapid eye movement (NREM) sleep at a frequency of ≥5 per hour
D. The disorder is not better explained by another current sleep disorder, medical or neurologic disorder, medication use (e.g., narcotics), or substance use disorders

*High altitude means typically at least 2500 meters (8202 feet), although some individuals may exhibit the disorder at altitudes as low as 1500 meters.

Central Sleep Apnea Caused by High-Altitude Periodic Breathing

High-altitude periodic breathing is characterized by alternating periods of central apnea and hyperpnea associated with recent ascent to high altitude (Box F29-2). Periodic breathing is a common response to ascent to high altitude. Associated symptoms are required to make the diagnosis of a disorder. No level of the central apnea–hypopnea index (AHI) separates a normal and abnormal response to high altitude. The cycle length of the periodic breathing is commonly less than 40 seconds and often as short as 12 to 20 seconds. The percentage of individuals exhibiting periodic breathing during sleep increases at higher altitudes. Approximately 25% exhibit periodic breathing at 2500 meters (m) (8202 feet) and virtually 100% demonstrate periodic breathing at 4000 m (13,123 feet). Periodic breathing has been described at altitudes as low as 1500 m (4900 feet).

With acclimatization, sleep quality tends to improve, even though the amount of periodic breathing may actually increase in some individuals. Treatment includes a return to lower altitudes, supplemental oxygen, and acetazolamide. Hypnotics may decrease sleep disturbance.

Treatment-Emergent Central Sleep Apnea

The terms *complex sleep apnea* and *treatment-emergent central sleep apnea* are often used to designate the same condition. However, in this book *complex sleep apnea* (complex SA) will refer to any circumstance in which a patient has predominantly obstructive events during a diagnostic study but exhibits the emergence or persistence of CSA on PAP after obstructive events have resolved with a central AHI ≥ 5/hour and more than 50% of the residual events being central (Figure F29-3; see Table F29-3). This is the

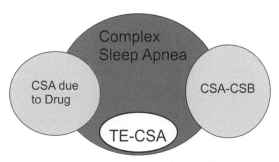

FIGURE F29-3 ■ Some patients with central apnea with Cheyne-Stokes breathing (CSA-CSB) or CSA due to drug or substance will exhibit central apneas primarily when placed on positive airway pressure. In treatment-emergent central sleep apnea (TE-CSA) the central apnea is NOT better explained by another central sleep apnea disorder.

definition used by the Centers of Medicare and Medicaid Services (CMS) except that their wording specifies obstructive and mixed apneas rather than obstructive events). TE-CSA will follow the ICSD-3 diagnostic criteria and refer to those patients with complex sleep apnea in whom the *central sleep apnea is **not** better explained by another CSA disorder*. In this sense TE-CSA is "idiopathic" complex SA. The diagnostic criteria for TE-CSA are summarized in Table F29-3 and discussed in more detail in Patients 71 and 72.

Central Sleep Apnea Caused Due to Medication or Substance

In this disorder, the central apneas are believed to be caused by potent long-acting opioids or other respiratory-depressant medications. A number a potent long-acting opioids, including methadone, long-acting forms of morphine or oxycodone, a fentanyl patch, the combination of buprenorphine and naloxone (Suboxone), and constant narcotic infusions may cause the disorder. The ICSD-3 diagnostic criteria (see Table F29-3) state that five or more central apneas or hypopneas per hour of sleep with more than 50% of respiratory events being central must be present during a diagnostic or PAP titration PSG. The central events do *not* meet *AASM Scoring Manual* criteria for CSB. Patients commonly have other abnormalities of respiration, including a low respiratory rate, OSA, and ataxic breathing (variation in respiratory rate/cycle length and magnitude of flow). A diagnosis of CSA caused by drug or substance use does not exclude a diagnosis of OSA. Awake hypoventilation, sleep-related hypoventilation, or both may occur, and in this case, a diagnosis of "Sleep-Related Hypoventilation Due to Drug or Substance" may also be made. Patients may also have predominantly obstructive apneas during a diagnostic PSG but when placed on PAP have mainly central apneas after the obstructive events have resolved (complex SA). In this case,

a diagnosis of "OSA and CSA Due to Drug or Substance" may be made. Further discussion is available in Patients 71 and 74.

Central Apnea Due to a Medical Disorder without Cheyne-Stokes Breathing

In this group of disorders, CSA is attributed to a medical or neurologic condition (and does not have the pattern of CSB) (see Table F29-3). The ICSD-3 diagnostic criteria include requirements for five or more central apneas and/or central hypopneas per hour of sleep, >50% of respiratory events being central, and absence of CSB. The central apneas must be attributed to a medical or neurologic condition. A mixture of obstructive and central apneas may be present, and a simultaneous diagnosis of OSA is not excluded. Sleep-related hypoventilation may or may not be present. If present, a diagnosis of both CSA and sleep-related hypoventilation may be made. The majority of these patients have brainstem lesions of developmental, vascular, neoplastic, degenerative, demyelinating, or traumatic origin. Patients generally present with sleep fragmentation, excessive daytime sleepiness, or insomnia. Other signs and symptoms that are often, but not invariably, present include snoring, witnessed apnea, and awakening with shortness of breath. The presentation varies with the cause of central apnea and may include neurologic findings. The inclusion of a Chiari malformation (CM) in this group is important to note. Patients with CM may be relatively asymptomatic and surgical treatment may be curative.

Primary Central Sleep Apnea of Infancy

Primary central sleep apnea of infancy is characterized by prolonged central, mixed, or obstructive apneas or hypopneas associated with physiologic compromise (hypoxemia, bradycardia, or the need for intervention such as stimulation or resuscitation) (Table F29-4). The predominant feature is central apnea. It is a disorder of respiratory control that may be either a developmental problem associated with immaturity of the brainstem respiratory centers or secondary to other medical conditions that produce direct depression of central respiratory control or lung function. Apnea in the neonate or infant may be exacerbated or precipitated by a variety of medical conditions that must be recognized and treated to stabilize the apnea, for example, anemia, infection, hypoxemia, metabolic disease. The terms *sudden infant death syndrome (SIDS)* and *apparent life-threatening event (ALTE)* should ***not*** be used. If another medical

TABLE F29-4	**Apnea of Prematurity and Infancy (Adapted from ICSD-3 Criteria)**	
	Apnea of Prematurity	**Apnea of Infancy**
Age	Conceptional age <37 weeks at the time of onset of symptoms	Conceptional age ≥37 weeks at the time of onset of symptoms
Manifestations	Apnea or cyanosis is noted by an observer, or sleep-related central apnea, desaturation or bradycardia detected by hospital monitoring in the postnatal period	Apnea or cyanosis is noted by an observer, or sleep-related central apnea or desaturation is detected by monitoring
Polysomnography/ Monitoring	PSG or alternative monitoring such as hospital or home apnea monitoring shows either: • Frequent prolonged (>20 seconds duration) CAs • Periodic breathing for ≥5% of total sleep time	PSG or alternative monitoring such as hospital or home apnea monitoring shows either • Frequent prolonged (>20 seconds duration) CAs • Periodic breathing for ≥5% of total sleep time
Exclusions	Disorder is not better explained by another current sleep disorder, medical or neurological disorder, or medication	Disorder is not better explained by another current sleep disorder, medical or neurological disorder, or medication

Central apnea (CA) or periodic breathing as defined by the *AASM Scoring Manual*.
Obstructive and mixed apneas may also be present, but central apneas are predominant.
Normative data concerning the number of prolonged central apneas per hour are not well established.
PSG, Polysomnography.

condition appears to be the cause rather than an exacerbating factor for the CSA, then the condition should be classified as "Central Sleep Apnea due to a Medical Disorder," or "Central Sleep Apnea due to Drug or Substance." Despite the heterogeneity of infant risk groups and underlying pathophysiology, most studies report a progressive decrease in frequency of apneas and risk of symptomatic apnea secondary to other medical conditions after the early weeks of life.

Primary Central Sleep Apnea of Prematurity

Apnea is very common in preterm infants, and the prevalence varies inversely with gestational age. In the preterm infant, sleep apnea may be anticipated, is primarily related to immaturity, may require supportive ventilatory and pharmacologic treatment, and will improve with maturation unless extenuating conditions such as hypoxemia caused by chronic lung disease or gastroesophageal reflux, are present. Apneas may be central, mixed, or obstructive apneas or hypopneas associated with physiologic compromise (hypoxemia, bradycardia) or the need for intervention such as stimulation or resuscitation, although the predominant feature is central apnea. The ICSD-3 diagnostic criteria are listed in (Table F29-4). Apnea in the preterm infant is commonly associated with bradycardia. Primary CSA of prematurity is state dependent, and the frequency of respiratory events increases during active (REM) sleep. Paradoxic chest wall movements are common during active sleep in neonates and may cause a fall in arterial oxygen saturation (SaO_2)

because of ventilation or perfusion defects associated with a decrease in functional residual capacity (FRC). Underlying comorbidities (e.g., lung disease or abnormal neurologic status) may predispose the infant to having a more severe or prolonged course for apnea. Treatment is with supportive measures and caffeine or theophylline. Exacerbating factors such as infection or medical or neurologic disorders should be ruled out.

SLEEP-RELATED HYPOVENTILATION DISORDERS

Recall that the *AASM Scoring Manual* criteria for scoring hypoventilation during sleep in adults state than hypoventilation is scored with an increase in the arterial $PaCO_2$ (or surrogate) to a value >55 mm Hg for ≥10 minutes or with ≥10 mm Hg increase in $PaCO_2$ (or surrogate) during sleep (in comparison with an awake supine value) to a value exceeding 50 mm Hg for ≥10 minutes. For children, the $PaCO_2$ or surrogate is >50 mm Hg for >25% of total sleep time. *The general criterion for sleep-related hypoventilation syndromes is that hypoventilation is present during sleep.* In these disorders, OSA or CSA may be present but is not believed to be the main cause of sleep-related hypoventilation. Instead, the periods of reduced tidal volume and or respiratory rate that occur during sleep are not sufficient to maintain a normal $PaCO_2$. In normal individuals, the $PaCO_2$ typically increases 2 to 8 mm Hg. If pulmonary disease is present, an increase in physiologic dead space ventilation is often present, and this requires that a higher minute ventilation is needed to maintain a normal alveolar ventilation. Note that the obesity hypoventilation syndrome is the only sleep-related hypoventilation disorder in which demonstration of *awake hypoventilation* is required for a diagnosis. Patients with *other sleep-related hypoventilation syndromes may or may not also have awake hypoventilation.*

Congenital Central Alveolar Hypoventilation (CCAHS)

In this disorder (also known as congenital central hypoventilation syndrome), sleep-related hypoventilation is present because of failure of automatic ventilatory control associated with a mutation of the *PHOX2B* gene. Sleep-related hypoventilation may be associated with either daytime hypoventilation ($PaCO_2 > 45$ mm Hg) or normal daytime $PaCO_2$ levels. In either case, the $PaCO_2$ is higher during sleep and meets the criteria for sleep-related hypoventilation. PSG monitoring demonstrates severe hypercapnia and arterial oxygen desaturation. Some central apneas may occur, but *the predominant pattern is reduced flow or tidal volume.* The usual clinical presentation is the onset of hypoventilation at birth. The hypoventilation is worse during sleep than during wakefulness and is unexplained by primary pulmonary, neurologic, or metabolic disease. Although the condition is deemed congenital, some patients with a *PHOX2B* genotype may present phenotypically later in life (and even in adulthood), especially in the presence of a stressor such as general anesthesia or a severe respiratory illness. Congenital central alveolar hypoventilation syndrome (CCAHS) is discussed in detail in Patient 75.

Late-Onset Central Hypoventilation with Hypothalamic Dysfunction

In this disorder, sleep-related hypoventilation caused by dysfunction of the central control of ventilation is present, but symptoms are absent during the first few years of life. Dysfunction of the hypothalamic control of endocrine function also is present. The patient has at least two of the following: obesity, endocrine abnormalities of hypothalamic origin, severe emotional or behavioral disturbances, or a tumor of neural origin. A mutation of the *PHOX2B* gene is NOT present. On PSG, central apneas may occur but the predominant pattern is reduced flow or tidal volume associated with hypoventilation and arterial oxygen desaturation. Another name for this disorder is *rapid-onset obesity with hypothalamic dysfunction, hypoventilation, and autonomic dysregulation (ROHHAD).* Patients are usually healthy until early childhood (often 2 to

3 years of age) when they develop hyperphagia and severe obesity, followed by central hypoventilation, which often presents as respiratory failure. Patients require ventilatory support during sleep; most patients breathe adequately during wakefulness, but some need ventilatory support during both wakefulness and sleep. The hypoventilation persists even if the patient loses weight, differentiating the condition from OHS. The hypothalamic endocrine dysfunction is characterized by increased or decreased hormone levels, which may include one or more of the following: diabetes, inadequate antidiuretic hormone hypersecretion (diabetes insipidus), precocious puberty, hypogonadism, hyperprolactinemia, hypothyroidism, and decreased growth hormone secretion. Tumors of neural origin such as ganglioneuroma may occur.

Idiopathic Central Alveolar Hypoventilation

In this disorder, sleep-related hypoventilation is present. Hypoventilation is not primarily caused by lung parenchymal or airway disease, pulmonary vascular pathology, chest wall disorder, medication use, neurologic disorder, muscle weakness, obesity, or congenital hypoventilation syndromes. That is, as the name implies, the disorder is idiopathic. Although OSA may be present, it is not believed to be the major cause of hypoventilation, and the predominant respiratory pattern is one of reduced tidal volume or ataxic breathing and associated arterial oxygen desaturation. If sufficient obstructive events occur, a diagnosis of both OSA and idiopathic central alveolar hypoventilation may be made. Of note, arterial oxygen desaturation is often present but is not required for the diagnosis. Awake hypoventilation may also be present and, if so, worsens during sleep. The disorder is caused by dysfunction of the central control of ventilation, likely because of blunted chemoresponsiveness to CO_2 and O_2. However, a structural abnormality of the central nervous system cannot be found. *The diagnosis is one of exclusion.* This disorder is rare and may represent a mixed group of patients with varied underlying conditions erroneously deemed idiopathic as a result of incomplete diagnostic workup. Patients may complain of morning headaches, fatigue, neurocognitive decline and sleep disturbance or may be entirely asymptomatic.

Sleep-Related Hypoventilation Due to Medication or Substance

In this disorder, sleep-related hypoventilation is present and is believed to be caused by a medication or substance known to inhibit respiration, ventilatory drive, or both. Hypoventilation is not primarily caused by lung parenchymal or airway disease, pulmonary vascular pathology, chest wall disorder, neurologic disorder, muscle weakness, obesity hypoventilation syndrome, or a known congenital or idiopathic central alveolar hypoventilation syndrome. The offending agents include all of the potent long-acting opioids that cause CSA. Daytime hypoventilation may or may not be present. If present, hypoventilation worsens with sleep. This diagnosis does not exclude a diagnosis of "CSA Due to Drug or Substance." Hypoventilation may be caused by long periods of low tidal volume and low respiratory rate with superimposed central apneas of variable frequency.

Sleep-Related Hypoventilation Due to a Medical Disorder

Sleep-related hypoventilation is present and is believed to be caused by a lung parenchymal or airway disease, pulmonary vascular pathology, chest wall disorder (other than mass loading from obesity), neurologic disorder, or muscle weakness. Hypoventilation is *not* primarily caused by OHS, medication use, or a known congenital or idiopathic central alveolar hypoventilation syndrome.

Common causes of this disorder include chronic obstructive pulmonary disease (COPD), parenchymal restrictive disorders (interstitial lung disease), pulmonary vascular disease, neuromuscular disorders (myopathies, neuromuscular junction disorders, motor neuron disease, and traumatic, vascular or malignant damage to the spinal cord, ventilatory control centers, or peripheral nerves), and myopathies. OHS is classified under a separate diagnostic category, but chest wall disorders such as kyphoscoliosis are included here. Awake hypoventilation may or may not be present. A common characteristic of these disorders is that *gas exchange is the worse during rapid eye movement sleep.* This is in contrast to CCHS, in which the worse gas exchange occurs during NREM sleep.

Sleep-Related Hypoxemia

In this disorder, PSG or nocturnal oximetry shows the arterial oxygen saturation (SpO_2) of $\leq 88\%$ in adults or $\leq 90\%$ in children for ≥ 5 minutes during sleep. Sleep-related hypoventilation is not documented. If sleep-related hypoventilation is documented as measured by arterial blood gas, transcutaneous PCO_2 or end-tidal CO_2 sensors, the disorder is classified as sleep-related hypoventilation. OSA or CSA may be present, but these are not believed to be the major cause of hypoxemia. Many of these patients actually have a combination of hypoventilation and ventilation–perfusion mismatch. The diagnosis is made when hypoxemia is documented but a diagnosis of OSA or hypoventilation cannot be made. This is usually arises from oximetry monitoring that documents hypoxemia but not apnea, hypopnea, or hypoventilation (e.g., monitoring with end-tidal PCO_2 or transcutaneous PCO_2 is not preformed).

BIBLIOGRAPHY

American Academy of Sleep Medicine: *International classification of sleep disorders,* ed 3, Darien, IL, 2014, American Academy of Sleep Medicine.

Anholm J, Powles A, Downey R, et al: Operation Everest II: arterial oxygen saturation and sleep at extreme simulated altitude, *Am Rev Respir Dis* 145:817–826, 1992.

Aurora RN, Chowdhuri S, Ramar K, et al: The treatment of central sleep apnea syndromes in adults: practice parameters with an evidence-based literature review and meta-analyses, *Sleep* 35(1):17–40, 2012.

Bloch KE, Latshand TD, Turk AJ, et al: Nocturnal periodic breathing during Acclimatization at very high altitude at Mount Muztach Ata (7,546 m), *Am J Respir Crit Care Med* 182:562–568, 2010.

Bradley TD, McNicholas WT, Rutherford R, et al: Clinical and physiologic heterogeneity of the central sleep apnea syndrome, *Am Rev Respir Dis* 134:217–221, 1986.

Dempsey J: Crossing the apneic threshold. Causes and consequences, *Exp Physiol* 90:13–24, 2004.

Eckert DJ, Jordan AS, Merchia P, Malhotra A: Central sleep apnea, *Chest* 131:595–607, 2007.

Goldberg S, Schoene R, Haynor D, et al: Brain tissue pH and ventilatory acclimatization to high altitude, *J Appl Physiol* 72:58–63, 1992.

Johnson P, Edwards N, Burgess KR, Sullivan CE: Sleep architecture changes during a trek from 1400 to 500 m in the Nepal Himalaya, *J Sleep Res* 19:148–156, 2010.

Manisty CH, Willson K, Wensel R, et al: Development of respiratory control instability in heart failure: a novel approach to dissect the pathophysiological mechanisms, *J Physiol* 577(Pt 1):387–401, 2006.

Mathew OP: Apnea of prematurity: pathogenesis and management strategies, *J Perinatol* 31(5):302–310, 2011.

Nickol AH, Leverment J, Richards P, et al: Temazepam at high altitude reduces periodic breathing without impairing next-day performance: a randomized cross-over double-blind study, *J Sleep Res* 15(4):445–454, 2006.

Nussbaumer-Ochsner Y, Ursprung J, Siebenmann C, et al: Effect of short-term acclimatization to high altitude on sleep and nocturnal breathing, *Sleep* 35(3):419–423, 2012.

Schmidt B, Roberts RS, Davis P, et al., for the Caffeine for Apnea of Prematurity Trial Group: Long-term effects of caffeine therapy for apnea of prematurity, *N Engl J Med* 357(19):1893–1902, 2007.

Selim BJ, Junna MR, Morgenthaler TI: Therapy for sleep hypoventilation syndromes, *Curr Treat Options Neurol* 14:427–437, 2012.

Skatrud JB, Dempsey JA: Interaction of sleep state and chemical stimuli in sustaining rhythmic ventilation, *J Appl Physiol* 55:813–822, 1983.

White DP: Pathogenesis of obstructive and central sleep apnea, *Am J Respir Crit Care Med* 172:1363–1370, 2005.

A Man with Unexplained Central Sleep Apnea

A 55-year-old man complained of daytime sleepiness of a 2-year duration. His wife reported that he occasionally snored and was a "restless sleeper." No history of muscle weakness, orthopnea, pedal edema, or respiratory failure was present. The patient was not taking narcotics.

Sleep study: apnea–hypopnea index (AHI) 35 per hour; 80% of the respiratory events were similar to the one in Figure P70-1.

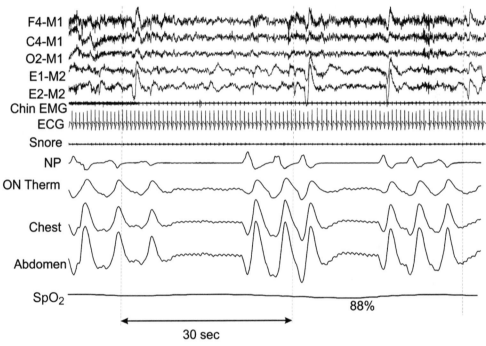

FIGURE P70-1 ■ Sleep tracing. *NP,* nasal pressure; *ON Therm,* Oronasal thermal sensor.

QUESTION

1. What is the cause of the patient's daytime sleepiness?

ANSWER

1. **Answer:** Primary central sleep apnea (CSA), also known as idiopathic CSA

   Discussion: Hypocapnic CSA occurs because the arterial partial pressure of carbon dioxide ($PaCO_2$) is below the apneic threshold —the level of $PaCO_2$ during sleep below which ventilatory effort is absent. The apneic threshold is usually within 2 to 4 mm Hg of the awake PCO_2 values. Most patients in stable sleep have PCO_2 levels around 5 mm Hg higher than the awake values. Hyperventilation during wakefulness does not cause apnea because of the presence of the wakefulness stimulus—a poorly defined but important component of ventilatory drive that is lost during sleep. During

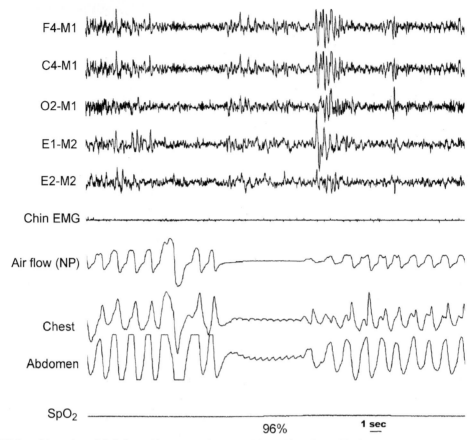

FIGURE P70-2 ■ A large breath is followed by a central apnea. Adapted from Berry RB: *Sleep medicine pearls,* Philadelphia, 2003, Hanley & Belfus, p 237.

non–rapid eye movement (NREM) sleep, ventilation depends on metabolic control. If the $PaCO_2$ falls below the apneic threshold for any reason (even in normal individuals), CSA is the result. Patients with primary CSA are believed to have an increased hypercapnic ventilatory response, a normal to decreased awake $PaCO_2$, and a small difference between the apneic threshold and the sleeping $PaCO_2$ level. The small difference between the sleeping $PaCO_2$ and the AT is due to a high ventilatory drive. Central apneas often follow periods of increased ventilation (Figure P70-2). The periods of increased ventilation triggering central apneas are often associated with a preceding arousal. Arousal may trigger a transient increase in ventilation and a fall in $PaCO_2$. This transient fall in PCO_2 is then associated with a central apnea as the patient returns to sleep ($PaCO_2$ below the apneic threshold). Thus, arousal may initiate or predispose to continuation of central apnea. Because ventilatory drive is lower during REM sleep than during NREM sleep, hypocapnic central apnea is much less common during that sleep stage.

In research studies, the addition of dead space or inhalation of CO_2 with the goal of stabilizing the $PaCO_2$ has been shown to reduce central apnea in primary CSA patients. However, these interventions have not been tried for long-term treatment, nor are they practical.

The presentation of primary CSA is somewhat variable, including complaints of insomnia, daytime sleepiness, or choking during the night. In one series, the symptom of excessive daytime sleepiness was the major presenting complaint. Snoring may occur in idiopathic CSA but is less prominent than in OSA. Patients with primary CSA also tend to be thinner than those with OSA. Primary CSA is believed to be rare and much less common than Cheyne-Stokes breathing (CSB), which is another form of hypocapnic CSA. In one study, only 5% of >300 patients with sleep apnea had idiopathic CSA.

Polysomnography (PSG) in primary CSA typically reveals frequent, isolated central apneas or runs of central apneas (one form of periodic breathing). A run of central apneas may follow arousal from a nonrespiratory stimulus. Central apneas occur mainly during stages N1 and N2 and are uncommon in stage N3. This form of CSA usually does not occur during REM sleep, possibly because of a reduced ventilatory drive in that sleep stage. Of note, the morphology of primary

BOX P70-1	Primary Central Sleep Apnea (Idiopathic CSA)—ICSD 3 Diagnostic Criteria

A. The presence of at least one of the following:
   i. Sleepiness
   ii. Difficulty initiating or maintaining sleep, frequent awakenings, or nonrestorative sleep
   iii. Awakening short of breath
   iv. Snoring
   v. Witnessed apnea
B. Polysomnography (PSG) demonstrates all of the following:
   i. Five or more central apneas or central hypopneas per hour of sleep

   ii. The total number of central apneas and/or central hypopneas is >50% of the total number of apneas and hypopneas
   iii. Absence of Cheyne-Stokes Breathing
C. There is no evidence of daytime or nocturnal hypoventilation
D. The disorder is not better explained by another current sleep disorder, medical or neurologic disorder, medication use, or substance use disorder

In children, symptoms may not be evident.

CSA differs from CSA-CSB in several ways: (1) short ventilatory phase between central apneas, (2) shorter cycle time, (3) the ventilatory phase not having the crescendo–decrescendo pattern, and (4) arousals occurring at event termination rather than at the zenith of effort. The diagnosis of primary CSA is one of exclusion. Many other forms of CSA may have central apneas with similar morphology, including narcotic-associated CSA, treatment-emergent CSA, and CSA caused by a medical disorder without CSB. See Box P70-1 for the *International Classification of Sleep Disorders*, 3rd Edition (ICSD-3) diagnostic criteria for primary CSA.

No controlled studies of treatments of primary CSA have been performed. Treatments have included respiratory stimulants (acetazolamide), benzodiazepine receptor agonists (to reduce arousal), supplemental oxygen, continuous positive airway pressure (CPAP), and adaptive servoventilation (ASV). The addition of supplemental oxygen may decrease ventilatory drive, thereby stabilizing ventilation. Of interest, CPAP is also effective in some patients with primary CSA. This is probably the treatment of choice if patients also have significant obstructive sleep apnea (OSA). The reason CPAP works in patients with primary CSA is unknown, but it may result in a slight increase in $PaCO_2$ or prevent triggering of arousal by high upper airway resistance. One study found that central apnea occurred mainly in the supine position. High upper airway resistance may trigger an arousal, resulting in subsequent central apnea in patients with an instability in ventilatory control caused by high ventilatory drive and a low arousal threshold. If CPAP does not work use of ASV should be tried. Case series report effective treatment with ASV for a wide variety of hypocapnic CSA disorders. Another approach would be use of both CPAP and oxygen.

In the present patient, over 70% of the respiratory events were central apnea (see Figure P70-1). Note the absence of movement in the chest and the abdominal tracings (small deflections are from cardiac pulsations). As the events were not of the Cheyne-Stokes morphology, and no indication congestive heart failure, a neurological disorder, or ingestion of respiratory depressants was present, a diagnosis of primary CSA was made. Magnetic resonance imaging to rule out Chiari malformation and other central nervous system pathology was negative. As the patient did snore and have some obstructive events, a trial of nasal CPAP was ordered. On this treatment, the AHI fell to 10/hr and treatment with CPAP resulted in the alleviation of symptoms.

CLINICAL PEARLS

1. Primary CSA is a form of hypocapnic central apnea that occurs in patients with a normal or low awake $PaCO_2$, that have no obvious an obvious associated disease (neurologic disorder or congestive heart failure), and are not being treated with respiratory-depressant medications (narcotics).

2. The morphology of the central apneas differs from that of CSB (short cycle time, lack of crescendo-decrescendo ventilatory pattern between events).

3. Some patients with primary CSA complain of excessive daytime sleepiness and have a history of snoring, but some complain mainly of insomnia (frequent awakenings).

4. Primary CSA is uncommon, and patients with this condition comprise less than 5% of patients with sleep apnea. A diagnosis of primary CSA is a diagnosis of exclusion.

5. As patients with idiopathic CSA have low daytime PCO_2 levels, arousal from sleep may trigger several large breaths with a subsequent central apnea.

6. The best treatment for primary CSA is unknown. Possible treatments include supplemental oxygen, acetazolamide, hypnotics, and PAP. An initial trial of CPAP is probably the treatment of choice for most patients. If CPAP is not effective, ASV to stabilize breathing will likely be effective.

BIBLIOGRAPHY

American Academy of Sleep Medicine: *International classification of sleep disorders*, ed 3, Darien, IL, 2014, American Academy of Sleep Medicine.

Aurora RN, Chowdhuri S, Ramar K, et al: The treatment of central sleep apnea syndromes in adults: practice parameters with an evidence-based literature review and meta-analyses, *Sleep* 35(1):17–40, 2012.

Banno K, Okamura K, Kryger MH: Adaptive servo-ventilation in patients with idiopathic Cheyne-Stokes breathing, *J Clin Sleep Med* 2(2):181–186, 2006.

Bonnet MH, Dexter JR, Arand DL: The effect of triazolam on arousal and respiration in central sleep apnea patients, *Sleep* 13:31–41, 1990.

Carnevale C, Georges M, Rabec C, et al: Effectiveness of adaptive servo ventilation in the treatment of hypocapnic central sleep apnea of various etiologies, *Sleep Med* 12(10):952–958, 2011.

Chowdhuri S, Ghabsha A, Sinha P, et al: Treatment of central sleep apnea in U.S. veterans, *J Clin Sleep Med* 8(5):555–563, 2012.

DeBacker WA, Verbacken J, Willemen M, et al: Central apnea index decreases after prolonged treatment with acetazolamide, *Am J Respir Crit Care Med* 151:87–91, 1995.

Dempsey JA, Skatrud JB: A sleep-induced apneic threshold and its consequences, *Am Rev Respir Dis* 133:1163–1170, 1986.

Dempsey JA, Smith CA, Przybylowski T, et al: The ventilatory responsiveness to CO_2 below eupnoea as a determinant of ventilatory stability in sleep, *J Physiol* 560(Pt 1):1–11, 2004.

Eckert DJ, Jordan AS, Merchia P, Malhotra A: Central sleep apnea: pathophysiology and treatment, *Chest* 131(2):595–607, 2007.

Grimaldi D, Provini F, Vertrugno R, et al: Idiopathic central sleep apnea syndrome treated with zolpidem, *Neurol Sci* 29:255–257, 2008.

Quadri S, Drake C, Hudgel DW: Improvement of idiopathic central sleep apnea with zolpidem, *J Clin Sleep Med* 15:122–129, 2009.

White DP, Zwillich CW, Pickett CK, et al: Central sleep apnea. Improvement with acetazolamide therapy, *Arch Intern Med* 142:1816–1819, 1982.

Xie A, Rankin F, Rutherford R, et al: Effects of inhaled CO_2 and added dead space on idiopathic central sleep apnea, *Am Rev Respir Dis* 82:918–926, 1997.

Xie A, Rutherford R, Rankin F, et al: Hypocapnia and increased ventilatory responsiveness in patients with idiopathic central sleep apnea, *Am J Respir Crit Care Med* 152:1950–1955, 1995.

Xie A, Wong B, Phillipson EA, et al: Interaction of hyperventilation and arousal in pathogenesis of idiopathic central sleep apnea, *Am J Respir Crit Care Med* 150:489–495, 1994.

Advanced PAP Modes and NPPV Titration

ADVANCED PAP MODES

The modes of positive airway pressure (PAP) to be discussed in this chapter include bilevel PAP (BPAP) in the spontaneous (S), spontaneous-timed (ST), and timed (T) modes, adaptive servo-ventilation, (ASV) and volume-assured pressure support (VAPS) (Table F30-1).

BPAP-ST AND BPAP-T

BPAP in the (S) mode does not have a backup rate and is usually sufficient for treatment of obstructive sleep apnea. BPAP in the ST and T modes is used to deliver noninvasive positive airway pressure ventilation (NPPV) in patients with chronic hypoventilation syndromes. Patients with chronic hypoventilation include those with the obesity hypoventilation syndrome (OHS; usually the S mode suffices), neuromuscular weakness, chest wall disease, or disorders of the central control of ventilation. Expiratory PAP (EPAP) and inspiratory PAP (IPAP) are specified by the clinician. BPAP delivers pressure support (PS) equal to IPAP-EPAP. PS is adjusted to augment ventilation. With BPAP-ST, a backup rate is available, and the PAP device initiates a breath if no spontaneous breath occurs during a time window that depends on the backup rate. The duration of the timed breaths must be specified. BPAP-ST may be used to treat central sleep apnea (CSA)—both hypocapnic and hypercapnic. Adaptive servoventilation is usually preferred over BPAP-ST for treatment with hypocapnic CSA, as ventilation can be stabilized with fewer device-triggered breaths and may be better tolerated. A polysomnography (PSG) titration is used to determine the settings needed for effective BPAP-ST treatment (IPAP, EPAP, backup rate, inspiratory time). An alternative used for some patients with neuromuscular disease is to start with lower pressure (BPAP 8/4 centimeters of water [cm H_2O]) on an outpatient basis, with adjustment of settings based on information the devices stores (tidal volume, respiratory rate) as well as nocturnal oximetry. A PSG titration has the advantage of allowing adjustment

---

TABLE F30-1 Advanced Modes of Positive Airway Pressure Devices

PAP Mode	Method	Use
BPAP with backup rate NPPV	BPAP modes o ST (spontaneous-timed) o Timed PS=pressure support=IPAP −EPAP	NPPV— hypoventilation syndromes Central sleep apnea
Volume-assured PS AVAPS, IVAPS	Adjusts pressure support to meet tidal volume or ventilation target	NPPV— hypoventilation syndromes Central sleep apnea
ASV	PS support varies to stabilize breathing EPAP set or varies to eliminate airway obstruction. Backup rate available (see Table F30-2).	Hypocapnic CSA Complex SA Cheyne-Stokes breathing Narcotic-associated central apnea Primary central sleep apnea

ASV, Adaptive servo-ventilation; *AVPAP*, average volume assured pressure support; *BPAP*, bilevel positive airway pressure; *EPAP*, expiratory positive airway pressure; *IPAP*, inspiratory positive airway pressure; *iVAPS*, intelligent assured pressure support; *NPPV*, noninvasive positive pressure ventilation; *PAP*, positive airway pressure; *PS*, pressure support; *S mode*, spontaneous mode; *ST*, spontaneous timed.
I/E ratio=IPAPtime/EPAPtime expressed with IPAPtime=1. If IPAPtime=1.2, EPAP time=1.8, I/E=1.2/1.8=1/1.5.

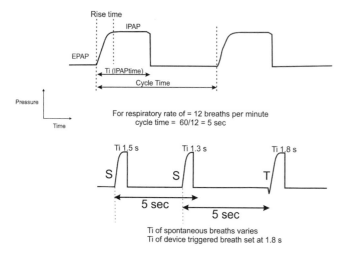

FIGURE F30-1 ■ *Top,* Definitions of IPAPtime, rise time, and cycle time. The IPAP-time is sometimes referred to as the inspiratory time (Ti). *Bottom,* A spontaneous breath (*S*) occurs because it followed the previous breath by less than 5 seconds. A breath did not occur within the next 5 seconds, and a machine-triggered breath (T) is delivered. The small downward pressure spike marks a machine-triggered breath. In this case, the Ti was set at 1.8 second. The spontaneous breath has a short Ti of 1.3 seconds.

of the EPAP to prevent obstructive apnea, optimize mask fit, intervene for patient issues, and determine if the addition of supplemental oxygen is needed. In all BPAP modes, the rise time can be adjusted. The rise time is the time from the start of the IPAP cycle until the IPAP is reached (usually 300 milliseconds [msec]) (Figure F30-1). The rise time is adjusted for patient comfort. Patients needing a long time for exhalation may like a short rise time (shortens inspiratory time), and those with pressure intolerance may like a longer rise time.

The ST mode is used to provide NPPV to patients who unreliably cycle the device between IPAP and EPAP because of muscle weakness or to those who have abnormal central ventilatory control (central apnea, inadequate respiratory rate). The effect of a backup rate is illustrated in Figure F30-1. If the patient does not initiate a breath within a time window (the cycle time in seconds equal to 60/backup rate in breaths per minute) the device will provide a device triggered breath with an IPAP duration (IPAPtime) set by the clinician. For example, if the backup rate is 12 breaths per minute, a 5-second window exists following the start of the last breath (see Figure F30-1). If no spontaneous breath (S) occurs during the time window, the machine with deliver a timed breath (T) for the IPAPtime specified by the clinician. For BPAP-ST, the clinician must specify the IPAP, EPAP, rise time, and IPAP time. The IPAPtime is often referred to as the *inspiratory time (Ti)*. The term *IPAPtime* is more accurate, as the actual inspiratory time is defined by flow, not the pressure the device delivers. However, the term *Ti* is commonly used. In Philips-Respironics BPAP devices (BiPAP), a Ti must be set in the ST mode, and 1.5 seconds is the recommended time as an initial Ti value for titration (machine default 1 second). In ResMed BPAP devices

(VPAP-ST), a fixed Ti is not specified; rather, a *minimum IPAPtime (TImin)* and *maximum IPAPtime (TImax)* are specified. The device cycles from IPAP to EPAP between those time limits based on patient flow.

In the timed mode, BPAP devices deliver the set PS at the rate and Ti set by the clinician. The patient cannot trigger a breath and does not determine the duration of IPAP during each cycle (set time of Ti for all breaths).

In both the ST and T modes the Ti (IPAP-time) is usually 1.2 to 1.6 seconds, depending on the backup rate. A %IPAP time = IPAPtime ×100/cycle time can be defined. The IPAPtime (Ti) is usually between 30% and 40% of the cycle time. Patients with obstructive lung disease need a long exhalation time, and a %IPAPtime of 30% is recommended for them. Patients with restrictive lung disease may need a longer inhalation time, and a %IPAPtime of 40% is recommend for them (Table F30-2). For example, with a respiratory rate of 12 per minute, the cycle time is 5 seconds. The Ti for a 30% IPAPtime is 0.3 × 5 = 1.5 seconds.

BPAP devices must determine the appropriate time to cycle from EPAP to IPAP and IPAP to EPAP. The decision is based on pressure and flow. If flow drops during the IPAP cycle because of a stiff chest wall, the device may cycle to EPAP prematurely (Figure 30-2, *B*). These patients would benefit from a longer IPAPtime. Conversely, patients who require a long exhalation time may benefit from a shorter IPAPtime. If flow continues during the IPAP cycle because of leak or high inspiratory resistance, the IPAP-time may be excessively long and will shorten the time for exhalation (Figure F30-2, *C*). Patients with chronic lung disease who require a long time for exhalation may benefit from a shorter IPAPtime. As noted above, BPAP devices by ResMed (VPAP) require the setting of the

TABLE F30-2 **IPAPtime (Ti, Inspiratory Time) at Different Respiratory Rates and %IPAPtime**

%IPAPtime (Seconds)	RR	Cycle Time (Seconds)	Inspiratory time (Ti) (Seconds) (Ti also known as IPAPtime)	Inspiratory/Expiratory (I/E) Ratio
30%	12	5	1.5	1/2.3
	15	4	1.2	1/2.3
	20	3	0.9	1/2.3
40%	12	5	2.0	1/1.5
	15	4	1.6	1/1.5
	20	3	1.2	1/1.5

Cycle time = 60/ respiratory rate in breaths per minute. Cycle time = IPAPtime + EPAPtime.
%IPAPtime = IPAPtime × 100 ÷ cycle time.
EPAP time = Cycle time − IPAP time.
EPAP, Expiratory positive airway pressure; *IPAP*, Inspiratory positive airway pressure; *RR*, respiratory rate.
I/E ratio = IPAPtime/EPAPtime expressed with IPAPtime = 1. If IPAPtime = 1.2, EPAP time = 1.8, I/E = 1.2/1.8 = 1/1.5.

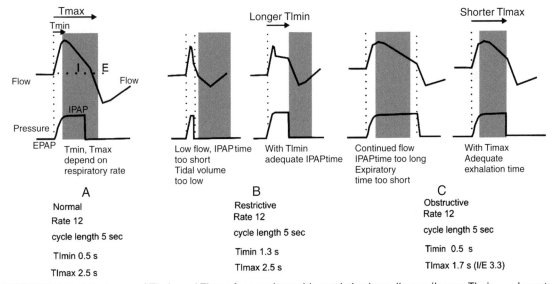

FIGURE F30-2 ■ Adjustment of TImin and TImax for a patient with restrictive lung disease (longer TImin − adequate inspiratory time) and a patient with obstructive lung disease (shorter TImax − more expiratory time).

IPAPtime–minimum (TImin) and IPAPtime–maximum (TImax) durations (see Figure F30-2) and not a fixed Ti. It should be noted that TImin and TImax constrain every breath (spontaneous and device-triggered breaths). In the Philips-Respironics BPAP-ST, the set Ti affects only machine-triggered breaths. The recommended TImin and TImax values depend on the respiratory rate and the type of patient being treated. TImin is set to a higher-than-normal value to ensure adequate time for delivery of the tidal volume if a patient has a restrictive chest wall disorder or low respiratory compliance. A shorter-than-normal TImax is useful to prevent excessive time in the IPAP cycle for patients with chronic obstructive pulmonary disease (COPD). ResMed devices also allow adjustment of sensitivity of transitions from EPAP to IPAP and IPAP to

EPAP. Another method of specifying the relationship between IPAPtime and cycle time is the inspiratory to expiratory ratio (I/E ratio). For example, If the IPAPtime is 1 second and the cycle time is 3 seconds, the I/E ratio = IPAPtime/EPAPtime = 1/2. An I/E ratio of 1/2 to 1/3 is usually optimal for most patients. %IPAPtime of 30% or 40% corresponds to I/E ratios of 1/2.3 and 1/1.5. The TImax is usually chosen to give an I/E ratio of 1/3 to 1/2 in patients with COPD and 1/1 in patients with restrictive lung disease. For normal individuals TImin = 0.5 seconds and TImax is 2.0 and 1.5 seconds for respiratory rates of 15 and 20 per minute, respectively. For restrictive disease the TImin/TImax = 1.0/2.0 seconds for a respiratory rate of 15 per minute and TImin/TImax = 0.8/1.5 for a respiratory rate of 20 breaths per minute. For COPD patients the TImin = 0.5 and for a respiratory rate of 15 and 20 per minute the recommended TImax is 1.3 and 1.0 seconds, respectively. It should be noted that the BiPAP-ST (Philips Respironics) and VPAP-ST (ResMed) devices have a maximum pressure of 25 cm H_2O.

ADAPTIVE SERVOVENTILATION

ASV was developed for treatment of Cheyne-Stokes breathing (CSB) but may be used for any patient with hypocapnic CSA. Such patients have high ventilatory drive and ventilatory control instability. The PS adapts by providing higher support when flow and tidal volume are decreased and lower support when flow and tidal volume are increased (Figure F30-3). The goal is to stabilize ventilation. By preventing excessive ventilation and hypocapnia, central apnea is eliminated. Examples of disorders suitable for ASV treatment include CSA with CSB, primary CSA, and treatment-emergent CSA. ASV may also be used in patients with narcotic-induced CSA, but a sufficient minimum PS must be used to deal with hypoventilation (if present). Two brands of ASV devices are available in the United States. They work differently, and the setup is also different

(Tables F30-3 and F30-4). The recommended and available settings for these devices are frequently revised, and the reader should check the most current information from the manufacturer. The BiPAP Auto SV advanced device (Philips-Respironics) automatically adjusts the EPAP between EPAPmin and EPAPmax to eliminate upper airway obstruction and narrowing (APAP algorithm). The PS is adjusted by the device between minimum and maximum PS settings (between PSmin and PSmax) to stabilize ventilation by delivering a target *peak flow* based on the average of peak flow values of preceding breaths determined over a moving time window. The PS is adjusted within each breath based on the early flow rate to reach the peak flow target. A fixed backup rate or the auto-rate option may be used. In the auto-rate mode, the backup rate, rise time, and Ti are automatically determined by the device based on the patient's breathing pattern. If a backup rate is specified, a Ti and rise time must be specified. The recommended Ti is 1.5 seconds. The PS is constrained by the maximum pressure (Pmax), adjustable up to 25 cm H_2O.

The VPAP Adapt SV (ResMed) delivers PS and a backup rate based on the previous *minute ventilation* computed from a moving time window (target = 90% of average minute ventilation

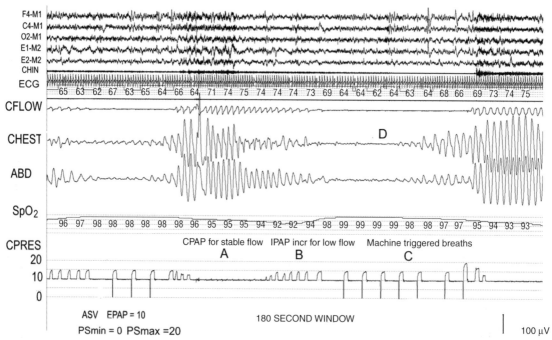

FIGURE F30-3 ■ A patient with Cheyne-Stokes breathing on an older BiPAP Auto SV device (Philips-Respironics, with manually adjusted EPAP). **A,** CPAP is delivered as minimum pressure support (PSmin) was set at 0 cm H_2O and flow is high. **B,** PS increases as flow is low. **C,** Machine-triggered breaths during a central apnea. **D,** The machine-triggered PS was not effective because of a closed upper airway. An increase in expiratory positive airway pressure (EPAP) is needed. *ABD,* Abdomen; *ASV,* adaptive servoventilation; *BPAP,* bilevel positive airway pressure; *CPAP,* continuous positive airway pressure; *Cpress,* delivered pressure; *ECG,* electrocardiography; *IPAP,* inspiratory positive airway pressure; *PS,* pressure support; *SpO2,* pulse oximetry. Inspiration is upward. (From Brown LK: Adaptive servoventilation for sleep apnea: technology, titration protocols, and treatment efficacy, *Sleep Med Clin* 5:433, 2010.)

TABLE F30-3 **Adaptive Servoventilation Characteristics**

	ResMed VPAP Adapt SV	Philips-Respironics BiPAP Auto SV Advanced
Target	90% of previous average ventilation (moving time window)	Target: computed fraction of previous average peak flow (moving time window)
EPAP	EPP (EPAP) titrated manually EPAP adjusted automatically (ASV auto-mode)	EPAP automatically adjusted between EPAPmin and EPAP max to prevent upper airway obstruction or narrowing
PS	Max pressure available = 25 cm H_2O IPAP varies between PSmin and PSmax to deliver target minute ventilation PS Limits: PSmin to PSmax, constrained by EPP and maximum machine pressure (PSmax) New devices PSmin 0-6 cm H_2O, formerly PSmin $\geq$ 3 cm H_2O	Max Pressure up to 25 cm H_2O IPAP varies between PSmin and PSmax to deliver target peak flow PS Limits: PSmin (can be 0) to PSmax, constrained by EPAP and PSmax
Backup rate	Automatic Approximately 15 breaths per minute, Ti set automatically	Auto rate (Ti chosen automatically) 0 or fixed rate (if fixed rate must specify Ti)

ASV, Adaptive servoventilation; *BiPAP*, bilevel positive airway pressure; *cm H_2O*, centimeters of water; *EPAP*, expiratory positive airway pressure; *EPP*, manual EPAP; *IPAP*, inspiratory positive airway pressure; *PS*, pressure support.

TABLE F30-4 **Adaptive Servoventilation Setting Range and Defaults or Recommended Values**

BiPAP Auto SV Advanced (System One)	Range	Default
Pmax	25 cm H_2O	25 cm H_2O
PS	PSmin 0 to 20 PSmax 0 to 20 Constrained by EPAP and Pmax	PSmin = 0, PSmax = 20
EPAPmin	4–25	4
EPAPmax	4–25	15
Rate and inspiratory time (Ti = IPAPtime)	0–25 Auto-rate	With fixed rate, Ti = 1.5 recommended (Ti must be specified) With auto-rate the Ti is automatically determined

VPAP Adapt SV	Range	Default
Pmax	Up to 25 cm H_2O	25 cm H_2O
PSmin	3–6 older 0–6 new[†]	3 3
PSmax	9–16 older 5–20 new[†]	15 15
EPAP manual	4–15	adjusted manually
EPAPmin*	4–15	4
EPAPmax*	4–15	15
Rate, Ti (sec)	Automatic	15 per minute

BiPAP, Bilevel positive airway pressure; *cm H_2O*, centimeters of water; *EPAP*, expiratory positive airway pressure.
*ASV auto mode, pressures in cm H_2O, time in seconds.
[†]Latest devices.

over about a 3-minute window). The device automatically adjusts the backup rate and Ti. In the past, EPAP was manually set (EPP), but current models now allow the option of automatic adjustment between EPAPmin and EPAPmax values (ASV auto-mode). The algorithms used to adjust the backup rate in the Adapt SV in auto-mode or the BiPAP Auto SV Advanced are proprietary. However, the decision to provide a machine triggered breath depends on the average expiratory time of preceding breaths, the time since the last breath, and the recent respiratory rate.

When using ASV, it is important to consider the possibility of closed airway central apnea. During central apnea, the upper airway may close. For example, during mixed apnea, the airway has closed during the central portion. If a closed airway central apnea occurs, the machine-triggered PS will not effectively deliver flow (or tidal volume). In this case, higher EPAP is needed (see Figure F30-3). In the past, this depended on the sleep technologist recognizing that closed airway central apnea was occurring and increasing the EPAP. With automatic adjustment of EPAP, this may be less of an issue. The exact algorithms for EPAP adjustment are proprietary. However, EPAP may increase automatically in the absence of closed airway apnea if increases in PS are not effective in increasing flow or tidal volume (narrowed but not closed upper airway).

The default PSmin is 0 cm H_2O in the BiPAP Auto SV device and 3 cm H_2O for the VPAP Adapt SV. For patients with ventilatory instability caused by high loop gain, delivering CPAP (PSmin = 0) during periods of stable ventilation is desirable to avoid overshoots in ventilation following arousals. However, a PSmin > 0 is desirable in several situations. A pressure intolerant patient may benefit from EPAP of 10 and PSmin of 4 (equivalent to BPAP 14/10) versus EPAP of 12 with a PSmin of 0 cm H_2O. ASV devices were not specifically designed for patients with nocturnal hypoventilation. However, some patients with complex sleep apnea caused by narcotics have both hypoventilation and instability in breathing. A higher PSmin ($\geq$ 6 to 8 cm H_2O) may be needed if the arterial oxygen saturation (SaO_2) remains low but breathing is regular (e.g., in patients with hypoventilation). A proposed update of the algorithm for the BiPAP Auto SV Advanced may automatically adjust the PSmin and the backup rate if minute ventilation is low. Note that if a patient requires high EPAP, significantly high IPAP values may be needed to deliver an adequate PS. As patient triggered breaths typically require less PS than machine triggered breaths, stabilizing breathing and avoiding the need for machine triggered breaths will reduce the need for high pressures.

VOLUME-ASSURED PRESSURE SUPPORT

The PS required for an adequate tidal volume may vary in a given patient during the night or from night to night, depending on changes in the muscle strength or function (including changes during rapid eye movement [REM] sleep) and respiratory system compliance. To meet this challenge, Volume Assured Pressure Support (VAPS) devices have been developed to automatically adjust the PS to deliver an adequate tidal volume. At present, the two devices available in the United States for VAPS (Table F30-5) are Average Volume-Assured Pressure Support (AVAPS, Phillips Respironics) and Intelligent Volume-Assured Pressure Support (iVAPS, Res Med). The AVAPS device may be used in the S, ST, PC, or T modes. The S, ST, and T modes are as discussed for BPAP except that *the pressure support varies to deliver the target tidal volume* (Figure F30-4). The PC (pressure control) mode differs from the ST and T modes because an IPAP cycle may be triggered by the patient or the machine, but the Ti of all breaths is fixed (including spontaneous breaths). The PC mode is used when the IPAPtime during spontaneous breaths is too short for effective ventilation. PS varies automatically in the PC mode.

The VPAP-STA devices by ResMed with iVAPS capability may operate in the iVAPS, VPAP-ST. VPAP-T, or VPAP-PAC (pressure assist-control) modes. PS varies automatically only in the iVAPS mode. In the PAC mode both PS and Ti are fixed (specified by the clinician). Unlike VPAP-T, in the PAC mode the patient or the device may trigger a breath, but, like the VPAP-T mode, the Ti for all breaths is fixed (specified).

Both AVAPS devices and VPAP-STA devices have a maximum pressure of 30 cm H_2O. According to the recommendations of Philips-Respironics for AVAPS, a target **tidal volume** of 8 mL per kilogram (mL/kg, based on ideal body weight) is selected. Initial settings are EPAP = 4 cm H_2O, IPAP minimum = EPAP + 4 cm H_2O, and IPAP max = 25 to 30 cm H_2O. If AVAPS is used in the ST or T mode, the backup rate and Ti must also be specified. The recommended Ti (IPAPtime) for AVAPS is 1.5 seconds, but a different Ti may be chosen as for BPAP-ST (see Table F30-5). *The backup rate is set to 1 to 2 breaths per minute below the spontaneous respiratory rate.*

For VPAP-STA devices in the iVAPS mode, both pressure support and the device intelligent backup rate (iBR) vary to deliver the target alveolar ventilation. The anatomic dead space (Vd) is estimated from the patient's height (specified by the clinician, see Hart et al, Vd versus height). The alveolar ventilation is computed by subtracting the dead space ventilation (Vd X respiratory rate) from the minute ventilation (tidal volume X respiratory rate). The patient's height and the patient's desired respiratory rate must be specified. The target alveolar ventilation can be specified, or the default can be used

TABLE F30-5	**Volume-Assured Pressure Support Devices**	
Device	VPAP with iVAPs (Res Med) intelligent Volume Assured Pressure Support	AVAPS (Philips-Respironics) Average volume assured pressure support
Target	Alveolar ventilation Computed from specified minute ventilation and calculated dead space ventilation (based on height) For a set backup rate and height, as the alveolar ventilation is varied the delivered alveolar volume is displayed. Target alveolar ventilation adjusted so alevolar volume is 6 mL/kg.	Tidal volume (8 ml/kg of ideal body weight) IPAPmax varies to meet goals IPAPmin = EPAP + 4 cm H_2O
EPAP	Set to maintain an open airway	same
PS	Varies to deliver needed tidal volume	Varies to deliver target tidal volume
Backup Rate	The iBR (intelligent backup rate) varies from 2/3 the set backup rate to the backup rate to deliver the target alveolar ventilation. Set back up rate = spontaneous breathing rate	Fixed, set based on spontaneous rate (usually 1 or 2 breaths lower)
Modes	iVAPS - both PS and rate (iBR) vary	AVAPS S, ST, or T (PS varies), PC (pressure control) - PS varies but all breaths have a set Ti
Settings:	Clinician specifies height, backup rate, and alveolar ventilation target (device displays calculated target minute ventilation, tidal volume goal, and tidal volume as ml/Kg ideal body weight Back up rate = actual spontaneous breathing rate This serves as an upper limit for iBR	Set target tidal volume to 110% of displayed patient tidal volume in the S/T mode or 8 ml per kg of ideal body weight. IPAP Max = 25-30 cm H_2O IPAPmin = EPAP + 4 cm H_2O Respiratory rate 2 breaths below spontaneous Ti 1.5 sec, rise time 1 to 3 for patient comfort EPAP set to eliminate obstructive apnea

AVAPS, Average volume-assured pressure support; *EPAP*, expiratory positive airway pressure; *IPAP*, inspiratory positive airway pressure; *iVAPS*, intelligent volume-assured pressure support; *PS*, pressure support.

(5.2 L/min). For a given height and respiratory rate, the device displays the corresponding computed minute ventilation, tidal volume, and tidal volume in mL/kg ideal body weight (IBW). If the *target alveolar ventilation* is changed, the device displays adjusted values for these 3 parameters. Note that the patients actual desired respiratory rate is specified. Unlike the backup rate in AVAPS the intelligent backup rate (iBR) varies. The iBR is 2/3 the set patient respiratory rate unless no effort (central apnea) is detected. Then the iBR slowly increases to the set patient backup rate unless spontaneous breaths occur (the iBR falls to two thirds of the backup rate when spontaneous breathing returns) (see Figure F30-4). The speed at which the iBR increases toward the set backup rate following apnea depends on previous the ventilation (faster if ventilation is low).

A number of studies have compared BPAP-ST and VAPS in patients with OHS, neuromuscular disorders, and chest wall disorders. VAPS resulted in slightly lower partial pressure of arterial carbon dioxide ($PaCO_2$) in some studies, but sleep quality was either not improved or was worse compared with BPAP-ST. Thus, a clear advantage of VAPS compared with BPAP-ST has not been demonstrated. However, VAPS units may avoid the need for frequent PAP titrations. When VAPS is used, a major purpose of a PSG PAP titration is to select a level of EPAP that eliminates obstructive events (obstructive apnea and hypopnea) and document that the device does deliver adequate tidal volumes. In the future, VAPS devices will automatically adjust EPAP (as in ASV). For AVAPS devices this mode will be called AVAPS-AE.

USE OF AVAPS VERSUS ASV VERSUS BPAP-ST

Some overlap exists in the patient populations that may benefit from AVAPS, ASV, and BPAP-ST devices. However, ASV uses a relatively long window to determine a target (ventilation or peak flow) and varies with the main goal of stabilizing ventilation. Patients with hypocapnic CSA, including CSB, primary CSA, and treatment-emergent CSA, are candidates for ASV. Of note, a considerable percentage of these patients may actually respond to continuous PAP (CPAP) (especially chronic treatment). Patients with narcotic-induced CSA without sleep-related hypoventilation often respond to ASV. However, if mild hypoventilation is present, ASV with PSmin 6 to 8 cm H_2O (to augment ventilation) is usually needed. If moderate to severe hypoventilation is present, BPAP-ST or VAPS should

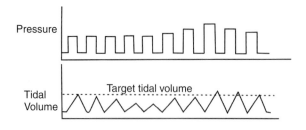

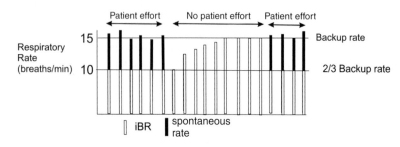

FIGURE F30-4 ■ *Upper panel*, The schematic illustrates the Average Volume-Assured Pressure Support (AVAPS) with an increase in pressure support to deliver the target tidal volume. *Lower panel*, The function of the intelligent backup rate (iBR) is shown. The iBr stays at two thirds the backup rate (inactive) unless patient effort is absent. Then the iBR slowly increases to the set backup rate and stays there until spontaneous effort is again noted.

be used. With the use of BPAP-ST, more machine-triggered breaths and higher average pressure tend to be required compared with treatment with ASV. Patients with sleep-related hypoventilation—COPD, neuromuscular disorders, restrictive chest wall disorders, ventilatory control disorders, and the OHS (if not adequately controlled with CPAP or BPAP in the S mode)—are candidates for BPAP-ST or VAPS. The advance of VAPS is adjustment to changes in the patient's condition over time. In summary, if hypoventilation is the most prominent feature, BPAP-ST or VAPS is used. If ventilatory instability is the major feature, ASV is used. BPAP-ST can be used in patients with ventilatory instability, but a large majority of the breaths are often machine-triggered breaths.

NPPV TITRATION AND TREATMENT

The titration of NPPV focuses on providing ventilatory support in addition to maintaining an open airway. Some of the basics of PAP titration were covered in Fundamentals 24. IPAP and EPAP are titrated as per the protocol, discussed previously in Fundamentals 24, to eliminate obstructive events. The EPAP is set to prevent obstructive apnea. The goal in NPPV is to use as low an EPAP as possible so that adequate PS can be delivered without requiring very high IPAP. Patients with neuromuscular disorders, thoracic cage disorders, or disorders of inadequate ventilatory control may not be obese and may not require as high an EPAP as patients with OSA or OHS. When titrating BPAP for OSA usually pressure support is 4 to 6 cm H_2O. However, to provide sufficient pressure support to

augment tidal volume, much higher pressure support is usually needed (6 to 12 cm H_2O). Typical pressures for a thin patient with neuromuscular disease might be IPAP/EPAP of 12/4 to 14/4 cm H_2O. If patients have underlying sleep apnea, higher EPAP is usually needed. A lower pressure support may be needed when treatment is started to allow adaptation to PAP. The ST mode is used in most patients with neuromuscular disorders and thoracic cage disorders and in those with central ventilatory control disorders. It is also needed if central apneas are noted during the NPPV titration. For BPAP-ST the backup rate is usually set 1 to 2 breaths below the sleeping spontaneous breathing rate (8 to 10 breaths per minute minimum). Information on choosing the appropriate IPAPtime (Ti) has been discussed above. As discussed previously, when using VPAP-ST-A in the iVAPS mode, the backup rate is set to the patient's actual spontaneous respiratory rate (unless very low).

If NPPV is titrated in the sleep center, recording of pressure, flow, tidal volume, and leak are recommended (Figure F30-5). The pressure tracings help the clinician determine what the PAP device is delivering (how much pressure and for low long). As adequate minute ventilation is a goal, recording the tidal volume may help determine if sufficient pressure support is being delivered. As shown in Figure F30-5, recording tidal volume is useful because tidal volume depends on both flow and Ti (IPAPtime). Although the computer programs used to control PAP devices in the sleep laboratory may display the tidal volume on a breath-to-breath basis, having the information recorded is of great help to the clinician.

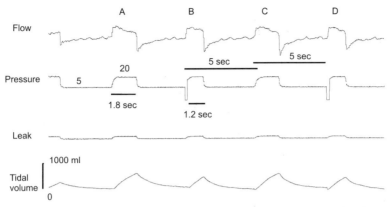

FIGURE F30-5 ■ Tracings of flow (inspiration is upward), pressure, leak, and tidal volume signals provided by the positive airway pressure (PAP) device while a patient is breathing on bilevel PAP (BPAP) in the spontaneous time (ST) mode with a backup rate of 12 breaths per minute. Breaths A and C are patient initiated, and breaths B and D are machine-cycled breaths. If the patient does not cycle the device from expiratory positive airway pressure (EPAP) to inspiratory positive airway pressure (IPAP) within a 5-second window, a machine breath (IPAPcycle) for the chosen inspiratory time (IPAPtime) occurs (breath B). The particular noninvasive positive airway pressure (NPPV) device used supplies a negative pressure spike signifying a machine-triggered breath. Note the shorter inspiratory time in breath B compared with breath A. Although the peak flow rates are similar, the tidal volume differs between breaths A and B due to a different IPAPtime. This illustrates the utility of recording tidal volume as well as flow. (From Berry RB: *Fundamentals of sleep medicine*, Philadelphia, 2012, Saunders, p 316.)

GOALS OF NPPV TITRATION AND TREATMENT

The goals of the NPPV treatment vary between patients but generally include (1) improving sleep quality and preventing nocturnal dyspnea, (2) prevention of nocturnal hypoventilation (or worsening of hypoventilation during sleep if daytime hypoventilation is present), and (3) providing rest for respiratory muscles. In patients with daytime hypoventilation, use of NPPV may improve the quality of life and delay the development of respiratory failure. The goal of nocturnal $PaCO_2$ is a value equal to or less than the daytime $PaCO_2$. However, sufficient PS may not be tolerated initially. NPPV may be started on an outpatient basis at low pressure (BPAP 8/4) and increased as tolerated, depending on patient symptoms and oximetry, daytime end-tidal PCO_2 measurements, or daytime arterial blood gas measurements. However, NPPV PSG titration is recommended, as it allows the correct choice of treatment (IPAP, EPAP, backup rate) that will eliminate obstructive apnea or hypopnea and deliver the optimal PS. Some patients will also require the addition of supplemental oxygen. Close follow-up is needed, as the prescribed level of pressure support may prove inadequate if respiratory muscles weaken.

NPPV TITRATION PROTOCOL

A best clinical practices NPPV titration protocol has been published by the American Academy of Sleep Medicine (AASM) and is a useful guide to NPPV titration. Some of the titration recommendations are listed in Table F30-6.

Generally, a starting pressure BPAP of 8/4 cm H_2O is used. The IPAP and EPAP are increased if obstructive apneas are noted. Otherwise, the IPAP is increased to deliver an adequate tidal volume. The effectiveness of ventilatory support may be assessed by monitoring the SaO_2 and the delivered tidal volume. If available in the sleep center, the ability to monitor transcutaneous PCO_2 (TcPCO2) may help guide the titration (if device is calibrated and validated). A goal of delivering a tidal volume of 6 to 8 cc/kg ideal body weight is recommended. PS is increased if the PCO_2 remains above goal. If desaturation persists, a slightly higher tidal volume goal may be chosen. If the further increases in ventilation are desired but the patient does not tolerate high PS, use of a higher backup rate may be tried. Supplemental oxygen may be added if desaturation persists despite optimization of NPPV. A schematic of NPPV titration is shown in Figure F30-6.

REIMBURSEMENT FOR NPPV DEVICES

NPPV devices are called *respiratory-assist devices* (RADs) and are classified on the basis of their ability to deliver a backup rate—E0470 (BPAP) and E0471 (BPAP ST). RADs have specific criteria for reimbursement depending on the type of patient. Of note VAPS and ASV devices are considered to be RADS. The different categories

TABLE F30-6	**Recommendations for Adjustment of Pressure Support During Noninvasive Positive Pressure Ventilation Titration**		
Pressure Change	**Trigger**	**Duration Between Changes**	**Goal**
IPAP/EPAP increased	Obstructive apnea, hypopnea RERA	≥5 min	Eliminate obstructive events: IPAP and EPAP both increased for apnea, IPAP increased for hypopnea, RERAs, and snoring
PS increased 1–2 cm H_2O	Low tidal volume (<6–8 cc/kg IBW)	≥5 min	Adequate tidal volume
PS increased 1–2 cm H_2O	$PaCO_2 > 10$ mm Hg above goal	≥10 min	Adequate ventilation and $PaCO_2$
PS increased 1–2 cm H_2O	Respiratory muscle rest not achieved	≥10 min	Adequate respiratory muscle rest Reduction of respiratory rate with higher tidal volumes, reduction in inspiratory respiratory EMG activity, or both
PS increased 1–2 cm H_2O	$SaO_2 < 90\%$ with tidal volume <8 cc/kg (assumes discrete apnea, hypopnea, RERAs not present)	≥5 min	Adequate oxygenation

cc/kg, Cubic centimeter per kilogram; *EMG*, electromyography; *EPAP*, expiratory positive airway pressure; *IBW*, ideal body weight; *IPAP*, inspiratory positive airway pressure; *min*, minutes; *PaCO₂*, arterial carbon dioxide pressure; *PS*, pressure support; *RERA*, respiratory effort–related arousal; *SaO₂*, arterial oxygen saturation.

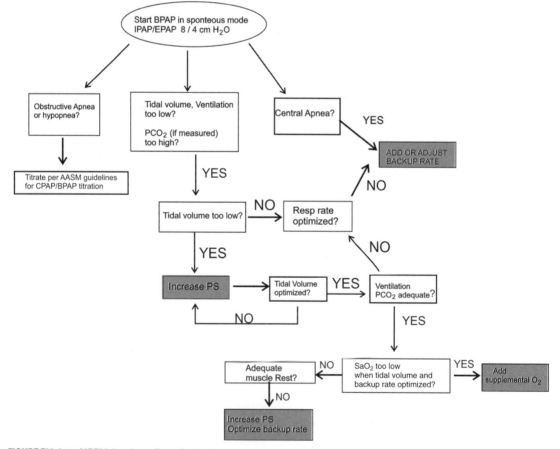

FIGURE F30-6 ■ NPPV titration. Even if a backup rate is not needed during the NPPV titration, BPAP-ST is usually prescribed in patients with neuromuscular disorders and abnormal ventilatory control. (Adapted from Berry RB, Chediak A, Brown LK, et al: NPPV Titration Task Force of the American Academy of Sleep Medicine. Best clinical practices for the sleep center adjustment of noninvasive positive pressure ventilation [NPPV] in stable chronic alveolar hypoventilation syndromes, *J Clin Sleep Med* 6[5]:491-509, 2010.)

include neuromuscular disease or chest wall disorders, hypoventilation, central apnea or complex sleep apnea, and COPD. A summary of the major Medicare criteria is provided in Appendix 3 at the end of the book. The criteria may vary, depending on the local carrier, private health providers, or both.

BIBLIOGRAPHY

Ambrogio C, Lowman X, Kuo M, et al: Sleep and non-invasive ventilation in patients with chronic respiratory insufficiency, *Intensive Care Med* 35(2):306–313, 2009.

Berry RB: Initiating NPPV treatment with patients with chronic hypoventilation, *Sleep Med Clin* 5:485–505, 2010.

Berry RB, Chediak A, Brown LK, et al., NPPV Titration Task Force of the American Academy of Sleep Medicine: Best clinical practices for the sleep center adjustment of noninvasive positive pressure ventilation (NPPV) in stable chronic alveolar hypoventilation syndromes, *J Clin Sleep Med* 6(5):491–509, 2010.

Brown LK: Adpative servo-ventilation for sleep apnea: technology, titration protocols, and treatment efficacy, *Sleep Med Clin* 5:419–439, 2010.

Hart MC Orzalesi, Cook CD: Relationship between anatomic respiratory dead space and body size and lung volume, *J Appl Physiol* 18(3):519–522, 1963.

Janssens JP, Metzger M, Sforza E: Impact of volume targeting on efficacy of bi-level non-invasive ventilation and sleep in obesity hypoventilation syndrome, *Respir Med* 103:165–172, 2009.

Javaheri S: positive airway pressure treatment of central sleep apnea and emphasis on heart failure, opioids, and complex sleep apnea, *Sleep Med Clin* 5(3):407–418, 2010.

Javaheri S, Malik A, Smith J, Chung E: Adaptive pressure support servoventilation: a novel treatment for sleep apnea associated with use of opioids, *J Clin Sleep Med* 4:305–310, 2008.

Jaye J, Chatwin M, Dayer M, et al: Autotitration versus standard noninvasive ventilation: a randomized crossover trial, *Eur Respir J* 33:566–573, 2009.

Selim BJ, Junna MR, Morgenthaler TI: Therapy for sleep hypoventilation and central apnea syndromes, *Curr Treat Options Neurol* 14(5):427–437, 2012.

Storre JH, Seuthe B, Fiechter R, et al: Average volume-assured pressure support in obesity hypoventilation: a randomized crossover trial, *Chest* 130:815–821, 2006.

PATIENT 71

Three Patients with Central Apneas on CPAP

Patient A: An 82-year-old man was evaluated for a history of snoring and frequent awakenings. About 6 months before the current sleep study, he was diagnosed with congestive heart failure (CHF) and atrial fibrillation. The patient underwent a split-night sleep study, and the results are shown in Table P71-1. Figures P71-1 and P71-2 display tracings from the diagnostic and titration portions, respectively.

TABLE P71-1 Patient A: Split-Night Sleep Study Results—Patient A

	Diagnostic Portion	PAP Titration Portion
Total sleep time (min)	108.5	314
Rapid eye movement (min)	0	123
Apnea–hypopnea index (AHI) (#/hr)	66.3	40.1
AHI non-REM (NREM) (#/hr)	66.3	47.0
AHI REM (#/hr)	N/A	30.7
Obstructive apnea (#)	106	17
Mixed apnea (#)	10	5
Central apnea (#)	3	152
Hypopnea (#)	1	36
Desaturations (#)	120	210
Low SaO$_2$	87	87

(#),= Number, SaO$_2$ arterial oxygen saturation.

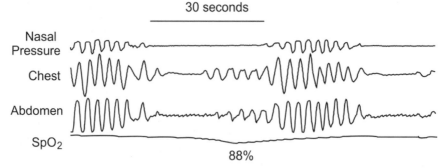

FIGURE P71-1 ■ A 90-second tracing during the diagnostic portion (Patient A).

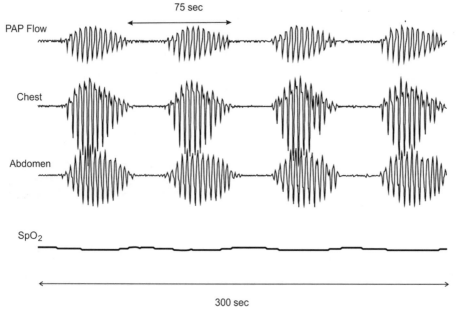

FIGURE P71-2 ■ A 300-second tracing from patient A while on continuous positive airway pressure of 12 centimeters of water (cm H_2O).

Question 1: What is your diagnosis for Patient A?
A. Obstructive sleep apnea (OSA)
B. Treatment-emergent central sleep apnea (TE-CSA)
C. CSA with Cheyne-Stokes breathing (CSB)
D. A + C

Patient B: A 40-year-old woman was evaluated for daytime sleepiness. She had a history of snoring, frequent awakenings, and severe chronic back pain. She was using a fentanyl patch for pain control. The results of a split-night study are shown in Table P71-2. A tracing from the diagnostic portion of the study is shown in Figure P71-2. A tracing from the positive airway pressure (PAP) titration is shown in Figure P71-3.

TABLE P71-2   **Split-Night Sleep Study Results—Patient B**

Respiratory Events	Diagnostic	Treatment
Total sleep time (minutes [min])	130	329.0
Rapid eye movement (REM) (min)	0	67
Apnea–hypopnea index (AHI) (#/hr)	60.9	71.6
AHI non-REM (NREM) (/hr)	60.9	82.0
AHI REM (/hr)	0.0	15.2
Obstructive apnea (#):	27	62
Mixed apnea (#):	1	24
Central apnea (#)	17	227
Hypopneas (#)	87	80
Desats(#)	132	393

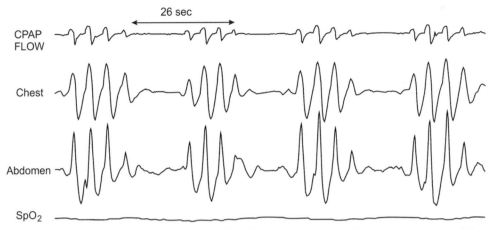

FIGURE P71-3 ▪ A tracing from the titration of patient B while on continuous positive airway pressure of 10 centimeters of water (cm H_2O).

Question 2: What is your diagnosis for Patient B?

A. OSA
B. TE-CSA
C. CSA caused by drug or substance
D. A + C

Patient C: A 55-year-old male was evaluated for complaints of loud snoring and daytime sleepiness. He had no history of CHF and was not taking narcotics. The results of a split-night sleep study are shown in Table P71-3. A tracing from the PAP titration is shown in Figure P71-4.

TABLE P71-3 Split Sleep Study Results - Patient C

	Diagnostic	Treatment
Monitoring time (min)	143	342.4
Total sleep time (min)	120	166.5
Rapid eye movement (REM) (min)	4.5	14.5
Apnea–hypopnea index (AHI) (#/hr)	45.2	33.1
AHI non-REM (NREM) (#/hr)	45.0	35.8
AHI REM (#/hr)	50	4.1
Obstructive apneas (#)	50	0
Mixed apneas (#)	0	0
Central apneas (#)	0	**71**
Hypopneas (#)	40	21
Central AHI (#/hr)	0	25.5
Obstructive AHI (#/hr)	45.2	7.5

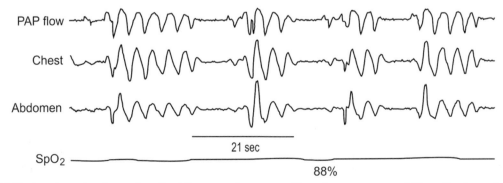

FIGURE P71-4 ▪ A tracing for patient C while on continuous positive airway pressure of 11 centimeters of water (cm H_2O).

TABLE P71-4   **PAP Titration Treatment Table for Patient C**

PAP	TST	REM	TST sup	AHI	AHI-REM	OA	MA	CA	HYP
Level (cm H$_2$O)	(min)	(min)	(min)	(#/hr)	(#/hr)	(#)	(#)	(#)	(#)
4	2.5	0	0	0	n/a	0	0	0	0
5	41.5	0	0	0	n/a	0	0	0	0
6	17	0	9.6	21.2	n/a	0	0	4	2
7	4.5	0	2.9	40	n/a	0	0	0	3
8	35	15	35.0	24.0	4	0	0	13	1
9	28.5	9.5	27.5	46.3	0	0	0	21	1
10	60	3	49.3	34	0	0	0	26	8

AHI, Apnea–hypopnea index; *CA*, central apnea; *cm H$_2$O*, centimeters of water; *HYP*, hypopnea, *MA*, mixed apnea; *OA*, obstructive apnea; *REM*, rapid eye movement; amount of stage R on that pressure; *TST*, total sleep time; *TSTsup*, supine TST on that pressure.

Question 3: What is your diagnosis for Patient C?
A. OSA + complex sleep apnea
B. OSA and TE-CSA
C. TE-CSA

ANSWERS

1. **Answer for Patient A:** D. Both OSA and CSA with CSB are present.

   Discussion: Patients with CHF often have variable amounts of both OSA and CSA-CSB. Some may manifest mainly OSA during the diagnostic portion of a split-night sleep study but on PAP manifest CSA-CSB (during non–rapid eye movement [NREM] sleep). In Figure P71-1, note a mixed apnea with an underlying crescendo–decrescendo pattern. Also, note the saturation of peripheral oxygen (SpO$_2$) nadir is in the middle of the apnea. The delay in the position of the nadir is caused by an increased circulation time (decreased cardiac output). When this patient was exposed to PAP, the upper airway obstruction was eliminated and pure CSA-CSB was noted (Figure P71-2). On PAP, CSA-CSB was the predominant residual event. This scenario meets the definition of complex sleep apnea, as used by the Centers for Medicare and Medicaid Services (CMS) and many clinicians. Although the CSA-CSB was "treatment emergent" using the *International Classification of Sleep Disorders*, 3rd Edition (ICSD-3), patient A should be diagnosed with both OSA and CSA-CSB, as the latter diagnosis explains the appearance of central apnea. In the ICSD-3 diagnostic criteria for CSA with CSB, central apneas may occur during diagnostic study *or PAP titration* (Box P71-1). A diagnosis of treatment emergent central sleep apnea (TE-CSA) in the ICSD-3 is reserved for patients without an obvious cause of CSA. About 50% of patients with CSA-CSB will respond to CPAP either acutely or with chronic treatment. Thus, a trial with CPAP is indicated. CPAP is usually increased until obstructive events are eliminated with pressures of at least 10 to 12 centimeters of water (cm H$_2$O). If the CSA-CSB does not respond to CPAP, adaptive servoventilation (ASV) will usually be effective for both the obstructive and central events. Supplemental oxygen and bilevel PAP (BPAP) with a backup rate (BPAP-ST) are other treatment options. The first intervention in patients with CSA-CSB is always to optimize treatment for the underlying problem (CHF).

   In patient A, CPAP was not effective for central events. A subsequent titration with ASV reduced the apnea–hypopnea index (AHI) to less than 3 per hour.

2. **Answer for Patient B:** D. Both OSA (diagnostic portion) and CSA due to a drug or substance are present.

   Discussion: Patients on potent narcotics may exhibit a variety of respiratory events including severe OSA, ataxic breathing, hypoventilation, and CSA (either on a diagnostic study, PAP titration, or both). Figure P71-3 shows central apneas with a short cycle length—not of the Cheyne-Stokes type. Note that some of the respiratory phases between central apneas do have a crescendo–decrescendo pattern but the cycle length is too short (21 seconds, must be ≥ 40 seconds to score CSB) (see Fundamentals 13 for scoring criteria for CSB). In this patient, CPAP at a level of 10 cm

---

BOX P71-1	**CSA with Cheyne-Stokes Breathing (CSB)—ICSD-3 Diagnostic Criteria**

(A+C+D or B+C+D satisfy the criteria)
A. The presence of one or more of the following:
   Sleepiness:
   i. Difficulty initiating or maintaining sleep, frequent awakenings, or nonrestorative sleep.
   ii. Awakening short of breath
   iii. Snoring
   iv. Witnessed apneas
B. The presence of atrial fibrillation or flutter, congestive heart failure, or a neurologic disorder
C. Polysomnography (PSG) (during **diagnostic or PAP titration**) shows all of the following:

i. Five or more central apneas or central hypopneas per hour of sleep*
ii. The total number of central apneas, central hypopneas, or a combination of both is >50% of the total number of apneas and hypopneas
iii. The pattern of ventilation meets criteria for CSB*
D. The disorder is not better explained by another current sleep disorder, medication use (e.g., narcotics), or substance use disorders

Adapted from the American Academy of Sleep Medicine: International classification of sleep disorders, ed 3, Darien, IL, 2014, American Academy of Sleep Medicine.
*Central apnea and CSB as defined by the most recent version of the *AASM Scoring Manual*.

BOX P71-2	**Central Sleep Apnea Due to a Medication or Substance — ICSD-3 Diagnostic Criteria (Criteria A+B+C+D must be met)**

A. The patient is taking an opioid or other respiratory depressant
B. The presence of one or more of the following:
   i. Sleepiness
   ii. Difficulty initiating or maintaining sleep, frequent awakenings or nonrestorative sleep
   iii. Frequent pauses in breathing
   iv. Awakening short of breath
   v. Witnessed snoring
C. Polysomnography (PSG) (**diagnostic or on positive airway pressure**) shows all of the following:

i. Five or more central apneas and/or or central hypopneas* per hour of sleep (PSG)
ii. The number of central apneas and/or central hypopneas is >50% of the total number of apneas and hypopneas
iii. Absence of Cheyne-Stokes breathing*
D. The disorder occurs as a consequence of an opioid or other respiratory depressant and is not better explained by another current sleep disorder

Notes:
1. Ataxic breathing (irregular variations in respiratory cycle time and tidal volume) may be noted.
2. As defined by the most recent version of the *AASM Manual for the Scoring of Sleep and Associated Events*.
3. Nocturnal and/or daytime hypoventilation may be present but is not required. If sleep-related hypoventilation is present, a diagnosis of "Sleep-Related Hypoventilation Due to Medication or Substance Use" can be made as well as a diagnosis of "Central Sleep Apnea Due to Drug or Substance."
4. A diagnosis of "CSA Due to a Medication or Substance" Does not exclude a diagnosis of obstructive sleep apnea.
Adapted from the American Academy of Sleep Medicine: *International classification of sleep disorders*, ed 3, Darien, IL, 2014, American Academy of Sleep Medicine.
*Table Adapted from American Academy of Sleep Medicine: *International classification of sleep disorders*, ed 3, Darien, IL, 2013, American Academy of Sleep Medicine.

H_2O was effective at eliminating most obstructive events, but many central apneas were still present (see Figure P71-3). This scenario meets the criteria for complex sleep apnea, as used by CMS and others. However, in the ICSD-3, the scenario does not meet criteria for TE-CSA as a known cause of the CSA exists (CSA due to fentanyl). A diagnosis of both OSA and CSA due to a medication or substance is appropriate (see Box P71-2). In this patient, a subsequent titration with ASV reduced the AHI to less than 10/hr.

3. **Answer for Patient C: B:** OSA (diagnostic portion), TE-CSA (PAP titration portion)

Discussion: This patient had predominantly obstructive events during the diagnostic study but developed frequent central apneas on the PAP titration. No history of congestive heart failure was present, and the central apneas did not have a Cheyne-Stokes morphology. The patient did not take narcotics. Therefore, he has TE-CSA, according to the ICSD-3 diagnostic criteria (see Box P71-3). Note the CPAP treatment summarized in Table P71-4. The patient developed frequent central apneas on CPAP of 8 cm H_2O or higher. He was treated with CPAP of 8 cm

H_2O, as most obstructive events (1 residual obstructive hypopnea) were eliminated on that pressure. A CPAP device download after 1 month of treatment showed an AHI of 5/hr with no clear airway events, and the patient felt much improved on CPAP. In patients without an obvious cause of central apneas, TE-CSAs often resolve simply with chronic CPAP treatment. However, 2% to 4% of patients may not have resolution of central apneas and will benefit from ASV. In some studies of the natural course of TE-CSAs, many patients were lost to follow-up. Therefore, the true percentage of those with residual central apnea on CPAP treatment is unknown. A difficulty with these observational studies is that patients not doing well on CPAP (residual central apneas) may not return for follow-up.

BOX P71-3   **Treatment-Emergent CSA—ICSD-3 Diagnostic Criteria (Criteria A-D must be met)**

A. Diagnostic polysomnography (PSG) shows five or more predominantly obstructive respiratory events (apneas, hypopneas or respiratory–effort related arousals [RERAs]) per hour of sleep*
B. PSG during use of positive airway pressure without a backup rate shows significant resolution **of obstructive events and emergence or persistence of central apnea or central hypopnea** with all of the following:
   i. Apnea–hypopnea index (AHI) ≥ 5/hr

   ii. Central AHI [CAHI] ≥ 5/hr;
   iii. Number of central apneas and central hypopneas is ≥ 50% of total number of apneas and hypopneas.[†]
D. *The central sleep apnea is not better explained by another central sleep apnea disorder* (e.g., central sleep apnea with Cheyne-Stokes breathing* or "Central Sleep Apnea Due to Drug or Substance").

Adapted from the American Academy of Sleep Medicine: *International classification of sleep disorders*, ed 3, Darien, IL, 2014, American Academy of Sleep Medicine.
*As defined by the most recent version of the *AASM Manual for the Scoring of Sleep and Associated Events*.
[†]A diagnosis of "Treatment Emergent Central Sleep Apnea" does not exclude a diagnosis of obstructive sleep apnea. That is, a diagnosis of obstructive sleep apnea can be made based on the diagnostic sleep study.

CLINICAL PEARLS

1. The term *complex sleep apnea* is often used to denote patients with predominantly obstructive events during a diagnostic study that develop primarily central events on PAP once obstructive events have resolved. This is definition of complex sleep apnea used by the Centers for Medicare and Medicaid Services. Patients with CHF and CSA-CSB or those on narcotics may exhibit this pattern. However, in the ICSD-3, the diagnostic criteria for TE-CSA state that "the central apnea is not better explained by another central sleep apnea disorder." TE-CSA is used for patient with "idiopathic" complex sleep apnea, that is CSA is not explained by another central sleep apnea disorder. The term *complex sleep apnea* is not used in the ICSD-3.

2. The CSA in patients with TE-CSA, as defined by the ICSD-3, often resolves with chronic CPAP treatment. However, a small proportion of patients continue to exhibit central apneas and usually do not experience benefit from CPAP alone. The exact fraction of patients with TE-CSA and residual central events on CPAP treatment is unknown but probably has been underestimated as many patients were lost to follow-up in observational studies. Use of ASV is appropriate in patients with significant persistent central apnea on chronic CPAP treatment.

BIBLIOGRAPHY

American Academy of Sleep Medicine: *International classification of sleep disorders*, ed 3, Darien, IL, 2013, American Academy of Sleep Medicine.

Aurora RN, Chowdhuri S, Ramar K, et al: The treatment of central sleep apnea syndromes in adults: practice parameters with an evidence-based literature review and meta-analyses, *Sleep* 35(1):17–40, 2012.

Dernaika T, Tawk M, Nazir S, et al: The significance and outcome of continuous positive airway pressure–related central sleep apnea during split-night sleep studies, *Chest* 132:81–87, 2007.

Dowdell WT, Javaheri S, McGinnis W: Cheyne-Stokes respiration presenting as a sleep apnea syndrome, *Am Rev Respir Dis* 141:874, 1990.

Javaheri S, Smith J, Chung E: The prevalence and natural history of complex sleep apnea, *J Clin Sleep Med* 5:205–211, 2009.

Lehman S, Antic NA, Thompson C, et al: Central sleep apnea on commencement of continuous positive airway pressure in patients with a primary diagnosis of obstructive sleep apnea-hypopnea, *J Clin Sleep Med* 3:462–466, 2007.

Morgenthaler TI, Gay PC, Gordon N, Brown LK: Adaptive servoventilation versus noninvasive positive pressure ventilation for central, mixed, and complex sleep apnea syndromes, *Sleep* 30:468–475, 2007.

Selim BJ, Junna MR, Morgenthaler TI: Therapy for sleep hypoventilation and central apnea syndromes, *Curr Treat Options Neurol* 14(5):427–437, 2012.

Treatment-Emergent Central Sleep Apnea

A 40-year-old man with a history of snoring and daytime sleepiness underwent a split-night sleep study (Tables P72-1 and P72-2). During the diagnostic portion, the apnea–hypopnea index (AHI) was severely increased, but the arterial oxygen saturation was mild. During the titration portion of the study, the AHI remained elevated because of central apneas that did not have a Cheyne-Stokes morphology. No history of congestive heart failure (CHF) or opioid use was present. The only medications the patient was taking were levothyroxine and bupropion. The patient was started on continuous positive airway pressure (CPAP) of 8 cm H_2O as this was the lowest pressure on which most obstructive events resolved. It was presumed that the central apneas would resolve on chronic treatment. The patient returned to the clinic, and the machine download is shown in Table P72-3. The patient reported still having many awakenings, and his daytime sleepiness had not improved. He also reported difficulty sleeping on CPAP.

TABLE P72-1 Split-Night Study Results

	Diagnostic	Treatment
TST	120	220
REM (minutes)	24	44
AHI	36	32.2
AHI NREM	30	39
AHI REM	60	7
OA	30	7
MA	0	0
CA	5	81
Hypopnea	37	30
Desaturations	72	118
Low SaO$_2$	85	88

AHI, Apnea–hypopnea index; *CA*, central apnea; *OA*, obstructive apnea; *MA*, mixed apnea; *NREM*, non– rapid eye movement; *REM*, rapid eye movement; *SaO$_2$*, saturation of arterial oxygen; *TST*, total sleep time.

TABLE P72-2 PAP Treatment Table

PAP	TST	REM	AHI	AHI REM	OA	CA	MA	Hypopnea
5	20	0	36	0	8	0	0	4
6	30	0	34	0	5	0	0	12
7	20	6	32	40	5	3	0	3
8	60	18	10	7	0	9	0	1
9	20	0	60	0	0	24	0	6
10	30	10	38	0	0	15	0	4
12	30	10	40	0	0	15	0	5

AHI, Apnea–hypopnea index; *CA*, central apnea; *OA*, obstructive apnea; *MA*, mixed apnea; *PAP*, positive airway pressure; *REM*, rapid eye movement; *TST*, total sleep time.

TABLE P72-3	Download from CPAP Device After 1 Month of Treatment
Used 20/30 days	
Average use (days used)	4 hours
Apnea–hypopnea index (#/hr)	20
Clear airway apnea index (#/hr)	18
Obstructive airway apnea index (#/hr)	2
Hypopnea index (#/hr)	0
Large leak (min)	3 minutes

CPAP, Continuous positive airway pressure.

QUESTION

1. What is your diagnosis, and what intervention do you recommend?

ANSWER

1. **Answer:** Treatment-emergent central sleep apnea (TE-CSA); titration with adaptive servoventilation (ASV)

    Discussion: This patient meets the *International Classification of Sleep Disorders,* Third Edition (ICSD-3) criteria for TE-CSA. He had ≥ 5 predominantly obstructive events per hour on the diagnostic portion of the polysomnography (PSG). During the PAP PSG, obstructive events were eliminated by CPAP or bilevel PAP (BPAP) without a backup rate, but central events emerged with a CAHI >5 per hour (hr), and more than 50% of residual events were central. In addition the CSA was not better explained by another CSA syndrome (no CSA-CSB or CSA due to narcotics.).

    TE-CSA, as defined by the ICSD-3, also meets commonly used criteria for complex sleep apnea (CompSA) as defined by the Centers for Medicare and Medicaid Services (CMS) (Box P72-1). CompSA is defined as a form of CSA identified by the persistence or emergence of CSAs or central sleep hypopneas upon exposure to CPAP or BPAP without a backup rate when obstructive events have disappeared. These patients have predominantly obstructive or mixed apneas (most studies have also included obstructive hypopneas) during a diagnostic occurring at ≥ 5 per hour. With the use of CPAP or BPAP without a backup rate, they show a pattern of apneas and hypopneas that meets the definition of CSA. The CMS definition of CSA is an AHI ≥ 5/hr, central AHI ≥ 5/hr, and with more than 50% of the events being central. CompSA includes patients with TE-CSA (as defined by the ICSD-3), patients with CSA-CSB who have mainly obstructive events on a diagnostic study, and patients with CSA on opioids who also often have persistence and emergence of central apneas on PAP. In what follows, most of the discussion applies to all forms of CompSA. It should also be emphasized that a diagnosis of both OSA and TE-CSA may be made. See also Patient 71-C.

BOX P72-1	Complex Sleep Apnea

1. Symptoms of daytime sleepiness or disrupted sleep
2. Diagnostic study or diagnostic portion of a split sleep study ≥ 5 per hour predominantly obstructive or mixed apneas (Most studies of complex sleep apnea have included obstructive hypopneas as well.)
3. On CPAP or BPAP without a backup rate after obstructive events have resolved:
   - AHI ≥ 5/hour
   - Central AHI ≥ 5/hour (central apneas or central hypopneas)
   - >50% of events are central

AHI, Apnea–hypopnea index; *BPAP,* bilevel positive airway pressure; *CPAP,* continuous positive airway pressure.
Note: Exact definitions of complex sleep apnea vary between studies.

Patients with TE-CSA are thought to have an instability in ventilatory control or a sleep state instability. The underling instability is believed to be exacerbated by CPAP or BPAP. CPAP or BPAP could result in a lower sleeping partial pressure of arterial oxygen ($PaCO_2$) by decreasing upper airway resistance. A lower PCO_2 during sleep narrows the difference between the PCO_2 and the apneic threshold (AT). Recall that the apneic threshold in the value of PCO_2 below which central apnea occurs during sleep. Patients with TE-CSA are believed to have a small difference between the sleeping PCO_2 and the AT (likely due to high ventilatory drive), as well as difficulty reaching stable sleep (frequent arousals). Arousal results in a lower PCO_2 on return to sleep and increases the risk for CSA. Risk factors for TE-CSA have varied (Box P72-2) but include NREM > REM, men > women, high altitude, high levels of CPAP or BPAP without a backup rate, higher AHI or presence of central apneas on the diagnostic portion, supine > nonsupine position, and use of a split-night sleep study. Johnson and Johnson found that BPAP without a backup rate was more likely to be associated with central apneas than CPAP. If central apneas appear on CPAP, a switch to BPAP *without* a backup rate is likely to increase the amount of central apnea. The same risk factors for CompSA are noted as for TE-CSA with the addition of CHF or opioid medication as risk factors. TE-CSA has also been demonstrated after treatment of OSA with an oral appliance and after upper airway surgery.

The incidence of CompSA and TE-CSA has varied tremendously between studies (Table P72-4). On the first titration, 1.5% to 20% had TE-CSA and after chronic treatment with

BOX P72-2	Risk Factors for Treatment-Emergent Central Sleep Apnea*

NREM (stages N1, N2) > stage R	Split-night study > a separate night for PSG titration
Men > women	High CPAP (overtitration), BPAP without a backup
Supine position > nonsupine position	rate
High AHI	High altitude, oral breathing
Central apneas during the diagnostic study	

AHI, Apnea–hypopnea index; *BPAP*, bilevel positive airway pressure; *CPAP*, continuous positive airway pressure; *NREM*, non–rapid eye movement; *PSG*, polysomnography.
*Opioids and congestive heart failure are additional risk factors for CompSA.

TABLE P72-4	Percentage with CompSA on the First Titration and After Treatment		

Author	Patient Number	CompSA on First Titration	Titration After Chronic Treatment (3 to 6 month)
Javaheri (2009)	1286	6.5% (84)	N = 42 studied, 9 still had CSA Estimated 18 out of 84 had all come for study assuming those lost to follow-up had the same proportion of persistent CSA (1.4% of 84) Javaheri quoted estimate 1.5%
Dernaika (2007)	116	N = 23 (19.8%)	N = 14 studied, 2 had persistent CSA 14% of 14 or estimated 2.5% of 116
Lehman (2007)	99	N = 13 13%	
Morgenthaler[1] (2006)	223 consecutive With OSA 4 had CHF	33 (15% of 223) Or 31/219 If 4 excluded for CHF 14% had CompSA	
Cassel (2011)	675	82 (12.8%)	28 lost to follow-up, 14 of 54 had persistent CSA (estimate of 3.1% of original 675) 16/382 without CSA on the first titration now had CSA
Westhoff (2012)	1776	28 (normal BNP levels), 1.57%	

See bibliography for reference to these studies.
BNP, Brain natriuretic peptide; *CHF*, congestive heart failure; *CompSA*, complex sleep apnea; *CSA*, central sleep apnea; *OSA*, obstructive sleep apnea.

CPAP about 1.5% to 3% had persistent CSA. Some studies were performed in community-based sleep centers and some in referral centers. Most used the definition of CompSA similar to CMS and therefore included some patients with CHF and patients on opioids. In studies that looked for persistence of CSA with chronic CPAP, a high number of subjects dropped out or were lost to follow-up. A large proportion of these patients may not have accepted CPAP because of persistent CSA.

Of interest, a study by Cassel et al. comparing the results of an initial CPAP study with one performed after 6 months of CPAP therapy found some patients who did not meet criteria for CompSA on the initial study met the criteria on the second study. Those patients with TE-CSA who do not experience resolution of central apneas on chronic PAP treatment are found to have a high number of residual events on PAP machine interrogation in clinical follow-up. Nocturnal oximetry at home on PAP treatment may show persistent arterial oxygen desaturation. Sleep fragmentation and daytime sleepiness may persist if a significant number of central apneas remain. The potential for poor adherence and acceptance of PAP treatment exists.

Treatment of CompSA is still controversial. In patients with CSA-CSB or CSA-opioids on CPAP, most clinicians would immediately proceed with ASV treatment if the central AHI is high, sleep was poor on the initial CPAP titration, or both. In TE-CSA (no explanation for CSA), a large proportion of patients will respond to CPAP (see Patient 71C). A CPAP pressure that will eliminate most obstructive events (avoiding high pressures associated with frequent central apneas, see Patient 71C) is chosen. However, those with a high central AHI or poor sleep on CPAP may benefit from immediate ASV treatment. If CPAP is used for patients with TE-CSA, close follow-up is needed. If they do not respond to CPAP treatment, ASV titration should be ordered. An alternative treatment for TE-CSA is a combination of oxygen and CPAP. In one study of patients with treatment emergent CSA, use of CPAP and oxygen was effective at reducing central apnea in those not responding to CPAP alone.

The current patient had not done well on CPAP. The overall AHI on CPAP remained quite elevated due to central apneas (see Table P72-3). The patient was started on a level of CPAP that was associated with abolition of obstructive events. However, his CPAP adherence was poor and his residual AHI high, with most events being clear airway apneas (see Table P27-3). He was referred for PSG titration with ASV. On this treatment, his AHI was reduced to 5/hr. He tolerated the pressure well and was started on treatment. A download in 1 month showed excellent adherence and the patient reported much better sleep on treatment.

CLINICAL PEARLS

1. CompSA includes patients with predominantly OSA on a diagnostic study but predominantly CSA-CSB, CSA-opioids, or TE-CSA (CSA of unknown cause) on a PAP titration study.

2. Risk factors for TE-CSA include a high AHI or presence of central apneas during the diagnostic study, NREM > REM, men > women (some studies), high altitude, split-night studies, use of high levels of CPAP, use of BPAP without a backup rate, and the supine position.

3. The percentage of patients with CSA on the first CPAP titration for OSA has varied from 1.5% to 20%. The percentage of patients with persistent CSA on CPAP treatment has been estimated to be 1.5% to 3%. However, this may underestimate the true frequency of this phenomenon. Current published studies had a significant proportion of patients lost to follow-up.

4. The great majority of patients with TE-CSA will have resolution of CSA with chronic CPAP. However, those that do not are at risk for CPAP treatment failure.

5. One treatment approach for TE-CSA is to use a level of CPAP eliminating obstructive events and closely monitor the patient. Those having persistent central events, poor response to CPAP, or both should undergo ASV titration.

6. Many clinicians would immediately proceed with ASV titration and treatment in patients with CompSA associated with CSA-CSB or opioids when the central AHI is high and sleep quality poor on the initial CPAP titration.

BIBLIOGRAPHY

Allam JS, Olson EJ, Gay PC, Morgenthaler TI: Efficacy of adaptive servoventilation in treatment of complex and central sleep apnea syndromes, *Chest* 132(6):1839–1846, 2007.

Aurora RN, Chowdhuri S, Ramar K, et al: The treatment of central sleep apnea syndromes in adults: practice parameters with an evidence-based literature review and meta-analyses, *Sleep* 35(1):17–40, 2012.

Cassel W, Canisius S, Becker HF, et al: A prospective polysomnographic study on the evolution of complex sleep apnea, *Eur Respir J* 38(2):329–337, 2011.

Chowdhuri S, Ghabsha A, Sinha P, et al: Treatment of central sleep apnea in U.S. veterans, *J Clin Sleep Med* 8(5):555–563, 2012.

Dernaika T, Tawk M, Nazir S, et al: The significance and outcome of continuous positive airway pressure-related central sleep apnea during split-night sleep studies, *Chest* 132(1):81–87, 2007.

Gay PC: Complex sleep apnea: it really is a disease, *J Clin Sleep Med* 4(5):403–405, 2008.

Gilmartin GS, Daly RW, Thomas RJ: Recognition and management of complex sleep-disordered breathing, *Curr Opin Pulm Med* 11(6):485–493, 2005.

Javaheri S, Smith J, Chung E: The prevalence and natural history of complex sleep apnea, *J Clin Sleep Med* 5(3):205–211, 2009.

Johnson KG, Johnson DC: Bilevel positive airway pressure worsens central apneas during sleep, *Chest* 128(4):2141–2150, 2005.

Lehman S, Antic NA, Thompson C, et al: Central sleep apnea on commencement of continuous positive airway pressure in patients with a primary diagnosis of obstructive sleep apnea-hypopnea, *J Clin Sleep Med* 3(5):462–466, 2007.

Malhotra A, Bertisch S, Wellman A: Complex sleep apnea: it isn't really a disease, *J Clin Sleep Med* 4(5):406–408, 2008.

Morgenthaler TI, Kagramanov V, Hanak V, et al: Complex sleep apnea syndrome: is it a unique clinical syndrome? *Sleep* 29 (9):1203–1209, 2006.

Selim BJ, Junna MR, Morgenthaler TI: Therapy for sleep hypoventilation syndromes, *Curr Treat Opt Neurol* 14:427–437, 2012.

Thomas RJ, Terzano MG, Parrino L, Weiss JW: Obstructive sleep-disordered breathing with a dominant cyclic alternating pattern–a recognizable polysomnographic variant with practical clinical implications, *Sleep* 27(2):229–234, 2004.

Westhoff M, Arzt M, Litterst P: Prevalence and treatment of central sleep apnoea emerging after initiation of continuous positive airway pressure in patients with obstructive sleep apnoea without evidence of heart failure, *Sleep Breath* 16 (1):71–78, 2012.

Xie A, Bedekar A, Skatrud J, et al: The heterogeneity of obstructive sleep apnea (predominant obstructive vs pure obstructive apnea), *Sleep* 34:745–750, 2011.

PATIENT 73

A Patient with CHF and Central Apnea

A patient with congestive heart failure (CHF) and breathing pauses was found to have obstructive sleep apnea (OSA) during the diagnostic portion of the study. On continuous positive airway pressure (CPAP) of 12 centimeters of water (cm H_2O) the tracing in Figure P73-1 was noted.

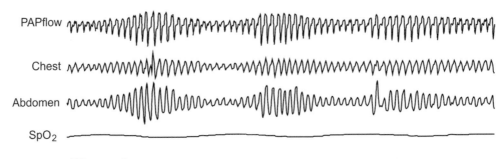

FIGURE P73-1 ■ A tracing on continuous positive airway pressure (CPAP) of 12 centimeters of water (cm H_2O). PAP flow is the flow signal from the PAP device.

QUESTIONS

1. What type of breathing is depicted in Figure P73-1?

2. Does Figure P73-2 depict Cheyne-Stokes breathing (CSB)?

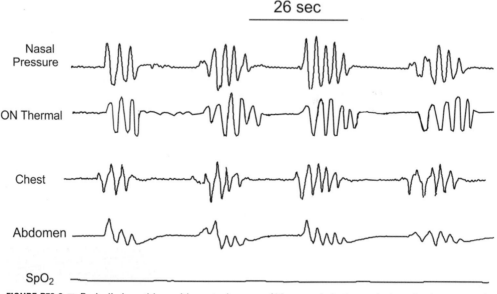

FIGURE P73-2 ■ Periodic breathing with central apneas (26 seconds is the cycle length of one event).

ANSWERS

1. **Answer:** CSB with central hypopneas

2. **Answer:** This is NOT CSB. The tracing shows periodic breathing with central apneas, but the cycle length is <40 seconds, and the ventilatory pattern between apneas does not always have a crescendo-decrescendo pattern.

Discussion (Questions 1 and 2): CSB with central sleep apnea (CSB-CSA) is characterized by recurrent central apneas separately by a crescendo–decrescendo pattern of breathing between the apneas. The key features of CSB-CSA are listed in Box P73-1. The minimum cycle length as defined in the *AASM Scoring Manual* is 40 seconds. However, CSB may also be composed of central hypopneas at the nadirs of respiratory effort as shown in Figure P73-1. In this case cycle length is measures for zenith to zenith in respiration. CSB-CSA occurs most commonly in patients with left ventricular systolic dysfunction but also may occur in patients with *diastolic* CHF or neurologic disorders. In the case of diastolic CHF, the cycle length of CSB-CSA is shorter, as the ejection fraction is normal. The *worse the systolic function, the longer is the cycle length* (because of a longer ventilatory portion between central apneas and hypopneas). The neurologic disorders associated with CSB include a prior cerebrovascular accident (CVA) and neurodegenerative disorders (multiple system atrophy). Although OSA is the predominant form of sleep apnea present in patients after CVA, CSB-CSA may be present in up to 30% of patients in the first few days after stroke. Central apnea tends to resolve and is less commonly seen in studies of patients studied several months after stroke. CSB-CSA caused by systolic CHF is probably the most common cause of CSA seen today. Javaheri and colleagues found occult sleep-disordered breathing (SDB) in 45% of a group with stable CHF and an ejection fraction <45%, and CSA was common in the affected individuals. MacDonald and associates studied a group of patients in stable CHF with maximal modern medical management and found 61% to have some form of sleep apnea (31% central apnea and 30% OSA). Oldenburg and coworkers studied 700 patients with CHF and found similar results. It should be noted that many patients in these studies had variable amounts of both CSA and OSA.

BOX P73-1	Key Features of CSA-CSB in Congestive Heart Failure (CHF)

- Common in stages N1, N2
- Uncommon in rapid eye movement (REM) sleep (stage R)
- Worse in the supine position
- Longer cycle length is correlated with lower ejection fraction. Cycle length > 40 seconds
- Low or normal daytime partial pressure of arterial oxygen (PaO$_2$)
- High ventilatory drive

- Small difference between sleeping PCO$_2$ and apneic (low CO$_2$ reserve)
- Relative amount of central versus obstructive apnea may increase during the night as PaCO$_2$ decreases (likely due to increased ventilatory drive caused by pulmonary congestion)
- Arousals at zenith of inspiratory effort between central apnea rather than at apnea termination

In these studies defining what percent of events qualified the patient for the central apnea group was somewhat arbitrary. In addition, *the percentage of central events may increase overnight, increase in the supine position, or vary or from night to night.* In any case, the prevalence of CSB-CSA is high in patients with significant systolic heart failure. As noted above, patients with diastolic heart failure may also have CSA-CSB, but the cycle length is shorter.

Patients with CSA-CSB may complain of the typical symptoms of sleep apnea, including disturbed sleep or daytime sleepiness. However, in most studies, the majority of patients do not complain of subjective excessive daytime sleepiness. Thus, a high index of suspicion is needed to suspect the presence of CSA-CSB. Nocturnal sleep complaints are often assumed to be secondary to CHF rather than to comorbid sleep apnea. Despite the lack of subjective sleepiness complaints in CSA-CSB patients, studies have documented improvement in sleep quality and objective daytime sleepiness with successful treatment.

Polysomnography in CSA-CSB: The crescendo–decrescendo morphology of breathing between central apneas in CSA-CSB has been discussed in Fundamentals 13. The minimum cycle length of 40 seconds is somewhat arbitrary, but most patients with CSB-CSA and systolic heart failure will have a cycle length of 60 to 90 seconds. Another characteristic to appreciate is the long delay in the nadir in the saturation of arterial oxygen (SaO$_2$) tracing after event termination because of a prolonged circulation time (low cardiac output). Another finding distinguishing CSA-CSB compared to other forms of CSA is that arousals usually occur at the zenith of effort rather than at apnea termination. If central hypopneas rather than central apneas are present, this may also make CSB more difficult to recognize. CSA-CSB is *most common in stages N1 and N2 and uncommon in stage R.* In stage R, the ventilatory response to hypercapnia is lower, and less overshoot in ventilation tends to occur. Often, a patient manifesting CSA-CSB will suddenly show resolution of central apneas when entering rapid eye movement (REM) sleep. Some patients with severe CHF will have CSA-CSB while awake. See Patient 71 for a Table listing the ICSD-3 diagnostic criteria for CSA-CSB.

Pathophysiology of CSA-CSB: The factors contributing to CSB include high ventilatory drive (high sympathetic tone, pulmonary congestion), long circulation time, and a small difference between the sleeping PaCO$_2$ and the AT. Patients with CSB have low daytime partial pressure of arterial oxygen (PaCO$_2$) compared with patients with CHF but without CSB (because of increased ventilatory drive). High drive is thought to be caused by increased sympathetic tone and stimulation of lung J receptors by pulmonary interstitial edema. In patients with CHF, the higher the pulmonary capillary wedge pressure, the lower is the awake PaCO$_2$ and the higher is the central apnea–hypopnea index (AHI). Some patients with mixtures of OSA and CSA tend to have more CSA at the end of the night as the pulmonary capillary wedge increases and the PaCO$_2$ decreases. CSA-CSB is also more likely in the supine position. Sin and colleagues in a study published in 1999 evaluated patients with CHF and identified risk factors for CSA compared to OSA to include male gender, atrial fibrillation, age older than 60, and hypocapnia (PaCO$_2$ < 38 mm Hg) during wakefulness. Risk factors for OSA compared to CSA included a high body mass index (BMI) in men and an increase in age in women. The presence of CSA-CSB also has prognostic implications. Studies have suggested that the presence of CSA in patients with CHF is associated with a worse prognosis.

Treatment of CSA-CSB: Possible treatments of CSA-CSB are listed in Table P73-1. Most would also pertain to patients with CSA-CSB due to neurologic disorders. A recent large systematic review by Aurora et al. contains many pertinent references for treatment of CSA associated with heart failure. Medical treatment of heart failure may reduce CSA-CSB. Transplantation may also

TABLE P73-1 **Treatment Options for CSB-CSA Due to CHF**

Treatment of CSB-CSA	Comments	AASM Practice Parameters for Treatment of CSA Due to CHF (Level of Recommendation) Standard > Guideline > Option
Optimize treatment of CHF	AHI correlated with wedge pressure	N/A
CPAP	Effective in about 50% of CSB-CSA	Standard
ASV	Effective in most patients AHI <10/hour is common Also treats obstructive events	Standard
Oxygen	Prevents desaturation May reduce central apnea Can be used with CPAP (CPAP for obstructive events)	Standard
BPAP-ST	If CPAP, ASV, oxygen are not effective	Option
Aminophylline	Consider if PAP therapy not successful Can worsen ventricular arrhythmias	Limited Evidence (Option)
Acetazolamide	Consider if PAP therapy not successful	Limited Evidence (Option)

Adapted from Aurora RN, Chowdhuri S, Ramar K, et al: The treatment of central sleep apnea syndromes in adults: practice parameters with an evidence-based literature review and meta-analyses, *Sleep* 35(1):17-40, 2012.
AHI, Apnea–hypopnea index; *ASV*, adaptive servoventilation; *BPAP-ST*, bilevel positive airway pressure (spontaneous timed mode); *CHF*, congestive heart failure; *CPAP*, continuous positive airway pressure; *CSB-CSA*, Cheyne-Stokes breathing with central sleep apnea; *N/A*, not applicable.

cure CSA-CSB. A number of treatments for CSA-CSB have been tried, including aminophylline, acetazolamide, hypnotics, oxygen, and PAP. Neither aminophylline (may increase arrhythmias) nor acetazolamide has been widely used. Treatment with CPAP is effective in about 50% of patients with CSA-CSB. If effective, CPAP may improve sleep quality and ejection fraction and reduce sympathetic activity. Titration of CPAP in CSA-CSB patients differs from that in OSA patients. On a given titration night, a pressure that eliminates CSA cannot usually be found. Typically, pressure is increased until obstructive events are eliminated and then increased to 8 to 10 cm H_2O (if pressure is not already above that level). In some studies of CPAP treatment for CSA-CSB, CPAP was started on an outpatient basis and increased slowly, with a goal of 8 to 10 cm H_2O commonly recommended. A large multicenter randomized controlled trial comparing CPAP and standard treatment did not show an improvement in survival with CPAP (CAN-PAP trial, Bradley et al 2005). The trial provided evidence that about 50% of patients will respond to CPAP (50% had AHI <15/hour). A study by Teschler and coworkers compared CPAP, oxygen, bilevel PAP with a backup rate (BPAP-ST [spontaneous-timed mode]), and adaptive servoventilation (ASV) with each used for a single night (Figure P73-3). This study showed a modest improvement in the AHI with oxygen and CPAP. BPAP-ST was more effective. ASV reduced the AHI to very low levels typical of CPAP titrations in OSA patients. ASV treatment of CSA-CSB often reduces the AHI to less than 5/hr on the first night and is generally well tolerated. An initial trial of CPAP with a switch to ASV if CPAP is not effective is one approach. Nocturnal supplemental oxygen with or without CPAP (for obstructive events) is an option if PAP is not tolerated. Trials of the effects of ASV on CHF outcomes are ongoing. To date, no treatment has been demonstrated to improve survival. However, treatment with ASV and CPAP may improve sleep quality, increase the ejection fraction, and reduce measures of sympathetic tone.

If a patient with CHF has predominantly OSA on a diagnostic study, then CPAP titration is certainly indicated. If underlying CSB is suspected in a patient with predominantly obstructive events, CPAP titration would still be indicated as a study must demonstrate that the patient has complex sleep apnea (emergence of frequent central apneas on CPAP) before a device with a backup rate (ASV) is reimbursed by most insurance carriers. On the other hand, if a patient has predominately CSA-CSB on the diagnostic study, one may proceed directly with an ASV titration unless reimbursement issues mandate an initial trial of CPAP. The Centers for Medicare and Medicaid (CMS) and many insurance carriers no longer require an attempt at CPAP if a patient meets criteria for central sleep apnea on the diagnostic study (http://www.cms.gov/mcd/viewlcd.asp?lcd_id=5023&lcd_version=56&show=all) (see Appendix 3).

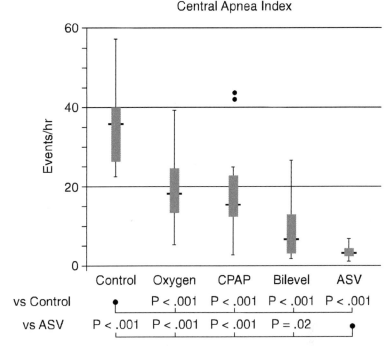

Central Apnea Index

FIGURE P73-3 ■ Effectiveness in reducing the central apnea index by oxygen, continuous positive airway pressure (CPAP), bilevel positive airway pressure (BPAP-ST) with a backup rate, and adaptive servoventilation (ASV). ASV was the most successful at lowering the central apnea index. The figure shows box plots: median (*horizontal bar*); interquartile range (*thick vertical bar*); range excluding outliers (*thin bar*); outliers (*circles*). (From Teschler H, Döhring J, Wang YM, Berthon-Jones M: Adaptive pressure support servo-ventilation: a novel treatment for Cheyne-Stokes respiration in heart failure, *Am J Respir Crit Care Med* 164:614-619, 2001.)

The CMS criteria for central sleep apnea include:
1. AHI ≥ 5/hr
2. Central apneas or hypopneas >50% of the total apneas and hypopneas
3. Central apneas or hypopneas ≥ 5/hour
4. Symptoms of excessive daytime sleepiness or disrupted sleep

Of note, some clinicians would still order a titration with CPAP (at least during the initial part of the titration). The rationale is some patients with CSA-CSB will respond to CPAP. Failure of CPAP would then trigger ASV titration during the rest of the study. A problem with this approach is that time for an optimal ASV titration may be more limited.

In summary, although the best treatment for patients with CSA-CSB remains controversial, most clinicians would use ASV unless a patient has a satisfactory response to CPAP. Of note, BPAP *without* a backup rate is unlikely to be effective if CPAP is not effective. BPAP-ST (with backup rate) may be effective in patients failing ASV. Attempts to optimize treatment of CHF are the first line of treatment in patients with CSA-CSB caused by heart failure.

CLINICAL PEARLS

1. CSA-CSB is uncommon in stage R and is common in stages N1 and N2.

2. CSA-CSB is often reduced with sleep in the lateral position.

3. About 50% of patients with CSA-CSB will respond to CPAP (AHI <15/hr).

4. ASV is an effective treatment for patients with CSA-CSB.

5. Oxygen treatment is also a recommended treatment of CSA-CSB but is less likely to reduce the AHI to low levels. Most clinicians would not use this as a first-line treatment.

6. CSB may be associated with central hypopneas as well as central apneas.

7. In CSA-CSB, the lower the ejection fraction the longer the cycle length (because of a longer period of ventilation between central respiratory events).

8. Patients with both OSA and CSA-CSB may manifest more central apneas at the end of the night or when placed on positive airway pressure.

BIBLIOGRAPHY

Arzt M, Floras JS, Logan AG, et al: CANPAP Investigators: Suppression of central sleep apnea by continuous positive airway pressure and transplant-free survival in heart failure: a post hoc analysis of the Canadian Continuous Positive Airway Pressure for Patients with Central Sleep Apnea and Heart Failure Trial (CANPAP), *Circulation* 115:3173–3180, 2007.

Aurora RN, Chowdhuri S, Ramar K, et al: The treatment of central sleep apnea syndromes in adults: practice parameters with an evidence -based literature review and meta-analyses, *Sleep* 35(1):17–40, 2012.

Bitter T, Faber L, Hering D, et al: Sleep-disordered breathing in heart failure with normal left ventricular ejection fraction, *Eur J Heart Fail* 11:602–608, 2009.

Bradley TD, Logan AG, Kimoff RJ, et al: CANPAP Investigators: Continuous positive airway pressure for central sleep apnea and heart failure, *N Engl J Med* 353:2025–2033, 2005.

Braver HM, Brandes WC, Kubiet MA, et al: Effect of cardiac transplantation on Cheyne-Stokes respiration occurring during sleep, *Am J Cardiol* 76:632–634, 1995.

Dark DS, Pingleton SK, Kerby GR, et al: Breathing pattern abnormalities and arterial oxygen desaturation during sleep in the congestive heart failure syndrome: improvement following medical therapy, *Chest* 91:833–836, 1987.

Hanly PJ, Zuberi-Khokhar NS: Increased mortality associated with Cheyne-Stokes respiration in patients with congestive heart failure, *Am J Respir Crit Care Med* 153:272–276, 1996.

Hermann DM, Siccoli M, Kirov P, et al: Central periodic breathing during sleep in ischemic stroke, *Stroke* 38:1082–1084, 2007.

Javaheri S, Ahmend M, Parker TJ: Effects of nasal O_2 on sleep-related disordered breathing in ambulatory patients with stable heart failure, *Sleep* 22:1101–1106, 1999.

Javaheri S, Parker TJ, Wexler L, et al: Occult sleep-disordered breathing in stable congestion heart failure, *Ann Intern Med* 122:487–492, 1995.

Lorenzi-Filho G, Azevedo ER, Parker JD, Bradley TD: Relationship of carbon dioxide tension in arterial blood to pulmonary wedge pressure in heart failure, *Eur Respir J* 19:37–40, 2002.

MacDonald M, Fang J, Pittman SD, et al: The current prevalence of sleep disordered breathing in congestive heart failure patients treated with beta-blockers, *J Clin Sleep Med* 4:38–42, 2008.

Oldenburg O, Lamp B, Faber L, et al: Sleep-disordered breathing in patients with symptomatic heart failure: a contemporary study of prevalence in and characteristics of 700 patients, *Eur J Heart Fail* 9:251–257, 2007.

Oldenburg O, Schmidt A, Lamp B, et al: Adaptive servoventilation improves cardiac function in patients with chronic heart failure and Cheyne-Stokes respiration, *Eur J Heart Fail* 10:581–586, 2008.

Philippe C, Stoïca-Herman M, Drouot X, et al: Compliance with and effectiveness of adaptive servoventilation versus continuous positive airway pressure in the treatment of Cheyne-Stokes respiration in heart failure over a six-month period, *Heart* 92:337–342, 2006.

Sin DD, Fitzgerald F, Parker JD, et al: Risk factors for central and obstructive sleep apnea in 450 men and women with congestive heart failure, *Am J Respir Crit Care Med* 160:1101–1106, 1999.

Sin DD, Logan AG, Fitzgerald FS, et al: Effects of continuous positive airway pressure on cardiovascular outcomes in heart failure patients with and without Cheyne-Stokes respiration, *Circulation* 102:61–66, 2000.

Solin P, Bergin P, Richardson M, et al: Influence of pulmonary capillary wedge pressure on central apnea in heart failure, *Circulation* 99:1574–1579, 1999.

Szollosi I, Roebuck T, Thompson B, Naughton MT: Lateral sleeping position reduces severity of central sleep apnea / Cheyne-Stokes respiration, *Sleep* 29(8):1045–1051, 2006.

Teschler H, Döhring J, Wang YM, Berthon-Jones M: Adaptive pressure support servo-ventilation: a novel treatment for Cheyne-Stokes respiration in heart failure, *Am J Respir Crit Care Med* 164:614–619, 2001.

Tkacova R, Niroumand M, Lorenzi-Filho G, Bradley TD: Overnight shift from obstructive to central apneas in patients with heart failure: role of PCO_2 and circulatory delay, *Circulation* 103:238–243, 2001.

PATIENT 74

A Patient with Sleep Apnea on Pain Medications

A 40-year-old man was evaluated for daytime sleepiness and snoring at night. His Epworth Sleepiness Scale (ESS) score was 16/24. He was taking medications for pain. A sleep study was performed, and a sample tracing is shown in Figure P74-1

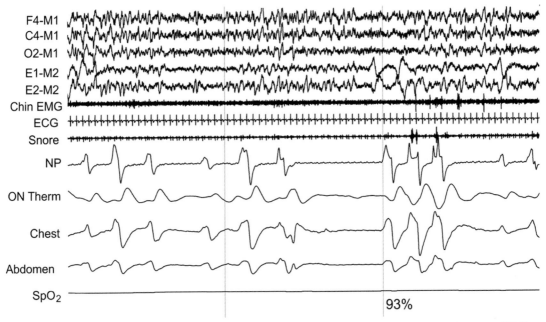

FIGURE P74-1 ■ A 90-second tracing. Note the slow respiratory rate, ataxic breathing and central apneas. *NP*, Nasal pressure; *ON Therm*, oronasal thermal air flow sensor. Ataxic breathing is characterized by a chaotic variation in cycle length and magnitude of flow (tidal volume).

QUESTION

1. What medication is the patient likely taking?
   A. Pregabalin
   B. Gabapentin
   C. Tramadol
   D. Methadone

BOX P74-1	Opioid-Induced Sleep-Related Breathing Disorders

Low respiratory rate
Ataxic breathing—variations in cycle length and air flow magnitude
Obstructive sleep apnea—long events
Central sleep apnea—intermittent events or as form of periodic breathing

Complex sleep apnea
Sleep-related hypoventilation (with or without awake hypoventilation)
Excessive daytime sleepiness

Note: Obstructive sleep apnea (OSA) is the most common form of breathing disorder in patients taking narcotics.

ANSWER

1. **Answer:** Methadone, opioid-induced sleep-related breathing disorder (OISRBDs)

   Discussion: OISRBDs are becoming increasingly common with more aggressive treatment of chronic pain with potent narcotics such as oxycodone, morphine (including sustained-release formulation), fentanyl patch, the combination of buprenorphine and naloxone (Suboxone), and methadone, often in very high doses. Affected patients may manifest obstructive apneas—often of long duration; ataxic breathing; low respiratory rates during sleep; central apneas, either intermittent or in the form of periodic breathing; and daytime and sleep-related hypoventilation (Box P74-1). *Ataxic breathing* is a unique breathing pattern characterized by variations in tidal volume and

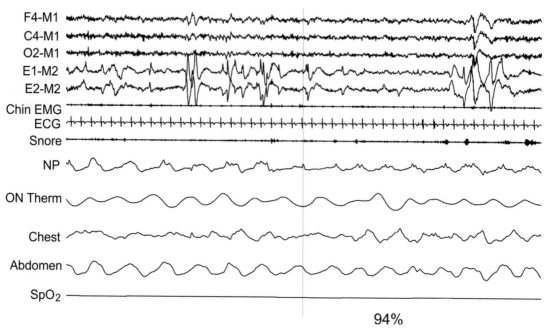

FIGURE P74-2 ■ A 60-second tracing during stage R in the patient illustrated in Figure P74-1.

respiratory rate (Figure P74-1). Webster et al evaluated a group of patients on narcotics for pain and found an apnea–hypopnea index (AHI) ≥ 5 per hour (hr) in 75% of patients (39% had obstructive sleep apnea [OSA], 4% had sleep apnea of indeterminate type, 24% had central sleep apnea [CSA], and 8% had both CSA and OSA). They found a direct relationship between the AHI and the daily dosage of methadone ($p = 0.002$).

Opioids also may be one cause of complex sleep apnea, that is, predominantly obstructive events during a diagnostic study and predominantly central apneas on CPAP once obstructive events have resolved. The etiology of the OISRBDs is believed to be depression of the central drive by the opioid medications. Although opioid-induced CSA is typically placed in the hypercapnic CSA group, patients often have either normal or only mildly increased awake partial pressure of arterial oxygen ($PaCO_2$) values (45–50 mm Hg). During sleep, patients may develop sleep-related hypoventilation even if the awake $PaCO_2$ is normal. Patients with awake hypoventilation experience a further increase in $PaCO_2$ during sleep. Of interest, in some patients with OISRBD, the AHI in non–rapid eye movement (NREM) sleep is greater than the AHI in REM sleep. *That is, central apneas are more common in NREM sleep than in REM sleep* (Figure P74-2). A level of continuous positive airway pressure (CPAP) effective during stage R may not be effective in NREM sleep (high number of residual central apneas).

Patients with an OISRBD may have relatively few arousals and an increase in stage N3. Despite a normal total sleep time with few arousals, patients often complain of *severe daytime sleepiness, which may not improve with PAP treatment*. This is likely caused by the sedative effect of medication. Effective treatment of daytime sleepiness may require the addition of stimulants or a reduction in narcotic dose. In contrast, daytime sleepiness is uncommon in patients on methadone maintenance for addiction (lower dose than used for pain).

The OISRBD often improves with a reduction in the narcotic dose, but this is rarely acceptable to the patient. Some patients with mainly obstructive events may respond to CPAP. However, central apneas either persist or emerge on CPAP in a significant number of patients. Treatment with either bilevel PAP (BPAP) with a backup rate or adaptive servoventilation (ASV) may be successful in narcotic-induced complex sleep apnea. When using ASV, it is essential to increase EPAP sufficiently to prevent upper airway closure. Javaheri and associates found ASV to be an effective treatment for both CSA and OSA in narcotic-induced CSA. In the current patient, Figure P74-1 shows a pattern of ataxic breathing, slow respiratory rate, and central apneas during NREM sleep. Figure P74-2 shows relatively normal breathing pattern during REM sleep. The patient had obstructive and central apneas during the diagnostic study and predominantly central apnea during a CPAP titration. An ASV titration was subsequently performed showing good control of obstructive and central events. The patient was treated with ASV, and device download showed good adherence with an AHI of 10/hr. However, severe sleepiness persisted (ESS score of 14). The patient has declined an attempt at a reduction in the dose of methadone.

CLINICAL PEARLS

1. Patients taking potent narcotics may exhibit a wide variety of sleep-related respiratory events, including a low respiratory rate, ataxic breathing, long obstructive apneas, periodic breathing with central apneas (not of the Cheyne-Stokes type), hypoventilation during wake or only during sleep, and complex sleep apnea.

2. The first-line treatment of OISRBD is a reduction in narcotic dose, if possible.

3. Opioids may be a cause of sleep-related hypoventilation with or without daytime hypoventilation.

4. Opioids may be a cause of complex sleep apnea (e.g., "Central Sleep Apnea Due to Drug or Substance" on PAP treatment).

5. Treatment with CPAP will suffice for many patients taking opiates who manifest primarily obstructive apnea. However, those with predominantly CSA on a diagnostic study or those with complex sleep apnea will require either BPAP with a backup rate or ASV (also with backup rate).

6. Some patients have a prominent component of hypoventilation and will require either BPAP with adequate pressure support (8 to 10 centimeters of water [cm H$_2$O]) and a backup rate or ASV using a high minimum pressure support (Psmin; 6 to 8 cm H$_2$O) to provide a baseline amount of pressure support.

7. OISRBD patients with predominantly central apneas during a diagnosis study may have a higher AHI in NREM sleep than AHI in REM sleep.

8. Patients with narcotic-associated complex sleep apnea may have better control with CPAP during stage R compared with that during NREM sleep.

9. Patients with narcotic-induced sleep apnea may exhibit profound daytime sleepiness that may persist after successful treatment of the sleep-related breathing disorder and may require alerting/stimulant medications.

BIBLIOGRAPHY

Farney RJ, Walker JM, Boyle KM, et al: Adaptive servoventilation (ASV) in patients with sleep disordered breathing associated with chronic opioid medications for non-malignant pain, *J Clin Sleep Med* 4:311–319, 2008.

Farney RJ, Walker JM, Cloward TV, Rhondeau S: Sleep-disordered breathing associated with long-term opioid therapy, *Chest* 123:632–639, 2003.

Glidewell RN, Orr WC, Imes N: Acetazolamide as an adjunct to CPAP treatment: a case of complex sleep apnea in a patient on long-acting opioid therapy, *J Clin Sleep Med* 5:63–64, 2009.

Javaheri S, Malik A, Smith J, Chung E: Adaptive pressure support servoventilation: a novel treatment for sleep apnea associated with use of opioids, *J Clin Sleep Med* 4:305–310, 2008.

Morgenthaler TI: The quest for stability in an unstable world: adaptive servoventilation in opioid induced complex sleep apnea syndrome, *J Clin Sleep Med* 4:321–323, 2008.

Wang D, Teichtahl H, Drummer O, et al: Central sleep apnea in stable methadone maintenance treatment patients, *Chest* 1238:1348–1356, 2005.

Webster LR, Choi Y, Desai H, et al: Sleep-disordered breathing and chronic opioid therapy, *Pain Med* 9(4):425–432, 2008.

PATIENT 75

A Newborn with Cyanosis and a Young Child with Hypoventilation

Patient A: A sleep study was requested to evaluate a full-term infant at 5 weeks of age. No problems had occurred during delivery, but the child developed arterial oxygen desaturation to 60% during sleep in the nursery until aroused by a nurse. During these episodes, the infant had shallow breathing. The awake saturation of arterial oxygen (SaO$_2$) was 96%. Physical examination was normal for age.

Question 1: What genetic test would you order in this patient?

Patient B: A 3-year-old male child had an uneventful birth, and the first 3 years of his life were normal. However, he developed hyperphagia and obesity rather suddenly. One year after the development of obesity, he was admitted for respiratory failure following an upper respiratory infection (URI) and was found to have unexplained hypoventilation. Laboratory testing revealed low free thyroxine (T4) associated with a low thyroid-stimulating hormone (TSH). After recovering from the illness, the patients was able to maintain a normal partial pressure of arterial oxygen (PaCO$_2$) and SaO$_2$ during wakefulness but had severe oxygen desaturations during sleep. Monitoring with end-tidal PCO$_2$ revealed an increase of 20 mm Hg during sleep. The main pattern of ventilation was low tidal volume and a normal respiratory rate that did not respond to arterial oxygen desaturation.

Question 2: What disorder is causing manifestations exhibited by Patient B?

ANSWER

1. **Answer for Patient A:** Testing for the *PHOX2B* gene

Discussion: The congenital central hypoventilation syndrome (CCHS) is a rare disorder affecting approximately 1 per 200,000 live births,[1] Although the condition is termed *congenital*, some patients with the *PHOX2B* genotype may present phenotypically later in life (and even in adulthood) following the presence of a stressor such as general anesthesia or a severe respiratory illness. However, most CCHS is present from birth and is characterized by alveolar hypoventilation without evidence of pulmonary, neuromuscular, or structural brainstem abnormalities. A typical presentation is an infant who is noted to have cyanosis, feeding difficulties, hypotonia or, occasionally, central apnea. The infant may require intubation and mechanical ventilation, but chest radiography is normal. During wakefulness, many CCHS patients have normal ventilation (approximately 15% hypoventilate during wakefulness), but all patients with the disorder manifest hypoventilation during sleep. Those with hypoventilation during wakefulness have worsening of hypoventilation during sleep and require continuous ventilatory support. Ventilatory responses to hypercapnia or hypoxemia by the rebreathing method are absent or blunted, and dyspnea is absent. As noted above, the most severely affected patients with CCHS also have hypoventilation during wakefulness. Those patients with normal awake ventilation do have peripheral chemoreceptor responses to hypoxemia or hypercapnia.[2] It has been hypothesized that the central integration of chemoreceptor information, rather than the chemoreceptors themselves, is the abnormality in patients with CCHS. One study found that CCHS patients did have intact arousal responses to hypercapnia.[3] However, such arousals do not reliably result in an appropriate ventilatory response and rapid reversal of hypoxemia.

During sleep, all patients with CCHS have worsening of ventilation with profound hypoxemia and hypercapnia on polysomnography (PSG). Central apneas may occur, but hypoventilation is exhibited by diminished tidal volume and normal or decreased respiratory rates.[1,4] In contrast to most types of sleep-disordered breathing (SDB) in children, *abnormalities may be more severe during non–rapid eye movement (NREM) sleep than during REM sleep.* Patients may not arouse from sleep despite severe gas exchange abnormalities.

Other forms of autonomic dysregulation may be seen in these patients. These abnormalities may include Hirschsprung disease (20%) usually presenting with constipation, esophageal dysmotility presenting with feeding difficulty, tumors of neural crest origin (6%) such as neuroblastoma or ganglioneuroma, decreased heart rate variability, decreased heart rate response to exercise, decreased papillary light response, intermittent profuse sweating, and dysregulation of body temperature with decreased baseline body temperature.[1,5] Patients with CCHS are at risk for adverse outcomes from respiratory infections because they may not exhibit a fever or complain of dyspnea, even if severely hypoxemic.

The diagnosis of CCHS should be considered in an infant or young child with apneic or cyanotic spells that especially occur during sleep. The most severe cases occur in patients who do not breathe after birth and require immediate ventilatory support. In others, the abnormalities are noted when the infants sleep. Milder cases may present later with signs of cor pulmonale or hypoxic damage to central nervous system (CNS) structures. Some cases may not present until late childhood, and a few present in adulthood.[6,7] The diagnosis of CCHS depends on exclusion of other causes of hypoventilation such as brainstem malformation, inborn errors of metabolism, myopathy, diaphragmatic paralysis, lung or respiratory pump abnormalities. PSG with end-tidal PCO_2 monitoring usually reveals high end-tidal PCO_2 and low tidal volume (Figure P75-1).[1,5]

Diagnosis is confirmed by genetic testing for mutations in the *PHOX2B* gene.[1,8,9] Most persons with CCHS are heterozygous for a polyalanine repeat expansion mutations in exon 3 of *PHOX2B*. The expansion results in lengthening the normal 20-repeat polyalanine tract to 25-33 repeats. Those with more polyalanine repeats are more likely to have severe disease, including waking hypoventilation. Patients with a point mutation or frame shift mutations are at greater risk for neural tumors. Most mutations occur de novo, but in families with CCHS, it is inherited as an autosomal dominant trait. Research suggests that severity of illness is related to the type of mutation present.

Treatment includes lifelong ventilatory support for all patients during sleep. Some patients will require ventilatory support while awake as well. Ventilatory support for severe cases is usually provided by a volume-cycled ventilator via a tracheostomy tube. In older patients and in those with milder symptoms, noninvasive mask ventilation may suffice.[1,6] Diaphragmatic pacing has also been

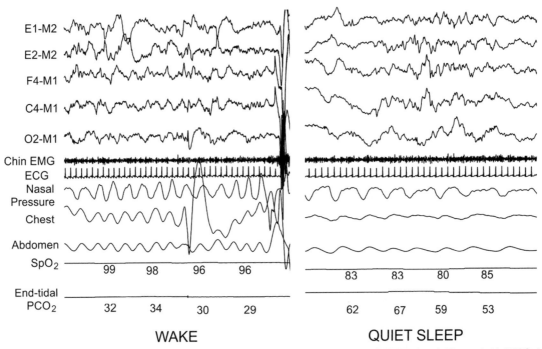

FIGURE P75-1 ■ Tracings (15 seconds each) during wakefulness and quiet sleep (NREM sleep). The end-tidal PCO_2 is not a capnogram but rather tracking the most recent end-tidal value (maximum value).

used during the day. Diaphragmatic pacing at night requires the presence of a tracheostomy tube because obstructive events usually occur when the upper airway muscles do not contract in synchrony with the diaphragm. Infants in CCHS must be closely monitored because they are at risk for hypoventilation or apnea at sleep onset. Noninvasive positive pressure ventilation (NPPV) with bilevel PAP (BPAP) with a backup rate has been successfully used in infants when parents have refused tracheostomy.[10,11] Appropriate alarms are essential. Older children may be transitioned to NPPV if their symptoms are milder and they are adherent to treatment.

In the present case, the patient required mechanical ventilation and ultimately tracheostomy. Genetic testing revealed a mutation of the *PHOX2B* gene manifested by a large number of polyalanine repeats. Chest radiography was normal, and no evidence of a metabolic disorder was observed. Fluoroscopy revealed a mobile diaphragm. Ultimately, the patient was managed with a home ventilator with appropriate alarms.

2. **Answer for Patient B:** Late-onset central hypoventilation with hypothalamic dysfunction is also called rapid-onset obesity with hypothalamic dysfunction, hypoventilation, and autonomic dysregulation (ROHHAD).

Discussion: Late-onset central hypoventilation with hypothalamic dysfunction is a disorder of central control of ventilation. Patients are usually healthy until early childhood (often 2–3 years of age) when they develop hyperphagia and severe obesity, followed by central hypoventilation,[12,13] which often presents as respiratory failure. The respiratory failure may be precipitated by a mild respiratory illness or anesthesia. Patients require ventilatory support during sleep; most patients breathe adequately during wakefulness, but some hypoventilate during wakefulness, especially during periods of stress (infections) or after exercise. The hypoventilation persists even if the patient loses weight, differentiating the condition from obesity hypoventilation syndrome. Manifestations of hypothalamic endocrine dysfunction are characterized by increased or decreased hormone levels, which may include one or more of the following: diabetes insipidus, precocious puberty, hypogonadism, hyperprolactinemia, hypothyroidism, and decreased growth hormone secretion. Other symptoms of hypothalamic dysfunction such as temperature dysregulation have been reported. Mood and behavior abnormalities, sometimes severe, have been reported frequently.

Hypoxemia and hypercapnia are present on PSG during sleep. Central apneas may be present, but hypoventilation associated with decreased tidal volume and respiratory rate is more common.

Patients have flat hypoxic and hypercapnic responses. Arterial blood gases may be normal during wakefulness but will be abnormal if obtained from an arterial line during sleep. In patients with chronically untreated or poorly controlled hypoventilation, compensated respiratory acidosis may be present, with elevated serum bicarbonate levels. In these patients, polycythemia may be present. Serum tests may show evidence of endocrine abnormalities; hypernatremia is common (diabetes insipidus). Computed tomography and magnetic resonance imaging of the head are normal. The current patient had sudden-onset obesity followed by hypoventilation and evidence of hypopituitary hypothyroidism. There was no evidence of a *PHOX2B* genetic abnormality. The patient was treated with noninvasive positive pressure ventilation during sleep with a mask.

CLINICAL PEARLS

1. CCHS should be suspected if an infant develops unexplained cyanosis and desaturation with apparently normal lung (normal chest radiography), normal diaphragmatic mobility, and no evidence of a CNS lesion or metabolic abnormality.

2. CCHS requires ventilatory support during sleep, and the most severely affected (about 15%) require support during wakefulness as well.

3. Diagnosis of CCHS is based on genetic testing for a mutation in the *PHOX2B* gene, usually with polyalanine repeats. Patients with a point mutation or frame shift mutations are at greater risk for neural crest tumors.

4. Arterial oxygen desaturation is often worse during NREM sleep than in REM sleep in patients with CCHS.

5. Central apneas may occur, but the main pattern is one of reduced tidal volume and a normal or decreased respiratory rate.

6. When a young child develops rapid-onset obesity and evidence of hypothalamic dysfunction with respiratory failure, a diagnosis of late-onset central hypoventilation with hypothalamic dysfunction should be considered.

REFERENCES

1. Weese-Mayer DE, Berry-Kravis EM, Ceccherini I, et al: ATS Congenital Central Hypoventilation Syndrome Subcommittee: An official ATS clinical policy statement: congenital central hypoventilation syndrome: genetic basis, diagnosis, and management, *Am J Respir Crit Care Med* 181:626–644, 2010.
2. Gozal D, Marcus CL, Shoseyov D, Keens TB: Peripheral chemoreceptor function in children with the congenital hypoventilation syndrome, *J Appl Physiol* 74:379–387, 1993.
3. Marcus CL, Bautista DB, Amihyia A, et al: Hypercapnic arousal responses in children with congenital central hypoventilation syndrome, *Pediatrics* 88:993–998, 1991.
4. Wagner MH, Berry RB: A full term infant with cyanotic episodes. Congenital central hypoventilation syndrome, *J Clin Sleep Med* 3:425–426, 2007.
5. Grigg-Damberger M, Wells A: Central congenital hypoventilation syndrome: changing face of a less mysterious but more complex genetic disorder, *Semin Respir Crit Care Med* 30:262–274, 2009.
6. Weese-Mayer DE, Berry-Kravis EM, Zhou L: Adult identified with congenital central hypoventilation syndrome—mutation in PHOX2b gene and late-onset CHS, *Am J Respir Crit Care Med* 171:88, 2005.
7. Katz ES, McGrath S, Marcus CL: Late-onset central hypoventilation with hypothalamic dysfunction: a distinct clinical syndrome, *Pediatr Pulmonol* 29:62–88, 2000.
8. Berry-Kravis EM, Zhou L, Rand CM, Weese-Mayer DE: Congenital central hypoventilation syndrome *PHOX2b* mutations and phenotype, *Am J Respir Crit Care Med* 174:1139–1144, 2006.
9. Amiel J, Laudier B, Attie-Bitach T, et al: Polyalanine expansion and frameshift mutations of the paired-like homeobox gene *PHOX2B* in congenital central hypoventilation syndrome, *Nat Genet* 33(4):459–461, 2003.
10. Tibballs J, Henning RD: Noninvasive ventilatory strategies in the management of a newborn infant and three children with congenital central hypoventilation syndrome, *Pediatr Pulmonol* 36:544–548, 2003.
11. Ramesh P, Boit P, Samuels M: Mask ventilation in the early management of congenital central hypoventilation syndrome, *Arch Dis Child Fetal Neonatal Ed* 93:F400–F403, 2008.
12. Ize-Ludlow D, Gray JA, Sperling MA, et al: Rapid-onset obesity with hypothalamic dysfunction, hypoventilation, and autonomic dysregulation presenting in childhood, *Pediatrics* 120(1):e179–e188, 2007.
13. Lesser DJ, Ward SL, Kun SS, Keens TG: Congenital hypoventilation syndromes, *Semin Respir Crit Care Med* 30(3):339–347, 2009.

A Young Woman with Headaches and Central Apnea and a Man with Breathing Pauses After Stroke

Patient A: A 25-year-old woman began to experience snoring and increased headaches with mild sleepiness. The headaches tended to occur in the morning or with exertion. She denied any other neurologic symptoms (no problems with balance, strength, sensation, or intellectual function). Although she was thin, she had mildly enlarged tonsils and a high arched palate. A sleep study was ordered to determine if obstructive sleep apnea (OSA) could be causing her symptoms. Sleep study results are listed in Table P76-1, and a typical tracing is shown in Figure P76-1.

TABLE P76-1 **Sleep Study**			
Total sleep time (min)	400	Apnea–hypopnea index (AHI) (#/hr)	16.5
Rapid eye movement (min)	60	AHI non-REM (NREM) (#/hr)	16.5
Obstructive apnea (#)	25	AHI REM (#/hr)	0
Mixed apnea (#)	5	Desaturations (#)	110
Central apnea (#)	70	Low saturation of arterial oxygen	88%
Hypopnea (#)	10		

(#), Number; *min*, minutes.

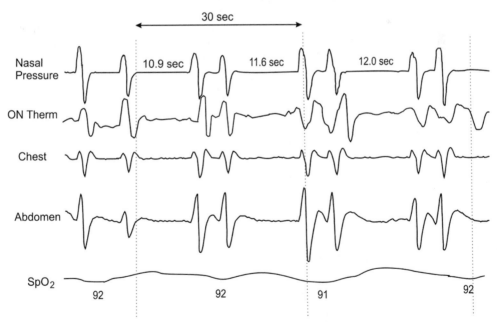

FIGURE P76-1 ■ Patient A: Tracing during non–rapid eye movement (NREM) sleep. ON Therm is an oronasal thermal airflow sensor. Inspiration is upward in this tracing.

Question 1: For patient A, what radiologic evaluation do you recommend?

Patient B: A 60-year-old man suffered a cerebrovascular accident (CVA). During recovery, he was noted to have repeated desaturations during the night. No history of prior snoring or witnessed apnea was present. The patient did not report daytime sleepiness.

Question 2: Is Patient B more likely to have OSA or central sleep apnea (CSA)? If CSA is present, will it have a Cheyne-Stokes morphology?

ANSWER

1. **Answer for Patient A:** Magnetic resonance imaging (MRI) to diagnose Chiari malformation (CM)

   Discussion: Sleep-related breathing disorders (SBDs) are common in both children and adults with CM. With the increased use of MRI, cases are often detected before symptoms begin. CM type I (CM-I) is defined as herniation of the cerebellar tonsils through the foramen magnum. CM-II involves caudal displacement of the vermis and is usually associated with myelodysplasia and meningomyelocele. In CM-I, obstructive apneas, central apneas, or a combination may occur. Nocturnal hypoventilation without discrete apneas may also be noted. A small minority of patients with CM-I have daytime hypercapnia. Presenting symptoms of CM include worsening of snoring, breathing pauses, headaches, neck pain, ataxia, occulomotor disturbances, scoliosis, and lower cranial nerve palsies. Although CM-I may present in infancy and childhood, the *most common presentation is in young adulthood between 20 and 40 years*. In many cases of CM, the neurologic examination is completely normal and often the only symptom is unexplained headache, especially with exertion. In some cases, after initial improvement with surgery, brainstem compression recurred, with recurrent sleep apnea being the only manifestation.

   Sleep apnea is believed to be caused by pressure on the medullary structures controlling the ventilation and upper airway muscles. Surgical decompression (posterior fossa decompression, duraplasty, and cervical laminectomy) often improves the degree of sleep apnea, although significant apnea may be present in the postoperative period. Some reports have described patients treated for obstructive hydrocephalus with shunts who experienced an acute worsening of sleep apnea as the only manifestation of shunt failure.

   CSA caused by CM is classified under "Central Apnea Due to a Medical Disorder without Cheyne-Stokes Breathing (CSB)" (Box P76-1). Other causes of CSA in this group include brainstem neoplasms and neurodegenerative disorders. In the current patient, the central apneas (see Figure P76-1) were unexpected, given the history of snoring. Although some obstructive apneas were present, central apneas *not* of the Cheyne-Stokes type were the most frequent events. MRI showed evidence of CM-1 malformation. After surgical decompression, a repeat sleep study showed an apnea–hypopnea index (AHI) of <5 per hour (hr), and the patient's headaches improved.

2. **Answer for Patient B:** Sleep apnea is common following a CVA, with OSA being more common than CSA. If CSA is present, a Cheyne-Stokes morphology is most commonly present.

   Discussion: Sleep apnea (obstructive or central) is present in 50% to 70% of patients during recovery following a stroke. It is unknown how many patients had sleep apnea before the stroke. OSA is the most common finding. CSA-CSB may be are present in up to 30% of patients in the first few days after the stroke. Central apnea tends to resolve and is less commonly seen in patients studied several months after stroke. Of interest, a recent study suggested that a significant proportion of CSA-CSB in patients after a stroke was caused by occult cardiovascular disease. CSA-CSB has been

---

BOX P76-1	**Central Apnea Due to a Medical Disorder without Cheyne-Stokes Breathing—ICSD-3 Diagnostic Criteria**

Criteria A-C must be met
A. The presence of one or more of the following
   i. Sleepiness
   ii. Difficulty initiating or maintaining sleep, frequent awakenings, or nonrestorative sleep
   iii. Awakening short of breath
   iv. Witnessed snoring
B. Polysomnography (PSG) shows all of the following:

   i. Five or more central apneas and/or or central hypopneas per hour of sleep
   ii. The number of central apneas and/or central hypopneas is >50% of the total number of apneas and hypopneas
   iii. Absence of Cheyne-Stokes breathing
C. The disorder occurs as a consequence of a *medical or neurologic* disorder but is not caused by medication use or substance use.

noted after damage to different portions of the brain, including lacunar strokes. Screening of all patients for sleep apnea following a CVA has been recommended by some authors, whereas others recommend a clinical evaluation for symptoms or signs of OSA and polysomnography (PSG) if clinical suspicion of sleep apnea exists. One study of continuous positive airway pressure (CPAP) in patients with CVA and OSA found improved survival with CPAP treatment. However, CPAP adherence tends to be low in patients with CVA and OSA. Further studies in this area are needed.

CLINICAL PEARLS

1. A diagnosis of CM should be considered in patients with unexplained CSA or a combination of OSA and CSA.

2. The appearance of headache (especially worsened with exertion) in young adults should alert the clinician to the possibility of CM.

3. In CM, the neurologic examination is frequently normal.

4. CSA in patients with CM often resolves are surgical decompression.

5. OSA is the most commonly observed type of sleep apnea following a stroke. However, CSA-CSB may be present in up to 30% of patients after a stroke. Central apneas tend to resolve with time.

BIBLIOGRAPHY

Chiari Malformation

Aarts LA, Willemsen MA, Vandenbussche NL, van Gent R: Nocturnal apnea in Chiari type I malformation, *Eur J Pediatr* 170 (10):1349–1352, 2011.

Cormican LJ, Higgins AC, Davidson R, et al: Multisystem atrophy presenting as central sleep apnea, *Eur Respir J* 24:323–325, 2004.

Dauvilleriers Y, Stal V, Coubes P, et al: Chiari malformation and sleep related breathing disorders, *J Neurol Neurosurg Psychiatry* 78:1344–1348, 2007.

Fernández AA(1), Guerrero AI, Martínez MI, et al: Malformations of the craniocervical junction (Chiari type I and syringomyelia: classification, diagnosis and treatment), *BMC Musculoskelet Disord* 10(1):S1, 2009.

Gagnadoux F, Meslier N, Svab I, et al: Sleep-disordered breathing in patients with Chiari malformation: improvement after surgery, *Neurology* 66(1):136–138, 2006.

Herschberger ML, Chidekel A: Arnold-Chiari malformation type I and sleep disordered breathing, *J Pediatr Health Care* 17:190–197, 2003.

Kesler R, Mendizabal JE: Headache in Chiari malformation: a distinct clinical entity? *J Am Osteopath Assoc* 99(3):153–156, 1999.

Murray C, Seton C, Prelog K, Fitzgerald DA: Arnold Chiari type 1 malformation presenting with sleep disordered breathing in well children, *Arch Dis Child* 91(4):342–343, 2006.

Zolty P, Sanders MH, Pollack IF: Chiari malformation and sleep-disordered breathing: a review of diagnostic and management issues, *Sleep* 23(5):637–643, 2000.

Cerebrovascular Accidents and Sleep Apnea

Bassetti CL, Milanova M, Gugger M: Sleep-disordered breathing and acute ischemic stroke: diagnosis, risk factors, treatment, evolution, and long-term clinical outcome, *Stroke* 37(4):967–972, 2006.

Bonnin-Vilaplana M, Arboix A, Parra O, et al: Cheyne-stokes respiration in patients with first-ever lacunar stroke, *Sleep Disord* 2012:257890, 2012.

Hermann DM, Siccoli M, Kirov P, et al: Central periodic breathing during sleep in ischemic stroke, *Stroke* 38:1082–1084, 2007.

Hermann DM, Bassetti CL: Sleep-related breathing and sleep-wake disturbances in ischemic stroke, *Neurology* 73 (16):1313–1322, 2009.

Martínez-García MA, Soler-Cataluña JJ, Ejarque-Martínez L, et al: Continuous positive airway pressure treatment reduces mortality in patients with ischemic stroke and obstructive sleep apnea: a 5-year follow-up study, *Am J Respir Crit Care Med* 180 (1):36–41, 2009.

Nopmaneejumruslers C, Kaneko Y, Hajek V, et al: Cheyne-Stokes respiration in stroke: relationship to hypocapnia and occult cardiac dysfunction, *Am J Respir Crit Care Med* 171:1048–1052, 2005.

Parra O, Arboix A, Bechich S, et al: Time course of sleep-related breathing disorders in first-ever stroke or transient ischemic attack, *Am J Respir Crit Care Med* 161(2 Pt 1):375–380, 2000.

Siccoli MM, Valko PO, Herman DM, Bassetti CL: Central periodic breathing during sleep in 74 patients with acute ischemic stroke, *J Neurol* 255:1687–1692, 2008.

Bilevel Positive Airway Pressure (BPAP) and Adaptive Servoventilation (ASV)

Patient A: A patient with a neuromuscular disorder is being treated with bilevel positive airway pressure (BPAP) in the spontaneous timed (ST) mode. The patient weights about 70 kilograms (kg) and is using a full-face mask. Nocturnal oximetry on BPAP showed that the arterial oxygen saturation (SaO_2) was less than 88% for 20 minutes. The patient comes to clinic for further evaluation with complaints of morning headache, and the following data are obtained from his BPAP (Table P77-1).

TABLE P77-1	**BPAP Download for Patient A**
IPAP/EPAP (cm H_2O)	10/4
Backup rate	12
Inspiratory time	1.6 seconds
Average use	6 hours 30 minutes
Average patient triggered breaths	95%
AHI	2.0
Average tidal volume	350 milliliters (mL)
Average respiratory rate	20
Average minute ventilation	7.0 liters per minute (L/min)

AHI, Apnea–hypopnea index; *cm H_2O*, centimeters of water; *EPAP*, expiratory positive airway pressure; *IPAP*, inspiratory positive airway pressure.

Question 1: At this point, which intervention is most appropriate?
  A. Increase EPAP
  B. Increase IPAP
  C. Increase backup rate
  D. Add supplemental oxygen to BPAP

Patients B: Patients B1, B2, and B3 are started on adaptive servoventilation (ASV). The device is to function in the mode in which EPAP is automatically adjusted. You are asked to supply treatment settings.

Patient B1. A 50-year-old man was diagnosed with obstructive sleep apnea (OSA) and central sleep apnea with Cheyne-Stokes breathing (CSA-CSB) resulting from congestive heart failure (CHF). He had severe OSA on the diagnostic portion of the study. During titration, continuous positive airway pressure (CPAP) of 12 cm H_2O was needed to maintain or eliminate obstructive events during rapid eye movement (REM) sleep. During non-REM (NREM) sleep, frequent CSA-CSB was noted.

Patient B2. A 50-year-old man was diagnosed with OSA and CSA-CSB resulting from CHF. During PAP titration, he had many central events of the CSB morphology. He was very pressure intolerant.

Patient B3. A 50-year-old man had OSA on the diagnostic portion of a sleep study and many central apneas during CPAP titration. The patient was on methadone for chronic pain. He also had a low sleeping SaO_2 on CPAP 90% to 92% even during periods when central apneas were not present. Awake arterial blood gas showed a partial pressure of carbon dioxide (PCO_2) of 48 mm Hg.

Question 2: Match the clinical scenario B1, B2, and B3 with reasonable ASV settings #1, #2, #3 (Table P77-2). Assume the maximum pressure (Pmax) = 25 cm H_2O, and rate setting is auto-rate.

TABLE P77-2 Possible ASV Setting for Patients B1, B2, and B3

Settings:	Default	#1	#2	#3
EPAPmin	4	4	8	4
EPAPmax	15	10	15	15
PSmin	0	4	0	8
PSmax	20	10	20	20

ASV, Adaptive servoventilation; *EPAP*, expiratory positive airway pressure; *PSmax*, maximum pressure support; *PSmin*, minimum pressure support.

Patients C:

Patient C1 has a neuromuscular disorder and is undergoing noninvasive positive pressure ventilation (NPPV). His awake respiratory rate is 12 breaths per minute. BPAP-ST is being used.

Patient C2 has kyphoscoliosis. He is being titrated with BPAP-ST. Assuming he will breathe 15 times per minute.

Patient C3 has both muscle weakness and moderate chronic obstructive pulmonary disease (COPD). He is being titrated with BPAP-ST. Assuming he will breathe 15 times per minute.

Question 3: What backup rate would you order for Patient C1? What Ti will you order for Patient C2? What Ti will you order for Patient C3?

ANSWERS

1. **Answer for Patient A:** B: Increase IPAP

   Discussion: The major findings are a low tidal volume and high respiratory rate. Although the arterial PCO_2 was not measured, the nocturnal desaturation and low tidal volume suggest sleep-related hypoventilation. Assuming the ideal body weight is 70 kg, the recommended tidal volume for NPPV should be at least 420 to 560 mL (6–8 mL/kg). An increase in tidal volume requires an increase in pressure support (IPAP-EPAP). Therefore, answer B is correct (increase IPAP). An increase in EPAP might be needed if the AHI were elevated but the machine estimate of the AHI is low, and therefore A is not correct. Answer C is not correct as an increase in tidal volume is the most efficient approach to increasing alveolar ventilation. The patient's respiratory rate is well above the backup rate and already quite high. Rapid shallow breathing is associated with large dead space ventilation. An increase in tidal volume will likely be associated with a fall in the spontaneous respiratory rate. The addition of supplemental oxygen may improve nocturnal oxygen saturation but does not address the need for support of ventilation (prevention of hypoventilation) in this patient. Therefore, answer C is not the best choice. In patient A, a PSG NPPV titration was ordered to determine the appropriate IPAP (Pressure Support). An alternative approach would be an empiric increase in IPAP (PS) with a repeat BPAP download (has tidal volume adequately increased) and nocturnal oximetry to determine if treatment was effective.

2. **Answers for Patient B:** B1: setting #2; B2: setting #1; B3: setting #3

   Discussion: The settings for ASV may be modified for individual patients. What follows are general guidelines. Sometimes, patients will not tolerate a pressure that theoretically should be effective.

   Patient B1 likely requires a high EPAP to maintain an open upper airway. Therefore, setting #2 (EPAPmin = 8 cm H_2O) is a reasonable initial setting. If PS = 0 and EPAPmin = 4 cm H_2O, the patient will actually start on CPAP of 4 cm H_2O. This may also be too low to be comfortable. If information about a prior titration is available and CPAP of <10 cm H_2O eliminated obstructive apneas, EPAPmin of 4 to 6 cm H_2O may be used. If CPAP >10 cm H_2O eliminated obstructive events on a previous study, EPAPmin of 6 to 8 cm H_2O may be used. If a previous study is not available, a higher EPAPmin may still be used for patients likely to need higher EPAP (large neck circumference). The choice of CPAP of 10 cm H_2O as the dividing line to make the EPAPmin determination is somewhat arbitrary.

Patient B2 is pressure intolerant so use of setting #1 (EPAPmin=4, PSmin=4 cm H_2O) is a reasonable approach. Use of PSmin=4 cm H_2O will allow use of a lower EPAP to keep the upper airway open. His starting pressure will be essentially BPAP 8/4 cm H_2O.

Patient B3 is on methadone and has mild daytime hypoventilation and suspected sleep-related hypoventilation on CPAP (low baseline SaO_2 when central apneas were not present). Use of setting #3 (PSmin=8 cm H_2O) is a reasonable approach. Using a high PSmin will help augment tidal volume and address hypoventilation. If the patient has a low baseline respiratory rate, hopefully the auto-rate will provide an effective backup rate. If this does not occur, one could switch to a fixed rate. If a fixed rate is used one needs to set a Ti (IPAPtime) when using the Philips-Respironics BiPAP AutoSV Advanced.

3. **Answers for Patients C:** C1: 10 breaths per minute; C2: Ti=1.6 seconds; C3: Ti=1.2 seconds

Discussion: These are merely guidelines for illustration, and the Ti may be adjusted during the study to match a patient's preferred inspiratory (IPAP) time and actual respiratory rate. The usual recommendation is to use a backup rate 1 to 2 breaths per minute lower than the spontaneous rate. However, should one use the awake or sleeping spontaneous rate? These are usually similar but could vary. A minimum backup rate of 8 to 10 is recommended when using BPAP-ST.

For Patient C1: Given a spontaneous rate of 12 breaths per minute, a backup rate of 10 for C1 is recommended.

For Patient C2: The IPAPtime or Ti depends on the cycle time (60/respiratory rate) and the %IPAPtime used for the particular patient type. The %IPAPtime = IPAPtime ×100/cycle time. A patient with a respiratory rate of 15 has a cycle time of 4 seconds (60/15). The %IPAP time is usually 30% to 40%. A %IPAPtime of 40% is used for chest wall disorders or for anyone with low respiratory system compliance. It may take time to deliver an adequate tidal volume. Patient C2 has a chest wall disorder; therefore the Ti = 0.4 × 4 = 1.6 seconds. A typical recommended value is 1.5 seconds.

Patient C3 has COPD. For patients with prolonged exhalation caused by chronic obstructive airway disease, a %IPAPtime of 30% is recommended to allow more time for exhalation.

For patient C3: This patient has COPD, and a longer expiratory time is needed. Ti = 0.3 × 4 = 1.2 seconds. These are merely guidelines for the clinical examples, and the Ti may be adjusted during the study to match a patient's preferred inspiratory (IPAP) time. These are merely guidelines and the Ti may be adjusted during the study to match a patient's preferred inspiratory (IPAP) time and actual respiratory rate.

BIBLIOGRAPHY

Berry RB, Chediak A, Brown LK, et al: NPPV Titration Task Force of the American Academy of Sleep Medicine: Best clinical practices for the sleep center adjustment of noninvasive positive pressure ventilation (NPPV) in stable chronic alveolar hypoventilation syndromes, *J Clin Sleep Med* 6(5):491–509, 2010.

Brown LK: Adpative servo-ventilation for sleep apnea: technology, titration protocols, and treatment efficacy, *Sleep Med Clin* 5 (30):419–439, 2010.

Javaheri S: Positive airway pressure treatment of central sleep apnea and emphasis on heart failure, opioids, and complex sleep apnea, *Sleep Med Clin* 5(3):407–418, 2010.

PATIENTS 78

Patients with a Neuromuscular Disorder

Patient A: A patient with a progressive neuromuscular disorder reported mild snoring and had a daytime partial pressure of arterial carbon dioxide ($PaCO_2$) of 42 mm Hg. However, nocturnal oximetry revealed an arterial oxygen saturation (SaO_2) $\leq 88\%$ for 15 minutes. Forced vital capacity (FVC) was 60% of predicted, and the maximum inspiratory force was 70 centimeters of water (cm H_2O).

Question 1: What do you recommend for Patient A?
A. Nocturnal supplemental oxygen
B. Diagnostic PSG and PSG for titration with continuous PAP (CPAP)
C. Diagnostic PSG and PSG for titration with BPAP
D. Diagnostic PSG and PSG for titration with BPAP-ST
E. Empiric treatment with BPAP-ST 8/4 cm H_2O and backup rate of 12 breaths per minute

Patient B: A patient with a progressive neuromuscular disorder is being treated with bilevel positive airway pressure (BPAP) in the spontaneous timed (ST) mode. The current treatment was chosen on the basis of a previous polysomnography (PSG) titration about 1 year ago. The patient weighs about 70 kilograms (kg) and is using a full-face mask. Nocturnal oximetry on bilevel positive airway pressure (BPAP) showed that the SaO_2 was less than 88% for 30 minutes. The patient came to the clinic for further evaluation with complaints of morning headaches, and the following data are obtained from his BPAP (Table P78-1).

TABLE P78-1 **BPAP-ST Download for Patient B**	
IPAP/EPAP (cm H_2O)	10/4
Backup rate	12
Inspiratory time	1.6 seconds
Average use	6 hours 30 minutes
Average patient triggered breaths	95%
AHI	2.0
Average tidal volume	300 milliliters (mL)
Average respiratory rate	25
Average minute ventilation	7.5 liters per minute (L/min)

AHI, Apnea–hypopnea index; *cm H_2O*, centimeters of water; *EPAP*, expiratory positive airway pressure; *IPAP*, inspiratory positive airway pressure.

Question 2: Would treatment with BPAP using the volume assured pressure mode be useful in for Patient B? If so, assuming a 70 kg ideal body weight, what initial AVAPS settings would you use during a NPPV titration?

ANSWERS

1. **Answer for Patient A:** D. Diagnostic PSG and PSG for titration with BPAP-ST

Discussion: The patient may have nocturnal hypoventilation, and noninvasive positive pressure ventilation (NPPV), rather than supplemental oxygen, is indicated for treatment of nocturnal hypoventilation. The patient also meets consensus criteria for the initiation of NPPV (Box P78-1). Some clinicians would begin empiric BPAP 8/4 cm H_2O, with upward titration, as indicated. However, diagnostic PSG is indicated to determine if obstructive sleep apnea (OSA), nocturnal hypoventilation, or both are present. If the nocturnal arterial oxygen desaturation is caused by OSA alone, treatment with CPAP may be considered. However, given that NPPV initiation is indicated, titration and treatment with BPAP, rather than CPAP, is probably the best answer. A titration with NPPV (BPAP-ST) may determine settings that would eliminate OSA events and effectively treat nocturnal hypoventilation as well as providing respiratory muscle rest. BPAP with a backup rate is recommended for patients with neuromuscular disorders, as they may not trigger IPAP/EPAP cycles because of weak muscles (especially during rapid eye movement [REM] sleep). A backup rate will also provide intervention for central apneas. When nocturnal oximetry is used to screen a patient with neuromuscular disease for abnormal nocturnal gas exchange, the presence of a sawtooth pattern, would suggest that sleep apnea is present (discrete events).

In the Box P78-1, consensus indications for use of NPPV in restrictive thoracic chest wall disease and neuromuscular disorders are listed. For both classes of the disorder, either an SaO_2 ≤88% for 5 or more minutes or evidence of awake hypoventilation ($PaCO_2 > 45$ mm Hg) is an indication for NPPV. For neuromuscular disorders, an inspiratory force less than 60 cm H_2O or forced vital

BOX P78-1	**Indications for Noninvasive Positive Pressure Ventilation Treatment in Restrictive Thoracic Chest Wall Disease (RTCD) and Neuromuscular Disease (NMD)**
RTCD	Symptoms of hypoventilation (morning headache, daytime somnolence) AND one of the following physiological criteria: Partial pressure of arterial carbon dioxide ($PaCO_2$) > 45 mm Hg (daytime) Nocturnal oximetry demonstrating an arterial oxygen saturation $\leq 88\%$ for 5 consecutive minutes or more
NMD	Symptoms of hypoventilation (morning headache, daytime somnolence) AND one of the following physiological criteria: $PaCO_2$ > 45 mm Hg (daytime) Nocturnal oximetry $SaO_2 \leq 88\%$ for 5 consecutive minutes or more Forced vital capacity (FVC) <50% of predicted Maximal inspiratory pressure <60 centimeters of water (cm H_2O)

Adapted from American College of Chest Physicians: Clinical indications for noninvasive positive pressure ventilation in chronic respiratory failure due to restrictive lung disease, COPD, and nocturnal hypoventilation—a consensus conference report, *Chest* 116:521–534, 1999.
Note: Today most clinicians use a cumulative time with a SaO_2 <=88% rather than a consecutive time.

capacity (FVC) <50% of predicted is also an indication NPPV. In both cases, a requirement of symptoms (morning headache, daytime sleepiness, nocturnal dyspnea) also exists. Clinical judgment is needed for the best time to start NPPV and depends on the prognosis for disease progression and patient preferences. An FVC <50% of predicted is considered severe, and some degree of nocturnal hypoventilation or arterial oxygen desaturation would be expected. However, studies have shown that considerable nocturnal desaturation may occur in patients with FVC >50% of predicted (Figure P78-1).

Other factors such as obesity, coexistent sleep apnea, or underlying lung disease likely have a role in the etiology of nocturnal oxygen desaturation. In patients who have bulbar muscle involvement, making an effective mouth seal for FVC or an inspiratory force maneuver may be difficult. In these patients, a sniff nasal inspiratory force (SNIF) is measured with a pressure catheter inserted into one nostril through the center of a soft plug that occludes the nostril. The catheter is attached to a pressure transducer and the other nostril occluded (with the help of the individual taking the measurement). The SNIF has been found to be useful in predicting outcome. In a study by Morgan et al, a SNIF less than 40 cm H_2O was significantly related to nocturnal hypoxemia. When SNIF was less than 40 cm H_2O, the hazard ratio for death was 9.1 times higher, and median survival was 6 months. A study by Bourke et al is widely quoted as showing a survival advantage with the use of NPPV in patients with amyotrophic lateral sclerosis (ALS). However, careful review of the study shows that the control group (standard of care group) had a very high early mortality, raising doubts about the

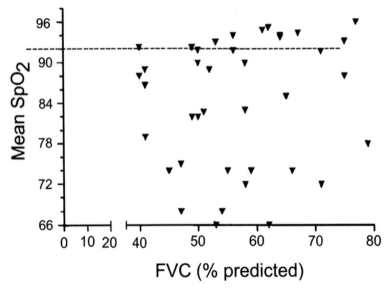

FIGURE P78-1 ■ Mean nocturnal saturation of arterial oxygen (SpO_2) versus forced vital capacity (FVC) as a percent of predicted in patients with amyotrophic lateral sclerosis (ALS). Considerable arterial oxygen desaturation can be seen at FVC values above 50% of predicted. (From Morgan RS, McNally S, Alexander M, et al: Use of sniff nasal inspiratory force to predict survival in amyotrophic lateral sclerosis, *Am J Respir Crit Care Med* 171:269-274, 2005.)

validity of the findings. However, even if NPPV does not prolong survival, it certainly may improve the quality of life in patients with ALS.

In chest wall disorders such as kyphoscoliosis, very high pressure support may be needed to provide recommended tidal volumes of 6 to 8 mL/kg (e.g., pressure support (PS) = 20 cm H_2O). In some patients, using a lower tidal volume and a higher-than-spontaneous backup rate may prove more effective. In patients with neuromuscular and chest wall disorders, the most severe desaturations invariably occur during REM sleep (Figure P78-2).

Early in the course of the disease, patients with disorders associated with chronic hypoventilation may have sleep-related hypoventilation with a normal awake $PaCO_2$. As the disease progresses, daytime hypoventilation may develop. The goal of NPPV is to intervene early before daytime hypoventilation develops. Although oximetry is a useful screening tool, PSG provides considerably more information about the presence or absence of sleep apnea. Use of end-tidal PCO_2 or transcutaneous PCO_2 monitoring may detect sleep-related hypoventilation. Attended NPPV PSG titration allows adjustment of mask, pressure, and backup rate to treat both OSA and nocturnal hypoventilation.

In the current patient, the FVC was >50% of predicted, but SaO_2 was ≤88% for 31 minutes, suggesting both desaturation and the possibility of hypoventilation. During the diagnostic portion, the SaO_2 fell to 80% during NREM sleep and 75% during REM sleep. No discrete events were noted, except during REM sleep. Transcutaneous PCO_2 during wake was 43 mm Hg and >55 mm Hg for 90 minutes during sleep in the diagnostic portion. At this point, an NPPV titration was initiated, and on BPAP of 16/4 cm H_2O, the SaO_2 normalized, and the transcutaneous PCO_2 dropped to 50 mm Hg.

2. **Answer for Patient B:** Volume Assured Pressure Support would be reasonable. Initial settings for AVAPS might include a target tidal volume of 560 mL, EPAP 4 cm H_2O, IPAPmin = 8 cm H_2O, IPAPmax = 25 cm H_2O, ST mode, and Ti = 1.5 seconds would be reasonable initial settings.

Discussion: The major finding in Table P78-1 is a *low tidal volume and high respiratory rate*. Rapid shallow breathing is associated with large dead space ventilation (inefficient mode of breathing) (Table P78-2) and is often a sign of respiratory muscle weakness or high respiratory system impedance (stiff chest wall or massive obesity). Although the arterial PCO_2 was not measured during sleep, the nocturnal desaturation and low tidal volume suggested the presence of sleep-related hypoventilation. Assuming the ideal body weight is 70 kg, the recommended tidal volume for NPPV should be at least 420 to 560 mL (6 to 8 mL/kg). An increase in tidal volume requires an increase in pressure support (IPAP-EPAP). In patient B one approach during an NPPV titration would be to increase the IPAP to 12 cm H_2O, then progressively higher as needed. As the AHI was not elevated (Table P78-1), a starting EPAP of 4 cm H_2O (current level) would be reasonable.

As the major goal of treatment in NPPV is to augment tidal volume and alveolar ventilation, it is desirable to keep the EPAP is low as possible so that an adequate PS will not result in a very high peak pressure. For example, 15/5 might be better tolerated that 20/10 cm H_2O. The initial setting for the backup rate in a NPPV titration is usually 1 to 2 breaths per minute below the spontaneous rate. The respiratory rate on download in Patient B was 25 per minute. One would expect the

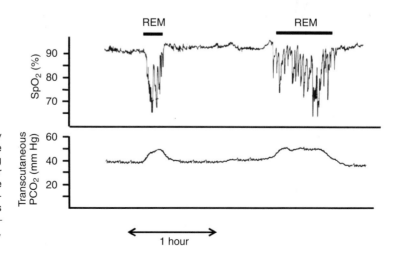

FIGURE P78-2 ■ Nocturnal oximetry and transcutaneous partial pressure of carbon dioxide (PCO_2) monitoring in a patient with a neuromuscular disorder. During non–rapid eye movement (NREM) sleep the saturation of arterial oxygen (SpO_2) was normal. (From Berry RB: *Fundamentals of sleep medicine*, Philadelphia, 2012, Saunders, p 400.)

respiratory rate to decrease considerably if tidal volume increased with higher pressures support. Therefore a backup rate of 12 to 15 bpm might be a reasonable starting point. The rate could be adjusted during a NPPV titration.

In patients who are likely to undergo a progressive deterioration of muscle strength, use of volume assured pressure support (AVAPS, Philips Respironics) or Intelligent Volume Pressure Support (iVAPs, ResMed) are viable options. Using AVAPS, the target tidal volume (8 mL/kg ideal weight), EPAP, mode S, ST, T and IPAP range (IPAPmin = EPAP + 4, IPAPmax) are specified (see Fundamentals 30). For Patient B, a tidal volume of 560 mL, EPAP 4 cm H_2O, IPAPmin 8 cm H_2O, IPAPmax 25 cm H_2O, and the ST mode (backup rate 15 breaths per minute) with Ti 1.5 seconds would be reasonable initial titration settings (see Table P78-2). During the titration the EPAP and backup rate could be adjusted. If pressure intolerance is noted, the target tidal volume could be reduced. From the current download, we know that EPAP of 4 cm H_2O was effective (AHI 2/hr).

Patient B was offered a PSG AVAPS titration but declined. Empirical treatment with AVAPS-ST was initiated using the above settings. However, the patient complained of excessive pressure and the target tidal volume was reduced to 510 mL. A download after 1 month showed that tidal volumes were near the target, and the average pressure support was 8 cm H_2O. The average rate was 14 breaths per minute. The backup rate was reduced to 12 breaths per minute. Table P78-2 shows that the use of a higher tidal volume and lower respiratory rate delivered a higher alveolar ventilation with a lower minute ventilation and lower dead space ventilation. Nocturnal oximetry on AVAPS revealed no time with a SaO_2 at or below 88%. Rather than use of AVAPS one could have progressively increased the pressure support on an outpatient basis until the tidal volume reached the desired range.

TABLE P78-2   **Minute and Alveolar Ventilation at Different Tidal Volumes and Rates**

	Tidal Volume	Respiratory Rate	Minute Ventilation (MV)	Dead Space Vd (mL)	Dead Space Ventilation (mL/min) (DMV)	Alveolar Ventilation (mL/min) = MV − DMV
On BPAP 10/4	300	25	7500	150 ml	3750	3750
On AVAPS	510	14	7140	150	2100	5340

Alveolar ventilation = Minute ventilation − Dead space ventilation. Minute ventilation = Tidal volume × RR. Dead space ventilation = Dead space volume × RR.
Vd (dead space volume) is assumed to be equal to the person's weight in pounds.
RR, Respiratory rate.

CLINICAL PEARLS

1. The standard indications for initiation of noninvasive positive pressure ventilation (NPPV) in a patient with neuromuscular weakness are FVC <50% of predicted or a maximum inspiratory pressure <60 cm H_2O. However, a considerable number of patients not meeting these criteria will have significant nocturnal desaturation. Nocturnal oximetry may be a useful screening tool. If the nocturnal oximetry reveals $SaO_2 \leq 88$ for more than 5 minutes, NPPV is also "indicated." However, the initiation of NPPV depends on the clinical situation and the patient's preferences.

2. The goal of NPPV is to improve alveolar ventilation and oxygenation during sleep while reducing the work of breathing and providing respiratory muscle rest. Ideally NPPV should be begun before daytime hypoventilation develops.

3. PS should be adjusted to augment tidal volume. The usual goal is 6 to 8 mL/kg of ideal body weight.

4. A ventilatory pattern of rapid shallow breathing produces a low alveolar ventilation for a given minute ventilation. This pattern of breathing results in a large amount of dead space ventilation.

5. Evidence of improvement following an increase in PS is an increase in tidal volume to an acceptable level (6 to 8 mL/kg) and a decrease in respiratory rate.

6. Volume-assured pressure support (VAPS) modes of BPAP are potentially useful in treating patients with progressive hypoventilation disorders. The level of pressure support adapts to the changing condition of the patient.

7. Daytime hypoventilation would also be an indication to begin NPPV in a patient with neuromuscular disease, but ideally NPPV should be initiated before daytime hypoventilation has developed.

BIBLIOGRAPHY

American College of Chest Physicians: Clinical indications for noninvasive positive pressure ventilation in chronic respiratory failure due to restrictive lung disease, COPD, and nocturnal hypoventilation—a consensus conference report, *Chest* 116:521–534, 1999.

Berry RB, Chediak A, Brown LK, et al: NPPV Titration Task Force of the American Academy of Sleep Medicine: Best clinical practices for the sleep center adjustment of noninvasive positive pressure ventilation (NPPV) in stable chronic alveolar hypoventilation syndromes, *J Clin Sleep Med* 6(5):491–509, 2010.

Bourke SC, Tomlinson M, Williams TL, et al: Effects of non-invasive ventilation on survival and quality of life in patients with amyotrophic lateral sclerosis: a randomized controlled trial, *Lancet Neurol* 5:140–147, 2006.

Budweiser S, Heinemann F, Fischer W, et al: Impact of ventilation parameters and duration of ventilator use on non-invasive home ventilation in restrictive thoracic disorders, *Respiration* 73:488–494, 2006.

Gonzalez C, Ferris G, Diaz J, et al: Kyphoscoliotic ventilatory insufficiency: effects of long-term intermittent positive-pressure ventilation, *Chest* 124:857–862, 2003.

Gruis KL, Brown DL, Lisabeth LD, et al: Longitudinal assessment of noninvasive positive pressure ventilation adjustments in ALS patients, *J Neurol Sci* 247:59–63, 2006.

Morgan RS, McNally S, Alexander M, et al: Use of sniff nasal inspiratory force to predict survival in amyotrophic lateral sclerosis, *Am J Respir Crit Care Med* 171:269–274, 2005.

Perrin C, D'Ambrosio C, White A, Hill NS: Sleep in restrictive and neuromuscular respiratory disorders, *Semin Respir Crit Care Med* 26:117–130, 2005.

Storre JH, Seuthe B, Fiechter R, et al: Average volume-assured pressure support in obesity hypoventilation: a randomized crossover trial, *Chest* 130(3):815–821, 2006.

Diagnosis of RLS and PLMD

RESTLESS LEG SYNDROME (WILLIS-EKBOM DISEASE), PERIODIC LIMB MOVEMENTS IN SLEEP, AND THE PERIODIC LIMB MOVEMENT DISORDER—DIAGNOSIS

The restless legs syndrome (RLS), periodic limb movements in sleep (PLMS), and the periodic limb movement disorder (PLMD) are three distinct but related entities.[1-5] (Table F31-1). A diagnosis of RLS is based on clinical history. PLMS is a polysomnography (PSG) finding that may or may not be clinically important. PLMD is diagnosed in patients with PLMS on PSG, who have a sleep complaint (sleep-onset or maintenance insomnia or, less commonly, daytime sleepiness) that is not better explained by another sleep disorder. A diagnosis of RLS excludes a diagnosis of PLMD. PLMS is a very common finding especially in older patients and is often asymptomatic.[3] Approximately 80% to 90% of patients with RLS will have findings of PLMS on PSG.[1] The percentage of patients with PLMS who have RLS has not been

well defined, but the vast majority of patients with PLMS do not have RLS. PLMS has been associated with narcolepsy, the rapid eye movement (REM) sleep behavior disorder, and obstructive sleep apnea (OSA). PLMS is very common, RLS is common, and PLMD is thought to be rare. Fundamentals 16 outlined the criteria for scoring PLMS with illustrative tracings. This chapter emphasizes the clinical significance of PLMS and discusses RLS and PLMD.

RESTLESS LEGS SYNDROME

The four essential diagnostic criteria for RLS are known by the acronym URGE = **U**rge to move, **R**est induced, **G**ets better with activity, **E**vening and night worse.

The Essential RLS Diagnostic Criteria (Box F31-1 and F31-2)[2,4,5]

1. An *urge to move the legs* is usually accompanied or caused by uncomfortable and unpleasant sensations in the legs. Of note,

TABLE F31-1	Different Leg Movement Conditions		
	RLS	**PLMS**	**PLMD**
Diagnosis	History	PSG	PSG + History
Prevalence	Common	Very common Asymptomatic individuals Narcolepsy REM sleep behavior disorder OSA	Rare
PSG findings	~80% have PLMS	PLMS present	PLMS index >5/hr children >15/hour adults
Relationship with other leg movement conditions	A diagnosis of RLS excludes a diagnosis of PLMD	PSG finding not a disorder Usually asymptomatic or symptoms are not due to PLMS RLS not reported by many patients but a clue to explore RLS symptoms	Not diagnosed if RLS is present Must exclude other causes of insomnia or daytime sleepiness

OSA, Obstructive sleep disorder; *PLMD*, periodic limb movement disorder; *PLMS*, periodic limb movement during sleep; *PSG*, polysomnography; *REM*, rapid eye movement; *RLS*, restless leg syndrome.

the urge to move may be present without associated symptoms. Commonly reported RLS sensations are listed in Box F31-1. Although called *restless legs syndrome*, symptoms may occur in the arms as well as the legs in 30% to 50% of the patients.[2,4,5] Although RLS symptoms are usually bilateral, some patients report symptoms mainly in one extremity. About 20% of patients with RLS report the leg sensations to be painful. Involuntary leg movements may also be reported without an urge to move ("the legs just move on their own").

2. RLS symptoms *begin or worsen* during periods of inactivity such as lying or sitting. Being stationary and having decreased mental activity appear to worsen symptoms.

3. The urge to move or unpleasant sensations are totally or partially relieved by movements such as walking or stretching as long as the activity continues (temporary relief). Rubbing the legs or taking hot or cold baths may improve symptoms in some patients. Of note, increased mental activity or eating may improve the symptoms ("popcorn therapy" while watching a movie).

4. The urge to move or unpleasant sensations are worse in the evening or night. If RLS has become very severe, nocturnal worsening may not be reported but should have been present earlier in the disease course. When RLS is severe, daytime symptoms may occur especially during periods of inactivity.

The *International Classification of Sleep Disorders*, 3rd Edition (ICSD-3) diagnostic criteria for RLS[4] (see Box F31-2) added the additional stipulation that the symptoms of RLS are not *solely accounted for* as symptoms primary to another medical or a behavioral condition (e.g., leg cramps, positional discomfort, myalgia, venous stasis, leg edema, arthritis, habitual foot tapping). The addition was based in part on a study by Hening et al[6] that found 16% of RLS "mimics" could satisfy all four RLS diagnostic criteria. If patients describe their symptoms entirely associated with leg cramps, it is not RLS. If symptoms are present only in certain body positions such as crossed legs, it is more likely to be positional discomfort and less likely to be RLS. If patients describe symptoms as

---

BOX F31-1	Common Descriptions of Abnormal Sensations in Restless Legs Syndrome

- Creepy, crawly
- Ants crawling under the skin
- Worms crawling in the veins
- Pepsi-Cola in the veins
- Nervous feet "gotta move"
- Itching under the skin, itchy bones
- Crazy legs/Elvis legs
- Tooth ache feeling— can't leave it alone
- Excited nerves, electric-like shocks
- Painful sensation in 20%
- Sensation involves arms in 50%

BOX F31-2	ICSD-3 Diagnostic Criteria for RLS (Willis-Ekbom Disease)

The diagnosis of restless legs syndrome (RLS) requires the report of a strong, nearly irresistible urge to move the legs (criterion A) that must have all of the characteristics of criterion A (i-iii). In addition, the sensory symptoms cannot be solely attributable to another condition (criterion B). Clinical significance is specified by criterion C.

A. An urge to move the legs, usually but not always accompanied by or felt to be caused by uncomfortable and unpleasant sensations in the legs.* These symptoms must:
  i. begin or worsen during periods of rest or inactivity such as lying down or sitting; and

  ii. be partially or totally relieved by movement, such as walking or stretching, at least as long as the activity continues[†]; and
  iii. occur exclusively or predominantly in the evening or night rather than during the day.[‡]
B. The occurrence of the above features are not *solely accounted for* as symptoms primary to another medical or a behavioral condition (e.g., leg cramps, positional discomfort, myalgia, venous stasis, leg edema, arthritis, habitual foot tapping).
C. The symptoms of RLS cause concern, distress, sleep disturbance, or impairment in mental, physical, social, occupational, educational, behavioral, or other important areas of functioning.[§]

Adapted from American Academy of Sleep Medicine: *International classification of sleep disorders*, ed 3, Darien, IL, 2014, American Academy of Sleep Medicine.

Notes:

*Sometimes the urge to move the legs is present without the uncomfortable sensations, and sometimes the arms or other parts of the body are involved in addition to the legs. For children, the description of these symptoms should be in the child's own words.

†When symptoms are very severe, relief by activity may not be noticeable but must have been previously present.

‡With treatment or treatment-induced augmentation, or when symptoms are very severe, the worsening in the evening or night may not be noticeable but must have been previously present.

§For certain research applications such as genetic or epidemiologic studies, it may be appropriate to omit criterion C. If so, this should be clearly stated in the research report.

painful and associated with a localized problem area (painful joint, leg edema) or painful in a pattern consistent with a radiculopathy or neuropathy (numbness in specific area), it is less likely to be RLS. Individuals with RLS are very aware of leg movements. If individuals report pronounced or frequent unconscious foot or leg movements (e.g., hypnic jerks, habitual foot taping, leg shaking, general nervous movements) it is likely not RLS. RLS symptoms are more likely to be described as *irresistible* or a cause of sleep disturbance. Patients with RLS to not tolerate confinement (e.g., long airplane journey). Some mimics of RLS may get better with walking. Table F31-2 lists a series of questions (Cambridge-Hopkins RLS questionnaire) that have been shown to be sensitive and specific for a diagnosis of RLS.[7]

Supportive Clinical Features

Supportive clinical features of RLS including (1) a family history of RLS (reported in 30% to 50% of patients), (2) a response to dopaminergic treatment, and (3) the presence of PLMS may help resolve diagnostic uncertainty but are not required for a diagnosis. An improvement with a trial of dopaminergic treatment is evidence that symptoms represent the RLS. However, placebo-controlled studies in RLS report considerable improvement in symptoms with

inactive medication. The PLMS index (PLMSI) is defined as the number of periodic limb movements per hour (hr) of sleep. It is difficult to define a normal PLMSI. In the past, some sleep centers considered a PLMSI >5/hr to be abnormal. However, many asymptomatic individuals have much higher PLMSI values.[3,8] One study employing a PLMSI cutoff of 5/hr reported that 80.2% of patients with RLS had PLMS (87% if two nights were monitored).[1] Patients with RLS often report repetitive involuntary leg movements during wakefulness when at rest, especially at night. This is a manifestation of periodic limb movement during wakefulness (PLMW).

Causes of RLS

RLS is often divided into primary RLS (independent of other disorders, cause unknown) and secondary RLS (caused by an identifiable factor such as a medical disorder, condition, or medication). The common causes of secondary RLS are listed in Box F31-3. RLS associated with renal failure is not helped by dialysis and is cured by renal transplantation. RLS of pregnancy commonly vanishes or improves following delivery. If the onset of RLS is associated with the start of a given medication, a switch to an alternate medication may be tried. For example, if a selective serotonin reuptake inhibitor (SSRI) is

---

TABLE F31-2 **Critical Diagnostic Questions from the Cambridge Hopkins Restless Legs Questionnaire CH-RLSq**

Questions:	Answers	Definite RLS
1. Do you have, or have you had, recurrent uncomfortable feelings or sensations in your legs while you are sitting or lying down?	_ Yes _ No	Yes
2. Do you, or have you had, a recurrent need or urge to move your legs while you were sitting or lying down?	_ Yes _ No	Yes
3. Are you more likely to have these feelings when you are resting (either sitting or lying down) or when you are physically active?	_ Resting _ Active	Resting
4. If you get up or move around when you have these feelings do these feelings get any better while you actually keep moving?	Yes _ No _ Don't know	Yes
5. Which times of day are these feelings in your legs **least** likely to occur?	(Please circle one or more than one) _ Morning _ Mid-day _ Afternoon _ Evening _ Night _ About equal at all times	NOT equal or morning
6. Will simply changing leg position by itself once without continuing to move usually relieve these feelings?	_ Usually relieves _ Does not usually relieve _ Don't know	Does not usually relieve
7a. Are these feelings ever due to muscle cramps?	_ Yes _ No _ Don't know	NO (or 7b)
7b. If so, are they always due to muscle cramps?	_ Yes _ No _ Don't know	NO

Allen RP, Burchell BJ, Ben MacDonald B, et al: Validation of the self-completed Cambridge-Hopkins questionnaire (CH-RLSq) for ascertainment of restless legs syndrome (RLS) in a population survey, *Sleep Med* 10:1097–1100, 2009.

BOX F31-3	Causes of RLS

- Primary RLS (idiopathic, often familial)
- Secondary RLS
  - Iron deficiency
  - Pregnancy
  - Neuropathy—diabetic and others
  - Multiple sclerosis
  - Renal failure
  - Parkinson disease
- Medications
  - First-generation (sedating) antihistamines (e.g., diphenhydramine)
  - Antinausea medication—prochlorperazine
  - Dopamine receptor blockers—metoclopramide
  - Antidepressants (SSRIs, SNRIs)—exception is bupropion

RLS, Restless legs syndrome; *SNRI*, serotonin–norepinephrine reuptake inhibitor; *SSRI*, selective serotonin reuptake inhibitor.

believed to worsen RLS, switching to bupropion, an antidepressant that does not worsen RLS, may be considered.[9] Of interest, first-generation antihistamines such as diphenhydramine (contained in many over-the-counter [OTC] sleep aids) may worsen RLS.

Epidemiology of RLS

The prevalence of RLS in adults has been estimated at approximately 5% to 10%. RLS is approximately *1.5 to 2 times more common in women than in men*. It is believed that most of the increased incidence may be attributed to the increase in RLS during pregnancy. RLS may begin at any age and the clinical course is variable. One pattern is an early onset (age <50 years) characterized by insidious onset, less severity, and higher familial association. A late onset RLS (age >50 years) is characterized by a more abrupt onset and more severe manifestations. Patients with late-onset RLS also tend to have lower ferritin levels compared with patients with early-onset RLS.

Sleep Disturbance Associated with RLS

The two most common complaints that cause patients with RLS to seek medical attention are the *uncomfortable leg sensations* and the *disturbance of sleep*. Beyond the significant discomfort caused by RLS symptoms, the disorder may cause difficulty with sleep initiation and maintenance. In a group of patients with RLS and symptoms on at least two nights a week, sleep-related symptoms (prolonged sleep latency or awakenings) were present in 43.4%, but only 6% complained of daytime sleepiness.[10] RLS symptoms may prolong sleep latency. If the patient awakens, return to sleep may also be delayed by RLS symptoms. Because the majority of patients with RLS have PLMS, it might be assumed that patients with a higher PLMSI or PLMS arousal index might have more sleep disturbance. However, the PLMSI is not highly correlated with any measure of sleep disturbance in most studies of patients with RLS.

Medical Evaluation in RLS

The diagnostic evaluation should include a history to elicit the essential and associated features of RLS. A detailed medication history including OTC medications (sedating antihistamines worsen RLS) is very important. Physical examination should look for signs of neuropathy. Laboratory studies should check renal and thyroid function. A serum iron level, total iron-binding capacity (TIBC), % iron saturation, and ferritin levels should be checked. Ferritin is the most useful single test. However, ferritin may be elevated by inflammatory processes, and ordering both ferritin level and % iron saturation and TIBC is recommended.[11-13] If the ferritin level is less than 45 to 50 micrograms (mcg), or the iron saturation is less than 20%, iron supplementation may improve symptoms and/or treatment efficacy.[11-13] PSG is *not* required in most cases of RLS unless sleep apnea or another sleep disorder is suspected. Of note, abnormal movements during sleep, including leg kicks, may occur with OSA, epilepsy, and the REM sleep behavior disorder. As noted previously, daytime sleepiness is *not* a common symptom of RLS, and the presence of this symptom should prompt consideration of disorders other than RLS. A combination of sleep disorders, for example, RLS and sleep apnea, is common.

PSG Findings in Patients with RLS

In a study of 133 patients with RLS, it was found that the PLMSI was greater than 5/hr in 80.2% of RLS patients.[1] The *PLMSI did increase with RLS severity*. A significant correlation also existed between the PLMSI and the PLMW index (PLMWI). However, no correlation existed between the PLMSI and measures of sleep disturbance such as sleep efficiency and nocturnal awakenings. Another study found a weak correlation between the PLMS arousal index and RLS severity in only one of two groups of unmedicated patients with RLS.[14] Therefore, PLMS does not appear to be a major cause of sleep disturbance in most patients with RLS. *The major importance of an elevated PLMSI is to alert the clinician to the possibility of RLS.*

RLS in Children

RLS may be difficult to diagnose in children.[15,16] In some children, the complaint is the presence of typical RLS symptoms and in others "growing pains" or simply difficulty "sitting still." The Peds REST study found criteria for definite RLS in 1.9% of children age 8 to 11 years and 2% in adolescents age 12 to 17 years.[16] Of note, PLMS is less common in children, and a PLMSI of ≥5/hr is considered abnormal. Some children with attention deficit hyperactivity disorder (ADHD) have PLMS and possible RLS, and vice versa. The relationship of RLS and ADHD remains to be determined.

PERIODIC LIMB MOVEMENTS IN SLEEP

In the earlier descriptions of PLMS, the phenomenon was referred to as *nocturnal myoclonus*, but this terminology is no longer used. The diagnostic criteria for scoring PLMS in presented in Fundamental 16.

The ICSD, first edition[17], listed the following grading of the severity of PLMs: PLMSI <5/hr normal, 5–24/hr mild, 25–49/hr moderate, and ≥50/hr severe. However, these cutoffs are entirely arbitrary and are not based on any outcome data. Given the high prevalence of PLMS in asymptomatic individuals, an absolute separating the asymptomatic population from the symptomatic population is not available. In the ICSD-3, a PLMSI >15/hr in adults and >5/hr in children is part of the diagnostic criteria for PLMD. However, asymptomatic individuals may have quite high PLMSI values (Figure F31-1). PLMs occur most commonly in stage N1 and N2 but may also occur in stage N3 or, less commonly, during stage R sleep.[18,19] The PLMSI is often higher during the first part of the night. Culpepper and colleagues[19] described two patterns of PLMS. In one pattern, PLMS was much more common in the first part of the night. In the second pattern, PLMS was more evenly distributed through the night. The interval between individual PLMs increases from stage N1 to stage N3. PLMs are less likely to cause arousal from stage N3 sleep. Frequent *PLMs have been described during REM sleep in patients with the REM sleep behavior disorder (RBD) and narcolepsy.*[20,21]

PLMS and Arousals

An individual PLM and an arousal are considered to be associated with each other if they are overlapping or if there is 0.5 seconds or less from the end of one event to the onset of the

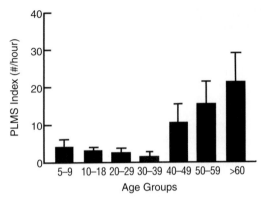

FIGURE F31-1 ■ Mean periodic limb movements during sleep (PLMS) index (# events/hr of sleep) at different ages for normal healthy individuals. The average PLMS index increases in older individuals. (From Pennestri M, Whittom S, Adam B, et al: PLMS and PLMW in healthy subjects as a function of age: prevalence and interval distribution, Sleep 29:1183-1187, 2006.)

other event regardless of which is first.[22] The PLMS arousal index is the number of PLMS arousals per hour of sleep. No widely accepted normal values exist for the PLMS arousal index. The ICSD-1[16] listed a PLMS arousal index of ≥25/hr as severe. One study looking at the association of PLMs and arousals found that 49% of electroencephalography (EEG) arousals occurred before PLMs, 30.6% simultaneously, and 23.2% occurred just after the limb movements.[23] PLMs may often be associated with K-complexes or delta-bursts that do not meet the criteria for cortical arousal. Of note, autonomic changes (increase in heart rate, increase in blood pressure, change in pulse transit time) may occur in association with the PLMs with and without cortical arousals.

Differential Diagnosis of PLMS

The differential of other periodic movements includes hypnagogic foot tremor (HFT), alternating leg movement activities (ALMAs), excessive fragmentary myoclonus, and the rhythmic movement disorder. The reader is referred to Fundamental 16 for more details on these entities.

Clinical Significance of the PLMSI and the PLMS Arousal Index

The clinical significance of PLMS and the utility of monitoring limb movements have been the subject of controversy.[24,25] The utility of counting PLMS arousals has also been questioned because the index does not appear to correlate with subjective measures of disturbed sleep, daytime sleepiness, or the sense of nonrestorative sleep. Claman and associates[8] studied 455 community-dwelling older women and found that 66% had a PLMSI >5/hr and 52% >15/hr. The associations between the PLMSI and the PLMS arousal index with measures of sleep quality were determined. The associations were adjusted for age, body mass index (BMI), apnea–hypopnea index (AHI), and antidepressant medication use. An increased PLMSI was associated with a statistically significant higher total arousal index but not impairment of other indices of sleep quality. A higher PLMS arousal index was associated with lower total sleep time, less stage N3, and a higher total arousal index. However, neither a higher PLMSI nor the PLMS arousal index was associated with worse subjective daytime sleepiness by Epworth Sleepiness Scale (ESS). It remains to be determined whether determination of the PLMS arousal index really adds anything of clinical significance to other measures of sleep quality.

PLMS and Other Disorders

PLMS is common in a number of disorders other than RLS including narcolepsy, RBD, neuropathy of diverse etiology, and OSA.[20,21,26] An increase in the PLMSI on continuous positive airway pressure (CPAP) compared with baseline was noted in a study of patients with OSA by Fry et al.[27] Chervin and colleagues[28] evaluated 1124 patients with suspected or confirmed OSA and found that 24% of the patients with OSA had a PLMSI >5/hr. In most patients diagnosed with OSA on a sleep study, the incidental finding of PLMS is usually of no or limited clinical significance. *It should prompt the clinician to check for symptoms of RLS.*

PERIODIC LIMB MOVEMENT DISORDER

In this disorder, PLMS, as described previously, results in clinical sleep disturbance (sleep maintenance insomnia), daytime sleepiness, or fatigue. The clinical symptoms are not better explained by another primary sleep disorder. Thus, the diagnosis depends on PSG to demonstrate PLMS and exclusion of other causes of the symptoms by a clinical history and PSG (Box F31-4). Recall that a diagnosis of RLS excludes a diagnosis of PLMD. The mere presence of a sleep complaint and PLMS does not make a diagnosis of PLMD. Symptoms and PLMS must be causally related and other causes of sleep disturbance ruled out. The reader should carefully read the noted in Box F31-4.

Prevalence and Manifestations of PLMD

Although PLMS is common, PLMD is thought to be rare. The exact prevalence of the PLMD is unknown.[14] Patients rarely are aware that they have PLMS until informed by their bed partner. The disturbance of the bed partner's sleep because of the other person's PLMS is thought

---

BOX F31-4	ICSD-3 Diagnostic Criteria: Periodic Limb Movement Disorder

A. Polysomnography demonstrates PLMS, as defined in the most recent version of the American Academy of Sleep Medicine (AASM) Manual for the Scoring of Sleep and Associated Events.

B. The frequency is >5/hour in children or >15/hour in adults.

C. The PLMS cause clinically significant sleep disturbance or impairment in mental, physical, social, occupational, educational, behavioral, or other important areas of functioning.

D. The PLMS and the symptoms are not better explained by another current sleep disorder, medical or neurological disorder, or mental disorder (e.g., PLMS occurring with apneas or hypopneas should not be scored).

Notes:

1. The PLMS Index must be interpreted in the context of a patient's sleep related complaint. In adults, normative values greater than five per hour have been found in studies that did not exclude respiratory event-related arousals (using sensitive respiratory monitoring) and other causes for PLMS. Data suggest a partial overlap of PLMS Index values between symptomatic and asymptomatic individuals, emphasizing the importance of clinical context over an absolute cutoff value.

2. If PLMS are present without clinical sleep disturbance or daytime impairment, the PLMS can be noted as a polysomnographic finding, but criteria are not met for a diagnosis of PLMD.

3. The presence of insomnia or hypersomnia with PLMS is not sufficient to establish the diagnosis of PLMD. Studies have shown that in most cases the cause of the accompanying insomnia or hypersomnia is something other than the PLMS. To establish the diagnosis of PLMD, it is essential to establish a reasonable cause-and-effect relationship between the insomnia or hypersomnia and the PLMS. This requires that other causes of insomnia such as anxiety or other causes of hypersomnia such as obstructive sleep apnea or narcolepsy are ruled out. PLMS are common, but PLMD is thought to be rare in adults.

4. **PLMD cannot be diagnosed in the context of RLS, narcolepsy, untreated obstructive sleep apnea, or REM sleep behavior disorder;** PLMS occur commonly in these conditions but the sleep complaint is more readily ascribed to the accompanying disorder. The diagnosis of RLS takes precedence over that of PLMD when potentially sleep-disrupting PLMS occur in the context of RLS. In such cases, the diagnosis of RLS is made and the PLMS are noted.

5. When it is reasonably certain that the PLMS have been induced by medication, and full criteria for PLMD are met, it is preferred that the more specific diagnosis of PLMD be used, rather than "Sleep related movement disorder due to a medication or substance."

to be more common than PLMD. Some of the patients previously thought to have PLMD on the basis of sleep studies that monitored air flow with a thermal device rather than nasal pressure may have actually had respiratory effort–related arousal (RERA) or hypopnea-associated PLMS. In these patients, the symptoms of daytime sleepiness may have been caused by mild OSA rather than PLMD.[29] Other patients with PLMD may have had somewhat atypical of RLS without prominent sensations. The ICSD-3 states: "PLMD cannot be diagnosed in the context of RLS, narcolepsy, untreated obstructive sleep apnea, or REM sleep behavior disorder"; PLMS occur commonly in these conditions but the sleep complaint is more readily ascribed to the accompanying disorder. The diagnosis of RLS takes precedence over that of PLMD when potentially sleep-disrupting PLMS occur in the context of RLS. In such cases, the diagnosis of RLS is made and the PLMS are noted.

The finding of PLMS in children may be especially helpful because RLS symptoms are often difficult to elicit. It has also been proposed that in children, PLMD (PLMS with sleep disturbance) may precede the development of symptoms of RLS.

PSG Findings in PLMD

The PLMSI in asymptomatic patients and in those with PLMD overlap. The ICSD-3 criteria for PLMD include the requirement of a PLMSI of >15/hr in adults and >5/hr in children. However, many asymptomatic individuals have a PLMSI >15/hr. Mendelson[25] evaluated a group of 67 patients thought to have PLMD. The patients had undergone both PSG and multiple sleep latency test (MSLT). The overall sleep latency was around 10 minutes (near normal). No significant correlation existed between the PLM arousal index and sleep latency or a measure of objective sleepiness.

CLINICAL PEARLS

1. A diagnosis of RLS is based on clinical history. PSG is needed only if another sleep disorder such as OSA or parasomnia is suspected (both may cause leg movements during sleep).

2. Daytime sleepiness is an uncommon complaint in patients with RLS alone. The presence of prominent daytime sleepiness should prompt consideration of other disorders.

3. Use the acronym "URGE" to make the diagnosis of RLS. Patients with leg cramps, unconscious foot tapping, positional discomfort, and pain caused by identifiable conditions (e.g., arthritis, leg edema) should not be diagnosed as having RLS.

4. In severe RLS, worsening of symptoms in the evening may not be present but should have been present at the start of RLS.

5. Abnormal RLS sensations may be absent (only the urge to move the legs is present). The abnormal sensations may be painful and involve the arms.

6. Diagnosis of RLS excludes a diagnosis of PLMD.

7. An elevated PLMSI on a sleep study should prompt evaluation for RLS (evaluation by history).

8. PLMS is present in 80% to 90% of patients with RLS.

9. An elevated PLMSI in children (>5/hr) should prompt consideration of a diagnosis of PLMD. Children may not report RLS symptoms.

REFERENCES

1. Montplasir J, Boucher S, Poirer G, et al: Clinical, polysomnographic, and genetic characteristics of restless legs syndrome: a study of 133 patients diagnosed with new standard criteria, *Mov Disord* 12:61–65, 1997.
2. Allen RP, Picchietti D, Hening W, et al: Restless legs syndrome: diagnostic criteria, special considerations, and epidemiology. A report from the restless legs syndrome diagnosis and epidemiology workshop at the National Institutes of Health, *Sleep Med* 4:101–119, 2003.
3. Pennestri M, Whittom S, Adam B, et al: PLMS and PLMW in healthy subjects as a function of age: prevalence and interval distribution, *Sleep* 29:1183–1187, 2006.
4. American Academy of Sleep Medicine: *International classification of sleep disorders*, ed 3, Darien, IL, 2014, American Academy of Sleep Medicine.
5. Zucconi M, Ferri R, Allen R, et al: The official World Association of Sleep Medicine (WASM) standards for recording and scoring periodic leg movements in sleep (PLMS) and wakefulness (PLMW) developed in collaboration with a task force from the International Restless Legs Syndrome Study Group (IRLSSG), *Sleep Med* 7:175–183, 2006.
6. Hening WA, Allen RP, Washburn M, Lesage SR, Earley CJ: The four diagnostic criteria for Restless Legs Syndrome are unable to exclude confounding conditions ("mimics"), *Sleep Med* 10(9):976–981, 2009.
7. Allen RP, Burchell BJ, Ben MacDonald B, et al: Validation of the self-completed Cambridge-Hopkins questionnaire (CH-RLSq) for ascertainment of restless legs syndrome (RLS) in a population survey, *Sleep Med* 10:1097–1100, 2009.
8. Claman DM, Redline S, Blackwell T, et al: Prevalence and correlates of periodic limb movements in older women, *J Clin Sleep Med* 2(4):438–445, 2006.
9. Nofzinger EA, Fasiczka A, Berman S, Thase ME: Bupropion SR reduces periodic limb movements associated with arousal from sleep in depressed patients with period limb movement disorder, *J Clin Psychiatry* 61:858–862, 2000.
10. Hening W, Walters AS, Allen RP, et al: Impact, diagnosis and management of restless legs syndrome in a primary care population: the REST (RLS Epidemiology,

Symptoms, and Treatment) Primary Care Study, *Sleep Med* 5:237–246, 2004.

11. Sun ER, Chen CA, Ho G, et al: Iron and the restless legs syndrome, *Sleep* 21:381–387, 1998.

12. Mackie S, Winkelman JW: Normal ferritin in a patient with iron deficiency and RLS, *J Clin Sleep Med* 9 (5):511–513, 2013.

13. Wang J, O'Reilly B, Venkataraman R, et al: Efficacy of oral iron in patients with restless legs syndrome and a low-normal ferritin: A randomized, double-blind, placebo-controlled study, *Sleep Med* 10(9):973–975, 2009.

14. Horynak M, Feige B, Riemann B, et al: Periodic leg movements in sleep and periodic limb movement disorder: prevalence, clinical significance, and treatment, *Sleep Med Rev* 10:169–177, 2006.

15. Picchietti MA, Picchietti DL: Advances in pediatric restless legs syndrome: iron, genetics, diagnosis and treatment, *Sleep Med* 11:643–651, 2010.

16. Picchietti D, Allen RP, Walters AS, et al: Restless legs syndrome: prevalence and impact in children and adolescents—The Peds REST Study, *Pediatrics* 120:253–266, 2007.

17. American Sleep Disorders Association: *International classification of sleep disorders*, ed 1, Rochester, MN, 1990, American Sleep Disorders Association.

18. Pollmacher T, Schulz H: Periodic leg movements: their relationship to sleep stages, *Sleep* 16:572–577, 1993.

19. Culpepper WJ, Badia P, Shaffer JI: Time of night patterns in PLMS activity, *Sleep* 15:306–311, 1992.

20. Fantini ML, Michaud M, Gosseline N, et al: Periodic leg movements in REM sleep behavior disorder and related autonomic and EEG activation, *Neurology* 59:1889–1894, 2002.

21. Dauvilliers Y, Pennestri MH, Petit D, et al: Periodic leg movements during sleep and wakefulness in narcolepsy, *J Sleep Res* 16(3):333–339, 2007.

22. Berry RB, Brooks R, Gamaldo CE, et al: for the American Academy of Sleep Medicine: *The AASM manual for the scoring of sleep and associated events: rules, terminology and technical specifications*, Version 2.0.3, www.aasmnet.org, Darien, IL, 2014, American Academy of Sleep Medicine.

23. Karadeniz D, Ondze B, Besset A, Billiard M: EEG arousals and awakenings in relations with periodic leg movements during sleep, *J Sleep Res* 9:273–277, 2000.

24. Montplasir J, Michaud M, Denesle R, Gosseline A: Periodic leg movements are not more prevalent in insomnia of hypersomnia but are specifically associated with sleep disorders involving a dopaminergic impairment, *Sleep Med* 1:163–167, 2000.

25. Mendelson WB: Are periodic leg movements associated with clinical sleep disturbance? *Sleep* 19:219–223, 1996.

26. Pizza F, Tartarotti S, Poryazova R, et al: Sleep-disordered breathing and periodic limb movements in narcolepsy with cataplexy: a systematic analysis of 35 consecutive patients, *Eur Neurol* 70(1–2):22–26, 2013.

27. Fry JM, DiPhillipo MA, Pressman MR: Periodic leg movements in sleep following treatment of obstructive sleep apnea with nasal continuous positive airway pressure, *Chest* 96:89–91, 1989.

28. Chervin RD: Periodic leg movements and sleepiness in patients evaluated for sleep-disordered breathing, *Am J Respir Crit Care Med* 164:1454–1458, 2001.

29. Exner EN, Collop NA: The association of upper airway resistance with periodic limb movement, *Sleep* 24:188–192, 2000.

PATIENTS 79

Patients with Leg Kicks on a Sleep Study

Patient A: A 40-year-old woman had a sleep study ordered by her primary care physician. The history and physical examination information provided for the physician interpreting the sleep study included only the following information. The patient reported mild daytime sleepiness (Epworth Sleepiness Scale [ESS] score of 12/24) and sleeping about 7.5 hours per night. Her husband reported that the patient snored loudly with intermittent gasping. He also reported that she sometimes kicked her legs. The patient was taking hydrochlorothiazide for hypertension. Sleep study results are listed in Table P79-1.

TABLE P79-1	**Sleep Study Results**		
AHI	25.7/hour	Obstructive apneas	65
AHI REM	65/hour	Mixed apneas	3
PLMS index	40/hour	Central apneas	2
PLMS arousal index	5/hour	Hypopneas	110

AHI, Apnea–hypopnea index; *PLMS*, periodic limb movement in sleep; *REM*, rapid eye movement.

QUESTIONS

1. What do you recommend for Patient A?
   A. Treatment of obstructive sleep apnea (OSA) and periodic limb movement in sleep (PLMS)
   B. Continuous positive airway pressure (CPAP) titration
   C. CPAP titration and further clinical history
   D. Treatment of OSA and restless legs syndrome (RLS)

2. If the PLMS index (PLMSI) in Patient A was >10 per hour (hr) during rapid eye movement (REM) sleep, what disorders would you consider?

Patient B: A 30-second tracing is shown in Figure P79-1. This patient has a prolonged sleep latency of 60 minutes.

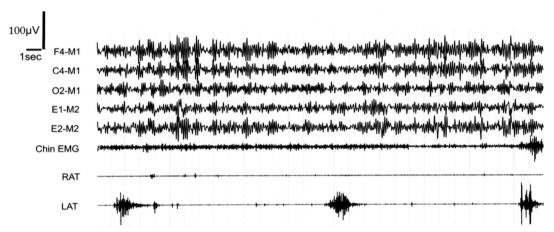

FIGURE P79-1 ■ A 30-second epoch is shown, *LAT*, Left anterior tibial electromyogram; *RAT*, right anterior tibial electromyogram.

3. What diagnosis is suspected in Patient B?

ANSWERS

1. **Answer:** CPAP titration and further clinical inquiry of history ("Are symptoms of the restless legs syndrome present?")

2. **Answer:** The PLMSI is usually much higher during non-REM (NREM) sleep than during REM sleep unless the patient has narcolepsy or REM sleep behavior disorder (RBD).

   Discussion (Patient A, questions 1 and 2): A diagnosis of RLS is based on clinical history, not polysomnography (PSG) findings. Although 80% to 90% of patients with RLS do have PLMS, most patients with PLMS do not have RLS. PLMS is found in asymptomatic populations, and the PLMSI increases with age.[1-4] The presence of PLMS should alert the clinician to determine if RLS is present and if the symptoms are significant. PLMS is also common in patients with OSA, narcolepsy, and RBD.[5-7] The presence of PLMs on PSG does not mandate that they be treated. The significance of PLMS in the absence of RLS is debated. Period limb movement disorder (PLMD) requires that RLS not be present and that the PLMSI is >15/hr in adults and >5/hr in children.[8] The sleep complaints (insomnia, poor sleep) must **NOT** be caused by another sleep disorder (e.g., OSA).

   PLMs occur most commonly in stage N1 and N2 but may also occur in stage N3 or, less commonly, during stage R sleep.[9,10] The PLMSI in NREM is usually much greater than during REM

TABLE P79-2	**PLMS in Narcolepsy**	
	Narcolepsy	**Controls**
PLMSI	20.9	6.7
PLMS NREM	21.1	8.2
PLMS REM	18.3	3.2

Data from Dauvilliers Y, Pennestri MH, et al: Periodic leg movements during sleep and wakefulness in narcolepsy, *J Sleep Res* 16(3):333–339, 2007.
PLMS, Periodic limb movement in sleep; *PLMSI*, periodic limb movement in sleep index; *NREM*, non–rapid eye movement; *REM*, rapid eye movement.

sleep. The PLMSI is often higher during the first part of the night. Culpepper and colleagues[10] described two patterns of PLMS. In one pattern, PLMS was much more common in the first part of the night. In the second pattern, PLMS was more evenly distributed across the night. The interval between individual PLMs increases from stage N1 to stage N3. PLMs are less likely to cause arousal from stage N3 sleep. The PLMSI during REM sleep is usually quite low. If a significant number of PLMs are present during REM sleep (Table P79-2), it should alert the clinician to the possibility of narcolepsy or RBD.[6,7]

3. **Answer (Question 3):** Restless legs syndrome. Periodic leg movements in wakefulness are shown in the figure.

Discussion: The *AASM Scoring Manual* does not define PLMs in wakefulness (PLMW).[11,12] However, diagnostic criteria for PLMW do exist.[13] The criteria for PLMW are similar to those used for PLMS (except that patients are awake). In PLMW, the periodicity is less regular and shorter than typical of PLMS. It was found that PLMW events tend to be longer (5–10 seconds in duration) compared with typical PLMS events. Recognizing the presence of PLMW is important, as this is highly suggestive of RLS and should alert the clinician reading a sleep study to review the patient history carefully for symptoms of RLS. The diagnosis of RLS is based on clinical history. In the tracing in Figure P79-1 alpha-activity is shown for the entire epoch (stage W). This is not PLMS, as sleep is not present. PLMW is present, and although not scored per AASM recommendations, the presence of leg activity during wakefulness suggests that RLS is present. Review of the history supplied with the sleep study request documented that the patient reported severe symptoms of RLS. The patient also reported on the poststudy questionnaire that leg symptoms were responsible for his difficulty falling asleep. The clinical interpretation of the sleep study report suggested that the patient be evaluated and treated for RLS, if clinically indicated.

CLINICAL PEARLS

1. The presence of PLMS should trigger inquiry to determine if RLS is present (diagnosis based on clinical history).
2. Frequent or periodic leg movement during wakefulness suggests the possibility that RLS is present. However, the diagnosis of RLS is based on history.
3. The PLMSI either tends to decrease across the night or remain relatively stable with a peak at the middle of the night.
4. The PLMSI of NREM sleep is greater than the PLMSI of REM sleep.
5. PLMS may be associated with narcolepsy, RBD, or OSA.
6. A diagnosis of PLMD requires that RLS not be present and that the sleep complaint is not better explained by another disorder or medication.
7. A high PLMSI during stage R is uncommon except in patients with narcolepsy or RBD.

REFERENCES

1. Carrier J, Frenette S, Montplaisir J, et al: Effects of periodic leg movements during sleep in middle-aged subjects without sleep complaints, *Mov Disord* 20:1127–1132, 2005.
2. Claman DM, Redline S, Blackwell T, et al: Prevalence and correlates of periodic limb movements in older women, *J Clin Sleep Med* 2:438–445, 2006.
3. Scofield H, Roth T, Drake C: Periodic limb movements during sleep: population, prevalence, clinical correlates and racial differences, *Sleep* 3:1221–1227, 2008.

4. Pennestri M, Whittom S, Adam B, et al: PLMS and PLMW in healthy subjects as a function of age: prevalence and interval distribution, *Sleep* 29:1183–1187, 2006.
5. Fantini ML, Michaud M, Gosseline N, et al: Periodic leg movements in REM sleep behavior disorder and related autonomic and EEG activation, *Neurology* 59:1889–1894, 2002.
6. Manconi M, Ferri R, Zucconi M, et al: Time structure analysis of leg movements during sleep in REM sleep behavior disorder, *Sleep* 30:1779–1785, 2007.
7. Dauvilliers Y, Pennestri MH, Petit D, et al: Periodic leg movements during sleep and wakefulness in narcolepsy, *J Sleep Res* 16(3):333–339, 2007.
8. American Academy of Sleep Medicine: *International classification of sleep disorders*, ed 3, Darien, IL, 2014, American Academy of Sleep Medicine.
9. Pollmacher T, Schulz H: Periodic leg movements: their relationship to sleep stages, *Sleep* 16:572–577, 1993.
10. Culpepper WJ, Badia P, Shaffer JI: Time of night patterns in PLMS activity, *Sleep* 15:306–311, 1992.
11. Walters AS, Lavigne G, Hening W, et al: The scoring of movements in sleep, *J Clin Sleep Med* 3(2):155–167, 2007.
12. Iber C, Ancoli-Israel S, Chesson A, Quan SF: for the American Academy of Sleep Medicine: *The AASM manual for the scoring of sleep and associated events: rules, terminology and technical specification*, ed 1, Westchester, IL, 2007, American Academy of Sleep Medicine, pp 41–42.
13. Zucconi M, Ferri R, Allen R, et al: The official World Association of Sleep Medicine (WASM) standards for recording and scoring periodic leg movements in sleep (PLMS) and wakefulness (PLMW) developed in collaboration with a task force from the International Restless Legs Syndrome Study Group (IRLSSG), *Sleep Med* 7:175–183, 2006.

PATIENT 80

A 58-Year-Old Man with Sleep Apnea and Leg Jerks on CPAP

A 58-year-old man was diagnosed as having severe obstructive sleep apnea (OSA) on an initial sleep study. He then underwent nasal continuous positive airway pressure (CPAP) titration, after which he remarked that he had had the "best night of sleep in years." However, a drastic change occurred in his periodic limb movement in sleep index (PLMSI) on CPAP (Table P80-1 and Figure P80-1).

TABLE P80-1	**PLMS during Polysomnography**	
Sleep Studies	**Diagnostic**	**CPAP Titration**
AHI	66/hr	10/hr (5/hr on CPAP of 12 cm H$_2$O)
PLMSI	10/hr	60/hr
PLM arousal index	5/hr	5/hr
Total arousal index	50/hr	10/hr

AHI, Apnea–hypopnea index; *cm H$_2$O*, centimeters of water; *CPAP*, continuous positive airway pressure; *hr*, hour; *PLMSI*, periodic limb movement in sleep index. All indices are the number of events per hour of sleep.

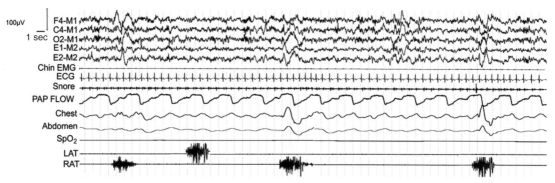

FIGURE P80-1 ■ A 60-second tracing of the patient on continuous positive airway pressure (CPAP) of 12 centimeters of water (cm H_2O).

TABLE P80-2	Periodic Limb Movement in Sleep Index with Possible Scenarios	
	Diagnostic Study	**Treatment Study**
Scenario #1	Zero or low	High
Scenario #2	High	Low
Scenario #3	High	High

QUESTION

1. What is your diagnosis?

ANSWER

1. **Answer:** PLMS associated with nasal CPAP treatment for OSA.

Discussion: The finding of both OSA and PLMS on polysomnography (PSG) may simply represent the coexistence of two common entities. Treatment with CPAP may decrease or increase the PLMSI compared with the diagnostic night (or diagnostic portion of a split sleep study) (Table P80-2). In a study by Baran et al patients with a high apnea–hypopnea index (AHI) during the diagnostic study tended to have an increase in PLMS during the CPAP titration. The CPAP treatment was hypothesized to "unmask" PLMS. That is, severe fragmentation of sleep by apnea (pre-CPAP) did not allow manifestation of the PLMS, and treatment with CPAP unmasked the PLMS by allowing continuous sleep. Another explanation of this scenario is that the rebound in sleep during the initial CPAP treatment results in less spontaneous patient movement, and the stasis or pressure on the nerves caused by immobility leads to PLMS. Many patients with sleep apnea spend more time supine when treated with CPAP than in the untreated state. In the study by Baran et al patients with mild AHI values tended to have a decrease in the PLMSI during the CPAP titration. Their hypothesis was that high upper airway resistance may be triggering periodic limb movements (PLMs) as a surrogate of arousal. Although these hypotheses are interesting, they are difficult to prove, and the real question for the clinician is whether or not the PLMs significantly contribute to the patient's sleep disturbance and sleepiness. The first consideration in a patient with an elevated PLMSI is to determine if the restless legs syndrome (RLS) is present and if symptoms warrant treatment (diagnosis by history). If RLS is not present, is periodic limb movement disorder (PLMD) present? Recall that a diagnosis of PLMD requires that RLS be excluded and that symptoms of sleep disturbance or fatigue are felt to be due to PLMS rather than other sleep disorders (e.g., OSA) or medications. As PLMD is felt to be uncommon in adults, in most OSA patients with a high PLMS index, initial treatment with PAP alone is sufficient in most cases. Typically, the PLM arousal index is low. Haba-Rubio prospectively studied a group of patients starting CPAP treatment. Those with PLMS and those without PLMS during CPAP titration were compared. The study did not find a link between PLMS and increased objective or self-evaluated sleepiness in patients with OSA before or after treatment with CPAP.

If symptoms of daytime sleepiness resolve on CPAP treatment, no additional treatment is necessary (even if PLMS persist). However, if daytime sleepiness persists or returns after treatment of OSA is initiated, PLMD could be one cause of treatment failure. Note that the mere presence of PLMS during CPAP titration should not exclude consideration of other causes of persistent daytime sleepiness such as inadequate pressure, poor compliance, inadequate sleep, and narcolepsy (which often coexists with PLMS). The patient's bed partner should be questioned about the frequency of body movements while the patient is on nasal CPAP. However, the body movements noted by the bed partner could also be caused by persistent apnea (insufficient pressure or mask leak). Repeat sleep monitoring on CPAP to determine the adequacy of treatment and determination of the PLMSI and PLM arousal index could be considered. If PLMD is thought to be present, a trial of a dopamine agonist may be considered. If leg movements and symptoms improve this supports a diagnosis of PLMD.

In the present case, the patient denied RLS symptoms. The PLM arousal index on CPAP was modest. The patient noted a marked improvement in daytime sleepiness almost immediately with CPAP treatment. His wife reported that he did not kick at night and was "as cool as a cucumber." Good control of his symptoms persisted on nasal CPAP therapy, and no treatment for the PLMS was initiated.

CLINICAL PEARLS

1. A large increase in the PLMSI may follow initiation of nasal CPAP therapy in some patients with OSA. The increase may be transient. Often, the PLM arousal index remains low.
2. An elevated PLMS index should always trigger evaluation for possible RLS (history).
3. In most patients with OSA and PLMS, treatment of the OSA alone may result in complete resolution of symptoms. Unless RLS is present, no intervention associated with the presence of PLMS is usually needed.
4. When adequate treatment of OSA (nasal CPAP) fails to abolish symptoms of daytime sleepiness, PLMD may be one cause of persistent sleepiness. As PLMD is thought to be rare, the mere presence of PLMS during CPAP titration should not discourage the clinician from excluding other causes of persistent daytime sleepiness such as inadequate PAP adherence.
5. If treatment of PLMD is indicated, use of a dopamine agonist or alpha-2-delta ligand (e.g., gabapentin) are treatment options.

BIBLIOGRAPHY

Aritake-Okada S, Namba K, Hidano N, et al: Change in frequency of periodic limb movements during sleep with usage of continuous positive airway pressure in obstructive sleep apnea syndrome, *J Neurol Sci* 317(1–2):13–16, 2012.

Baran AS, Richert AC, Douglass AB, et al: Change in periodic limb movement index during treatment of obstructive sleep apnea with continuous positive airway pressure, *Sleep* 26(6):717–720, 2003.

Fry JM, Diphillip MA, Pressman MR: Periodic leg movements in sleep following treatment of obstructive sleep apnea with nasal CPAP, *Chest* 96:89–91, 1989.

Haba-Rubio J, Staner L, Krieger J, Macher JP: Periodic limb movements and sleepiness in obstructive sleep apnea patients, *Sleep Med* 6(3):225–229, 2005.

Hedli LC, Christos P, Krieger AC: Unmasking of periodic limb movements with the resolution of obstructive sleep apnea during continuous positive airway pressure application, *J Clin Neurophysiol* 29(4):339–344, 2012.

Skomro R, Silva R, Alves R, et al: The prevalence and significance of periodic leg movements during sleep in patients with congestive heart failure, *Sleep Breath* 13(1):43–47, 2009.

Treatment of RLS and PLMD

The major medication groups (Table F32-1) for the treatment of restless legs syndrome (RLS) include dopaminergic medications (the dopamine precursor levodopa and dopamine agonists), opioids, anticonvulsant medications (alpha-2-delta receptor ligands), and sedative-hypnotic medications (usually benzodiazepine receptor agonists [BZRAs]).[1-3] Similar medications have been used to treat periodic limb movement disorder (PLMD), with the exception that opioids have not been well studied for this indication. Of note, three dopamine agonists (DAs) (ropinirole, pramipexole, and a rotigitine patch) and gabapentin encarbil are the only medications that have been approved by the U.S. Food and Drug Administration (FDA) for RLS treatment (in adults).

Few studies concerning treatment of PLMD and RLS in children have been published. No medication is FDA approved for the treatment of PLMD or RLS in children. However, it appears that dopaminergic therapy is effective treatment for PLMD or RLS in children.[4,5]

NONPHARMACOLOGIC TREATMENTS

In mild and intermittent RLS, nonpharmacologic treatments may be useful. These include stretching, heating or cooling of the extremities (warm bath), and avoidance of alcohol and

TABLE F32-1   Treatments for RLS and PLMD

Class	Interventions	Comments
Nonpharmacologic	Exercise, stretching, warm baths Avoid caffeine Avoid first-generation antihistamines Iron supplementation (po or IV) if ferritin <50 ng/mL (mcg/L) (325 mg iron sulfate three times daily with 100 to 200 mg vitamin C)	Low iron stores increase risk for DA augmentation

Dopaminergic medications	Carbidopa/Levodopa—intermittent RLS
	Dopamine agonist (DA)-daily RLS
	    Pramipexole*
	    Ropinirole*
	    Rotigitine patch (NeuPro*)
		Generic forms of CD/LD, ropinirole, and pramipexole available
		Use over alpha-2-delta 2 ligands if weight gain an issue

Anticonvulsants (alpha-2-delta ligands)	Gabapentin (Neurontin, generic) Gabapentin encarbil (Horizant)* Pregabalin (Lyrica)	Treatment of choice when RLS associated with pain, insomnia, anxiety. Combination with a DA effective option Use if DA intolerance
Narcotics	Tramadol Hydrocodone or APAP Oxycodone Methadone	Intractable RLS Augmentation with DA Cannot tolerate DA Opioids contraindicated if history of substance abuse or dependence
Hypnotics	Adjunctive or mild RLS May not reduce PLMS index	Clonazepam most studied

APAP, acetaminophen; PLMD, periodic limb movement disorder; PLMS, periodic limb movement in sleep; po, orally; RLS, restless legs syndrome.
*FDA approved for treatment of RLS in adults, all except narcotics have been used to treat PLMD, DA dopamine agonists.

caffeine. Antidepressant treatment may sometimes be associated with initiation or worsening of RLS.[6] However, if antidepressant treatment is deemed necessary, RLS may be treated as if primary RLS is present and antidepressant treatment continued. Studies have suggested that bupropion either improves or does not worsen PLMS and RLS,[7,8] so use of this medication could be considered in a patient with depression and RLS. However, concerns about RLS should not limit effective treatment of depression. Iron deficiency may cause or worsen RLS. Checking a ferritin level[9-11] is recommended in patients with RLS because this disorder may be the only indication of low iron stores. The ferritin level may be elevated in patients with inflammation, so the total iron binding capacity (TIBC) and the iron saturation should also be tested.[10] Most clinicians recommend that a ferritin level above 45 to 50 micrograms per milliliter (mcg/mL) be achieved in patients with RLS.[2,9-11] Patients should also be evaluated for occult gastrointestinal blood loss if clinically indicated. Typical iron supplementation is ferrous sulfate 325 milligrams (mg) three times daily with the addition of 100 to 200 mg of ascorbic acid with each dose (to improve absorption). Iron absorption is best achieved on an empty stomach, but iron usually must be taken with food to avoid severe gastrointestinal upset. Monitoring of ferritin levels is recommended to ensure adequate replenishment of iron stores and to avoid inducing iron overload. Studies of the use of intravenous (IV) administration of iron for RLS treatment have shown conflicting results.[12] However, some RLS patients with low iron stores will show considerable improvement after IV iron administration. The main indication for IV iron administration is patients who cannot tolerate oral administration of iron or have iron malabsorption. Use of IV iron gluconate or iron sucrose is recommended, as use of iron dextran has a high frequency of allergic reactions. When ferritin levels exceed the goal, iron supplementation may be stopped. It is important to note that iron supplementation alone does not always improve RLS. However, many patients will have better results from treatment from standard RLS medications if iron stores are adequate.

DOPAMINERGIC MEDICATIONS

Levodopa (LD) is a precursor that is converted to dopamine by dopa decarboxylase (DDC). Carbidopa (CD) does not penetrate the blood–brain barrier but acts as an inhibitor of DDC outside the central nervous system (CNS). Therefore, using the CD/LD combination there is less peripheral conversion of LD to dopamine. This results in fewer side effects and an increased amount of LD reaching the brain. The CD/LD combination (Sinemet or generic CD/LD) is very effective in RLS treatment and has a quick onset of action. The starting dose is half to one pill of the CD/LD 100/25 mg preparation with the usual effective dose range of 100 to 200 mg of LD (maximum 200 mg LD). The CD/LD combination is available as 10/100, 25/100, and 25/250 mg tablets. Two problems exist with the use of CD/LD in treating RLS. First, the drug has a short duration of action, and a rebound in symptoms may occur in the early morning hours. The patient could take another dose at that time. Longer-acting forms of CD/LD are available, but they have a slower onset of action. The second problem is that continued use of CD/LD especially at high doses (LD >200 mg/day), commonly results in augmentation (a change in the effectiveness of dopaminergic medications, discussed later). In some studies, up to 80% of patients taking CD/LD for RLS develop augmentation.[13]

The nonergotamine DAs pramipexole, ropinirole, and rotigitine are considered first-line medications for the treatment of daily moderate to severe RLS.[2,14-20] Randomized, controlled studies have documented the efficacy of these medications for treating RLS and PLMD. They have a sufficiently long duration of action such that rebound does usually not occur. Augmentation, discussed in detail later, may occur in up to 30% of patients during short-term follow-up but is usually mild and may be controlled for ropinirole and pramipexole by taking a portion of the dose at an earlier time (split dose).[21] *However, long-term follow-up studies have shown that a large proportion of patients ultimately stop taking DAs because of augmentation or loss of effectiveness.*[22,23] Both augmentation and side effects from the DAs may be minimized by starting at a low dose (0.125 mg for pramipexole and 0.25 mg for ropinirole) with a slow upward titration, as needed (Table F32-2). It is important to note that with both drugs, the effect has a long time of onset, so they should be taken several hours before symptoms are expected (2 to 3 hours for pramipexole, 1 to 2 hours for ropinirole). If patients have symptoms in the morning, treatment with twice or three times a day dosing or ropinirole or pramipexole may be tried. Of note, some patients will respond better to pramipexole than to ropinirole, and vice versa. Studies have suggested that the equivalent dose of ropinirole is about four times the dose of pramipexole. Switching DAs is also an intervention that may be tried if augmentation develops.

In the manufacturer's drug prescribing information, the maximum recommended doses of

TABLE F32-2   **Dopamine Agonists Approved for RLS Treatment**

Medication	Pramipexole	Ropinirole	Rotigotine
	Non-ergot DA	Non-ergotamine DA	Non-ergotamine DA
Brand/generic	Mirapex, generic available	Requip, generic available	NeuPro, no generic
Time to max blood level	2 hours	1-1.5 hours	Transdermal Patch 15-18 hours, variable Terminal half-life 5-7 hours
Elimination half life	8–12 hours	6 hours	
Metabolism and excretion	Renal excretion	Hepatic metabolism, renal excretion	Hepatic metabolism; renal excretion
Starting dose/ titration	0.125 milligram (mg) 2-3 hours before bedtime Step 1: 0.125 mg Step 2: 0.25 mg Step 3: 0.5 mg Increase to next step every 4-7 days Max dose 0.75 mg*	0.25 mg 1 to 2 hours before bedtime Increase by 0.5 mg weekly, if needed Max dose 4 mg	1 mg/24 hours Increase by 1 mg/24 hours to maximum of 3 mg/24 hours

DA, Dopamine agonists; *RLS*, restless legs syndrome.
*Prescribing information: 0.5 mg max for RLS.

TABLE F32-3   **Dopamine Agonist Side Effects**

Acute	Subacute or Severe	Parkinsons Disorders
Nausea, less commonly vomiting Light-headedness, rarely syncope Headache Somnolence Insomnia Local site reactions (Rotigotine patch) Peripheral edema Nasal congestion Constipation	Augmentation Hypersomnia, including sleep attacks Dopamine dysregulation syndrome Impulse control disorders • Hypersexuality • Pathologic gambling • Excessive shopping • Punding Rotigitine patch—allergic (metabisulfite)	(Higher doses) Dyskinesias Hallucinations Psychosis

0.5 mg pramipexole and 4 mg ropinirole are listed. The drug labeling states pramipexole doses up to 0.75 mg has been used in studies, but little additional benefit resulted from doses above 0.5 mg. The rotigitine transdermal patch is potentially useful for patients with daytime RLS symptoms or augmentation. The starting dose of the rotigitine patch is 1 mg and the maximum dose for RLS is 3 mg.

Dopaminergic Side Effects

All dopaminergic medications share similar side effects (Table F32-3). All dopamine agonists are category C and not recommended for use during pregnancy. Nausea is the most common side effect, but headache, light-headedness, somnolence, peripheral edema, and nasal congestion may occur. Severe side effects include severe hypersomnia (including sudden sleep attacks), augmentation, and dopamine dysregulation syndrome or impulse control disorders. Long-term studies of patients using DAs have shown that a significant proportion of patients stop taking the medications because of augmentation or side effects. *Dopamine dysregulation syndrome* is a dysfunction of the rewards system in patients taking dopamine treatment. The most common symptom is craving for the dopaminergic medication, sometimes associated with taking extra doses even in the absence of symptoms that indicate the need for additional medication. DAs may also be associated with defects in *impulse control (compulsive gambling, hypersexuality, punding, or compulsive shopping)*. *Punding* is characterized by compulsive fascination with and performance of repetitive, mechanical tasks such as assembling and disassembling, collecting, or sorting household objects. Impulse control disorders are more common during DA treatment of Parkinson disease than DA treatment of RLS, but the problem is increasingly reported as complication of DA

RLS treatment.[24,25] When DAs are used to treat Parkinson disease much higher doses than those used to treat RLS are used, DA treatment of Parkinson disease may be associated with dyskinesias, hallucinations, or psychosis.

The rotigitine patch is associated with a significant number of local site reactions. The location patch placement should be changed with each application. The rotigitine patch contains sodium metabisulfite, a substance that may cause allergy-type reactions, including anaphylactic symptoms and life-threatening or less severe asthmatic episodes in certain susceptible people. The overall prevalence of sulfite sensitivity in the general population is 30% to 60%. Sulfite sensitivity is seen more frequently in persons with asthma than in those without asthma. Of note, allergy to metabisulfites is not the same as sulfa allergy. Use of the rotigitine patch is contraindicated if a patient is allergic to metabisulfites.

Augmentation

Augmentation is defined as a change in the efficacy of RLS treatment with dopaminergic medications[2,21,26] (Box F32-1). It is characterized by one or more of the following: (1) earlier symptom onset; (2) greater severity of symptoms at the same dose (assuming prior response to the dose); (3) paradoxical response to treatment: RLS symptom severity increases sometime after a dose increase, and improves sometime after a dose decrease; (4) reduced latency to onset of symptoms with rest; and (5) spread of symptoms to involve new body parts (arms as well as legs). Patients with severe augmentation are usually on CD/LD or a high dose of a DA. As noted previously, augmentation is common with daily CD/LD treatment of RLS (80%) but also occurs in around 30% of RLS patients treated with a DA during the first year or two of treatment. DA augmentation may be milder than with CD/LD but can be severe, especially if high doses of DAs are used. More recent studies have suggested augmentation with DAs is more of a problem than realized and that a substantial percentage of patients stop DA treatment because of augmentation when monitored over 5 to 10 years.[22,23] When using a DA, it is imperative to be certain the patient is taking the DA *early enough* before increasing the dose. Using the lowest effective dose of DA is prudent to minimize augmentation.

Approaches to augmentation are listed in Box F32-2. Low iron stores appear to increase the frequency or severity of augmentation so a ferritin should be checked[27] if augmentation is present. If the patient is on CD/LD the first approach would be to change to a DA. If the patient is on a DA and symptoms occur earlier

---

BOX F32-1 **Diagnostic Criteria for Augmentation***

Augmentation requires criteria: A+B, A+C, or A+B+C to be met.
A. Basic features (all of which need to be met):
  1. The increase in symptom severity was experienced on 5 out of 7 days during the previous week.
  2. The increase in symptom severity is not accounted for by other factors such as a change in medical status, lifestyle, or the natural progression of the disorder.
  3. It is assumed that a prior positive response to treatment had occurred.
B. Persisting (although not immediate) paradoxical response to treatment: restless legs syndrome (RLS) symptom severity increases sometime after a dose increase, and improves sometime after a dose decrease.
  OR
C. Earlier onset of symptoms:
  1. An earlier onset by at least 4 hours.
  OR
  2. An earlier onset (between 2 and 4 hours) occurs with one of the following compared to symptom status before treatment:
    a. Shorter latency to symptoms when at rest
    b. Extension of symptoms to other body parts
    c. Greater intensity of symptoms (or increase in periodic limb movements [PLM] if measured by polysomnography [PSG] or the suggested immobilization test [SIT])
    d. Shorter duration of relief from treatment

*From Max Planck conference.

BOX F32-2 **Approaches to Augmentation**

1. If on CD/LD, stop and change to a DA (avoid CD/LD in daily RLS, avoid dose >200 milligrams [mg] LD).
2. If on a DA and earlier symptom onset is the problem, split the dose and give half of the dose earlier.
3. Change to a different DA medication.
4. If morning symptoms are a problem, try an evening and morning dose of medication (or use rotigitine patch).
5. If patient is taking a DA and has moderate augmentation, reduce dose and add gabapentin or an opioid.
6. If very severe augmentation, stop (wean) the DA or CD/LD and add high-potency opioid.
7. **Avoid high doses of DAs**, use combination therapy (add opiate, gabapentin, or BZRA).
8. Low iron stores may predispose to augmentation, correct low iron stores.

BZRA, Benzodiazepine receptor agonists; *CD,* carbidopa; *DA,* dopamine agonist; *LD,* levodopa.

in the evening, the medication dose could be split or another dose added earlier (e.g., pramipexole 0.125 mg at 6 PM and 9 PM). If the problem is morning symptoms, a morning dose could be added (two to three times daily dosing). Sometimes, a midday dose is not needed because of the "RLS protected period" in the middle of the day. If RLS symptoms become more intense on the current dose of the DA, approaches include a cautious increase in dose (unless already on a high dose) or a switch to another DA. Sometimes, patients respond better to one DA than to another. Many physicians would rather add another class of medication (an opioid or gabapentin) rather than increase the DA dose above a moderate level.

If augmentation is severe or the current DA dose is high, the best approach is weaning off or stopping the DA (although severe exacerbation of RLS may occur) and adding a high-potency opiate with or without another class of medication. Clearly, the best approach is to not use CD/LD for daily RLS, use the lowest dose possible of the DA with slow upward titration, and correct low iron stores (goal ferritin >45–50 micrograms per liter [mcg/L]).

OPIOIDS OR OPIATES

Opiates, opioids, and opioid receptor agonists (tramadol) may be effective treatment for RLS.[2,27–32] They are rapid acting and may be used either singly or in combination with other medication groups such as DAs. Except with tramadol, augmentation has not been described with opioid treatment of RLS. Milder RLS may respond to low-potency opiates (propoxyphene, codeine) or the opioid agonist (tramadol).

Moderate to severe RLS may respond to high-potency opiates (hydrocodone, oxycodone, methadone). Hydrocodone is available in the United States in combination with acetaminophen (APAP). One must be cautious not to prescribe an excessive dose of APAP. For example, it is preferable to use hydrocodone/APAP 10/325 mg, rather than two tablets of 5/325 mg. A maximum of 2 grams (g) of APAP per day may be used, although lower doses could be harmful if liver disease is present. Side effects of opiates include nausea, itching, and constipation. These medications should not be used with alcohol and should be used with caution in patients with OSA, central sleep apnea (CSA), or hypoventilation. Because of the risk for abuse and dependence, opiates are not the drugs of choice for treating daily RLS. However, studies and clinical experience suggest that dependence is not a problem if patients do not have a history of opioid dependence. Typical doses of opiates or opioid agonists include tramadol 50 to 100 mg, propoxyphene napsylate 100 mg, hydrocodone 5 to 15 mg, oxycodone 5 to 15 mg, and methadone 5 to 15 mg (see Patient 84). Long-term follow-up studies[22] have shown that fewer patients discontinue opioids compared with DAs for RLS treatment. In very severe RLS, opioids may need to be taken during the day and at bedtime.

ANTICONVULSANT MEDICATIONS (ALPHA-2-DELTA LIGANDS)

Three alpha-2-delta receptor ligands have been shown to be effective for use in RLS (Table F32-4). Of these medications, only a form of gabapentin (gabapentin encarbil, Horizant) is

TABLE F32-4	Anticonvulsant Medications (Alpha-2-Delta) for Restless Legs Syndrome			
Medication	**Structure**	**FDA approved for RLS or Cost**	**Bioavailability**	**Dose**
Gabapentin (Neurontin, Generics)	Structural analog of GABA*	No/inexpensive	Unpredictable	Start 100 to 300 milligrams (mg) (100 mg older adults) Usual effective dose 900–1200 mg
Gabapentin encarbil (Horizant)	Prodrug of Gabapentin Undergoes rapid hydrolysis to gabapentin	Yes/expensive	Predictable (Dose proportional absorption) Better absorbed with food	600 (1200 mg) at 5 PM
Pregabalin (Lyrica)	Structural analog of GABA*	No/expensive	Predictable	75 mg every night at bed time (qhs) or 2 to 3 hours before bed (50 mg older adults) Effective dose 300–450 mg qhs (Maximum daily does 600 mg)

*Binds alpha-2-delta subunit of voltage gated calcium channels and not gamma-aminobutyric acid (GABA) receptors. Class side effects: sleepiness, dizziness, unsteadiness, weight, gain, depression.

FDA approved for the treatment of RLS. These medications are an alternative to dopamine agonists for the treatment of daily moderate to severe RLS. Gabapentin is an analog of gamma-aminobutyric acid (GABA) but binds to the alpha-2-delta subunit of voltage-gated calcium channels in the CNS. It is FDA approved for the treatment of the pain of herpetic neuralgia and as an adjunct for patient with partial seizures. Some consider gabapentin the drug of choice for patients when RLS is associated with pain.[2] The efficacy of gabapentin treatment for RLS has been demonstrated by a number of trials.[33–36] One of these studies also reported a decrease in the periodic limb movement in sleep index (PLMSI) compared with that for placebo.[34] Patients reporting symptoms of pain received the most benefit from gabapentin. A study by Saletu et al[35] comparing gabapentin and ropinirole found that both improved RLS but gabapentin improved sleep quality more, whereas ropinirole decreased PLMS to a greater degree. The usual starting dose of gabapentin is 300 mg administered at night 30 minutes to 1 hour before symptoms (100 to 200 mg in older adults). The average effective dose is quite high (900–1200 mg). Side effects include sedation, fatigue, ataxia, nausea, weight gain, and peripheral edema. Serious reactions include leukopenia, thrombocytopenia, and depression. A slow upward titration has been used in studies of gabapentin with an increase of 300 to 600 mg every 1 to 2 weeks. This may improve tolerance to relatively high doses of gabapentin. A controlled cross-over study demonstrated that gabapentin was effective treatment of RLS in patients with renal failure who were on hemodialysis.[36] In this study, a dose of 200 to 300 mg was given after each dialysis session. Gabapentin is cleared by the kidney, so a reduced dose is needed in patients with renal insufficiency. One problem with gabapentin is that large variability in absorption and plasma levels exists because of saturable absorption in the upper intestine. The prodrug gabapentin encarbil (GEn) is rapidly absorbed throughout the gastrointestinal tract and, once absorbed, is converted to gabapentin. This drug delays the time to peak gabapentin plasma levels and provides dose-proportional exposure. The efficacy of GEn for RLS treatment has been documented by double-blind, placebo-controlled studies.[37,38]

Pregabalin (Lyrica) is a ligand that binds to the alpha-2-delta subunit of the voltage-dependent calcium channel in the CNS. Pregabalin was developed as an anticonvulsant, but it has the FDA approval for treatment of neuropathic pain and fibromyalgia. A recent double-blind, placebo-controlled study found that pregabalin in a mean dose of 333 mg was an effective treatment for RLS.[39] Treatment was started at 150 mg and increased as needed. Side effects include dizziness, drowsiness, blurred vision, and ataxia. It is more expensive that gabapentin but could be considered if a patient does not tolerate or improve with a DA and does not tolerate gabapentin.

SEDATIVE HYPNOTICS

The BZRAs, including both benzodiazepines (triazolam, temazepam, clonazepam) and non-benzodiazepines (zolpidem, zaleplon, eszopiclone) may be used for the treatment of RLS or PLMD.[40-44] The BZRAs work mainly by reducing sleep latency, increasing sleep efficiency, and reducing arousals caused by PLMS. Most studies have *not* found a decrease in the PLMSI. Some studies found clonazepam to be effective, but this medication may cause profound morning grogginess because of its long half-life.[40,41] The BZRAs with a short duration of action (triazolam),[42,43] zaleplon or zolpidem) or intermediate duration of action (zolpidem-CR, eszopiclone, temazepam) are likely to be as effective and better tolerated. In patients with early morning awakening, a change from the shorter-acting medication to a medium-duration medication may be helpful. This class of medications should be used with caution in patients with OSA or severe lung disease. The BZRAs are generally used as adjunctive treatment unless RLS is mild, insomnia is an independent problem only worsened by RLS, or both. BZRAs should not be used in patients with a history of alcohol or drug dependence.

RLS TREATMENT ALGORITHM

In choosing treatment (Table F32-5), it is useful to classify the patient using the approach of Silber and coworkers[2] into the following groups: (1) mild or intermittent RLS symptoms, (2) daily RLS symptoms, and (3) refractory RLS symptoms. The mild or intermittent group may be treated with conservative measures such as avoiding precipitating medications (sedating antihistamines) and substances (alcohol, caffeine), use of warm baths, and iron supplementation if irons stores are low. If an RLS medication is used, it should be a rapid-acting one because the patient often cannot predict that symptoms will occur. CD/LD in the short-acting form

TABLE F32-5 Restless Legs Syndrome (RLS) Treatment Algorithm

Type of RLS	Agents	Comments
Intermittent RLS RLS that is troublesome enough to require treatment but occurs on an average less than twice weekly	• Nonpharmacologic treatment • Benzodiazepines • Levodopa or carbidopa • Low potency opioids	• Need rapid onset of action • Normalize iron stores • Stop medications that worsen RLS, if possible
Chronic RLS RLS which is frequent and troublesome enough to require daily therapy, usually at least twice a week causing moderate or severe distress	Dopamine agonists*	• Very severe RLS • Co-morbid depression • Obesity/metabolic syndrome
	Alpha-2-delta ligands	• Comorbid pain or anxiety • Side effects with dopamine agonists (DAs) • Impulse control disorder on DA
Refractory RLS RLS unresponsive to monotherapy with tolerable doses of first-line agents because of reduced efficacy, augmentation or side effects	• Switch to another medication in the same class (e.g., pramipexole to ropinirole) • Combination therapy (DA +alpha-2-delta drug) • Opioid alone or in combination	• Add agent from another class with or without reduction of dose of first agent • Add benzodiazepine if RLS present at night

Adapted for Silber MH, Ehrenberg BL, Allen RP, et al: An algorithm for the management of restless legs syndrome, Mayo Clin Proc 79:916-922, 2004.
*Notes 1. If one DA does not work or is not tolerated, try other DA. 2. Consider rotigitine patch if RLS during the day

is active within a half hour and, therefore, is a good choice for the treatment of intermittent RLS (that may not be predictable). A DA will be effective, although the time to onset of effect is delayed for 1 to 3 hours. Ropinirole has a more rapid effect than pramipexole. Other choices are low-potency opiates such as propoxyphene or codeine. Sedative-hypnotics may also be effective is patients with mild or intermittent RLS.

Daily RLS of moderate severity requires a different approach. CD/LD while effective, has a short duration of action and high likelihood of augmentation and is not recommended. One of the nonergotamine DAs (ropinirole, pramipexole, or rotigitine) or an alpha-2-delta ligand are recommended for treatment of choice for daily or moderate to severe RLS. The enthusiasm for the use of DAs has diminished somewhat with the recognition that long-term follow-up reveals high rates of discontinuation of treatment. However, starting with a DA is suggested in most cases of moderate RLS. If a given DA is not effective or not tolerated, another should be tried because some patients respond better to either pramipexole or ropinirole. If daytime symptoms are a problem, use of rotigitine should be considered. *If comorbid pain, anxiety, or insomnia is present, use of an alpha-2-delta ligand should be considered as the first agent rather than a DA.* If the clinical response to a DA is inadequate or side effects prevent the use of

the DA, a low- to moderate-potency opiate, gabapentin, or a sedative-hypnotic should be tried. If side effects are noted at higher doses of a DA, a lower dose of DA may be combined with a medication from another class (e.g., lower dose of DA +gabapentin).

Refractory or severe RLS is defined as (1) inadequate initial response despite adequate dose (and timing of dose), (2) response has become inadequate over time, (3) intolerable side effects have occurred, or (4) augmentation is present. The approach to augmentation has already been discussed (see also Patient 82). Treatment approaches to refractory or severe RLS include (1) switching to another first-line agent in the same class (e.g., from ropinirole to pramipexole); (2) combination treatment (e.g., adding an opioid, alpha-2-delta ligand, or BZRA to DA treatment) with or without a reduction in the dose of the first agent; (3) changing to another class (e.g., from a DA to gabapentin), or (4) changing to a high-potency opioid. Because of the difficulty in treating severe augmentation, it is best to avoid high-doses of DAs, if possible. If combination treatment is used in a patient with mild augmentation, a reduction in the DA dose should be considered. If combination treatment for moderate to severe augmentation is used, withdrawal (weaning) of the DA is recommended after the other agent (usually an opioid) has been titrated to an effective dose.

CLINICAL PEARLS

1. Treatment options for RLS included conservative measures, dopaminergic medications (carbidopa/levodopa and dopamine agonists), anticonvulsants (alpha-2-delta ligands such as gabapentin or pregabalin), opioids, and sedative hypnotics.

2. Carbidopa/Levodopa is a rapidly absorbed dopaminergic medication (levodopa is a precursor of dopamine) that is an effective treatment of RLS. It is a good option for intermittent RLS. However, the medication has a short duration of action and continued use results in augmentation in up to 80% of cases (especially with doses of levodopa >200 mg daily).

3. The dopamine agonists ropinirole, pramipexole, and rotigitine patch are FDA approved for the treatment of RLS in adults and are considered as the treatment of choice for daily RLS. Pramipexole and ropinirole must be given several hours before symptoms to be most effective. The rotigitine transdermal patch is useful for patients with daytime RLS symptoms, augmentation associated with the other DAs, or both.

4. Anticonvulsants (gabapentin, gabapentin encarbil, pregabalin) are also effective for daily RLS or PLMD and are considered first-line agents if comorbid insomnia, anxiety, or pain exists. Gabapentin encarbil has more reliable absorption and requires less dose titration than gabapentin but is expensive. For gabapentin, a slow upward titration of the dose starting at 300 mg (100 to 200 mg in older adults) may improve tolerance to use. The effective dose range is 900 to 1200 mg in many patients. Gabapentin is considered a first-line medication by some clinicians if RLS is associated with pain.

5. Narcotics are effective treatment for RLS. They may be especially useful in patients who develop severe augmentation or do not tolerate dopamine agonists. If given only at bedtime they usually do not result in dependence. For milder cases, codeine, propoxyphene, or tramadol may be effective. For moderate RLS hydrocodone (combined with acetaminophen in the United States) or oxycodone are often used. For severe RLS, oxycodone or methadone has been used with success.

6. Sedative hypnotics may be useful in milder RLS associated with insomnia or may be combined with other classes of medications. Most of the published treatment trials used clonazepam (long half-life) but other benzodiazepine receptor agonists may also be effective.

7. Augmentation describes a phenomenon that is characterized by one or more of the following: (1) earlier symptom onset, (2) greater severity of symptoms at the same dose or escalating dose, (3) reduced latency to onset of symptoms with rest, and (4) spread of symptoms to involve new body parts (arms as well as legs).

8. Low serum ferritin is a risk factor for development of augmentation.

9. Patients with RLS who have ferritin levels <45 to 50 mcg/mL may improve with iron supplementation. The usual dose is ferrous sulfate 325 mg three times daily with each dose given with 100 to 200 mg of ascorbic acid to improve absorption. Patients with augmentation may improve with iron supplementation.

10. Impulse control disorders are more common in patients on DAs than previously recognized, but symptoms are often not reported by patients.

REFERENCES

1. Littner MR, Kushida C, Anderson WM, et al: Practice parameters for the dopaminergic treatment of restless legs syndrome and periodic limb movement disorder, *Sleep* 27:557–559, 2004.
2. Silber MH, Ehrenberg BL, Allen RP, et al: An algorithm for the management of restless legs syndrome, *Mayo Clin Proc* 79:916–922, 2004.
3. Aurora RN, Kristo DA, Bista SR, et al: The treatment of restless legs syndrome and periodic limb movement disorder in adults-an update for 2012: practice parameters with an evidence-based systematic review and meta-analyses: an American Academy of Sleep Medicine Clinical Practice Guideline, *Sleep* 35(8):1039–1062, 2012.
4. Picchietti MA, Picchietti DL: Advances in pediatric restless legs syndrome: iron, genetics, diagnosis and treatment, *Sleep Med* 11:643–651, 2010.
5. Walters AS, Mandelbaum DE, Lewin DS, et al: Dopaminergic therapy in children with restless legs/periodic limb movements in sleep and ADHD. Dopaminergic Therapy Study Group, *Pediatr Neurol* 22:182–186, 2000.
6. Hoque R, Chesson Jr AL: Pharmacologically induced/exacerbated restless legs syndrome, periodic limb movements of sleep, and REM behavior disorder/REM sleep without atonia: literature review, qualitative scoring, and comparative analysis, *J Clin Sleep Med* 6(1):79–83, 2010.
7. Nofzinger EA, Fasiczka A, Berman S, Thase ME: Bupropion SR reduces periodic limb movements associated with arousal from sleep in depressed patients with period limb movement disorder, *J Clin Psychiatry* 61:858–862, 2000.

8. Bayard M, Bailey B, Acharya D, et al: Bupropion and restless legs syndrome: a randomized controlled trial, *J Am Board Fam Med* 24(4):422–428, 2011.
9. Sun ER, Chen CA, Ho G, et al: Iron and the restless legs syndrome, *Sleep* 21:381–387, 1998.
10. Mackie S, Winkelman JW: Normal ferritin in a patient with iron deficiency and RLS, *J Clin Sleep Med* 9(5):511–513, 2013.
11. Wang J, O'Reilly B, Venkataraman R, et al: Efficacy of oral iron in patients with restless legs syndrome and a low-normal ferritin: A randomized, double-blind, placebo-controlled study, *Sleep Med* 10(9):973–975, 2009.
12. Cho YW, Allen RP, Earley CJ: Lower molecular weight intravenous iron dextran for restless legs syndrome, *Sleep Med* 14(3):274–277, 2013.
13. Earley CJ, Allen RP: Pergolide and carbidopa/levodopa periodic leg movements in sleep in a consecutive series of patients, *Sleep* 19:801–810, 1996.
14. Montplaisir J, Nicolas A, Denesle R, et al: Restless leg syndrome improved by pramipexole: a double-blind randomized trial, *Neurology* 52:938–943, 1999.
15. Montplaisir J, Denesle R, Petit D: Pramipexole in the treatment of restless leg syndrome: a follow-up study, *Eur J Neurol* 1:27–31, 2000.
16. Adler CH, Hauser RA, Sethi K, et al: Ropinirole for restless legs syndrome, *Neurology* 62:1405–1407, 2004.
17. Allen R, Becker PM, Bogan R, et al: Ropinirole decreases periodic leg movements and improves sleep parameters in patients with restless legs syndrome, *Sleep* 27:907–914, 2004.
18. Saletu M, Anderer P, Saletu B, et al: Sleep laboratory studies in periodic limb movement disorder (PLMD) patients as compared to normals and acute effects of ropinirole, *Hum Psychopharmacol Clin Exp* 16:177–187, 2001.

19. Inoue Y, Hirata K, Hayashida K, et al: Rotigotine Study Group: Efficacy, safety and risk of augmentation of rotigotine for treating restless legs syndrome, *Prog Neuropsychopharmacol Biol Psychiatry* 40:326–333, 2013.
20. Hening WA, Allen RP, Ondo WG, et al: SP792 Study Group: Rotigotine improves restless legs syndrome: a 6-month randomized, double-blind, placebo-controlled trial in the United States, *Mov Disord* 25(11):1675–1683, 2010.
21. Winkleman JW, Johnson L: Augmentation and tolerance with long-term pramipexole treatment of restless legs syndrome, *Sleep Med* 5:9–14, 2004.
22. Silver N, Allen RP, Senerth J, Earley CJ: A 10-year, longitudinal assessment of dopamine agonists and methadone in the treatment of restless legs syndrome, *Sleep Med* 12(5):440–444, 2011.
23. Lipford MC, Silber MH: Long-term use of pramipexole in the management of restless legs syndrome, *Sleep Med* 13(10):1280–1285, 2012.
24. Cornelius JR, Tippmann-Peikert M, Slocumb NL, et al: Impulse control disorders with the use of dopaminergic agents in restless legs syndrome: a case-control study, *Sleep* 33:81–87, 2010.
25. Voon V, Schoerling A, Wenzel S, et al: Frequency of impulse control behaviours associated with dopaminergic therapy in restless legs syndrome, *BMC Neurol* 11:117, 2011.
26. García-Borreguero D, Allen RP, Kohnen R, et al: International Restless Legs Syndrome Study Group: Diagnostic standards for dopaminergic augmentation of restless legs syndrome: report from a World Association of Sleep Medicine-International Restless Legs Syndrome Study Group consensus conference at the Max Planck Institute, *Sleep Med* 8(5):520–530, 2007.
27. Trenkwalder C, Hogl B, Benes H, et al: Augmentation in restless legs syndrome is associated with low ferritin, *Sleep Med* 9:572–574, 2008.
28. Walters AS, Wagner ML, Hening WA, et al: Successful treatment of the idiopathic restless leg syndrome in a randomized double-blind trial of oxycodone versus placebo, *Sleep* 16:327–332, 1993.
29. Kaplan PW, Allen RP, Bucholz DW, Walters JK: A double-blind, placebo-controlled study of the treatment of periodic limb movements in sleep using carbidopa/levodopa and propoxyphene, *Sleep* 16:717–723, 1993.
30. Walters AS, Winkelmann J, Trenkwalder C, et al: Long-term follow-up on restless legs syndrome patients treated with opioids, *Mov Disord* 16(6):1105–1109, 2001.
31. Ondo WG: Methadone for refractory restless legs syndrome, *Mov Disord* 20(3):345–348, 2005.
32. Walters AS: Review of receptor agonist and antagonist studies relevant to the opiate system in restless legs syndrome, *Sleep Med* 3(4):301–304, 2002.
33. Happe S, Sauter C, Klosch G, et al: Gabapentin versus ropinirole in the treatment of idiopathic restless legs syndrome, *Neuropsychobiology* 48:82–86, 2003.
34. Garcia-Borreguero D, Larrosa O, de la Llave Y, et al: Treatment of restless legs syndrome with gabapentin, *Neurology* 59:1573–1579, 2002.
35. Saletu M, Anderer P, Saletu-Zyhlarz GM, et al: Comparative placebo-controlled polysomnographic and psychometric studies on the acute effects of gabapentin versus ropinirole in restless legs syndrome, *J Neural Transm* 117(4):463–473, 2010.
36. Thorp ML, Morris CD, Bagby SP: A crossover study of gabapentin in treatment of restless legs syndrome among hemodialysis patients, *Am J Kidney Dis* 38:104–108, 2001.
37. Kushida CA, Becker PM, Ellengoben AL, et al: Randomized, double-blind, placebo-controlled study of XP135412/GSK1838262 in patients with RLS, *Neurology* 72:439–446, 2009.
38. Lee DO, Ziman RB, Perkins AT, et al: XP053 Study Group: A randomized, double-blind, placebo-controlled study to assess the efficacy and tolerability of gabapentin enacarbil in subjects with restless legs syndrome, *J Clin Sleep Med* 7(3):282–292, 2011.
39. Garcia-Borreguero D, Larrosa O, Williams AM, et al: Treatment of restless legs syndrome with pregabalin: a double-blind, placebo-controlled study, *Neurology* 74:1897–1904, 2010.
40. Mitler MM, Browman CP, Menn SJ, et al: Nocturnal myoclonus: treatment efficacy of clonazepam and temazepam, *Sleep* 9:385–392, 1986.
41. Peled R, Lavie P: Double-blind evaluation of clonazepam on periodic leg movements in sleep, *J Neurol Neurosurg Psychiatry* 50:1679–1681, 1987.
42. Bonnet MH, Arand DL: The use of triazolam in older patients with periodic leg movements, fragmented sleep, and daytime sleepiness, *J Gerontol* 45:M139–M144, 1990.
43. Doghramji K, Browman CP, Gaddy JR, et al: Triazolam diminishes daytime sleepiness and sleep fragmentation in patients with periodic leg movements in sleep, *J Clin Psychopharmacol* 11:284–290, 1991.
44. Saletu M, Anderer P, Saletu-Zyhalrz G, et al: Restless legs syndrome (RLS) and periodic limb movement disorder (PLMD): acute placebo-controlled sleep laboratory study with clonazepam, *Eur Neuropsychopharmacol* 11:153–161, 2001.

PATIENT 81

Problems with Dopamine Agonist Treatment for RLS

Patient A: A 35-year-old woman was evaluated for severe restless legs syndrome (RLS) that typically occurred every night and prevented her from going to sleep for at least 1 or 2 hours. The patient was treated with ropinirole at bedtime, and the dose was progressively increased to 1 milligram (mg) without any improvement in symptoms. She had declined use of an opioid. Clonazepam was added but did not dramatically improve her symptoms and caused severe morning sedation. She was also tried on gabapentin but developed severe dizziness and headache. The patient was taking bupropion for depression and had no other active health problems except for menorrhagia.

Question A: What treatment options do you suggest for Patient A? What laboratory tests might be helpful?

Patient B: A 50-year-old man was being monitored for the RLS. His condition had been fairly well controlled with pramipexole 0.50 mg, but recently, the dose had been increased to pramipexole 1 mg. The patient did not report any side effects following the increase in the dosage of the medication. However, his wife reported that she had noted some very uncharacteristic changes in his behavior. For example, he had charged over $2000 on his credit card with purchases from the shopping television channel. He also traded in his car for a more expensive luxury model and had gained 20 pounds from uncharacteristic eating.

Question B: How do you explain the change in behavior in Patient B?

ANSWERS

1. **Answer (Patient A):** Pramipexole should be taken 2 to 3 before bedtime. Obtaining serum ferritin and iron saturation levels is important as low iron stores may worsen RLS. Patients with resistant RLS or augmentation often have low iron stores.

Discussion: The dopamine agonists (DAs) pramipexole and ropinirole are approved by the U.S. Food and Drug Administration (FDA) for treatment of RLS. As the duration of action of these drugs is fairly long, adequate control of symptoms for the entire night is usually possible without the need for dosing for the middle of the night. The DAs are very effective in the treatment for RLS, but a number of considerations exist in using the medications. It is important to note that the onset of action of the DAs is delayed following drug ingestion. The manufacturers recommend taking ropinirole 1 to 2 hours and pramipexole 2 to 3 hours before bedtime (or symptoms). If both are taken 2 hours before bedtime, they should be effective. Ropinirole has a slightly faster onset of action than pramipexole. Failure to observe the need for an early medication administration may result in an unnecessary increase in dose or in the conclusion that the medications are not effective. Using higher than needed doses of DAs predispose patients to the risk of augmentation (worse RLS control at current dose, need to continually escalate the dose, symptoms earlier in the day, or symptoms in the arms as well as the legs). See Patient 82 for a detailed discussion of augmentation. Avoiding excessive doses of DAs may reduce the risk of this problem. Rotigitine is a DA available as a transdermal patch and is especially useful if treatment of RLS is needed during the day.

Iron deficiency may cause or worsen RLS. A ferritin level is recommended in patients with RLS because this disorder may be the only indication that iron stores are low. Most clinicians recommend that a ferritin level above 45 to 50 nanograms per milliliter (ng/mL) be achieved in patients with RLS. As ferritin may be elevated by inflammation, most clinicians recommend determining iron saturation and total iron binding capacity (TIBC) as well. If iron saturation is reduced and TIBC increased, iron supplementation may be beneficial, even if the ferritin is not decreased. Patients should also be evaluated for occult gastrointestinal blood loss, if clinically indicated. Typical iron supplementation is ferrous sulfate 325 mg three times daily with 100 to 200 mg of ascorbic acid (to improve absorption). Iron absorption is best achieved on an empty stomach, but the supplement may need to be taken with food to avoid severe gastrointestinal upset. Monitoring of ferritin levels is recommended to ensure adequate replenishment of iron stores and to avoid inducing iron overload. When ferritin levels exceed the goal, iron supplementation may be stopped. It is important to note that iron supplementation alone does not always improve RLS. However, many patients will have better results with treatment with standard RLS medications. It has also been observed that low iron levels are a risk factor for augmentation. Some patients have difficulty replenishing iron stores because of ongoing bleeding, poor absorption of iron, or intolerance to oral iron. In such cases, intravenous (IV) iron replacement could be considered. Newer forms of IV iron are associated with fewer side effects.

Patient A was instructed to take the pramipexole 2 hours before bedtime. A lower dose of 0.75 mg was effective when taken earlier. On a few nights, an extra dose of pramipexole was still needed. Laboratory results revealed serum ferritin level to be 5 ng/mL, and the patient was referred to a gynecologist for her menorrhagia and started on oral iron therapy. With control of excessive menstrual bleeding and iron supplementation, the ferritin level reached 40 ng/mL after 3 months. At that time, the symptoms of RLS were reliably controlled with a dose of 0.75 mg.

2. **Answer (Patient B):** Impulse control disorder (ICD) caused by a dopamine agonist

Discussion: Dopamine dysregulation syndrome (DDS) is a relatively recently described iatrogenic disturbance that may complicate long-term treatment with dopaminergic medications. It is more common in patients with Parkinson disease but not uncommon in patients with RLS. In Parkinson disease, patients with DDS develop an addictive pattern of dopamine replacement therapy (DRT) use, administering doses in excess of those required to control their motor symptoms as well as impulse control disorders (ICDs). The prevalence of DDS in patients attending specialist Parkinson disease centers is 3% to 4%. The hallmark of ICDs is a "failure to resist an impulse, drive, or temptation to perform an act that is harmful to the person or to others." *ICDs include punding, pathologic gambling, hypersexuality, compulsive shopping, and compulsive (binge) eating.* Punding is characterized by compulsive fascination with and performance of repetitive, mechanical tasks such as assembling and disassembling, collecting, or sorting household objects. Cornelius et al used a questionnaire followed by a telephone interview and found an increased incidence of ICDs in populations of patients with OSA and patients with RLS not on dopaminergic treatment (case-controlled study). The incidence of specific types of ICDs in patients with RLS on dopaminergic treatment was found to be: 9% compulsive shopping, 5% pathologic gambling, 11% compulsive eating, 3% hypersexuality, 7% punding, and 17% any ICD. In this study, a higher dose of pramipexole was associated with an increased risk for the ICDs. The treatment of ICDs in patients with RLS usually involves stopping the dopaminergic medication and switching to another class of medications. Some authors have hypothesized that the use of a transdermal dopamine agonist (constant lower dose) might prevent ICDs. However, a recent study by Schreglmann et al found ICDs were present in a group of patients using transdermal rotigotine. In the current patient, the problematic behavior and likely cause were discussed with the patient and his wife. Pramipexole was stopped, and the patient was started on gabapentin enacarbil 600 mg to be taken at 5 PM. On this mediation, RLS symptoms were controlled. The patient and his wife reported that the symptoms of poor impulse control had resolved.

CLINICAL PEARLS

1. The onset of action of the DAs ropinirole and pramipexole is delayed, and they should be taken 2 hours before bedtime (or onset of symptoms).
2. The dose of dopamine agonists should be escalated slowly to avoid using an excessive dose. Higher doses may cause more side effects and increase the risk of augmentation.
3. Iron deficiency may worsen RLS and probably decrease the effectiveness of medication treatment. Iron deficiency also increases the risk of augmentation. Laboratory evaluation of ferritin, total iron binding capacity, and the iron saturation is suggested in all patients with RLS.
4. Although the normal range for ferritin is often listed as >12 to 20 ng/mL, the desired range for a patient with RLS is >45 to 50 ng/mL (some clinicians use 70).
5. ICDs are more common than previously thought in patients being treated with dopaminergic medications for RLS. Patients should be questioned carefully about symptoms of the ICDs and informed of the risk before starting medications. Manifestations of impulse control include compulsive gambling, compulsive shopping, risky sexual behaviors, and compulsive eating. The treatment of choice is stopping the dopaminergic medication and switching to another class of medications to treat RLS.

BIBLIOGRAPHY

Aurora RN, Kristo DA, Bista SR, et al: The treatment of restless legs syndrome and periodic limb movement disorder in adults—an update for 2012: practice parameters with an evidence-based systematic review and meta-analyses, *Sleep* 35(8):1039–1062, 2012.
Cho YW, Allen RP, Earley CJ: Lower molecular weight intravenous iron dextran for restless legs syndrome, *Sleep Med* 14 (3):274–277, 2013.
Cornelius JR, Tippmann-Peikert M, Slocumb NL, et al: Impulse control disorders with the use of dopaminergic agents in restless legs syndrome: a case–control study, *Sleep* 33(1):81–87, 2010.
Dang D, Cunnington D, Swieca J: The emergence of devastating impulse control disorders during dopamine agonist therapy of the restless legs syndrome, *Clin Neuropharmacol* 34(2):66–70, 2011.
Garcia-Borreguero D(1), Kohnen R, Silber MH, et al: The long-term treatment of restless legs syndrome/Willis-Ekbom disease: evidence-based guidelines and clinical consensus best practice guidance: a report from the International Restless Legs Syndrome Study Group, *Sleep Med* 14(7):675–684, 2013.
O'Sullivan SS, Evans AH, Lees AJ: Dopamine dysregulation syndrome: an overview of its epidemiology, mechanisms and management, *CNS Drugs* 23(2):157–170, 2009.

Schreglmann SR, Gantenbein AR, Eisele G, et al: Transdermal rotigotine causes impulse control disorders in patients with restless legs syndrome, *Parkinsonism Relat Disord* 18(2):207–209, 2012.

Silber MH, Ehrenberg BL, Allen RP, et al, Medical Advisory Board of the Restless Legs Syndrome Foundation: An algorithm for the management of restless legs syndrome, *Mayo Clin Proc* 79(7):916–922.

Tippmann-Peikert M, Park JG, Boeve BF, et al: Pathologic gambling in patients with restless legs syndrome treated with dopaminergic agonists, *Neurology* 68(4):301–303, 2007.

Transdermal rotigotine causes impulse control disorders in patients with restless legs syndrome, *Parkinsonism Relat Disord* 18 (2):207–209, 2012.

Trenkwalder C, Hogl B, Benes H, et al: Augmentation in restless legs syndrome is associated with low ferritin, *Sleep Med* 9:572–574, 2008.

Voon V, Schoerling A, Wenzel S, et al: Frequency of impulse control behaviours associated with dopaminergic therapy in restless legs syndrome, *BMC Neurol* 11:117, 2011.

Wang J, O'Reilly B, Venkataraman R, et al: Efficacy of oral iron in patients with restless legs syndrome and a low-normal ferritin: A randomized, double-blind, placebo-controlled study, *Sleep Med* 10(9):973–975, 2009.

PATIENT 82

Patients on Dopamine Agonists with Worsening RLS

Patient A: A 50-year-old woman complained of worsening of her restless legs syndrome (RLS). Her condition was initially well controlled on pramipexole 0.5 milligram (mg) given 2 hours before her usual bedtime (11PM). Then she developed RLS symptoms at 7 PM, and the dose was split (0.25 mg at 5 PM and 0.5 mg at 9 PM). This alleviated the symptoms for a few months, but the symptoms began to worsen again. Over the next month, her dose of pramipexole was increased to 0.5 mg at 5 PM and 0.75 mg at 9 PM. However, her symptoms continued to worsen, and she began to experience her familiar RLS sensations in her arms.

Patient B: A 45-year-old man was evaluated for difficult-to-control RLS. He had been on pramipexole at high doses (2 mg), but his symptoms worsened. His physician asked him to stop taking the medication. This caused such severe symptoms that he was up most of the night. He was started on oxycodone 10 to 15 mg, which provided good relief of his symptoms. At the time of evaluation, his dose of pramipexole was down to 1 mg. He is very concerned about taking narcotics for the rest of his life.

Patient C: A 35-year-old woman with RLS had her symptoms well controlled on ropinirole 0.5 mg at 5 PM and 1.5 mg taken 2 hours before bedtime. Recently, she noted nights when her symptoms were not in good control. Her iron stores were checked and were normal.

QUESTIONS

1. What interventions do you suggest for Patient A? Why is her RLS worsening?

2. What treatment do you suggest for Patient B?

3. What treatment do you suggest for Patient C?

ANSWERS

1. **Answer (Patient A):** The patient has severe augmentation with worsening of RLS. Interventions include starting a potent opioid, weaning off from pramipexole, and checking iron stores.

Discussion: Augmentation occurs in the short term (months to a year) in up to 30% of patients started on a dopamine agonist (DA) (Box P82-1). Although generally milder than augmentation with carbidopa/levodopa, augmentation may be severe. If patients experience symptoms starting earlier in the evening using a split dose (e.g., half the total dose at 6 PM and the other half give 2 hours before bedtime) may be successful (Box P82-2). This was tried in this patient and did work for a few months. Another approach if augmentation is mild is to change to another DA (e.g., from pramipexole to ropinirole or the rotigotine patch) (Figure P82-1). If symptoms worsen on a given dose after a period of good control, rather than escalating the dose of the DA, a medication from another class may be added, for example, the addition of gabapentin to the current dose (or a reduced dose) of the DA. Low iron stores predispose patients to augmentation, so ferritin and iron saturation levels should be checked. If iron stores are low, iron supplementation may help control RLS symptoms without having to escalate the dose of DA. When augmentation is severe, withdrawal of the DA is indicated. This usually results in a significant worsening of symptoms if done without the addition of another effective medication. A potent opioid or an alpha-2-delta ligand (e.g., gabapentin) is added at an effective dose before the DA is weaned. In the setting of severe augmentation most clinicians would add a potent opioid and wean the DA. Opioid medications

---

BOX P82-1	**Characteristics of Augmentation**

- Previous response to a dopamine agonist (DA) followed by need for dose escalation
- Paradoxical response—symptoms worsen when DA dose increased (although not necessarily immediately) and improve when dose decreased

- Symptoms earlier in the day
- Symptoms in the arms
- Shorter latency to symptoms when at rest
- Shorter duration of benefit from medication

BOX P82-2	**Approaches to Augmentation**

1. If on LD/CD, stop and change to a DA (avoid LD/CD in daily RLS, avoid dose >200 milligrams [mg] LD).
2. If on a DA and earlier symptom onset is the problem, split the dose and give half of the dose earlier.
3. Change to a different DA medication.
4. If morning symptoms are a problem, try an evening and morning dose of medication (or use rotigotine patch).

5. If patient is taking a DA and has moderate augmentation, reduce dose and add gabapentin or an opioid.
6. If augmentation is very severe, stop (wean) the DA or LD/CD, and add high-potency opioid.
7. Avoid high doses of DAs; use combination therapy (add opiate, gabapentin, or BZRA).
8. Low iron stores may predispose to augmentation, correct low iron stores.

BZRA, Benzodiazepine receptor agonist; *DA*, dopamine agonist; *LD/CD*, levodopa/carbidopa, *RLS*, restless legs syndrome.

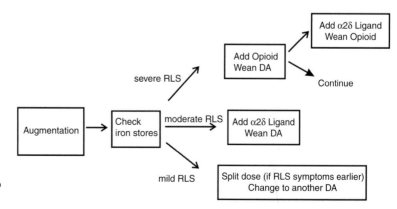

FIGURE P82-1 ■ Approaches to treating augmentation.

do not need to be titrated slowly and are very effective. If a patient has a history of drug abuse or dependence, then an alpha-2-delta medication would be a better choice. Use of gabapentin enacarbil instead of gabapentin could be considered as the period of titration is quicker. Most patients respond to either 600 mg or 1200 mg at 5 PM.

Patient A was started on oxycodone 10 mg given 1 hour before bedtime and the pramipexole weaned off over 2 weeks. During the first week, an additional 5-mg dose of oxycodone at 5 PM was needed for early symptoms. The ferritin level was checked (20 micrograms per liter [mcg/L]) and found to be lower than desired (>45 to 50 mcg/L). Iron supplementation was started. The patient continued on oxycodone 10 mg nightly with good control of her RLS.

2. **Answer (Patient B):** For the short term, continue to wean the DA with simultaneous treatment with an opioid. Once the patient is weaned off the DA, start an alpha-2-delta ligand medication, and taper the opioid, if possible.

Discussion: When patients have severe RLS and augmentation on DA treatment, tapering or stopping the DA is often associated with intolerable symptoms. Potent opioids (methadone, oxycodone) are rapidly effective in this setting. Once the patient is weaned off the DA, the opioid may be continued as monotherapy. If continued use of an opioid is not desired, an alpha-2-delta ligand medication may be tried (see Figure P82-1). This usually requires combination therapy as the dose of gabapentin is slowly increased to improve tolerance to the medication. Typically, dose of the alpha-2-delta ligand medication is increased and the dose of the opioid medication decreased. Some patients with severe RLS may require continued combination therapy (both opioid and alpha-2-delta medication). When augmentation is milder, the patient can be started on an alpha-2-delta medication and weaned off the DA. As the dose of DA is reduced, the dose of the alpha-2-delta medication is increased, if needed. The option of simply reducing the DA dose and adding an alpha-2-delta medication or opioid is also available. Some patients with significant side effects from high doses of DAs, alpha-2-delta ligands, or opioids may benefit from combination therapy (lower dose of each agent).

In patient B, oxycodone was continued, and the patient was weaned off pramipexole over 2 weeks. Once the DA medication was stopped, gabapentin was started at 300 mg at night and increased to 900 mg before bedtime. Gabapentin was well tolerated, and the dose of oxycodone was reduced to 5 mg. After 1 week on this combination, oxycodone was stopped. Unfortunately, RLS control was not satisfactory on a few nights each week. Gabapentin was increased to 1200 mg, but this dose was not tolerated. The patient was agreeable to the use of gabapentin 900 mg nightly with an as-needed 5-mg dose of oxycodone for breakthrough symptoms. On this treatment regimen, his RLS was in good control.

3. **Answer (C):** Add an agent from another class of medications rather than further increasing the DA.

Discussion: If a patient is on a relatively high dose of a DA and continues to have RLS symptoms, use of combination therapy may be effective and reduce the risk of augmentation. It may be possible to actually reduce the dose of the DA once the second agent is started. An opioid, an alpha-2-delta ligand, or a benzodiazepine receptor agonist may be added. In Patient C, oxycodone was started and increased to 10 mg. The RLS symptoms were in good control on combination therapy. The dose of ropinirole was decreased to 0.5 mg at 5 PM and 0.5 mg at bedtime along with oxycodone 10 mg. On this treatment regimen, the RLS symptoms remained in good control.

CLINICAL PEARLS

1. It is important to recognize the signs of augmentation to avoid continuing escalation of the dose of a DA medication, which will only worsen the augmentation.

2. In patients with severe augmentation, weaning off the patient from the DA with coverage with an opioid is an effective approach. An alternative is to use an alpha-2-delta receptor ligand (e.g., gabapentin), but this may not control the symptoms if RLS is severe.

3. Use of combination therapy to avoid excessive doses of DAs is a useful approach. The combination of a DA and an alpha-2-delta ligand is an effective option. If alpha-2-delta agonists are not tolerated, the combination of a DA and an opioid may be effective.

4. In patients with augmentation or inadequate control of symptoms, it is important to normalize iron stores. The goal is a ferritin level of >50 nanograms per milliliter (ng/mL).

BIBLIOGRAPHY

Aurora RN, Kristo DA, Bista SR, et al: The treatment of restless legs syndrome and periodic limb movement disorder in adults-an update for 2012: practice parameters with an evidence-based systematic review and meta-analyses: an American Academy of Sleep Medicine Clinical Practice Guideline, *Sleep* 35(8):1039–1062, 2012.

Garcia-Borreguero D(1), Kohnen R, Silber MH, et al: The long-term treatment of restless legs syndrome/Willis-Ekbom disease: evidence-based guidelines and clinical consensus best practice guidance: a report from the International Restless Legs Syndrome Study Group, *Sleep Med* 14(7):675–684, 2013.

Lipford MC, Silber MH: Long-term use of pramipexole in the management of restless legs syndrome, *Sleep Med* 13 (10):1280–1285, 2012.

Silber MH, Ehrenberg BL, Allen RP, et al: An algorithm for the management of restless legs syndrome, *Mayo Clin Proc* 79:916–922, 2004.

Silver N, Allen RP, Senerth J, Earley CJ: A 10-year, longitudinal assessment of dopamine agonists and methadone in the treatment of restless legs syndrome, *Sleep Med* 12(5):440–444, 2011.

Trenkwalder C, Hogl B, Benes H, et al: Augmentation in restless legs syndrome is associated with low ferritin, *Sleep Med* 9:572–574, 2008.

Winkleman JW, Johnson L: Augmentation and tolerance with long-term pramipexole treatment of restless legs syndrome, *Sleep Med* 5:9–14, 2004.

PATIENT 83

A Patient with RLS and Pain and a Patient with Ropinirole-Induced Nausea

Patient A: A 60-year-old man with diabetes complained of uncomfortable sensations in his legs nearly every night. The sensations were painful (burning and tingling) and started about 9 PM while he was watching television. The sensations were associated with an urge to move the legs and were temporarily improved by walking. He also had numbness in his legs during the day, but the sensations at night were different and much more intense. The patient was being treated for diabetes and was taking metformin and lisinopril (angiotensin-converting enzyme [ACE] inhibitor). He denied snoring or daytime sleepiness. However, about three nights per week, the leg pain resulted in a very prolonged time to fall asleep.

Patient B: A 40-year-old woman was being seen at the request of her primary physician for assistance in treatment of her restless legs syndrome (RLS). The patient was tried on ropinirole but developed severe nausea when the dose was increased from 0.5 milligrams (mg) to 0.75 mg. The dose increase had been prompted by incomplete control of her symptoms. She had been on escitalopram for many years for recurrent depression. The patient's primary care physician started her on gabapentin 300 mg at bedtime, but this did not improve her RLS symptoms.

QUESTIONS

1. What treatment to you recommend for Patient A?

2. What treatment do you recommend for Patient B?

ANSWERS

1. **Answer (Patient A):** Treatment with gabapentin (or gabapentin enacarbil, pregabalin)

   Discussion: In patients with significant daily RLS symptoms, the treatment of choice is usually a dopamine agonist (DA). However, because of reports of long-term decreases in efficacy with DAs, some now consider use of an alpha-2-delta medication (gabapentin, gabapentin enacarbil, pregabalin) as alternative first-line treatment (Table P83-1). If the patient has comorbid insomnia, pain, or anxiety, alpha-2-delta medications are probably the treatment of choice. These agents bind to alpha-2-delta subunits of voltage-gated calcium channels in the central nervous system.

   Gabapentin has been approved by the U.S. Food and Drug Administration (FDA) for treatment of herpetic neuralgia and as an adjunct treatment for partial seizures. It has also been used for diabetic neuropathy (not FDA approved for this indication). It is excreted unchanged in urine with a half-life of 5 to 7 hours. The dose must be reduced in patients with decreased renal function. Coadministration with antacids reduces absorption of gabapentin, whereas some medications (methadone, morphine, hydrocodone) increase the plasma levels of gabapentin. On the other hand, gabapentin lowers the levels of hydrocodone. A major problem with the use of gabapentin is that it has a dose-dependent bioavailability (as the dose increases the proportion absorbed decreases). In addition, the ability to absorb gabapentin varies between individuals. Because gabapentin is mildly sedating, it also tends to improve sleep quality and may increase stage N3 sleep. Unlike RLS treatment with DAs, augmentation has not been described. A slow dose escalation is needed to improve tolerance to gabapentin. Typically, the starting dose is 300 mg (100 to 200 mg in older adults), with progressive increases as tolerated or needed. The usual effective dose is between 900 and 1200 mg. Some patients will benefit from lower doses, and some need a higher dose.

   Gabapentin enacarbil (Horizant) is the first nonDA that is FDA approved treatment for moderate to severe RLS. It is a prodrug of gabapentin with reliable absorption. The drug is absorbed via high capacity rapid intestinal transporters. The drug undergoes rapid hydrolysis to gabapentin. Side effects are similar to gabapentin (e.g., headaches, dizziness, weight gain, somnolence). No significant drug interactions exist. The usual dose is 600 mg at 5 PM. As no generic formulation is available, the medication is more expensive than gabapentin. On the other hand, the need for dose titration, which is needed with gabapentin, may be avoided with this drug.

   Pregabalin (Lyrica) is a structural analog to gamma-aminobutyric acid (GABA) and an alpha-2-delta receptor ligand. It is FDA approved for pain caused by herpetic or diabetic neuropathy, for treatment of fibromyalgia, and as adjunct medication for partial seizures. It has primarily renal elimination, with a half-life of 1.5 hours. No significant drug interactions are noted in pregabalin.

2. **Answer:** Try pramipexole rather than ropinirole, use a lower dose of ropinirole and add gabapentin, or increase the dose of gabapentin.

   Discussion: Some patients who experience intolerable side effects from one DA will tolerate another medication (e.g., ropinirole if pramipexole is not tolerated). The same is true for patients

TABLE P83-1   Alpha-2-Delta Ligands for Restless Legs Syndrome Treatment

Medication	Starting Dose	Usual Effective Dose Range	Side Effects
Gabapentin 100-, 300-, 400-milligram (mg) tablets Category C	Start 300 mg in adults 100–200 mg in older adults	900–1200 mg	Dizziness or ataxia Somnolence or drowsiness Tremor Headache Constipation or diarrhea Edema Dry mouth Weight gain
Gabapentin enacarbil (Horizant)*	600 gm at 5 PM	600–1200 mg	Same as gabapentin
Pregabalin (Lyrica) (25-, 50-, 75-, 100-, 150-, 200-, 225-, 300-mg capsules)	75 mg in early afternoon or evening	150–300 mg	Same as gabapentin Impaired mentation

Note: Gabapentin, gabapentin enacarbil, and pregabalin are Category C.
*FDA approved for RLS treatment.

experiencing lack of efficacy. If side effects from a DA are experienced after an increase in the dose of the DA, another approach is a return to the lower tolerated dose with the addition of an agent from another class (e.g., a narcotic or gabapentin). If a patient has intolerable side effects at the starting dose of a DA, then an immediate switch to another DA, an alpha-2-delta ligand (gabapentin), or a narcotic is a reasonable approach. Gabapentin may require a period of dose escalation, so if symptoms are severe, use of an opioid may be a better choice. Another approach would be to use gabapentin enacarbil, which is often effective at the starting dose.

In the current patient, a dose of 300 mg of gabapentin was not effective. The dose was increased slowly to 900 mg. However, on this dose, the patient noted ataxia when she got out of bed during the night. The dose was reduced to 600 mg and ropinirole restarted at 0.25 mg taken 2 hours before bedtime. The combination was effective without intolerable side effects.

CLINICAL PEARLS

1. Alpha-2-delta ligand medications (gabapentin, gabapentin enacarbil, pregabalin) are effective treatment options for RLS. In comparison with DAs, they are often as effective and may improve sleep quality in addition to decreasing RLS. Augmentation has not been described with these medications.

2. Alpha-2-delta medications should be considered in patients with moderate to severe RLS who have pain, anxiety, or insomnia as prominent symptoms.

3. Alpha-2-delta medications are useful in patients with DA side effects or augmentation. They may be used either as substitutes or as combination therapy with a lower dose of DA.

4. Failure of alpha-2-delta RLS treatment is often attributed to an insufficient dose or not slowly titrating the dose upward (intolerable side effects).

5. Gabapentin has unpredictable bioavailability, and gabapentin enacarbil has predictable bioavailability but a higher cost.

BIBLIOGRAPHY

Aurora RN, Kristo DA, Bista SR, et al: The treatment of restless legs syndrome and periodic limb movement disorder in adults—an update for 2012: practice parameters with an evidence-based systematic review and meta-analyses, *Sleep* 35(8):1039–1062, 2012.

Bogan RK, Bornemann MA, Kushida CA, et al: XP060 Study Group: Long-term maintenance treatment of restless legs syndrome with gabapentin enacarbil: a randomized controlled study, *Mayo Clin Proc* 85(6):512–521, 2010.

Garcia-Borreguero D, Larrosa O, Williams AM, et al: Treatment of restless legs syndrome with pregabalin: a double-blind, placebo-controlled study, *Neurology* 74:1897–1904, 2010.

Garcia-Borreguero D, Larrosa O, de la Llave Y, et al: Treatment of restless legs syndrome with gabapentin, *Neurology* 59:1573–1579, 2002.

Happe S, Sauter C, Klosch G, et al: Gabapentin versus ropinirole in the treatment of idiopathic restless legs syndrome, *Neuropsychobiology* 48:82–86, 2003.

Kushida CA, Becker PM, Ellengoben AL, et al: Randomized, double-blind, placebo-controlled study of XP135412/GSK1838262 in patients with RLS, *Neurology* 72:439–446, 2009.

Lee DO, Ziman RB, Perkins AT, et al: XP053 Study Group: A randomized, double-blind, placebo-controlled study to assess the efficacy and tolerability of gabapentin enacarbil in subjects with restless legs syndrome, *J Clin Sleep Med* 7(3):282–292, 2011.

Thorp ML, Morris CD, Bagby SP: A crossover study of gabapentin in treatment of restless legs syndrome among hemodialysis patients, *Am J Kidney Dis* 38:104–108, 2001.

PATIENT 84

Patients with RLS and Treatment Challenges

Patient A: A 40-year-old male was evaluated for severe restless legs syndrome (RLS) symptoms. He developed severe nausea on ropinirole and pramipexole at the starting doses (neither significantly reduced the RLS symptoms). He was tried on gabapentin starting at 300 milligrams (mg) every night at bed time and titrated up to 900 mg with little benefit. On 1200 mg, he developed severe dizziness. The patient had no history of medication abuse or dependence.

Patient B: A 30-year-old woman was in the third trimester of a pregnancy. She began to develop significant symptoms of RLS. Her iron stores had been checked and were normal. Warm baths helped her alleviate the symptoms, but on some nights, the symptoms were intolerable.

Patient C: A 40-year-old woman had only fair control of RLS with pramipexole. She initially responded to 0.25 mg given 2 hours before bed time (bed time 11 PM). Then she developed symptoms at 6 PM. The early symptoms improved with 0.125 mg at 4 PM and 0.250 mg at 9 PM. However, on some nights, the symptoms were still bothersome before bed time.

QUESTIONS

1. What treatment do you recommend for Patient A?

2. What treatment do you recommend for Patient B?

3. What treatment do you recommend for Patient C?

ANSWERS

1. **Answer (Patient A):** Treatment with a potent opioid and checking the ferritin level

   Discussion: Opioids and opioid receptor agonists (tramadol) may be effective treatment options for RLS (Table P84-1). They are fairly rapid acting and may be used either singly or in combination with other medication groups such as dopamine agonists (DAs). Milder RLS may respond to low-potency opiates (propoxyphene, codeine) or the opioid agonists (tramadol). Moderate to severe RLS may respond to high-potency opiates (hydrocodone, oxycodone, methadone). Methadone has a long duration of action and may be used when patients have significant RLS symptoms during the day. Hydrocodone is available in the United States in combination with acetaminophen (APAP). One must be cautious not to prescribe an excessive dose of APAP. For example, it is preferable to using hydrocodone/APAP 10/325 rather than 2 tablets of 5/325 mg. A maximum of 2 grams (g) of APAP/day can be used, although lower doses can be harmful if liver disease is present. Side effects of opiates include nausea and constipation. These medications should not be used with alcohol and should be used with caution in patients with obstructive sleep apnea (OSA). Because of the potential for abuse and dependence, opiates are not the drugs of choice for daily treatment of RLS. However, studies and clinical experience suggest that dependence is not a problem if patients

TABLE P84-1	Opioids Treatment of Restless Leg Syndrome					
	Dose Forms	Initial Dose (mg)	Usual Effective Dose (milligram [mg])	Max Dose (24-hour [hr])	Time to Onset of Action	Half-Life (Elimination)
Propoxyphene napsylate (Darvon) Propoxyphene hydrochloride	100 32, 65	100 65	100 65	100 mg every 4 hours (q4h) 600/24-hr 65 mg q4h 390/24-hr	15–60 minutes (min) peak level 2–2.5 hr	4–6 H, R
HC/APAP (Lortab, Vicodin)	5, 7.5, 10/325 5, 7.5, 10/500	5	5–20 mg HC	20–30 mg/day in 2 or 3 divided doses	1.3 hr	3–4
Oxycodone Oxycodone/APAP (Percocet)	5, 10, 15	5	5–20 mg	5–30 q4h	10–15 min 30–60 min peak level	3–6 hr H, R
Methadone	5, 10	2.5–5	5–20 mg	15	30–60 min	8–59 hr
Tramadol*	50	50	50–100 mg	50–100 q4h 400 mg/24h	1 hr, peak level 2–3 hr	6–7 hr

APAP, Acetaminophen; *HC*, hydrocodone.
*Augmentation and seizure risk reported.

TABLE P84-2   Opioids for Restless Leg Syndrome

Advantages	Disadvantages/Side Effects
Rapid action Quick titration of dose No augmentation (except tramadol) No evidence of decreased effect with time	Abuse potential Dependence potential Side effects: - Drowsiness - Exacerbation of obstructive or central sleep apnea - Itch - Nausea - Constipation

do not have a history of opiate dependence and take medication only at night. Patients with a history of alcohol or other drug dependence or abuse are not candidates for opioid treatment. Long-term studies of patients on narcotic medications for RLS have shown that many fewer patients stop taking these medications compared with those taking DAs. Augmentation usually does not occur (except for tramadol), but an increase in dose is sometimes needed. Typical doses of opiates or opioid agonists include tramadol 50 to 100 mg, propoxyphene napsylate 100 mg, hydrocodone 5 to 15 mg, oxycodone 5 to 15 mg, and methadone 5 to 15 mg. Potential advantages and problems with narcotic treatment of RLS are listed in Table P84-2. Of note, narcotics are not approved by the U.S. Food and Drug Administration (FDA) for treatment of RLS. In addition, no studies have addressed treatment of periodic limb movement disorder (PLMD) with narcotics. In patient A, the ferritin and percentage of iron saturation studies were normal. Oxycodone was started at 5 mg at night with rapid increase of several days to 15 mg. At this dose, RLS symptoms were controlled. During follow-up at 1 year, adequate control of RLS was still present.

2. **Answer (Patient B):** Nonpharmacologic measures and iron replacement are recommended. If medications are absolutely necessary, oxycodone, which has been classified as category B, may be used.

   Discussion: RLS occurs in up to one third of patients during the third trimester of pregnancy. In the majority, RLS resolves within a few weeks after delivery. If patients have RLS before pregnancy, the severity may worsen. Nonpharmacologic treatments and replacement of iron stores is recommended. No RLS medication has been proven to be safe in pregnancy. DAs and gabapentin are category C drugs (animal reproduction studies have shown an adverse effect on the fetus, and no adequate and well-controlled studies have been performed in humans), and clonazepam is a category D drug (positive evidence of human fetal risk is based on adverse reaction data from investigational or marketing experience or studies in humans). Oxycodone is a category B drug (animal reproduction studies have failed to demonstrate a risk to the fetus, and no adequate and well-controlled studies have been performed in pregnant women) and could be used, if absolutely necessary. Near delivery, depression of fetal respiration is a concern. Although one small prospective study has documented the safety of DAs for RLS in pregnancy, most clinicians would recommend avoiding such medications, if possible. In the current patient, the risks and advantages of medications were discussed with the patient, and she opted to continue her nightly warm baths and not take medications.

3. **Answer:** Consider addition of opioid on an as-needed basis, rather than increasing the dose of pramipexole; check iron stores.

   Discussion: The maximum dose of pramipexole recommended for RLS treatment is 0.5 mg daily (although some clinician use higher doses). Higher doses are used when given over 24 hours for treatment of Parkinson disease. One option for this patient is pramipexole 0.125 mg early and 0.375 mg given 2 hours before bedtime. To avoid augmentation, it is prudent to try to use the lowest dose of the DA that is effective. Therefore, one option is the addition of an as-needed dose of an opioid on nights when RLS is not controlled. Instead, an additional 0.125 mg of pramipexole may be taken only on nights when RLS is not controlled, but the onset of an effect may be delayed for hours. Opioids are rapid acting. Checking iron stores is always indicated if RLS control is not adequate and no recent iron testing results are available. Sometimes, improved control of RLS at the current dose of a DA will occur once iron stores are >50 nanograms per milliliter (ng/mL). This takes time (unless iron is given intravenously), but some improvement may occur before iron stores are optimized. A switch from pramipexole to ropinirole is another option. The equivalent dose of ropinirole is about four times higher than the current dose of pramipexole (1 mg of pramipexole = 4 mg of ropinirole). Other approaches are use of the current dose of pramipexole and addition of an alpha-2-delta ligand medication or a benzodiazepine receptor agonist. If one of these approaches does not work or is not tolerated, another approach could be tried. In the current patient, oxycodone 5 mg was added to the patient's current regimen on nights the RLS was not in good control. Laboratory testing revealed a serum ferritin level of 20 ng/mL and iron supplementation was started. After 3 months of iron replacement, the addition of oxycodone was rarely needed.

CLINICAL PEARLS

1. Opioids are effective treatment for moderate to severe RLS.
2. Opioids may be used in patients who cannot tolerate DAs or alpha-2-delta ligands (eg gabapentin, pregabalin).
3. Opioids may be used as combination therapy with DAs or gabapentin.
4. Opioids may be used as a treatment for severe augmentation from DAs.
5. Augmentation and decreased effectiveness with time are not usually problems with most opioid medications used for the treatment of the RLS. Augmentation has been reported with tramadol.
6. Patients with a history of drug abuse or dependence are not good candidates for opioid treatment.
7. RLS is common during pregnancy, most physicians recommend iron replacement if needed and nonpharmacologic treatment. Most RLS medications with the exception of some narcotics are Category C or D.

BIBLIOGRAPHY

Kaplan PW, Allen RP, Bucholz DW, Walters JK: A double-blind, placebo-controlled study of the treatment of periodic limb movements in sleep using carbidopa/levodopa and propoxyphene, *Sleep* 16:717–723, 1993.
Lyons KE, Pahwa R: An open-label conversion study of pramipexole to ropinirole prolonged release in Parkinson's disease, *Mov Disord* 24(14):2121–2127, 2009.
Ondo WG: Methadone for refractory restless legs syndrome, *Mov Disord* 20(3):345–348, 2005.
Silver N, Allen RP, Senerth J, Earley CJ: A 10-year, longitudinal assessment of dopamine agonists and methadone in the treatment of restless legs syndrome, *Sleep Med* 12(5):440–444, 2011.
Vetrugno R, La Morgia C, D'Angelo R, et al: Augmentation of restless legs syndrome with long-term tramadol treatment, *Mov Disord* 22(3):424–427, 2007.
Walters AS: Review of receptor agonist and antagonist studies relevant to the opiate system in restless legs syndrome, *Sleep Med* 3 (4):301–304, 2002.
Walters AS, Wagner ML, Hening WA, et al: Successful treatment of the idiopathic restless leg syndrome in a randomized double-blind trial of oxycodone versus placebo, *Sleep* 16:327–332, 1993.
Walters AS, Winkelmann J, Trenkwalder C, et al: Long-term follow-up on restless legs syndrome patients treated with opioids, *Mov Disord* 16(6):1105–1109, 2001.

PATIENT 85

A Child with Difficulty Staying Asleep and Leg Kicks

A 6-year-old boy was brought for evaluation by his parents over concerns that he slept poorly and had behavioral problems in school. The parents reported that he had difficulty getting to sleep or staying asleep. He frequently got out of bed and came to sleep in his parent's bed. He also had frequent nightmares and sometimes complained that his legs hurt. Because he snored, the patients were concerned about the possibility of sleep apnea. Eliciting symptoms from the boy was difficult. His parents reported that sitting still in school or church was very difficult for the patient. The patient said his legs did not feel funny nor did he feel that he had to move them. He said that his legs just hurt at night sometimes.

Physical examination was normal BMI, 3 + enlarged tonsils (see Table P85-1).

TABLE P85-1   Sleep Study Results

Total recording time (min)	540 min		
Total sleep time (min)	451 min	Stage N1 (%TST)	7
Sleep efficiency (%)	83.8	Stage N2 (%TST)	58
Sleep latency (min)	41.7	Stage N3 (%TST)	23
REM latency (min)	166	Stage R (%TST)	15
WASO (min)	45.4		
AHI (#/hr)	0.2/hr	PLMS index (#/hr)	15
		PLMS arousal index (#/hr)	9

AHI, Apnea–hypopnea index; *min*, minutes; *PLMS*, periodic limb movement in sleep; *REM*, rapid eye movement; *TST*, total sleep time; *WASO*, wakefulness after sleep onset.

BOX P85-1   ICSD-3 Diagnostic Criteria: Periodic Limb Movement Disorder

Criteria A-D must be met
A. Polysomnography demonstrates PLMS, as defined in the most recent version of the American Academy of Sleep Medicine (AASM) Manual for the Scoring of Sleep and Associated Events.
B. The frequency is >5/hour in children or >15/hour in adults.
C. The PLMS cause clinically significant sleep disturbance or impairment in mental, physical, social, occupational, educational, behavioral, or other important areas of functioning.
D. The PLMS and the symptoms are not better explained by another current sleep disorder, medical or neurological disorder, or mental disorder (e.g., PLMS occurring with apneas or hypopneas should not be scored).

Note: PLMD cannot be diagnosed in the context of RLS, narcolepsy, untreated obstructive sleep apnea, or REM sleep behavior disorder; PLMS occur commonly in these conditions but the sleep complaint is more readily ascribed to the accompanying disorder. The diagnosis of RLS takes precedence over that of PLMD when potentially sleep-disrupting PLMS occur in the context of RLS. In such cases, the diagnosis of RLS is made and the PLMS are noted.

QUESTION

1. What is your diagnosis?

ANSWER

1. **Answer:** Periodic limb movement disorder (PLMD)

   Discussion: PLMD is diagnosed when the following are present (Box P85-1): (1) PLMS documented by polysomnography (PLMS index >5 per hour [hr] for children, 15/hr for adults); (2) a sleep complaint or daytime fatigue is attributable to periodic limb movement in sleep (PLMS), and (3) PLMS and symptoms are not better explained by another sleep disorder, medical or neurologic disorder, medication, or substance use.[1] A diagnosis of restless legs syndrome (RLS) excludes a diagnosis of PLMD.

   Because it is often difficult to obtain a history of typical RLS symptoms in children, a diagnosis of PLMD is much more likely in children than adults.[2] It has been said that childhood PLMD may be a precursor to RLS, but this may simply occur partly because of the dependence of a diagnosis of RLS on clinical history.

   A study by Gingras et al[3] found a PLMD prevalence of 14% in a clinic population of children. The study compared children with PLMD and those with OSA. When compared with children with OSA, children with PLMD were more likely to refuse to go to bed, have difficulty falling and staying asleep, have difficulty awakening in the morning, have a family history of RLS, complain of leg pain or discomfort at night, refuse to go to bed, and be more likely to get out of bed and go to the parents' bed. Children with PLMD were also more likely to report nightmares or sleep terrors. In this study, the PLMS index (PLMSI) was 23.5/hr in patients with PLMD versus 1.3/hr in patients with OSA. The PLMS arousal index was 9.6 versus 0.8/hr in the two groups. *At least 50% of patients were NOT reported by their parents to kick or jerk during sleep, showing that history in this regard is not reliable.* Most of the patients were treated successfully with a dopamine agonist. No published randomized trials of dopaminergic medications in children have been performed, but dopamine agonists (DAs) have been reported to be effective. Normalization of iron stores (checking ferritin and replacement, if needed) may often be effective and alleviate symptoms.

A diagnosis of PLMD requires that RLS be excluded. However, the accurate diagnosis of RLS in children and adolescents requires understanding of their age-appropriate language and cognitive skills. Adequate verbal skills are needed for children to communicate the sensory component of RLS and description must be in "the child's own words," rather than in the words of a parent or caregiver. Children rarely use or understand the word "urge." Instead, they describe that their legs "need to," "have to," "got to," or " want to" kick. A significant subset of children does not report worsening at evening or night, yet they meet all other diagnostic criteria and have supportive features for RLS, including a positive family history. Children who are 6 years or older and developmentally normal have been shown to report detailed, adequate descriptors for RLS symptoms. In children who are too young to adequately describe RLS sensations or are developmentally delayed, PLMD diagnosis may be the initial diagnosis, and full RLS symptomatology may become evident over time.[1]

In the present patient, iron stores were checked and the ferritin was 30 nanograms per milliliter (ng/mL). Iron supplementation was started, along with ropinirole 0.25 mg given at 6 PM (bedtime 8 PM). On this treatment, the patient began to sleep much better, and his teacher noted an improvement in his behavior in school.

CLINICAL PEARLS

1. A diagnosis of PLMD is more frequent in children than in adults, likely because the diagnosis of RLS is dependent on history and the difficulty of eliciting symptoms from children.

2. PLMD in children is a cause of sleep difficulty and difficulty functioning during the day. Some patients have great difficulty sitting still for any length of time during both day and night.

3. No medications are approved by the U.S. Food and Drug Administration (FDA) for the treatment of pediatric RLS. DAs have been used successfully. Normalization of iron stores is also indicated and may alleviate the symptoms.

4. A diagnosis of pediatric RLS is based on the same criteria as in adults, but children must describe "in their own words" the symptoms to support a diagnosis of RLS.

5. Parental report fails to endorse leg movements during sleep in patients ultimately found to have PLMD in about 50% of cases.

REFERENCES

1. American Academy of Sleep Medicine: *International classification of sleep disorders*, ed 3, Darien, IL, 2013, American Academy of Sleep Medicine.
2. Picchietti MA, Picchietti DL: Advances in pediatric restless legs syndrome: Iron, genetics, diagnosis and treatment, *Sleep Med* 11(7):643–651, 2010.
3. Gingras JL, Gaultney JF, Picchietti DL: Pediatric periodic limb movement disorder: sleep symptom and polysomnographic correlates compared to obstructive sleep apnea, *J Clin Sleep Med* 7(6):603–609, 2011.
4. Picchietti DL, Arbuckle RA, Abetz L, et al: Pediatric restless legs syndrome: analysis of symptom descriptions and drawings, *J Child Neurol* 26:1365–1376, 2011.
5. Picchietti MA, Picchietti DL, England SJ, et al: Children show individual night-to-night variability of periodic limb movements in sleep, *Sleep* 32(4):530–535, 2009.
6. Walters AS, Mandelbaum DE, Lewin DS, et al: Dopaminergic therapy in children with restless legs/periodic limb movements in sleep and ADHD. Dopaminergic Therapy Study Group, *Pediatr Neurol* 22(3):182–186, 2000.
7. Simakajornboon N, Kheirandish-Gozal L, Gozal D: Diagnosis and management of restless legs syndrome in children, *Sleep Med Rev* 13(2):149–156, 2009.
8. Mohri I, Kato-Nishimura K, Kagitani-Shimono K, et al: Evaluation of oral iron treatment in pediatric restless legs syndrome (RLS), *Sleep Med* 13(4):429–432, 2012.
9. England SJ, Picchietti DL, Couvadelli BV, et al: L-Dopa improves restless legs syndrome and periodic limb movements in sleep but not attention-deficit-hyperactivity disorder in a double-blind trial in children, *Sleep Med* 12:471–477, 2011.

Hypersomnolence of Central Origin—I

The disorders of hypersomnolence (hypersomnia) of central origin (Box F33-1) are an important part of the differential diagnosis in patients presenting with excessive daytime sleepiness (EDS). Of these disorders, insufficient sleep syndrome is likely the most common. In the *International Classification of Sleep Disorders*, Second Edition (ICSD-2), narcolepsy was divided into narcolepsy with cataplexy and narcolepsy without cataplexy (N+C, N−C).[1] Cataplexy (emotion-induced weakness) is the only symptoms specific for narcolepsy. In the ICSD-3, narcolepsy is classified as type 1 (N-T1) based on a low or absent level of cerebrospinal fluid (CSF) hypocretin-1 or type 2 (N-T2) if there is normal CSF hypocretin-1.[2] Neither classification (N+C, N−C or N-T1, N-T2) is completely satisfactory because hypocretin deficiency can currently be documented only by CSF sampling, and determining if cataplexy is truly present is often challenging. In the ICSD-2, idiopathic hypersomnia was divided into patients with and without long sleep time (< or >10 hours). In the ICSD-3, patients with idiopathic hypersomnia (IH) are no longer classified according to sleep time. This chapter discusses narcolepsy and IH. Other hypersomnias of central origin are discussed in Fundamentals 34.

NARCOLEPSY

Narcolepsy is a disorder characterized by EDS and symptoms related to the abnormal regulation of wakefulness and sleep.[1-7] A short rapid eye movement (REM) latency and intrusion of REM sleep features into wakefulness are characteristic of the disorder. As noted previously, narcolepsy may be classified on the basis of the presence or absence of cataplexy (N+C, N−C) or hypocretin deficiency (N-T1, N-T2). Diagnostic criteria for N-T1 and N-T2 are listed in Box F33-2 and Table F33-1. Hypocretin deficiency is documented by determining the level of hypocretin-1 in the CSF. The loss of hypocretin is caused by the destruction of the hypocretin-producing cells in the posterolateral hypothalamus. The destruction is thought to be autoimmune mediated. Hypocretin is believed to stabilize wakefulness and sleep transitions and prevent intrusion of the manifestations of REM sleep into wakefulness[4] A patient with daytime sleepiness for at least 3 months and a low or absent CSF hypocretin-1 level meets criteria for a diagnosis of N-T1. If hypocretin levels have not been measured, a diagnosis of N-T1 requires both the presence of cataplexy and a PSG/MSLT evaluation meeting diagnostic criteria for narcolepsy.

BOX F33-1	Hypersomnolence of Central Origin

1. Narcolepsy type 1 (N-T1, hypocretin deficiency)—usually with cataplexy
2. Narcolepsy type 2 (N-T2, normal hypocretin levels)—without cataplexy
3. Narcolepsy Due to Medical Condition (NDMC)—listed as subtype of 1 and 2 in ICSD-3
   - Type I NDMC
   - Type II NDMC
4. Idiopathic hypersomnia (IH)
5. Kleine-Levin syndrome (KLS)
6. Hypersomnia Due to a Medical Disorder (HDMD)
7. Hypersomnia Due to Medication or Substance (HDMS)
8. Hypersomnia Associated with a Psychiatric Disorder (HDPD)
9. Insufficient sleep syndrome

Adapted from the American Academy of Sleep Medicine: *International classification of sleep disorders*, ed. 3, Darien, IL, 2014, American Academy of Sleep Medicine.
ICSD-2, International Classification of Sleep Disorders, 2nd edition; ICSD-3, International Classification of Sleep Disorders, 3rd edition.

BOX F33-2 Narcolepsy ICSD-3 Diagnostic Criteria

NARCOLEPSY TYPE 1 (MOST N+C)

Criteria (A+B1 or A+B2) must be met
A. The patient has daily periods of irrepressible need to sleep or daytime lapses into sleep occurring for at least 3 months.*
B. The presence of one or both of the following:
1. Cataplexy *and* a mean sleep latency of ≤8 minutes **AND** 2 or more sleep-onset REM periods (SOREMP) on a multiple sleep latency test (MSLT) performed according to standard techniques. A SOREMP (within 15 minutes of sleep onset) on preceding nocturnal polysomnography (PSG) may replace one of the SOREMPs on the MSLT.†
2. Cerebrospinal fluid (CSF) hypocretin-1 concentration, measured by immunoreactivity, is either ≤110 picogram per milliliter (pg/mL) or <⅓ of mean values obtained in normal subjects with the same standardized assay.

NARCOLEPSY TYPE 2 (N−C)

Criteria A-E must be met

A. The patient has daily periods of irrepressible need to sleep or daytime lapses into sleep occurring for at least 3 months.
B. A mean sleep latency of ≤8 minutes and 2 or more SOREMPs are found on an MSLT performed according to standard techniques. A SOREMP (within 15 minutes of sleep onset) on preceding nocturnal PSG may replace one of the SOREMPs on the MSLT.
C. Cataplexy is absent.‡
D. *Either* CSF hypocretin-1 concentration has not been measured *or* CSF hypocretin-1 concentration measured by immunoreactivity is either >110 pg/mL or >⅓ of mean values obtained in normal subjects with the same standardized assay.§
E. The hypersomnolence and/or MSLT findings are not better explained by other causes such as insufficient sleep, obstructive sleep apnea, delayed sleep phase disorder or the effect of medication or substances or their withdrawal.

---

*In young children, narcolepsy may sometimes present as excessively long night sleep or by resumption of previously discontinued daytime napping.
†If narcolepsy type 1 is strongly suspected clinically but the MSLT criteria of B1 are not met, a possible strategy is to repeat the MSLT.
‡If cataplexy develops later, then the disorder should be reclassified as narcolepsy type 1.
§If the CSF hypocretin-1 concentration is tested at a later stage and found to be either ≤110 pg/mL or <⅓ of mean values obtained in normal subjects with the same assay, then the disorder should be reclassified as narcolepsy type 1.

TABLE F33-1 Summary of Diagnostic Criteria for Narcolepsy Types 1 and 2 and Characteristics – ICSD-3

	Narcolepsy Type 1 (Most N+C)	Narcolepsy Type 2 (N−C)
Sleepiness	≥3 months	≥3 months
Cataplexy	Usually present	Absent
Diagnostic criteria	Sleepiness for ≥3 mo + (1 or 2+3)	Sleepiness ≥3 months + 1 + 2 + 3+not better explained by other disorder
1. CSF hypocretin-1	Low (if measured)	Normal (or not measured)
2. Cataplexy	Present	Absent
3. PSG/MSLT	MSLT MSL ≤8 min, ≥2 SOREMPs A SOREMP on the PSG may be used as of the two SOREMPs	Same, required
MSL, # SOREMPs	N-T1 patients have lower MSL values and a greater number of SOREMPs compared to N-T2	Longer MSL, fewer SOREMPs compared to NT1
DQB1*0602	Virtually 100% +	About 45% (higher than general population)
SRH, SP	Yes	Yes
Obesity	Common	Less common

CSF, Cerebrospinal fluid; *MSL*, mean sleep latency; *MSLT*, multiple sleep latency test; *N+C*, narcolepsy with cataplexy; *N−C*, narcolepsy without cataplexy; *PSG*, polysomnography; *SOREMP*, sleep-onset rapid eye movement period; *SP*, sleep paralysis; *SRH*, sleep-related hallucinations (at sleep offset or onset).

1. If Type II patient develops cataplexy or if the CSF hypocretin-1 level is measured and is low, patient reclassified as having type 1.
2. In type 1, a low CSF hypocretin is present, but some patients may not have exhibited cataplexy.
3. If a patient has cataplexy, CSF hypocretin not measured, and the PSG-MSLT is not diagnostic for narcolepsy a repeat PSG/MSLT testing should be considered.

In patients without cataplexy or low CSF hypocretin-1, the diagnosis of N-T2 (N−C) is based on findings from the PSG/MSLT evaluation and exclusion of other explanations for the PSG/MSLT findings. The MSLT criteria for narcolepsy are short mean sleep latency (MSL) that is ≤8 minutes and two or more sleep onset REM periods. The short MSL documents excessive sleepiness, and the presence of two or more sleep-onset REM periods (SOREMPs) is specific for narcolepsy in the absence of other explanations for this finding (based on PSG and history). In the ICSD-3 diagnostic criteria for narcolepsy, a *SOREMP on the preceding PSG may count as one of the required two SOREMPs on the MSLT.* In fact, a nocturnal SOREMP (on PSG) alone has a high positive predictive value for the diagnosis of narcolepsy. Unfortunately, the MSLT is not absolutely sensitive (70% to 90% depending on the population studied). If a patient initially classified as N-T2 (no cataplexy, no CSF available) later develops cataplexy, the patient is reclassified as N-T1. If CSF hypocretin is low and sleepiness is present for more than 3 months, the patient is classified as N-T1, even if cataplexy is absent and the PSG and MSLT combination does not meet diagnostic criteria for narcolepsy. Many patients with low CSF hypocretin-1 and absent cataplexy will develop the symptom of cataplexy at a later time.

Core Symptoms of Narcolepsy

1. **Excessive sleepiness** is present in virtually 100% of patients (duration ≥ 3 months required) and is defined as an irrepressible need for sleep or unintended lapses into drowsiness or sleep. Sleepiness may vary in severity and is more likely if the individual is at rest or in monotonous situations. The sudden onset of sleepiness without a prodromal warning may occur (sleep attacks). *Sleepiness is usually the first initial symptom of narcolepsy (rarely, cataplexy may be the first symptom).*

2. Cataplexy is the only symptom specific for narcolepsy but is present in only 60% to 70% of patients defined by excessive sleepiness and a positive PSG/MSLT evaluation. In the ICSD-3, *cataplexy* is defined as more than one episode of generally brief (<2 minutes), usually bilaterally symmetrical sudden loss of muscle tone with retained consciousness. The episodes are precipitated by strong emotions, usually positive, with almost all patients reporting some episodes precipitated by emotions associated with laughter (laughing, telling a joke). *Cataplexy usually appears within a few years of the onset of sleepiness.* Cataplexy may be unilateral, involve the muscles of the neck (head bobbing), and be associated with muscle twitching. In children, cataplexy may be often more dramatic with total loss of postural muscle strength. In children, cataplexy may also present as facial (or generalized) hypotonia with droopy eyelids, mouth opening and protruded tongue, or gait unsteadiness. Not all events are clearly related to emotion. In children, cataplexy may be triggered in anticipation of a reward. *During cataplexy, deep tendon reflexes (DTRs) are absent.*

3. Sleep-related hallucinations (SRH) are vivid, often bizarre dreamlike images associated with sleep onset (hypnogogic) or offset/awakening (hypnopompic). The patient often is aware that the images are not real, but the experience is still frightening. A commonly described vision is an animal or a stranger in the room.

4. Sleep paralysis (SP) may be either partial or complete and usually is noted on awakening. The affected individual is awake but cannot move. SP may occur with sleep-related hallucinations. The diaphragm and extraocular muscles are not paralyzed. However, some patients experience dyspnea.

5. Other manifestations frequently associated with narcolepsy include poor nocturnal sleep (increased stage N1), automatic behavior (performing a seemingly purposeful task without memory of having preformed the activity), periodic limb movements in sleep (PLMS), and the REM sleep behavior disorder (RBD). PLMS during REM sleep is rare in most individuals but common in patients with narcolepsy.

HLA Typing, Genetics, and CSF Hypocretin

Nearly all patients with narcolepsy and cataplexy have low CSF hypocretin-1 and are positive for the human leukocyte antigen (HLA) DQB1*0602 (and DR2 or DRB1*1501 in Caucasians and Asians).[8–10] However, the presence of the DQB1*0602 antigen is not diagnostic of narcolepsy. Approximately 25% of the normal Caucasian population, 12% of the Japanese population, and 38% of the African American population are positive for the same antigen. Low CSF hypocretin in a patient negative for HLA DQB1*0602 is very rare (1/500). The results of HLA typing are useful when a spinal tap is contemplated to assess CSF hypocretin-1 values. If the patient is DQB1*0602 negative, hypocretin-1 levels are most likely normal (procedure not indicated). Of note, patients with a low CSF hypocretin-1 level but without cataplexy are invariably DQB1*0602 positive. Presumably, many in this group will eventually develop cataplexy. It has been estimated that about 45% of patients with N-T2 are HLA DQB1*0602 positive compared with 12% to 38% of controls. Presumably, the higher positivity is caused by those patients who are actually hypocretin deficient but who have not yet manifested cataplexy.

A genetic predisposition for narcolepsy seems to exist, but environmental factors also play a role. *If one member of identical twins has narcolepsy, the chance that the other twin will develop narcolepsy is only 30%.* The development of hypocretin-deficient narcolepsy is believed to be autoimmune mediated, and a genetic predisposition coupled with an antigen challenge (infection or vaccine) may trigger an immune response and damage to the cells in the lateral posterior hypothalamus that make hypocretin.[3-6,11]

PSG-MSLT Criteria for Diagnosis of Narcolepsy

For proper interpretation the MSLT is preceded by a PSG that does not demonstrate another sleep disorder believed to cause abnormal MSLT findings or sleepiness.[12,13] Medications that may affect sleep (including REM sleep) and alertness should be withdrawn for 2 weeks (or five half-life intervals) prior to testing. In the 2 weeks prior to the MSLT, the patient should have a normal sleep schedule and adequate sleep (>7 hours per night). Ideally actigraphy + sleep log should document adequate sleep for at least one week prior to the MSLT. If actigraphy is not available a sleep log can be used. The criteria for a positive MSLT are a MSL ≤8 minutes and 2 or more SOREMPs. A SOREMP on PSG (nocturnal REM latency ≤15 minutes) may be used as one of the two SOREMPs. It has been demonstrated that in the absence of sleep apnea a *nocturnal* SOREMP has a high positive predictive value but is not sensitive (nocturnal SOREMP in about 25%–50% of patients with narcolepsy, depending on the population studied).[14,15] The MSLT is not 100% sensitive for narcolepsy and false negatives may occur 7% to 30% of the time, depending on the population studied and the criteria used for the gold standard for the diagnosis of narcolepsy.[13-15] A repeat MSLT may be needed if a high clinical suspicion of narcolepsy exists and initial testing does not meet diagnostic criteria. The MSLT, although highly specific for the diagnosis of narcolepsy, may be associated with false positives (OSA, insufficient sleep).[13,14,16]

Narcolepsy Type I

The manifestations of N-T1 (hypocretin deficiency, most have N+C) generally begin between the ages of 15 and 30 years.[17] However, this form of narcolepsy may present in the pediatric age group or in patients older than 60 years. EDS alone or in combination with hypnagogic hallucinations, SP, or a combination of both is the presenting symptom in approximately 90% of patients.[17] Cataplexy may develop several years after symptoms begin. However, *most patients with N-T1 develop cataplexy within 3 to 5 years of the onset of EDS.*[17,18] Rarely, cataplexy may precede EDS.

The diagnostic criteria for N-T1 are listed in Box F33-2 and Table F33-1. Nearly all N-T1 patients have cataplexy and are positive for the HLA DQB1*0602. An exception is a patient with a low CSF hypocretin-1 and absent cataplexy (still classified as type I). In clinical practice, this is a very rare occurrence, as most patients will not have a CSF hypocretin-1 level available. The percentage of N-T2 (N − C) patients who would have a low hypocretin level, if measured, is unknown. One study found that 24% of a sample of N−C patients actually had low CSF hypocretin level (would be reclassified as N-T1). However, this was a select population seen at research centers in which CSF hypocretin levels were available.[19] Until an easier method for detecting hypocretin deficiency is available, the percentage of patients who would otherwise be classified as N-T2 (N−C) who have hypocretin deficiency will remain unknown. Patients with hypocretin deficiency and absent cataplexy may develop the symptom in the future. *In the ICSD-3, if a low CSF hypocretin has NOT been documented, a diagnosis of N-T1 requires BOTH the presence of cataplexy and a PSG-MSLT evaluation meeting the diagnostic criteria. The symptom of cataplexy alone is not sufficient for a diagnosis of N-T1.* The rationale is avoiding overdiagnosis, given the uncertainly of determining if cataplexy is really present. If PSG-MSLT evaluation does not meet criteria for narcolepsy in a patient with cataplexy, the studies could be repeated.

Of note, the ICSD-3 states "It is strongly recommended that the MSLT be preceded by at least one week of actigraphic recording with a sleep log to establish whether the results could be biased by insufficient sleep, shift work, or another circadian sleep disorder." *If a patient is negative for the DQB1*0602 antigen, a history of cataplexy should be considered doubtful, given the fact that virtually 100% of patients with a low CSF hypocretin and cataplexy are positive for this antigen.* If a patient has atypical cataplexy and a negative MSLT, determining the CSF hypocretin is an option. However, obtaining a CSF sample in a patient negative for DQB1*0602 is not indicated as the CSF hypocretin-1 level will almost always be normal. Patients with N-T1 tend to have a lower MSL and more SOREMPs than those with N-T2. The PSG will often show increased stage N1. Of interest, N-T1 patients have an increased incidence of obesity. In some series, SP and hypnagogic hallucinations are more common in patients with N-T1 compared with those with N-T2.

Narcolepsy Type II (N-T2)

These patients exhibit EDS in the absence of cataplexy. They may also manifest the other core symptoms of narcolepsy. The diagnosis of N-T2 is based on a symptom of EDS for at least 3 months and a PSG-MSLT evaluation meeting the criteria for narcolepsy, CSF hypocretin-1 levels being unavailable or normal, and the fact that the *hypersomnia and the MSLT findings are not better explained by insufficient sleep, OSA, delayed sleep phase disorder, or the use of medications or substances (or their withdrawal).* As noted above, the ICSD-3 recommends that "the MSLT be preceded by at least 1 week of actigraphic recording with a sleep log to establish whether the results could be biased by insufficient sleep, shift work, or another circadian sleep disorder." N-T2 patients, by definition, have N−C. Some patients with N−C actually have low CSF hypocretin, and if this is documented in the future, they are reclassified as having type N-T1. If a patient meeting diagnostic criteria for N-T2 later develops cataplexy, he or she is also reclassified as N-T1.

TREATMENT OF NARCOLEPSY

Treatment of Narcolepsy addresses (1) sleepiness, (2) cataplexy, (3) sleep-related hallucinations or paralysis, and (4) disturbed nocturnal sleep (see Table F33-2).[3,20,21]

Daytime Sleepiness

Modafinil and armodafinil (R enantiomer) are alerting agents that are FDA approved for treatment of sleepiness in patients with narcolepsy.[21–24] They are schedule IV medications, and refills are allowed. Unlike stimulants, these medications have limited abuse potential or problems with tolerance or rebound. The main side effects are headache, nausea, potential drug interactions (oral contraceptives possibly less effective), plavix possibly less effective, increased citalopram levels (possibly prolonged QT on high doses of citalopram). Stevens-Johnson syndrome is a very rare but potentially severe side effect. Provigil is usually given once daily (100 to 400 milligrams [mg]), but some patients respond better to a split dose (once every morning and once in the early afternoon (e.g., 1 PM). Armodafinil (NuVigil) is the R enantiomer of modafinil and has a longer half-life than L-modafinil.[25] The usual dose is 150 mg or 250 mg daily. Modafinil (Provigil) is the racemic form of the medication (L and R enantiomers), and after a few hours only R-modafinil remains in the circulation.

Stimulants (Schedule II) are effective for treating EDS, but monthly prescriptions are required and telephone prescriptions are not allowed. They are associated with a risk for abuse, tolerance, and rebound of symptoms.

TABLE F33-2 **Summary of Treatments for Narcolepsy**			
Excessive Sleepiness	**Cataplexy**	**Sleep-Related Hallucinations and Sleep Paralysis**	**Disturbed Sleep**
Alerting agents:	**Antidepressants**	Same as cataplexy	**Hypnotics**
*Modafinil	TCA		
*Armodafinil	SSRIs		
Stimulants:	Fluoxetine		
*Methylphenidate	SNRIs		
* Dextroamphetamine	Venlafaxine		
*Dextroamphetamine salts	NRIs		
Lisdextroamphetamine	Atomoxetine (Strattera)		
Methamphetamine	*Sodium Oxybate		
Other Treatments:			
*Sodium Oxybate (Xyrem)			
Scheduled naps			

NRIs, Norepinephrine reuptake inhibitors; *SNRIs,* serotonin norepinephrine reuptake inhibitors; *SSRIs,* selective serotonin reuptake inhibitors; *TCA,* tricyclic antidepressants.
*FDA approved for this indication.

Although direct head-to-head comparisons with modafinil are not available, stimulants are likely more effective than modafinil/armodafinil in some patients.[26] The main action of these medications is an increase in dopaminergic activity in the CNS (NE also increased). Methylphenidate, dextroamphetamine, and dextroamphetamine salts are FDA approved for EDS treatment. Methamphetamine and lisamphetamine (Vyvanse) are not FDA approved but may also be effective. Some patients respond to one stimulant medication better than to alternatives. Methylphenidate is probably the best tolerated stimulant but has a short duration of action requiring two to three times daily dosing. Long-acting (extended-release) forms of methylphenidate are available and may be better tolerated with a slower onset and offset of action. Dextroamphetamine has a longer half-life than methylphenidate. Extended release forms of dextroamphetamine are available and may be better tolerated and more effective than immediate release preparations. A combination of immediate-release and sustained-release medications may also be useful. For example, some immediate acting medications may be needed in the morning to help the patient get going and immediate release in the afternoon to avoid sleep disturbance from longer-acting preparations taken in the afternoon. An intermediate duration medication may be given in the early afternoon in patients requiring evening alertness but this risks sleep disturbance. Side effects of stimulants include anxiety, irritability, weight loss, palpitations, increased blood pressure, and disturbed sleep. Attacks of paranoia or hallucinations have been reported with amphetamines, but major psychiatric side effects are rare in the absence of underlying psychiatric disorders. However, use of very high doses of stimulants is associated with an increased risk of adverse outcomes.[27] For more information on dosing and use of stimulants, see Patient 92. Of note, stimulant medications (dextroamphetamine) may have a mildly beneficial effect on cataplexy (increase in norepinephrine), but modafinil has no effect on cataplexy.[28]

Cataplexy

Sodium oxybate (Xyrem) [gamma-hydroxy butyrate] is the only medication FDA approved for treatment of both sleepiness and cataplexy in patients with narcolepsy.[20,21] It is also known as the "date rape drug" and is dispensed only from one central pharmacy. It is a liquid with a short half-life and must be given in divided doses. The first dose is at bedtime and a repeated dose

is taken 2 to 3 hours (awakened by the alarm clock or spontaneous awakening). The starting nightly dose is 4.5 grams (g) (2.25 mg bedtime and repeated in 2–3 hours). The dose may be slowly increased by 0.5 to 1 g per night every 1 to 2 weeks to a maximum dose of 9 g per night (e.g., week 1: 4.5 g; week 2: 5 g). Side effects include confusion, enuresis, and sleep walking. Sodium oxybate (SBX) is rich in sodium and this medication is relatively contraindicated in patients with heart failure. In general, *higher doses are needed for improvement in sleepiness than for treatment of cataplexy*. Sodium oxybate (SBX) is effective for cataplexy in doses as low as 4.5 g nightly. The full effect on cataplexy from a given dose may require several weeks of use. Concurrent use of SBX and other sedatives, narcotics, or alcohol is potentially dangerous and is contraindicated. Of note, many patients require both SBX and an alerting agent for optimal control of EDS. Sodium oxybate may be used in patients with both narcolepsy and OSA, but caution is advised. Ideally, the patients should be on effective treatment (e.g., continuous positive airway pressure [CPAP]), and some type of monitoring should be performed to determine if significant desaturation is present when the patient takes sodium oxybate. More information on sodium oxybate is available in Patient 93.

For treatment of cataplexy, tricyclic antidepressants, selective serotonin reuptake inhibitors (SSRIs), serotonin–norepinephrine reuptake inhibitors (SNRIs), and norepinephrine reuptake inhibitors (NRIs) are effective but are not FDA approved for this indication. Medications that have both norepinephrine and serotonin effects are the most effective for treatment of cataplexy. Venlafaxine XR is a useful medication for treatment of cataplexy (37.5 to 75 mg daily). SSRIs must be given in full dose for effectiveness. Medications effective for the treatment of cataplexy are also effective in the treatment of hypnagogic hallucinations and SP.[20,21]

Narcolepsy in Children

This topic is discussed in detail in Patient 90. Modafinil, stimulants, and sodium oxybate have both been used with some success but are not FDA approved for treatment of narcolepsy in children.

Narcolepsy Due to Medical Condition (NDMC type 1 and type 2)

This group of disorders is also known as *secondary or symptomatic narcolepsy*.[1,29] The patient must report EDS and meet other criteria for the

TABLE F33-3	**Medical Disorders Causing Narcolepsy Due to a Medical Disorder**
Narcolepsy Type 1 (N+C)	**Narcolepsy Type 2 (N−C)**
Tumors, sarcoidosis, arteriovenous malformations affecting the hypothalamus	Head trauma
	Myotonic dystrophy
Multiple sclerosis plaques impairing the hypothalamus	Prader-Willi syndrome
Paraneoplastic syndrome anti-Ma2 antibodies	Parkinson disease
Neiman-Pick type C disease	Multiple system atrophy
Possibly Coffin-Lowry syndrome	

From American Academy of Sleep Medicine: *International classification of sleep disorders: diagnostic and coding manual*, ed 2, Westchester, IL, 2005, American Academy of Sleep Medicine.
N+C, narcolepsy with cataplexy; *N−C*, narcolepsy without cataplexy.

diagnosis of either N-T1 or N-T2. The disorder must be associated with a medical disorder (often a neurologic disorder) known to cause narcolepsy (see Table F33-3). Note that if hypersomnia is thought to be secondary to one of the listed medical conditions but *criteria for narcolepsy are not met*, the diagnosis is "*Hypersomnia* Due to a Medical Disorder (HDMD)." Note that some of the disorders causing HDMD may also cause NDMC. EDS following closed head injury is a well-known finding.[30] However, most patients with EDS following head trauma do not have narcolepsy. Patients with NDMC are *not* typically neurologically normal, and often structural abnormalities are noted with magnetic resonance imaging (MRI) of the CNS. Some of the disorders are associated with genetic abnormalities.

IDIOPATHIC HYPERSOMNIA

Patients with IH manifest EDS without cataplexy and do not meet diagnostic criteria for N-T2 (one or less SOREMP on the PSG-MSLT evaluation.[2,31–34] ICSD-3 diagnostic criteria are listed in Box F33-3, with notes in Box F33-4. Patients must exhibit a MSL ≤8 minutes on an MSLT, or a 24-hour PSG must show a total sleep time (TST) >660 minutes. *IH is a diagnosis of exclusion*, so other causes of sleepiness must be ruled out. The major exclusion is insufficient sleep. A trial of sleep extension prior to the MSLT or 24-hour PSG is needed if insufficient sleep is suspected. In any case, documentation of adequate sleep for at least 7 days by actigraphy and sleep log for 1 week prior to the MSLT or

BOX F33-3	**Idiopathic Hypersomnia: Diagnostic Criteria**

A. The patient has daily periods of irrepressible need to sleep or daytime lapses into sleep occurring for at least 3 months.*
B. **Cataplexy is absent**
C. A multiple sleep latency test (MSLT) performed according to standard techniques shows <2 sleep onset REM periods (SOREMPs) or no SOREMPs if the REM latency on preceding polysomnography (PSG) was ≤15 minutes.*
D. The presence of at least *one* of the following:
   1. The multiple sleep latency test shows a mean sleep latency of ≤8 minutes.
   2. Total 24 hour sleep time is ≥660 minutes (typically 12–14 hours)† on 24-hour PSG sleep monitoring (performed after correction for chronic sleep deprivation), *or* by wrist actigraphy in association with a sleep log (averaged over at least 7 days with unrestricted sleep).‡
E. Insufficient sleep syndrome is ruled out (if deemed necessary, by lack of improvement of sleepiness after an adequate trial of increased nocturnal time in bed, confirmed by at least a week of wrist actigraphy).
F. The hypersomnolence and/or MSLT findings are not better explained by another sleep disorder, other medical or psychiatric disorder, or use of drugs or medications.

*A high sleep efficiency (90%) on preceding polysomnography (PSG) is a supportive finding (as long as sleep insufficiency is ruled out).
†In children and adolescents, this may need to be adapted to account for normal changes in sleep time associated with stages of development as well as variability across cultures.
‡Occasionally, patients fulfilling other criteria may have a multiple sleep latency test (MSLT) mean sleep latency (MSL) >8 minutes and total 24-hour sleep time <660 minutes. Clinical judgment should be used in deciding if these patients should be considered to have idiopathic hypersomnia (IH). Great care should be exercised in excluding other conditions that might mimic the disorder. Another option is to repeat the MSLT if the clinical suspicion for IH remains high.

24-hour PSG is recommended. Patients classified here likely have a mixture of etiologies. *CSF hypocretin-1 levels are normal in patients with IH.* One study also found low CSF histamine[34] in patients with IH, but another study found no difference in CSF hypocretin levels between hypocretin-deficient narcolepsy and other causes of central hypersomnia (including IH).[35] The typical age of onset of IH is 16 to 20 years, and constant sleepiness for many years is typical. However, spontaneous remission has been reported in up to 14%. Important facts about IH are listed in Box F33-5.

The term *sleep drunkenness* is defined in the ICSD-3 as a prolonged and severe form of sleep

BOX F33-4	Notes on Diagnostic Criteria of Idiopathic Hypersomnia—ICSD-3

1. Severe and prolonged sleep inertia, known as *sleep drunkenness* (SD, defined as prolonged difficulty waking up with repeated returns to sleep, irritability, automatic behavior and confusion), long (>1 hour) unrefreshing naps, or both are additional supportive clinical features.
2. A high sleep efficiency (≥90%) on preceding polysomnography (PSG) is a supportive finding (as long as sleep insufficiency is ruled out).
3. In children and adolescents, this may need to be adapted to account for normal changes in sleep time associated with stages of development as well as variability across cultures.
4. Occasionally, patients fulfilling other criteria may have a multiple sleep latency test (MSLT) mean sleep latency (MSL) >8 minutes and total 24-hour sleep time <660 minutes. Clinical judgment should be used in deciding if these patients should be considered to have idiopathic hypersomnia (IH). Great care should be exercised in excluding other conditions that might mimic the disorder. Another option is to repeat the MSLT if the clinical suspicion for IH remains high.

BOX F33-5	Important Facts About Idiopathic Hypersomnia

- Long unrefreshing naps
- Sleep drunkenness (36%–66%)
- Difficulty waking up to alarms
- 24-hour sleep >10 hours reported in 30%
- Hypnagogic hallucinations and sleep paralysis are common
- Dysfunction of the autonomic nervous system may be present (especially in patients with a long sleep time), including headaches, orthostatic disturbances, perception of temperature dysregulation, and peripheral vascular complaints (Raynaud-type phenomena with cold hands and feet)
- PSG: high sleep efficiency
- PSG+MSLT ≤1 SOREMP
- MSLT mean sleep latency ≤8 minutes
- 24-hour PSG total sleep time >660 minutes

MSLT, Multiple sleep latency test; *PSG*, polysomnography; *SOREMP*, sleep-onset rapid eye movement period.

inertia, consisting of prolonged difficulty waking up, as well as repeated returns to sleep, irritability, automatic behavior, and confusion. It is reported in 36% to 66% of patients in different series (IH). The presence of sleep drunkenness provides support for a diagnosis of IH. Patients with IH typically do not easily awaken to alarms. Long (>60 minutes) naps are typical, and 46% to

78% of patients describe the naps as unrefreshing. This is in contrast to napping in patients with narcolepsy, which is often beneficial. Dysfunction of the autonomic nervous system may be present, and manifestations include headaches, orthostatic disturbances, temperature dysregulation, and peripheral vascular complaints (Raynaud-type phenomena with cold hands and feet). Of note, hypnogogic hallucinations and SP also may be present in patients with IH.

The PSG usually shows a high sleep efficiency. An MSLT may not be possible if the patient cannot be awakened. If a PSG-MSLT evaluation is performed, the MSL on the MSLT is ≤8 minutes and ≤1 SOREMP is observed on the PSG-MSLT combination. The MSL for IH was listed as 6.2 ± 3.0 minutes in a recent review of the literature.[13] If an MSLT is not possible, 24-hour PSG showing a TST >660 minutes is an alternative finding that helps with diagnosis. If a 24 hour PSG this is not possible, use of actigraphy could be considered (has not been validated). Sleep efficiency on PSG is usually high (mean 90%–94%). Self-reported TST is longer than in controls and is ≥10 hours in at least 30% of patients.

Diagnostic Approach for IH

After a thorough history and physical examination, a PSG and an MSLT should be ordered. It is imperative to document adequate sleep before the testing. A sleep diary and actigraphy for at least 7 days before testing should eliminate the possibility of insufficient sleep syndrome. The PSG should rule out OSA. The differential diagnosis of IH includes N-T2 with a false-negative PSG-MSLT evaluation, head trauma, occult drug abuse, and sleepiness associated with a psychiatric disorder (bipolar disorder–depressive phase), neurologic disorder, or structural CNS lesion. CNS imaging is suggested if any suspicion of a CNS lesion exists. Use of a urine drug screen may also be considered.

Subtype: IH with Long Sleep Time

In the ICSD-2, patients with IH were divided into two categories: those with long sleep time and those and without long sleep time (less than or more than 10 hours of sleep). However, the ICSD-3 dropped this division of patients, as the separation of patients into these two groups lacked validity. In comparing patients with ≥10 hours sleep to those with <10 hours, no differences were seen in the Epworth Sleepiness Scale (ESS) scores, MSLT mean sleep latencies, or percentage with sleep drunkenness.[32] The factor that complicates the use of a 10-hour TST to separate patients into categories is that patients with IH tend to overestimate their TST. The ICSD-3 mentions that some clinicians may elect to retain IH with long sleep time as a subtype.

Treatment of IH

The same medications indicated for the treatment of EDS in narcolepsy are effective in IH. However, no medication is FDA approved for the treatment of IH. Amphetamines, methylphenidate, and modafinil[20,21] have all been used with variable success for the treatment of EDS. The *AASM Practice Parameters for Treatment of Narcolepsy and Other Hypersomnias of Central Origin* states that "modafinil may be effective for treatment of idiopathic hypersomnia (Option)."[21] Amphetamine, methamphetamine, and methylphenidate were also listed as treatments for IH (Option).

REFERENCES

1. American Academy of Sleep Medicine: *International classification of sleep disorders: diagnostic and coding manual*, ed 2, Westchester, IL, 2005, American Academy of Sleep Medicine.
2. American Academy of Sleep Medicine: *International classification of sleep disorders: diagnostic and coding manual*, ed 3, Darien, IL, 2013, American Academy of Sleep Medicine.
3. Scammell TE: The neurobiology, diagnosis, and treatment of narcolepsy, *Ann Neurol* 53:154–166, 2003.
4. Burgess CR, Scammell TE: Narcolepsy: neural mechanisms of sleepiness and cataplexy, *J Neurosci* 32 (36):12305–12311, 2012.
5. Harris SF, Monderer RS, Thorpy M: Hypersomnias of central origin, *Neurol Clin* 30(4):1027–1044, 2012.
6. Frenette E, Kushida CA: Primary hypersomnia of central origin, *Semin Neurol* 29:354–267, 2009.
7. Bourgin P, Zeitzer JM, Mignot E: CSF hypocretin-1 assessment in sleep and neurological disorders, *Lancet Neurol* 7(7):649–662, 2008.
8. Mignot E, Chen W, Black J: On the value of measuring CSF hypocretin-1 in diagnosing narcolepsy, *Sleep* 26:646–649, 2003.
9. Krahn LE, Pankratz S, Oliver L, et al: Hypocretin (Orexin) levels in cerebrospinal fluid of patients with narcolepsy: relationship to cataplexy and HLADQB1*0602 status, *Sleep* 25:733–736, 2003.
10. Mignot E, Lin X, Arrigoni J, et al: DBQ1*602 and DQA1*0102 are better markers than DR2 for narcolepsy in Caucasians and Black Americans, *Sleep* 17(8 Suppl): S60–S67, 1994.
11. Mahlios J, De la Herrán-Arita AK, Mignot E: The autoimmune basis of narcolepsy, *Curr Opin Neurobiol* 23(5):767–773, 2013.
12. Littner MR, Kushida C, Wise M, et al: Practice parameters for clinical use of the multiple sleep latency test and the maintenance of wakefulness test, *Sleep* 28:113–121, 2005.
13. Arand D, Bonnet M, Hurwitz T, et al: The clinical use of the MSLT and MWT, *Sleep* 28:123–144, 2005.
14. Aldrich MS, Chervin RD, Malow BA: Value of the multiple sleep latency test (MSLT) for the diagnosis of narcolepsy, *Sleep* 20:620–629, 1997.
15. Andlauer O, Moore H, Jouhier L, et al: Nocturnal rapid eye movement sleep latency for identifying patients with narcolepsy/hypocretin deficiency, *JAMA Neurol* 6:1–12, 2013.
16. Chervin RD, Aldrich MS: Sleep onset REM periods during multiple sleep latency tests in patients evaluated for sleep apnea, *Am J Respir Crit Care Med* 161:426–431, 2000.
17. Dauvilliers Y, Montplasir J, Molinari N, et al: Age of onset of narcolepsy in two large populations of patients in France and Quebec, *Neurology* 57:2029–2033, 2001.
18. Okun ML, Lin L, Pelin Z, et al: Clinical aspects of narcolepsy-cataplexy across ethnic groups, *Sleep* 25:27–35, 2002.
19. Andlauer O, Moore H 4th, Hong SC, et al: Predictors of hypocretin (orexin) deficiency in narcolepsy without cataplexy, *Sleep* 35(9):1247–1255, 2012.
20. Mignot EJ: A practical guide to the therapy of narcolepsy and hypersomnia syndromes, *Neurotherapeutics* 9 (4):739–752, 2012.
21. Morgenthaler TI, Kapur VK, Brown TM, et al: Practice parameters for the treatment of narcolepsy and other hypersomnias of central origin, *Sleep* 30:1705–1711, 2007.
22. U.S. Modafinil in Narcolepsy Study Group: Randomized trial of modafinil for the treatment of pathological somnolence in narcolepsy, *Ann Neurol* 43:88–97, 1998.
23. U.S. Modafinil in Narcolepsy Study Group: Randomized trial of modafinil as a treatment for the excessive daytime somnolence of narcolepsy, *Neurology* 53:1166–1175, 2000.
24. Harsh JR, Hayduk R, Rosenberg R, et al: The efficacy and safety of armodafinil as treatment for adults with excessive sleepiness associated with narcolepsy, *Curr Med Res Opin* 22:761–774, 2006.
25. Darwish M, Kirby M, D'Andrea DM, et al: Pharmacokinetics of armodafinil and modafinil after single and multiple doses in patients with excessive sleepiness associated with treated obstructive sleep apnea: a randomized, open-label, crossover study, *Clin Ther* 32 (12):2074–2087, 2010.
26. Mitler M, Aldrich MS, Koob GF, et al: ASDA standards of practice: narcolepsy and its treatment with stimulants, *Sleep* 17:352–371, 1994.
27. Auger RR, Goodman SH, Silber MH: Risks of high-dose stimulants in treatment of disorders of excessive somnolence: a case control study, *Sleep* 28:667–672, 2005.
28. Guilleminault C, Aftab FA, Karadeniz D, et al: Problems associated with switch to modafinil—a novel alerting agent in narcolepsy, *Eur J Neurol* 7:381–384, 2000.
29. Nishino S, Kanbayashi T: Symptomatic narcolepsy, cataplexy, and hypersomnia, and their implications in the hypothalamic/hypocretin/orexin system, *Sleep Med Rev* 9:269–310, 2005.
30. Castriotta RJ, Atanasov S, Wilde MC, et al: Treatment of sleep disorders after traumatic brain injury, *J Clin Sleep Med* 5(2):137–144, 2009.
31. Anderson KN, Pilsworth S, Sharples LD, et al: Idiopathic hypersomnia: a study of 77 cases, *Sleep* 30:1274–1281, 2007.
32. Vernet C, Arnuf I: Idiopathic hypersomnia with and without long sleep time: a controlled series of 75 patients, *Sleep* 32:753–759, 2009.
33. Ali M, Auger RR, Slocumb NL, Morgenthaler TI: Idiopathic hypersomnia: clinical features and response to treatment, *J Clin Sleep Med* 5:562–568, 2009.
34. Kanbayashi T, Kodama T, Kondo H, et al: CSH histamine contents in narcolepsy, idiopathic hypersomnia and obstructive sleep apnea syndrome, *Sleep* 32:181–187, 2009.
35. Dauvilliers Y, Delallée N, Jaussent I, et al: Normal cerebrospinal fluid histamine and tele-methylhistamine levels in hypersomnia conditions, *Sleep* 35(10):1359–1366, 2012.

A 20-Year-Old Woman with Emotion-Induced Weakness

Patient A: A 20-year-old woman reported severe daytime sleepiness for over 6 months and definite bilateral leg weakness lasting for 1 to 2 minutes when she heard or told a joke or was embarrassed. The episodes of leg weakness were present virtually every day. As they came on slowly, she was able to sit down or support herself and had never fallen. The patient was taking no medications except for oral contraceptives. While she normally slept for 7 hours, sleeping longer did not improve the daytime sleepiness. The patient often fell asleep in class. She did report waking up and being weak for a few seconds, but this sensation was not a problem. No history of sleep associated hallucinations or dreams or snoring was present. The results of a sleep study (PSG) and the following MSLT are shown in Table P86-1.

TABLE P86-1 Sleep Study and MSLT

Total recording time (min)	450		
Total sleep time (TST) (min)	400	Stage N1 (%TST)	7
Sleep efficiency (%)	83.8	Stage N2 (%TST)	58
Sleep latency (min)	5.0	Stage N3 (%TST)	23
REM latency (min)	10	Stage R (%TST)	22
Wakefulness after sleep onset (WASO) (min)	20.0		
Apnea–hypopnea index (AHI)	0.2/hour	Periodic limb movement in sleep (PLMS) index	15
		PLMS arousal index	9
Multiple sleep latency test (MSLT)			
Mean sleep latency (MSL)	3.0 min		
Sleep-onset REM periods (SOREMPs)	1 of 5 naps		

Laboratory findings: Positive for HLA DQB1*602 human leukocyte antigen (HLA)

QUESTIONS

1. What is your diagnosis for Patient A?
   Patient B: Identical history as Patient A's.
   Polysomnography (PSG): Identical to Patient A, except the rapid eye movement (REM) latency was 60 minutes
   Multiple sleep latency test (MSLT): mean sleep latency (MSL) 3 minutes; 1 sleep-onset REM period (SOREMP) in 5 naps
   Laboratory findings: positive for DQB1*602 HLA

2. What is your diagnosis for Patient B?

ANSWERS

1. **Answer for Patient A:** Narcolepsy type 2.

   Discussion: The *International Classification of Sleep Disorders*, Third Edition (ICSD-3) diagnostic criteria for narcolepsy type I (N-T1) (Box P86-1) require the following: (1) excessive sleepiness

BOX P86-1	Narcolepsy Type I—ICSD-3 Diagnostic Criteria

A. The patient has daily periods of irrepressible need to sleep or daytime lapses into sleep occurring for at least 3 months.*

B. The presence of one or both of the following:
  1. Cataplexy (as defined under Essential Features) *and* a mean sleep latency of ≤8 minutes and ≥2 sleep onset REM periods (SOREMP) on a multiple sleep latency test (MSLT) performed according to standard techniques. A SOREMP (within 15 minutes of sleep onset) on the preceding nocturnal polysomnography (PSG) may replace one of the SOREMPs on the MSLT.†
  2. Cerebrospinal fluid (CSF) hypocretin-1 concentration, measured by immunoreactivity, is either ≤110 picogram per milliliter (pg/mL) or < ⅓ of mean values obtained in normal subjects with the same standardized assay.

Notes:

*In young children narcolepsy may sometimes present as excessively long night sleep or by resumption of previously discontinued daytime napping.

†If narcolepsy type I is strongly suspected clinically but the MSLT criteria of B1 are not met, a possible strategy is to repeat the MSLT.

for at least 3 months and (2) either a low cerebrospinal fluid (CSF) hypocretin OR both the presence of cataplexy AND a PSG-MSLT evaluation meeting the criteria for narcolepsy. In addition, there is an *absence* of other disorders, which could explain the sleepiness and MSLT findings (e.g., obstructive sleep apnea [OSA], insufficient sleep, medication use or stimulant withdrawal). Here, PSG-MSLT evaluation meeting the criteria for narcolepsy means that the MSL is ≤8 minutes with ≥2 SOREMPs. A SOREMP on the nocturnal study (PSG SOREMP) may count as one of the two required SOREMPs on the MSLT. In the ICSD-2, a diagnosis of narcolepsy with cataplexy (N+C) was possible on the basis of the presence of sleepiness and cataplexy alone. Confirmation with an MSLT was suggested but not required. This approach emphasized that cataplexy is the only narcolepsy symptom specific for narcolepsy and that false-negative MSLT findings do occur. In the study of Aldrich et al about 30% of patients with definite cataplexy and sleepiness did not have an MSLT meeting the criteria of (MSL ≤8 minutes and 2 or more SOREMPs). The systematic review of the MSLT by Arand et al found a sensitivity of 78% with respect to the presence of two SOREMPs for making the diagnosis of narcolepsy. A recent study by Andlauer et al using either a low CSF hypocretin-1 or the presence of both cataplexy and the HLA DQB1*602 antigen as the gold standard for N-T1 found a much higher sensitivity of 92%. The ICSD-3 requirement of additional evidence for narcolepsy beyond a history of a cataplexy recognizes that in many patients, the history of cataplexy is atypical, uncertain, or both. The goal is to avoid a false positive of narcolepsy given the lifelong implications. It is possible that patients could provide a spurious history of cataplexy because of their desire for disability or stimulant medications.

As noted above per the ICSD-3, a SOREMP on the nocturnal PSG may be used as one of the two required sleep onset REM periods. In the study by of Aldrich et al of the utility of the MSLT for diagnosing narcolepsy, a PSG SOREMP was present in 33% of N+C patients and 24% of N−C patients (not sensitive) but had a high positive predictive value. In that study, only 1% of patients with sleep-related breathing disorders (SBDs) has a PSG SOREMP. In the study by Andlauer and coworkers, a PSG SOREMP was present in 35% of N-T1 and about 50% of a group composed of N-T1 and N-T2. In this study, the finding of a PSG SOREMP also had a high positive predictive value for a diagnosis of narcolepsy.

It is worth noting that virtually 100% of patients with cataplexy and a low CSF hypocretin-1 are positive for the DQB1*602 HLA antigen. About 12% to 20% of normal population is also positive for the antigen. Therefore, testing is not clinically useful in most situations. However, if a patient is negative for the DBQ1*602 antigen, then the CSF hypocretin level is virtually always normal. Obtaining CSF will not be clinically useful in a HLA DQB1*602 negative individual, as almost all such patients will have a normal CSF hypocretin level. Patients with a history of cataplexy in whom CSF hypocretin has not be measured will not meet diagnostic criteria for N-T1 if the PSG-MSLT evaluation documents <2 SOREMPs (including the PSG). If the patient is DQB1*602 negative, the presence of true cataplexy may be doubted. However, such a patient could have N-T2 and "atypical cataplexy." In any case, if a strong clinical suspicion of narcolepsy exists, and the initial PSG-MSLT does not meet the diagnostic criteria, repeat PSG-MSLT testing is indicated.

In the current patient, with the use of the PSG SOREMP as one of the two required SOREMPs, the patient met criteria for NT-1 (sleepiness + cataplexy + positive PSG-MSLT). She was treated with modafinil for daytime sleepiness and venlafaxine XR 37.5 mg for cataplexy. Use of sodium oxybate was considered, but the patient declined this treatment.

2. **Answer for Patient B:** Narcolepsy type 1 is possible; consider repeat MSLT.

Discussion: This patient has a history of typical cataplexy, but in the absence of a low CSF hypocretin or PSG-MSLT evaluation meeting criteria, the patient does not meet the ICSD-3 criteria for N-T1. The nocturnal REM latency was mildly reduced but not within 15 minutes. A PSG SOREMP is defined as a REM latency ≤15 minutes. Given the strong history for cataplexy and the fact that the patient was positive for the DQB1*602 antigen (supporting the history of cataplexy), a false-negative MSLT is a possibility. One approach is a repeat PSG-MSLT, which is medically indicated but costly. Another approach would be to obtain a CSF hypocretin-1 level. This would *not* be a viable option if the patient were DQB1*602 negative, as the CSF would invariably show normal levels of hypocretin. A third approach would be to empirically make a diagnosis of NT-1 on the basis of a strong history of typical cataplexy. The diagnostic criteria for narcolepsy in the *Diagnostic and Statistical Manual of Mental Disorders (DSM-V)* allows a diagnosis of narcolepsy based entirely on the presence of cataplexy as one of the criteria. A fourth approach would be to consider a diagnosis of idiopathic hypersomnia (IH). The PSG-MSLT findings do meet the criteria for IH (MSL ≤8 minutes, <2 SOREMPs on PSG-MSLT). However, the diagnostic criteria for IH mandate *the absence of cataplexy*. In summary, unless the patient is willing to undergo a lumbar puncture, the two choices are to make a diagnosis of N+C on the basis of the clinical history or to repeat the PSG-MSLT.

CLINICAL PEARLS

1. The ICSD-3 criteria for narcolepsy N-T1 (most with cataplexy) requires more than a history of daytime sleepiness and cataplexy. Either a low CSF hypocretin level or the combination of cataplexy AND a PSG-MSLT evaluation meeting the diagnostic criteria must also be present.

2. The presence of the DQB1*602 antigen is not diagnostic for narcolepsy. Approximately 25% of the normal Caucasian population, 12% of the Japanese population, and 38% of the African American population is positive for the same antigen.

3. If a patient with a history of cataplexy is DQB1*602 antigen negative, it causes one to question if cataplexy is truly present.

4. As virtually all narcolepsy patients with a low CSF hypocretin are positive for DQB1*602 antigen, a spinal tap in a DQB1*602-negative patient is not indicated, as the CSF hypocretin level will invariably be normal.

5. False-negative PSG-MSLT evaluations do occur, and if there is a high index of suspicion for narcolepsy, repeat testing is indicated.

6. The presence of a SOREMP on PSG preceding the MSLT has a high positive predictive value for the presence of narcolepsy. However, a PSG SOREMP is only present 24% to 50% of the time. A PSG SOREMP may be used as one of the two required SOREMPs on the MSLT in the ICSD-3 diagnostic criteria.

7. Most but not all N-T1 patients exhibit cataplexy. Excessive sleepiness and a low CSF hypocretin level fulfill the diagnostic criteria in the absence of cataplexy. The ICSD-3 lists narcoleptic patients without cataplexy but with a low CSF hypocretin-1 level as a subtype of N-T1. These patients will presumably exhibit cataplexy at a later time.

BIBLIOGRAPHY

Aldrich MS, Chervin RD, Malow BA: Value of the multiple sleep latency test (MSLT) for the diagnosis of narcolepsy, *Sleep* 20:620–629, 1997.

American Academy of Sleep Medicine: *International classification of sleep disorders: diagnostic and coding manual*, ed 3, Westchester, IL, 2005, American Academy of Sleep Medicine.

American Academy of Sleep Medicine: *International classification of sleep disorders: diagnostic and coding manual*, ed 3, Westchester, IL, 2013, American Academy of Sleep Medicine.

American Psychiatric Association: *Diagnostic and statistical manual of mental disorders*, ed 5, Arlington, VA, 2013, American Psychiatric Association.

Andlauer O, Moore H, Jouhier L, et al: Nocturnal rapid eye movement sleep latency for identifying patients with narcolepsy/hypocretin deficiency, *JAMA Neurol* 6:1–12, 2013.

Arand D, Bonnet M, Hurwitz T, et al: The clinical use of the MSLT and MWT, *Sleep* 28:123–144, 2005.

Burgess CR, Scammell TE: Narcolepsy: neural mechanisms of sleepiness and cataplexy, *J Neurosci* 32(36):12305–12311, 2012.

Bourgin P, Zeitzer JM, Mignot E: CSF hypocretin-1 assessment in sleep and neurological disorders, *Lancet Neurol* 7(7):649–662, 2008.

Littner MR, Kushida C, Wise M, et al: Practice parameters for clinical use of the multiple sleep latency test and the maintenance of wakefulness test, *Sleep* 28:113–121, 2005.

Scammell TE: The neurobiology, diagnosis, and treatment of narcolepsy, *Ann Neurol* 53:154–166, 2003.

A 45-Year-Old Male with Severe Sleepiness

A 45-year-old man was evaluated for severe sleepiness. He reported an Epworth Sleepiness Scale (ESS) score of 18/24 but denied cataplexy. The patient's bed partner did report mild snoring. The only medication the patient was taking was lisinopril for hypertension. No history of head trauma or symptoms of depression was present. The patient reported sleeping 6.5 hours every night. He was asked to extend the total sleep time, but this did not improve the sleepiness. He reported episodes of sleep paralysis. Given the severe sleepiness with a lower risk of obstructive sleep apnea (OSA), polysomnography (PSG) (Table P87-1) followed by a multiple sleep latency test (MSLT) (Table P87-2) was ordered.

Sleep log: Average of 7 hours of sleep per night

DQB1*602 antigen: positive

TABLE P87-1 Sleep Study Results

				(min)	%TST	
Total recording time (min)	450	(390–468)				
Total sleep time (min)	395.5	(343–436)				
Sleep efficiency (%)	88	(85–97)	Stage N1	19.5	5	(5–11)
Sleep latency (min)	5	(2–18)	Stage N2	217.5	55	(44–66)
REM latency (min)	15	(55–78)	Stages N3	79.5	20	(2–15)
WASO (min)	34.5		Stage REM	79.5	20	(19–27)
Apnea–hypopnea index (AHI)	2/hr					
Periodic limb movement in sleep (PLMS) index	10/hr					

( ), Normal values for age; min, minutes; REM, rapid eye movement; WASO, wake after sleep onset.

TABLE P87-2 Multiple Sleep Latency Test Results

	Sleep Latency (minutes)	SOREMPs
Nap 1	2	0
Nap 2	3	1
Nap 3	5	1
Nap 4	2	0
Nap 5	2	0
Mean sleep latency	2.8	

SOREMPs, Sleep-onset rapid eye movement periods.

QUESTIONS

1. What is your diagnosis?

2. Could this patient have a decreased cerebrospinal fluid (CSF) hypocretin-1 level?

ANSWERS

1. **Answer:** Narcolepsy type 2, or narcolepsy without cataplexy (N-T2 or N–C).

2. **Answer:** It is estimated that about 24% of patients with N−C have low CSF hypocretin levels. These patients are invariably positive for the DBQ1*602 antigen.

Discussion: The *International Classification of Sleep Disorders*, Third Edition (ICSD-3) diagnostic criteria for N-T2 are listed in Box P87-1. Patients must have excessive daytime sleepiness for ≥3 months. Cataplexy must be absent. The MSLT shows a mean sleep latency (MSL) of ≤8 minutes with ≥2 sleep-onset rapid eye movement periods (SOREMPs). A SOREMP on the preceding PSG may count for one of the two required SOREMPs. The CSF hypocretin-1 level has not been measured or, if measured, is not decreased. In addition, the hypersomnia, MSLT findings, or both are not better explained by other causes such as sleep insufficiency, OSA, delayed sleep phase disorder, or the effect of medication or substances or their withdrawal. The ICSD-3 recommends that a sleep log and actigraphy be obtained for at least 7 days before testing to rule out insufficient sleep or abnormal timing of the sleep period. In a study by Aldrich et al 6% of patients found to have a sleep-related breathing disorder (SBD) had an MSL of ≤8 minutes and ≥2 SOREMPs on the MSLT. If sleep apnea is present, it must be treated before the MSLT can reliably be used to diagnose narcolepsy. As the presence of cataplexy is an exclusion criteria for N-T2 the patients may also be characterized as N−C.

About 30% of patients with narcolepsy do not have cataplexy (N−C). Some will develop the symptom at a later time. The time from the onset of symptoms of daytime sleepiness to the onset of cataplexy has been studied (Figure P87-1). The onset of cataplexy is usually within 5 years, but wide variability exists. Some patients diagnosed with N−C will later develop cataplexy. If a patient with a diagnosis of N-T2 develops cataplexy, they will be reclassified as N-T1. In studies of CSF hypocretin-1 levels, a proportion of patients with low CSF hypocretin did not report cataplexy. In the ICSD-3, a patient with low CSF hypocretin would be classified as N-T1, even if cataplexy or a diagnostic PSG/MSLT combination or both were not present. The question arises as to how many patients with a diagnosis of N−C have a low CSF hypocretin level. The answer is not known, as CSF hypocretin levels are routinely obtained at only a few centers and a referral bias may exist. Bourgin et al estimated that about 20% of patients with N−C have low CSF hypocretin level. Virtually all of these patients are positive for the DQB1*602 antigen. A recent investigation sought to determine characteristics of this group. In the study by Andlauer and coworkers, 24% of patients diagnosed with N−C (in whom CSF samples were available) had low hypocretin. However, this finding may not be representative of a community based sample of N-C patients.

Patients with N−C tend to have longer sleep latencies and fewer SOREMPs compared with those with N+C. They may also have a lower incidence of sleep paralysis and hypnogogic hallucinations. Given that we do not know the pathophysiology of N−C, they may be a heterogeneous group with more than one etiology.

The diagnosis of N-T2 (N−C) depends entirely on the findings of PSG/MSLT combination and exclusion of other causes of abnormal MSLT findings. In the study of Aldrich et al., using repeat MSLT evaluations, it was determined that 91% of patients with N−C would have a MSLT meeting the current criteria of MSL of ≤8 minutes and ≥2 SOREMPs. Therefore, the MSLT is not 100% sensitive for a diagnosis of narcolepsy. If a sleepy patient without cataplexy has an MSL of

---

BOX P87-1   Narcolepsy Type 2 (Criteria A-E must be present)

A. The patient has daily periods of irrepressible need to sleep or daytime lapses into sleep occurring for *at least 3 months*.

B. Cataplexy is absent.
   Note: If cataplexy develops later, then the disorder should be reclassified as narcolepsy type 1.

C. A mean sleep latency of ≤8 minutes and ≥2 sleep onset REM periods (SOREMPs) are found on a multiple sleep latency test (MSLT) performed according to standard techniques. A SOREMP (within 15 minutes of sleep onset) on the preceding nocturnal polysomnography (PSG) may replace one of the SOREMPs on the MSLT.

D. *Either* CSF hypocretin-1 concentration *has not been measured* OR CSF hypocretin-1 concentration measured by immunoreactivity is either >110 picogram per milliliter (pg/mL) or > 1/3 of mean values obtained in normal subjects with the same assay.
   Note: If the CSF hypocretin-1 concentration is tested at a later stage and found to be either ≤110 pg/mL or < 1/3 of mean values obtained in normal subjects with the same assay, then the disorder should be reclassified as narcolepsy type 1.

E. The hypersomnia, MSLT findings, or both are not better explained by other causes such as sleep insufficiency, obstructive sleep apnea, delayed sleep phase disorder, or the effect of medication or substances or their withdrawal.

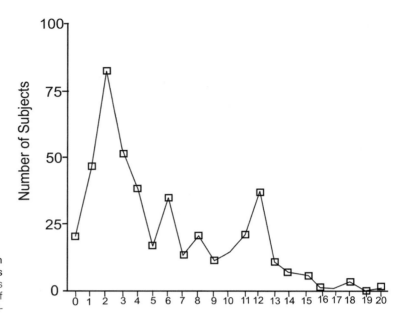

FIGURE P87-1 ■ Time of onset from excessive daytime sleepiness (EDS) to cataplexy. (From Dauvilliers Y, Montplasir J, Molinari N, et al: Age of onset of narcolepsy in two large populations of patients in France and Quebec, *Neurology* 57:2029–2033, 2001.)

Age Difference [onset EDS to cataplexy] (years)

≤8 minutes but has <2 SOREMPs (on PSG and MSLT combined), a diagnosis of idiopathic hypersomnia may be made. If the clinical suspicion of narcolepsy is high, repeat PSG or MSLT should be ordered. A study by Coelho et al. found that when the PSG-MSLT was repeated after a previously negative evaluation that narcolepsy was confirmed about 20% of the time.

In the ICSD-3, proper conditions for the performance of the MSLT are specified. "For the correct interpretation of MSLT findings, the recordings should be performed with the following conditions: the patient must be free of drugs that influence sleep for at least 14 days (or at least five times the half-life of the drug and longer-acting metabolite), confirmed by a urine drug screen; the sleep-wake schedule must have been standardized and, if necessary, extended to a minimum of 7 hours in bed each night (longer for children) for at least seven days before polysomnography (and documented by sleep log and actigraphy); and nocturnal polysomnography should be performed on the night immediately preceding the MSLT to rule out other sleep disorders that could mimic the diagnostic features of narcolepsy type 1. Sleep time during polysomnography should be curtailed as little as possible with the goal of at least 7 hours asleep."

In the current patient, who did not have a history of cataplexy, a diagnosis of N-T2 (e.g., N−C) was made on the basis of the PSG/MSLT findings and absence of another explanation for these finding. Of interest a SOREMP was also present on the PSG. The answer to the question about the possibility of the patient having a low hypocretin level is yes. Patients with N−C who are positive for the DBQ1*602 antigen may have low CSF hypocretin. Studies suggest that 20% to 24% of patients with N−C have low hypocretin and all are DBQ1*602 positive. They actually represent a subtype of N-T1 in the ICSD-3 classification (narcolepsy with low CSF hypocretin and absent cataplexy). These N-C patients would be reclassified as N-T1 if a low hypocretin level was documented or if they develop cataplexy.

CLINICAL PEARLS

1. Excessive daytime sleepiness is usually the first symptom of narcolepsy. Cataplexy usually appears within 5 years, but the range of time from the onset of sleepiness until the appearance of cataplexy is wide.
2. N-T2 is diagnosed on the basis of sleepiness for 3 months or more, absent cataplexy, CSF hypocretin level normal or not available, and a positive PSG/MSLT evaluation. If nocturnal PSG has a SOREMP, this may be used as one of the two required MSLT SOREMPs.
3. A diagnosis of N-T2 requires that another explanation for the sleepiness and MSLT findings not be present. If significant OSA is present, it must be treated before an MSLT evaluation for narcolepsy. It is imperative that adequate sleep for at least 7 days be documented before the PSG/MSLT. The ICSD-3 recommends documentation by actigraphy as well as a sleep log.
4. In one study, 6% of patients found to have a sleep related breathing disorder had an MSLT with an MSL of ≤8 minutes and ≥2 SOREMPs.

BIBLIOGRAPHY

Aldrich MS, Chervin RD, Malow BA: Value of the multiple sleep latency test (MSLT) for the diagnosis of narcolepsy, *Sleep* 20:620–629, 1997.

American Academy of Sleep Medicine: *International classification of sleep disorders: diagnostic and coding manual*, ed 2, Westchester, IL, 2005, American Academy of Sleep Medicine.

American Academy of Sleep Medicine: *International classification of sleep disorders*, ed 3, Darien, IL, 2014, American Academy of Sleep Medicine.

Andlauer O, Moore H 4th, Hong SC, et al: Predictors of hypocretin (orexin) deficiency in narcolepsy without cataplexy, *Sleep* 35 (9):1247–1255, 2012.

Arand D, Bonnet M, Hurwitz T, et al: The clinical use of the MSLT and MWT, *Sleep* 28:123–144, 2005.

Andlauer O, Moore H, Jouhier L, et al: Nocturnal rapid eye movement sleep latency for identifying patients with narcolepsy/hypocretin deficiency, *JAMA Neurol* 6:1–12, 2013.

Bourgin P, Zeitzer JM, Mignot E: CSF hypocretin-1 assessment in sleep and neurological disorders, *Lancet Neurol* 7(7):649–662, 2008.

Burgess CR, Scammell TE: Narcolepsy: neural mechanisms of sleepiness and cataplexy, *J Neurosci* 32(36):12305–12311, 2012.

Chervin RD, Aldrich MS: Sleep onset REM periods during multiple sleep latency tests in patients evaluated for sleep apnea, *Am J Respir Crit Care Med* 161:426–431, 2000.

Coelho FM, Georgsson H, Murray BJ: Benefit of repeat multiple sleep latency testing in confirming a possible narcolepsy diagnosis, *J Clin Neurophysiol* 28(4):412–414, 2011.

Dauvilliers Y, Montplasir J, Molinari N, et al: Age of onset of narcolepsy in two large populations of patients in France and Quebec, *Neurology* 57:2029–2033, 2001.

Frenette E, Kushida CA: Primary hypersomnia of central origin, *Semin Neurol* 29:354–267, 2009.

Harris SF, Monderer RS, Thorpy M: Hypersomnias of central origin, *Neurol Clin* 30(4):1027–1044, 2012.

Littner MR, Kushida C, Wise M, et al: Practice parameters for clinical use of the multiple sleep latency test and the maintenance of wakefulness test, *Sleep* 28:113–121, 2005.

Mignot E, Lin X, Arrigoni J, et al: DBQ1*602 and DQA1*0102 are better markers than DR2 for narcolepsy in Caucasians and Black Americans, *Sleep* 17(8 Suppl):S60–S67, 1994.

Scammell TE: The neurobiology, diagnosis, and treatment of narcolepsy, *Ann Neurol* 53:154–166, 2003.

PATIENT 88

A Patient with Frequent Cataplexy and Sleep Paralysis

Patient A: A 25-year-old woman was diagnosed with narcolepsy with cataplexy on the basis of symptoms of typical cataplexy and results of polysomnography (PSG) followed by a multiple sleep latency test (MSLT). The attacks of cataplexy occurred almost daily and followed laughter, surprise, or even the excitement of her college team scoring a touchdown during a football game. During the episodes, she was awake but noted bilateral leg weakness. Sometimes, the muscles of her face were also weak. In addition, she was bothered by episodes of sleep paralysis, during which she awakened but was unable to move for a minute. The episode would end if she moved her eyes during the episode or another person touched her. The episodes were also often associated with hallucinations, typically containing visions of a person or animal in the room. Although she knew these were not real, they were still frightening.

The daytime sleepiness experienced by the patient responded to modafinil, but the episodes of weakness and sleep paralysis were distressing. The patient was taking no medications other than modafinil. The patient was offered sodium oxybate, but she declined this treatment.

QUESTION

1. What treatment do you recommend for Patient A's cataplexy?

Patient B: A 30-year-old woman was evaluated for recurrent episodes of being unable to move when she awakened from sleep. Some of the episodes were associated with visions of a stranger in the room. The episodes were noted several times per week. They were actually more likely on awakening from naps and also were worse if she had a poor night of sleep. No history of daytime sleepiness or cataplexy was present. The patient denied symptoms of depression and was otherwise healthy.

2. What is the problem with Patient B? What treatment do you recommend?

ANSWERS

1. **Answer for Patient A:** Antidepressants are effective treatment for cataplexy, sleep paralysis, and hypnagogic hallucinations.

   Discussion: Sodium oxybate is the only medication approved by the U.S. Food and Drug Administration (FDA) for treatment of cataplexy in patients with narcolepsy. The medication also is effective at preventing sleep paralysis and hypnagogic hallucination. However, sodium oxybate is not acceptable or appropriate for every patient. Other treatment options are available. The American Academy of Sleep Medicine (AASM) practice parameters and recommendations for the treatment of cataplexy and associated phenomena are listed in Box P88-1.

   Antidepressants with the ability to increase norepinephrine (NE) neurotransmission are the most effective treatment for cataplexy. The tricyclic antidepressants (TCAs) were the first group used to treat cataplexy. The first agent used was imipramine, but other TCAs, including protriptyline, desipramine, and clomipramine, have been used. They are commonly effective in doses *less* than those used for antidepressant action. Protriptyline, desipramine, and imipramine block reuptake of NE, and clomipramine is a more potent blocker of serotonin reuptake. The major problem with these medications is their anticholinergic side effects (TCAs are also lethal in overdose). For this reason, these drugs are not the first choice for treatment of cataplexy. The selective serotonin reuptake inhibitors (SSRIs) such as fluoxetine have also been found useful in treating cataplexy. The SSRIs are used in typical antidepressant doses (often high doses needed) and their effect may be more delayed than that of the TCAs (perhaps because of the time required for titration up to an effective dose). However, because the SSRIs generally are better tolerated and safer in overdose than TCAs, they are widely used. The more specific SSRIs (e.g., escitalopram) have less effect on NE and would be expected to be less effective. Fluoxetine does increase NE as well as serotonin and has the advantage of a long half-life. Skipping a dose has fewer consequences. The selective serotonin and NE reuptake inhibitors (SNRIs) such as venlafaxine, desvenlafaxine, and duloxetine block the reuptake of both serotonin and NE. They have been shown to be particularly effective as a treatment for cataplexy. The extended-release formulation of venlafaxine is preferred because the drug has a short half-life. Venlafaxine XR 37.5 milligrams (mg) is the starting dose with upward titration to 75 to 150 mg daily. In some patients a dose as low as 37.5 mg may be effective.

BOX P88-1	**AASM Recommendations for Treatment of Cataplexy and Sleep Paralysis**
CATAPLEXY Sodium oxybate (Standard) Tricyclic antidepressants (Guideline) SSRIs (Guideline) Venlafaxine (Guideline) Selegiline (Option)	**SLEEP PARALYSIS, HYPNAGOGIC HALLUCINATIONS DUE TO NARCOLEPSY** Sodium oxybate (Option) Tricyclic antidepressants (Option) SSRIs (Option) Venlafaxine (Option)

Adapted from Morgenthaler TI, Kapur VK, Brown TM, et al: Practice parameters for the treatment of narcolepsy and other hypersomnias of central origin, *Sleep* 30:1705–1711, 2007.
AASM, American Academy of Sleep Medicine; *SSRIs,* selective serotonin reuptake inhibitors.
Strength of recommendations: standard>guideline>option.

Although less commonly used bupropion (NE and dopamine activity) might be effective in some patients. Atomoxetine (Strattera), an adrenergic reuptake blocker used for attention deficit hyperactivity disorder, has also been used as a treatment for cataplexy. Both venlafaxine and atomoxetine may increase blood pressure. Of note, the effect on cataplexy of these antidepressant medications occurs immediately once an effective dose is reached. This is in contrast to the antidepressant activity which may take 4 to 8 weeks. Selegiline, a selective inhibitor of MAO-B (at high doses MAO-A as well) can be used for treatment of cataplexy. However, given the many alternatives and potential side effects, the medication is rarely used to treat cataplexy.

Of note, skipping a dose of medication of an antidepressant may be associated with a rebound in the severity of cataplexy. Status cataplecticus (recurrent cataplexy) has been described with abrupt discontinuation of venlafaxine. This medication is associated with a well-known withdrawal syndrome. The medication should not be abruptly stopped, if possible. Of interest, an increase in cataplexy in patients started on the alpha-blocker prazosin has been reported. It is not known if other alpha-blockers have similar effects on cataplexy.

Obtaining adequate sleep in essential for patients with narcolepsy both for control of daytime sleepiness and cataplexy. Narcolepsy is characterized by fragmented nighttime sleep and frequent arousals often with an increase in stage N1. The 24-hour duration of sleep is typically normal but in untreated patients is scattered throughout both the night and day. One treatment approach to improve daytime symptoms is to consolidate nighttime sleep through decreasing arousals. In some narcolepsy patients, *use of a hypnotic may improve sleep and daytime symptoms*. Improvement of sleep quality may be one mechanism by which sodium oxybate works to decrease sleepiness and cataplexy. A few studies suggest that both daytime sleepiness and cataplexy might improve with improved nocturnal sleep. A single study found clonazepam improved cataplexy in 10 of 14 patients with narcolepsy, although no improvement in daytime sleepiness was reported. In another retrospective review of a few patients on temazepam, an improvement in subjective daytime sleepiness and cataplexy was reported.

In the current patient, venlafaxine 37.5 mg XR was started. Cataplexy improved, but episodes were still present. At a dose of 75 mg daily, attacks of cataplexy and sleep paralysis were essentially eliminated. The patient was also encouraged to improve sleep hygiene and obtain at least 7 hours of sleep each night.

2. **Answer:** Recurrent isolated sleep paralysis, obtaining an adequate amount of sleep each night.

Discussion: This syndrome if often classified under parasomnias but is discussed here, given the discussion about sleep paralysis in narcolepsy. Recurrent isolated sleep paralysis is characterized by an inability to perform voluntary movements at sleep onset (hypnagogic or predormital form) or on waking from sleep (hypnopompic or postdormital form) in the absence of a diagnosis of narcolepsy. The event is characterized by an inability to speak or to move the limbs, trunk, and head. Respiration is usually unaffected. Consciousness is preserved, and full recall is present. An episode of sleep paralysis lasts seconds to minutes. It usually resolves spontaneously but may be aborted by sensory stimulation such as being touched or spoken to or by the patient making intense efforts to move (moving the eyes vigorously). Patients feel that they are awake and aware of their surroundings and have total recall of the event. The experience may be distressful and is sometimes accompanied by visual, auditory, or tactile hallucinations (commonly a stranger or animal in the room). The other symptoms of narcolepsy are absent (no sleepiness or cataplexy). The episodes usually happen after a period of disrupted or curtailed sleep. Students often experience an episode after reducing sleep during examinations. In some studies of younger individuals, 15% to 40% have experienced one episode of sleep paralysis in their lifetime. The reason some patients have recurrent episodes in unknown. Improved sleep is the first intervention. If this is not successful, the medications used for cataplexy in patients with narcolepsy can be used (except for sodium oxybate).

In patient B, once the association of poor sleep and the episodes were explained to the patient she was very motivated to establish good sleep habits. In addition, because the phenomenon was well known and had no long-term consequences, the patient was much less fearful. On follow-up, she reported only one episode in 6 months and that the episode was not frightening, as she understood what was happening.

CLINICAL PEARLS

1. Improving sleep quantity and quality is important for treatment of patients with narcolepsy.

2. Treatments for cataplexy include sodium oxybate (only FDA-approved medication for this indication) and antidepressants.

3. Antidepressants with the ability to increase NE are most useful for treatment of cataplexy. In particular, venlafaxine XR in relatively low doses has been effective.

4. SSRIs in relatively high doses are also effective treatment for cataplexy. Those with some ability to increase NE are more effective. Fluoxetine has some NE activity and has a long half-life that makes skipping a dose less problematic.

5. Abrupt withdrawal of antidepressants (skipping a dose) may trigger a rebound in cataplexy—best described with venlafaxine.

6. Medications effective for treatment of cataplexy are also effective treatments for sleep paralysis and sleep-related hallucinations.

7. Isolated sleep paralysis is common in normal individuals. The treatment of choice is improved sleep quality and regularity.

BIBLIOGRAPHY

Aldrich M, Rogers AE: Exacerbation of human cataplexy by prazosin, *Sleep* 12:254–256, 1989.

Frey J, Darbonne C: Fluoxetine suppresses human cataplexy, *Neurology* 44:707–709, 1994.

Guilleminault C, Aftab FA, Karadeniz D, et al: Problems associated with switch to modafinil—a novel alerting agent in narcolepsy, *Eur J Neurol* 7:381–384, 2000.

Kansagra S, Walter R, Vaughn B: Nocturnal temazepam in the treatment of narcolepsy, *J Clin Sleep Med* 9(5):499–500, 2013.

McCarty DE, Chesson AL Jr.: A case of sleep paralysis with hypnopompic hallucinations. Recurrent isolated sleep paralysis associated with hypnopompic hallucinations, precipitated by behaviorally induced insufficient sleep syndrome, *J Clin Sleep Med* 5 (1):83–84, 2009.

Mignot EJ: A practical guide to the therapy of narcolepsy and hypersomnia syndromes, *Neurotherapeutics* 9(4):739–752, 2012.

Mignot E: An update on the pharmacotherapy of excessive daytime sleepiness and cataplexy, *Sleep Med Rev* 333–338, 2004.

Morgenthaler TI, Kapur VK, Brown TM, et al: Practice parameters for the treatment of narcolepsy and other hypersomnias of central origin, *Sleep* 30:1705–1711, 2007.

Ohayon M, Zulley J, Guilleminault C, Smirne S: Prevalence and pathologic associations of sleep paralysis in the general population, *Neurology* 52:1194–1200, 1999.

Parkes JD, Schachter M: Clomipramine and clonazepam in cataplexy, *Lancet* 2:1085–1086, 1979.

Takeuchi T, Fukuda K, Sasaki Y, et al: Factors related to the occurrence of isolated sleep paralysis elicited during a multi-phasic sleep-wake schedule, *Sleep* 25:89–96, 2002.

Takeuchi T, Miyasita A, Sasaki Y, et al: Isolated sleep paralysis elicited by sleep interruption, *Sleep* 15:217–225, 1992.

Wang J, Greenberg H: Status cataplecticus precipitated by abrupt withdrawal of venlafaxine, *J Clin Sleep Med* 9(7):715–716, 2013.

A Patient with Sleep Apnea and Possible Narcolepsy

Patient A: A 40-year-old man with excessive daytime sleepiness since age 20 was diagnosed as having obstructive sleep apnea (OSA) (apnea–hypopnea index [AHI] 80 per hour [hr]) at another hospital about 1 year ago. Nasal continuous positive airway pressure (CPAP) at 12 centimeters of water (cm H_2O) reduced the AHI to 3/hr. However, significant daytime sleepiness persisted despite using CPAP for at least 7 hours a night (documented by CPAP download) and treatment with modafinil 400 milligrams (mg) daily. No history of cataplexy or sleep paralysis was present. Medications included lisinopril and modafinil. A sleep study on CPAP and a multiple sleep latency test (MSLT) on CPAP were ordered. The patient had not taken modafinil for 1 week preceding the studies (Table P89-1).

TABLE P89-1 PSG and MSLT on CPAP of 12 cm H_2O (Patient A)

		Normal		(min)	%TST	Normal
Total Recording Time (min)	450	(390–468)	Stage N1	19.5	5	(5–11)
Total sleep time (min)	395.5	(343–436)	Stage N2	217.5	55	(44–66)
Sleep efficiency %	88	(85–97)	Stages N3	79.5	20	(2–15)
Sleep latency (min)	10	(2–18)	Stage R	79.5	20	(19–27)
REM latency (min)	10	(55–78)				
WASO (min)	34.5					
AHI (#/hr)	3/hour					
PLM index (#/hr)	10					

( ), Normal values for age, *AHI*, apnea + hypopnea index; *cm H_2O*, centimeters of water; *PLM*, periodic limb movement; *REM*, rapid eye movement; *TST*, total sleep time; *WASO*, wakefulness after sleep onset.
MSLT = on nasal CPAP (12 cm H_2O).
Mean sleep latency = 4 minutes.
SOREMPs = 3 of 5 naps.

Question 1: What is causing Patient A's persistent sleepiness on CPAP Treatment.
Patient B: A 30-year-old woman with loud snoring underwent sleep testing (Table P89-2). She denied cataplexy but reported severe sleepiness (Epworth Sleepiness Scale [ESS] score of 16/24).

TABLE P89-2 Sleep Study and MSLT Results

	Time (min)	Normal range		Time (min)	%TST	Normal range
Total Recording Time	470 min	(425–462)	Stage N1	43.0	9.9	(3–6)
Total sleep time	434.5 min	(394–457)	Stage N2	226.0	52.0	(46–62)
Sleep efficiency	91.5 %	(90–100)	Stage N3	83.0	19.1	(7–21)
Sleep latency	5 min	(0–19)	Stage REM	82.5	19.0	(21–31)
REM latency	10 min	(69–88)				
WASO	29.5 min	(0–26)				
AHI (#/hr)	30/hr					
Obst Apneas (#)	60		PLMS index	10/hr		
Mixed Apneas (#)	1		Desaturations	200		
Central Apneas (#)	3		Low SaO₂	75%		
Hypopnea (#)	60					

( ), Normal values for age; *AHI*, apnea + hypopnea index; *PLMs*, periodic limb movement in sleep; *REM*, rapid eye movement; *SaO₂*, saturation of arterial oxygen; *TST*, total sleep time; *WASO*, wakefulness after sleep onset.

Question 2: In patient B, is narcolepsy present in addition to OSA?

ANSWERS

1. **Answer for Patient A:** Narcolepsy type 2 (N-T2; narcolepsy without cataplexy [N−C]).

   Discussion: Patients with a combination of narcolepsy and OSA are not rare. Adequate treatment of both disorders is required for control of daytime sleepiness. If cataplexy is unequivocal, a diagnosis of narcolepsy as well as OSA is likely. However, according to the diagnostic criteria in the *International Classification of Sleep Disorders*, Third Edition (ICSD-3), a diagnosis of narcolepsy type 1 requires both the presence of cataplexy and a PSG-MSLT evaluation meeting the diagnostic criteria. Cataplexy is present in 60% to 70% of patients with narcolepsy. However, cataplexy makes a delayed appearance in many patients with narcolepsy—sometimes years after the daytime sleepiness begins. In OSA patients with suspected narcolepsy type 1 and type 2 a PSG-MSLT evaluation can support a diagnosis. The first step in all of these cases is successful treatment of the OSA. A repeat sleep study (on treatment) is then followed by an MSLT (also on treatment). The sleep study documents adequate treatment (and adequate sleep), and the MSLT provides objective evidence of continued daytime sleepiness (mean sleep latency [MSL] of ≤8 minutes) and the presence of ≥2 sleep-onset REM periods (SOREMPs). The ICSD-3 allows a SOREMP on nocturnal PSG (REM latency ≤15 min) to count as one of the two required MSLT SOREMPs. Although not addressed in the recent MSLT practice parameters, the 1992 AASM MSLT guidelines stated: "To determine the concurrent presence of narcolepsy after treatment of the obstructive sleep apnea syndrome by CPAP, the MSLT should be performed with the patient using the CPAP device." The differential diagnosis of a patient with OSA still sleepy on CPAP includes inadequate adherence, inadequate CPAP pressure, narcolepsy, periodic limb movement disorder (PLMD), medication side effects, idiopathic hypersomnia, insufficient sleep, and depression. Before a PSG and MSLT are ordered, good objective PAP adherence must be documented. Some patients require 7 hours or more of CPAP use nightly for improvement in sleepiness.

   In Patient A, the early age of onset of symptoms is consistent with narcolepsy. The sleep study on CPAP showed excellent treatment of his sleep apnea and sleep of fairly good quality (no evidence of REM rebound). The MSLT documented both severe daytime sleepiness and SOREMPs in three of five naps. The absence of other reasons to explain these MSLT findings makes a diagnosis of narcolepsy without cataplexy highly likely. In addition, a short REM latency was evident on PSG. Given the diagnosis and the inadequate response to modafinil, this medication was stopped and the patient was treated with methylphenidate 20 mg ER in the morning and methylphenidate 20 mg immediate release at 1 PM with improvement in his symptoms of daytime sleepiness. Of note, had the MSLT been negative, the switch from modafinil to methylphenidate could still have been made, but this would be an off-label treatment of the medication for daytime sleepiness. Some patients with OSA without narcolepsy have persistent daytime sleepiness on both CPAP and modafinil. In such patients, a trial of a stimulant is a viable treatment option. In OSA with persistent sleepiness despite adequate treatment who do NOT meet criteria for narcolepsy a diagnosis of Hypersomnia due to a Medical Disorder is appropriate if other causes of sleepiness are ruled out.

2. **Answer for Patient B:** A diagnosis of narcolepsy without cataplexy cannot be made until sleep apnea is adequately treated. However, a nocturnal SOREMP is very uncommon in patients with OSA alone.

   Discussion: Untreated sleep apnea may be associated with a short nocturnal REM latency or ≥2 SOREMPs on an MSLT. Studies have found that about 5% to 6% of patients with sleep apnea have ≥2 SOREMPs on the MSLT. In a study by Aldrich et al, *only 1% of 1251 patients had a nocturnal SOREMP*. In this study, 33% of patients with narcolepsy with cataplexy has a nocturnal SOREMP, as did 24% of patients with narcolepsy without cataplexy. Other causes of a short REM latency on PSG are depression, schizophrenia, withdrawal from an REM sleep suppressant or prior REM sleep deprivation. Therefore, if a patient with untreated sleep apnea is suspected of having possible narcolepsy, adequate treatment of the sleep apnea is essential before further evaluation with another sleep study and MSLT. It is essential to objectively document PAP adherence. After effective treatment documented for several months, PSG on CPAP and an MSLT on CPAP may be ordered.

   Although daytime sleepiness is a core symptom in patients with OSA, the degree of sleepiness, as assessed by the mean sleep latency (MSL) on the MSLT, is much lower in patients with narcolepsy than

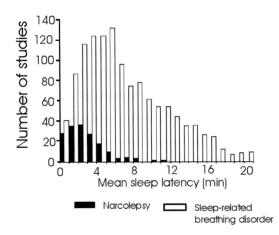

FIGURE P89-1 ■ Distribution of mean sleep latency (MSL) results for groups of patients with narcolepsy and sleep-related breathing disorders. Although considerable overlap is noted, patients with narcolepsy tend to have much lower MSL (more sleepy). (From Aldrich MS, Chervin RD, Malow BA: Value of the multiple sleep latency test [MSLT] for the diagnosis of narcolepsy, *Sleep* 20:620–629, 1997.)

in patients with sleep apnea. Considerable overlap exists, but the great majority of patients with OSA alone have MSL values above 5 minutes (Figure P89-1).

Patient B underwent CPAP titration and was started on effective treatment. Daytime sleepiness dramatically improved. As the ESS score was normal, further evaluation was not indicated. It is assumed the short nocturnal REM latency was an uncommon manifestation of OSA.

CLINICAL PEARLS

1. When daytime sleepiness persists on nasal CPAP, consider the possibility of other sleep disorders as well as inadequate adherence, inadequate pressure, or insufficient sleep (sleep on CPAP <7.5 hours).
2. An MSLT can provide objective evidence of persistent sleepiness on nasal CPAP and help support a diagnosis of narcolepsy. Such a study should be performed only after optimizing PAP treatment and ensuring adequate adherence. PSG on CPAP should precede the MSLT (also on CPAP).
3. If narcolepsy is suspected in a patient with significant OSA, first treat the OSA. Then, a sleep study and MSLT on treatment may be ordered to support a diagnosis of narcolepsy as well as OSA.
4. The presence of a SOREMP on PSG has a high positive predictive value for narcolepsy. However, such a finding may very rarely be caused by OSA alone. However, a nocturnal SOREMP should alert the clinician that narcolepsy as well as OSA could be present.

BIBLIOGRAPHY

Aldrich MS, Chervin RD, Malow BA: Value of the multiple sleep latency test (MSLT) for the diagnosis of narcolepsy, *Sleep* 20:620–629, 1997.

American Academy of Sleep Medicine: *International classification of sleep disorders*, ed 3, Darien, IL, 2013, American Academy of Sleep Medicine.

Arand D, Bonnet M, Hurwitz T, et al: A review by the MSLT and MWT Task Force of the Standards of Practice Committee of the AASM. The clinical use of the MSLT and MWT, *Sleep* 28:123–144, 2005.

Carskadon MA: Guidelines for the multiple sleep latency test, *Sleep* 9:519–524, 1986.

Chervin RD, Aldrich MS: Sleep onset REM periods during multiple sleep latency tests in patients evaluated for sleep apnea, *Am J Respir Crit Care Med* 161:426–431, 2000.

Littner MR, Kushida C, Wise M, et al: Practice parameters for clinical use of the multiple sleep latency test and the maintenance of wakefulness test, *Sleep* 28:113–121, 2005.

Standards of Practice Committee, American Sleep Disorders Association: The clinical use of the multiple sleep latency test, *Sleep* 15:268–276, 1992.

A Child with Sleepiness and "Syncope"

An 8-year-old boy was evaluated for poor performance in school (inattention and irritability), a return to napping during the day, and episodes of syncope (falling to the ground) on during recess. On further questioning, he reported that he was awake during the fainting spells but felt that he could not talk during these episodes. The patient's parents also reported a notable weight gain of 10 pounds associated with the development of the other symptoms. No history of seizure activity, head trauma, or problems with coordination was present. Also, a history of loud snoring or labored breathing during sleep was not reported. The boy's typical bedtime was 9 PM and wake time was 6 AM.

Physical examination showed a cooperative child with droopy eyelids and mild obesity. The tonsils were only slightly enlarged.

Polysomnography (PSG): normal sleep architecture, rapid eye movement (REM) latency was normal and the apnea–hypopnea index (AHI) was 0 per hour (hr) without arterial oxygen desaturations.

Multiple sleep latency test (MSLT): mean sleep latency (MSL) 4 minutes; 1 sleep-onset REM period (SOREMP).

QUESTION

1. What is your diagnosis? What other testing would you consider?

ANSWER

1. **Answer:** Narcolepsy with cataplexy (N + C) (although the patient does not meet ICSD-3 diagnostic criteria).

Discussion: Approximately 30% to 50% of patients diagnosed with narcolepsy have the onset of symptoms before age 15 (although diagnosis may be delayed). A meta-analysis of 235 pediatric cases derived from three studies by Challamel et al found that 34% of all patients with narcolepsy experienced onset of symptoms before age 15 years, 16% before the age 10 years, and 4.5% before age 5 years.[1] In another databank of patients, only 2% had the onset of narcolepsy before age 5. Therefore, the onset of narcolepsy before age 5 is felt to be rare. Detection of excessive sleepiness may be more challenging in children than adults.[2,3] *Excessive sleepiness may manifest as a return to taking daytime naps in a child that previously discontinued napping or as an increase in sleep duration.* In older children, daytime sleepiness may sometimes manifest as symptoms similar to those of attention-deficit hyperactivity disorder (ADHD) with irritability, mood swings, and inattentiveness. It should be noted that normal prepubertal children have an MSL around 19 minutes on an MSLT.[4,5] Cataplexy is present in about two thirds of pediatric patients with narcolepsy. *In children, not all cataplexy is associated with a clearly identifiable emotional trigger.* Because cataplexy may be subtle, the examiner might need to ask leading questions about sudden muscle weakness in the lower extremities, neck, facial muscles, or trunk in response to laughter, fright, excitement, anger, or the anticipation of a reward. Cataplexy may be confused with syncope (except the child is awake during an attack of cataplexy) or seizurelike activity. Serra et al[6] reported on cataplexy in 23 patients diagnosed before the age of 18 years. Forty-three percent of patients had falls as part of their attacks. During cataplexy knees, head, and jaw were the most frequently compromised body segments; eyelids, arms, and trunk being less commonly involved. More rarely, blurred vision, slurred speech, irregular breathing, and a sudden loss of smiling were reported. One third of the sample presented with a previously unrecognized description of cataplexy that they termed "cataplectic facies," consisting of a state of semipermanent eyelid and jaw weakness (droopy eyelids, mouth open), on which partial or complete cataplectic attacks were superimposed. This last pattern was often present soon after the onset of the disorder. The usual triggering emotions for cataplexy such as laughter, amusement, or anger were not always present, especially when temporally adjacent to an often abrupt onset of narcolepsy. In children with narcolepsy, cataplexy may sometimes be the first symptom and often the most prominent. If cataplexy is the first symptom of narcolepsy, an evaluation of narcolepsy caused by medical condition (secondary narcolepsy) is indicated, including central nervous system (CNS) imaging and genetic testing (if indicated). In one study of children with N + C, the onset of narcolepsy was often associated with the rapid development of obesity. In general, *obesity is present in up to 25% of cases with childhood narcolepsy*, and nocturnal eating syndrome may be present. The development of precocious puberty associated with the onset of narcolepsy has also been reported.

In children, as in adults, the MSLT is used to diagnose narcolepsy, although in younger children, normative values for the MSLT are less well defined.[5] As noted above, prepubertal children tend to have long sleep latencies on the MSLT. For example, the MSL on the MSLT in one study by Carskadon et al of normal prepubertal children was 19 ± 16 minutes (in adults, 10.4 ± 4.3).[6] Therefore, use of sleep latency criteria of 8 minutes for narcolepsy could potentially be problematic (e.g., 12 minutes might indicate significant sleepiness). Some clinicians consider an MSL <12 minutes as consistent with daytime sleepiness in children.[5] Fortunately, published studies of children with narcolepsy show very short sleep latencies (Table P90-1) well below 8 minutes.[3] However, false-negative MSLT evaluations may occur in prepubertal children (see Table P90-1), mainly because of the lack of 2 SOREMPs. If the clinical suspicion is high, a repeat MSLT could be considered. A lumbar puncture for cerebrospinal fluid (CSF) sampling (hypocretin-1) could be considered (in a patient positive for the human leukocyte antigen [HLA] DQB1*0602) if the diagnosis is uncertain (e.g., atypical cataplexy), if the patient does not respond to treatment, or both. In summary, in children, narcolepsy is often misdiagnosed as epilepsy (cataplexy confused as epileptic seizures), syncope, neuromuscular disorders (muscle weakness), conversion disorder, ADHD (sleepiness manifested an inattention or irritability), depression (inattention, loss of focus, behavioral problems), or psychosis (when hypnagogic hallucinations are a prominent feature), leading to inadequate pharmacotherapy and further complications. Of interest, studies have associated certain influenza vaccines with an increase in development of narcolepsy in children.[7]

Treatment of narcolepsy in children with standard medications is "off label," as no medication is FDA approved for narcolepsy treatment in children. The AASM Practice Parameters for Treatment of Narcolepsy and Other Hypersomnias of Central Origin stated that "methylphenidate or modafinil in children 6 to 15 years appears to be relatively safe in the treatment of hypersomnias of central origin (Option)."[8] However, modafinil and armodafinil are not approved by the U.S. Food and Drug Administration (FDA) for treatment of children. Modafinil appears to be well tolerated in children (typical doses 50 to 400 milligrams [mg]).[9,10] The most common side effect is headache. Stevens-Johnson syndrome may have developed in a few children on modafinil (very rare), and parents should be informed to immediately notify their physician if a rash develops while taking the medication. The AASM practice

TABLE P90-1	**Results of Hypocretin-Deficient Narcolepsy with Cataplexy in Children**			
	All	**Prepubertal**	**Peripubertal**	**Postpubertal**
Excessive daytime sleepiness (%)	100	100	100	100
Cataplexy (%)	100	100	100	100
Hypnagogic hallucinations (%)	66	62	67	89
Sleep paralysis (%)	55	44	60	78
% low CSF hypocretin (%)	100	100	100	100
DQB1*0602 positive (%)	100	100	100	100
Presenting symptom: excessive daytime sleepiness (%)	85	85	92	71
Cataplexy with 2 months of onset (%)	82	85	75	86
MSLT MSL (min)	2.5	2.8	2.4	1.5
Positive MSLT (%) (MSL ≤ 8 min + 2 or more SOREMPs)	92	85	100	100

From Aran A, Einen M, Lin L, et al: Clinical and therapeutic aspects of childhood narcolepsy-cataplexy: a retrospective study of 51 children, *Sleep* 33:1457–1464, 2010.
CSF, Cerebrospinal fluid; *EDS*, excessive daytime sleepiness; *MSL*, mean sleep latency; *MSLT*, multiple sleep latency test; *SOREMPs*, sleep-onset rapid eye movement periods.

parameters made no recommendation for the treatment of cataplexy in children. Venlafaxine and fluoxetine have used for cataplexy in this age group.[11] Finally, sodium oxybate has been used in children when both excessive sleepiness and cataplexy are prominent symptoms.[3]

As sodium oxybate may be associated with weight loss, this may be beneficial in obese children. A study of children with narcolepsy by Aran et al reported successful use of modafinil, venlafaxine, and sodium oxybate.[3] The authors recommended starting dose of sodium oxybate of 60 to 90 mg/kg per day (on an empty stomach, divided into two doses—the first at bedtime and the second 2.5 hours later). As in adults, caution is advised in patients with sleep-related breathing disorders (SBDs), and enuresis is a common side effect.

In the current patient, the episodes of "syncope" with maintained consciousness were highly suggestive of cataplexy, as is the finding of droopy eyelids. PSG did not document sleep apnea, and the MSLT showed severe sleepiness for an 8-year-old but only 1 SOREMP. As noted above, false-negative MSLT evaluations may occur in prepubertal patients with N-T2 (N+C). Obtaining a CSF sample was considered, as the patient was positive for the HLA DQB1*0602 allele, but the parents declined the procedure. A repeat MSLT was also proposed, but the patient's parents felt that some treatment would be necessary, even if the repeat study was negative. Given convincing cataplexy, a diagnosis of narcolepsy type 1 was made (although the patient did not meet ICSD-3 criteria). The patient would meet diagnostic criteria of the diagnostic and statistical manual of mental disorders (DSM-5)12 which accepts sleepiness and cataplexy as meeting diagnostic criteria.[12] The patient was treated with modafinil but developed severe headaches and was switched to dextro-amphetamine 5 mg ER in the morning and scheduled naps. Later the dose of dextro-amphetamine was increased to 10 mg ER in the AM. The patient's sleepiness decreased and his behavior improved, and cataplexy was rarely noted (dextro-amphetamine has some anticataplexy activity).

CLINICAL PEARLS

1. Daytime sleepiness and cataplexy may be difficult to identify in children.
2. In children, cataplexy may be more likely to result in falls and may not always be associated with an emotional trigger. Attacks of cataplexy may be mistaken for a seizure or an episode of syncope. Some patients may develop a "cataplectic facies" with droopy eyelids and open mouth.
3. While the MSLT mean sleep latency (MSL) is longer in prepubertal children than in adults, children with narcolepsy have a very short MSL (much less than 8 minutes). The criterion of a MSL <8 minutes can still be used to diagnose narcolepsy in children.
4. Sudden weight gain (10 pounds or more) has been associated with the onset of hypocretin-deficient narcolepsy (N-T1) in children.
5. Pharmacologic treatment of narcolepsy in children is "off label," as no medications have been approved for treatment of narcolepsy in this age group. Modafinil, stimulants, fluoxetine, venlafaxine, and sodium oxybate have all been used in children with narcolepsy and appear to be effective. The use of scheduled naps may also be beneficial in some patients.

REFERENCES

1. Challamel MJ, Mazzola ME, Nevsimalova S, et al: Narcolepsy in children, *Sleep* 17:S17–S20, 1994.
2. Nevsimalova S: Narcolepsy in childhood, *Sleep Med Rev* 13:169–180, 2009.
3. Aran A, Einen M, Lin L, et al: Clinical and therapeutic aspects of childhood narcolepsy-cataplexy: a retrospective study of 51 children, *Sleep* 33:1457–1464, 2010.
4. Serra L, Montagna P, Mignot E, et al: Cataplexy features in childhood narcolepsy, *Mov Disord* 23(6):858–865, 2008.
5. Aurora RN, Lamm CI, Zak RS, et al: Practice parameters for the non-respiratory indications for polysomnography and multiple sleep latency testing for children, *Sleep* 35(11):1467–1473, 2012.
6. Carskadon MA, Harvey K, Duke P, et al: Pubertal changes in daytime sleepiness, *Sleep* 2:453–460, 1980.
7. Miller E, Andrews N, Stellitano L, et al: Risk of narcolepsy in children and young people receiving AS03 adjuvanted pandemic A/H1N1 2009 influenza vaccine: retrospective analysis, *Br Med J* 346:f794, 2013.
8. Morgenthaler TI, Kapur VK, Brown TM, et al: Practice parameters for the treatment of narcolepsy and other hypersomnias of central origin, *Sleep* 30:1705–1711, 2007.
9. Ivanenko A, Tauman R, Gozal D: Modafinil in the treatment of excessive daytime sleepiness in children, *Sleep Med* 4:579–582, 2003.
10. Lecendreux M, Bruni O, Franco P, et al: Clinical experience suggests that modafinil is an effective and safe treatment for paediatric narcolepsy, *J Sleep Res* 21(4):481–483, 2012.
11. Møller LR, Østergaard JR: Treatment with venlafaxine in six cases of children with narcolepsy and with cataplexy and hypnagogic hallucinations, *J Child Adolesc Psychopharmacol* 19:197–201, 2009.
12. American Psychiatric Association: Diagnostic and statistical manual of mental disorders, ed 5, Arlington, VA, 2013, American Psychiatric Association.

Modafinil and Narcolepsy

Patient A: A 30-year-old woman was diagnosed as having narcolepsy without cataplexy (Type 2). She was started on modafinil 200 milligrams (mg) daily, and the dose was slowly increased to 400 mg daily in the morning. The medication was effective until about 1 to 2 PM, at which time a significant return of daytime sleepiness occurred.

Question 1: What change in treatment do you recommend for Patient A?

Patient B: A 25-year-old woman with narcolepsy is using an oral contraceptive. She is to be started on modafinil 200 mg in the morning.

Question 2: What information do you give Patient B concerning modafinil?

Patient C: You are considering starting modafinil in a 30-year-old man with narcolepsy to treat his symptom of daytime sleepiness. While looking over his medical record, you notice that he frequently suffers from headaches.

Question 3: If you decide to start modafinil, what intervention do you recommend for Patient C?

ANSWERS

1. **Answer for Patient A:** Modafinil 200 mg every morning and 200 mg at 1 PM. Although once-daily dosing of modafinil is the usual recommendation, some patients will benefit from a split dose. An alternative is the use of armodafinil, the R enantiomer of modafinil with a longer half-life.

2. **Answer for Patient B:** Modafinil may potentially reduce the effectiveness of oral contraceptives by altering hepatic metabolism (increased). Consider other contraceptive methods.

3. **Answer for Patient C:** Headache is the most common side effect of modafinil. This may be minimized by starting at a low dose and slow upward titration. Of note, some patients with severe headaches may experience fewer problems with stimulants (although they may also worsen headaches).

Discussion (Patients A-C): Modafinil (racemic R, L modafinil) and armodafinil (R enantiomer of modafinil) are non-amphetamine wakefulness-promoting medications that are Schedule IV medications (refills and telephone orders are allowed). They are considered to have less abuse potential compared with stimulant medications. Modafinil is considered the first-line medication for the treatment of excessive daytime sleepiness (EDS) associated with narcolepsy.[1,2] Randomized, placebo-controlled trials have documented the effectiveness of modafinil in patients with narcolepsy.[3,4]

The elimination half-life of modafinil is 9 to 14 hours, permitting once-daily administration for most patients. Modafinil is usually administered once daily in the morning (200–400 mg). Modafinil is available in 100- and 200-mg tablets. A typical starting dose is 100 mg, with increase to 200 mg over a few days. A considerable number of patients taking modafinil only in the morning may experience poor control of daytime sleepiness in the afternoon or early evening. They may respond to split dosing (200 mg in the morning, 200 mg at 1–2 PM).[5,6] Although the maximum recommended daily dose of modafinil is 400 mg, higher doses have been used. In some patients, adequate control of sleepiness may require a slightly higher dose than 400 mg (400 mg in the morning and 200 mg in the early afternoon).[5,6]

The mechanism of action of modafinil is still debated, but it is likely that binding the *dopamine active transporter (DAT)* and increasing dopaminergic transmission is the main effect.[1,7] Of note, L-modafinil has a lower binding affinity for the DAT. The L enantiomer of modafinil has a shorter half-life (3–4 hr) than the R enantiomer (10–14 hours). Modafinil (racemic, containing both L and R enantiomers) has a similar terminal half-life as armodafinil, as within a few hours, the only form of modafinil present in the blood is armodafinil.[8–10] If the same dose of modafinil and armodafinil is given in the morning, by the afternoon blood levels of armodafinil are considerably higher. For this reason, a morning dose of armodafinil (150 or 250 mg) may control afternoon sleepiness better than modafinil. The starting dose of armodafinil is 50 to 150 mg. The available dose forms are 50, 150, and 250 mg. A double-blind study by Harsh and associates[11] documented the efficacy and safety of armodafinil for treatment of sleepiness in narcolepsy. Armodafinil is about twice as potent as modafinil.

No evidence suggests that tolerance develops to modafinil or that the drug impairs sleep quality (if taken in the morning). It has a number of advantages compared with traditional stimulants, including once-daily dosing, low abuse potential, and the fact that it is not a Schedule II medication. No head-to-head studies have compared the effectiveness of modafinil and stimulant medications. However, when compared for the ability to normalize sleep latency, stimulant medications appear more effective.[12] Thus, although modafinil is considered the drug of choice for daytime sleepiness in patients with narcolepsy, many patients will respond better to a stimulant.

The most common side effects of modafinil include headache, nausea, and nervousness. Headache may be minimized by a slow increase in dose. Modafinil may rarely induce mania in a patient with bipolar disorder. A few cases of severe skin rash (Stevens-Johnson syndrome) have been reported in patients taking modafinil (very low prevalence). Modafinil is metabolized in the liver by the cytochrome P-450 (CYP450) system. It may induce CYP450 3A4 and reduce the levels of certain drugs metabolized by this enzyme (e.g., ethynyl estradiol). The main interaction of significance is that certain oral contraceptives may be less effective after modafinil is started (and for up to 1 month after the drug is stopped). The clinical significance of the interaction in unknown, but female patients of reproductive age who are taking oral contraceptives should use additional (or alternative) methods of contraception. Pregnancy occurring in patients on modafinil and oral contraceptives has been documented.[13] Modafinil may also potentially reduce the effectiveness of clopidogrel (Plavix). It may also increase the levels of citalopram. When citalopram used at a high dose (40 mg daily), sufficiently high levels of citalopram may exist and significantly increase the Q–T interval in some patients. This problem is avoided by using the L isomer of citalopram (escitalopram), which is equally effective (or more effective) at a lower dose of 20 mg. Modafinil should also be used with caution in patients with an arrhythmia or cardiac disease.

Unlike the indirect sympathomimetics, withdrawal of modafinil does not result in a rebound of rapid eye movement (REM) and slow wave sleep. Patients may be switched from stimulants to modafinil without a washout period. However, because stimulant medications have some anticataplectic action, patients changed from dextroamphetamine to modafinil may require the addition of specific medications for cataplexy.[14]

CLINICAL PEARLS

1. Modafinil is the medication of choice for the treatment of daytime sleepiness in narcolepsy because of its low abuse potential, lack of tolerance, and lack of withdrawal side effects. Although no head-to-head comparison with stimulants has been made, clinical experience suggest that it is less effective than stimulants at improving daytime sleepiness.
2. Patient not responding to modafinil often respond to a stimulant (e.g., methylphenidate, dextroamphetamine).
3. Racemic modafinil (R and L isomers, Provigil) and armodafinil (R isomer, NuVigil) are available. L modafinil has a much shorter half-life than armodafinil and also has less affinity for the DAT.
4. Although once a day modafinil dosing is recommended, many patients taking only a morning dose of modafinil experience worsening of sleepiness in the early afternoon and respond better to a split dose (e.g., 200 mg in the morning, 100–200 mg at 1 PM). An alternative is to use armodafinil, which has a longer duration of action.
5. The most common side effect of modafinil is headache. This may be minimized by starting at a low dose and increasing gradually.
6. Modafinil may potentially render oral contraceptives less effective, so women of reproductive age should not depend on an oral contraceptive alone for contraception when taking modafinil
7. Modafinil has no anticataplectic activity.

REFERENCES

1. Mignot EJ: A practical guide to the therapy of narcolepsy and hypersomnia syndromes, *Neurotherapeutics* 9(4):739–752, 2012.
2. Morgenthaler TI, Kapur VK, Brown TM, et al: Practice parameters for the treatment of narcolepsy and other hypersomnias of central origin, *Sleep* 30:1705–1711, 2007, in narcolepsy-cataplexy, *Sleep* 16:444–456, 1993.

3. U.S. Modafinil in Narcolepsy Study Group: Randomized trial of modafinil for the treatment of pathological somnolence in narcolepsy, *Ann Neurol* 43:88–97, 1998.
4. U.S. Modafinil in Narcolepsy Study Group: Randomized trial of modafinil as a treatment for the excessive daytime somnolence of narcolepsy, *Neurology* 53:1166–1175, 2000.
5. Schwartz JRL, Feldman NT, Bogan RK: Dose effects of modafinil in sustaining wakefulness in narcolepsy patients with residual evening sleepiness, *J Neuropsychiatry Clin Neurosci* 7:405–412, 2005.
6. Schwartz JRL, Feldman NT, Bogan RK, et al: Dosing regimen effects of modafinil for improving daytime wakefulness in patients with narcolepsy, *Clin Neuropharmacol* 26:252–257, 2003.
7. Mignot E, Nishino S, Guilleminault C, et al: Modafinil binds to the dopamine uptake carrier site with low affinity, *Sleep* 17:436–437, 1994.
8. Darwish M, Kirby M, Hellriegel ET: Comparison of steady-state plasma concentrations of armodafinil and modafinil late in the day following morning administration: post hoc analysis of two randomized, double-blind, placebo-controlled, multiple-dose studies in healthy male subjects, *Clin Drug Investig* 29:601–612, 2009.
9. Darwish M, Kirby M, Hellriegel ET, Robertson P Jr.: Armodafinil and modafinil have substantially different pharmacokinetic profiles despite having the same terminal half-lives: analysis of data from three randomized, single-dose, pharmacokinetic studies, *Clin Drug Investig* 29:613–623, 2009.
10. Darwish M, Kirby M, D'Andrea DM, et al: Pharmacokinetics of armodafinil and modafinil after single and multiple doses in patients with excessive sleepiness associated with treated obstructive sleep apnea: a randomized, open-label, crossover study, *Clin Ther* 32(12):2074–2087, 2010.
11. Harsh JR, Hayduk R, Rosenberg R, et al: The efficacy and safety of armodafinil as treatment for adults with excessive sleepiness associated with narcolepsy, *Curr Med Res Opin* 22:761–774, 2006.
12. Mitler M, Harsch J, Hirshkowitz M, et al: Long-term efficacy and safety of modafinil for the treatment of excessive daytime sleepiness associated with narcolepsy, *Sleep* 17:352–371, 1994.
13. Davies M, Wilton L, Shakir S: Safety profile of modafinil across a range of prescribing indications, including off-label use, in a primary care setting in England: results of a modified prescription-event monitoring study, *Drug Saf* 36(4):237–246, 2013.
14. Guilleminault C, Aftab FA, Karadeniz D, et al: Problems associated with switch to modafinil—a novel alerting agent in narcolepsy, *Eur J Neurol* 7:381–384, 2000.

PATIENT 92

A 25-Year-Old Woman with Narcolepsy Who Is Still Sleepy on Medication

A 20-year-old woman was evaluated for narcolepsy on the basis of symptoms of excessive daytime sleepiness (EDS) and cataplexy. Polysomnography (PSG) revealed no sleep apnea, and the multiple sleep latency test (MSLT) showed a mean sleep latency (MSL) of 2 minutes and 3 sleep-onset rapid eye movement periods (SOREMPs). Cataplexy was an infrequent problem, but daytime sleepiness was severe. The patient was started on modafinil and the dose increased to 400 mg daily with minimal improvement in her symptoms. The patient was changed to dextroamphetamine (D-AMP) 10 milligrams (mg) three times daily, which significantly alleviated the sleepiness but also caused nervousness and a jittery feeling. In addition her sleep was impaired. The patient declined a trial of sodium oxybate therapy.

QUESTION

1. What treatment do you recommend?

ANSWER

1. **Answer:** Sustained-release preparation of methylphenidate (MPH) or D-AMP.

   Discussion: Alerting agents (modafinil and armodafinil) and stimulants (D-AMP, mixed amphetamine salts [MAS; e.g., Adderall]), and methylphenidate are approved by the U.S. Food and Drug Administration (FDA) for the treatment of the EDS of narcolepsy. Only two long-acting forms of methylphenidate are FDA approved for narcolepsy treatment (metadate ER, Ritalin SR), but the others are useful for off-label treatment. Methamphetamine and lisdexamfetamine are also effective in the treatment of narcolepsy but are not FDA approved for this indication. In general, the potency of the alerting or stimulant medications is:

   methamphetamine > D-AMP > MPH > modafinil/armodafinil

   Methamphetamine is potent and long-acting but has the greatest abuse potential. MPH and D-AMP are available as immediate release (IR) or longer acting forms (sustained release [SR], extended release [ER], long-acting [LA]). MPH is probably the best tolerated stimulant with relatively few peripheral effects. However, MPH-IR has a very short duration of action. MPH is best used in a sustained action preparation. D-AMP-IR (duration of action 3 to 4 hours) and MAS are more effective than MPH in some patients and have a slightly longer duration of action. However, D-AMP may be associated with more significant side effects. The amphetamines are available as D-AMP (d isomer, D-AMP sulfate) or mixed amphetamine salts (MAS) (e.g., Adderall or generic MAS). MAS contains 1 part D-AMP saccharate, 1 part D-AMP sulfate, 1 part D,L-AMP aspartate, and 1 part D,L-AMP sulfate [D/L isomer 3 to 1]. It has been hypothesized that D-AMP has more action on dopamine than norepinephrine (NE), whereas L-AMP has a balanced action. In any case, some patients will respond to MAS better than to D-AMP. D-AMP and MAS are also available in a longer-acting preparation (MAS XR, Adderall XR). Lisdexamfetamine is a prodrug of D-AMP and is not effective until absorbed and converted to D-AMP and L-lysine. It has a long duration of action and this is very helpful in some patients in whom side effects with other D-AMP preparations are problematic. Some patients not responding to one of the stimulants (e.g., MPH) will respond to another (D-AMP). The terminology of the stimulant medications is confusing (SR versus ER versus LA). Table P92-1 shows most of the available MPH preparations and Table P92-2 the D-AMP and methamphetamine preparations. Higher doses than listed have been used in some patients. In general, above a total dose of 60 to 80 mg daily, additional efficacy is minimal and side effects increase.

TABLE P92-1   Methylphenidate (MPH) Preparations

Generic (Brand Name)	Generic Available	Duration of Action	How Supplied	Dose
MPH IR (Ritalin)*	Yes	3–4 hours	5-,10-, 20-mg tablet	5–20 mg tid (max. 60 mg)
MPH IR (Methylin)	Yes	3–4 hours	10 mg chewable 2.5, 5, 10 mg	Same
MPH SR (Ritalin SR)*	Yes	8 hours	20 mg, generic 10-, 20-mg tablet	10–30 mg bid
MPH ER (Metadate ER)*	Yes	8 hours	10-, 20-mg tablet	10–30 mg bid
MPH ER QD or MPH CD (Metadate CD)	Yes	8 hours	10, 20, 30, 40, 50, 60 mg capsules	10–30 mg bid or 10 to 60 mg qd
MPH LA (Ritalin LA)	Yes	8–10 hours	10-, 20-, 30-, 40- (generic), 20-, 30-, 40-mg capsules	10–60 mg qd
MPH ER OSM (Concerta)	Yes	12 hours	18-, 27-, 36-, 54-mg capsules	18–54 mg qd

Bid, Two times daily; *CD,* continuous delivery uses two types of beads, 30% quick and 70% delayed delivery; *ER,* extended release; *LA,* long-acting; *qd,* once a day; *SR,* sustained release; *tid,* three times daily; ( ) Brand names; *OSM,* osmotic release.
*FDA approved for narcolepsy.

TABLE P92-2	**Amphetamine (AMP) Preparations**			
	Generic Available	**Duration of Action (hours)**	**How Supplied**	**Dose**
D-AMP IR (Dexedrine)*,†	Yes	4–5	5-mg tablets, Generic 5-, 10-, 20-mg tablets	bid to tid; 10–60 mg total
D-AMP IR (Dextrostat)	Yes	4–5	5-, 10-mg tablets	bid to tid; 10–60 mg total
D-AMP ER (Dexedrine ER)	Yes	8	5-, 10-, 15-mg spansules	Bid; 5–30 bid
MAS (Adderall)†	Yes	4–6	5-, 7.5-, 10-, 12.5-, 15-, 30-mg tablets	bid to tid; 5–30 mg bid
MAS XR (Adderall XR)	Yes	10–12	5-, 10-, 15-, 20-, 25-, 30-mg capsules	5–60 mg qd
Lisdexamfetamine (Vyvanse)	yes	12	20-, 30-, 40-, 50-, 60-, 70-mg capsules	20–70 mg qd
Methamphetamine (Desoxyn)	Yes	12	5-mg tablets	5–25 daily; qd or bid dosing

Bid, Two times daily; *ER*, extended release; *IR*, immediate release; *MAS*, mixed amphetamine salts; *qd*, once a day; *tid*, three times daily; *XR*, extended release.
*Brand name IR not available.
†FDA approved for narcolepsy.

BOX P92-1	**Examples of Combination of Sustained Duration and Immediate Release Forms of Stimulants**

1. MPH ER 20 milligrams (mg) in AM; MPH IR 20 mg at 1 PM
2. MPH ER 20 mg and MPH IR 10 mg in AM; MPH IR 10 to 20 mg at 1 PM
3. MPH ER 20 mg in AM; MPH IR 10 mg before lunch; MPH IR 10 mg 3 PM
4. MPH ER 20 mg in AM ;MPH 20 mg at 2 PM
5. D-AMP ER 20 mg in the AM; D-AMP 20 mg early afternoon
6. Adderall XR 20 mg in AM; Adderall IR 10 mg at 1 to 2 PM

D-AMP, Dextro-amphetamine; *ER*, extended release; *IR*, immediate release; *MAS*, mixed amphetamine salts; *MPH*, methylphenidate; *qd*, once a day; *tid*, three times daily; *XR*, extended release.

The most important intervention is dosing so that medication is available when the patient feels sleepiest. It is also important to avoid late dosing because stimulants may disturb sleep, and this may be a significant problem. Most clinicians would start with MPH and if not effective change to D-AMP or MAS. Finally, if patients do not respond to these medications, methamphetamine may be tried.

Not all of the extended preparations work the same in a given patient. They also differ in the time course of the serum level of the medication. The formulations differ in the way the dose of medication is released. For example, Metadate CD has 30% rapid release and 70% slow release of the dose. Ritalin SR and Metadate ER utilize slow release for the entire dose of medication. Ritalin LA preparations have half IR beads and half SR beads. The ER, SR, LA medications should not be chewed. All of the stimulant medications are more effective if taken on an empty stomach. The forms of MPH and AMP with *longer duration of action* are preferred, as they avoid the sudden onset of effect "rush" and offset of effect "crash." *Some patients who cannot tolerate the IR forms may tolerate the sustained action forms.* In Box P92-1, some examples of dosing with sustained action stimulants are illustrated. Sometimes, a small dose of IR medication is paired with sustained action medication in morning if the patient has trouble starting the day. Other patients will need sustained-action medication in the morning and short-acting medication in the early afternoon. Patients who have trouble with alertness in the early evening may take a sustained-action medication in the morning and very early afternoon. The caution for using sustained-action medications later in the day is that sleep may be impaired. While sustained action preparations are useful, individual patients seem to respond better to frequent dosing of IR mediations (e.g., D-AMP IR 20 mg three times daily). Having some IR medication available may help patients cope with special situations (e.g., driving at night). The side effects of stimulant medication are listed in Box P92-2. Patients should rarely need

BOX P92-2	Side Effects of Stimulants

Nervousness	Growth retardation in children
Palpitations	Headache
Diaphoresis	Anxiety
Increased blood pressure or heart rate	Insomnia
Decreased appetite (and rebound when medications wears off)	

a total dose of AMP or MPH over 60 to 80 mg per day. However, an occasional large patient does require and tolerate higher doses. Very high doses may predispose to complications. One study compared groups of patients taking stimulant doses higher than the recommended dose with those taking doses within the normal recommendations. The study demonstrated a significantly higher occurrence of psychosis, substance misuse, and psychiatric hospitalizations in patients using high-dose stimulants compared with those using standard doses. In this study, the maximum doses were considered to be 100 mg methylphenidate, 80 mg methamphetamine, and 100 mg D-AMP (all would be considered very high by most clinicians). Tachyarrhythmias and anorexia or weight loss were also more common in the group with very high doses compared with those taking more standard doses. Clinicians should be very cautious in prescribing dosages that exceed maximum guidelines.

Before increasing doses, check if the medication is being taken on an empty stomach. Check the amount of sleep the patient is actually getting, and consider interventions to improve nocturnal sleep. Scheduled naps may also be very useful. In addition, the possibility of the development of another sleep disorder such as obstructive sleep apnea should also be considered.

Of interest, D-AMP appears to have some activity against cataplexy. In one study, when patients with narcolepsy were withdrawn from amphetamine and switched to modafinil, the reappearance or worsening of cataplexy was noted. In our experience, some patients with mild cataplexy and significant daytime sleepiness have a response in both symptoms to D-AMP. The reason possibly is that the medication increase NE as well as dopamine in the central nervous system (CNS). In contrast, modafinil has no activity against cataplexy. If modafinil and/or stimulants are not effective or tolerated, use of sodium oxybate for daytime sleepiness should be considered. Many patients continue to take a stimulant or alerting agent with sodium oxybate. Sodium oxybate would also have the advantage of treating cataplexy if this symptoms is present.

The current patient was tried on MPH, but the medication was not as effective, although the patient was less nervous on this medication than on D-AMP. She was switched to Vyvanse lisdexamfetamine (Vyvanse), a medication with a long duration of action, and the dose slowly increased to 60 mg daily. On this dose and with scheduled naps, her sleepiness was in good control and she was not anxious.

CLINICAL PEARLS

1. The general order of potency of stimulants and alerting medications is:
   Modafinil < MPH < D-AMP < methamphetamine

2. Use of sustained-action forms of stimulant medication will often minimize side effects and avoid a roller-coaster pattern of alertness resulting from taking multiple doses of a shorter-acting medication. A small amount of immediate-release medication may be added in the morning or afternoon if worsening sleepiness is noted at those time points.

3. Most stimulants have generic formulations but all may not be equally effective.

4. If daytime sleepiness does not respond to one type of stimulant, the patient may respond to another. For example, if methylphenidate is not effective, try D-AMP. A rare patient will respond only to methamphetamine. Despite the abuse potential, methamphetamine is probably the most potent of the stimulants.

5. Very high doses of stimulants are associated with increased risk of side effects and should be avoided. Patients should be warned about the risk of stimulants and their abuse and dependence potential.

6. Nonpharmacologic measures such as good sleep hygiene, adequate sleep, and daytime naps are an essential part of treatment of daytime sleepiness in patients with narcolepsy.

7. With proper dose titration, stimulant medication may control symptoms of daytime sleepiness in 60% to 80% of patients with narcolepsy. If patients do not have good control of sleepiness with stimulants, consider using sodium oxybate. Other sleep disorders or inadequate sleep duration should be ruled out.

BIBLIOGRAPHY

Auger RR, Goodman SH, Silber MH, et al: Risks of high-dose stimulants in the treatment of disorders of excessive somnolence: a case–control study, *Sleep* 28(6):667–672, 2005.

Chavez B, Sopko MA Jr., Ehret MJ, et al: An update on central nervous system stimulant formulations in children and adolescents with attention-deficit/hyperactivity disorder, *Ann Pharmacother* 43(6):1084–1095, 2009.

Connor DF, Steingard RJ: New formulations of stimulants for attention-deficit hyperactivity disorder: therapeutic potential, *CNS Drugs* 18:1011–1030, 2004.

Guilleminault C, Aftab FA, Karadeniz D, et al: Problems associated with switch to modafinil—a novel alerting agent in narcolepsy, *Eur J Neurol* 7:381–384, 2000.

López FA, Leroux JR: Long-acting stimulants for treatment of attention-deficit/hyperactivity disorder: a focus on extended-release formulations and the prodrug lisdexamfetamine dimesylate to address continuing clinical challenges, *Atten Defic Hyperact Disord* 5(3):249–265, 2013.

Mignot EJ: A practical guide to the therapy of narcolepsy and hypersomnia syndromes, *Neurotherapeutics* 9(4):739–752, 2012.

Mitler M, Aldrich MS, Koob GF, et al: ASDA standards of practice: narcolepsy and its treatment with stimulants, *Sleep* 17:352–371, 1994.

Morgenthaler TI, Kapur VK, Brown TM, et al: Practice parameters for the treatment of narcolepsy and other hypersomnias of central origin, *Sleep* 30:1705–1711, 2007.

Wise MS, Arand DL, Auger RR, et al: American Academy of Sleep Medicine: Treatment of narcolepsy and other hypersomnias of central origin, *Sleep* 30(12):1712–1727, 2007.

PATIENT 93

Patients with Daytime Sleepiness and Cataplexy

A 25-year-old woman presented with complaints of severe daytime sleepiness. (Epworth Sleepiness Scale [ESS] score of 18/24). She was falling asleep during her classes in graduate school. In addition, she reported episodes of leg weakness associated with hearing jokes. She underwent testing with polysomnography (PSG) and a multiple sleep latency test (MSLT). The results were consistent with narcolepsy, and a diagnosis of narcolepsy with cataplexy (type 1) was made. Treatment was begun with modafinil with only partial improvement in sleepiness (ESS score of 14/24). The patient was switched to dextro-amphetamine, which was more effective for maintenance of wakefulness but caused significant anxiety and difficulty with sleep. She was switched back to modafinil and started on venlafaxine 75 milligrams (mg) extended release (XR) for cataplexy, as this symptom was becoming more significant. Unfortunately, venlafaxine also worsened her anxiety. She reported difficulty sleeping at night with venlafaxine as well.

QUESTIONS

1. What treatment do you recommend?

2. Does modafinil have activity against cataplexy?

3. Is sudden withdrawal of venlafaxine in this patient potentially problematic?

ANSWERS

1. **Answer:** Addition of sodium oxybate to modafinil.

2. **Answer:** Modafinil has no anticataplectic activity.

3. **Answer:** Sudden withdrawal of venlafaxine may cause an exacerbation of cataplexy. Nearly continuous cataplexy is called *status cataplecticus*.

Discussion: Sodium oxybate (SXB) (Xyrem) is the only medication that is approved by the U.S. Food and Drug Administration (FDA) for BOTH daytime sleepiness and cataplexy. Generally, higher doses are needed for improvement in daytime sleepiness than for cataplexy (Figures P93-1 and P93-2). SXB is also effective for the treatment of other symptoms of narcolepsy, including sleep paralysis, hypnagogic hallucinations, and disturbed nocturnal sleep. Improvement in symptoms of cataplexy may take weeks to months of treatment. The patient should be informed that often progressive improvement occurs with time. In Figure P93-1, note that the effect of a given dose of SXB improves over time, although the greatest improvement occurs in the first 4 weeks. In addition, significant activity of cataplexy was noted at the starting nightly dose of 4.5 grams (g) per night. SXB is also effective for improvement of daytime sleepiness. It is the only medication that can restore near-normal alertness. In Figure P93-2, at 9 g per night, the median ESS score was nearly

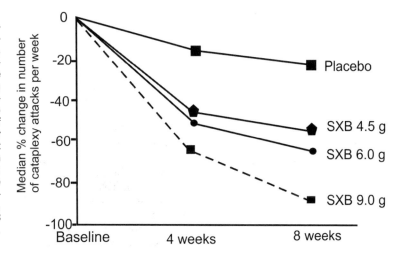

FIGURE P93-1 ■ Reduction in cataplexy attacks per week (% of baseline) in groups treated with 4, 6, and 9 grams (g) of sodium oxybate (SXB). A significant decrease was seen even with the 4.5-g dose, and the improvement continued increased from 4 to 8 weeks. Thus, the full benefit of SXB for the treatment of cataplexy may require at least 8 weeks (at least at 9 g total dose). (From Xyrem International Study Group: Further evidence supporting the use of sodium oxybate for the treatment of cataplexy: a double-blind, placebo-controlled study in 228 patients, *Sleep Med* 6:415–421, 2005.)

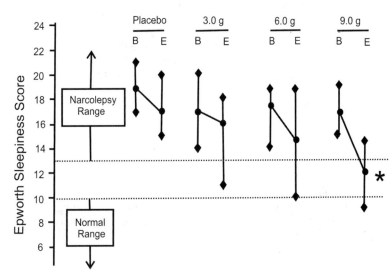

FIGURE P93-2 ■ Effect of sodium oxybate on subjective sleepiness in narcolepsy. Lines are median (*solid circle*) and 25th and 75th percentile values (*solid diamond*). At 9 grams (g), the reduction was significant and the median was just above the normal range. *B,* Baseline; *E,* end of the study. Note that patients were allowed to stay on their stimulant medications (83% did so). (From U.S. Xyrem Multicenter Study Group: A randomized, double-blind, placebo-controlled multicenter trial comparing the effects of three doses of orally administered sodium oxybate with placebo for the treatment of narcolepsy, *Sleep* 25:42–49, 2002.)

in the normal range. It is important to note that 83% of patients were also taking their prestudy stimulant medication (modafinil, methylphenidate, etc.). However, the addition of SXB led to significant improvement.

As the half-life of SXB is 30 minutes and the duration of action is only 2 to 4 hours, SXB must be administered twice during the night (at bedtime and 2 to 3 hours later). The medication is not potent and grams instead of milligrams are needed. Xyrem is available as a liquid (500 milligrams per milliliter [mg/mL]) and is diluted to reduce the salty taste. Before getting into bed, the patient prepares the two doses carefully and puts them in childproof containers. The patient then gets into bed and takes the first dose. Usually, the patient awakens spontaneously or with an alarm clock and takes the second dose 2 to 3 hours after the first dose. The starting dose of SXB is 2.25 g at bedtime and 2.25 g administered 2 to 3 hours later (total of 4.5 g nightly). The total dose is increased by 0.5 to 1.5 g per night every week until symptoms improve or side effects are intolerable. Effective doses are in the range of 6 to 9 g (9 g is the maximum recommended dose). Dizziness may occur following SXB ingestion, and the sedative effect is potent and rapid, so it is strongly recommended that the patient be in bed before taking the first dose. Some clinicians also advice that someone observe the patient the first night (for snoring or gasping) and be available if the patients awakens confused. The sedative effects of SXB lessens as the patient adapts to the medication with time. Some patients awaken spontaneously for the second dose, and some others use an alarm clock. Side effects of SXB include nausea, dizziness, confusion, enuresis, sleep walking, anxiety, and night eating. Weight loss may also occur, but this side effect is beneficial in patients who develop obesity associated with narcolepsy. If nausea is severe, some patients will respond to odansetron or cyproheptadine. Most side effects are dose related, and tolerance may develop with time. When significant side effects occur, the SXB dose should be temporarily reduced until the symptoms abate. Then a slower increase in dose may be attempted. As noted above, symptoms may improve at a lower dose, with time. For example, if 5 g, not 6 g, is tolerated, with time 5 g may actually be sufficient. In general, sleep quality improves with SXB, which is often associated with an increase in stage N3 sleep. In most studies, an alerting agent (modafinil or stimulant) was continued with SXB. The combination appears to be more effective at alleviating sleepiness. Recall that modafinil has no activity against cataplexy.

SXB is active at gamma-aminobutyric acid class B (GABA-B) and gamma-hydroxybutyrate acid (GHB) receptors. The mechanism of action in narcolepsy is unknown. In overdose, SXB causes respiratory depression and may cause death. It is also a drug with the potential for abuse ("date rape drug"), and for this reason, it is available only from a single central pharmacy. Both physicians and patients must undergo training in the use of the medication. Taking SXB after eating may significantly delay the onset of action, so SXB should be taken on an empty stomach. The simultaneous use of SXB and other sedatives, including alcohol, is not recommended (contraindicated) to avoid oversedation or respiratory depression. Although SXB has been safely used in patients with obstructive sleep apnea (OSA), caution is advised. Patients with moderate to severe OSA should be on effective treatment (e.g., continuous positive airway pressure [CPAP]) before SXB is started. The safety of administration of SXB in patients with severe OSA may be documented in the sleep center, with the patient taking SXB and using CPAP. As doses are increased, nocturnal oximetry could be performed at home. Some physicians also monitor carbon dioxide (CO_2) in sleep centers to document that hypoventilation does not occur with use of SXB. When SXB is used in high doses as a drug of abuse, a significant withdrawal syndrome may occur. However, when SXB is used within the recommended dose range and only at night, abrupt cessation does not lead to significant rebound or withdrawal effects. Some patients take an SXB holiday 1 day a week so that they can consume alcohol safely. Skipping a dose does not usually result in an exacerbation of symptoms. In contrast, skipping a dose of venlafaxine may be associated with a rebound in cataplexy. If venlafaxine is to be stopped, the patient should be weaned off this medication slowly.

In a recent review, Mignot addressed the fact that SXB has been associated with an increase in anxiety as observed in some studies. In susceptible patients, SXB may cause significant anxiety. The dose may be temporarily reduced or SXB withheld and a selective serotonin reuptake inhibitor (SSRI) started for this problem. After several weeks of SSRI treatment, the SXB dose may be restarted (or increased) again. Some patients also report paradoxical insomnia with SXB. If early morning awakening is a problem and the patient is able to fall asleep easily without medication, the patient may be allowed to sleep for 1 to 2 hours before the first dose of SXB is administered followed by the second dose 2 to 3 hours later. Using this approach, the entire night of sleep could be consolidated without exceeding the maximum recommended dose of 9 g. This assumes that at least 4 hours of sleep time remain when the second dose is taken. Other patients wake up after the first dose fairly rapidly and remain awake for an hour or more before it is time for the second dose. One approach would be to take a slightly higher dose at the start of the night (e.g., with a 7-g nightly dose, the first dose is 4 g followed by 3 g).

In the current patient, SXB was started at a total nightly dose of 4.5 g and titrated up slowly to 6 g per night. A higher dose (6.5 g per night) caused one episode of sleep walking, so a maximum dose of 6 g was used. At 6 g per night, cataplexy episodes were virtually eliminated. Over a 2-month period, a treatment combination of modafinil 400 mg daily and SXB 6 g nightly improved daytime sleepiness until the ESS score was in the 10-to-12 range.

CLINICAL PEARLS

1. Sodium oxybate (SXB) is the only medication that is FDA approved for the treatment of BOTH daytime sleepiness *and* cataplexy in patients with narcolepsy.

2. Sodium oxybate is the only medication that is FDA approved for the treatment of cataplexy. The medication is also effective for treating sleep paralysis and hypnagogic hallucinations.

3. Side effects of sodium oxybate include nausea, dizziness, enuresis, sleep walking, sleep-related eating, confusion, and anxiety. A reduction in the dose may help alleviate the side effects. Patients may develop tolerance to side effects with time, which allows retitration back to the dose that caused the side effect.

4. Sodium oxybate must be used with caution in patients with OSA.

5. Many studies of the effects of sodium oxybate on daytime sleepiness in narcolepsy allowed patients to continue the use of stimulants. Patients may benefit from a combination of modafinil and sodium oxybate (at least at the lower doses of sodium oxybate).

6. The typical effective nightly dose of sodium oxybate is 6 to 9 g. Cataplexy may respond to doses as low as 4.5 g per night.

7. Stopping SXB does not cause an immediate rebound in the severity of cataplexy. This is in contrast to stopping antidepressants used for cataplexy. Abruptly stopping venlafaxine may result in status cataplecticus.

8. Patients taking SXB may experience sleep maintenance insomnia and this may require adjustment in the medication dosing.

BIBLIOGRAPHY

Mignot EJ: A practical guide to the therapy of narcolepsy and hypersomnia syndromes, *Neurotherapeutics* 9(4):739–752, 2012.

U.S. Xyrem Multicenter Study Group: A randomized, double-blind, placebo-controlled multicenter trial comparing the effects of three doses of orally administered sodium oxybate with placebo for the treatment of narcolepsy, *Sleep* 25:42–49, 2002.

U.S. Xyrem Multicenter Study Group: A 12-month open-label, multi-center extension trial of orally administered sodium oxybate for the treatment of narcolepsy, *Sleep* 1:31–35, 2003.

The Xyrem International Study Group: A double-blind, placebo-controlled study demonstrates sodium oxybate is effective for treatment of excessive daytime sleepiness in narcolepsy, *J Clin Sleep Med* 1:391–397, 2005.

Black J, Houghton WC: Sodium oxybate improves excessive daytime sleepiness in narcolepsy, *Sleep* 29:939–946, 2006.

Black J, Pardi D, Hornfledt, Inhaber N: The nightly administration of sodium oxybate results in significant reduction in the nocturnal sleep disruption of patients with narcolepsy, *Sleep Med* 10:829–835, 2009.

U.S. Xyrem Multicenter Study Group: Sodium oxybate demonstrates long-term efficacy for the treatment of cataplexy in patients with narcolepsy, *Sleep Med* 5:119–123, 2004.

Xyrem International Study Group: Further evidence supporting the use of sodium oxybate for the treatment of cataplexy: a double-blind, placebo-controlled study in 228 patients, *Sleep Med* 6:415–421, 2005.

George CFP, Feldman N, Inaber N, et al: A safety trial of sodium oxybate in patients with obstructive sleep apnea, *Sleep Med* 11:38–42, 2010.

Wang J, Greenberg H: Status cataplecticus precipitated by abrupt withdrawal of venlafaxine, *J Clin Sleep Med* 9(7):715–716, 2013.

A Patient with Extreme Difficulty Getting Out of Bed in the Morning

A 25-year-old woman was evaluated for complaints of severe sleepiness present for the last 3 years. The Epworth Sleepiness Scale (ESS) score was 14/24. The patient denied cataplexy but did report both sleep paralysis and hypnagogic hallucinations. She snored only when she had nasal congestion. The only medication the patient was taking was an oral contraceptive. The patient reported sleeping up to 10 hours per day without improvement in her symptoms. She did take naps, but they were not refreshing. Getting out of bed in the morning was very difficult, and she felt in a daze until after drinking several cups of coffee. The patient denied a history of depression, mania, hypomania, or head trauma.

Actigraphy for 1 week: estimated total sleep time 9 hours per night
Urine drug screen: negative
Polysomnography and MSLT: See Table P94-1.

TABLE P94-1 **Polysomnography and MSLT Results**

Lights out 9:00 AM						
Lights on 6:00 AM		**Normal Range**		**min**	**%TST**	**Normal**
Total Recording Time (min)	540	(410-454)	Stage N1	10	2	(2–7)
Total sleep time (min)	510	(408-452)	Stage N2	275.5	53	(40–55)
Sleep efficiency (%)	98%	(94-98)	Stage N3	130	25	(15–28)
Sleep Latency (min)	2	(3-23)	Stage R	104	20	(22–29)
REM Latency (min)	85	(75-115)				
WASO (min)	17	(0–10)				
AHI (#/hr)	2					
PLM index (#/hr)	3					
MSLT						
Mean sleep latency (min)	6					
SOREMPs	1/5 naps					

SOREMP, Sleep onset REM periods.

QUESTION

1. What is your diagnosis?

ANSWER

1. **Answer:** Idiopathic hypersomnia.

Discussion: Idiopathic hypersomnia (IH) describes a heterogeneous group of patients and may well have multiple etiologies. Patients with IH complain of excessive daytime sleepiness (EDS) but do not report cataplexy. The typical age of onset is around 20 years. The sleep of patients with IH is usually normal or increased in duration. About 30% reports sleep durations over 9 to 10 hours. However, even after a normal or prolonged sleep duration, patients with IH have a difficult time awakening in the morning.

The diagnostic criteria and differential diagnosis of IH are listed in Boxes P94-1 and P94-2. The main entity to exclude is the insufficient sleep syndrome (ISS). Daytime sleepiness must be present for ≥ 3 months. Sleep drunkenness is defined in the *International Classification of Sleep Disorders*, Third Edition (ICSD-3) as "a prolonged and severe form of sleep inertia, consisting of prolonged difficulty waking up with repeated returns to sleep, irritability, automatic behavior and confusion." This symptom is present in

BOX P94-1	Diagnostic Criteria for Idiopathic Hypersomnia—ICSD-3

A. The patient has daily periods of irrepressible need to sleep or daytime lapses into sleep occurring for at least 3 months.*
B. Cataplexy is absent.
C. A multiple sleep latency test (MSLT) performed according to standard techniques shows fewer than 2 sleep-onset REM periods (SOREMPs) or no SOREMPs if the REM latency on the preceding polysomnography (PSG) was ≤15 minutes.†
D. The presence of at least *one* of the following:
  1. The MSLT shows a mean sleep latency (MSL) of ≤8 minutes.
  2. Total 24-hour sleep time is ≥660 minutes (typically 12–14 hours)‡ on 24-hour PSG

sleep monitoring (performed after correction for chronic sleep deprivation), *or* by wrist actigraphy in association with a sleep log (averaged over at least 7 days with unrestricted sleep).§
E. Insufficient sleep syndrome is ruled out (if deemed necessary, by lack of improvement of sleepiness after an adequate trial of increased nocturnal time in bed, confirmed by at least a week of wrist actigraphy).
F. The hypersomnolence and/or MSLT findings are not better explained by another sleep disorder, other medical or psychiatric disorder, or use of drugs or medications.

Adapted from American Academy of Sleep Medicine: *International classification of sleep disorders*, ed 3, Darien, IL, 2014, American Academy of Sleep Medicine.
*Severe and prolonged sleep inertia, known as *sleep drunkenness* (defined as prolonged difficulty waking up with repeated returns to sleep, irritability, automatic behavior and confusion) and/or long (>1 hour) unrefreshing naps are additional supportive clinical features.
†A high sleep efficiency (≥90%) on the preceding PSG is a supportive finding (as long as sleep insufficiency is ruled out).
‡In children and adolescents, this criterion may need to be adapted to account for normal changes in sleep time associated with stages of development as well as variability across cultures.
§Occasionally, patients fulfilling other criteria may have an MSLT MSL >8 minutes and total 24-hour sleep time <660 minutes. Clinical judgment should be used in deciding if these patients should be considered to have idiopathic hypersomnia. Great care should be exercised in excluding other conditions that might mimic the disorder. Another option is to repeat the MSLT if the clinical suspicion for idiopathic hypersomnia remains high.

BOX P94-2	Differential Diagnosis of Idiopathic Hypersomnia

Insufficient sleep syndrome
Narcolepsy type 2 (narcolepsy without cataplexy)
Occult obstructive sleep apnea

Hypersomnia caused by medication or substance (occult drug abuse)
Atypical or bipolar depression
Hypersomnia caused by medical condition

36% to 66% of patients with IH and is supportive of a diagnosis of IH. Hypnagogic hallucinations and sleep paralysis may occur. Long (>1 hour) naps are common and usually nonrestorative. In contrast, naps are usually helpful in patients with narcolepsy. Cataplexy is absent. Dysfunction of the autonomic nervous system may be present, manifesting as headaches, orthostatic disturbances, temperature dysregulation, and peripheral vascular complaints (Raynaud-type phenomena with cold hands and feet). The cerebrospinal fluid (CSF) hypocretin-1 level is normal, and the cause of the sleepiness is unknown.

Insufficient sleep should be ruled out by sleep logs and, if possible, by actigraphy. A trial of sleep extension to determine if daytime sleepiness improves should also be performed. A sleep diary or actigraphy for at least 7 days before sleep testing is recommended eliminate the possibility of ISS. PSG followed by an MSLT is performed to rule out other causes of daytime sleepiness (obstructive sleep apnea [OSA]). The PSG usually shows a high sleep efficiency (>90% to 95%) and normal or increased total sleep time (TST) without significant sleep apnea. The PSG-MSLT combination shows <2 sleep-onset rapid eye movement periods (SOREMPs), including a PSG SOREMPs if present. For example, if the nocturnal REM latency was 10 minutes, the MSLT could have no SOREMPs. Of note, while a PSG SOREMP alone does not meet the present ICSD-3 diagnostic criteria for narcolepsy, this finding has a high positive predictive value for the presence of narcolepsy. A nocturnal SOREMP is defined as a PSG REM latency ≤15 minutes). Objective evidence of sleepiness is present (MSLT mean sleep latency [MSL] ≤8 minutes). *The MSL on the MSLT for patients with IH is around 6 minutes (in contrast to 3 minutes in narcolepsy).* If an MSLT is not possible because of a long sleep period, a 24-hour PSG should show >660 minutes of sleep). The findings should not be better explained by another medical or psychiatric disorder or medication or substance. It is common practice in most sleep centers to include a urine drug screen with the MSLT. It is necessary that the MSLT be performed after 2 weeks of withdrawal of medications that might affect the sleep latency or REM latency. It is important to recall that the atypical depression or depression associated with a bipolar disorder may present with complaints of hypersomnia (although MSL is usually

>10 minutes). Patients should be questioned about previous manic or hypomanic episodes, which would raise the suspicion of a current depressive phase of bipolar disorder.

In the ICSD-2, IH was divided into less than 10 hours of sleep and more than10 hours of sleep (IH with or without a long sleep time). However, the ICSD-3 dropped this categorization, as it lacks validity. In a study by Vernet et al, in which patients with ≥ 10 hours sleep were compared with those with <10 hours, no differences in ESS scores, MSLT mean sleep latencies, or percentage with sleep drunkenness were noted. Nevertheless, some clinicians may continue to consider the group with very long sleep time to be a distinct subgroup.

The differential diagnosis of IH is wide and includes insufficient sleep, NT-2 with a false-negative PSG-MSLT evaluation, bipolar disorder in the depressive phase, conditions listed under hypersomnia caused by medial disorders (including head trauma), medications, and substance abuse. A drug screen and imaging of the central nervous system (CNS) should be considered. If the patient has bipolar depression it is important to recognize this condition, as treatment differs from unipolar depression. Patients may focus on the fatigue and sleepiness rather than the depressed mood. IH is essentially a diagnosis of exclusion, and the concern that a definite cause has been overlooked is always present.

The treatment of IH includes modafinil and stimulants. These medications have variable effectiveness. *Lack of improvement may be a clue that a medical, neurologic, or psychiatric disorder may have been overlooked.* The American Academy of Sleep Medicine (AASM) practice parameters for the treatment of central hypersomnia lists modafinil and stimulants (amphetamine, methamphetamine, dextroamphetamine, and methylphenidate) as treatments for the daytime sleepiness of IH (Option).

In this patient, cataplexy was absent and extreme difficulty awakening with prolonged confusion was reported consistent with IH. The findings on PSG and the MSLT met the diagnostic criteria. Note the increased total sleep time and high sleep efficiency. No evidence of a drug or substance causing sleepiness was present. The patient denied depression. The neurologic examination was normal, and a reason to suspect a medical neurologic cause of sleepiness (no history of head trauma) did not exist. A diagnosis of IH was made, and treatment with modafinil was started. Unfortunately, this was not effective. After trying several stimulants, methamphetamine, 10 mg two times daily, was moderately effective. The patient continued to require long periods of sleep but arranged her schedule to accommodate this requirement.

CLINICAL PEARLS

1. Patients with IH experience excessive sleepiness despite either normal or increased total sleep time. They do not report cataplexy but often report sleep drunkenness—extreme difficulty waking up in the morning

2. The MSLT criteria are an MSL of ≤ 8 minutes and 0 or 1 SOREMP during PSG-MSLT evaluation. If a SOREMP is noted on the nocturnal PSG, no SOREMPs can be present on the MSLT. In some patients, an MSLT is not possible because of a long sleep time. In such cases, 24-hour PSG showing >660 minutes (typically 11 to 12 hours) is diagnostic.

3. The previous division of IH into groups with and without long sleep time has been dropped in the ICSD-3.

4. A sleep diary and actigraphy for at least 7 days before testing should verify adequate sleep.

5. The differential diagnosis of IH includes insufficient sleep, patients with narcolepsy without cataplexy (N-T2) with a false-negative PSG-MSLT evaluation, bipolar depression, and medical and neurologic disorders that may be associated with hypersomnia. However, the insufficient sleep syndrome is the most important exclusion in many cases.

BIBLIOGRAPHY

American Academy of Sleep Medicine: *International classification of sleep disorders: diagnostic and coding manual*, ed 2, Westchester, IL, 2005, American Academy of Sleep Medicine.

American Academy of Sleep Medicine: *International classification of sleep disorders: diagnostic and coding manual*, ed 3, Westchester, IL, 2013, American Academy of Sleep Medicine.

American Academy of Sleep Medicine: *International classification of sleep disorders*, ed 3, Darien, IL, 2014, American Academy of Sleep Medicine.

Bassetti C, Aldrich MS: Idiopathic hypersomnia, *Brain* 120:1423–1435, 1997.

Anderson KN, Pilsworth S, Sharples LD, et al: Idiopathic hypersomnia: a study of 77 cases, *Sleep* 30:1274–1281, 2007.

Vernet C, Arnuf I: Idiopathic hypersomnia with and without long sleep time: a controlled series of 75 patients, *Sleep* 32:753–759, 2009.

Ali M, Auger RR, Slocumb NL, Morgenthaler TI: Idiopathic hypersomnia: clinical features and response to treatment, *J Clin Sleep Med* 5:562–568, 2009.

Bastujii H, Jouvet M: Successful treatment of idiopathic hypersomnia and narcolepsy with modafinil, *Prog Neuropsychopharmacol Biol Psychiatry* 12:695–700, 1988.

Pizza F, Ferri R, Poli F, et al: Polysomnographic study of nocturnal sleep in idiopathic hypersomnia without long sleep time, *J Sleep Res* 22(2):185–196, 2013.

Morgenthaler TI, Kapur VK, Brown TM, et al: Practice parameters for the treatment of narcolepsy and other hypersomnias of central origin, *Sleep* 30:1705–1711, 2007.

Hypersomnolence of Central Origin II

The disorders of hypersomnolence (hypersomnia) of central origin discussed in this section are listed in Box F34-1.

KLEINE-LEVIN SYNDROME (KLS)

Kleine-Levin syndrome (KLS), also known as *recurrent hypersomnia*, is a rare disorder (1 or 2 per million) that is characterized by episodes of severe hypersomnia in association with cognitive, psychiatric, and behavioral disturbances (hyperphagia, hypersexuality), which are recurrent, with periods of remission (normal function) between episodes (Box F34-2).[1-4] A typical episode has a median duration of 10 days (rarely several weeks to months). Episodes reoccur every 1 to 12 months (median interval 3 months). The first episode is often triggered by an upper respiratory tract infection or alcohol intake. The episodes are characterized by hypersomnia (sleep up to 16 hours to 20 hours per day) with waking or getting out of bed only eat or go to the bathroom. It is possible to awaken the patients, but they are very irritable. When they are awake during episodes, most patients are confused, are slow in speaking and answering, and have anterograde amnesia. Almost all report a dreamlike, altered perception of the environment (derealization). The most common manifestation of KLS is hyperphagia, which occurs in about two thirds, and one third of the patients eat less than normal. Other manifestations include hypersexuality (about 50%, typically men), depression (about 50%, predominantly women), anxiety at being left alone and seeing strangers. Patients may experience hallucinations and delusions (30%). Patients are *remarkably normal between episodes* with regard to sleep, cognition, mood, and eating attitude. Typically, hypersomnia is present at episode onset. All the associated behavioral disturbances may not occur during each episode. The male-to-female ratio in KLS is 2:1, and the age of onset is typically early adolescence (second decade). Several long-term studies suggest that

BOX F34-1	Hypersomnolence of Central Origin (ICSD-3)

1. Kleine-Levin Syndrome (KLS)
2. Hypersomnia Due to Medical Disorder (HDMD)
3. Hypersomnia Due to a Medication or Substance (HDMS)
4. Hypersomnia Associated with a Psychiatric Disorder (HAPD)
5. Insufficient Sleep Syndrome (ISS)

Adapted from American Academy of Sleep Medicine: *International classification of sleep disorders*, ed 3, Darien, IL, 2014, American Academy of Sleep Medicine.

BOX F34-2	Kleine-Levine Syndrome Diagnostic Criteria: ICSD-3

Criteria A-E must be met
A. The patient experiences at least two recurrent episodes of excessive sleepiness and sleep duration, each persisting for two days to five weeks.
B. Episodes recur usually more than once a year and at least once every 18 months.
C. The patient has normal alertness, cognitive function, behavior, and mood between episodes.
D. The patient must demonstrate at least one of the following during episodes:
    1. Cognitive dysfunction.
    2. Altered perception.
    3. Eating disorder (anorexia or hyperphagia).
    4. Disinhibited behavior (such as hypersexuality).
E. The hypersomnolence and related symptoms are not better explained by another sleep disorder, other medical, neurologic, or psychiatric disorder (especially bipolar disorder), or use of drugs or medications.

Adapted from American Academy of Sleep Medicine: *International classification of sleep disorders*, ed 3, Darien, IL, 2014, American Academy of Sleep Medicine.

KLS often has a benign course, with episodes lessening in duration, severity, and frequency over a median course of 14 years. The disease typically resolves after 14 years on average except when the onset is in adulthood. Birth and developmental problems, as well as Jewish heritage, are risk factors for developing the syndrome. Head computed tomography (CT) and magnetic resonance imaging (MRI) are normal. The cerebrospinal fluid (CSF) hypocretin-1 level is normal. Brain function imaging is abnormal in most cases, with hypoperfusion of the left or right temporal frontal lobes as well as the diencephalon. These abnormalities are present both during the episode of hypersomnolence and sometimes between episodes. The differential diagnosis of KLS includes mainly psychiatric disorders such as depression, bipolar disorder, seasonal affective disorder, and somatoform disorder.

The best treatment for KLS is not known because of the limited number of patients, and no large well-controlled study has been performed. Improvement has been reported with treatment with lithium, amantadine, lamotrigine, and valproic acid.[3,5] The American Academy of Sleep Medicine (AASM) *Standard of Practice Paper on Treatment of Narcolepsy and Other Hypersomnias of Central Origin* listed lithium as possibly effective.[5]Lithium may reduce the duration of episodes and reduce undesirable behaviors. Methylphenidate and modafinil could be used for daytime sleepiness.

HYPERSOMNIA DUE TO A MEDICATION OR SUBSTANCE

Patients with this disorder have excessive nocturnal sleep, daytime sleepiness, or excessive napping that is believed to be caused by (1) sedating medications, (2) substance abuse (alcohol or drugs of abuse), or (3) withdrawal from amphetamines and other drugs.[2,6] See Fundamentals 8 for a list of medications that cause sleepiness. In those who regularly consume coffee or other sources of caffeine, discontinuation may produce sleepiness, fatigue, and inattentiveness for 2 to 9 days. Polysomnography (PSG) is generally unnecessary unless a concomitant sleep disorder is suspected. PSG and multiple sleep latency test (MSLT) results vary, depending on the specific substance in question and on the timing of the most recent intake. With stimulant withdrawal, nocturnal PSG may show normal sleep, whereas the MSLT typically demonstrates a short mean sleep latency (MSL) with or without multiple sleep-onset rapid eye movement periods (SOREMPs). Urine toxicology screen may be positive for the suspected substance.

The diagnosis is often confirmed if symptoms resolve after the causal agent is removed.

INSUFFICIENT SLEEP SYNDROME (ISS)

Patients with the induced insufficient sleep syndrome (ISS) fail to obtain sufficient nocturnal sleep to maintain daytime alertness and mental functioning (Box F34-3).[7] Patients may not be aware that insufficient sleep is responsible for their symptoms. The diagnosis depends on patient report or sleep logs but may also be documented by actigraphy. Patients characteristically sleep longer on weekends and vacations. They usually report feeling more refreshed with a longer sleep period. The evening chronotype may predispose to insufficient sleep.

A sleep study is not needed for diagnosis but, if performed because of suspicion of other disorders, will often show a short sleep latency, high sleep efficiency, and long total sleep time. Sometimes evidence of stage N3 or stage R rebound (high amount of those sleep stages) is present.[7] Note that up to 30% of the normal population

---

BOX F34-3	**Insufficient Sleep Syndrome—ICSD-3**

Criteria A-F must be met
A. The patient has daily periods of irrepressible need to sleep or daytime lapses into sleep or, in the case of prepubertal children, a complaint of behavioral abnormalities attributable to sleepiness is present.
B. The abnormal sleep pattern is present most days (in the case of workers, on at least working days) for at least 3 months.
C. The patient's sleep time, established by personal or collateral history, sleep logs or actigraphy*, is usually shorter than expected taking age into account[†].
D. The patient usually curtails sleep time by such measures as an alarm clock or being woken up by another person and generally sleeps longer when such measures are not used, such as on weekends or vacations.
E. Extending total sleep time results in resolution of the symptoms of sleepiness.
F. The symptoms are not better explained by another untreated sleep disorder, the effects of medications or drugs or other medical, neurologic, or mental illnesses.

---

*If there is doubt about the accuracy of personal history or sleep logs, then actigraphy should be performed, preferably for at least two weeks.
[†]In the case of long sleepers, reported habitual sleep periods may be normal based on age. However, these sleep periods may be insufficient for these patients.

has an MSL <8 minutes.[8] The complaint of daytime sleepiness and documentation of inadequate sleep are more important than the MSLT finding. SOREMPs may occur.

HYPERSOMNIA DUE TO A MEDICAL DISORDER (HDMD)

In these patients, hypersomnolence is believed to be caused by a medical condition.[9–14] The sleepiness may be mild to severe. Symptoms associated with either narcolepsy or idiopathic hypersomnia may be present including sleep paralysis, hypnagogic hallucinations, or automatic behavior may occur. If the patient meets the diagnostic criteria for narcolepsy type 1 or type 2 (N-T1, N-T2), then narcolepsy due to a medical condition (NDMC) should be the diagnosis. If the MSLT documents sleepiness but does not meet the criteria for narcolepsy, HDMD should be the diagnosis. In patients with both sleep-related breathing disorders (SBDs) and HDMD, *a diagnosis of the latter should be made only if the hypersomnolence persists after adequate treatment of the SBD.* HDMD is only diagnosed if the medical condition is judged to be directly causing the hypersomnolence. Hypersomnolence has been described in association with a large range of conditions (Box F34-4), including metabolic encephalopathy, head trauma, stroke, brain tumors, encephalitis, systemic inflammation (e.g., chronic infections, rheumatologic disorders, cancer), genetic

---

BOX F34-4	Disorders Associated with Hypersomnia Due to Medical Disorder

A. Posttraumatic hypersomnia
B. Hypersomnia due to Parkinson disease
C. Genetic disorders associated with central hypersomnia (Niemann-Pick type C, myotonic dystrophy, Norrie disease, Prader-Willi syndrome, Moebius syndrome)
D. Genetic disorders associated with central hypersomnia and SBDs (Prader-Willi syndrome, Mytonic Dystrophy)
E. Hypersomnia due to endocrine disorder (hypothyroidism)
F. Hypersomnia due to central nervous system lesion (infection, tumor)
G. Hypersomnia due to metabolic encephalopathy (liver or kidney failure)
I. Residual hypersomnia in obstructive sleep apnea despite adequate treatment

---

Adapted from American Academy of Sleep Medicine: *International classification of sleep disorders*, ed 3, Darien, IL, 2014, American Academy of Sleep Medicine. *SBD*, Sleep-related breathing disorders.

disorders, and neurodegenerative diseases. A diagnosis of HDMD assumes that a complaint of daytime sleepiness exists and that this is not simply the result of a decreased amount of sleep.

Selected HDMD Conditions

Posttraumatic Hypersomnia

Cases of hypersomnia secondary to head trauma have been documented and in some cases may be caused by injury to the hypocretin neurons or other wakefulness-promoting neural systems.[9,10] However, head trauma has also been reported to be associated with obstructive sleep apnea. Therefore, diagnosis and control of other potential sleep disorders is necessary prior to making this diagnosis.

Residual Hypersomnia in Patients with Adequately Treated Obstructive Sleep Apnea

Some patients with obstructive sleep apnea (OSA) report persistent sleepiness despite apparently adequate amounts of sleep and optimal treatment of their sleep apnea and other obvious sleep disorders.[11] This problem is discussed under medical treatments for sleep apnea (see Fundamentals 22). The patients may have moderately elevated Epworth Sleepiness Scale (ESS) scores, but most have a mean sleep latency of >8 minutes on the MSLT. They also report more fatigue, apathy, and depression. It is essential that SBD be fully treated, confirmed by a download of continuous positive airway pressure (CPAP) machine compliance data demonstrating optimal usage, preferably at least 7 hours a night, and a PSG demonstrating elimination of essentially all SBD. Other causes of sleepiness such as insufficient sleep syndrome, psychiatric disorders, or hypersomnia related to medications should be ruled out. Modafinil and armodafinil are approved by the U.S. Food and Drug Administration (FDA) for treatment of this condition.

Parkinson Disease (PD)

Excessive daytime sleepiness (EDS) not caused by OSA or medications is a well-known phenomenon in PD. Sleepiness was once thought to be caused by side effects from dopamine agonists (DAs) used to treat PD. Most recent studies suggest that medications used to treat PD may worsen EDS but that the underlying disease process is the most common cause of EDS in PD. Studies have reported 50% loss of hypocretin neurons in patients with PD.[12,13] Treatment of EDS not caused by OSA in patients with

PD includes modafinil, bupropion, and traditional stimulants. Fatigue may also be a major complaint. The AASM practice parameters for treatment of central hypersomnia state that modafinil may be an effective treatment of daytime sleepiness in PD. However, the evidence from studies of the effects of modafinil in PD is somewhat conflicting.[14–16] Sudden attacks of sleepiness is a major side effect of DAs. A case report by Hauser found that the addition of modafinil to DA therapy reduced the severity of this DA side effect.[17]

Myotonic Dystrophy (MD)

Myotonic dystrophy type 1 (MD1) is an autosomal dominant inherited disorder characterized by myotonia and muscle weakness. The incidence is estimated to by about 1/10,000, so it is a much rarer disorder than narcolepsy. Myotonia is described as repetitive muscle depolarization resulting in muscle stiffness and impaired relaxation. The muscles usually involved include facial, masseter, levator palprebra, forearm, hand, pretibial, and sternocleidomastoid muscles. Pharyngeal and laryngeal muscles and muscles of respiration, including the diaphragm, may be involved. Dysfunction of the hypothalamic region may result in daytime sleepiness or daytime sleepiness with SOREMPs (NDMC).[18–21] Adult-onset MD usually appears in individuals age 20 to 40 and tends to be slowly progressive. Daytime sleepiness is a common complaint and may be caused by MD (HDMD), MD as a cause of secondary narcolepsy (NDMC), or OSA. Thus, several mechanisms may cause daytime sleepiness in patients with MD.

Physical examination findings include a narrow face, premature frontal balding, distal weakness, and myotonia. Patients with MD have decreased strength on hand grip and are slow to relax the grip. Wasting of hand and forearm muscles is seen. PSG may reveal OSA, and PSG+MSLT may meet the criteria for narcolepsy or simply document EDS without SOREMPs. Modafinil has been used for the sleepiness associated with MD with variable results.[21]

HYPERSOMNIA ASSOCIATED WITH A PSYCHIATRIC DISORDER (HAPD)

Patients with hypersomnia associated with a psychiatric disorder may report excessive nocturnal sleep, daytime sleepiness, or excessive napping.[22–26] In addition, they often feel their sleep is of poor quality and nonrestorative. Patients may focus on hypersomnia and ignore the psychiatric symptoms and even deny depression. The ICSD-3 diagnostic criteria for HAPD require

(1) daytime sleepiness for at least 3 months, (2) the daytime sleepiness occurs in association with a concurrent psychiatric disorder, and (3) the sleepiness is not better explained by another untreated sleep, medical, or neurological disorder or from the effects of medications. Hypersomnia associated with psychiatric disorders accounts for 5% to 7% of hypersomnia cases. Women are more susceptible than men, and the typical age range is between 20 and 50 years. In patients with major depression, the prevalence of hypersomnia is around 30%, varying from 5% to over 50%, depending on how hypersomnia is defined. Hypersomnia affects over 50% of patients with seasonal affective disorder (SAD).

Hypersomnia Associated with Mood Disorder

Although insomnia, rather than hypersomnia, is more common in depression, hypersomnia may occur in up to one third of cases and is often noted in atypical depression and depression associated with bipolar II disorder (recurrent major depressive episodes with at least one hypomanic episode and no manic episodes). The MSLT results are usually normal,[23] *but long hours spent in bed are reported.* Twenty-four-hour continuous sleep-recording studies typically show considerable time spent in bed during day and night, a behavior sometime referred to as *clinophilia*. With major depression, hypersomnia may persist even after the depressive episode ceases, and persistent hypersomnia is associated with increased risk of recurrent depression in some (but not all) studies.

REFERENCES

1. American Academy of Sleep Medicine: *International classification of sleep disorders: diagnostic and coding manual*, ed 2, Westchester, IL, 2005, American Academy of Sleep Medicine.
2. American Academy of Sleep Medicine: *International classification of sleep disorders: diagnostic and coding manual*, ed 3, Darien, IL, 2013, American Academy of Sleep Medicine.
3. Arnulf I, Rico TJ, Mignot E: Diagnosis, disease course, and management of patients with Kleine-Levin syndrome, *Lancet Neurol* 11(10):918–928, 2012.
4. Billiard M, Jaussent I, Dauvilliers Y, Besset A: Recurrent hypersomnia: a review of 339 cases, *Sleep Med Rev* 15:247–257, 2011.
5. Morgenthaler TI, Kapur VK, Brown TM, et al: Practice parameters for the treatment of narcolepsy and other hypersomnias of central origin, *Sleep* 30:1705–1711, 2007.
6. Schweitzer P: Drugs that disturb sleep and wakefulness. In Kryger MH, Roth T, Dement WC, editors: *Principles and practice of sleep medicine*, ed 5, St. Louis, 2011, Saunders, pp 542–560.
7. Roehrs T, Zorick F, Sicklesteel J, et al: Excessive daytime sleepiness associated with insufficient sleep, *Sleep* 6:319–325, 1983.
8. Arand D, Bonnet M, Hurwitz T, et al: The clinical use of the MSLT and MWT, *Sleep* 28:123–144, 2005.

9. Kempf J, Werth E, Kaiser PR, et al: Sleep-wake disturbances 3 years after traumatic brain injury, *J Neurol Neurosurg Psychiatry* 81:1402–1405, 2010.

10. Castriotta RJ, Atanasov S, Wilde MC, et al: Treatment of sleep disorders after traumatic brain injury, *J Clin Sleep Med* 5(2):137–144, 2009.

11. Vernet C, Redolfi S, Attali V, et al: Residual sleepiness in obstructive sleep apnoea: phenotype and related symptoms, *Eur Respir J* 38:98–105, 2011.

12. Arnulf I, Leu S, Oudiette D: Abnormal sleep and sleepiness in Parkinson's disease, *Curr Opin Neurol* 21:472–477, 2008.

13. Bruin VM, Bittencourt LR, Tufik S: Sleep-wake disturbances in Parkinson's disease: current evidence regarding diagnostic and therapeutic decisions, *Eur Neurol* 67:257–267, 2012.

14. Ondo WG, Fayle F, Atassi F, Jankovic J: Modafinil for daytime somnolence in Parkinson's disease: double-blind, placebo-controlled parallel trial, *J Neurol Neurosurg Psychiatry* 76:1636–1639, 2005.

15. Hogl B, Saletu M, Brandauer E, et al: Modafinil for the treatment of daytime sleepiness in Parkinson's disease: a double-blind, randomized, crossover, placebo-controlled polygraphic trial, *Sleep* 25:905–909, 2002.

16. Nieves AV, Lang AE: Treatment of excessive daytime sleepiness in patients with Parkinson's disease with modafinil, *Clin Neuropharmacol* 25:111–114, 2002.

17. Hauser RA, Walha MN, Anderson WM: Modafinil treatment of pramipexole associated somnolence, *Mov Disord* 15:1269–1271, 2000.

18. Martinez-Rodriguez JE, Lin L, Iranzo A, et al: Decreased hypocretin-1 (orexin-A) levels in the cerebrospinal fluid of patients with myotonic dystrophy and excessive daytime sleepiness, *Sleep* 26:287–290, 2003.

19. Romigi A, Izzi F, Pisani V, et al: Sleep disorders in adult-onset myotonic dystrophy type 1: a controlled polysomnographic study, *Eur J Neurol* 18(9):1139–1145, 2011.

20. Dauvilliers YA, Laberge L: Myotonic dystrophy type 1, daytime sleepiness and REM sleep dysregulation, *Sleep Med Rev* 16(6):539–545, 2012.

21. Orlikowski D, Chevret S, Quera-Salva MA, et al: Modafinil for the treatment of hypersomnia associated with myotonic muscular dystrophy in adults: a multicenter, prospective, randomized, double-blind, placebo-controlled, 4-week trial, *Clin Ther* 31:1765–1773, 2009.

22. Plante DT, Winkleman JW: Sleep disturbance in bipolar disorders, *Am J Psychiatry* 165:830–843, 2008.

23. Nofzinger EA, Thase ME, Reynolds CF, III, et al: Hypersomnia in bipolar depression: a comparison with narcolepsy using the multiple sleep latency test, *Am J Psychiatry* 148:1177–1181, 1991.

24. Kaplan KA, Harvey AG: Hypersomnia across mood disorders: a review and synthesis, *Sleep Med Rev* 13:275–285, 2009.

25. Kotagal S: Hypersomnia in children: interface with psychiatric disorders, *Child Adolesc Psychiatr Clin N Am* 18:967–977, 2009.

26. Vgontzas AN, Bixler EO, Kales A, et al: Differences in nocturnal and daytime sleep between primary and psychiatric hypersomnia: diagnosis and treatment implications, *Psychosom Med* 62:220–226, 2000.

PATIENT 95

A 35-Year-Old Man Requesting Stimulant Medication

A 35-year-old man was evaluated for complaints of excessive daytime sleepiness for 6 years. He had been diagnosed with idiopathic hypersomnia by another physician and had been receiving stimulant medications for more than 2 years. After having recently moved, he sought medical attention for medication refills. For the previous 2 months he had not taken stimulant medications, and at work he drank large amounts of coffee to combat sleepiness. His usual bedtime was 11:00 PM, and he awoke at 4:30 AM by alarm. The early awake time was necessary because of a lengthy commute to work. On the weekends, he slept till 9:00 AM and felt somewhat less sleepy. The patient denied a history of cataplexy, hypnagogic hallucinations, sleep paralysis, head trauma, or depression. No history of snoring was present. His previous evaluations included a normal nocturnal polysomnography (PSG), and a multiple sleep latency test (MSLT) showed short sleep latency (7 minutes) with no episodes of rapid eye movement (REM) sleep. The patient was asked to keep a sleep log and actigraphy and to obtain at least 7 hours of sleep nightly before repeat PSG and MSLT.

Physical examination: normal.

Laboratory findings: normal thyroid function.

Sleep logs and actigraphy: average sleep duration of about 7 hours.

Sleep study and MSLT: Table P95-1

TABLE P95-1 **Sleep Study and MSLT Results**

PSG Results

Total recording time	440 (min)	(414–455)		**%TST**		
TST	422 min	(400–443)	Stage N1	13	(2–9)
Sleep efficiency	96 (95–99) %	(95–99)	Stage N2	49	(50–64)
Sleep latency	5 min (2–10 min)	(2–10)	Stage N3	15	(7–18)
REM latency	110 min	(70–100)	Stage R	20	(20–27)
WASO	30 min	(0–20)			
Arousal index	10 (#/hr)		PLMS index	0/hr	
AHI	2 /hr		PLMS arousal index	0/hr	
( ) normal for age					

AHI, Apnea–hypopnea index; *MSL*, mean sleep latency; *PLMS*, periodic limb movement in sleep; *REM*, rapid eye movement; *TST*, total sleep time; *WASO*, wakefulness after sleep onset; ( ), normal for age.

MSLT Results
MSL = 12 min, no SOREMPs in 5 naps

QUESTION

1. What is your diagnosis?

ANSWER

1. **Answer:** Insufficient sleep syndrome (ISS; behaviorally induced insufficient sleep).

Discussion: In ISS, an **inadequate** amount of time is allotted for sleep by the patient because of personal or societal (work) schedules. The amount of sleep required for normal function varies considerably among individuals, with a population mean around 7.5 hours. The *International Classification of Sleep Disorders*, Third Edition (ICSD-3) diagnostic criteria for ISS are listed in Box P95-1. The sleep need of an individual is genetically determined. When less sleep is obtained, a sleep debt accumulates. Commonly, such patients sleep considerably more on weekends. A study of patients with ISS by Roehrs et al found that this disparity between the amounts of sleep obtained on weekday nights and on weekends was an important clinical clue. These patients had normal-to-high sleep efficiencies during nocturnal sleep testing, with greater total sleep times than reported for a typical night, and they showed moderate reductions in sleep latency without REM periods on an MSLT.

One study by Rosenthal and coworkers in normal subjects found that a reduction of the time in bed from 8 to 6 hours reduced the mean sleep latency (MSL) from approximately 12.5 to 8.5 minutes. Thus, a mild reduction in nocturnal sleep may increase daytime sleepiness, although usually not to a severe degree (i.e., sleep latency <5 minutes). Remember, however, that any reduction in nocturnal sleep magnifies the sleepiness associated with other sleep disorders such as narcolepsy or sleep apnea.

BOX P95-1 **Diagnostic Criteria—Insufficient Sleep Syndrome**

Criteria A-F must be met

A. The patient has daily periods of irrepressible need to sleep or daytime lapses into sleep; or in the case of prepubertal children, a complaint of behavioral abnormalities attributable to sleepiness is present.

B. The patient's sleep time, established by personal or collateral history, sleep logs or actigraphy,[1] is usually shorter than expected for age.[2]

C. The curtailed sleep pattern is present most days for at least 3 months.

D. The patient curtails sleep time by such measures as an alarm clock or being woken by another person and generally sleeps longer when such measures are not used, for example, on weekends or vacations.

E. Extension of total sleep time results in resolution of the symptoms of sleepiness.

F. The symptoms are not better explained by another untreated sleep disorder; the effects of medications or drugs; or other medical, neurologic, or mental illnesses.

Notes:
1. If doubt exists about the accuracy of personal history or sleep logs, actigraphy should be performed, preferably for at least 2 weeks.

Although having the patient keep a sleep log was optional on the basis of the most recent practice parameters for the MSLT, most sleep centers require a sleep log for at least 7 days. Unfortunately, sleep logs may not be accurate. The ICSD-3 states "It is strongly recommended that the MSLT be preceded by at least one week of actigraphic recording with a sleep log to establish whether the results could be biased by insufficient sleep, shift work, or another circadian sleep disorder." A study by Bradshaw et al obtained self-report of average sleep duration, sleep logs and actigraphy before an MSLT. The study found sleep logs overestimated the total nightly sleep (compared with both self-report and actigraphy) by almost an hour. Only the TST by actigraphy correlated with the mean sleep latency (MSL) on the MSLT (the shorter total sleep time, the shorter the MSL).

Further recommendations in the ICSD-3 were made concerning the MSLT: "For the correct interpretation of MSLT findings, the recordings should be performed with the following conditions: the patient must be free of drugs that influence sleep for at least 14 days (or at least five times the half-life of the drug and longer-acting metabolite), confirmed by a urine drug screen; the sleep-wake schedule must have been standardized and, if necessary, extended to a minimum of 7 hours in bed each night (longer for children) for at least 7 days before polysomnography (and documented by sleep log and actigraphy); and nocturnal polysomnography should be performed on the night immediately preceding the MSLT to rule out other sleep disorders that could mimic the diagnostic features of narcolepsy." Several studies have analyzed the sequence of sleep before sleep onset REM periods (SOREMPs). A study by Dakotas et al found the sleep stage sequences stage N1→ stage R → stage N2 or stage W → stage R to be more common in narcolepsy, whereas the sequence stage N1 → stage N2 → stage R was more common in the insufficient sleep syndrome. The clinical importance of this observation remains to be established.

The present patient's normal duration of sleep was, at most, 5.5 hours. Thus the possibility of insufficient sleep was considered. This short sleep time would make interpretation of an MSLT difficult, which is why the patient was asked to sleep for at least 7 hours and keep a sleep log before testing. Nocturnal PSG documented fairly normal sleep. The MSLT revealed sleep latency in the "gray" zone: traditionally; sleep latency >15 minutes is considered normal, <10 minutes abnormal, and 10 to 15 minutes could be either (mildsleepiness). The MSL criterion for diagnosis of narcolepsy or idiopathic hypersomnia is a mean sleep latency of 8 minutes. Certainly, sleep latency of 12 minutes is inconsistent with the severe symptoms reported by this patient. A recent meta-analysis by Arand et al found that up to 30% of normal individuals have an MSL of <8 minutes. When confronted with the results of his testing, the patient admitted that he thinks "sleep is a waste of time" and that he always tries to function on as little sleep as possible. Although he could not remember his sleep habits before the previous sleep testing at the other facility, he believed he had allotted the usual short amount of time. Although not entirely happy with the physician's decision not to prescribe stimulants, the patient did understand that the test proved he would be less sleepy during the day if he had more nocturnal sleep.

CLINICAL PEARLS

1. Proper interpretation of the MSLT depends on the patient having an adequate amount of sleep (ideally 7-7.5 hours a night) for at least 1 week before testing. Ideally, the sleep period should be regular and normalized compared to the planned schedule of PSG and the MSLT.
2. An accurate sleep log for at least the last 7 days preceding the PSG and the MSLT is an essential part of the evaluation of daytime sleepiness. It is helpful in interpreting the results of both the nocturnal sleep study and the MSLT. The ICSD-3 recommends actigraphy be performed with the sleep log.
3. A modest shortening of nocturnal sleep (to about 6 hours) may shorten the MSL on the MSLT to <10 minutes.
4. ISS should be considered in the differential diagnosis of excessive daytime sleepiness. It is the most common cause of daytime sleepiness. Insufficient sleep may also worsen the impact of other disorders such as narcolepsy and obstructive sleep apnea.

BIBLIOGRAPHY

Aldrich MS: The clinical spectrum of narcolepsy and idiopathic hypersomnia, *Neurology* 46:383–401, 1996.
American Academy of Sleep Medicine: *International classification of sleep disorders*, ed 3, Darien, IL, 2013, American Academy of Sleep Medicine.
American Sleep Disorders Association: The clinical use of the multiple sleep latency test, *Sleep* 15:268–276, 1992.
Arand D, Bonnet M, Hurwitz T, et al: The clinical use of the MSLT and MWT, *Sleep* 28:123–144, 2005.
Bradshaw DA, Yanagi MA, Pak ES, et al: Nightly sleep duration in the 2-week period preceding multiple sleep latency testing, *J Clin Sleep Med* 3(6):613–619, 2007.
Drakatos P, Kosky CA, Higgins SE: First rapid eye movement sleep periods and sleep-onset rapid eye movement periods in sleep-stage sequencing of hypersomnias, *Sleep Med* 14(9):897–901, 2013.

522

Littner MR, Kushida C, Wise M, et al: Practice parameters for clinical use of the multiple sleep latency test and the maintenance of wakefulness test, *Sleep* 28:113–121, 2005.

Marti I, Valko PO, Khatami R, et al: Multiple sleep latency measures in narcolepsy and behaviourally induced insufficient sleep syndrome, *Sleep Med* 10(10):1146–1150, 2009.

Roehrs T, Zorick F, Sicklesteel J, et al: Excessive daytime sleepiness associated with insufficient sleep, *Sleep* 6:319–325, 1983.

Rosenthal L, Roehrs TA, Rosen A, et al: Level of sleepiness and total sleep time following various time in bed conditions, *Sleep* 16:226–232, 1993.

PATIENT 96

Insufficient Sleep

A 23-year-old female college student was evaluated for complaints of sleepiness and fatigue. Her Epworth Sleepiness Scale (ESS) score was 12 to 14 (mild to moderate sleepiness). She was on no medications and denied cataplexy. When she arrived for polysomnography (PSG) and multiple sleep latency test (MSLT), she stated that she forgot to bring her sleep log. However, she did bring the actigraph she had been wearing. Her usual bedtime was reported as 12:30 AM and wake time 7:30 AM to 9:30 AM (during summer break). She admitted to enjoying social media past midnight nearly every night. The 7:30 AM awakening was on days she had early morning tennis lessons (3 days a week). The patient reported infrequent episodes of both sleep paralysis and hypnogogic hallucinations.

Urine drug screen: negative.
Actigraphy: Figure P96-1
Polysomnography: Table P96-1
MSLT: Table P96-2

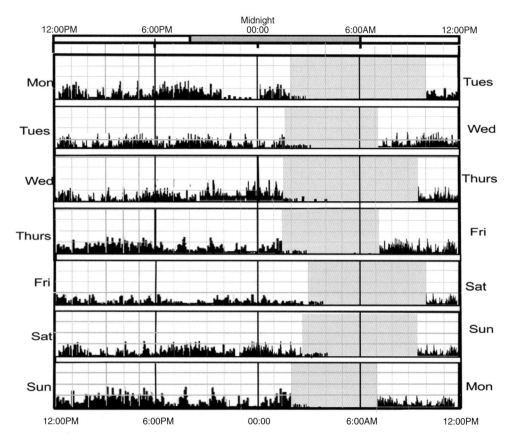

FIGURE P96-1 ■ Sleep actigraphy prior to sleep study. The patient forgot to bring the corresponding sleep log.

TABLE P96-1 **Polysomnography**

		Normal Range			Normal Range
Total recording time (min)	470	(422–470)	%TST		
Total sleep time (min)	460	(408–452)	Stage N1	5	(2–7)
Sleep efficiency (%)	98	(94–98)	Stage N2	40	(46–58)
Sleep latency (min)	2	(3–20)	Stage N3	20	(11–24)
REM latency (min)	75	(78–122)	Stage R	35	(22–29)
WASO (min)	8	(0–15)			
AHI (#/hr)	1				
PLM index (#/hr)	5				

AHI, Apnea–hypopnea index; *PLM*, periodic limb movement; *REM*, rapid eye movement; *TST*, total sleep time; *WASO*, wakefulness after sleep onset.

TABLE P96-2 **Multiple Sleep Latency Test**

	Sleep Latency	SOREMP
Nap 1	2	1
Nap 2	5	0
Nap 3	10	0
Nap 4	12	0
Nap 5	20	0
Mean sleep latency	9.8	

SOREMP, Sleep-onset rapid eye movement period.

QUESTION

1. Does the patient have idiopathic hypersomnia?

ANSWER

1. **Answer:** Insufficient sleep syndrome and delayed sleep period.
Discussion: In this patient, although a total sleep period of 7 hours was reported, it was not substantiated by actigraphy, and a chronically short (many nights of the week) and delayed sleep period was documented (Figure P96-1). The fact that sleep latency was short (see Table P96-1), even at an earlier that habitual bedtime, is evidence of against a true intrinsic circadian rhythm disorder (delayed sleep-wake disorder). Rather, the patient behaviorally delays her sleep period. The high amount of rapid eye movement (REM) sleep (see Table P96-1) suggests a rebound effect and could be caused by curtailment of the last part of her sleep when the most REM sleep occurs. On the MSLT (see Table P96-2), it was interesting to note that sleep latency was short only on the first two naps and the only sleep-onset REM period (SOREMP) was on nap 1. This suggested a chronically delayed sleep period. The patient reported an earlier sleep time and rise time during the school semester. In any case, her mean sleep latency (MSL) of 9.8 minutes did not meet the diagnostic criterion for idiopathic hypersomnia (IH) (MSL ≤8 minutes). In addition, the ability to stay awake for the entire 20 minutes on nap 4 is strong evidence against IH. The patient was confronted with the actigraphy information, and she admitted that she had not followed instructions to normalize her sleep pattern. The patient also reported that she had a "secret" boyfriend and texting at night was their major interaction when she was staying at home. Even with the pattern of very insufficient sleep for at least 3 nights per week, she did not meet the criteria for narcolepsy and IH. Sleep paralysis and hypnagogic hallucinations may occur in IH and in normal individuals as well as in patients with narcolepsy. Sleep paralysis often occurs in normal individuals during periods of sleep restriction.

BIBLIOGRAPHY

American Academy of Sleep Medicine: *International classification of sleep disorders*, ed 3, Darien, IL, 2014, American Academy of Sleep Medicine.

Roehrs T, Zorick F, Sicklesteel J, et al: Excessive daytime sleepiness associated with insufficient sleep, *Sleep* 6:319–235, 1983.

Taylor DJ, Bramoweth AD: Patterns and consequences of inadequate sleep among college students: substance use and motor vehicle accidents, *J Adolesc Health* 46:610–612, 2010.

Tucker AM, Whitney P, Belenky G, et al: Effects of sleep deprivation on dissociated components of executive functioning, *Sleep* 33:47–57, 2010.

Van Dongen HP, Maislin G, Mullington JM, et al: The cumulative cost of additional wakefulness: dose-response effects on neurobehavioral functions and sleep physiology from chronic sleep restriction and total sleep deprivation, *Sleep* 26:117–126, 2003.

PATIENT 97

A Patient with Prader-Willi Syndrome and Daytime Sleepiness

A 25-year-old male with Prader-Willi syndrome (PWS) is sent for evaluation for severe daytime sleepiness. Before entering a group home with strict dietary management, he was morbidly obese and had obstructive sleep apnea (OSA) with hypoventilation. He was placed on a strict diet and received growth hormone replacement therapy. He lost 100 pounds and no longer snored or used continuous positive airway pressure (CPAP). The attendants in the group home verified that he sleeps at least 8 hours per night. He was currently not taking any sedating medication.

Physical examination: body mass index (BMI) 31 kilograms per square meter (kg/m^2); typical PWS appearance, with small hands and feet; HEENT: Mallampati 4; chest: clear to auscultation, cardiovascular regular rhythm; extremities: no edema

Awake arterial oxygen saturation (SaO$_2$) on room air 96%.

TABLE P97-1   **Sleep Study Results**

Sleep Architecture			**Normal Range**
Total recording time	(min)	464.3	(430–454)
Total sleep time	(min)	438.0	(405–434)
Sleep efficiency	(%)	94.2	(91–99)
Sleep latency	(min)	3.5	(3–26)
REM latency	(min)	42.0	(78–99)
Sleep Stages			
WASO	(min)	23.5	(0–5)
		(% of TST)	
Stage N1	(min)	29.5	6.7	(3–6)%
Stage N2	(min)	191.0	43.6	(40–51)%
Stage N3	(min)	115.5	26.4	(16–26)%
Stage R	(min)	102.0	23.3	(22–34)%

Respiratory Events (AHI)					
AHI (/hour [hr])	7.0	Obstructive apneas (#):	3	Minimum SaO_2 NREM (%)	89
AHI NREM (/hr)	6.0	Mixed apneas (#):	0	Minimum SaO_2 REM (%)	86
AHI REM (/hr)	8.6	Central apneas (#):	6	Desaturations TST (#)	60
AHI supine (/hr)	7.5	Hypopnea (#):	62	Average SaO_2 at Desaturation (%)	86
AHI nonsupine (/hr)	2.0				
% TST on back (%)	90.2				

AHI, Apnea–hypopnea index; *NREM*, non–rapid eye movement; *REM*, rapid eye movement; SaO_2, saturation of arterial oxygen; *TST*, total sleep time; *WASO*, wakefulness after sleep onset.

TABLE P97-2   **Multiple Sleep Latency Test**

	Sleep Latency (min)	SOREMP
Nap 1	2.5	1
Nap 2	2.4	0
Nap 3	0.5	0
Nap 4	0.9	0
Nap 5	1.5	0
Mean	1.6	

SOREMP, Sleep-onset rapid eye movement period.

Sleep study and MSLT: Tables P97-1 and P97-2

QUESTION

1. What is causing the severe sleepiness?

ANSWER

1. **Answer:** Hypersomnia due to a medical disorder (HDMD)-Prader Willi Syndrome (PWS).

   Discussion: PWS is a genetic disorder usually associated with a deletion of the long arm of chromosome 15 and is characterized by hyperphagia, obesity, hypogonadotrophic hypogonadism, behavioral disorders, and sleep disorders. Abnormal growth hormone secretion results in short stature, reduced muscle mass, and low bone density (scoliosis is common). The characteristic appearance of PWS includes a high narrow forehead, almond-shaped eyes, turned-down lips, a prominent nasal bridge, and small hands and feet. Intelligence is variable but usually ranges from low-normal to mild to moderately decreased. Growth hormone deficiency is a major etiology of a number of medical problems. Growth hormone injections are commonly used to increase lean body mass and bone density. PWS typically is associated with low muscle tone, short stature if not treated with growth hormone and incomplete sexual development. A chronic feeling of hunger, coupled with decreased metabolism that utilizes drastically fewer calories than normal, may lead to excessive eating and life-threatening obesity.

Patients with PWS may have daytime sleepiness from a number of etiologies, including sleep apnea, narcolepsy, or the PWS itself. Sleep related breathing disorders associated with PWS include sleep apnea with both obstructive and central events and hypoventilation. Unless strict dietary control is imposed, morbid obesity is common and may be associated with hypoventilation. Excessive daytime sleepiness (EDS) is reported commonly in persons with PWS, may begin early in life, and has been correlated with daytime behavioral issues. In fact, EDS has been reported independent of nocturnal sleep problems (sleep apnea), suggesting that it is a primary feature of PWS. Some persons with excessive sleepiness and PWS meet the diagnostic criteria for narcolepsy, and PWS is considered a cause of narcolepsy due to medical condition (NDMC). Abnormal sleep architecture has been reported in persons with PWS, including reduced rapid eye movement (REM) latency and sleep-onset REM periods (SOREMPs). These findings may be present in patients with PWS but without significant sleep-related breathing problems. Although PWS is thought to most commonly cause NDMC *without* cataplexy, patients with PWS may have cataplexy (accurate history is often difficult to obtain in these patients). Nevsimalova and associates found reduced levels of cerebrospinal fluid (CSF) hypocretin levels in four patients with PWS. However, none had cataplexy. Fronczek and coworkers found no difference in the total number of hypocretin-containing neurons in seven PWS patients compared with age-matched controls. If sleepiness is present in PWS but the criteria for narcolepsy are not met and sleepiness is *not* thought to be caused by sleep apnea, a diagnosis of hypersomnia due to a medical disorder is appropriate.

In this patient, the sleep apnea was very mild and was not thought to be the major cause of the severe sleepiness noted. Polysomnography (PSG) and the multiple sleep latency test (MSLT) did not meet criteria for a diagnosis of narcolepsy without cataplexy. A mildly decreased REM latency was noted but no nocturnal SOREMP (<15 minutes). Therefore, the most likely cause of the sleepiness is hypersomnia due to a medical disorder. The patient was treated with modafinil 200 milligrams (mg) and showed improvement but not normalization in sleepiness. More effort was made in the supervision of the diet with the goal of a reduction in the BMI to address the mild OSA.

CLINICAL PEARLS

1. PWS is a genetic disorder associated with excessive sleepiness. Etiologies of the excessive sleepiness include sleep apnea, narcolepsy due to a medical condition (usually Type 2), and hypersomnia due to a medical disorder (e.g., sleepiness due to PWS).
2. Morbid obesity due to hyperphagia is common unless stringent dietary controls are in place.
3. The hypocretin level in CSF appears to be normal in the majority of patients with PWS and sleepiness. Daytime sleepiness due to OSA and hypersomnia due to PWS are much more common than narcolepsy due to PWS.

BIBLIOGRAPHY

Bruni O, Verrillo E, Novelli L, Ferri R: Prader-Willi syndrome: sorting out the relationships between obesity, hypersomnia, and sleep apnea, *Curr Opin Pulm Med* 16(6):568–573, 2010.

Camfferman D, McEvoy RD, O'Donoghue F, Lushington K: Prader Willi syndrome and excessive daytime sleepiness, *Sleep Med Rev* 12(1):65–75, 2008.

De Cock VC, Diene G, Molinas C, et al: Efficacy of modafinil on excessive daytime sleepiness in Prader-Willi syndrome, *Am J Med Genet A* 155A(7):1552–1557, 2011.

Fronczek R, Lammers GJ, Balesar R, et al: The number of hypothalamic hypocretin orexin neurons is not affectd in PWS, *J Clin Endocrinol Metab* 90:5466–5470, 2005.

Manni R, Politini L, Nobili L, et al: Hypersomnia in the Prader-Willi syndrome: clinical, electrophysiological features, and underlying factors, *Clin Neurophysiol* 112:800–805, 2001.

Nevsimalova S, Vankova J, Stepanova I, et al: Hypocretin deficiency in Prader-Willi syndrome, *Eur J Neurol* 12:70–72, 2005.

Tobias ES, Tolmie GJ, Stephenson JBP: Cataplexy in Prader-Willi syndrome, *Arch Dis Child* 87:170, 2002.

Wagner MH, Berry RB: An obese female with Prader Willi syndrome, *J Clin Sleep Med* 3(6):645–647, 2007.

Williams K, Scheimann A, Sutton V, et al: Sleepiness and sleep disordered breathing in Prader-Willi syndrome: relationship to genotype, growth hormone therapy, and body composition, *J Clin Sleep Med* 4(2):111–118, 2008.

PATIENT 98

Sleepiness After Head Trauma

Patient A: A 20-year-old man was referred for evaluation of daytime sleepiness. He was involved in a motor vehicle accident and suffered head trauma about 6 months before referral. He was unconscious for 24 hours. Since recovery he has complained of headache and some difficulty with memory and intellectual function. However, his major difficulty has been excessive daytime sleepiness (Epworth Sleepiness Scale [ESS] score of 18/24). No history of snoring was present. The patient reported sleeping 7 hours per night and denied cataplexy. He also denied nightmares or significant depression.

Polysomnography (PSG): Normal sleep architecture except for a mild decrease in sleep efficiency; total sleep time 425 minutes; sleep latency 5 minutes; rapid eye movement (REM) latency 70 minutes; apnea–hypopnea index (AHI) = 3/hour

Multiple sleep latency test (MSLT): mean sleep latency 6 minutes; 1 sleep-onset rapid eye movement period (SOREMP) out of 5 naps

Patient B: A 25-year-old man suffered severe whiplash injury when his car was hit from the rear by another vehicle. He had persistent headaches and neck pain. Over the 3 months after recovery, his wife noted progressive snoring and breathing pauses. He had only a 5-pound weight gain. Prior to the automobile accident, the patient had no history of snoring before the motor vehicle accident. Moderate daytime sleepiness was present (ESS score of 14/24).

PSG followed by an MSLT was ordered. The MSLT was cancelled after PSG revealed significant sleep apnea.

PSG: AHI 30/hour (hr), 30% of events obstructive apneas, 70% hypopneas, 200 desaturations, low SaO_2 85%.

QUESTIONS

1. What is your diagnosis?

2. Was the development of obstructive sleep apnea (OSA) a coincidence or associated with head trauma?

ANSWER

1. **Answer for Patient A:** Hypersomnia due to medical disorder (posttraumatic hypersomnia).

2. **Answer for Patient B:** OSA may develop after traumatic brain or spinal cord injury. It is especially common after whiplash injury.

   Discussion: The ICSD-3 diagnostic criteria for hypersomnia due to medical disorder are shown in Box P98-1. If criteria for narcolepsy are met a diagnosis of narcolepsy due to medication condition (Type 1 or Type 2) should be made. Traumatic brain injury (TBI) is a major problem and cause of long-term disability in millions of individuals in both the military and civilian populations. Sleep disturbances after TBI are estimated to occur in 30% to 70% of patients with head injuries, often preventing the resumption of normal activities. The prevalence of sleep disorders in individuals with TBI is very high, yet often unrecognized. Civilian closed head injuries are typically caused by falls (28%); motor vehicle accidents (20%); impact from an object (19%); and assaults (11%). These injuries often occur in the context of construction or industrial accidents and domestic or child abuse. Awareness of TBI in military personnel returning from conflicts abroad is increasing. Among those deployed, 11% to 23% have suffered mild TBI, often from improvised explosive device blasts. Theodorou and Rice noted that 59% of blast-exposed veterans of the Afghanistan or Iraq conflict had TBI.

   Up to 50% of all patients with chronic TBI have sleep disorders, which require nocturnal PSG and the MSLT for diagnosis. These disorders include sleep apnea (23% of all TBI patients), posttraumatic hypersomnia (11%), narcolepsy (6%) and periodic limb movement disorder (PLMD) (7%). Over half of all patients with TBI will have insomnia complaints, most often with less severe injury and after personal assault, and half of these may be related to a circadian rhythm disorder. A delayed sleep phase and non–24-hour sleep-wake disorder have been described.

   Sleep disorders following head trauma may depend on the area of brain that is injured. Posttraumatic hypersomnia is seen when areas involved in the maintenance of wakefulness are damaged. These regions include the brainstem reticular formation, posterior hypothalamus, and the area surrounding the third ventricle. Hypothalamic injury with decreased levels of wakefulness-promoting neurotransmitters such as hypocretin (orexin) may be involved in the pathophysiology of daytime sleepiness. Low cerebrospinal fluid (CSF) hypocretin-1 levels are found in most cases of narcolepsy with cataplexy following head trauma, but normal levels are typically seen in hypersomnia due to trauma (posttraumatic hypersomnia). Most patients with moderate-to-severe TBI have low or intermediate hypocretin-1 levels in the acute injury phase. Hypocretin levels tend to normalize (become >200 picograms per milliliter [pg/mL]) 6 months after the injury, which may explain why post-TBI sleepiness resolves in many over time. High cervical cord lesions have also been known to cause sleepiness and OSA. In addition, whiplash injury may cause hypersomnia by precipitating sleep-disordered breathing. Coup-contre-coup brain injury after head trauma occurs most frequently at the base of the skull in areas of bony irregularities (especially the sphenoid ridges), with consequent damage to the inferior frontal and anterior temporal regions, including the basal

---

BOX P98-1 **Hypersomnia Due to Medical Disorder (ICSD-3)**

Criteria A-D must be met

A. The patient has daily periods of irrepressible need to sleep or daytime lapses into sleep occurring for at least three months.

B. The daytime sleepiness occurs as a consequence of a significant underlying medical or neurological condition.

C. If an MSLT is performed, the mean sleep latency is ≤8 minutes, and fewer than two sleep onset REM periods (SOREMPs) are observed.*

D. The symptoms are not better explained by another untreated sleep disorder,† a mental disorder, or the effects of medications or drugs.

From American Academy of Sleep Medicine: *International classification of sleep disorders*, ed 3, Darien, IL, 2014, American Academy of Sleep Medicine.

*In the subtype of residual hypersomnolence after treatment of obstructive sleep apnea, the MSLT mean latency may be >8 minutes.

†Should criteria for narcolepsy be fulfilled, a diagnosis of narcolepsy type 1 or type 2 due to a medical condition should be used rather than hypersomnia due to a medical condition.

Note: In patients with severe neurological or medical disorders in whom it is not possible or desirable to perform sleep studies, the diagnosis can be made by clinical criteria.

forebrain (an area involved in sleep initiation). As a result, insomnia is a common symptom after injuries of this mechanism. Closed head injury may involve the suprachiasmatic nucleus or its output tracts, leading to disturbance of circadian rhythmicity with concomitant hypersomnia and insomnia.

Common sleep disorders associated with head trauma are listed in Box P98-2. Castriotta and colleagues prospectively studied 87 adults at least 3 months after TBI. PSG and the MSLT were administered to all subjects; 46% had abnormal sleep studies. The authors diagnosed 23% with OSA, 11% with posttraumatic hypersomnia, 7% with periodic limb movements in sleep (PLMS), and 6% with narcolepsy. Although hypersomnia after TBI is most commonly associated with OSA, less common causes are hypersomnia due to a medical condition (posttraumatic hypersomnia) and narcolepsy due to a medical condition (NDMC). In posttraumatic hypersomnia, the symptoms are not believed to be caused by OSA, and MSLT findings document short mean sleep latency ($\leq$ 8 minutes) but 0 to 1 SOREMP. The diagnosis of narcolepsy due to TBI requires that patients meet the usual diagnostic criteria for narcolepsy. In both conditions, hypersomnia must be present for at least 3 months. Head trauma has been reported to precipitate a few cases of Kleine-Levin syndrome, a rare disorder consisting of recurrent hypersomnia and cognitive or behavioral disturbances, hypersexuality, and compulsive eating. Head trauma occasionally triggers parasomnia, including sleepwalking, sleep terrors, and REM sleep behavior disorder.

Fatigue and depression are also common after TBI. It is often difficult to differentiate fatigue and sleepiness. Objective testing with PSG and the MSLT may be useful in objectively documenting sleepiness. Fatigue after TBI is more common in women than in men. Posttraumatic stress disorder (PTSD) is also common, but whether this is caused by TBI or the incident that caused the TBI is difficult to determine. The usual treatments for PTSD are often effective. Most standard treatment regimens of sleep disorders appear to be effective in these patients, including continuous positive airway pressure (CPAP) for sleep apnea, pramipexole for periodic limb movements, and cognitive behavioral therapy for insomnia. The role of wakefulness-promoting agents and central nervous system (CNS) stimulants for the sleepiness involved in TBI is still evolving. One study found modafinil to be useful in patients with hypersomnia following TBI.

In Patient A, PSG and the MSLT revealed objective daytime sleepiness but did not meet the criteria for narcolepsy. A diagnosis of hypersomnia due to a medical disorder was made. The patient was started on modafinil 200 milligrams (mg) daily, and this dose was increased to 400 mg daily. The complaints of sleepiness improved but the ESS score remained abnormal (12/24). In Patient B, a diagnosis of OSA was made, and the patient was ultimately started on CPAP. Although pre-trauma PSG was not performed, given the history absent snoring preTBI, the OSA probably was the result of head trauma.

BOX P98-2 | **Sleep Disorders After Traumatic Brain Injury**

Obstructive sleep apnea	Circadian rhythm sleep wake disorder (delayed
Central sleep apnea	sleep phase, non-24-hour disorder)
Complex sleep apnea	Insomnia
Hypersomnia due to a medical disorder	Parasomnia
Narcolepsy due to a medical condition	Periodic limb movement disorder

Adapted from Viola-Saltzman M, Watson NF: Traumatic brain injury and sleep disorders, *Neurol Clin* 30(4):1299-1312, 2012.

CLINICAL PEARLS

1. The entire range of sleep disorders may follow TBI and may depend on the area of the brain that is injured.

2. Hypersomnia after TBI is most commonly associated with OSA but may be caused by posttraumatic hypersomnia (a type of hypersomnia due to medical disorder) or narcolepsy due to medication condition (NDMC).

3. The CSF hypocretin level is reduced following TBI but tends to normalize over the next 6 months. Daytime sleepiness also resolves in the majority of patients. However, daytime sleepiness persists in a significant proportion of patients with TBI and is associated with significant morbidity.

4. The diagnosis of NDMC requires that patients meet the usual diagnostic criteria for narcolepsy. If objective evidence for daytime sleepiness exists but the criteria for narcolepsy are not met, a diagnosis of hypersomnia due to medical condition (posttraumatic hypersomnia) is appropriate. This assumes that OSA, medications, or insufficient sleep are not the predominant cause of sleepiness.

BIBLIOGRAPHY

Ayalon L, Borodkin K, Dishon L, et al: Circadian rhythm sleep disorders following mild traumatic brain injury, *Neurology* 68(14):1136–1140, 2007.

Baumann CR, Stocker R, Imhof HG, et al: Hypocretin-1 (orexin A) deficiency in acute traumatic brain injury, *Neurology* 65(1):147–149, 2005.

Carter KA, Lettieri CJ, Pena JM: An unusual cause of insomnia following IED induced traumatic brain injury, *J Clin Sleep Med* 6 (2):205–206, 2010.

Castriotta RJ, Atanasov S, Wilde MC, et al: Treatment of sleep disorders after traumatic brain injury, *J Clin Sleep Med* 5(2):137–144, 2009.

Castriotta RJ, Murthy JN: Sleep disorders in patients with traumatic brain injury: a review, *CNS Drugs* 25(3):175–185, 2011.

Castriotta RJ, Wilde MC, Lai JM, et al: Prevalence and consequences of sleep disorders in traumatic brain injury, *J Clin Sleep Med* 3(4):349–356, 2007.

Dauvilliers Y, Baumann CR, Carlander B, et al: CSF hypocretin-1 levels in narcolepsy, Kleine-Levin syndrome, and other hypersomnias and neurological conditions, *J Neurol Neurosurg Psychiatry* 74(12):1667–1673, 2003.

Guilleminault C, Yuen KM, Gulevich MG, et al: Hypersomnia after head-neck trauma: a medicolegal dilemma, *Neurology* 54(3):653–659, 2000.

Kaiser PR, Valko PO, Werth E, et al: Modafinil ameliorates excessive daytime sleepiness after traumatic brain injury, *Neurology* 75(20):1780–1785, 2010.

Ouellet MC, Savard J, Morin CM: Insomnia following traumatic brain injury: a review, *Neurorehabil Neural Repair* 18(4):187–198, 2004.

Shekleton JA, Parcell DL, Redman JR, et al: Sleep disturbance and melatonin levels following traumatic brain injury, *Neurology* 74(21):1732–1738, 2010.

Theodorou AA, Rice SA: Is the silent epidemic keeping patients awake? *J Clin Sleep Med* 3(4):347–348, 2007.

Viola-Saltzman M, Watson NF: Traumatic brain injury and sleep disorders, *Neurol Clin* 30(4):1299–1312, 2012.

Watson NF, Dikmen S, Machamer J, et al: Hypersomnia following traumatic brain injury, *J Clin Sleep Med* 3(4):363–368, 2007.

PATIENT 99

A Patient with Possible Narcolepsy and Weakness in the Hands

A 32-year-old male was referred for treatment for possible narcolepsy. No history of cataplexy was present. The Epworth Sleepiness Scale (ESS) score was 12/24. The patient had responded to methylphenidate, but his physician had left the area. He was currently on no medications. He reported sleeping 7 to 8 hours each night, and his wife did not report that he snored or stopped breathing. The patient's only other complaint was slowly progressive weakness in his hands (difficulty opening jars).

Physical examination:
General: thin male with body mass index (BMI) 24
Head: high forehead, thin face, frontal balding
HEENT: Mallampati 1
Chest: clear to auscultation
Neurologic: some wasting noted in the hand and forearm muscles; hand grip was weak but the patient had difficulty letting go
Polysomnography (PSG): unremarkable
Multiple sleep latency test (MSLT): mean sleep latency (MSL) 2.5 minutes; 1 sleep-onset rapid eye movement period (SOREMP)

QUESTION

1. What is causing the daytime sleepiness?

ANSWER

1. **Answer:** Myotonic dystrophy (MD).

Discussion: MD type 1 (MD1, Steinert disease) is an autosomal dominant inherited disorder characterized by myotonia, distal muscle weakness, premature cataracts, hypogonadism, and cardiac arrhythmias. The genetic defect in MD1 results from an amplified trinucleotide CTG repeat in the 3-prime untranslated region of a protein kinase gene (*DMPK*) on chromosome 19. The pathogenesis of myotonic dystrophy is related to trinucleotide repeat expansions that produce toxic mutant messenger ribonucleic acid (mRNA) with subsequent interference of RNA-splicing mechanisms. Definitive diagnosis is by genetic testing of the deoxyribonucleic acid (DNA) of leukocytes. The incidence is estimated to be about 1 per 10,000, so it is a much rarer disorder than narcolepsy. *Myotonia* is defined as repetitive muscle depolarization resulting in muscle stiffness and impaired relaxation. The muscles usually involved in MD include the facial, masseter, levator palprebra, forearm, hand, pretibial, and sternocleidomastoid muscles. Pharyngeal and laryngeal muscles and the muscles of respiration, including the diaphragm, may be involved. Dysfunction of the hypothalamic region may result in daytime sleepiness or in daytime sleepiness with SOREMPs, which may lead to the additional diagnosis of narcolepsy due to a medical condition (NDMC). If criteria for narcolepsy are not met, a diagnosis of hypersomnia due to a medical condition could be considered. Involvement of the upper airway muscles may result in sleep apnea. Some patients have abnormal ventilatory control and hypoventilation. Involvement of the cardiac system may occur (heart block, prolonged QRS or P–R intervals). In one case-controlled study comparing age-matched groups of patients with and without MD, the patients with MD had a greater frequency of severe obstructive sleep apnea (OSA), an elevated periodic limb movement in sleep (PLMS) index, shorter MSL on the MSLT, and more frequent SOREMPs. One and two SOREMPs being present in 47.5% and 32.5%. More stage N3 and stage R and a higher REM density were noted in MD-1.

Differences in MD presentation depend on the age of onset. Congenital MD is apparent at birth and often severe. Juvenile MD is characterized by symptoms that appear between birth and adolescence. Adult-onset MD usually appears in individuals age 20 to 40 and tends to be slowly progressive. Late-onset MD occurs after 40 and has mild symptoms.

On physical examination, findings in MD1 include a narrow face, temporal wasting, premature frontal balding, distal weakness, and myotonia. Patients with MD have decreased strength on hand grip but then are slow to relax ("distal myopathy with myotonia"). Symptomatic myotonia typically precedes muscle weakness in MD1. Individuals describe muscle stiffness or difficulty releasing their grip. Patients may observe a delayed ability to open their eyes after a forceful closure or a delayed ability to extend their fingers after a firm handshake. Wasting of hand and forearm muscles (especially hand flexors) is seen. As noted above, PSG may reveal OSA. PSG + MSLT findings may meet the criteria for narcolepsy or simply document excessive daytime without two SOREMPs. The *American Academy of Sleep Medicine (AASM) Practice Parameter on the Treatment of Narcolepsy and Other Hypersomnias of Central Origin* stated: "Methylphenidate and modafinil may be effective treatment for myotonic dystrophy" (Option—the lowest recommendation level). Two studies found modafinil to be effective (Talbot et al; MacDonald et al) but a more recent study (Orlikowski et al) did not show a benefit.

In the current patient, clues on the physical examination that MD was present included frontal balding, distal muscle wasting, and myotonia (weak hand grip but difficulty letting go). The diagnostic criteria for narcolepsy were not met on the PSG + MSLT. Significant sleep apnea was not present. A diagnosis of hypersomnia due to a medical disorder was made. The patient's insurance would not pay for modafinil. He was continued on methylphenidate with good control of his daytime sleepiness. Given the association of MD with premature cataracts and ECG abnormalities, the patient was referred for a slit lamp examination of his eyes and electrocardiography (ECG).

CLINICAL PEARLS

1. Consider a diagnosis of MD if a patient presents with complaints of muscle weakness in the hands or arms and daytime sleepiness.
2. Physical examination results that clearly indicate myotonia include a delay in the ability to open the eyes after a forceful closure or a delayed ability to extend the fingers that is, relaxation, after a firm handshake.
3. The sleepiness associated with MD may be caused by sleep apnea, narcolepsy due to a medication condition, or hypersomnia due to a medical condition.
4. Excessive daytime sleepiness in patients with myotonic dystrophy may respond to treatment with modafinil or traditional stimulants.

BIBLIOGRAPHY

Dauvilliers YA, Laberge L: Myotonic dystrophy type 1, daytime sleepiness and REM sleep dysregulation, *Sleep Med Rev* 16(6):539–545, 2012.

Johnson NE, Heatwole CR: Myotonic dystrophy: from bench to bedside, *Semin Neurol* 32(3):246–254, 2012.

MacDonald JR, Hill JD, Tarnopolsky MA: Modafinil reduces excessive somnolence and enhances mood in patients with myotonic dystrophy, *Neurology* 59:1876–1880, 2002.

Orlikowski D, Chevret S, Quera-Salva MA, et al: Modafinil for the treatment of hypersomnia associated with myotonic muscular dystrophy in adults: a multicenter, prospective, randomized, double-blind, placebo-controlled, 4-week trial, *Clin Ther* 31:1765–1773, 2009.

Talbot K, Stradling J, Crosby J, et al: Reduction in excess daytime sleepiness by modafinil in patients with myotonic dystrophy, *Neuromuscul Disord* 13:357–364, 2003.

Yu H, Laberge L, Jaussent I, et al: Daytime sleepiness and REM sleep characteristics in myotonic dystrophy: a case-control study, *Sleep* 34(2):165–170, 2011.

Parasomnia

Parasomnia is a motor, verbal, or experiential phenomenon that occurs in association with sleep (at sleep onset, during sleep, or after arousal from sleep) and is often undesirable. The term *parasomnia* comes from the Greek prefix *para* meaning "alongside of" and the Latin word *somnus* meaning "sleep." In the usual clinical setting, the term refers to undesirable events. Some types of parasomnia are associated with non–rapid eye movement (NREM) sleep and some with REM sleep, and some are classified as "other parasomnias (e.g., enuresis)" because they may occur during either NREM or REM sleep or during wakefulness soon after arousal from sleep.

EVALUATION OF PARASOMNIAS

Evaluation of nocturnal "spells or unusual behavior" begins with a detailed history of the nature, age of onset, and time of night of the episodes. Factors (sleep deprivation and medications) that may have affected the behaviors should be explored. A neurologic examination should be performed to rule out associated neurologic disorders. Not all parasomnias require evaluation by polysomnography (PSG). The indications for evaluation with PSG include (1) potentially violent or injurious behavior, (2) behavior is extremely disruptive to household members, (3) parasomnia resulting in a complaint of excessive sleepiness, and (4) parasomnia associated with medical, psychiatric, or neurologic symptoms or findings.

Video PSG (usually with synchronized video and audio) is the recommended method of evaluating parasomnias. Today, virtually all digital PSG equipment manufacturers offer synchronized video and audio with their digital PSG recording systems. Additional electrodes beyond those used to score sleep (T3, T4) are commonly recorded in patients with suspected parasomnia to improve the ability to detect interictal or seizure activity. Additional arm electromyography (EMG) (flexor digitorum superficialis) is often performed in addition to right and left tibialis anterior (leg) EMG to detect transient muscle activity (TMA; phasic muscle activity) during REM sleep. One problem with monitoring a patient for a suspected parasomnia is that the events frequently do not occur every night. Multiple nights of video PSG may be needed.

NREM PARASOMNIA

The traditional classification of NREM parasomnia includes (1) confusional arousals, (2) sleepwalking, (3) sleep terrors. Considerable overlap exists in these types of parasomnia (Box F35-1 and Table F35-1), and individual patients may manifest behaviors consistent with all three subtypes of NREM parasomnia on different nights. The disorders are considered disorders of arousal with the physiologic state being and a mixture of wakefulness and NREM sleep. The ICSD-3 diagnostic criteria for NREM parasomnias (confusional arousal, sleep walking, night terrors) are show in Box F35-2 In the ICSD-3 the sleep related eating disorder (SRED) is included as a NREM parasomnia. SRED will be discussed in a Patient 103 and diagnostic criteria are shown on p. 551

BOX F35-1	Common Characteristics of Non–Rapid Eye Movement (NREM) Parasomnia Types

- Impaired cognition during event (eyes open but "glassy")
- Amnesia about the preceding event
- In children NREM parasomnias occur in stage N3; in adults stages N1, N2 or N3
- In adults with NREM parasomnia—a high percentage (e.g., two thirds) experienced episode in childhood
- Familial tendency
- Not usually associated with psychiatric disorders or head injury
- Precipitating events—stress, sleep deprivation, obstructive sleep apnea, fever in children, medications
- May be precipitated by a loud noise, touch, or other stimuli

TABLE F35-1	Comparison of the Characteristics of Non–Rapid Eye Movement Parasomnia Types		
	Confusional Arousal	**Sleep Walking**	**Sleep Terrors**
Sleep stage at onset	Stage N3 children Stage N1, N2, N3 adults	Same	Same
Autonomic hyperactivity	No	No	Prominent
Loud scream	No	No	Yes
Ambulation out of bed	No	Yes	No
Confusion during episode	Yes	Yes	Yes
Amnesia (partial or complete)	Yes	Yes	Yes

A given episode may be a mixture of these three types.

BOX F35-2	ICSD-3 Diagnostic Criteria for Disorders of Arousal from Non–Rapid Eye Movement Sleep*

GENERAL DIAGNOSTIC CRITERIA (CRITERIA A-E MUST BE MET)

A. Recurrent episodes of incomplete awakening from sleep (The events usually occur during the first third of the major sleep episode, in adults anytime)
B. Inappropriate or absent responsiveness to efforts of others to intervene or redirect the person during the episode
C. Limited (e.g., a single visual scene) or no associated cognition or dream imagery
D. Partial or complete amnesia for the episode
E. The disturbance not better explained by another sleep disorder, mental disorder, medical condition, or medication or substance use
    Note: The individual may continue to appear confused and disoriented for several minutes or longer following the episode.

DIAGNOSTIC CRITERIA FOR CONFUSIONAL AROUSAL (CRITERIA A-C MUST BE MET)

A. The disorder meets general criteria for NREM disorders of arousal.
B. The episodes are characterized by mental confusion of confused behavior which occurs while the patient is in bed

C. Absence of terror or ambulation outside of the bed
    Note: There is typically a lack of autonomic arousal such as mydriasis, tachycardia, tachypnea, and diaphoresis during an episode.

DIAGNOSTIC CRITERIA FOR SLEEP WALKING (CRITERIA A AND B MUST BE MET)

A. The disorder meets general criteria for NREM disorders of arousal.
B. The arousals are associated with ambulation and other complex behaviors out of bed.
    Note: There is typically a lack of autonomic arousal such as mydriasis, tachycardia, tachypnea, and diaphoresis during an episode.

SLEEP TERRORS DIAGNOSTIC CRITERIA (CRITERIA A-C MUST BE MET)

A. The disorder meets general criteria for NREM disorders of arousal.
B. The arousals are characterized by episodes of abrupt terror, typically beginning with an alarming vocalization such as a frightening scream
C. There is intense fear and signs of autonomic arousal including mydriasis, tachycardia, tachypnea, and diaphoresis during an episode.

From American Academy of Sleep Medicine: *International classification of sleep disorders,* ed 3, Darien, IL, 2014, American Academy of Sleep Medicine.
*For Diagnostic criteria for the Sleep Related Eating Disorder see Patient 101.

Common Characteristics of NREM Parasomnia

The disorders share similar genetic and familial patterns and similar pathophysiology (partial arousals from NREM sleep). NREM parasomnias are generally not secondary to neuropathology or head injury. The episodes may be triggered by sound, touch, or other stimuli. The events occur out of stage N3 in children but in stages N1, N2, and N3 in adults. During the event, cognition (eyes open but glassy) is impaired, and communication with the individual is difficult. If the patients are "awakened" (returned to totally awake state), they are confused. Amnesia is present with regard to the preceding event. Stress, sleep deprivation, and treatment of sleep apnea (stage N3 rebound) may precipitate the event. Adults with a NREM parasomnia typically have a history of similar events as a child. However, *the onset of NREM parasomnia may occur in adulthood in up to one third of cases.* NREM parasomnia is not thought to be caused by psychopathology. One study of patients with sleep terrors or sleep walking evaluated for sleep-related injury found that only 48% had evidence of current or prior psychopathology. Thus, adults with sleep terrors are just as likely not to have related psychopathology as to have this problem. In addition, sleep terrors or sleepwalking and any concurrent psychopathology are usually not closely associated with respect to their onset, clinical course, or treatment response. In contrast to REM parasomnia, dream mentation is uncommonly reported in NREM parasomnia.

Types of NREM Parasomnia

A. **Confusional arousals (CAs)** are brief episodes of partial arousal from sleep that are characterized by awakening with mental confusion in bed and often go unnoticed unless reported by the bed partner. Ambulation out of bed is absent and autonomic arousal (tachycardia, tachypnea, and diaphoresis) does not occur. During awakening, behavior may be inappropriate (especially forced awakening) and even violent. Although behaviors are usually simple (movements in bed, thrashing about, vocalization, or inconsolable crying), they may be more complex. Frequently, an overlap exists between confusional arousals and sleepwalking. In contrast to sleep terrors, patients with confusional arousals do *not* exhibit autonomic hyperactivity or signs of fear or emit a blood-curdling scream. Confusional arousals are common in children with a prevalence of 17% and usually resolve by age 5.

B. **Sleepwalking (somnambulism)** is defined as a series of complex behaviors that are initiated during sleep and result in ambulation. Activity may range from simply sitting up in bed and picking at the covers to walking. Abnormal behaviors include routine behaviors that occur at inappropriate times, inappropriate or nonsensical behaviors, and dangerous or potentially dangerous behaviors. Of interest, *the eyes are usually open (wide open and "glassy-eyed") during sleepwalking*, but patients may be clumsy in their movements. Talking during sleep (somniloquy) may occur simultaneously.

In addition to ambulation, the episodes have evidence of persistent sleep, altered consciousness, or *impaired judgment during ambulation*. Evidence for an altered state of consciousness includes difficulty in arousing the person, mental confusion when awakened from an episode, amnesia (complete

or partial) about the episode, and abnormal behaviors. Episodes of sleep walking in children are rarely violent, and movements often are slow. In adults, sleepwalking episodes may be more complex, frenzied, violent, and longer in duration. Episodes of sleepwalking may be terminated by the patient returning to bed or simply lying down and continuing sleep out of bed. Patients are difficult to arouse during sleepwalking episodes. When aroused during sleepwalking, patients are typically very confused. Sleepwalking occurs in 10 to 20% of children and the incidence peaks between the ages of 4 and 8. *The onset of sleepwalking can also occur in adulthood in up to 1/3 of affected individuals.* However, *most adult sleepwalkers had episodes during childhood* (60% to 70% of adults with sleepwalking exhibited this parasomnia during childhood). Sleepwalking usually disappears in adolescence. One study of 100 adult patients with sleep-related injury found that 33% with sleepwalking had an age of onset after age 16, and 70% had episodes arising from both stages N1 and N2, as well as stage N3. The sleepwalking behaviors were variable in duration and intensity. There is a definite *familial role in the development of sleepwalking*. If one or both parents have a history of sleepwalking, the risk of a child developing sleepwalking episodes is greatly increased. Fever, sleep deprivation, and certain medications (e.g., zolpidem and other benzodiazepine receptor agonists [BZRAs], phenothiazines, tricyclic antidepressants [TCAs], lithium) may precipitate the sleep walking events.

C. **Sleep terrors (STs)** consist of sudden arousal from sleep accompanied by a blood-curdling scream or cry and manifestations of severe fear (behavioral and autonomic). The affected individual typically is confused, diaphoretic, and tachycardic, and he or she frequently sits up in bed. It is difficult or impossible to communicate with a person having a sleep terror, and total amnesia about the event is usual. Patients may sleepwalk during episodes of night terrors. Sleep terrors typically occur in prepubertal children ($\leq 3\%$) and subside by adolescence; they are uncommon in adults. Sleep terrors rarely begin in adulthood.

PSG in NREM Parasomnia

PSG is not required for diagnosis or evaluation unless the episodes are recurrent and bothersome, are atypical (sterotypical, many per night), if treatment is being considered, and if the episodes have resulted in injury or the potential for injury. During arousal, EEG may show persistent slow wave activity with increased chin EMG activity and muscle artifact on EEG. At the onset the heart rate increases, but no pre-event increase in heart rate occurs.

Treatment of NREM Parasomnia

Treatment includes avoiding precipitating factors (e.g., sleep deprivation) and environmental precautions. Medication is usually not needed. No randomized, controlled trials of treatments for NREM parasomnia have been conducted. Medications that have been used include benzodiazepines (clonazepam 0.5 to 2.0 milligrams [mg] at bed time [qhs], or temazepam 30 mg qhs), TCAs, or selective serotonin reuptake inhibitors (SSRIs). If medications are used, they should be given early enough to prevent sleepwalking in the first cycle of NREM sleep. Of note, zolpidem has been associated with sleepwalking and complex behaviors during sleep. In one study of patients with self-injurious behavior, bedtime clonazepam was successful in controlling sleep terrors or sleepwalking in >80% of cases. However, not all studies have found clonazepam to be this effective. Another study of treatment of patients with sleepwalking found that those with any degree of a sleep apnea had fewer sleepwalking episodes if sleep apnea was effectively treated. A recent systematic review of sleepwalking treatments found that no large controlled studies of treatment for sleepwalking have been reported.

Sleep-Related Sexual Behavior and Sleep-Related Violence

The main complications of sleepwalking are social embarrassment and danger of self-injury or injury to others. Violent behavior (self-mutilation or homicide) and sexual assault (sleep sex) have been reported in association with sleepwalking episodes. **Sleep-related sexual behavior** or **sexsomnia** is a type of parasomnia in which sexual behavior occurs with limited awareness during the act, relative unresponsivenss to the external environment, and amnesia about the event. The behaviors range from sexual vocalizations to intercourse. These actions may include behaviors highly atypical of the individual (e.g., anal intercourse). In contrast to typical sleepwalking, these events may exceed 30 minutes.

Sleep-related violence occurs in a state consistent with sleepwalking or sleep terrors and is associated with an emotion of fear or anger. The violent behavior may be directed at individuals in proximity or those who confront the individual during the parasomnia. The patient may either awaken or go back to sleep but typically has amnesia for the event. The violence is often atypical of the individual. Most cases of sleep-related violence occur in middle-aged men with a history of prior sleepwalking.

Parasomnia Usually Associated with REM Sleep

Parasomnia types usually associated with REM sleep (stage R) include the REM sleep behavior disorder (RBD), recurrent isolated sleep paralysis, and nightmare disorders. RBD has two variants: overlap parasomnia and status dissociatus (SD). Discussion of SD is beyond the scope of this chapter.

REM SLEEP BEHAVIOR DISORDER (RBD) (INCLUDING VARIANTS)

RBD is characterized by a loss of the normal muscle atonia associated with REM sleep with dream-enactment behavior (oneirism) that is often violent in nature. Limb and body movements often are violent (e.g., hitting a wall, kicking) and may be associated with emotionally charged utterances. The movements may be related to dream content ("kicking an attacker"), but the patient *may* or *may not* remember associated dream material when awakened during an episode. Serious injury to the patient or the bed partner may result from these episodes, which typically occur one to four times a week. Because the episodes occur during REM sleep, they are most common during the early morning hours (the second half of the night). A strong male predominance exists, and the median age of onset is about 50 years. A milder prodrome of sleeptalking, simple limb-jerking, or vividly violent dreams may precede the full-blown syndrome. The pathophysiology of RBD includes dysfunction of areas of the brain responsible for atonia during REM sleep and also other areas of the brain (limbic system and others) involved with the generation of the violent dreams.

RBD—Causes and Associations

An acute form of RBD may occur after withdrawal from REM suppressants such as ethanol. Even after extensive evaluation, about 60% of cases of chronic RBD are idiopathic (iRBD). Causes of chronic RBD include multiple sclerosis, subarachnoid hemorrhage, dementia, ischemic cerebrovascular disease, and brainstem neoplasms. RBD may be associated with a number of neurologic disorders, including narcolepsy and alpha-synucleopathies, including Parkinson disease, Lewy body dementia, and multiple system atrophy. A recent update found that 81% of patients originally diagnosed with idiopathic RBD later developed Parkinson disease or an atypical Parkinson syndrome with a mean time interval of 13 years. Some studies have found that development of an abnormality in olfaction or color vision was associated a risk of developing Parkinson disease. A strong male predominance exists in RBD. The acute onset of RBD in a middle-aged woman with other neurologic complaints should raise the possibility of multiple sclerosis. Drug-induced or exacerbated cases of RBD have been reported with the use of monoamine oxidase inhibitors, TCAs (e.g., imipramine), SSRIs (e.g., fluoxetine), selective serotonin norepinephrine reuptake inhibitors (venlafaxine), and other antidepressants (mirtazapine). Bupropion has not been associated with RBD. Beta-blockers (bisoprolol, atenolol), anticholinesterase inhibitors, and selegiline may also trigger RBD. A sudden exacerbation of RBD may also occur when the dose of medications associated with RBD are increased. Some clinicians feel that drug associated RBD is really the result of the effects of a medication on a patient with latent RBD who would later develop idiopathic RBD.

Pseudo-RBD

A group of patients with a history of dreamenactment behavior and daytime sleepiness was found to have obstructive sleep apnea (OSA) on PSG but no evidence of REM sleep without atonia. Treatment with continuous positive airway pressure (CPAP) eliminated the behaviors. It is possible that increased pressure for REM sleep (prior REM sleep fragmentation) overwhelmed normal REM atonia processes in these cases. Of note, patients with both true RBD and OSA may also exhibit fewer RBD episodes when adequately treated with CPAP.

PSG in RBD

Video PSG, including both leg and arm EMG, is recommended. A given PSG study may or may not reveal an episode of abnormal behavior or body movements because most patients do not have nightly attacks. For this reason, some sleep centers perform multiple sleep studies if the diagnosis remains unclear. However, even if abnormal behavior is not documented by a given PSG study, evidence of REM sleep without atonia (tonic or phasic EMG abnormality during REM sleep) is usually present. The *American Academy of Sleep Medicine (AASM) Scoring Manual* provides criteria for scoring the EMG activity associated with RBD (Box F35-3). Sustained chin EMG activity may be noted. Excessive phasic activity (transient muscle activity [TMA]) may be noted on chin EMG, limb EMG (anterior tibial, flexor digitorum superficialis, extensor digitorum), or both. Some studies suggest that increased EMG activity in the arm muscles is more useful than leg EMG activity for distinguishing patients with RBD from normal individuals. When the chin EMG muscle activity is not reduced (e.g., in RBD), identification of REM sleep (versus stage W) may be challenging. Epochs could potentially be scored as stage W (REMs + increased chin EMG). Clues that abnormal REM sleep is present include the presence of sawtooth waves on EEG, excessive TMA on chin EMG, limb EMG, or both and alterations in air flow associated with bursts of eye movements. The heart rate also may remain constant despite the sudden appearance of increased EMG tone (as opposed to an awakening). TMA may also be mistaken for periodic limb movement in sleep (PLMS) activity. However, TMA usually contains many more brief spikes of activity. Of interest, during RBD body movements, video monitoring of the face will often show closed eyes but obvious movements of the eyes under the eyelids consistent with REMs. In contrast, during confusional arousals

BOX F35-3	Scoring Rules for the Electromyographic Activity Associated with the Rapid Eye Movement Sleep Behavior Disorder (RBD)

1. Polysomnography (PSG) findings of RBD are characterized by either or both of the following features:
   a. Sustained muscle activity in REM sleep on **chin electromyography (EMG).**
   b. Excessive transient muscle activity during REM on **chin or limb EMG.**

DEFINITIONS

Sustained muscle activity in REM sleep—an epoch of REM sleep with at least 50% of the duration of the epoch having a chin EMG amplitude greater than the minimum amplitude in non-REM (NREM) sleep.

Excessive transient muscle activity in REM sleep—in a 30-second epoch of REM sleep divided into 10 sequential 3-second mini-epochs, at least 5 (50%) of the mini-epochs contain bursts of transient muscle activity. In RBD, excessive transient muscle activity bursts are 0.1 to 5.0 seconds in duration and at least four times as high in amplitude as the background EMG activity.

or sleepwalking, the eyes are typically open, with a blank stare and dilated pupils (affected individual are minimally responsive).

The *AASM Scoring Manual* provides criteria to determine if a given epoch has sufficient activity on chin and limb EMG during REM sleep to be classified as abnormal or excessive (e.g., REM sleep without atonia [RSWA]). However, the number of such epochs (as a percentage of the total amount of REM sleep) that should be considered to be abnormal (sufficient supporting a diagnosis of RBD) was not specified. To date, no widely accepted method of defining the amount of RSWA to diagnose RBD exists. A study by Monteplasir et al published in 2010 suggested that RBD is supported by PSG findings of either (1) tonic chin EMG activity in >30% of REM sleep or (2) phasic chin EMG activity in >15% REM sleep, scored in 20-second epochs. An analysis by Frauscher et al published in 2012 suggested that any (tonic/phasic) chin EMG activity combined with bilateral phasic activity of the flexor digitorum superficialis muscles in >32% of REM sleep, scored in 3-second mini-epochs (or 27% scored in 30 second epochs) is evidence of sufficient RSWA to support a diagnosis of RBD. However, in these studies, some normal individuals showed abnormal activity, and some RBD individuals did not exhibit sufficient RSWA for their condition to be classified as abnormal. The ICSD-3 quotes the work of Frauscher et al and states that the most current evidence-based data for detecting RSWA in the evaluation of RBD indicate that any (tonic/phasic) chin EMG activity combined with bilateral phasic activity of the flexor digitorum superficialis muscles in >27% of REM sleep (scored in 30-second epochs) reliably distinguishes RBD patients from controls. Best criteria for determining sufficient RSWA to make a diagnosis of RBD have yet to be determined.

Diagnosis of RBD

The ICSD-3 criteria for RBD are listed in Box F35-4. The major points are demonstration of vocalization or complex motor behaviors (usually violent) during REM sleep (as recorded on video PSG or based on clinical history), demonstration of RSWA, and absence of EEG epileptiform activity during REM sleep. Seizure disorders may present with manifestations virtually identical to those of RBD. Therefore, making a diagnosis of RBD without PSG monitoring is not recommended. Absence of RSWA, body movements out of NREM sleep, or both would be inconsistent with RBD. Nocturnal epilepsy occurs most commonly out of NREM sleep but may rarely occur out of REM sleep (NREM > wake > REM). A detailed neurologic

---

BOX F35-4	Rapid Eye Movement Sleep Behavior Disorder (RBD)— Diagnostic Criteria

Criteria A-D must be met
A. Repeated episodes of sleep related vocalization and/or complex motor behaviors. (observation of repetitive episodes during a single night of video polysomnography).
B. These behaviors are documented by polysomnography to occur during REM sleep or, based on clinical history of dream enactment, are presumed to occur during REM sleep.
C. Polysomnographic recording demonstrates REM sleep without atonia (RSWA)
D. The disturbance is not better explained by another sleep disorder, mental disorder, or the sleep related eating disorder medication, or substance use.
Notes: observed vocalizations or behaviors often correlate with simultaneously occurring dream mentation, leading to the frequent report of "acting out one's dreams.")

From Adapted from American Academy of Sleep Medicine: *International classification of sleep disorders*, ed 3, Darien, IL, 2014, American Academy of Sleep Medicine.

---

evaluation of patients suspected of having RBD is indicated with attention to symptoms and signs of associated neurologic disorders such as Parkinson disease. Magnetic resonance imaging (MRI) of the brain (to rule out structural causes) and full clinical EEG (preferably during sleep) are usually performed if manifestations are atypical or patients do not respond to therapy.

Variants of RBD

REM Sleep without Atonia

This variant includes findings of RSWA without a clinical history of RBD. Limb twitching may occur without overt body movements. This is common in patients taking SSRIs. Some evidence suggests that some of these patients go on to develop RBD.

Parasomnia Overlap Disorder

Parasomnia overlap disorder consists of a combination of RBD and NREM parasomnia (i.e., confusional arousals, sleepwalking, sleep terrors, or the sleep related eating disorder). Diagnostic criteria for both RBD and one or more of the NREM parasomnias must be met. Most patients with overlap parasomnia had some manifestation of some type of NREM parasomnia in childhood. Overlap parasomnia may be idiopathic or associated with narcolepsy, multiple sclerosis, brain tumor, and psychiatric disorders. The disorder may respond to treatments used for RBD, for example, clonazepam.

Treatment of RBD

No randomized, controlled clinical trials for the treatment of RBD have been performed. Best clinical practice guidelines for the treatment of RBD developed by the Standards of Practice Committee of the AASM have been published following a systematic review of the published literature. Environmental precautions are an essential first step in RBD treatment because even with effective treatment with medications, breakthrough episodes do occur. Environmental precautions include having the bedmate sleep in a separate room or bed, closed and locked windows and doors, removal of furniture with sharp edges, and use of mattresses or pads on the floor near the bed.

The strongest evidence for effective RBD treatment is for the use of clonazepam. Successful treatment of RBD has been achieved in approximately 80% to 90% of patients with clonazepam 0.5 to 2 mg ($\leq$4 mg) given 30 minutes before bedtime. Clonazepam dramatically reduces episode frequency or severity but is some studies did not eliminate the finding of RSWA. The medication also does not work by decreasing the amount of REM sleep. Clonazepam may modify dream content or inhibit the brainstem locomotor pattern generators. Clonazepam has a half-life of 30 to 40 hours and may cause early morning sedation, confusion, motor incoordination, or memory dysfunction. It may also increase the risk of falls or worsen OSA. A response hierarchy with increasing doses has been described: vigorous violent behavior > complex nonvigorous behavior > simple limb jerking > excessive EMG twitching in stage R. Unfortunately, a significant proportion of RBD patients treated with clonazepam have one or more significant side effects. Melatonin in doses of 3 to 12 mg has also been found to be effective treatment for RBD either as a sole agent or as an add-on to clonazepam. Side effects of melatonin include hallucinations, morning headaches, nightmares, and morning sleepiness. Some studies suggest that in contrast to clonazepam, melatonin decreases the number of stage R epochs without atonia. Successful treatment of RBD has also been reported (case reports with small patient numbers) with pramipexole (total dose 0.75–1.5 mg), paroxetine, acetylcholinesterase inhibitors, BZRAs other than clonazepam (temazepam, triazolam, alprazolam), clozapine, Yi-Gan San (a herbal medication), and carbamazepine.

RECURRENT ISOLATED SLEEP PARALYSIS

Recurrent isolated sleep paralysis is characterized by inability to move at sleep onset (hypnogogic) or on awakening (hypnopompic). Patients are awake and have full recall of the event. Although diaphragmatic function is not affected, a sensation of dyspnea is common. Episodes may be aborted by touching or speaking to the affected individual or by the individual making intense efforts to move. Sleep paralysis is also common in patients with narcolepsy and idiopathic hypersomnia. The term *isolated* refers to the fact that other sleep disorders such as narcolepsy or idiopathic hypersomnia are not present. The frequency of sleep paralysis episodes is very variable—once per lifetime to several per month. Hallucinatory experiences accompany sleep paralysis in 25% to 75% of individuals. Studies of students suggested that 15% to 40% had experienced as least one episode of sleep paralysis. Sleep disruption, irregular sleep periods, sleep deprivation, and stress are known triggers. In most cases, treatment with medications is not needed. Avoiding sleep deprivation and following a regular sleep pattern may help prevent isolated sleep paralysis: SSRIs (in antidepressant doses) and TCAs (low doses) are usually effective treatment for isolated sleep paralysis. None of these medications are approved for this indication by the U.S. Food and Drug Administration (FDA).

NIGHTMARE DISORDER

Nightmare disorder (dream anxiety attacks) are characterized by recurrent nightmares, which are disturbing mental experiences that usually occur during REM sleep and often result in awakening. Nightmares may follow acute trauma (acute stress disorder [ASD]) or occur 1 month or more after trauma (posttraumatic stress disorder [PTSD]). The dreams of PTSD may occur out of NREM stages N2 or N3, during REM sleep, and at sleep onset. A number of medications may also be associated with nightmares (see Fundamentals 8), including efavirenez, pramipexole, donezepril, and varenicline. About 50% to 80% of adults reports one or more nightmares.[1] In 10% to 50% of children age 3 to 5, the experience of nightmares is severe enough to awaken their parents from sleep. Nightmares within 3 months of trauma are present in up to 80% patients with PTSD. Few PSG studies of nightmares exist, but typically, accelerated heart rate and respiratory rate precede awakening from REM sleep with report of a nightmare.

Diagnosis of Nightmare Disorder

The *International Classification of Sleep Disorders*, Third Edition (ICSD-3) diagnostic criteria for the nightmare disorder are listed in Box F35-5.

BOX F35-5	Nightmare Disorder Diagnostic Criteria (ICSD-3)

A. **Repeated occurrences** of extended, extremely dysphoric, and well-remembered dreams that usually involve threats to survival, security or physical integrity.

B. The episodes generally occur during the second half of the major sleep episode.

C. On awakening from the dysphoric dreams, the person rapidly becomes oriented and alert.

D. The dream experience, or the sleep disturbance produced by awakening from it, causes clinically significant distress or impairment in social, occupational, or other important areas of functioning as indicated by the report of ***at least one*** of the following:

1. Mood disturbance (i.e., persistence of nightmare effect, anxiety, dysphoria)
2. Sleep resistance (i.e., bedtime anxiety, fear of sleep or subsequent nightmares)
3. Cognitive impairments (i.e., intrusive nightmare imagery, concentration, impaired memory)
4. Negative impact on caregiver or family functioning (i.e., nighttime disruption)
5. Behavioral problems (i.e., bedtime avoidance, fear of the dark)
6. Daytime sleepiness
7. Fatigue or low energy
8. Impaired occupational or educational function
9. Impaired interpersonal or social function

Note that repeated episodes and adverse consequences are both required to meet the criteria for the diagnosis. One would probably not classify the rare occurrence of a nightmare as a disorder given the high percentage of normal individuals experiencing an occasional nightmare. A diagnosis of nightmare disorder requires that the dream or awakening must cause significant distress or impairment of social function, including mood disturbance and resistance to going to sleep.

Treatment of Nightmare Disorder

If a medication is temporally associated with nightmares, a trial of medication discontinuation or change is prudent. Cognitive behavioral treatments have been used to treat nightmares with some success. One behavioral technique called *imagery rehearsal therapy* has proved successful in several studies. Patients are asked to rewrite their previous dreams with a positive outcome. In the past, use of medications for nightmares had limited success. Recently, several studies report success with the alpha₁-blocker prazosin

in nightmares associated with PTSD. Doses of 2 to 12 mg have been used (usually 3 to 6 mg). Note that when prazosin is started, the drug should be initiated with a dose of 1 mg at bedtime to avoid severe first-dose hypotension (often orthostatic hypotension). The drug may then be titrated upward slowly over several nights.

BIBLIOGRAPHY

American Academy of Sleep Medicine: *International classification of sleep disorders: diagnostic and coding manual*, ed 3, Darien, IL, 2013, American Academy of Sleep Medicine.

American Academy of Sleep Medicine: *International classification of sleep disorders: diagnostic and coding manual*, ed 2, Westchester, IL, 2005, American Academy of Sleep Medicine.

Aurora RN, Zak RS, Maganti RK, et al: Best practice guidelines for the treatment of REM sleep behavior disorder (RBD), *J Clin Sleep Med* 6:85–95, 2010.

Aurora RN, Zak RS, Auerbach SH, et al: Best practice guide for the treatment of nightmare disorder in adults, *J Clin Sleep Med* 6(4):389–401, 2010.

Boeve BF, Silber MH, Ferman TJ: Melatonin for treatment of REM sleep behavior disorder in neurological disorders: results in 14 patients, *Sleep Med* 4:281–284, 2003.

Boeve BF, Silber MH, Saper CB, et al: Pathophysiology of REM sleep behavior disorder and relevance to neurodegenerative disease, *Brain* 130:2770–2788, 2007.

Frauscher B, Iranzo A, Gaig C, et al: Normative EMG values during REM sleep for the diagnosis of REM sleep behavior disorder, *Sleep* 35(6):835–847, 2012.

Guilleminault C, Kirisogluc C, Bao G, et al: Adult chronic sleepwalking and its treatment based on polysomnography, *Brain* 128:1062–1069, 2005.

Harris M, Grunstein RR: Treatments for somnabulism in adults: assessing the evidence, *Sleep Med Rev* 13:295–297, 2009.

Iber C, Ancoli-Israel S, Chesson A, Quan SF: for the American Academy of Sleep Medicine: *The AASM manual for the scoring of sleep and associated events: rules, terminology and technical specification*, ed 1, Westchester, IL, 2007, American Academy of Sleep Medicine.

Iranzo A, Santamaria J: Severe obstructive sleep apnea/hypopnea mimicking REM sleep behavior disorder, *Sleep* 28:203–206, 2005.

Krakow B, Hollifield M, Johnston L, et al: Imagery rehearsal therapy for chronic nightmares in sexual assault survivors with post-traumatic stress disorder, *JAMA* 286:537–545, 2001.

Millman RP, Kipp GJ, Carskadon MA: Sleepwalking precipitated by treatment of sleep apnea with nasal CPAP, *Chest* 99:750–751, 1991.

Montplaisir J, Gagnon JF, Fantini ML, et al: Polysomnographic diagnosis of idiopathic REM sleep behavior disorder, *Mov Disord* 25(13):2044–2051, 2010.

Pagel JF, Helfter P: Drug-induced nightmares—an etiology-based review, *Hum Psychopharmacol Clin Exp* 18:59–67, 2003.

Pressman MR, Meyer TJ, Kendrick-Mohamed J, et al: Night terrors in adults precipitated by sleep apnea, *Sleep* 18:773–775, 1995.

Raskind MA, Peskind ER, Hoff DJ, et al: A parallel group placebo-controlled study of prazosin for trauma nightmares and sleep disturbance in combat veterans with post-traumatic stress disorder, *Biol Psychiatry* 61:928–934, 2007.

Schenck CH, Arnulf I, Mahowald MW: Sleep and sex: what can go wrong? A review of the literature on sleep related disorders and abnormal sexual behaviors and experiences, *Sleep* 30:683–702, 2007.

Schenck CH, Bundlie SR, Patterson AL, et al: Rapid eye movement sleep behavior disorder: a treatable parasomnia affecting older males, *JAMA* 257:1786–1789, 1987.

Schenck CH, Mahowald MW: On the reported association of psychopathology with sleep terrors in adults, *Sleep* 23:1–2, 2000.

Schenck CH, Mahowald MW: REM sleep behavior disorder: clinical, developmental, and neuroscience perspective 16 years after its formal identification in sleep, *Sleep* 25:120–138, 2002.

Schenck CH, Milner DM, Hurwitz TD, et al: A polysomnographic and clinical report of sleep related injury in 100 adult patients, *Am J Psychiatry* 146:1166–1172, 1989.

Schenck CH, Boeve BF, Mahowald MW: Delayed emergence of a parkinsonian disorder or dementia in 81% of older males initially diagnosed with idiopathic REM sleep behavior disorder (RBD): 16 year update on a previously reported series, *Sleep Med* 14:744–748, 2013.

Winkleman JW, James L: Serotonergic antidepressants are associated with REM sleep without atonia, *Sleep* 27:317–321, 2004.

PATIENT 100

A 20-Year-Old Student with Severe "Nightmares"

A 20-year-old male college student was evaluated for disturbing behavior during sleep. His roommate was awakened about once a month to find the patient sitting up in bed screaming. During these episodes, the patient was awake, confused, sweaty, and very fearful. The patient's roommate attempted to calm him down, but he usually did not respond or answer questions. At other times, the patient was noted to awaken abruptly, sit up, look around, mumble something, and then return to sleep without screaming. These less severe events happened almost every night. The patient reported sleepwalking as a child, but this problem had resolved by the time he was an adolescent. Although most of the screaming episodes were noted during the first one third of the night, a few happened during the early morning hours. The patient denied symptoms of anxiety or depression and had not started any new medications recently. The patient had gained about 10 pounds over 3 months and did snore loudly when supine. Figure P100-1 is a 30-second tracing. Following arousal, the patient sat up and looked around in a confused state. On audio, he was heard to mumble something about his car.

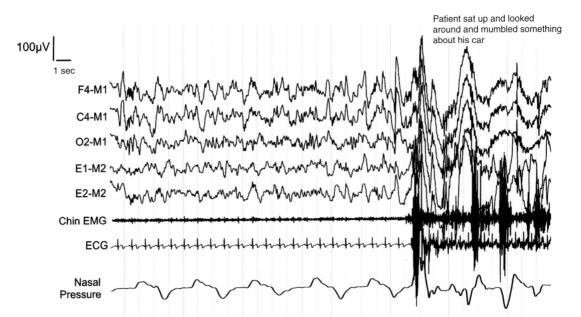

FIGURE P100-1 ■ A 30-second tracing. At the end of the epoch, the patient sat up abruptly, looked around, and mumbled something about his car.

QUESTION

1. What is your diagnosis?

ANSWER

1. **Answer:** Non– rapid eye movement (NREM) parasomnia: sleep terror and confusional arousals.

Discussion: The traditional classification of the types of NREM parasomnia includes (1) confusional arousals, (2) sleepwalking, and (3) sleep terrors. Considerable overlap exists in these types of parasomnia, and individual patients may manifest behaviors consistent with all three types on different nights (Table P100-1). Sleep terrors, also called *night terrors* or *pavor nocturnus*, consist of sudden arousal from NREM sleep, accompanied by a scream or cry and manifestations of severe fear (behavioral and autonomic). The affected individual typically is confused, diaphoretic, and tachycardic, and he or she frequently sits up in bed. It is difficult or impossible to communicate with a person having a sleep terror, and total amnesia about the event is usual. Confusional arousals are also somewhat similar to night terrors. Individuals are very confused following spontaneous or forced arousals from sleep (e.g., on hearing a noise). However, in contrast to night terrors, no autonomic hyperactivity, signs of fear, and blood curdling scream are observed. Although about two thirds of adults manifesting NREM parasomnia report a history or similar episodes during childhood, about one third experience onset of these behaviors in adulthood. Sleep terrors occur in about 3% of children but usually resolve by adolescence. Although sleep terrors are less common than confusional arousals in adults, this type of NREM parasomnia may occur and does not imply psychopathology or a neurologic disorder. Often, a period of stress or sleep deprivation triggers the return of the episodes in a patient who had them in childhood. For example, college students may experience a return of sleepwalking, confusional arousals, or sleep terrors during periods of stress and reduced sleep. In children, fever, acute illness, or any stressful event or new sleep environment may trigger NREM parasomnia. Slow-wave sleep rebound, as occurs with nasal continuous positive airway pressure (CPAP) treatment of obstructive sleep apnea (OSA), also has been associated with episodes sleep terrors.

In children, NREM parasomnia occurs during stage N3 sleep (in the first one third of the night) but in adults may occur during stage N1, N2, or N3 at any time during the night.

The differential diagnosis of night terrors includes nightmares, nocturnal seizure activity, the REM behavior disorder (RBD), and posttraumatic stress syndrome. Nightmares (dream anxiety attacks) and RBD occur during REM sleep and are more common in the second part of the night. RBD usually does not begin until after age 40. Definitive differentiation of NREM parasomnia from partial complex seizures is difficult without complete video and electroencephalography (EEG) monitoring. Seizures tend to be more stereotypical and may occur during the day (Table P100-2). Nocturnal frontal lobe epilepsy (NFLE) is the seizure disorder most likely to mimic an NREM parasomnia. Provini and colleagues described three general manifestations of NFLE, including paroxysmal arousals (PAs), nocturnal paroxysmal dystonia (NPD), and episodic

TABLE P100-1 **Comparison of the Characteristics of Non–Rapid Eye Movement Parasomnia Types**

	Confusional Arousal	Sleep Walking	Sleep Terrors
Onset in children	Stage N3	Same	Same
Onset in adults	N1, N2, N3	Same	Same
Autonomic hyperactivity	No	No	Prominent
Loud scream	No	No	Yes
Confusion during episode	Yes	Yes	Yes
Amnesia (partial or complete)	Yes	Yes	Yes

TABLE P100-2	Comparison of Characteristics of Nocturnal Frontal Lobe Epilepsy and Non–Rapid Eye Movement (NREM) Parasomnia	
	Nocturnal Frontal Lobe Epilepsy	**NREM Parasomnia**
Age of onset	14 ± 10	< 10 in two thirds About one third onset in adulthood
Movement seminology	Often violent, stereotypical	Complex, nonsterotypical
Episodes per night	Three or more common (especially paroxysmal arousal and nocturnal paroxysmal dystonia types)	1
Event duration	2 seconds to 3 minutes	15 sec–30 min
Autonomic activation	Very common (tachycardia)	Only in Sleep terror
Electroencephalography (EEG)	Episodes during NREM sleep Ictal: normal 50% with scalp electrodes Interictal EEG: normal in about 50%	Stage N3 children Stages N2, N3 adults NREM sleep with arousal
Clinical course	Increasing frequency	Tends to resolve

Adapted from Provini F, Plazzi G, Tinuper P, et al: Nocturnal frontal lobe epilepsy, *Brain* 122:1017-1031, 1999.

nocturnal wandering (ENW). *Paroxysmal arousals* (PAs) typically present during NREM sleep and consist of a stereotypical series of movements lasting 2 to 20 seconds in which the individuals raise the head, sit up, and look around confused with a frightened expression and then scream. Unlike typical sleep terrors, *PAs can occur many times during the night and are very sterotypical*. NPD is characterized by nocturnal coarse movements associated with tonic spasms that often occur multiple times per night. The episodes may be violent or be associated with vocalization. Patients often move the arms and legs with cycling or kicking movements and sometimes adopt a dystonic posture of the limbs. *Episodic nocturnal wanderings* (ENWs) may present with symptoms similar to sleepwalking and sleep terrors. Patients may jump out of bed, wander, vocalize, and exhibit violent behavior during sleep. In summary, PAs mimic sleep terrors and ENWs mimic sleepwalking. Classically, treatment with older-generation anticonvulsants (in particular, carbamazepine) or newer-generation anticonvulsants such as levetiracetam at bedtime is generally effective. However, some patients are refractory to antiepileptic medications. The facts that multiple episodes occur in one might and that they are all very similar differentiates these events from an NREM parasomia. Episodes of NFLE often occur out of NREM sleep (more common in stage N2), and frequently no EEG abnormality other than muscle artifact is noted (in over 50%, no ictal activity can be detected). Patients with nightmares, the posttraumatic stress syndrome, and RBD typically may relate complex dream mentation that promoted the event.

Polysomnography (PSG) usually is not required to evaluate sleep terrors unless the episodes are frequent, are violent, or have the potential to result in self-injury. When PSG is performed, inclusion of video monitoring (synchronized if possible) is ideal. If seizures are suspected, a complete clinical EEG montage is needed. When a night terror is captured, it appears as a sudden arousal from slow-wave sleep. Electromyography (EMG) amplitude is greatly increased, and alpha-waves are present; however, persistent slow-wave activity also is often noted.

If the episodes of night terrors are infrequent, treatment beyond simple environmental precautions is unnecessary. Several medications, including benzodiazepines (clonazepam 0.5 to 2 milligrams at bed time [mg qhs]), tricyclic antidepressants, and selective serotonin reuptake inhibitors, have been used with some success. Avoidance of inciting agents is recommended.

In the present case, PSG was preformed to rule out sleep apnea (loud snoring) and because the episodes were extremely worrisome to the patient. PSG recorded a confusional arousal out of stage N3 sleep (Figure P100-1), but no significant sleep apnea was present. The patient seemed well adjusted emotionally. He was told that irregular sleep patterns were probably responsible for the reappearance of the episodes. As he wanted to avoid medication at all costs, the patient diligently maintained good sleep habits and reported only one minor episode every 6 months.

CLINICAL PEARLS

1. Sleep terrors and characterized by awakening from NREM sleep with a loud scream and manifestations of intense fear. Complete amnesia about the event is usually present.
2. About two thirds of adults experiencing NREM parasomnia had a history of similar events during childhood.
3. Patients may exhibit all three variations of the NREM parasomnias (sleep terrors, confusional arousals, and sleep walking) or a combination of them on a given night.
4. NREM parasomnia occurs during stage N3 in the first one third of the night in children. In adults, NREM parasomnia may occur during stages N1, N2, or N3 in any part of the night.
5. The persistence of NREM parasomnia into adulthood or onset in adulthood is not necessarily evidence that psychopathology is present.
6. Unlike nightmares and RBD, patients with night terrors cannot relate dream mentation associated with the event.
7. Night terrors have been described in adults during nasal CPAP treatment for OSA.
8. NFLE may mimic NREM parasomnia. Video PSG as well as a complete set of EEG electrodes is needed. However, EEG may not show ictal activity in over 50% of cases. In contrast to NREM parasomnia, events tend to be sterotypical, and multiple episodes may occur in a single night.

BIBLIOGRAPHY

American Academy of Sleep Medicine: *International classification of sleep disorders: diagnostic and coding manual*, ed 2, Westchester, IL, 2005, American Academy of Sleep Medicine.

Derry CP, Harvey AS, Walker MC, et al: NREM arousal parasomnias and their distinction from nocturnal frontal lobe epilepsy: a video EEG analysis, *Sleep* 32:1637–1644, 2009.

Guilleminault C, Kirisogluc C, Bao G, et al: Adult chronic sleepwalking and its treatment based on polysomnography, *Brain* 128:1062–1069, 2005.

Harris M, Grunstein RR: Treatments for somnabulism in adults: assessing the evidence, *Sleep Med Rev* 13:295–297, 2009.

Mahowald MW, Ettinger MG: Things that go bump in the night—parasomnias revisited, *J Clin Neurophysiol* 7:119–143, 1990.

Millman RP, Kipp GJ, Carskadon MA: Sleepwalking precipitated by treatment of sleep apnea with nasal CPAP, *Chest* 99:750–751, 1991.

Pressman MR, Meyer TJ, Kendrick-Mohamed J, et al: Night terrors in adults precipitated by sleep apnea, *Sleep* 18:773–775, 1995.

Provini F, Plazzi G, Montagna P, Lugaresi E: The wide spectrum of nocturnal frontal lobe epilepsy, *Sleep Med Rev* 4:375–386, 2000.

Provini F, Plazzi G, Tinuper P, et al: Nocturnal frontal lobe epilepsy, *Brain* 122:1017–1031, 1999.

Schenck C, Pareja JA, Patterson AL, Mahowald MW: Analysis of polysomnographic events surrounding 252 slow wave sleep arousals in thirty-eight adults with injurious sleep walking and sleep terrors, *J Clin Neurophysiol* 15:159–166, 1998.

Schenck CH, Mahowald MW: On the reported association of psychopathology with sleep terrors in adults, *Sleep* 23:1–2, 2000.

Schenck CH, Milner DM, Hurwitz TD, et al: A polysomnographic and clinical report of sleep related injury in 100 adult patients, *Am J Psychiatry* 146:1166–1172, 1989.

Shapiro CM, Trajanovic NN, Fedoroff JP: Sex-somnia: a new parasomnia? *Can J Psychiatry* 48:311–317, 2003.

Tachiban N, Shinde A, Ikeda A, et al: Supplementary motor area seizure resembling sleep disorder, *Sleep* 19:811–816, 1996.

Violent Behavior During Sleep

Patient A: A 60-year-old man was evaluated because of violent behavior during sleep. During sleep, he sometimes appeared to be acting out a dream and hit his wife on several occasions. When she managed to awaken the patient, he reported that he was dreaming that he was fighting with an attacker. The episodes tend to occur about three times a week and usually in the last half of the night. The episodes had become more frequent and violent after the patient was started on venlafaxine for depression. Video polysomnography (PSG) was ordered, but no violent behavior was recorded. Figure P101-1 shows a typical epoch of stage R.

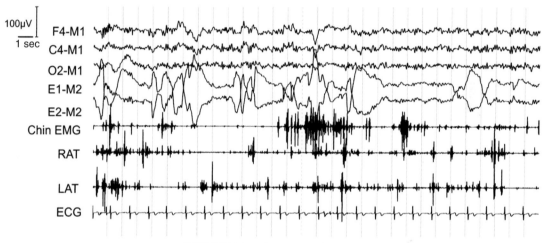

FIGURE P101-1 ■ A 30-second tracing.

Question 1: What is your diagnosis for Patient A? What neurologic disorder may develop in this patient?

Patient B: A 50-year-old man was evaluated for loud snoring, witnessed apnea, and daytime sleepiness. His wife also reported that he sometimes moved violently during sleep and once had hit her in the face. The patient was not taking an antidepressant and had no neurologic symptoms. Figure P101-2 shows a typical 30-second epoch of stage R.

Question 2: What is your diagnosis for Patient B?

ANSWERS

1. **Answer for Patient A:** Rapid eye movement (REM) sleep behavior disorder; risk of developing Parkinson disease or atypical Parkinson disease.

   Discussion: The diagnosis of REM sleep behavior disorder requires demonstration of REM sleep without atonia (RSWA) and either PSG video documenting body movement during stage R or a compatible history of violent dream enactment. RSWA alone is *not* sufficient (see Fundamentals 35). Patients taking selective serotonin reuptake inhibitors (SSRIs) may demonstrate phasic muscle activity during stage R. Recent studies by Frausher et al suggest that using a combination of chin, leg, and arm EMG is more sensitive for detection of RSWA than using only the chin and legs. The exact number of epochs with REM sleep without atonia needed for a diagnosis of RBD is not defined in the *American Academy of Sleep Medicine (AASM) Scoring Manual*. Criteria for what constitutes an epoch with RSWA have been established (see Fundamentals 16). The number of epochs with RSWA needed to make a diagnosis of RBD remains uncertain. The ICSD-3 states that "the

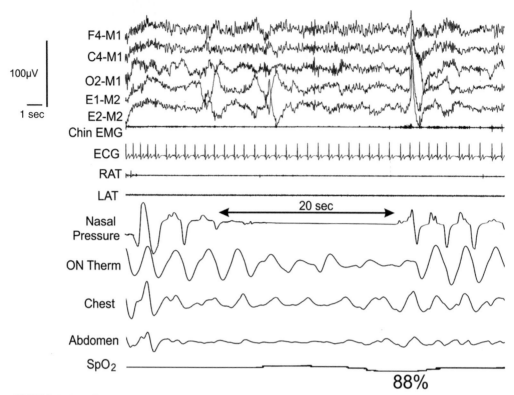

FIGURE P101-2 ■ A 30-second tracing. RAT and LAT are right and left anterior tibial (leg) EMG tracings.

most current evidence-based data for detecting RSWA in the evaluation of RBD indicate that any (tonic/phasic) chin EMG activity combined with bilateral phasic activity of the flexor digitorum superficialis muscles in >27% of REM sleep (scored in 30-second epochs) reliably distinguishes RBD patients from controls." In the current patient (see Figure P101-1), increased phasic muscle activity was noted on both leg electromyography (EMG) and chin EMG (both present for more than 50% of the epoch shown). Of note, 30% of REM epochs contained evidence of RSWA. In addition, the patient was noted to move his arms violently, and this was recorded on video.

Seizure disorders may present with manifestations virtually identical to those of RBD. Therefore, making a diagnosis of RBD without PSG monitoring is not recommended. *Absence* of RSWA, body movements out of REM sleep, or both would be *inconsistent* with RBD. Nocturnal epilepsy occurs most commonly during NREM sleep but may rarely occur during REM sleep (seizure occurrence: NREM sleep > wakefulness > REM sleep). A detailed neurologic evaluation of patients suspected of having RBD is indicated with attention to symptoms and signs of associated neurologic disorders such as Parkinson disease. Magnetic resonance imaging (MRI) of the brain (to rule out structural causes) and full clinical EEG (preferably during sleep) are usually performed especially if manifestations are atypical or patients do not respond to therapy.

Patients with RBD are at risk for developing Parkinson disease, but the interval between RBD and the onset of Parkinson disease may be up to 20 years. One recent series found 81% conversion rate from idiopathic RBD to parkinsonism or dementia with a mean interval of 13 years. Conversely, RBD is present in >90% of reported cases of multiple system atrophy (MSA) and in approximately 50% of reported cases of dementia with Lewy bodies (DLB). Patients with MSA or DLB often develop RBD concurrently with the manifestations of those disorders (see Patient 109). In the current patient, starting venlafaxine may have exacerbated the RBD, but history revealed that dream enactment was present before starting that medication.

2. **Answer (for Patient B):** Pseudo-RBD.

Discussion: A group of patients with a history of dream enactment behavior and daytime sleepiness was found to have obstructive sleep apnea (OSA) on PSG but no evidence of RSWA. Treatment with continuous positive airway pressure (CPAP) eliminated the behaviors. It is possible that increased pressure for REM sleep (prior REM sleep fragmentation) overwhelms normal REM atonia processes in these cases. Of note, patients with both *true RBD and OSA* may also exhibit fewer

RBD episodes when adequately treated with CPAP. In the present case, PSG showed an apnea–hypopnea index (AHI) of 25 per hour (hr) overall and 50/hr during REM sleep. The tracing in Figure P101-2 shows hypopnea, but chin EMG and the left and right anterior tibial EMG (LAT, RAT) do not show evidence of RSWA. Of note, a few patients with OSA may not clearly exhibit RSWA until treated with CPAP, as they may have very reduced amount of REM sleep in the untreated state. During the first night on CPAP, REM rebound and a high REM density may be seen in some patients. Caution must be exercised in making a diagnosis of pseudo-RBD and monitor the patient carefully. Repeat PSG after a period of CPAP treatment may document RSWA, and a diagnosis of both OSA an RBD may be appropriate. The current patient was treated with nasal CPAP, and the problem of violent dream enactment resolved. He and his bed partner were advised to take environmental precautions. The patient will be monitored closely for the possibility of manifestations of RBD in the future.

CLINICAL PEARLS

1. A diagnosis of RBD requires both evidence of RSWA *and* either video PSG confirmation of body movement during REM sleep or a compatible clinical history of violent dream enactment.

2. A significant proportion of patients with "idiopathic RBD" are at risk for development of Parkinson disease, but latency may be up to 20 years (mean 13 years). RBD is common in patients with multiple system atrophy or Lewy Body dementia.

3. Pseudo-RBD is defined as a violent dream enactment associated with untreated OSA in the absence of evidence for RSWA. Resolution of symptoms occurs with adequate treatment of OSA. However, the combination of OSA and RBD is not rare. Some patients with the combination improve with adequate treatment of OSA.

BIBLIOGRAPHY

American Academy of Sleep Medicine: *International classification of sleep disorders*, ed 3, Darien, IL, 2014, American Academy of Sleep Medicine.

Boeve BF, Silber MH, Saper CB, et al: Pathophysiology of REM sleep behavior disorder and relevance to neurodegenerative disease, *Brain* 130:2770–2788, 2007.

Frauscher B, Iranzo A, Högl B, et al: Quantification of EMG activity during REM sleep in multiple muscles in REM sleep behavior disorder, *Sleep* 31:724–731, 2008.

Frauscher B, Iranzo A, Gaig C, et al: Normative EMG values during REM sleep for the diagnosis of REM sleep behavior disorder, *SLEEP* 35(6):835–847, 2012.

Iranzo A, Santamaria J: Severe obstructive sleep apnea/hypopnea mimicking REM sleep behavior disorder, *Sleep* 28:203–206, 2005.

Mahowald MW, Ettinger MG: Things that go bump in the night—parasomnias revisited, *J Clin Neurophysiol* 7:119–143, 1990.

Schenck CH, Boyd JL, Mahowald MW: A parasomnia overlap disorder involving sleep walking, sleep terrors, and REM sleep behavior disorder in 33 polysomnographically confirmed cases, *Sleep* 20:972–981, 1997.

Schenck CH, Mahowald MW: REM sleep behavior disorder: clinical, developmental, and neuroscience perspective 16 years after its formal identification in sleep, *Sleep* 25:120–138, 2002.

Schenck CH, Milner DM, Hurwitz TD, et al: A polysomnographic and clinical report of sleep related injury in 100 adult patients, *Am J Psychiatry* 146:1166–1172, 1989.

Schenck CH, Boeve B, Mahowald MW: Delayed emergence of a parkinsonian disorder or dementia in 81% of older males initially diagnosed with idiopathic REM sleep behavior disorder (RBD): 16 year update on a previously reported series, *Sleep Med* 14:744–748, 2013.

PATIENT 102

Patients with Violent Dreams

Patient A: A 60-year-old man was diagnosed as having rapid eye movement (REM) sleep behavior disorder. The patient punched and kicked during sleep. His wife was hit in the face during one episode, so she moved to another bed in the same room. The patient was started on clonazepam 0.5 milligram (mg), with a progressive increase in dose until his symptoms were controlled. Unfortunately, on an effective dose of 1.5 mg at bedtime, he experienced unacceptable daytime sleepiness.

Question 1: What treatment do you recommend for Patient A?

Patient B: A 55-year-old man was evaluated for both violent dream enactment and episodes of sleepwalking. The patient had a history of sleepwalking as a child. The episodes persisted into adulthood but had been infrequent until the last 2 years. In addition to the sleepwalking episodes, the patient was reported to act out violent dreams of fighting. During one episode, he hit the bedside table, which resulted in fracture of two of his fingers. The patient's wife then started to sleep in another room adjoining the bedroom. However, on one occasion, the patient walked across the bedroom into the room where his wife was sleeping, got into her bed, and displayed violent sexual behavior that was completely different from his usual behavior. He had amnesia about the event the following day. His medications included lisinopril and levothyroxine. No history of tremor, rigidity, balance problems, or any psychiatric disorder was present.

Video polysomnography (PSG) revealed two confusional arousals during stage N3 and REM sleep without atonia (RSWA). During REM sleep, he was also noted to hit the bed on several occasions.

Question 2: What is your diagnosis for Patient B?

ANSWERS

1. **Answer (for Patient A):** Addition of melatonin and reduction in the dose of clonazepam.

   Discussion: No randomized, controlled clinical trials have been conducted on treatment of RBD. Evidence for treatment comes from case series or anecdotal case reports. A best clinical practice guideline for the treatment of RBD, developed by the Standards of Practice Committee of the American Academy of Sleep Medicine (AASM), was published following a systematic review of the published literature. Some of the recommendations are discussed here. Environmental precautions are an essential first step in RBD treatment because even with effective treatment with medications, breakthrough episodes do occur. Environmental precautions include having the bedmate sleep in a separate room or bed and removal of furniture with sharp edges (or having minimal furniture near the bed). If falling out of bed is an issue, sleeping on a mattress close to the floor or using pads on the floor near the bed are options.

   The most evidence for an effective medication for RBD treatment is for clonazepam. Successful treatment of RBD has been achieved with clonazepam 0.5 to 2 mg ($\leq$4 mg) given 30 minutes before bedtime in approximately 80% to 90% of patients. Clonazepam dramatically reduces episode frequency or severity but usually does not eliminate the findings of RSWA. Information in the literature on this subject is conflicting. Clonazepam does not work by decreasing the amount of REM sleep. The medication may modify dream content or inhibit the brainstem locomotor pattern generators. Clonazepam has a half-life of 30 to 40 hours and may cause early morning sedation, confusion, motor incoordination, depression, or memory dysfunction. It may also increase risk of falls or worsen obstructive sleep apnea (OSA). A response hierarchy with increasing doses has been described: vigorous violent behavior → complex nonvigorous behavior → simple limb jerking → excessive twitching in stage R, as shown by electromyography (EMG). Unfortunately, a significant proportion of patients with RBD treated with clonazepam have experienced one or more significant side effects.

   Melatonin in doses of 3 to 12 mg has also been found to be effective treatment for RBD, either as a sole agent or as an addition to clonazepam. Side effects of melatonin include hallucinations, morning headaches, nightmares, constipation, and morning sleepiness. In contrast to clonazepam, some studies suggest that melatonin decreases the number of stage R epochs without atonia (Kunz et al). Of note, melatonin has a short half-life. Sustained-action forms of melatonin are available, but their advantage over routine melatonin preparations in RBD has not been demonstrated.

   Successful treatment of RBD has also been reported (case reports with small patient numbers) with pramipexole (total dose 0.75–1.5 mg), paroxetine, acetylcholinesterase inhibitors, benzodiazepine receptor agonists (BZRAs) other than clonazepam (temazepam, triazolam, alprazolam), clozapine, Yi-Gan San (a herbal medication), and carbamazepine. Recently, Howell et al found that use of a customized bed alarm system that incorporates the reassuring voice of a loved one was effective at reducing episodes of RBD. If episodes of what appears to be RBD do *not* respond to clonazepam but *do* respond to an antiepileptic medication such as carbamazepine, it suggests that a seizure disorder, rather than RBD, may actually be present.

2. **Answer (Patient B):** The Parasomnia overlap disorder.

Discussion: The Parasomnia overlap disorder consists of the combination of RBD and a disorder of arousal (confusional arousals, sleepwalking, and sleep terrors). Some clinicians also use the term for the combination of RBD with either sleep-related eating disorder, sex-somnia, or rhythmic movement disorder. Diagnostic criteria for both RBD and one or more types of NREM parasomnia (or sleep-related eating disorder, etc.) must be met. Most patients with overlap parasomnia had some manifestation of NREM parasomnia in childhood. Parasomnia overlap disorder is male predominant but less so than isolated RBD. Most cases begin during childhood or adolescence. Virtually all age groups may be affected. It may be idiopathic or symptomatic of a broad set of disorders, including narcolepsy, multiple sclerosis, brain tumor (and therapy), rhomboencephalitis (pontine tegmentum or medullary lesion), brain trauma, various psychiatric disorders and their pharmacotherapies, and substance abuse disorders or withdrawal states. Note that in typical RBD, walking or leaving the bedroom is uncommon, *since the eyes are usually closed attending to dream action and not the environment.* In NREM parasomnia, the eyes are open but have a "glazed" look.

The sleepwalking episodes in overlap syndrome may be associated with violent or sexual behavior. Violent behavior (self-mutilation or homicide) and sexual assault ("sleep sex") have been reported in association with sleepwalking episodes. *Sleep-related sexual behavior* or *sex-somnia* is a type of parasomnia, in which sexual behavior occurs with limited awareness during the act, relative unresponsiveness to the external environment, and amnesia about the event. The behaviors range from sexual vocalizations to intercourse. In contrast to typical sleepwalking, these events may exceed 30 minutes.

Overlap syndrome usually responds to the treatments used for RBD such as clonazepam. In Patient B, environmental precautions and clonazepam 1 mg at bedtime were started and were fairly effective. However, the patient's wife started to sleep in a room on the other side of their house. The bedroom door was fitted with a difficult to open latch to decrease the chance that the patient would leave the bedroom.

CLINICAL PEARLS

1. Clonazepam is the first-line treatment for RBD, but an effective dose may not be tolerated. The addition of melatonin (3 to 12 mg) and a reduction in the dose of clonazepam may allow adequate RBD control without excessive morning sedation from clonazepam.

2. Melatonin may also be used as monotherapy for RBD.

3. Overlap parasomnia is a combination of RBD and another type of parasomnia—usually NREM parasomnia (sleepwalking, sleep terrors, confusional arousals). The sleep related eating disorder may also occur in patients with the overlap syndrome.

4. Most patients with overlap parasomnia had NREM parasomnia as a child.

5. In RBD episodes, the eyes are closed, and patients rarely leave the vicinity of the bed. In sleepwalking, the eyes are open, and ambulation out of the bedroom or out of the house may occur.

6. Sex-somnia is a variant of NREM parasomnia, in which sexual behavior occurs with limited awareness during the act, relative unresponsiveness to the external environment, and amnesia about the event.

BIBLIOGRAPHY

American Academy of Sleep Medicine: *International classification of sleep disorders*, ed 3, Darien, IL, 2013, American Academy of Sleep Medicine.

Anderson KN, Shneerson JM: Drug treatment of REM sleep behavior disorder: the use of drug therapies other than clonazepam, *J Clin Sleep Med* 5:235–239, 2009.

Aurora RN, Zak RS, Maganti RK, et al: Best practice guidelines for the treatment of REM sleep behavior disorder (RBD), *J Clin Sleep Med* 6:85–95, 2010.

Boeve BF, Silber MH, Ferman TJ: Melatonin for treatment of REM sleep behavior disorder in neurologic disorders: results in 14 patients, *Sleep Med* 4(4):281–284, 2003.

Cicolin A, Tribolo A, Giordano A, et al: Sexual behaviors during sleep associated with polysomnographically confirmed parasomnia overlap disorder, *Sleep Med* 12(5):523–528, 2011.

Howell MJ, Arneson PA, Schenck CH: A novel therapy for REM sleep behavior disorder (RBD), *J Clin Sleep Med* 7(6):639–644A, 2011.

Kunz D, Mahlberg R: A two-part, double-blind, placebo-controlled trial of exogenous melatonin in REM sleep behaviour disorder, *J Sleep Res* 19(4):591–596, 2010.

Sasai T, Matsuura M, Inoue Y: Factors associated with the effect of pramipexole on symptoms of idiopathic REM sleep behavior disorder, *Parkinsonism Relat Disord* 19(2):153–157, 2013.

Schenck CH, Boyd JL, Mahowald MW: A parasomnia overlap disorder involving sleep walking, sleep terrors, and REM sleep behavior disorder in 33 polysomnographically confirmed cases, *Sleep* 20:972–981, 1997.

Shapiro CM, Trajanovic NN, Fedoroff JP: Sex-somnia. A new parasomnia? *Can J Psychiatry* 48:311–317, 2003.

A Woman Who Eats During the Night and Does Not Remember

A 40-year-old woman complained of episodes of eating during night and not remembering it in the morning. The episodes started about 3 months ago when she was started on a new sleeping pill. In the morning, she found food containers scattered all around the kitchen. Her husband informed her that he heard her in the kitchen during the night. Some raw meat in a dish had been partially consumed. On other nights, the patient had eaten flour mixed with butter or vegetables directly from the freezer, without cooking them. On one occasion, her husband found her eating plain bread covered with salt. When he asked her what she was doing, she said that she was hungry. However, the next morning she did not remember the events. The patient had gained about 10 pounds since these eating episodes had started.

QUESTION

1. What is your diagnosis? What sleeping pill is commonly associated with this problem?

ANSWER

1. **Answer:** Sleep-related eating disorder (SRED). Any benzodiazepine receptor agonist (BZRA) may cause this behavior, but SRED most commonly associated with zolpidem.

   Discussion: The ICSD-3 Diagnostic Criteria SRED are listed in Box 103-1. SREDs are manifested by dysfunctional eating and drinking during the main sleep period after arousal from sleep. The behavior must be associated with one of the following: eating peculiar food items, sleep-related injury or potential for injury (cooking), or adverse consequences of recurrent nocturnal eating (weight gain, morning anorexia). In the past, SRED was differentiated from night eating syndrome (NES) by the level of alertness during the episodes and the degree of recall. SREDs were said to be associated with decreased awareness during the episodes, whereas NES was said to be characterized by full alertness. However, considerable overlap exists between SRED and NES. Some clinicians consider them to be two eating disorders at the opposite ends of the spectrum of awareness. The level of consciousness in SRED has typically spanned the range from virtual unconsciousness to various levels of partial consciousness despite a concurrent electroencephalography (EEG) pattern that is often predominantly wakefulness, suggesting dissociation between EEG and the level of

BOX P103-1	Sleep-Related Eating Disorder—Diagnostic Criteria (ICSD-3)

Criterial A-D must be met

A. *Recurrent* episodes of dysfunctional eating that occur after an arousal from sleep, during the main sleep period

B. The presence of one or more of the following in association with the recurrent episodes of involuntary eating:
   1. Consumption of peculiar forms or combinations of food or inedible or toxic substances
   2. Sleep-related injurious or potentially injurious behaviors performed while in seeking food or while cooking food

   3. Adverse health consequences from recurrent nocturnal eating

C. There is partial or complete loss of conscious awareness during the eating episode, with subsequent impaired recall.

D. The disturbance not better explained by another sleep disorder, mental disorder, medical disorder, medication, or substance use

Adapted from American Academy of Sleep Medicine: *International classification of sleep disorders*, ed 3, Darien, IL, 2014, American Academy of Sleep Medicine.

consciousness. A diagnosis of NES applies when excessive eating occurs between dinner and sleep onset, although SRED may be a comorbid condition with NES. This pattern of NES should not apply as an exclusion criterion for those patients who otherwise fulfill criteria for SRED and who consciously eat during the pre-bedtime period in a futile attempt to suppress the compulsion to eat after subsequently falling asleep.

The *International classification of sleep disorders*, Third Edition (ICSD-3) requires the following: "at least partial loss of conscious awareness during the eating episode with subsequent impaired recall." SRED episodes may occur during anytime of the night. The degree of alertness and recall for the eating behavior are variable. Some patients cannot be brought to full consciousness during the eating events and have no recall of the event. Others are relatively alert during the episode and have considerable recall of the event the next morning. The extent of alertness may even vary between episodes on a given night. A sensation of hunger is usually missing, and patients may eat in an "out of control" manner. Patients often eat peculiar, inedible, or even dangerous substances. These may include frozen food, coffee grounds, and cat food. Of interest, alcoholic beverages are rarely consumed. High-calorie foods are often chosen. Foods not typically eaten during the day are often consumed. Multiple episodes of eating during a single night may occur. Some patients attempt to control weight with severe daytime food restriction.

SRED is much more common in females than in males. Females make up 66% to 83% of affected individuals in most series. The prevalence is higher in patients with other eating disorders. Typical age of onset of SRED is 20 to 30 years. The cause of SRED is unknown, but more than 50% of patients have another type of parasomnia, and the strong female predominance is typical of eating disorders. An idiopathic form does exist, for which no obvious cause or association has been identified. SRED is most commonly associated with sleepwalking but may occur with periodic limb movement disorder (PLMD), restless leg syndrome (RLS), obstructive sleep apnea (OSA), narcolepsy, and circadian rhythm disorders (irregular sleep phase). Medication-induced SRED has been reported with BZRAs, including zolpidem and triazolam, and psychotropic medications (lithium, quetiapine, mirtazapine, risperidone). SRED episodes have also been reported in patients taking sodium oxybate. Zolpidem-associated SRED is especially common if patients escalate the dose of medication in an attempt to sleep. Patients also report triggering of SRED episodes by stress, cigarette smoking cessation, and cessation of alcohol or other drugs of abuse.

Sleepwalking is the most common sleep disorder associated with sleep-related eating, although once eating becomes part of the behavioral repertoire, it quickly becomes the predominant, if not the exclusive, nocturnal "sleepwalking" behavior. In a recent controlled study of 65 patients with narcolepsy+cataplexy, 32% of patients had SRED compared with 2% of controls.

The diagnosis of SRED is usually based on observations by a significant other, finding evidence of nocturnal eating behavior (e.g., open food packages, dirty plates), videotaping, and self-report (in patients with some recall).

If SRED is medication associated (zolpidem), the medication should be withdrawn. Patients may not exhibit the behavior when using another medication in the same class (e.g., switch from zolpidem to eszopiclone). Sometimes, medication-induced SRED will continue, at least temporarily, even with discontinuation of the offending medication. Topiramate appears to be the best-documented treatment, although sertraline, carbidopa or levodopa, and pramipexole have been used successfully. The dose of topiramate is 25 to 200 milligrams (mg) at bedtime. Many patients may note an improvement at a 100-mg dose. The side effects of topiramate include weight loss, paresthesia, renal calculi, cognitive dysfunction, and orthostasis. In one series, up to 41% of patients discontinued the medication because of side effects. If SRED is associated with sleepwalking, clonazepam has sometimes been effective.

CLINICAL PEARLS

1. In SRED the degree of alertness and recall are variable. The level of alertness may vary during multiple episodes in the same night.

2. At least one of the following is required: eating unusual or unhealthy foods, self-injury (or potential for sleep injury), or adverse consequence from eating.

3. SRED may be associated with sleep walking, RLS, narcolepsy, RBD, or medications.

4. Medication-induced SRED has been reported with BZRAs, including zolpidem and triazolam, and psychotropic medications (lithium, quetiapine, mirtazapine, risperidone).

5. Any benzodiazepine receptor agonist may cause SRED, but zolpidem is the medication most commonly reported.

6. SRED is more common in women than in men.

7. Treatment of SRED includes withdrawal of a causative medication or addition of topiramate. If associated with sleep walking, clonazepam may be effective.

BIBLIOGRAPHY

American Academy of Sleep Medicine: *International classification of sleep disorders*, ed 3, Darien, IL, 2014, American Academy of Sleep Medicine.

Brion A, Flamand M, Oudiette D, et al: Sleep-related eating disorder versus sleepwalking: a controlled study, *Sleep Med* 13:1094–1101, 2012.

Howell MJ, Schenck CH, Crow SJ: A review of nighttime eating disorders, *Sleep Med Rev* 13:23–34, 2009.

Howell MJ, Schenck CH: Restless nocturnal eating: a common feature of Willis-Ekbom syndrome (RLS), *J Clin Sleep Med* 8:413–419, 2012.

Howell MJ, Schenck CH: Treatment of nocturnal eating disorders, *Curr Treatment Options Neurol* 11:333–339, 2009.

O'Reardon JP, Allison KC, Martino NS, et al: A randomized, placebo-controlled trial of sertraline in the treatment of night eating syndrome, *Am J Psychiatry* 163:893–898, 2006.

Palaia V, Poli F, Pizz F, et al: Narcolepsy with cataplexy associated with nocturnal compulsive behaviors: a case-control study, *Sleep* 34:1365–1371, 2011.

Provini F, Albani R, Vetrugno R, et al: A pilot double-blind placebo-controlled trial of low-dose pramipexole in sleep-related eating disorder, *Eur J Neurol* 12:432–436, 2005.

Schenck CH, Hurwitz TD, Bundlie SR, Mahowald MW: Sleep-related eating disorders: polysomnographic correlates of a heterogeneous syndrome distinct from daytime eating disorders, *Sleep* 14:419–431, 1991.

Tamanna S, Ullah MI, Pope CR, et al: Quetiapine-induced sleep-related eating disorder-like behavior: a case series, *J Med Case Rep* 6(1):380, 2012.

Vetrugno R, Manconi M, Ferini-Strambi L, et al: Nocturnal eating: sleep-related eating disorder or night eating syndrome? A videopolysomnographic study, *Sleep* 29:949–954, 2006.

Vinai P, Ferri R, Ferini-Strambi L, et al: Defining the borders between sleep-related eating disorder and night eating syndrome, *Sleep Med* 13:686–690, 2012.

Wallace DM, Maze T, Shafazand S: Sodium oxybate-induced sleep driving and sleep-related eating disorder, *J Clin Sleep Med* 7(3):310–311, 2011.

Winkelman JW: Efficacy and tolerability of open-label topiramate in the treatment of sleep-related eating disorder: a retrospective case series, *J Clin Psychiatry* 67:1729–1734, 2006.

Winkelman JW: Treatment of nocturnal eating syndrome and sleep-related eating disorder with topirmate, *Sleep Med* 4:243–246, 2003.

PATIENT 104

A Woman Who Moans at Night and a Woman Who Experiences Jerks When Falling Asleep

Patient A: A 20-year-old woman was evaluated for periods of nocturnal groaning. The episodes occurred several times a week. The patient was unaware of the episodes but sought medical evaluation because her boyfriend refused to stay with her at night because the episodes disturbed his sleep. An oral contraceptive was the only medication the patient was taking. No history of snoring or daytime sleepiness was present. The patient typically awakened in the morning feeling refreshed. The groaning episodes were not associated with body movements.

Question 1: What is your diagnosis for Patient A?

Patient B: A 35-year-old woman complains of repeated episodes of jerks as she falls asleep. The episodes are not painful but are distressing as they delay sleep onset. The episodes occur nightly for the last 3 years. She has tried hypnotic medication but this does not help. No history of prior seizure disorder is present.

Question 2: What is your diagnosis for Patient B?

ANSWERS

1. **Answer for Patient A:** Catathrenia.

   Discussion: Sleep-related groaning (catathrenia) is a chronic (often nightly) disorder characterized by expiratory groaning during non–rapid eye movement (NREM) or REM sleep. The initial reports of catathrenia described groaning *during REM sleep* (especially in the REM episodes in the second part of the night). Others described catathrenia as occurring during both NREM and REM sleep or predominantly during NREM sleep. The sleep stage predominance may vary from patient to patient. Episodes may be associated with bradypneic episodes (slow respiratory rate) with *long exhalations*. Typically, a large inspiration is followed by protracted expiration during which a monotonous vocalization ("mournful moaning or groaning") is produced. Catathrenia events tend to occur in clusters and are often associated with bradycardia. Patients are usually unaware of the groaning. The disorder is thought to be benign, and its main complication is disturbance of the bed partner. Catathrenia is very rare, with onset usually in adolescence or early adulthood (mean age 19 years with a range of 5 to 36 years). The prevalence of catathrenia is *greater in men than in women*.

   Catathrenia events may occur in clusters and resemble a run of central apneas. Electroencephalography (EEG) arousal, with or without body movement, often marks the end of the event. Clusters of catathrenia events may be confused with central apneas. However, in central apneas, an exhalation precedes the long *inspiratory* pause. In contrast, in catathrenia, a deep inspiration precedes the long *expiratory* pause (Figure P104-1). Mild bradycardia during the exhalation is common. Of note, atypical catathrenia has been described consisting of expiratory groaning without prolonged inspiration or exhalation.

   The differential diagnosis of catathrenia includes stridor, sleep-related laryngospasm, and sleep talking. Stridor may be inspiratory or expiratory, typically occurs with every breath, and if inspiratory does not have a prolonged expiratory phase. *Sleep-related laryngospasm* is associated with a sense of suffocation. Sleep talking consists of words rather than groans. Not all cases of catathrenia require treatment. Multiple medications have been tried without success. Two cases of benefit from continuous positive airway pressure (CPAP) treatment have been reported by Iriarte et al and Songu and coworkers. However, another study did not find a benefit from CPAP.

2. **Answer for Patient B:** Propriospinal myoclonus at sleep onset (PSM).

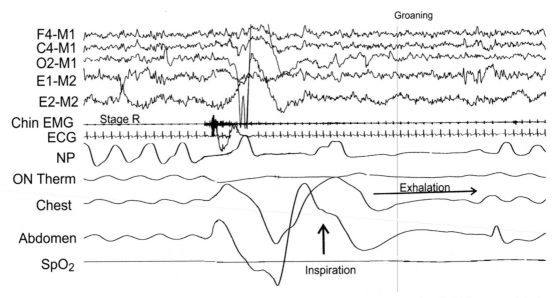

FIGURE P104-1 ■ A 30-second tracing during which time the patient was heard to groan loudly. This occurred during stage R sleep. Inspiration is upward.

Discussion: PSM consists of sudden myoclonic jerks occurring in the transition from wakefulness to sleep and, rarely, during intrasleep wakefulness and upon awakening in the morning. The jerks originate mainly in the axial muscles and spread rostrally and caudally according to propriospinal propagation. The jerks may be of variable intensity; they may be isolated, recurring in quasi-periodic fashion for variable durations, or may be repeated in brief clusters of a few movements, separated by longer intervals. Jerks involve the abdominal and truncal muscles first and are then propagated to proximal muscles of the limbs and the neck. The pattern of movement is usually flexor but may be an extension of the trunk. The jerks appear to be related to the lying-down position and a state of relaxed wakefulness, being present when the patient tries to fall asleep. Any mental activation makes the jerks disappear. The jerks eventually disappear at sleep onset and remain absent throughout all stages of sleep, even though sometimes the jerks reappear during intrasleep wakefulness. PSM is often associated with severe sleep-onset insomnia caused by the inability of the patient to fall asleep because of the recurrent disturbing muscular activity. Polysomnography (PSG) demonstrates brief myoclonic electromyography (EMG) bursts recurring nonperiodically with alpha-activity present on EEG and, in particular, when alpha-activity spreads from the posterior regions of the brain to the anterior regions. Epileptic EEG discharges are never found. Magnetic resonance imaging (MRI) of the brain is normal. MRI of the spine is also usually normal but may demonstrate a focal lesion in around 20% of the cases.

Symptomatic drug therapy of PSM is often disappointing. The most commonly reported effective treatment was clonazepam or other benzodiazepines. In a study by Roze et al, three patients that received zonisamide had significant improvements in myoclonus, without significant adverse effects, at daily doses ranging from 100 to 200 mg. Zonisamide has previously proven helpful, safe, and well tolerated as long-term antiepileptic therapy, in patients with various myoclonic epileptic syndromes. Studies with larger groups of patients are needed.

PSM should be differentiated from sleep starts, also known as *hypnic jerks*. Sleep starts are sudden, brief, simultaneous contractions of the body or one or more body segments occurring at sleep onset. Sleep starts (hypnic jerks) usually consist of a single contraction that often affects the body asymmetrically. The jerks may be either spontaneous or induced by stimuli. The motor activity is often associated with an impression of falling or less commonly pain or tingling; auditory stimuli such as banging, snapping, or crackling noises; or visual stimuli, including flashing lights, hypnagogic dreams, or hallucinations. A sharp cry may occur. The patient may not recall a jerk that was noted by a bed partner if the sleep start does not cause awakening. Multiple jerks occasionally occur in succession, usually early in the sleep.

CLINICAL PEARLS

1. Catathrenia consists of expiratory groaning. Typical events consist of a deep inspiration followed by a prolonged exhalation with groaning.

2. Catathrenia may occur during both NREM and REM sleep. Initial studies found predominance during REM sleep, whereas a few later studies found predominance during NREM sleep.

3. Catathrenia may not require treatment. It treatment is needed, CPAP has been used effectively in some patients.

4. Propriospinal myoclonus (PSM) consists of repeated jerks of the trunk with propagation caudally and rostrally at sleep onset. PSM may be associated with sleep-onset insomnia. The most effective treatment has yet to be determined. Clonazepam and zonisamide have been used.

5. PSM is eliminated by any mentation, and the jerks eventually disappear at sleep onset and remain absent throughout all stages of sleep (sometimes the jerks reappear during intrasleep wakefulness).

BIBLIOGRAPHY

Catathrenia

Abbasi AA, Morgenthaler TI, Slocumb NL, et al: Nocturnal moaning and groaning-catathrenia or nocturnal vocalizations, *Sleep Breath* 16:367–373, 2012.

Iriarte J, Alegre M, Urrestarazu E, et al: Continuous positive airway pressure as treatment for catathrenia (nocturnal groaning), *Neurology* 66:609–610, 2006.

Pevernagie DA, Boon PA, Mariman, et al: Vocalization during episodes of prolonged expiration: a parasomnia related to REM sleep, *Sleep Med* 2:19–30, 2001.

Poli F, Ricotta L, Vandi S, et al: Catathrenia under sodium oxybate in narcolepsy with cataplexy, *Sleep Breath* 16(2):427–434, 2012.

Ramar K, Olson EJ, Morgenthaler TI: Catathrenia, *Sleep Med* 9:457–459, 2008.

Siddiqui F, Walters AS, Chokroverty S: Catathrenia: a rare parasomnia which may mimic central sleep apnea on polysomnogram, *Sleep Med* 9:460–461, 2008.

Songu M, Yilmaz H, Uucetruk AV, et al: Effect of CPAP therapy on catathrenia and OSA: a case report and review of the literature, *Sleep Breath* 12:401–405, 2008.

Vetrugno R, Lugaresi E, Plazzi G, et al: Catathrenia (nocturnal groaning): an abnormal respiratory pattern during sleep, *Eur J Neurol* 14:1236–1243, 2007.

Vetrugno R, Provini F, Plazzi G, et al: Catathrenia (nocturnal groaning): a new type of parasomnia, *Neurology* 56:681–683, 2001.

Propriospinal Myoclonus

Montagna P, Provini F, Plazzi G, et al: Propriospinal myoclonus upon relaxation and drowsiness: a cause of severe insomnia, *Mov Disord* 12:66–72, 1997.

Montagna P, Provini F, Vetrugno R: Propriospinal myoclonus at sleep onset, *Neurophysiol Clin* 36:351–355, 2006.

Roze E, Bounolleau P, Ducreux D, et al: Propriospinal myclonus revisited. Clinical, neurophysiologic, and neuroradiologic findings, *Neurology* 72:1301–1309, 2009.

Tison F, Arne P, Dousset V, et al: Propriospinal myoclonus induced by relaxation and drowsiness, *Rev Neurol (Paris)* 154:423–425, 1998.

Vetrugno R, Provini F, Meletti S, et al: Propriospinal myoclonus at the sleep-wake transition: a new type of parasomnia, *Sleep* 24:835–843, 2001.

FUNDAMENTALS 36

Clinical Electroencephalography and Epilepsy

MONITORING WITH ELECTROENCEPHALOGRAPHY (EEG)

The location of EEG electrodes using the international 10-20 system is illustrated in Figures F36-1 and F36-2. Each electrode is represented by a letter that refers to the underlying area or lobe of the brain (Fp = frontopolar; F = frontal; P = parietal; C = central; O = occipital; T = temporal) and numerical subscripts that specify the electrode position. The nomenclature "10-20" refers to the fact that electrodes are positioned at 10% or 20% of the distance between landmarks such as nasion, inion,

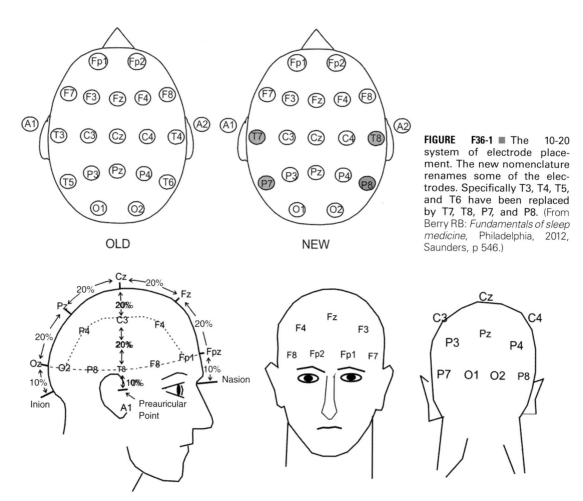

OLD   NEW

FIGURE F36-1 ■ The 10-20 system of electrode placement. The new nomenclature renames some of the electrodes. Specifically T3, T4, T5, and T6 have been replaced by T7, T8, P7, and P8. (From Berry RB: *Fundamentals of sleep medicine*, Philadelphia, 2012, Saunders, p 546.)

FIGURE F36-2 ■ The 10-20 system of electrode placement. All electrodes are placed either 10% or 20% of the distance between two standard landmarks. (From Berry RB: *Fundamentals of sleep medicine*, Philadelphia, 2012, Saunders, p 546.)

or the preauricular points (see Figure F36-2). The odd subscripts are on the left and the even on the right, and the "z" subscripts refer to electrodes in the midline. The left and right auricular (earlobe) electrodes are A_1 and A_2. In sleep monitoring, these are actually placed on the mastoids and appropriately called M1 and M2 [3]. Figure F36-1 illustrates the new electrode nomenclature, in which T3, T4, T5, and T6 have been replaced by T7, T8, P7, and P8. In the new nomenclature, all electrodes in a given sagittal plane have the same subscript (F_7, T_7, P_7), and most electrodes in the same coronal plane have the same letter (P7, P3, Pz, P4, P8). However, many EEG laboratories still use the old electrode nomenclature as does the majority of the published literature on epilepsy.

BIPOLAR MONITORING AND STANDARD MONTAGES

A *derivation* (also know as a channel in EEG monitoring) is the voltage difference between two electrodes: for example, Fp1 − F3 is the voltage difference between electrodes Fp1 and F3. By EEG convention, if Fp1 is more negative than F3, the deflection is up. A set of derivations is called a *montage*. Montages are designed with a particular purpose in mind. Standard clinical EEG montages are illustrated in Tables F36-1 and F36-2. *Bipolar*

longitudinal montages sequentially compare two adjacent electrodes in chains covering the head in an anteroposterior (AP) direction ("double banana"). In the most frequently used variant (LB-18.1), the chains start at the left temporal area and then progressively move toward the right (Figure F36-3). Bipolar transverse montages compare two electrodes in chains in the transverse directions (see Table F36-1). *Referential montages* compare multiple electrodes to a single electrode (or group of linked electrodes). The standard referential montages compare electrodes to the ipsilateral auricular electrodes A1 and A2 (see Table F36-2). In the sleep center M1 and M2 are used instead of A1 and A2. Different laboratories may display the electrodes in a given montage in different sequences. In modern digital EEG recording, all electrodes are usually recorded against a common reference electrode (REF). Any two electrodes may be compared by digitally subtracting the signals (F7-REF) − (P7-REF)= F7-P7. Thus, the display montage can be changed while recording or later during study review. In some EEG systems REF is an actual electrode often placed near Cz while others use a group of linked electrodes.

Digital recording also allows one to visualize multiple time scales. The polysomnography (PSG) window to stage sleep is 30 seconds but the clinical EEG window is 10 seconds. The 10-second time window allows detection of sharply

TABLE F36-1   Longitudinal Bipolar (AP Bipolar) 18-Channel "Double Banana"

LB-18.1		LB-18.2		LB-18.3	
Fp1-F7	Left temporal	Fz-Cz	Vertex	Fp1-F7	Left temporal
F7-T7		Cz-Pz		F7-T7	
T7-P7				T7-P7	
P7-O1		Fp1-F3	Left parasagittal	P7-O1	
		F3-C3			
Fp1-F3	Left parasagittal	C3-P3		Fp2-F8	Right temporal
F3-C3		P3-O1		F8-T8	
C3-P3				T8-P8	
P3-O1		Fp2-F4	Right parasagittal	P8-O2	
		F4-C4			
Fz-Cz	Vertex	C4-P4		Fp1-F3	Left parasagittal
Cz-Pz		P4-O2		F3-C3	
				C3-P3	
Fp2-F4	Right parasagittal	Fp1-F7	Left temporal	P3-O1	
F4-C4		F7-T7			
C4-P4		T7-P7		Fp2-F4	Right parasagittal
P4-O2		P7-O1		F4-C4	
				C4-P4	
Fp2-F8	Right temporal	Fp2-F8	Right temporal	P4-O2	
F8-T8		F8-T8			
T8-P8		T8-P8		Fz-Cz	Vertex
P_8-O_2		P_8-O_2		C_z-P_z	

American Clinical Neurophysiology Society: Guideline 6: a proposal for standard montages to be used in clinical EEG, *J Clin Neuophysiol* 23:111-117,2006.
See also Figure F36-3.

TABLE F36-2	Longitudinal and Transverse Bipolar and Referential	
A-P Bipolar "Double Banana" (LB 18.3)	Transverse - Bipolar (TB 18.1)	Referential (R-18.2)
Fp1-F7	F7-Fp1	FP1-A1
F7-T7	Fp1-Fp2	F7-A1
T7 – P7	Fp2-F8	T7-A1
P7-O1		P7-A1
Fp2-F8	F7-F3	FP2-A2
F8-T8	F3-Fz	F8- A2
T8-P8	Fz-F4	T8-A2
P8-O2	F4-F8	P8-A2
Fp1-F3	T7-C3	Fp1-A1
F3-C3	C3-Cz	F3-A1
C3-P3	Cz-C4	C3-A1
P3-O1	C4-T8	P3-A1
Fp2-F4	P7-P3	Fp2-A2
F4-C4	P3-Pz	F4-A2
C4-P4	Pz-P4	C4-A2
P4-O2	P4-P8	P4-A2
Fz-Cz	P7-O1	Fz-A2
Cz-Pz	O1-O2	Cz-A2
	O2-P8	

TABLE F36-3	Waveform Terminology
Spike	Transient with a pointed peak and duration of 20–70 msec
Polyspike	Transient with multiple spikes
Sharp wave	Transient with a pointed peak and duration of 70–120 msec
Spike and wave	Spike followed by a slow wave
Interictal discharge	Abnormal (epileptiform) EEG activity that occurs between seizures
Ictal activity	EEG correlate of a seizure

EEG, Electroencephalography; *msec,* milliseconds.

to 200 msec. A *spike and wave complex* is a spike followed by a slow wave (usually wide and often high amplitude). Polyspike complexes often consist of multiple spikes, which are sometimes followed by a slow wave. The term *epileptiform activity* literally means "EEG activity resembling that found in patients with epilepsy." This is a somewhat circular definition. Epileptiform activity includes spikes, spike and wave, and polyspike complexes. Abnormal sharp waves are also considered epileptiform or interictal activity. However, sharp waves may be normal (e.g., vertex sharp waves).

INTERICTAL AND ICTAL ACTIVITY

Interictal activity is defined as abnormal EEG activity (epileptiform) that occurs between seizures. In patients with known epilepsy (more than one seizure) only about 50% of EEG recordings will have abnormalities. Because seizures do not always appear during a given EEG recording (see Box F36-1), the physician reading an EEG or PSG looks for spikes, abnormal sharp waves, or a combination of both that may represent the interictal footprint of possible seizures activity. However, it should be noted that not all patients with spikes have seizures and not all patients with seizures have detectable interictal activity. Spikes represent abnormal brain activity that is seen as an area of negativity at the scalp. Spikes may be localized (negativity at the scalp over one area of the brain) or appear diffusely. Focal seizures usually, though not invariably, begin at the same location as the interictal spikes. The typical spike is followed by a *slow wave. Although most common postictally, spike and sharp waves may occur sporadically at any time, they may have a slight increase preictally.* Of note, artifacts may sometimes mimic spikes or spikes and waves. In general, true spike and wave complexes have a "field" (see Box F36-1). That is, a true spike and wave activity should be seen

contoured (narrow) waveforms that may signify seizure activity. If the capacity to add a few electrodes to traditional sleep monitoring exists, the ability to detect interictal epileptiform activity can be increased. For example, two electrodes (T7, T8) can be added. The derivations F3-T7, T7-O1, F4-T8, and T8-O2 would add coverage over much of the frontal and temporal areas. These areas are the predominant foci of seizures occurring mainly during sleep. The addition of synchronized digital video monitoring to nocturnal EEG or PSG recording greatly enhances the ability of the clinician to diagnose nocturnal events. As is discussed later, many nocturnal seizure disorders are not associated with scalp EEG findings, and the patient's actions during the seizure (seminology) may be very helpful in determining whether an episode is likely a parasomnia or nocturnal epilepsy.

WAVEFORM AND SEIZURE TERMINOLOGY

A *transient* is any isolated wave or complex that stands out compared with background activity. A *spike* is defined as a transient with a pointed peak and a duration of *20 to 70 milliseconds (msec)* (Table F36-3 and Figure F36-4). On a 30-second page, spikes look like a single vertical line. A *sharp wave* is a transient with a deflection of 70

FIGURE F36-3 ■ Three longitudinal bipolar chain displays. These are three methods of arranging the derivations for display. For example, in LB-18.1 the sequence is—left temporal→left parasagittal→vertex→right parasaggital→right temporal. (From Berry RB: *Fundamentals of sleep medicine*, Philadelphia, 2012, Saunders, p 547.)

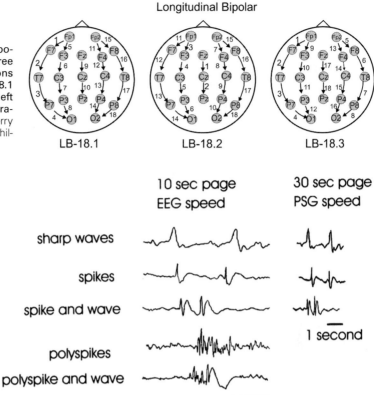

Longitudinal Bipolar

LB-18.1   LB-18.2   LB-18.3

10 sec page
EEG speed

30 sec page
PSG speed

sharp waves

spikes

spike and wave

1 second

polyspikes

polyspike and wave

1 second

FIGURE F36-4 ■ Sharp waves, spikes, spike and wave, polyspikes, and polyspikes and wave. *EEG*, Electroencephalography; *PSG*, polysomnography. (From Berry RB: *Fundamentals of sleep medicine*, Philadelphia, 2012, Saunders, p 546.)

BOX F36-1 | **Interictal and Ictal EEG and Epilepsy**

INTERICTAL EEG

- A true spike and wave is rarely confined to one derivation –i.e., has a "field" of involvement (especially true if a typical bipolar clinical EEG montage is used)
- A spike and wave confined to two derivations containing a common electrode is often an artifact

ICTAL EEG

- Typically ictal EEG activity "evolves" in:
  - Frequency—may increase then exhibit postictal slowing

- Field—amount of involved derivations increases
- Amplitude—may increase in amplitude
- Background rhythms often suppressed

EEG AND EPILEPSY

- A single EEG recording will show epileptiform abnormalities in about 50% of adult patients with epilepsy
- Diagnostic yield increased to 70% with repeated recordings and/or sleep EEGs
- A normal EEG does NOT rule out epilepsy
- A small percentage of normal individuals have epileptiform activity

EEG, Electroencephalography.

---

in derivations containing several contiguous electrodes. If a spike and wave are seen only in two derivations containing a common electrode, this may be an artifact.

PHASE REVERSAL

Localized EEG waveforms (including spikes and sharp waves) will show *phase reversal* if the bipolar

chain crosses the area of the localized EEG activity. That is, the spike or sharp wave in one derivation is out of phase with the corresponding waveform in the adjacent derivations (e.g., one down, the other up). *Phase reversal does not imply an abnormal waveform.* For example, K-complexes and vertex sharp waves show phase reversal in montages that cross the location of origin. Phase reversal may help differentiate epileptiform activity such as a spike from artifact. As

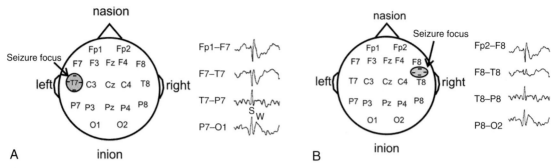

FIGURE F36-5 ■ Examples of phase reversal. **A,** A spike (s; negative) originates at electrode position T7 and a bipolar chain through the area shows phase reversal. *w,* Wave. **B,** Spike originated in between electrodes. The bipolar pair spanning the location show low amplitude because of cancellation effects (spike causes nearly equal voltage in F8 and T8) but bipolar pairs on either side show phase reversal. (From Berry RB: *Fundamentals of sleep medicine,* Philadelphia, 2012, Saunders, p 550.)

noted above, epileptiform activity is usually recorded as an electronegative potential. For example, in Figure F36-5A, negative spike activity is seen under electrode T7. This results in down-going deflections in F7-T7 because T7 is more negative than F7. This pattern reverses for T7-P7 because now P7 is more positive than T7. In this figure, "s" is for spike and "w" for wave. If the spike focus is located nearly equidistant between two monitoring electrodes (F8 and T8) (Figure F36-5B), the derivation containing these two electrodes may show little or no activity (F8-T8) and the derivations on either side will show phase reversal ([Fp2-F8] to [T8-P8]).

LOCALIZATION IN REFERENTIAL AND PSG MONTAGES

In referential montages, a spike will have greater activity in montages containing electrodes nearer to the location of the spike. In Figure F36-6, a spike focus is located between F8 and T8. On the bipolar montage, this results in the electrical activity being nearly equal in the two electrodes, resulting in minimal activity in F8-T8 but a phase reversal in adjacent bipolar pairs. However, in referential recording, the spike results in larger

and nearly equal activity in F8 and T8 with less activity in adjacent electrodes. In the usual PSG montage, electrodes are referenced to the opposite mastoid. Therefore, a spike located near F4 will result in greater deflection in F4-M1 compared with C4-M1 or O2-M1. *It is also important to recall that the mastoid electrodes M1 and M2 are close to the left and right temporal areas, respectively.* A right temporal spike may be better seen in C3-M2 (close proximity of M2 to spike focus) than C4-M1 although C3 is on the left side.

ICTAL ACTIVITY

Ictal (seizure) activity may be manifested by rhythmic activity of many types. The burst of activity is usually associated with an abnormality of movement or mentation. However, subclinical ictal activity can exist during sleep. Whereas the *spike and wave* activity is the most familiar waveform associated with ictal activity (Figure F36-7), the pattern of repetitive sharp waves or sinusoidal waves various frequencies is also common. On traditional sleep monitoring montages, ictal activity may even be mistaken for muscle artifact or normal theta (5-7 Hz), alpha (8-13 Hz), and beta (13-30 Hz) activity.

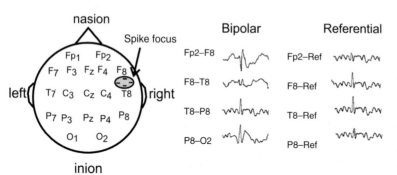

FIGURE F36-6 ■ Difference in localization with a bipolar or a referential montage. In referential montages, the electrode(s) nearest the activity in question has the largest deflection. (From Berry RB: *Fundamentals of sleep medicine,* Philadelphia, 2012, Saunders, p 550.)

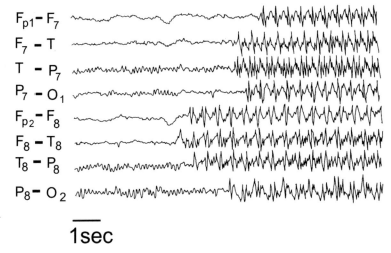

FIGURE F36-7 ■ A seizure beginning as focal activity in the right frontal-temporal areas with secondary generalization. The ictal activity has a spike and wave form. (From Berry RB: *Fundamentals of sleep medicine*, Philadelphia, 2012, Saunders, p 555.)

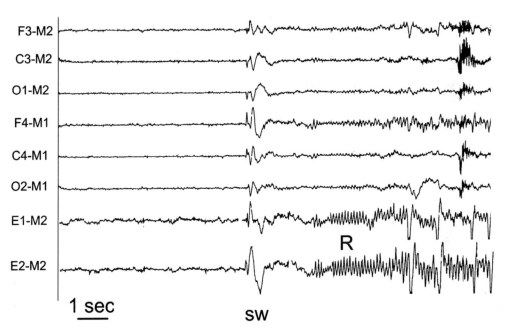

FIGURE F36-8 ■ A spike and wave (SW) complex is followed by rhythmic activity (R) in the alpha-frequency range that represents ictal activity in a patient with frontal lobe seizure. The origin is the right frontopolar area, and the largest amplitude is seen in the right eye derivation and F4-M1. (From Berry RB: *Fundamentals of sleep medicine*, Philadelphia, 2012, Saunders, p 555.)

In Figure F36-8, a portion of a tracing visualized in a 10-second window shows a spike and wave complex (SW) followed by rhythmic activity of 8 to 9 Hz (R). The rhythmic activity is differentiated from normal alpha rhythm by being more prominent in the eye derivations than in the occipital derivations. This is, in fact, a portion of a frontal lobe seizure manifested by oral automatisms and loss of responsiveness. One might suspect the frontal nature because the activity is higher amplitude in the eye leads (near the frontal lobes). Note in Figure F36-8 the slightly higher amplitude of the rhythmic activity

in E2-M1 than in E1-M2 as E2 is nearer the right frontal area. Indeed, a complete EEG montage localized the seizure activity to the right frontal lobe (or region).

It is important to note that ictal activity may not be seen in scalp EEG monitoring. Video recording is absolutely essential because the pattern of movements (seminology) is very important for helping differentiate nonepileptic movements (parasomnia) from epileptic movements. The type of movement and the focal or generalized distribution of ictal activity may help define the type of seizure, focus in partial or partial complex seizures, or both. High-resolution magnetic resonance imaging (MRI) or intracranial EEG monitoring may also identify the problem location in the brain. Ictal activity may be mistaken for a recording artifact, and vice versa. Some useful characteristics of true ictal activity are noted in Box F36-1. True ictal activity evolves; that is, it changes in frequency, amplitude, and spatial distribution during the episode. Often, the EEG activity slows after an ictal episode. As previously noted, synchronized video is very useful to determine if behavioral correlates (e.g., movements) temporally associated with ictal activity are present.

CLASSIFICATION OF SEIZURES AND TERMINOLOGY

A *seizure* is defined as an episode of disturbance of mental, motor, sensory, or autonomic activity caused by a paroxysmal cerebral neuronal malfunction. *Epilepsy* is defined as a disorder of recurrent seizures. The disorder is called *symptomatic* if an identifiable lesion exists or *idiopathic* if a discrete structural abnormality is not found. The term *idiopathic* is misleading because many seizure disorders classified as idiopathic have a genetic basis, and some have a known mechanism.

The most commonly used classification of seizures is based on their manifestations (see Box F36-2). Seizure disorders are divided into partial (focal) seizures that are caused by the initial involvement of a localized group of neurons limited to one hemisphere and generalized seizures beginning in both hemispheres. In Box F36-2, partial epilepsies are divided into simple partial (consciousness not impaired), complex partial (consciousness impaired), and focal seizures (simple or partial complex) that evolve into generalized seizures. The simple partial seizures are

---

BOX F36-2	**Classification of Seizures (Traditional Classification)**

PARTIAL (FOCAL, LOCAL) SEIZURES

A. Simple partial seizures (consciousness NOT impaired)
    i. Motor symptoms
        a. Focal motor without march—sustained tonic, intermittent clonic, or a sequence of tonic-clonic movements
        b. Focal motor with march (Jacksonian)—movements progressively involve adjacent parts of one side of the body
        c. Versive—turning of head or body, usually in a direction away from the side of the seizure discharge
        d. Postural—involuntary changes in body posture
        e. Aphasic—expressive or receptive, global loss of language
        f. Phonatory (vocalization or arrest of speech)
    ii. Somatosensory or special sensory symptoms
        a. Somatosensory
        b. Visual—hallucinations
        c. Auditory—hallucinations of simple or complex sounds
        d. Olfactory—hallucination of odors/ often precedes complex partial seizures
        e. Gustatory—hallucination of taste
        f. Vertiginous—transient vertigo
    iii. Autonomic symptoms or signs: epigastric, pallor, sweating
    iv. Psychic symptoms or signs (usually occur with impairment of consciousness and classified as complex partial)
        a. Dysphasic
        b. Cognitive
        c. Dysamnesic (déjà vu)
        d. Affective (fear)
        e. Illusions
        f. Hallucinations

B. Complex partial (with impairment of consciousness)
    i. Simple partial onset followed by impairment of consciousness
    ii. Impairment of consciousness at onset
        a. Impairment of consciousness only
        b. Automatisms

C. Partial seizures (simple or complex) evolving to generalized seizures

GENERALIZED SEIZURES

A. Nonconvulsive (absence)—petit mal
    i. Typical (3 per second spike and slow wave on EEG)
    ii. Atypical (<3 per second spike and slow wave complexes on EEG)

B. Convulsive
    i. Myoclonic seizures—brief jerks
    ii. Clonic seizures—jerking
    iii. Tonic seizures—tensing of muscles
    iv. Tonic-clonic seizures (grand mal)
    v. Atonic ("drop attacks")

UNCLASSIFIED SEIZURE

Adapted from Commission on Classification and Terminology of the International League Against Epilepsy: Proposal for revised classification of epilepsies and epileptic syndromes, *Epilepsia* 22:389-399, 1981.
EEG, Encephalography.

divided into those with (1) motor symptoms, (2) somatosensory symptoms, (3) autonomic symptoms, and (4) psychic symptoms or signs. The complex partial seizures are divided on the basis of whether or not impaired consciousness is apparent at the start of the seizure. *Auras* are subjective sensations such as déjà vu, epigastric sensation, and visual or olfactory disturbance that precedes the loss of awareness in complex partial seizure. Aura is actually a simple partial seizure that may or may not spread to areas that affect cognition resulting in subsequent loss of awareness. *Automatisms* are repetitive movements that may be purposeful but serve no obvious purpose in the actual situation. The *postictal state* is the state following ictal activity often associated with impaired sensorium or confusion. Partial seizures may show secondary generalization (see Figure F36-7) resulting in the ictal activity associated with generalized convulsive seizures. The focal seizures that commonly present at night are temporal lobe epilepsy (TLE) and frontal lobe epilepsy (FLE). TLE usually presents as a complex partial seizure with automatisms. FLE may be associated with dystonic posturing or violent movements, with consciousness often preserved. TLE most commonly presents during the day, and FLE more commonly presents at night. Nocturnal FLE may mimic confusional arousals or sleep terrors and sleepwalking. These disorders will be discussed in Patients 106 and 107.

Primary generalized seizures are ones in which ictal EEG activity and clinical manifestations involve both cerebral hemispheres at the onset. On EEG, simultaneous, bilateral, and diffuse ictal activity is present. Clinically, seizure activity results in loss of consciousness or loss of awareness. Generalized epilepsy is divided into nonconvulsive (absence or petit mal) epilepsy and convulsive epilepsy.

Nonconvulsive primary generalized epilepsy is divided into typical absence epilepsy (3 per second spike wave activity) and atypical absence epilepsy with slower frequency complexes and polyspikes. Nonconvulsive generalized epilepsy starts in childhood and may resolve by late adolescence to adulthood. Typical absence (petit mal) epilepsy is associated with impairment of consciousness (staring blankly) without loss of muscle tone or posture. Attacks are triggered by hyperventilation and photic stimuli. Atypical epilepsy is associated with spike and wave complexes of <3 per second frequency and may be associated with combinations of impaired consciousness and motor or autonomic changes.

Convulsive generalized epilepsy is divided into myoclonic, tonic, clonic, tonic-clonic, and atonic seizures. Myoclonic seizures are characterized by brief muscle jerking (muscle contraction then relaxation—often involving the shoulder muscles). An example of this type is juvenile myoclonic epilepsy (JME). Tonic seizures are associated with muscle tensing. Clonic seizures manifest with repeated jerking (repeated contraction and relaxation). Generalized tonic-clonic (GTC) seizures (grand mal) are characterized by initial tonic activity followed by clonic activity. Atonic seizures are characterized by a sudden loss of muscle tone (drop attacks). Unclassified seizures are ones in which the origin (focal or general) has not been determined.

It should be noted that the International League Against Epilepsy (ILAE) updated the previously described classification system in 2010 (see Berg et al 2010). However, the previous terminology is still widely used. The new classification uses the term *focal seizure* rather than *partial seizure* and the terms *simple* and *complex* are replaced by description of the manifestations of the seizure.

BIBLIOGRAPHY

American Clinical Neurophysiology Society: Guideline 5: Guidelines for standard electrode position nomenclature, *J Clin Neuophysiol* 23:107–110, 2006.

American Clinical Neurophysiology Society: Guideline 6: A proposal for standard montages to be used in clinical EEG, *J Clin Neuophysiol* 23:111–117, 2006.

Bazil CW: Nocturnal seizures, *Semin Neurol* 24:293–300, 2004.

Berg AT, Berkovic SF, Brodie MJ, et al: Revised terminology and concepts for organization of seizures and epilepsies: Report of the ILAE Commission on Classification and Terminology, 2005–2009, *Epilepsia* 51(4):676–685, 2010.

Commission on Classification and Terminology of the International League Against Epilepsy: Proposal for revised classification of epilepsies and epileptic syndromes, *Epilepsia* 30:389, 1989.

Foldvary-Schaefer N, Alsheikhtaha Z: Complex nocturnal behaviors: nocturnal seizures and parasomnias continuum, *Continuum (Minneap Minn)* 19(1):104–131, 2013.

Foldvary N, Caruso AC, Mascha E, et al: Identifying montages that best detect electrographic seizure activity during polysomnography, *Sleep* 23:1–9, 2000.

Foldvary-Schaefer N, Grigg-Damberger M: Sleep and epilepsy, *Sleep Med Clin* 3:443–454, 2008.

Herman ST, Walczak TS, Bazil CW: Distribution of partial seizures during the sleep-wake cycle: differences by seizure onset site, *Neurology* 56:1453–1459, 2001.

Hrachovy RA, Frost JD: The EEG in selected generalized seizures, *J Clin Neurophysiol* 23:312–332, 2006.

International Federation of Societies for Electroencephalography and Clinical Neurophysiology: Ten twenty electrode system, *EEG Clin Neurophysiol* 10:371–375, 1958.

Libenson MH, editor: *Practical approach to electroencephalography*, Philadelphia, 2010, Saunders.

Malow BA: Sleep and epilepsy, *Neurol Clin* 23:1127, 2005.

Vaughn BV, D'Cruz OF: Sleep and epilepsy, *Semin Neurol* 24:301–313, 2004.

Rhythmic Electroencephalography Pattern During Polysomnography

An obese 18-year-old college student was evaluated for snoring, daytime sleepiness, and awakening with body jerks during sleep. Until the patient entered college, he had always slept in a bedroom alone. The patient had gained about 20 pounds over the previous year and now snored very loudly at night. Obstructive sleep apnea (OSA) was noted during rapid eye movement (REM) sleep and in the supine position. On review of the study, episodes of paroxysmal activity lasting from a few to 30 seconds were noted. The technologist thought the finding might be artifact. He was viewing the data in a 120-second window during acquisition. Video showed that no patient activity of interest was noted during electroencephalography (EEG). *A 15-second segment as viewed in a 30-second window* is shown in Figure P105-1 (with an enlargement to the side).

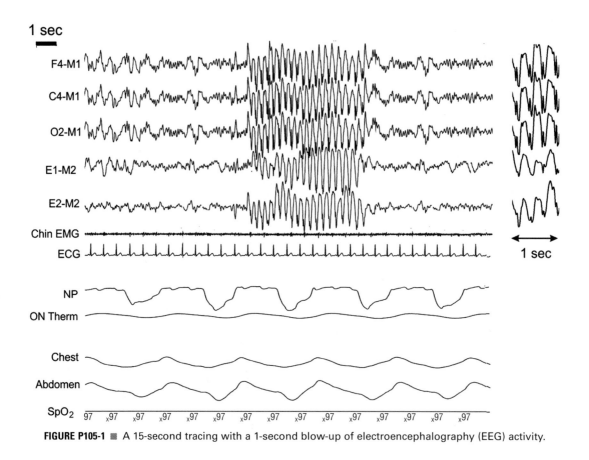

FIGURE P105-1 ■ A 15-second tracing with a 1-second blow-up of electroencephalography (EEG) activity.

QUESTION

1. What is your diagnosis?

ANSWER

1. **Answer:** Seizure activity (spike-and-wave activity).

Discussion: Spike-and-wave activity is a common form of ictal discharge. Spikes are transient waves that are 20 to 70 milliseconds (msec) in duration. Using a conventional polysomnography (PSG) time window (30 seconds), spikes appear as nearly vertical lines or may be difficult to separate from adjoining slow wave activity. They are usually surface negative (usually upward deflections) in frontal, central, or eye leads. Spikes are frequently followed by slow waves. Isolated spike discharges are often seen in patients with seizures (interictal activity) but may occasionally be seen in patients with a family history of seizures who never have clinical seizures.

About 10% to 40% of seizure activity occurs exclusively during sleep. Seizure thresholds are highest during REM sleep, followed by wakefulness, and then non-REM (NREM) sleep. Thus, the *likelihood of seizure activity* is NREM > Wake > REM. Generalized tonic clonic (GTC) seizures may be most common soon after awakening in many patients. Nocturnal seizures may present in many ways, including unusual behaviors or multiple arousals leading to complaints of insomnia or daytime sleepiness (Box P105-1). Seizure-associated behaviors are often recurrent, stereotypical, inappropriate, or all of these. Following generalized seizures, the patient usually has no recall of the events. Partial complex seizures from the temporal lobe commonly result in automatisms. Seizures from the frontal lobes may result in paroxysmal arousals, often with a cry (mimic of sleep terror), nocturnal wandering behavior (mimicking sleepwalking), or violent body movement (mimicking REM sleep behavior disorder). Screaming, vocalizations, and violent automatisms with the possibility of injury may also occur. Seizures may present as a recurrent nightmare or as isolated symptoms such as choking, nausea and vomiting, or laryngospasm. However, nocturnal seizures may also be entirely asymptomatic.

The non-neurologist may not be familiar with the elements of a clinical history that are important for differentiating seizures from other types of parasomnia. Abnormal focal movements, auras (a subjective sensation such as a smell or visual disturbance that precedes attacks), exact description of the attack, presence or absence of tongue laceration, nonresponsiveness during and following the episode, and the presence and absence of postictal confusion are all important historical elements. Unfortunately, if seizures occur only at night, the patient may not be observed doing anything unless body movements or sounds awaken the bedmate.

Distinguishing seizure activity from artifact on a polysomnogram may be difficult for the non-neurologist. The ability to view the tracing on a 10-second page is very helpful in determining the morphology and frequency of the activity. This is an advantage of digital recording systems. The presence of a spike-and-wave pattern during the rhythmic activity in question is virtually diagnostic of seizure activity. Bursts of delta- or theta-activity may look somewhat similar but do not have spikes. Such activity is also rarely as regular as seizure activity. Electrode popping may produce high-amplitude sharp waves but often involves a common bad electrode and has a slower periodicity. Ictal activity may present as rhythmic alpha, theta, or beta activity (13-30 Hz). Usually, changes precede the ictal activity such as a spikes or sharp wave, and postictally, slowing may be seen.

Of note, EEG findings may not be seen on surface EEG recording (temporal or frontal lobe epilepsy) during nocturnal spells. In such cases, video recording and technologist observation are essential in establishing the presence of subtle abnormal automatisms such as lip smacking or mouth movement. This may be an important clue that a seizure is occurring. In some cases in which no seizure activity can be documented despite extensive monitoring with additional leads, MRI will show a focal abnormality in the temporal or frontal lobe areas.

Even if seizure activity is seen during traditional PSG, identification of a focal onset or localization maybe difficult when the typical PSG EEG montage is used. Of note, frontal ictal activity is

BOX P105-1	Presentations of Nocturnal Seizures
• Frequent arousals • Daytime sleepiness • Complaints of insomnia	• Nocturnal "spells"—parasomnia • Unrecognized (asymptomatic) • Recurrent bad dreams

often seen in derivations containing E2 (close to the right frontal lobe, and temporal activity is often noted in the derivations containing the mastoid electrodes (M1, M2). This may cause confusion, as right temporal activity may be more prominent in E1-M2 and E2-M2 rather than in F4-M1 and C4-M1. Some focal seizures generalize extremely rapidly and therefore may appear at first glance as generalized seizures. Although frontal lobe seizures classically present as tonic posturing and temporal lobe seizures as partial complex seizures with automatisms or behavioral arrest, manifestations alone may not allow localization. For example, seizures originating from the orbitofrontal areas and the cingulate gyrus of the frontal lobes often resemble those originating from the temporal lobes with staring, nonresponsiveness, and automatisms.

In the current patient, nocturnal seizures were unrecognized by the roomate or the sleep lab technologist, as these seizures had no motor manifestations. The patient had many 15- to 20-second bursts of the above activity during sleep. A subsequent full clinical EEG montage study during the day also showed episodes of similar activity. The EEG technologist was able to document that the patient had a periods of unresponsiveness during the episodes. The seizure activity appeared to have a generalized onset, and a diagnosis of generalized seizure disorder of the absence type (no motor manifestations) was made. Onset of generalized seizures in an adult is distinctly rare. A generalized seizure disorder is usually diagnosed in childhood or adolescence. Although classic petit mal epilepsy is characterized by spike and wave of 3 hertz (Hz), the frequency may be faster in adults. It is always possible that this disorder was present from childhood and had been unrecognized. The patient was an only child who rarely slept in the same room with another individual until going to college. An alternative view is that the epilepsy was, in fact, a focal seizure with very rapid generalization. However, MRI results were within normal limits. The patient was treated with topiramate, an antiepileptic medication active against both focal and generalized seizures. The overall apnea–hypopnea index (AHI) was 20 per hour, and the patient was eventually started on continuous positive airway pressure (CPAP) treatment.

CLINICAL PEARLS

1. Rhythmic activity during sleep should be examined in a 10-second window to look for a spike-and-wave activity.
2. Spike-and-wave activity may be isolated (interictal) or may occur in bursts (ictal or seizure activity). Recognition of the characteristic shape helps differentiate a burst of seizure activity from artifact or EEG changes that mimic seizure activity. Use of the video to determine the behavioral correlates of the EEG activity is also very useful.
3. Ictal activity may consist of rhythmic activity with a frequency in the delta, theta, alpha, or beta ranges.
4. About 10% to 40% percent of seizures primarily occur only during sleep.
5. If seizures occur only or mostly during sleep and do not cause motor activity resulting in the patient moving the arms or legs or sitting up, they frequently remain unrecognized.
6. Using a complete seizure montage and video recording may assist in the diagnosis of seizures.
7. Nocturnal seizures may present with complaints of excessive daytime sleepiness or insomnia secondary to arousals during seizure activity.

BIBLIOGRAPHY

Aldrich MS, Jahnke B: Diagnostic value of video-EEG polysomnography, *Neurology* 41:1060–1066, 1991.
Bazil CW: Nocturnal seizures, *Semin Neurol* 24:293–300, 2004.
Chesson AL, DellaBadia J: Seizure disorders and sleep. In Lee-Chiong TL, Sateia MJ, Carsakadon MA, editors: *Sleep medicine*, Philadelphia, 2002, Hanley and Belfus, pp 521–531.
Foldvary-Schaefer N, Alsheikhtaha Z: Complex nocturnal behaviors: nocturnal seizures and parasomnias, *Continuum (Minneap Minn)* 19(1):104–131, 2013.
Foldvary-Schaefer N, Grigg-Damberger M: Sleep and epilepsy, *Sleep Med Clin* 3:443–454, 2008.
Hrachovy RA, Frost JD: The EEG in selected generalized seizures, *J Clin Neurophysiol* 23:312–332, 2006.
Libenson MH, editor: *Practical approach to electroencephalography*, Philadelphia, 2010, Saunders.
Maganti RK, Rutecki P: EEG and epilepsy monitoring, *Continuum (Minneap Minn)* 19(3):598–622, 2013.
Malow B, Fromes A, Gail A, et al: Usefulness of polysomnography in epilepsy patients, *Neurology* 48:1389–1394, 1997.
Vaughn BV, D'Cruz OF: Sleep and epilepsy, *Semin Neurol* 24:301–313, 2004.

A 55-Year-Old Man with Unusual Movements During Sleep

A 55-year-old man was evaluated for loud snoring and suspected sleep apnea. However, his wife also reported that he would sometimes sit up suddenly, exhibit repetitive mouth movements, grab at the bed sheets with his right hand. During the episodes, it was difficult to communicate with the patient, although he appeared to be awake. The episodes, which occurred once or twice weekly, had begun 1 year previously. After the episode, he would be responsive but groggy. In the morning, he had no recall of the events.

Physical examination: Unremarkable.

Sleep study: No overt body movements or periodic limb movements (PLMs) were noted. Figure P106-1 shows a 20-second tracing obtained when the patient had just fallen asleep.

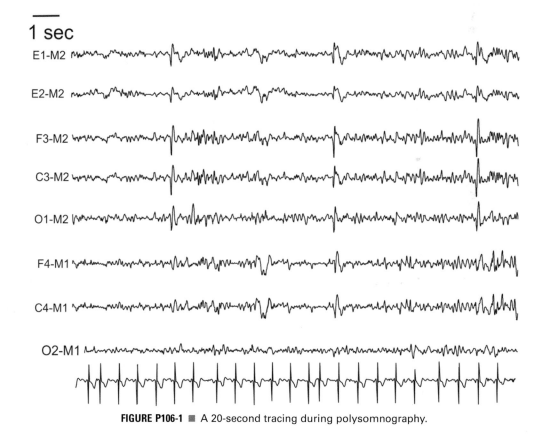

FIGURE P106-1 ■ A 20-second tracing during polysomnography.

QUESTION

1. What is causing the movements during sleep?

ANSWER

1. **Answer:** Seizure (complex partial; right temporal lobe), interictal spikes seen on electroencephalography (EEG).

Discussion: The 20-second tracing shows a spike (downward) in E1-M2, E2-M2, F3-M2, C3-M2, and O1-M2. Spikes are sharp transients with a duration of 20 to 70 milliseconds (msec). They appear to have a slightly narrower width than the electrocardiography (ECG) QRS complex. On 30-second windows, they appear as nearly straight lines. Spikes are often followed by waves. Note that the spike activity in Figure P106-1 is *not* ECG artifact, as the activity is not seen at the same time as ECG complexes. A spike-and-wave pattern usually indicates interictal activity rather than artifact. In Figure P106-1, the spikes are most prominent in the derivations that have M2 in common and are downward. This means that M2 is negative with respect to the other electrode (E1, F3, C3, and O1). Recall that spikes are usually electronegative. These findings suggest a seizure focus near M2 likely in the right temporal area. However, definite localization would require a more extensive montage. The complexes were not vertex sharp waves, which are associated with upward deflections in the usual sleep monitoring derivations and are wide-based (>70 msec) with central prominence and sporadic.

Seizure disorders are part of the differential diagnosis of "nocturnal spells"—episodes of abnormal motor activity during sleep. Depending on the type of patients studied, as many as 10% to 40% of seizures occur exclusively or mainly during sleep. The incidence of nocturnal seizures has two peaks: one about 2 hours after bedtime and another between 4 and 5 AM. Daytime seizures are most prevalent in the first hour after awakening. In general, all manifestations of nocturnal seizure disorders are much more common in non–rapid eye movement (NREM) sleep than in REM sleep. (NREM > Wake > REM). Prior sleep deprivation activates seizures; therefore, patients often undergo clinical EEG monitoring in a sleep-deprived state to increase the likelihood of recording seizure activity.

In Table P106-1, seizure disorders commonly associated with sleep or that typically occur soon after awakening are listed. Seizures are classified as partial (focal) onset, arising from a localized area of the brain (with or without subsequent generalization), and generalized onset, arising from both hemispheres simultaneously.

Partial seizures have a focal onset (localized part of the brain) but may become generalized and result in generalized tonic-clonic (GTC) seizures. Focal seizure disorders have higher incidence of interictal discharges or seizure activity in NREM sleep, particularly stage 2 sleep when brain activity is more synchronized. Simple partial seizures result in focal motor, sensory, autonomic, or psychic manifestations without a change of consciousness. Complex partial seizures usually arise from the mesial or lateral part of the temporal lobe or adjacent parts of the frontal lobe. The symptoms consist of changes in the content of consciousness that reduce the patient's ability to interact with the surroundings. They may occur with only a change in consciousness or also include *automatisms* (repetitive movements that may be purposeful but serve no obvious purpose in the actual situation). For example, lip smacking is a common automatism. Patients with complex partial seizures may have no recollection of the events or only partial memory. Patients may remember an aura, a subjective sensation such as déjà vu, epigastric sensation, and visual or olfactory disturbance that precedes the loss of awareness. The aura is actually a simple partial seizure that may sometimes spread to areas that affect cognition, resulting in subsequent loss of awareness.

TABLE P106-1   **Seizure Disorders Commonly Presenting During Sleep**

Partial Epilepsy (may be secondarily generalized)
1. Frontal lobe epilepsy (FLE)
   A. Nocturnal FLE (NFLE)
   B. Autosomal dominant FLE
2. Temporal lobe epilepsy (TLE)
3. Benign centrotemporal epilepsy with centrotemporal spikes (BECTS)

Generalized Epilepsy
1. Generalized tonic-clonic (GTC) seizures on awakening
2. Absence epilepsy (petit mal)
3. Juvenile myoclonic epilepsy (JME)

Primary generalized epilepsies include idiopathic GTC seizures, absence seizures (petit mal), and juvenile myoclonic seizures. GTC seizures consist of a sudden loss of consciousness, a tonic phase of intense muscle contraction and then a clonic phasic consisting of bilaterally synchronous jerking of the entire body. A postictal period after the seizure is characterized by disorientation lasting a variable amount of time. Absence seizures are manifested as a blank stare during which the patient is unresponsive typically for 10 to 30 seconds but immediately return to normal level of consciousness after the seizure. The characteristic waking electroencephalography (EEG) pattern is a 3-hertz (Hz) spike-and-wave pattern. Childhood absence seizures start in early childhood and rarely persist into adulthood. Juvenile absence seizures start later in childhood around age 8 to 12 years and persist throughout adulthood. Juvenile myoclonic epilepsy (JME), which typically starts in adolescence (12–18 years), is a genetically determined condition involving myoclonic jerks in the arms shortly after awakening. It may not be appreciated until the patient has a GTC. Primary generalized seizures are sometimes are called *awakening epilepsy* because the condition commonly occurs when the patient is in a drowsy state upon awakening from sleep. Patients with both juvenile absence and juvenile myoclonic seizures also may have GTC seizures. GTC seizures associated with these disorders usually occur on awakening. Sleep deprivation often precipitates these seizures.

Epileptiform activity is separated into interictal and ictal discharges (Table P106-2). Interictal refers to transient focal or generalized discharges between clinical seizures. Spikes (<70 msec), sharp waves (duration 70 to 120 msec), spike-and-wave complexes (Figure P106-2) are examples of interictal activity that may be isolated or repeated for several complexes. Ictal discharges refer to EEG rhythmic activity (delta, theta, alpha, or beta frequency) or runs of spike-and-wave complexes. Depending the location of onset of the seizure, the physiologic correlate of the ictal activity may be manifested by partial motor activity (limb jerking or dystonic posturing; frontal lobe partial seizure), staring and being nonresponsive for 1 to 3 minutes (temporal lobe partial seizure), GTC seizure, myoclonic jerking, absence seizure (brief period of unresponsiveness), or complex motor behavior. When these symptoms occur during sleep, they may not be recognized.

Temporal and frontal lobe epilepsies are often mislabeled as "other sleep-related conditions" (e.g., periodic limb movement in sleep [PLMS], sleepwalking). Video polysomnography (PSG)

TABLE P106-2 **Timing of Nocturnal Interictal and Ictal Activity—Effect of Sleep**					
	Interictal		**Ictal** AFTER		
	NREM	REM	AWAKENING	NREM	REM
Epilepsy with GTC on awakening	Common	Rare	Common	Less common	Uncommon
Focal	Common	Rare	Can occur	Common	Rare
Interictal activity	NREM > Wakefulness > REM				
Most common timing of nocturnal seizures	About 2 hours after bedtime Between 4 and 5 AM				
Incidence of nocturnal seizures	NREM > Wakefulness > REM				

GTC, General tonic-clonic; *NREM,* non–rapid eye movement; *REM,* rapid eye movement.

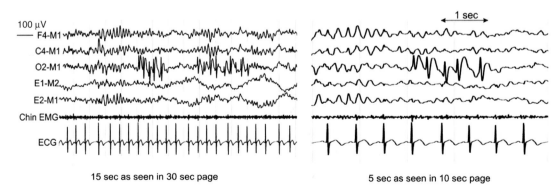

15 sec as seen in 30 sec page   5 sec as seen in 10 sec page

FIGURE P106-2 ■ Interictal activity consisting of bursts of three per second spike-and-wave complexes seen in the occipital derivation.

with synchronized video recording is very useful in making the correct diagnosis. Of note, some seizures are not associated with activity on scalp EEG. Therefore, capturing repetitive stereotypical events on video-EEG or even home videos is imperative to characterize seizure disorders, particularly those of frontal lobe origin. The type of movements that patients display during the "spell" (seminology) may be helpful. Although a full clinical EEG montage is optimal, it is helpful if additional electrodes such as T7 and T8 are added to electrodes typically recorded during routine PSG. It is then possible to have a display of the following bipolar chains mimicking the "double banana" (longitudinal) bipolar montage (Table P106-3).

Temporal lobe epilepsy (TLE) comprises about 70% to 80% of focal seizures. Temporal lobe seizures begin focally and impair consciousness (complex partial seizures). Staring, orofacial or limb automatisms, and head and body movements frequently occur. In TLE, limb automatisms are often ipsilateral and dystonic posturing occurs contralateral to the seizure focus. The ictal pattern is often a buildup of lateralized rhythmic theta activity (see Figure P106-3). Temporal lobe seizures are more common in NREM sleep but also occur during the transition from NREM sleep to REM sleep. Interictal activity may often be seen even when using traditional sleep EEG monitoring, as the mastoid electrodes are near the temporal lobes. Of note, no abnormal EEG activity may be observed in some patients with temporal lobe epilepsy when scalp electrodes are used in the study. Partial seizures with complex automatisms have been described in a few patients; unusual sleepwalking episodes, vocalization, and violent behavior were noted. The majority of patients with

TABLE P106-3	**Longitudinal Bipolar Montage with Addition of Two Temporal Electrodes**	
Additional Electrodes T3, T4		**No Additional Electrodes**
F3-T7		F3-M1
T7-M1		M1-O1
M1-O1		F3-C3
F3-C3		C3-O1
C3-O1		F4-C4
F4-C4		C4-O2
C4-O2		F4-M2
F4-T8		M2-O2
T8-M2		
M2-O2		

T7 and T8 are often labeled as T3 and T4, respectively.

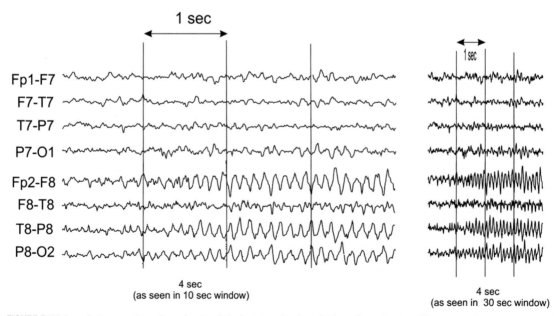

FIGURE P106-3 ■ A 4-second tracing obtained during monitoring during sleep in an epilepsy monitoring unit. 8 Hz ictal activity is noted in the right frontotemporal derivations.

TLE respond to antiepileptic medications. TLE is more common during wakefulness than during sleep. However, as TLE is more common that frontal lobe epilepsy (FLE), TLE is the most common nocturnal seizure type. TLE is more likely to generalize at night than during the day. FLE is more common at night than during the day. Daytime FLE is more likely to generalize.

Of focal seizure disorders, approximately 20% have an onset from the frontal lobes. The clinical manifestations of frontal lobe seizures may vary, depending on the localization of the epileptic focus. Typically, patients with EEG onset from the midline regions will have involvement of the supplementary motor area (SMA, also known as the supplemental sensorimotor area [SSMA]) eliciting complex motor manifestations such as dystonic posturing, vocalizations, or speech arrest with variable loss of consciousness and minimal postictal confusion. A classic manifestation is the "fencing posture" with the head turned toward an outstretched arm. Seizures arising from the supplemental sensorimotor area (SSMA) may involve thrashing with maintenance of consciousness and often are misdiagnosed as psychogenic seizures. Bicycling movements in the legs may occur. Seizures originating from the orbitofrontal areas and the cingulate gyrus often resemble those originating from the temporal lobes with staring, nonresponsiveness, and automatisms. Thus, the differentiation of frontal lobe and temporal lobe seizures, as listed in Table P106-4, is not absolute. In addition, seizures originating from the cingulate gyrus may also have autonomic features such as tachycardia, tachypnea, pallor, and sweating. Seizure onset from dorsolateral frontal lobes may result in behavioral arrest or aphasia or involve motor manifestations, depending on the extent of the spread of seizure activity (see Lee and Worrell 2012). In contrast, seizure onset in the posterior frontal lobes from the primary motor cortex may have discrete motor manifestation that have a jacksonian march, with muscle jerking that begins in the distal muscles of an extremity and moves up the extremity. Unfortunately, patients with frontal lobe seizures frequently do not exhibit interictal EEG activity. Patients with FLE often have multiple stereotypical events per night or per week, which helps differentiate them from parasomnia (which tends to have variable clinical manifestations that rarely occur more than twice per night).

Diagnosis of nocturnal seizures requires a full EEG montage and, ideally, simultaneous synchronized video recording. Temporal lobe epilepsy is especially difficult to document and often requires intracranial electrodes. Sometimes, a diagnosis is elusive, and an empiric trial of antiepileptic medications is needed. In routine clinical EEG monitoring, a 10-second window is typically used. In sleep monitoring, a 30-second window is used, and spikes appear as nearly a single vertical line. In sleep montages with a 30-second window, interictal activity appears sharper and often with a higher amplitude than on EEG monitoring (150 microvolts [μV] peak to peak versus 200 μV p-p on EEG). Unlike usual sleep patterns, interictal activity often manifests as repetitive occurrences of nearly identical patterns. If interictal activity is suspected, a switch to a 10-second window (the time window used in clinical EEG monitoring) and a bipolar montage should be made. The 10-second window allows improved recognition of spikes and other epileptiform waveforms. The differential of nocturnal seizures includes bruxism, PLMs, night terrors, sleepwalking, and REM sleep–related behavior disorder (RBD). General motor activity arising from seizures is simpler and more stereotypical than motor activity associated with sleepwalking, night terrors, and RBD.

In the present case, a routine sleep study was initially performed (see Figure P106-1) because of suspicion of sleep apnea. The patient had obstructive apnea during REM sleep, but frequent spike-and-wave complexes (S) also occurred during NREM sleep. The spike-and-wave complexes in the

TABLE P106-4	**Comparison of Frontal and Temporal Lobe Epilepsy***			
	Time of Occurrence	**Maintenance of Consciousness**	**Body Movements**	**Postictal Confusion**
Frontal lobe	More often during sleep	Often	Sudden onset and offset Sometimes violent dystonic posturing "fencing posture" Bicycling of legs or flipping to prone position Duration often <1 minute	Minimal
Temporal lobe	More often during wake	Consciousness impaired	Gradual onset and offset Oral (lip smacking) automatisms, ipsilateral limb automatisms, contralateral limb posturing Duration often >1 minute	Sometimes

*Note these differences are not absolute—see text.

figure occurred most prominently in derivations with M2 (near the right temporal lobe). The patient was referred to a neurologist, and full clinical EEG during sleep performed in the epilepsy monitoring unit confirmed the presence of ictal activity in the right temporal area during the patient's typical complex partial seizure (Figure P106-3). This shows ictal activity (about 8 Hz) on the right side. Activity at F8-T8 is minimal, suggesting a focus between electrodes F8 and T8 with phase reversal from Fp2-F8 to T8-P8, that is, a phase reversal in the frontotemporal area. The fact that the temporal leads are more involved than the frontocentral or frontopolar leads suggests an anterior temporal focus. When EEG shows 5 to 8 Hz theta- or alpha-activity from the temporal leads, it is classically from an anterior medial temporal lobe seizure focus involving the hippocampus. However, lateral frontal or orbitofrontal seizures may propagate to the temporal lobe. In focal seizures, the actual seizure focus may be at a location different from the one suggested by scalp EEG monitoring. Note that the ictal activity has a frequency in the high theta- to alpha-range but is not the typical-state alpha-rhythm associated with eyes-closed drowsiness, which is more prominent in occipital derivations. The patient was treated with levetiracetam, which resulted in the resolution of the episodes. MRI of the brain showed increased size of the temporal horn of the right lateral ventricle as well as atrophy of the right hippocampus.

CLINICAL PEARLS

1. Seizures are part of the differential diagnosis of abnormal motor behavior occurring during sleep. Some patients have seizures only at night associated with sleep or after awakening from sleep.
2. Optimal diagnosis of nocturnal seizures requires a full EEG montage, with simultaneous video recording. The ability of video PSG to detect and localize interictal activity is enhanced by addition of temporal electrodes T7, T8 (also known as T3 and T4).
3. Sharp EEG activity (spikes, sharp waves) noted during a routine sleep study could represent interictal epileptiform activity. It is recommended to switch to a 10-second page, a longitudinal bipolar montage, or a combination of both to more accurately access the activity. Remember, some sharp waves may be normal (vertex sharp waves). However, spike-and-wave activity is never normal. Epileptiform activity is usually electronegative and seen in more than one derivation.
4. Identification of interictal activity on PSG should prompt a more extensive evaluation for epilepsy, even if a clinical seizure is not recorded.
5. FLE is also called *sleeping epilepsy* because the seizures occur more frequently or only at night.
6. Complex partial seizures are associated with a focal onset and impairment of consciousness. Associated automatisms, dystonic posturing, thrashing of arms or legs, or complex automatisms mimicking sleepwalking may all occur.
7. TLE during sleep usually presents with complex partial seizures that may generalize.
8. Frontal lobe seizures originating in the supplementary sensorimotor cortex may be associated with maintenance of consciousness, bizarre dystonic movements (including a fencing posture or bicycling), with minimal postictal confusion. Such seizures are usually not associated with ictal activity on EEG (simply muscle artifact from movement).

BIBLIOGRAPHY

American Clinical Neurophysiology Society: Guideline 5: guidelines for standard electrode position nomenclature, *J Clin Neuophysiol* 23:107–110, 2006.
American Clinical Neurophysiology Society: Guideline 6: a proposal for standard montages to be used in clinical EEG, *J Clin Neuophysiol* 23:111–117, 2006.
Bazil CW: Nocturnal seizures, *Semin Neurol* 24:293–300, 2004.
Commission on Classification and Terminology of the International League Against Epilepsy: Proposal for revised classification of epilepsies and epileptic syndromes, *Epilepsia* 30:389, 1989.
Derry CP, Harvey AS, Walker MC, et al: NREM arousal parasomnias and their distinction from nocturnal frontal lobe epilepsy: a video EEG analysis, *Sleep* 32:1637–1644, 2009.
Foldvary-Schaefer N, Grigg-Damberger M: Sleep and epilepsy, *Sleep Med Clin* 3:443–454, 2008.
Herman ST, Walczak TS, Bazil CW: Distribution of partial seizures during the sleep-wake cycle: differences by seizure onset site, *Neurology* 56:1453–1459, 2001.
Hrachovy RA, Frost JD: The EEG in selected generalized seizures, *J Clin Neurophysiol* 23:312–332, 2006.
International Federation of Societies for Electroencephalography and Clinical Neurophysiology: Ten-twenty electrode system, *EEG Clin Neurophysiol* 10:371–375, 1958.
Lee RW, Worrell GA: Dorsolateral frontal lobe epilepsy, *J Clin Neurophysiol* 29(5):379–384, 2012.
Libenson MH, editor: *Practical approach to electroencephalography*, Philadelphia, 2010, Saunders.
Malow BA: Sleep and epilepsy, *Neurol Clin* 23:1127, 2005.
Tachiban N, Shinde A, Ikeda A, et al: Supplementary motor area seizure resembling sleep disorder, *Sleep* 19:811–816, 1996.
Vaught BV, D'Cruz OF: Sleep and epilepsy, *Semin Neurol* 24:301–313, 2004.

Abnormal Behavior During Sleep

Patient A: An 18-year-old male college student was referred for snoring, witnessed apnea, and possible confusional arousals. His roommate had witnessed only two of these episodes when he stayed up late studying while the patient was asleep. The patient would suddenly sit up in bed, groan, and stick out his right arm while turning his head to the right. The episode lasted about 30 seconds. The patient was awake but confused after the episode. He simply returned to the supine position and fell asleep. He did remember the episode the next morning when his roommate told him what he saw. The patient was aware of similar episodes which he attributed to severe muscle spasms and admitted that they often happened more than once a night. He did not take any medications. No history of head trauma was present. In his childhood, the patient did have sleepwalking episodes. However, he had slept in a bedroom by himself since age 13, and no similar episodes had been noted by his parents.

Physical examination: body mass index (BMI) 32 kilograms per square meter (kg/m^2); HEENT: normal except for Mallampati 4 upper airway; neurological examination: normal

Polysomnography (PSG): The apnea–hypopnea index (AHI) was 30 per hour (hr). A tracing obtained during an episode in the sleep center is shown in Figure P107-1. The patient sat up suddenly and extended the right arm and turned his head toward the right and groaned.

When the technologist entered the room, the patient was alert and said the felt like he had had muscle spasms in his arm and neck.

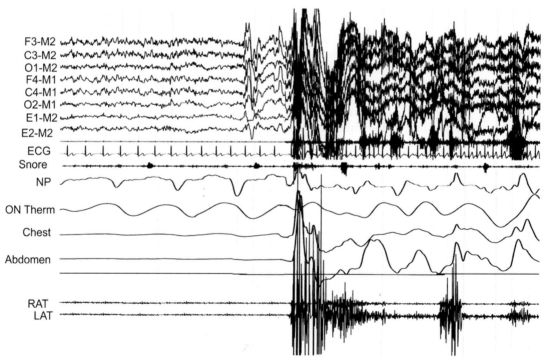

FIGURE P107-1 ■ A 30-second tracing. Patient A aroused from sleep, sat up, and extended his right arm for about 30 seconds.

QUESTION 1. What is causing the spells in Patient A?

Patient B: A 16-year-old male is referred for evaluation of recurrent sleep terrors. Although he usually slept in his own bedroom, during a trip, he had shared a room with his father. His father noted that at least four times during the night, the patient sat up in bed, screamed, and then quickly went back to sleep. The episodes lasted only 20 seconds. He asked his son what the problem was, but the patient had quickly returned to sleep without answering. The father remembered a few episodes when the patient was a young child, when he screamed during the night. The episodes had lasted longer and only one episode per night had been noted.

QUESTION 2. Why do so many "sleep terrors" occur in a single night in Patient B?

ANSWERS

1. **Answer for Patient A:** Nocturnal frontal lobe epilepsy (FLE)—supplemental motor cortex.

2. **Answer for Patient B:** Nocturnal FLE—paroxysmal arousal.

Discussion (Patients A and B): Nocturnal FLE (NFLE) is associated with a wide spectrum of manifestations and is the type of epilepsy most likely mistaken as a type of NREM or REM parasomnia. *In roughly half of the cases of NFLE, no abnormality is seen on scalp electroencephalography (EEG) during the episodes*, and many cases also have no interictal epileptiform activity. In some of the cases with normal scalp EEG, abnormalities may be demonstrated by invasive EEG monitoring. NFLE episodes are confined to sleep in most cases, so they are less well observed. Patients often remain conscious with minimal postictal confusion. Nocturnal ambulation such as walking and crying and autonomic activation may mimic sleepwalking and sleep terrors. NFLE exists in familial, sporadic, symptomatic (associated with identifiable structural lesion), and idiopathic forms.

Of focal seizure disorders, approximately 20% have an onset from the frontal lobes. The clinical manifestations of frontal lobe seizures may vary, depending on localization of the epileptic focus. Seizures originating from the orbitofrontal areas and the cingulate gyrus often resemble those originating from the temporal lobes, with staring, nonresponsiveness, and automatisms. Seizure onset in the posterior frontal lobes from the primary motor cortex may have discrete motor manifestations that have a jacksonian march that begins in the distal muscles of an extremity and moves up the extremity. Patients with a seizure focus located in the midline regions will often have involvement of the supplementary motor cortex, eliciting complex motor manifestations such as dystonic posturing, vocalizations, or speech arrest, with variable loss of consciousness and minimal postictal confusion. In addition, seizures originating from the cingulate gyrus may also have autonomic features such as tachycardia, tachypnea, pallor, and sweating. Seizure onset from dorsolateral frontal lobes may be (difficulty speaking or speech arrest) or involve motor manifestations such as tonic or clonic movements, depending on the extent of spread of the seizure activity. As noted above, patients with FLE seizures frequently do not exhibit interictal EEG activity.

NFLE SYNDROMES: Provinin and colleagues described three general manifestations of NFLE, including paroxysmal arousals (PAs), nocturnal paroxysmal dystonia (NPD), and episodic nocturnal wandering (ENW) (Table P107-1). PAs, which typically present during NREM sleep, consist of a stereotypical series of movements lasting 2 to 20 seconds, in which the individuals raise their head, sit up, and look around confused with a frightened expression and then scream. Unlike typical sleep terrors, *PAs may occur many times during the night and are very stereotypical.* Of note, vocalization during sleep terrors is usually a scream or other vocalization that may vary from episode to episode. Vocalization for PAs may include an obsenity and is the same every time (stereotypic). NPD is characterized by nocturnal coarse movements associated with tonic spasms that often occur multiple times per night. The episodes may be violent or be associated with vocalization. Patients often move the arms and legs with cycling or kicking movements and sometimes adopt a dystonic posture of the limbs. ENW may present with symptoms similar to sleepwalking and sleep terrors. Patients may jump out of bed, wander, vocalize, and show violent behavior during sleep. Classically, treatment with older anticonvulsants (in particular, carbamazepine) or newer anticonvulsants such as levetiracetam at bedtime is generally effective. However, some patients' conditions are refractory to antiepileptic medications. It is important to note that a significant proportion of patients with NFLE do have seizures during wakefulness, generalization to tonic-clonic seizures, and a demonstrable brain abnormality.

FAMILIAL NFLE: The original description was an autosomal dominant nocturnal frontal lobe epilepsy (ADNFLE) associated with a missense mutation of the neuronal nicotinic acetylcholine receptor (nAChR) alpha$_4$-subunit. Other mutations of the *nAChR* gene system have been found, and genetic heterogeneity has been observed in families with ADNFLE. Motor seizures are

TABLE P107-1 **Manifestations of Nocturnal Frontal Lobe Epilepsy**

	PA	NPD	ENW
Frequency	Multiple times per night (mean 2)	Multiple times per night (mean 3)	Multiple times (1 to 3 per night)
Duration of episodes	Short 20–40 seconds	More prolonged (25–98 seconds)	31–180 seconds
	Patients sit up, look around confused	Arm and leg movements Cycling Kicking Dystonic posture (fencing) Pelvic thrusting Vocalization Violence may occur	Jump out of bed Wander Vocalize Violent behavior
May communicate at end of seizure	100%	44% may communicate at end of episode	100%
May communicate during seizure	12/27	10/59 during episode	None
Stereotypical or varied	Stereotypical	Stereotypical	Stereotypical, agitated somnambulism
Daytime seizures	No	57% (49% secondarily generalized seizures)	13%
Brain structural abnormality	0%	24%	5%

Adapted from Provini F, Plazzi G, Tinuper P, et al: Nocturnal frontal lobe epilepsy, *Brain* 122:1017-1031, 1999.
ENW, Episodic nocturnal wandering; *NPD*, nocturnal paroxysmal dystonia; *PA*, paroxysmal arousal.

frequent (nearly every night), are often violent, occur in clusters, and are brief (<1 minute). The age of onset is variable (2 months to 56 years). About 90% of patients present by age 20 years.

SUPPLEMENTAL MOTOR AREA EPILEPSY: Focal seizures arising from the supplementary motor area (SMA), a region anterior to the motor cortex in the midline, is a type of FLE that typically involves unilateral or asymmetrical bilateral tonic posturing and may be associated with facial grimacing, vocalization, or speech arrest. SMA seizures may be preceded by a somatosensory aura. Complex automatisms such as kicking, laughing, vocal outbursts, or pelvic thrusting may be present with *responsiveness often preserved.* A classic manifestation of SMA epilepsy is the "fencing posture" with the head turned toward an outstretched arm (head turns away from side of seizure focus). *Because consciousness is often well preserved and postictal confusion is minimal, these episodes are sometime thought to be psychogenic.* However, unlike psychogenic movements, SMA epilepsy episodes are typically brief and stereotypical.

Patient A probably had manifestations of NFLE from the supplementary motor area (probably a left-sided focus). His movements during the episodes were similar to the classic fencing posture in which the arm is outstretched and head turned to the same side (contralateral to seizure focus). On the side ipsilateral to the focus, the arm may be flexed upward as in the fencing posture. The PSG tracing shows only muscle artifact, with the episode occurring out of stage N2. In this patient, full EEG with scalp electrodes failed to show interictal findings, and during his stay in the epilepsy monitoring unit, the episodes were documented, but no EEG ictal activity was noted (only muscle artifact). The patient was treated with levetiracetam, and the frequency of the episodes decreased.

Patient B exhibited behavior similar to paroxysmal arousal, as described by Provini. Of note, more than one were noted in a given night, and they were very brief.

PARASOMNIAS VERSUS NFLE: The differences between NFLE and NREM parasomnia are listed in Table P107-2. In general, NFLE is associated with greater frequency (episodes per month) and is more likely to consist of multiple episodes in a given night. The manifestations of NREM parasomnia also vary from night to night, whereas NFLE seizures have very stereotypical manifestations. They may be bizarre, but they always consist of the same activity. EEG is not that helpful in many cases because approximately 40% to 50% of patients with NFLE have no interictal or ictal EEG findings (apart from movement and muscle artifact associated with the spells).

TABLE P107-2 **Nocturnal Frontal Lobe Epilepsy (NFLE) Versus Non–Rapid Eye Movement (NREM) Parasomnia**

	NFLE	NREM Parasomnia (Confusional Arousals, Sleep Terrors, Sleepwalking)
Age at onset (year ± SD)	14 ± 10 (infancy to adolescence)	<10
Gender	Male/female 7/3	M = F
Ictal EEG	NREM: **sleep stage N2** Normal ictal EEG 44% (higher if only scalp electrodes used) Normal interictal EEG 51%	NREM sleep Stage N3 in children
Movement seminology	Violent, stereotypical	Complex, nonstereotypical
Family history of episodes	39%	62%–96%
Episode frequency per month	20 ± 11	<1–4
Episode frequency per night	3 ± 3 (higher with PA, NPD)	1
Episode duration	2 seconds to 3 minutes	15 sec–30 min
Clinical course	Increased frequency	Tends to resolve
Triggering factors	None in 78%	Sleep deprivation, alcohol, febrile illness
Autonomic activation	Very common (tachycardia)	Yes in sleep terrors
Episode onset after sleep onset	Any time	First third of night in children
Effect of treatment	Carbamazepine abolished (20%) or improved episodes (50%)	N/A

Adapted from Provini F, Plazzi G, Tinuper P, et al: Nocturnal frontal lobe epilepsy, *Brain* 122:1017-1031, 1999.
EEG, Electroencephalography; *N/A*, not applicable; *NFLE*, nocturnal frontal lobe epilepsy; *NPD*, nocturnal paroxysmal dystonia; *NREM*, non–rapid eye movement; *PA*, paroxysmal arousal; *SD*, standard deviation.

CLINICAL PEARLS

1. FLE may present with seizures only at night (NFLE). The manifestations vary, depending on the focus, but may include paroxysmal arousals that mimic sleep terrors, NPD (dystonic posturing) or ENW (mimics sleep walking) in which the patient leaves the bed and performs complex behaviors.

2. NFLE may manifest as very bizarre movements such as bicycling, pelvic thrusting with preserved consciousness, and partial to complete memory of the episodes.

3. In contrast to NREM parasomnia, NFLE episodes occur more frequently during stage N2 (versus stage N3), multiple short episodes may occur per night (versus one per night), and the behavior is stereotypical, whereas behavior in NREM parasomnia is variable from episode to episode.

4. In about 50% of cases of NFLE, scalp EEG will NOT show either interictal or ictal activity. EEG performed during the episode may simply show muscle and movement artifact.

BIBLIOGRAPHY

Bazil CW: Nocturnal seizures, *Semin Neurol* 24:293–300, 2004.
Derry CP, Harvey AS, Walker MC, et al: NREM arousal parasomnias and their distinction from nocturnal frontal lobe epilepsy: a video EEG analysis, *Sleep* 32:1637–1644, 2009.
Foldvary-Schaefer N, Alsheikhtaha Z: Complex nocturnal behaviors: nocturnal seizures and parasomnias, *Continuum (Minneap Minn)* 19(1):104–131, 2013.
Herman ST, Walczak TS, Bazil CW: Distribution of partial seizures during the sleep-wake cycle: differences by seizure onset site, *Neurology* 56:1453–1459, 2001.
Malow BA: Sleep and epilepsy, *Neurol Clin* 23:1127, 2005.
Provini F, Plazzi G, Montagna P, Lugaresi E: The wide spectrum of nocturnal frontal lobe epilepsy, *Sleep Med Rev* 4:375–386, 2000.
Provini F, Plazzi G, Tinuper P, et al: Nocturnal frontal lobe epilepsy, *Brain* 122:1017–1031, 1999.
Tachiban N, Shinde A, Ikeda A, et al: Supplementary motor area seizure resembling sleep disorder, *Sleep* 19:811–816, 1996.

A Child with Mouth Movements During Sleep and a Teenager with Jerks in the Morning After Awakening

Patient A: A 6-year-old male underwent sleep monitoring for loud snoring, labored breathing during sleep, and daytime behavioral problems. During the night, the boy's parents had noted that his arms sometimes jerked during sleep and that he had mouth movements and sometimes drooling.

Physical examination was normal for age except for enlarged tonsils.

Polysomnography (PSG) showed an apnea–hypopnea index (AHI) of 5 per hour (hr) with an arterial oxygen saturation (SAO_2) of 88%. A 15-second tracing from the sleep study performed soon after sleep onset is shown in Figure P108-1.

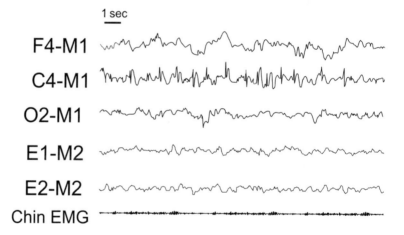

FIGURE P108-1 ■ A 15-second tracing from polysomnography performed in the 6-year-old boy undergoing a sleep study for suspected obstructive sleep apnea.

Patient B: A 16-year-old male was noted to have bilateral arm jerks soon after awakening in the morning while still in bed. These episodes also happened in the morning when he was out of bed (he threw his toothbrush across the bathroom). He also had difficulty handling objects when getting ready for school. The episodes were ignored until the patient had a generalized tonic-clonic (GTC) seizure.

QUESTIONS

1. What is your diagnosis for Patient A?

2. What seizure disorder in Patient B does this scenario suggest?

ANSWERS

1. **Answer:** Benign epilepsy of childhood with centrotemporal spikes (BECTS) also known as benign rolandic epilepsy (BRE).

   Discussion: Epileptiform discharges are found in 1% to 2% of patients on pediatric PSG, and the incidence may be higher in those with sleep-disordered breathing (SDB). BECTS, or BRE, accounts for 15% to 20% of childhood epilepsy. The average age of onset is 5 to 8 years (range 3–13 years), with a male predominance. The cardinal features of BRE are focal seizures consisting of unilateral facial sensory motor symptoms (numbness, tingling), oro-pharyngo-laryngeal symptoms (tingling or numbness of mouth, "death rattle," gargling, grunting, and guttural sounds), hypersalivation, tonic contractions of the ipsilateral arm and leg, and speech arrest. Hemifacial sensory motor seizures (tingling, numbness) are mainly localized in the lower lip and may spread to the ipsilateral hand. Motor manifestations are clonic contractions that are sometimes concurrent with ipsilateral tonic deviation of the mouth. In speech arrest, the child is actually anarthric, that is, unable to utter a single intelligible word, and attempts to communicate with gestures. Consciousness and recollection are fully retained in more than half (58%) of the cases of BREs. In the remainder, consciousness becomes impaired during the ictal EEG activity, and in one third, no recollection of ictal events exists. Three quarters of BREs occur during NREM sleep, mainly at sleep onset or just before awakening. The onset of seizure activity is about 20 minutes to 3 hours after bedtime. BREs are usually brief lasting for 1 to 3 minutes. By definition, centrotemporal spikes (CTS) are the hallmark of benign childhood epilepsy with CTS (see Figure P108-1). However, although called *centrotemporal*, these spikes are mainly localized in the C3 and C4, not in the temporal electrodes. The CTS EEG activity is often bilateral and typically activated by drowsiness and NREM sleep, but not by overbreathing. Generalized seizures may occur during sleep. Only those with cognitive impairment, very frequent epileptiform discharges on EEG, and history of generalized seizures are usually treated. Such patients should undergo neurologic evaluation.

   Panayiotopoulos syndrome (PS) is another "benign age-related focal seizure disorder" occurring in early and mid-childhood. It is characterized by seizures, often prolonged, with predominantly autonomic manifestations, including nausea, wretching, vomiting, pallor, syncope without convulsions, incontinence of urine, hypersalivation (10%), cyanosis (12%), and mydriasis. Unlike BECTS, the seizures can be prolonged, lasting 6 minutes to many hours. Prolonged seizures are called *autonomic status epilepticus*. EEG shows shifting and multiple foci, but usually with occipital predominance.

   In the current patient, spike-and-wave complexes were seen in the central derivation. The patient was referred to neurology and eventually had a tonsillectomy and adenoidectomy for obstructive sleep apnea (OSA). The nocturnal seizures decreased in number and eventually resolved without medication.

2. **Answer:** Juvenile myoclonic epilepsy (JME).

   Discussion: JME is idiopathic (i.e., no demonstrable brain lesion) and has a genetic basis, with an abnormality on the short arm of chromosome 6. Onset is in adolescence, peaking between ages 12 and 18. This is one of the more common forms of generalized epilepsy and consists of a combination of myoclonic seizures on awakening, generalized tonic-clonic (GTC) seizures, and absence seizures. The myoclonic seizures occur in clusters on awakening or shortly thereafter. Patients may not seek medical evaluation until after the first associated GTC seizure. The myoclonic seizure may subside during adulthood, but patients often have persistent GTC seizures and require lifelong treatment with antiepileptic medications. Interictal EEG in JME is characterized by diffuse polyspike and slow wave complexes of 4 to 6 hertz (Hz), usually maximal at the frontal electrodes (Figure P108-2). Neurologic examination and brain magnetic resonance imaging (MRI) are usually normal.

CLINICAL PEARLS
1. BECTS should be suspected when spike-and-wave activity is seen prominently in the central derivations and a history of abnormal mouth movements, hypersalivation, and unusual vocalizations is present in a young child with otherwise normal neurologic functioning.
2. The BECTS episodes are unilateral, and the patient responds but may not be able to speak.
3. Protracted episodes of vomiting that suddenly occur during sleep should suggest the possibility of PS.
4. Patients with JME commonly have myoclonic jerking soon after awakening. They may also have GTC seizures soon after awakening.

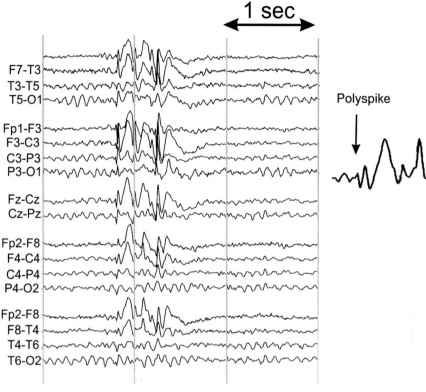

FIGURE P108-2 ■ Brief generalized spike-and-wave (some polyspikes) firing at about 4 hertz (Hz) in a patient with juvenile myoclonic epilepsy.

BIBLIOGRAPHY

Capdeila O, Dayyat E, Kheirandish-Gozal L, Gozal D: Prevalence of epileptiform activity in healthy children during sleep, *Sleep Med* 9(3):303–309, 2008.

Miano S, Bachiller C, Gutiérrez M, et al: Paroxysmal activity and seizures associated with sleep breathing disorder in children: a possible overlap between diurnal and nocturnal symptoms, *Seizure* 19(9):547–552, 2010.

Panayiotopoulos CP, Michael M, Sanders S, et al: Benign childhood focal epilepsies: assessment of established and newly recognized syndromes, *Brain* 131(9):2264–2286, 2008.

PATIENT 109

Patients with Parkinsonism and Sleep Problems

Patient A: A 50-year-old man is being treated with pramipexole for Parkinson disease. His wife reported that he snored loudly at night and had frequent breathing pauses. He was often awakened by nocturia or pain. During the day, he had increased daytime sleepiness. The sleepiness was usually constant throughout the day, but he had a few severe attacks of sleepiness that were unpredictable. One resulted in an automobile accident and the subsequent loss of his driver's license.

    Question:

1. Which of the following are possible causes daytime sleepiness in Patient A?
   A. Obstructive sleep apnea (OSA)
   B. Pramipexole use
   C. Parkinson disease (PD)
   D. All of the above

Patient B: A 60-year-old man is being evaluated for possible parkinsonism. He has symptoms of irregular hand tremor and slowed gait and falls. If he stood up quickly, he got dizzy, and he also reported erectile dysfunction and constipation. His wife reports that he has had at least a 5-year history of acting out violent dreams. He once hit her, and she now sleeps in another bed in the same room. The patient's intellectual function is intact. The patient has a long history of snoring and witnessed apnea but has refused polysomnography (PSG). Recently, the patient's wife has noted a high-pitched sound during his sleep when he breaths in (stridor). This has caused her great concern. The patient's primary physician referred the patient to an otolaryngologist for vocal cord evaluation, but this study was normal.

Physical examination showed a resting tremor and stooped shuffling gait.

Sleep study: Apnea-hypopea index 20 per hour. There were episodes of stridor noted during NREM. During REM sleep there was evidence of REM sleep without atonia, as well as movements of the arms and legs. However, no violent behavior was noted.

QUESTION

2. Which of the following conditions is likely present in Patient B?
   A. PD
   B. Multiple system atrophy (MSA)
   C. Lewy body dementia (LBD)
   D. Essential tremor

ANSWERS

1. **Answer for Patient A:** D. All of the above.

2. **Answer for Patient B:** Multiple system atrophy (MSA).

   Discussion (Patients A and B): Parkinsonism is a syndrome characterized by resting tremor, slowness of movement (bradykinesia), cogwheel rigidity, postural instability, or all of these symptoms. The differential diagnosis of parkinsonism (Table P109-1) includes Parkinson disease (PD), atypical parkinsonism disorders (formerly called *Parkinson plus*), and second parkinsonism (caused by medications, vascular injury). Atypical Parkinson disorders (APDs) include Lewy body dementia (LBD), MSA, progressive supranuclear palsy, and corticobasilar degeneration. Only PD, LBD, and MSA will be discussed here.

   Tremor is usually the first symptom of PD and is present in about 70% of patients. It is a resting tremor that is typically asymmetric, has a low frequency (4 to 6 hertz [Hz]), and is characterized by a pill-rolling movement (supination–pronation). Manifestations of bradykinesia (slow movement) include micrographia (small handwriting), hypophonia (quiet monotone speech), hypomimia (reduced facial expression) or masked facies (loss of facial expression), and the general lack of spontaneous movement. Mentation is normal early in the disease, but later, dementia, psychosis, and visual hallucinations occur. Gait instability may worsen with disease progression. Physical findings in PD include resting pill-rolling tremor, glabellar reflex (tapping of forehead elicits continued blinking [a frontal lobe sign]), and cogwheel rigidity (joint stiffness and increased muscle tone). Fewer blinks may occur, as well as less arm swinging with walking. Gait is often stooped and shuffling with pedestal-like turning. Early in the disease, distracting maneuvers may help detect rigidity, for example, having the patient tap on the table with the fingers of the contralateral hand while the tone of the ipsilateral arm is being tested. With progression of the disorder, urinary symptoms (nocturia and incontinence may occur).

   Patients with PD have abnormal sleep and daytime sleepiness (Box P109-1). They have frequent awakenings because of nocturia, discomfort from bradykinesia or rigidity (fewer position shifts in bed), and dyskinesia. Nocturnal hallucinations may occur in PD and disturb sleep. Antiparkinsonism medications may also produce hallucinations. A recent study compared sleep between groups of patients with PD who had visual hallucinations and those who did not. Although both groups slept

TABLE P109-1 **Causes of Parkinsonism**

Parkinson Disease (PD)

Resting tremor (pill rolling), bradykinesia, rigidity
Rapid eye movement sleep behavior disorder (RBD) common (20%–30%)
Dopamine responsive
Dementia or psychosis later (if present)
Postural instability later

Atypical Parkinsonism (Parkinson Plus)

Lewy body dementia (LBD)	Dementia early Bilateral No or poor response to dopamine RBD common (50%–70%)
Multiple system atrophy (MSA): 1. Striatonigral degeneration (MSA-P) 2. Olivopontocerebellar atrophy (MSA-C)	Postural instability often prominent early Autonomic dysfunction often s prominent early (erectile dysfunction, constipation, or postural hypotension/syncope) RBD common
3. Progressive supranuclear palsy (PSP)	Vertical gaze palsy, dementia, severe insomnia, RBD may occur
4. Corticobulbar degeneration (CBD)	Early postural instability + vertical gaze palsy Computed tomography abnormal Cortical deficits (apraxia)

Note: PD, LBD, MSA are alpha-synucleinopathies, and PSP and CBD are tau-synucleinopathies.

BOX P109-1 | **Sleep Problems Associated with Parkinson Disease**

- Insomnia
- Excessive daytime sleepiness
- Nightmares
- Sleep attacks (a sudden involuntary episode of sleep)
- Rapid eye movement (REM) sleep–related behavior disorder (acting out dreams during sleep)
- Periodic limb movement disorder (PLMD)
- Restless legs syndrome (RLS)
- Sleep apnea
- Nocturia (frequent nighttime urination)

poorly, the group with visual hallucinations had much poorer sleep. OSA is common in PD. Data about OSA being more common in PD than in age-matched controls are conflicting. A recent review of published evidence (da Silva-Júnior et al) concluded that OSA was *not* more common in patients with PD than in age-matched individuals without PD. In any case, OSA is common in patients with PD, and they often have a *normal BMI*. A study by Cochen De Cock concluded that OSA was not a significant cause of daytime sleepiness in *most* patients with PD. Daytime sleepiness in PD may be caused by treatment with dopamine agonists (DAs) or may be a direct manifestation of PD. Some evidence suggests that patients with PD may have partial loss of hypocretin-producing neurons. However, Patient A exhibited loud snoring and frequent breathing pauses, so sleep apnea could be a significant cause of daytime sleepiness.

Rapid eye movement sleep behavior disorder (RBD) is common in PD (30% to 60%, depending on the definition of RBD) and is often present for many years before onset of manifestations of PD. Patients with PD also have a high rate of restless leg syndrome (RLS) and periodic limb movement in sleep (PLMS). Dyskinesia, manifested by sudden jerky or uncontrolled movements of the limbs and neck, is a side effect of levodopa or carbidopa treatment and may disturb sleep. DAs are less likely to cause dyskinesia and may alleviate the rigidity but have some dose-dependent side effects of their own. In low doses, DAs tend to cause sleepiness or promote sleep. Although increased dopamine transmission usually increases wakefulness, ropinirole or pramipexole in low doses may stimulate the autoreceptors to decrease dopamine release and may cause sedation. In high doses, DAs may cause insomnia, frequent awakenings, and a reduction in the amount of stage N3 sleep. Another serious side effect of DA treatment of PD is the often unpredictable *sudden onset of severe daytime sleepiness.* Modafinil has been used for daytime sleepiness in PD. An attack of sudden sleepiness induced by pramipexole may have also been the cause of the "sleep attack" in Patient B.

In APDs, manifestations of parkinsonism are present, but certain symptoms that typically present late in the course of PD are present early in APDs. In general, tremor is less prominent. APDs should be suspected when dementia (LBD), gaze restriction (PSP), or autonomic dysfunction or postural instability (MSA) is present *early* in the disease course. For example, if dementia is noted within 1 year of the onset of parkinsonism symptoms, LBD is the likely diagnosis. In contrast to PD, APDs have a more rapid downhill course and have minimal or no response to DAs. Dopamine blockers (including antipsychotics and some antiemetics) may cause severe rigidity in some patients with APDs (especially LBD) and should be avoided. Quetiapine is an atypical antipsychotic that is used for psychosis in PD, LBD, and MSA and does not appear to worsen rigidity. RBD is very common in both MSA and LBD and may precede or start at the onset of other symptoms. As noted above, RBD may be present for many years before the onset of PD.

The major manifestations of LBD include (1) fluctuating cognition, with great variation in attention and alertness from day to day and hour to hour; (2) recurrent visual hallucinations (75% of patients with DLBD); (3) motor features of parkinsonism (tremor less common in DLBD than in PD); (4) RBD (50%–75%), and (5) problems with orthostasis, including repeated falls, syncope (fainting), and transient loss of consciousness. The onset of RBD may occur years before the other manifestations of DLBD (similar to PD).

An important characteristic of DLBD is *exquisite sensitivity to dopamine blockers.* When given dopamine blockers, patients with DLBD may develop life-threatening rigidity or malignant neuroleptic syndrome. Anticholinergic drugs such as diphenhydramine or terazosin (Hytrin) may worsen dementia.

MSA has traditionally been divided into three separate conditions: (1) striatonigral degeneration (MSA-P), (2) olivopontocerebellar degeneration (MSA-C), and (3) progressive autonomic failure (Shy-Drager syndrome). A recent consensus conference recommended new MSA terminology, and the term *Shy-Drager* is no longer used. MSA was divided into MSA-P (prominent parkinsonism) and MSA-C (prominent cerebellar or ataxic manifestations), with autonomic dysfunction being present in both. However, considerable overlap exists. In MSA, intellectual functioning is intact.

The manifestations of MSA include the following:
1. Autonomic dysfunction (erectile dysfunction; bladder control problems—urgency, incomplete emptying; constipation; abnormal breathing during sleep; orthostatic hypotension).
2. Parkinsonism = rigidity ± tremor, bradykinesia, and postural instability. The tremor of MSA is irregular and usually not a pill rolling tremor as seen in PD.
3. Ataxia (poor coordination or unsteady walking) may be a presenting symptom.
4. RBD is frequently present.
5. Central apnea, nocturnal hypoventilation, and Cheyne-Stokes breathing (CSB) have been reported in MSA, especially in patients with prominent autonomic features.

Stridor is a manifestation that sets MSA apart from PD and LBD. Stridor may occur in up to 30% of patients with MSA. It may be much worse during sleep. A *normal laryngeal examination during wakefulness does not rule out the problem.* The presence of stridor is associated with a poor prognosis (compared with patients with MSA without stridor) and has traditionally been managed by tracheostomy. Recently, continuous positive airway pressure (CPAP) has been used to alleviate stridor at night. Of note, patients with MSA often have OSA as well as worsening stridor during sleep. The etiology of stridor is controversial but is likely to be overactivity of the vocal cord adductors (close vocal cords) and underactivity of vocal cord abductors (posterior cricoarytenoid muscles [PCA]). Neuropathy of the recurrent laryngeal nerves that innervate the PCA muscles may be involved. However, the syndrome of stridor in many patients is a dystonia rather than vocal cord paralysis. In others, complete vocal cord immobility is present. Sudden death has been reported in patients with stridor in spite of treatment with tracheostomy or CPAP.

In Patient B, the presence of stridor, parkinsonism, RBD, and autonomic dysfunction are consistent with a diagnosis of MSA. In this patient, both OSA and stridor were present. The manifestations of tremor and autonomic dysfunction (erectile dysfunction, constipation, postural hypotension) were more prominent than ataxia. He was treated with CPAP, which alleviated both stridor and OSA.

CLINICAL PEARLS

1. The presence of nocturnal stridor and parkinsonism suggests that MSA is present. Nocturnal stridor may be present even if daytime vocal cord function is normal. The presence of stridor is a poor prognostic sign.
2. The differential of parkinsonism (tremor, bradykinesia, and rigidity or postural instability) includes PD and APDs, including LBD, MSA, progressive supranuclear palsy (PSP), and corticobasilar degeneration (CBD).
3. Sleep manifestations of PD include both insomnia (caused by rigidity, nocturia, dyskinesia, medication side effects) and daytime sleepiness (caused by DAs, OSA, PD itself).
4. APDs should be suspected when a patient with parkinsonism develops early dementia (LBD) or ataxia or autonomic dysfunction (MSA). APDs have a more rapid downhill course compared with PD and have no or minimal response to DAs.
5. RBD is common in PD, LBD, and MSA. RBD may precede the development of PD by ≥ 10 years. A significant fraction of patients with "idiopathic" RBD may develop PD in subsequent years.

BIBLIOGRAPHY

Barnes J, Connelly V, Wiggs L, et al: Sleep patterns in Parkinson's disease patients with visual hallucinations, *Int J Neurosci* 120:564–569, 2010.

Boeve BF: Idiopathic REM sleep behaviour disorder in the development of Parkinson's disease, *Lancet Neurol* 12(5):469–482, 2013.

Cochen De Cock V, Abouda M, Leu S, et al: Is obstructive sleep apnea a problem in Parkinson's disease? *Sleep Med* 11 (3):247–252, 2010.

Comella CL: Sleep disorders in Parkinson's disease, *Curr Treat Options Neurol* 10:215–221, 2008.

da Silva FP Jr, do Prado F, Barbosa ER: Sleep disordered breathing in Parkinson's disease: a critical appraisal, *Sleep Med Rev* 18(2):173–178, 2014.

Gagnon JF, Bédard MA, Fantini ML, et al: REM sleep behavior disorder and REM sleep without atonia in Parkinson's disease, *Neurology* 59(4):585–589, 2002.

Gillman S, Wenning P, Low PA, et al: Second consensus statement of the diagnosis of multiple system atrophy, *Neurology* 71:670–676, 2008.

Iranzo A: Management of sleep-disordered breathing in multiple system atrophy, *Sleep Med* 6:297–300, 2005.

Jankovic J: "Parkinson's disease": clinical features and diagnosis, *J Neurol Neurosurg Psychiatry* 79:368–376, 2008.

Juri C, Chana P, Tapia J, et al: Quetiapine for insomnia in Parkinson disease: results from an open label trial, *Clin Neuropharmacol* 28:185–187, 2005.

Kuźniar TJ, Morgenthaler TI, Prakash UBS, et al: Effects of continuous positive airway pressure on stridor in multiple system atrophy—sleep laryngoscopy, *J Clin Sleep Med* 5:65–67, 2009.

Louter M, Aarden WC, Lion J, et al: Recognition and diagnosis of sleep disorders in Parkinson's disease, *J Neurol* 259 (10):2031–2040, 2012.

Manni R, Terzaghi M, Repetto A, et al: Complex paroxysmal nocturnal behaviors in Parkinson's disease, *Mov Disord* 25:985–990, 2010.

McKeith JG, Galasko D, Kosaka K, et al: Consensus guideline for the clinical and pathological diagnosis of dementia with Lewy bodies: report of consortium on DLB international workshop, *Neurology* 47:1113–1124, 1996.

Ostrem JL, Galifianakis NB: Overview of common movement disorders, *Continuum (Minneap Minn)* 16(1 Movement Disorders):13–48, 2010.

Reichmann H: Clinical criteria for the diagnosis of Parkinson's disease, *Neurodegener Dis* 7:284–290, 2010.

Sadaoka T, Kakitsub N, Fujiwara Y, et al: Sleep-related breathing disorders in patients with multiple system atrophy and vocal fold palsy, *Sleep* 19:479–484, 1996.

Silber MH, Levine S: Stridor and death in multiple system atrophy, *Mov Disord* 15:699–714, 2000.

Swick TJ: Parkinson's disease and sleep/wake disturbances, *Parkinson's Dis* 2012:205471, 2012.

Thannickal TC, Lai YY, Siegel JM: Hypocretin (orexin) cell loss in Parkinson's disease, *Brain* 130:1586–1595, 2007.

FUNDAMENTALS 37

Evaluation of Insomnia

Insomnia is defined as *sleep difficulty* (difficulty initiating or maintaining sleep, early morning awakening, or both) that is associated *daytime consequences* because of night time sleep difficulty, with the proviso that the nighttime or daytime problems are not explained by an inadequate opportunity to sleep. The *International Classification of Sleep Disorders*, Second Edition (ICSD-2) defined eight insomnia disorders (Tables F37-1 and F37-2).[1] Other classifications such as that by *Diagnostic and Statistical Manual of Mental Disorders*, Fourth Edition (DSM-IV) classified insomnia as primary insomnia and secondary insomnia (insomnia associated with a mental disorder, medical disorder, or a drug or substance).[2] The term *comorbid insomnia* has often been used to refer to "secondary" insomnias, as it is often difficult to define the relationship between insomnia and the associated disorder (which disorder is primary and which is secondary?). For example, insomnia may precede depression, worsen during depression, and persist after remission from depression. The ICSD-3 defines only three insomnia disorders (see Table F37-1; Box F37-1),[3] and the ICSD-2 insomnia disorders have been consolidated into these three disorders. The rationale is that previously used subtypes could not reliably be diagnosed.[4] The same patient may be diagnosed with different subtypes by different experienced clinicians. This is not surprising, as many patients manifest overlapping symptoms.

Chronic insomnia disorder (CID) is defined in the ICSD-3 and encompasses elements of psychophysiologic insomnia, idiopathic insomnia, paradoxical insomnia, insomnia associated with mental disorder, inadequate sleep hygiene, as well the behavioral insomnias of childhood (limit setting or sleep association disorders) (Box F37-2 and see Table F37-2). The ICSD-3 states that CID is characterized by "frequent and persistent difficulty initiating or maintaining sleep that results in general sleep dissatisfaction." CID may occur in isolation or be a comorbid condition with a mental disorder, medical condition, or substance use. *Duration of at least 3 months* is required for the diagnosis of CID, and symptoms must occur on at least 3 nights per week. Note that in ICSD-2, only a 1-month duration was required for many of the insomnia disorders. More details on CID are provided below. A number of other sleep disorders are associated with insomnia complaints (Table F3-3). These included sleep apnea syndromes, circadian rhythm sleep-wake disorders, and the restless legs syndrome.

TABLE F37-1 Insomnia Disorders

International Classification of Sleep Disorders, 3rd Edition	International Classification of Sleep Disorders, 2nd Edition
Chronic insomnia disorder (CID) - Frequency: on at least 3 nights per week - Duration ≥3 months	Psychophysiologic insomnia Paradoxical insomnia Idiopathic insomnia Insomnia due to mental disorder Inadequate sleep hygiene Behavioral insomnia of childhood Insomnia due to drug or substance Insomnia due to medical condition
Short-term insomnia disorder (STID) - Duration <3 months	Adjustment insomnia (acute insomnia)
Other insomnia disorder - Difficulty initiating or maintaining sleep but does not meet criteria for CID or STID	

TABLE F37-2 **Major Characteristics of Insomnia Types in *International Classification of Sleep Disorders*, 2nd Edition**

Insomnia Types	Essential Features	Clinical Clues
Psychophysiologic	Duration at least 1 month Anxiety about sleep Heightened arousal when in bed Conditioned sleep-preventing associations (bedroom as a stimulus for wake not sleep)	Better sleep in novel environment (away from home) Can fall asleep outside bedroom or when not trying to sleep
Paradoxical	Duration at least 1 month Extreme and physiologically improbable complaints: "I never sleep." Despite report of little sleep, relatively minor daytime impairment	Objective sleep duration (PSG, actigraphy) is much greater than reported No or rare naps
Idiopathic	Onset in infancy or childhood No identifiable precipitant No period of sustained remission	Lifelong insomnia without remissions Insidious onset
Associated with a mental disorder	Insomnia present for at least 1 month Mental disorder has been diagnosed Temporally associated with mental disorder (may precede by a few days or weeks)	Insomnia waxes and wanes with mental disorder
Inadequate sleep hygiene	Improper sleep scheduling Use of products that disturb sleep near bedtime Stimulating activities near bedtime Use of the bed for nonsleep activities	Variable bedtime and wake times Napping
Behavioral insomnia of childhood sleep association type	Falling asleep is an extended process Sleep-onset associations demanded In absence of associated factors, sleep onset delayed	Nighttime awakenings require caregiver intervention for return to sleep
Behavioral insomnia of childhood limit-setting type	Difficulty initiating or maintaining sleep Refusal to go to bed or return to bed after awakening	Caregiver demonstrates insufficient limit setting to establish appropriate behavior
Adjustment Insomnia	Temporally associated with identifiable stressor Duration <3 months Expected to resolve	Recent psychological, psychosocial, environmental, or physical stressor

Adapted from Schutte-Rodin S, Broch L, Buysee D, et al: Clinical guideline for the evaluation and management of chronic insomnia in adults, *J Clin Sleep Med* 4:487-504, 2008.

SHORT-TERM INSOMNIA DISORDER

This disorder encompasses what was previously termed *adjustment insomnia*. The duration must be less that 3 months.

OTHER INSOMNIA DISORDER

This diagnosis is reserved for individuals who complain of difficulty initiating and maintaining sleep yet do not meet the full criteria for either CID or short-term insomnia disorder.

MAJOR COMPONENTS OF CHRONIC INSOMNIA DISORDER

1. **Sleep difficulty**: In adults, the major complaints are difficulty initiating sleep (sleep onset insomnia), difficulty maintaining sleep (frequent awakenings, sleep maintenance insomnia), and early morning awakening. In children, sleep difficulty is defined by caregiver observation of resistance to going to bed at an appropriate time and difficulty maintaining sleep without parent or caregiver intervention.

2. **Daytime difficulty caused by sleep difficulty**: Multiple complaints may be present, including fatigue, attention or concentration difficulty, impaired social or academic performance, irritability, daytime sleepiness, and reduced motivation. In children, behavioral problems such and hyperactivity, aggression, or impulsivity may be prominent. Often, patients express dissatisfaction with sleep or concerns about the effects of poor sleep on their health.

BOX F37-1 | **Chronic Insomnia Disorder—Diagnostic Criteria ICSD-3**

Criteria A-F must be met

A. The patient reports or the patient's parent or caregiver observes one or more of the following:
1. Difficulty initiating sleep
2. Difficulty maintaining sleep
3. Waking up earlier than desired
4. Resistance to going to bed on appropriate schedule
5. Difficulty sleeping without parent or caregiver intervention

B. The patient reports or the patient's parent or caregiver observes one or more of the following related to the nighttime sleep difficulty:
1. Fatigue/malaise
2. Attention, concentration, or memory impairment
3. Impaired social, family, occupational or academic performance
4. Mood disturbance/irritability

5. Daytime sleepiness
6. Behavioral problems (e.g., hyperactivity, impulsivity, aggression)
7. Reduced motivation/energy/initiative
8. Proneness for errors/accidents
9. Concerns about or dissatisfaction with sleep

C. The reported sleep/wake complaints cannot be explained purely by *inadequate opportunity* (i.e., enough time is allotted for sleep) or *inadequate circumstances* (i.e., the environment is safe, dark, quiet, and comfortable) for sleep.

D. **The sleep disturbance and associated daytime symptoms occur at least three times per week.**

E. The sleep disturbance and associated daytime symptoms have been present for at least 3 months.

F. The sleep/wake difficulty is not better explained by another primary sleep disorder.

Adapted from American Academy of Sleep Medicine: *International classification of sleep disorders*, ed 3, Darien, IL, 2014, American Academy of Sleep Medicine.

BOX F37-2 | **Short-Term Insomnia Disorder**

ICSD-3 DIAGNOSTIC CRITERIA

(Criteria A to E must be met)

A, B, C. As in Chronic Insomnia Disorder

D. The sleep disturbance and associated daytime symptoms have been *present for less than 3 months.*

E. The sleep/wake difficulty is not better explained by another primary sleep disorder.

---

3. **Frequency, duration, adequate sleep opportunity or environment**: A frequency of *at least 3 nights per week, a duration of ≥3 months*, and the requirement of an adequate opportunity and environment for sleep are requirements for the diagnosis of CID. The ICSD-3 states that patients with chronic insomnia characterized by recurrent episodes of sleep/wake difficulties lasting several weeks at a time (<3 months) over several years may also qualify for the CID diagnosis.

INSOMNIA EVALUATION

A detailed sleep history is the cornerstone of evaluation of insomnia.[5-9] First, the nature of the *primary sleep complaint* (problems with sleep onset, sleep maintenance, or quality) should be defined and the *duration of the complaint* determined. The history of the *origin* of the complaint, including age of onset should be explored, and particular life events or stressors at the start of the problem should be identified. For example, patients with the subtype idiopathic insomnia report problems since childhood or adolescence with an insidious onset. Patients with psychophysiologic subtype of insomnia may report that chronic insomnia began after a severe illness. *Presleep conditions* or activities that could affect sleep, including the bedroom environment, activities near bedtime, or mental state near bedtime should be explored. The *bedroom environment* should be characterized for factors that might disturb sleep (noise, clock easily seen from the bed, extreme hot or cold temperature). *Activities near bedtime*, including working late on the computer, drinking caffeinated beverages or alcohol in the evening, or exercise near bedtime, may impair the ability to sleep. The *mental status at bedtime* should be explored. Often, patients began worrying about their stresses and problems when retiring for the night. The presence or absence of *nocturnal symptoms*, including snoring, gasping during sleep, symptoms of restless legs syndrome (RLS), and body movements should be evaluated.

The *sleep-wake schedule* should be determined by report including variability of bedtime and rise time as well as the frequency and duration of naps. Factors that worsen or improve sleep should be detailed. For example, some patients with insomnia report sleeping better in a novel environment (reverse first-night effect).[10] Patient recall may be supplemented by sleep logs, actigraphy, or both, as discussed in a following section. *Daytime function* should be discussed with emphasis on possible consequences of insomnia. Reports of daytime fatigue or impaired cognition and mood are more common than true daytime sleepiness. *True daytime sleepiness should trigger suspicion for additional sleep problems such as sleep apnea, narcolepsy, or depression.* Daytime activities that may affect sleep such as the amount of caffeine, alcohol, exercise, sunlight exposure, and napping should be detailed. A general medical and psychiatric history is important to identify mental or medical conditions that may affect sleep. A detailed medication history including over-the-counter medications and substances of abuse is extremely important.

A physical examination and appropriate laboratory testing if not recently performed should rule out obvious medical causes of insomnia. Examination of the upper airway showing a high Mallampati score (upper airway narrowing)[11] might trigger suspicions of obstructive sleep apnea (OSA).

DIFFERENTIAL DIAGNOSIS

Major characteristics of the insomnia types listed in the ICSD-2 are listed in Table F37-2. Patients with CID often have characteristics of more than one type. A number of non CID sleep disorders may be associated with insomnia complaints (Box F37-3). Sleep apnea syndromes may be associated with repetitive arousal and sleep-maintenance problems. In patients with

BOX F37-3	Other Sleep Disorders Associated with Insomnia Complaints

1. Sleep apnea syndromes
2. Circadian rhythm sleep/wake disorders
   a. Delayed sleep/wake disorder type—sleep-onset insomnia
   b. Advanced sleep/wake disorder—early AM awakening
   c. Irregular sleep phase type—at least three sleep episodes per 24 hours
   d. Non-24 hour sleep phase type—alternating periods of insomnia and hypersomnia
3. Restless legs syndrome/periodic limb movement disorders

From American Academy of Sleep Medicine: *International classification of sleep disorders: diagnostic and coding manual*, ed 3, Darien, IL, 2013, American Academy of Sleep Medicine.

sleep apnea, insomnia symptoms are more likely to be present in women than in men.[1] The circadian sleep-wake rhythm disorders (CSWRDs) may also be associated with insomnia complaints, including delayed sleep phase syndrome (sleep-onset insomnia) and advanced sleep phase syndrome (early morning awakening). In delayed sleep phase syndrome, once the affected individuals are able to fall asleep, they have fairly normal sleep. In advanced sleep phase syndrome, individuals fall asleep early but then awaken in the early morning hours. In non–24-hour CSWRD, patients may report periods of insomnia alternating with hypersomnia.[1,3] RLS or periodic limb movement disorder (PLMD) may be associated with symptoms of insomnia or nonrestorative sleep. A number of medications may also disturb sleep quality (e.g., caffeine).

QUESTIONNAIRES, SLEEP LOGS, AND ACTIGRAPHY

Supporting information from questionnaires (mood, cognition about insomnia), sleep logs, and actigraphy may be helpful in evaluating patients with insomnia (Box F37-4 and Box F37-5). These may supplement other information obtained from the sleep history. Assessing the patient's attitudes about sleep and the sleep problem is as important as documenting the degree of sleep disturbance. In addition, some patients are hesitant to admit to feelings of depression. Sleep logs and actigraphy provide a more accurate estimate of the patient's sleep quantity than is possible from patient recall.

The Epworth Sleepiness Scale (ESS; see Fundamentals 17) is used to assess subjective estimates of the propensity to fall asleep in common situations.[12] The Pittsburgh Sleep Quality Index (PSQI) is a 24-item self-report measure of general sleep quality that specifically addresses the preceding 1-month period. The PSQI evaluates seven domains, including the duration of sleep, sleep disturbance, sleep-onset latency, daytime dysfunction because of sleepiness, sleep efficiency, need for medications to sleep, and overall sleep quality. The PSQI yields a global score and seven component scores (poor sleep: global score > 5).[13,14] The questionnaire has been shown to distinguish among healthy patients, patients with depression, and patients with sleep disorders. It was not designed specifically for insomnia but has been used in insomnia assessment and treatment studies. Detailed instructions for use and scoring of the PSQI are available at the

BOX F37-4	Evaluation of Insomnia

1 SLEEP HISTORY

A. Define primary complaint:
- Delayed sleep onset
- Sleep maintenance problems
- Frequent awakenings/early morning awakening
- Nonrestorative sleep

B. Define time course of complaint:
- Age of onset
- Precipitating event or stressor

C. Evaluate presleep conditions:
- Pre-bedtime activities
- Bedroom environment
- Physical and mental status before sleep

D. *Nocturnal symptoms* (awakenings, physical or mental symptoms, including snoring or body movements)

E. Sleep-wake schedule—by patient report including variability, naps

F. Daytime function—consequences of insomnia:
- Sleepiness versus fatigue
- Impairment of mood, cognitive dysfunction, quality of life

G. Daytime activities relevant for sleep:
- Sunlight exposure, exercise
- Napping

- Work schedule and disturbance
- Caffeine and alcohol intake

H. Medical and psychiatric conditions (e.g., chronic pain, depression) or medications that may affect sleep

2 PHYSICAL AND MENTAL STATUS EXAMINATION

A. Narrow upper airway (high Mallampati score), retrognathia

3 SUPPORTING INFORMATION

A. Sleep/mood questionnaires:
- Epworth Sleepiness Scale
- Dysfunctional Beliefs and Attitudes about Sleep
- Pittsburgh Sleep Quality Index

B. Sleep log for 2 weeks—attention to sleep and wake time variability, general patterns

C. Actigraphy

4 SLEEP STUDY—NOT ROUTINELY INDICATED

A. Indicated when another sleep disorder such as sleep apnea is suspected.

BOX F37-5	Questionnaires to Evaluate Patients with Insomnia

Epworth Sleepiness Scale	Propensity to fall asleep in eight situations (0 never, 1 slight, 2 moderate, 3 high chance) with a total score 0 to 24. Normal ≥ 10
Beck Depression Inventory	BDI or BDI-II is a 21-item self-report inventory used to measure depression. BDI-1 scores: Minimal or no depression BDI < 10, moderate to severe depression BDI ≥ 19 BDI-II scores: Minimal or no depression BDI < 14, moderate to severe depression BDI ≥ 20
Pittsburgh Sleep Quality Index	A 24-item self-report measure of sleep qualities (poor sleep: global score >5)
Dysfunctional Beliefs and Attitudes About Sleep Questionnaire	DBAS is a self-rating of 30 statements that is used to assess negative cognitions about sleep. Shorter version the DBAS-16 also exists (see Appendix 1).

BDI, Beck Depression Inventory; *DBAS*, Dysfunctional Beliefs and Attitudes about Sleep; *PSQI*, Pittsburgh Sleep Quality Index.

University of Pittsburgh Sleep Medicine Institute web site http://www.sleep.pitt.edu/content.asp?id=1484&subid=2316.

The Beck Depression Inventory (BDI-I or BDI-II) is a 21-item self-report inventory (Box F37-5) used to measure manifestations of depression, each item being scored from 0 to 3.[15,16] Higher total scores indicate more severe depressive symptoms. The BDI-II is a revision of the original BDI-I. Because primary insomnia and major depression share some daytime symptoms, the usual cutoff scores for the BDI might be less specific for depression in insomnia patients.[17] The Dysfunctional Beliefs and Attitudes about Sleep (DBAS) Questionnaire is a self-rating survey to assess negative cognitions about sleep.[18,19] Reversal of these cognitions is a goal of the cognitive component of cognitive behavioral therapy (CBT). The original DBAS was a 30-item questionnaire, in which patients responded using an analog scale (0, strongly disagree; 1, 2, 3..., to 10, strongly agree). A shorter version (DBAS-16)[19] has recently been validated and is less time-consuming for patients to complete (Figure F37-1).

SLEEP LOGS

A sleep log (sleep diary) for at least 2 weeks is recommended when evaluating patients with

Name	Strongly Disagree							Strongly Agree		
	1	2	3	4	5	6	7	8	9	10
1. I need 8 hours of sleep to feel refreshed and function well during the day.										
2. When I don't get a proper amount of sleep on a given night, I need to catch up on the next day by napping or on the next night by sleeping longer.										
3. I am concerned that chronic insomnia may have serious consequences on my physical health.										
4. I am worried that I may lose control over my abilities to sleep.										
5. After a poor nights sleep I know that it will interfere with my daily activities on the next day.										
6. In order to be alert and function well during the day, I believe would be better off taking a sleeping pill rather than having a poor nights sleep.										
7. When I feel irritable, depressed, or anxoius during the day it is mostly because I did not sleep well the night before.										
8. When I sleep poorly on one night, I know it will distrub my sleep schedule for the whole week.										
9. Without an adequate night's sleep I can hardly function the next day.										
10. I can't ever predict whether I'll have a good or poor night's sleep.										
11. I have little ability to manage the negative consequences of distrubed sleep.										
12. When I feel tired, have no energy, or just seem not to function well during the day, its generally because I did not sleep well the night before.										
13. I believe insomnia is essentially the result of a chemical imbalance.										
14. I feel insomnia is ruining my ability to enjoy life and prevents me from doing what I want										
15. Medication is probably the only solution to sleeplessness.										
16. I avoid or cancel obligations (social, family) after a poor night's sleep.										

FIGURE F37-1 ■ Dysfunctional Beliefs and Attitudes About Sleep (DBAS)-16. (From Morin CM, Vallières A, Ivers H: Dysfunctional beliefs and attitudes about sleep (DBAS): validation of a brief version (DBAS-16), *Sleep* 30:1547-1554, 2007.)

insomnia. Sleep logs are often more accurate and more reliable than patient recall of their chronic sleep patterns. Sleep logs usually follow a question format or time plot graphic format.[20] An adaptation of a basic consensus sleep log[20] is shown in Figure F37-2. The reader should look at Patient 111 for other examples. The essential elements of a sleep log include the ability to assess time in bed (TIB), sleep-onset latency (SOL), total sleep time (TST), and the amount of wakefulness after sleep onset (WASO). The TIB is the period from when the patient gets in bed until the final time the patient leaves the bed in the morning. WASO includes all wake from sleep onset until the patient leaves the bed in the morning. The patient need report only three of these four parameters because they are related (TIB = SOL + TST + WASO). Sleep efficiency can be computed (= TST × 100/TIB), with normal values exceeding 85%. Sleep logs

also typically provide space to record caffeine consumption, bedtime activities, or medications taken for sleep as well as estimates of sleep quality. *Sleep logs are very helpful in revealing general patterns of the sleep-wake cycle such as irregular bedtimes and wake times and the amount and frequency of napping.* A few characteristic patterns noted in sleep logs are listed in Box F37-6.

ACTIGRAPHY

Actigraphy involves use of a portable device (often resembling a watch and typically worn on the wrist) that collects movement information (activity) over an extended period (Figure F37-3). The absence of movement is assumed to be a surrogate of sleep.[21] The use of actigraphy is included in the ICSD-3 diagnostic criteria for several circadian sleep wake rhythm disorders.[3] Practice

	Sample	1	2	3	4	5	6	7
Today's date	4/5/12							
1. What time did you get into bed last night?	10:00 PM							
2. What time did you try go go to sleep last night?	10:30 PM							
3. How long did it take you to fall asleep last night?	60 min							
4. How many times did you wake up, not counting your final awakening?	5 times							
5. In total, how long were you awake last night?	60 min							
6. What time was your final awakening?	6:00 AM							
7. What time did you get out of bed for the day?	6:30 AM							
8. In total how long did you sleep last night?	5 hours 30 min							
9.How would you rate the quality of your sleep?	☐ Very poor ☒ Poor ☐ Fair ☐ Good ☐ Very good	☐ Very poor ☐ Poor ☐ Fair ☐ Good ☐ Very good	☐ Very poor ☐ Poor ☐ Fair ☐ Good ☐ Very good	☐ Very poor ☐ Poor ☐ Fair ☐ Good ☐ Very good	☐ Very poor ☐ Poor ☐ Fair ☐ Good ☐ Very good	☐ Very poor ☐ Poor ☐ Fair ☐ Good ☐ Very good	☐ Very poor ☐ Poor ☐ Fair ☐ Good ☐ Very good	☐ Very poor ☐ Poor ☐ Fair ☐ Good ☐ Very good
10. Comments								

Name _____

FIGURE F37-2 ■ Sleep log. (Adapted from Carney CE, Buysse DJ, Ancoli-Israel S, et al: The consensus sleep diary: standardizing prospective sleep self-monitoring, *Sleep* 35[2]:287-302, 2012.)

BOX F37-6	Some Typical Sleep Log Patterns
Delayed sleep phase	Late bedtime or long sleep latency, few awakenings, normal sleep duration on weekends or non-work/non-school days
Inadequate sleep hygiene	Irregular wake and rise times, naps
Psychophysiologic insomnia	Long sleep latency, decreased total sleep time, frequent awakenings Variability in sleep quality
Paradoxical insomnia	Nights of minimal or no sleep are reported followed by no or few naps the next day

parameters for use of actigraphy have been published by the American Academy of Sleep Medicine (AASM.[22,23] Although actigraphy is indicated for determining the circadian patterns of patients with insomnia, the AASM practice parameters did not state that actigraphy was indicated as a routine evaluation of patients with insomnia.

Actigraphy does not measure sleep as defined by electroencephalography (EEG), electrooculographic (EOG), or chin electromyographic (EMG) criteria or the subjective experience of sleep (as measured by sleep logs and questionnaires). Therefore, it is not surprising that estimates of TST, wake time, and sleep latency from sleep logs and actigraphy may differ from PSG findings.[24,25] Algorithms have been developed to estimate TST and WASO from the activity data. Actigraphy estimates of sleep duration, WASO, and sleep latency are more accurate in normal individuals than in patients with insomnia. Periods of low activity in which patients lie quietly in bed but are awake may be scored as sleep by actigraphy software. When performing actigraphy, it is essential to require patients to complete a sleep log (e.g., lights off, lights on, out of bed, actigraph off for shower; TST; sleep latency). This information enables

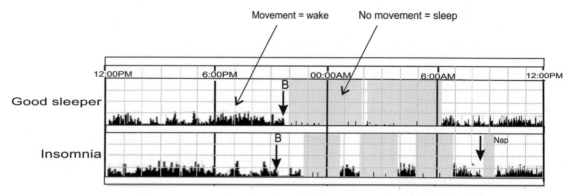

FIGURE F37-3 ■ Actigraphy from a good sleeper and a patient with insomnia. *B,* Bedtime ready to sleep. The patient with insomnia had long sleep latency and two prolonged awakenings as well as a nap.

a correct interpretation of actigraphy tracings. *If the actigraphy estimate of TST far exceeds patient estimates, this would suggest paradoxical insomnia.*

Sleep logs and actigraphy provide complementary information. Actigraphy is most valuable in determining the pattern of wake and sleep. It can detect irregular bedtimes and wake times and naps. Sleep logs are always filled out by patients wearing an actigraph. They provide complimentary information. Sleep logs may overestimate sleep latency while actigraphy underestimates sleep latency (lying still but awake). Sleep logs may underestimate total sleep time, and actigraphy overestimate total sleep. The relationship among PSG, actigraphy, and sleep log findings also may differ depending on the groups studied.

POLYSOMNOGRAPHY

PSG is not indicated for the routine assessment of insomnia. The 2003 AASM practice parameters for the role of PSG in insomnia state: *"PSG is indicated when the initial diagnosis (insomnia) is uncertain, treatment fails (either behavioral or pharmacologic), or precipitous arousals occur with violent of injurious behavior* (Guideline).[9] When PSG is performed, typical findings (Box F37-7) in patients with insomnia include long sleep latency (>30 minutes), reduced TST, increased WASO, and reduced sleep efficiency. Long rapid eye movement (REM) latency, a high arousal index, increased stage N1, and decreased stage N3 sleep may also be noted. In patients with paradoxical insomnia, objective sleep abnormality is much less severe than reported. It is not unusual for such patients to report little or no sleep following a PSG documenting only mild to moderate decrements in the TST. In some patients with

---

> **BOX F37-7** | **Typical Polysomnography Findings in Patients with Insomnia**
>
> - Increased sleep latency (>30 minutes)
> - Decreased TST
> - Decreased sleep efficiency
> - Increased stage N1 (%TST)
> - Decreased stage N3 (%TST)
> - Increased REM latency
> - Decreased REM latency (depression)

REM, Rapid eye movement; *TST,* total sleep time.

psychophysiologic insomnia, the "reverse first-night effect"[10] may be noted. In these patients, the sleep quality in the sleep center is better than that reported at home. It is essential to have all patients complete questionnaires assessing subjective sleep (estimate TST, sleep latency, sleep quality) after PSG.

CO-MORBID INSOMNIA

Many comorbid conditions such as chronic pain disorders may cause the sleep/wake complaints. If such conditions are the sole cause of the sleep difficulty, a separate insomnia diagnosis may not apply. The ICSD-3 states one should ask "How much of the time does the sleep difficulty arise as a result of factors directly attributable to the comorbid condition (e.g., pain ?)" or "Are there times that the sleep/wake complaints occur in the absence of these factors?" If there is evidence that the patient's sleep/wake complaints are not solely caused by the medical condition, and those sleep/wake complaints seem to merit separate treatment attention, then a diagnosis of chronic insomnia disorder should be made.

CLINICAL PEARLS

1. The diagnosis of CID requires the presence of (a) sleep difficulty, (b) daytime consequences, (c) difficulty for at least 3 nights per week for at least 3 months, and (d) adequate opportunity and environment for sleep.

2. Sleep difficulty may include problems initiating or maintaining sleep, and early morning awakening. In children, sleep difficulty includes resistance to going to bed and difficulty sleeping without caregiver intervention.

3. A good sleep history is the essential tool for evaluating insomnia. PSG has only a limited role in this evaluation.

4. Sleep logs and actigraphy provide complementary information, so the use of both can be valuable.

5. A number of insomnia disorders in ICSD-2 are now included in the ICSD-3 diagnosis of chronic insomnia disorder.

REFERENCES

1. American Academy of Sleep Medicine: *International classification of sleep disorders: diagnostic and coding manual*, ed 2, Westchester, IL, 2005, American Academy of Sleep Medicine.
2. American Psychiatric Association: *Diagnostic and statistical manual of mental disorders* (DSM-IV), ed 4, Washington, D.C, 1994, American Psychiatric Association.
3. American Academy of Sleep Medicine: *International classification of sleep disorders*, ed 3, Darien, IL, 2014, American Academy of Sleep Medicine.
4. Edinger JD, Wyatt JK, Stepanski EJ, et al: Testing the reliability and validity of DSM-IV-TR and ICSD-2 insomnia diagnoses. Results of a multitrait-multimethod analysis, *Arch Gen Psychiatry* 68(10):992–1002, 2011.
5. Schutte-Rodin S, Broch L, Buysee D, et al: Clinical guideline for the evaluation and management of chronic insomnia in adults, *J Clin Sleep Med* 4:487–504, 2008.
6. Sateia MJ, Doghramji K, Hauri P, Morin CM: Evaluation of chronic insomnia, *Sleep* 23:1–36, 2000.
7. Chesson A, Hartse K, McDowell Anderson W, et al: Practice parameters for the evaluation of chronic insomnia, *Sleep* 23:1–5, 2000.
8. Mai E, Buysee D: Insomnia, prevalence, impact, pathogenesis, differential diagnosis and evaluation, *Sleep Med Clin* 3:167–174, 2008.
9. Littner M, Hirshkowitz M, Kramer M: Standards of Practice Committee of the American Academy of Sleep Medicine: Practice parameters for using polysomnography to evaluate insomnia: an update for 2002, *Sleep* 26:754–760, 2003.
10. Agnew HW, Webb WB, Williams RL: The first night effect: an EEG study, *Psychophysiology* 2:263–266, 1966.
11. Nuckton TJ, Glidden DV, Browner WS, Claman DM: Physical Examination: Mallampati as an independent predictor of obstructive sleep apnea, *Sleep* 29:903–908, 2006.
12. Johns MW: Sleepiness in different situations measured by the Epworth Sleepiness Scale, *Sleep* 17:703–710, 1994.
13. Buysee DJ, Reynolds CF, Monk TH, et al: Quantification of subjective sleep quality in healthy elderly men and women using the Pittsburgh Sleep Quality Index (PSQI), *Sleep* 14:331–338, 1991.
14. Buysse DJ, Reynolds CF, Monk TH, et al: The Pittsburgh sleep quality index: a new instrument for psychiatric practice and research, *Psychiatry Res* 28:193–213, 1989.
15. Beck AT, Steer RA, Brown GK: *Manual for the beck depression inventory* (BDI-II), ed 2, San Antonio, 1996, The Psychological Association.
16. Beck AT, Ward CH, Mendelson M, et al: An inventory for measuring depression, *Arch Gen Psychiatry* 4:561–571, 1961.
17. Carney CE, Ulmer C, Edinger JD, et al: Assessing depression symptoms in those with insomnia: an examination of the beck depression inventory, 2nd edition (BDI-II), *J Psychiatr Res* 43:576–582, 2009.
18. Morin CM, Stone J, Trinkle D, et al: Dysfunctional beliefs and attitudes about sleep among older adults with and without insomnia complaints, *Psychol Aging* 8(3):463–467, 1993.
19. Morin CM, Vallières A, Ivers H: Dysfunctional beliefs and attitudes about sleep (DBAS): validation of a brief version (DBAS-16), *Sleep* 30:1547–1554, 2007.
20. Carney CE, Buysse DJ, Ancoli-Israel S, et al: The consensus sleep diary: standardizing prospective sleep self-monitoring, *Sleep* 35(2):287–302, 2012.
21. Lichstenin KL, Stone KC, Donaldson J, et al: Actigraphy validation with insomnia, *Sleep* 29:232–239, 2006.
22. Littner M, Kushida CA, McDowell Anderson W, et al: Practice parameters for the role of actigraphy in the study of sleep and circadian rhythms: an update for 2002, *Sleep* 26:337–341, 2003.
23. Morgenthaler T, Alessi C, Friedman L, et al: Practice parameters for the use of actigraphy in the assessment of sleep and sleep disorders: an update for 2007, *Sleep* 30:519–529, 2007.
24. Vallières A, Morin CM: Actigraphy in the assessment of insomnia, *Sleep* 26:902–906, 2003.
25. Sivertsen B, Omvik S, Havik OE, et al: A comparison of actigraphy and polysomnography in older adults treated for chronic primary insomnia, *Sleep* 29:1353–1358, 2006.

A 30-Year-Old Woman Having Difficulty Falling and Staying Asleep

A 30-year-old woman was referred for complaints of insomnia. This problem had been severe for more than 5 years (nearly every night of the week). The patient usually retired at 10 PM each night but did not fall asleep until midnight. She reported thoughts in her mind were "racing." Three to four awakenings occurred each night, with the final awakening at 6:30 AM (spontaneous). After each awakening, it took at least 30 minutes to fall asleep again. Self-medication with over-the-counter sleeping pills and alcohol were tried but were not effective. The patient had a good night of sleep only when she went on a vacation. The sleep environment at home was reported to be quiet and dark. The patient did keep a lighted clock at the bedside. During the day, fatigue was noted, but not definite sleepiness. No naps were taken. No symptoms of depression and no history of marital conflicts were present. The patient's husband reported that his wife did snore most nights.

Physical examination: General: thin and nervous; HEENT: Mallampati 3; otherwise unremarkable

A sleep study was ordered to rule out obstructive sleep apnea (OSA) (Table P110-1).

TABLE P110-1　Sleep Study

		Normal Range		%TST	Normal Range
Total recording time	460 minutes (min)	(425–462)	Stage N1	15	(3–6)
Total sleep time	395 min	(394–457)	Stage N	55	(46–62)
Sleep efficiency	85.8%	(90–100)%	Stages N3	10	(7–21)
Sleep latency	25 min	(0–19)	Stage R	20	(21–31)
REM latency	85 min	(69–88)	AHI	0/hour (hr)	
			PLM index	0/hr	

AHI, Apnea–hypopnea index; *PLM*, periodic limb movement; *REM*, rapid eye movement.

QUESTION

1. What is your diagnosis? Why is the sleep study relatively normal?

ANSWER

1. **Answer:** Chronic insomnia disorder (CID)—psychophysiologic insomnia subtype.

   Discussion: The patient meets the diagnostic criteria for chronic insomnia disorder (see Fundamentals 37). Sleep disturbance (difficulty with sleep onset and maintenance) has been present for >3 months and >3 nights per week. Daytime consequences (fatigue) are present. An adequate opportunity for sleep exists. The patient manifests many of the characteristics of the psychophysiologic insomnia subtype. She sleeps better in novel settings, lies in bed with her mind racing, and has a marked concern about the inability to sleep. Many patients with insomnia have somatized tension and learned sleep-preventing associations. The bedroom and lights-out time become stimuli for increased tension and anxiety. The insomnia usually is fairly fixed, although it may vary in severity. A precipitating event may have caused the onset of the problem, but it now has taken on a life of its own. Patients with this disorder frequently have a history of being "light sleepers" for many years. Inadequate sleep hygiene also may be present, but the problem persists even after correction. This diagnosis is not made if the patient can be classified as having an anxiety disorder, obsessive-compulsive neurosis, or major depression.

Polysomnography (PSG) is of limited utility in evaluating most cases of insomnia; therefore, it is not routinely recommended and often is not reimbursed by health insurance plans. When patients have not responded to behavioral and pharmacotherapy, PSG may be considered. The results usually corroborate the patient's complaints (long sleep latency, low sleep efficiency, frequent arousals, prolonged awakenings) and seldom reveal a specific reason for the sleep disturbance. However, identification of periodic limb movement in sleep (PLMS), a shortened rapid eye movement (REM) sleep latency (possible depression), or, rarely, OSA may be clues to the cause of the insomnia.

When PSG is performed to evaluate insomnia, the results may show better sleep than expected, considering the patients complaints. If the patient does report a fairly good night of sleep, the reason could be poor sleep environment at home or the problem could be a manifestation of the reverse first-night effect. Patients with the psychophysiologic subtype of CID may sleep better in a novel environment. Their bedroom has become a conditioned stimulus for sleep difficulty. If the total sleep time is much greater than the sleep time reported by the patient, this suggests the paradoxical insomnia subtype in which the patient may fail to experience a sensation of sleep. In this CID subtype, patients do not seem to recognize that they were asleep.

In the current case, the patient complained of both sleep-onset and sleep-maintenance insomnia. No historical information is available to suggest the restless legs syndrome or depression. A sleep study was performed because of the snoring and the physical examination showing a crowded upper airway. The study showed a near-normal night of sleep in the sleep laboratory and absence of evidence for other etiologies, making the chronic insomnia disorder (psychophysiologic subtype) the most likely diagnosis. The patient underwent cognitive behavioral treatment for the insomnia, and her sleep quality improved.

CLINICAL PEARLS

1. Diagnosis of the cause of insomnia usually is made on the basis of a careful history and review of a patient sleep diary (log), actigraphy, or both.

2. PSG generally is not indicated in the evaluation of insomnia. Three exceptions are (a) when there is a suspicion of sleep apnea and, (b) when the insomnia is severe and does not respond to pharmalogical or behavioral therapy, or (c) a PSG is needed for evaluation of nocturnal behavior (parasomnia).

3. A better-than-normal night of sleep in the sleep laboratory (a reverse first-night effect) suggests that the home sleep environment is suboptimal or has become a conditioned stimulus for sleep difficulty (chronic insomnia disorder— psychophysiologic type). In psychophysiologic insomnia, sleeping in a novel location may temporarily alleviate the insomnia.

4. If total sleep time by PSG greatly exceeds the time the patient reports being asleep, this suggests chronic insomnia disorder—paradoxical insomnia type.

BIBLIOGRAPHY

American Academy of Sleep Medicine: *International classification of sleep disorders: diagnostic and coding manual*, ed 2, Westchester, IL, 2005, American Academy of Sleep Medicine.

American Academy of Sleep Medicine: *International classification of sleep disorders*, ed 3, Darien, IL, 2014, American Academy of Sleep Medicine.

Chesson A, Hartse K, McDowell Anderson W, et al: Practice parameters for the evaluation of chronic insomnia, *Sleep* 23:1–5, 2000.

Mai E, Buysee D: Insomnia, prevalence, impact, pathogenesis, differential diagnosis and evaluation, *Sleep Med Clin* 3:167–174, 2008.

Sateia MJ, Doghramji K, Hauri P, Morin CM: Evaluation of chronic insomnia, *Sleep* 23:1–36, 2000.

Schutte-Rodin S, Broch L, Buysee D, et al: Clinical guideline for the evaluation and management of chronic insomnia in adults, *J Clin Sleep Med* 4:487–504, 2008.

A Patient with Insomnia and an Irregular Sleep Pattern

A patient being evaluated for insomnia completed a sleep diary, shown in Figure P111-1. The patient is a retired person and has minimal social obligations, but he frequently joins friends at a local bar for "happy hour." Some nights, he has noted sleep-onset insomnia, and on other nights, he reports that he falls asleep rapidly. Once asleep, the patient sleeps fairly soundly.

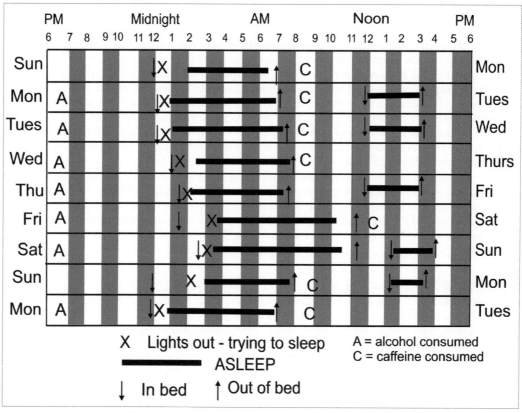

FIGURE P111-1 ■ Sleep diary from a patient with sleep difficulty.

QUESTION

1. What characteristics of the patient's sleep habits promote poor quality sleep?

ANSWER

1. **Answer**: Irregular bedtime and wake time, napping, spending time in bed without intending to sleep; nearly daily alcohol consumption.

Discussion: Inadequate Sleep Hygiene is not a diagnostic category in the International Classification of Sleep Disorders, edition 3 (ICSD-3). However, in the ICSD-2, one of the diagnostic categories for insomnia was "Inadequate Sleep Hygiene." This nomenclature is characterized by a number of behaviors that can potentially disrupt sleep, for example, exercise and ingestion of caffeine or alcohol near bedtime (Box P111-1). Patients with poor sleep habits often have irregular bedtimes and wake times and spend too much time in bed. Napping is another behavior that makes nocturnal sleep more difficult. Recommendations for good sleep hygiene are listed Box P111-2.

Although education about good sleep hygiene is a part of most behavioral treatment programs for insomnia, no evidence suggests that education about sleep hygiene alone is effective treatment for the insomnia syndromes. Insomnia caused by poor sleep hygiene occurs in approximately 5% to 10% of insomnia cases evaluated in a sleep center. The condition is present in 1% to 2% of adolescents and young adults.

A typical sleep log of a patient with poor sleep hygiene is shown in Figure P111-1. Findings include variation in bedtime and wake time, napping, and sleeping much longer (or later) on the weekend. Inappropriate use of caffeine and use of over-the-counter medications or alcohol may also be reported on sleep logs.

Inappropriate or excessive use of caffeine or alcohol may impair sleep. Caffeine is a widely used stimulant that may affect sleep for hours after ingestion. The half-life of caffeine varies from 3 to 7 hours and is longer at higher doses. One study found little difference in the effects of mild to moderate doses of caffeine consumed in the morning between normal sleepers and patients with insomnia. Overall few effects were seen. However, recent studies suggested that variants of certain genes (variant of the adenosine receptor) may predispose individuals to sensitivity to the effects of caffeine on sleep. Recall that caffeine is an adenosine receptor antagonist. In patients with insomnia, minimizing caffeine intake after the noon hour is recommended. Alcohol may also have a greater-than-expected effect on sleep in some individuals. Alcohol may aid sleep onset but tends to cause frequent awakenings in the second part of the night. A study of middle aged men by Landholt et al found that alcohol consumption 6 hours before bedtime (alcohol level at bedtime $= 0$) still caused sleep disturbance. Sleep efficiency, total sleep time, and stage 1 and rapid eye movement (REM) sleep were reduced. In the second half of the sleep episode, a twofold increase in wakefulness was observed. A study by Geoghegan and coworkers using actigraphy found low doses of alcohol in normal subjects to be disruptive, with decreased total sleep time caused by increased wakefulness in the second part of the night. Of note, not all studies have shown the dramatic effects of alcohol on sleep, but the reason may be the age of the subjects. Younger individuals may be less affected by alcohol.

BOX P111-1	**Essentials Aspects of Inadequate Sleep Hygiene**

Inadequate sleep hygiene practices include one or more of the following:

i. *Improper sleep scheduling* consistent with frequent daytime napping, selecting highly variable bedtimes or rising times, or spending excessive amount of time in bed

ii. Routine use of products containing alcohol, nicotine, or caffeine, especially in periods preceding bedtime

iii. Engagement in mentally stimulating, physically activating, or emotionally upsetting activities too close to bedtime

iv. Frequent use of the bed for activities other than sleep (TV watching, reading, studying, snacking, thinking, planning)

v. Failure to maintain a comfortable sleeping environment

BOX P111-2	**Good Sleep Hygiene Practices**

- Limited caffeine consumption until noon
- No exercise within 2 hours of bedtime
- Use of the bed only for sleep and sex (avoid excessive time in bed)
- Maintaining regular waking times
- Quiet and cool environment in the bedroom
- Avoidance of stimulating activity near bedtime
- Avoidance of napping if sleep maintenance is a problem
- Face of alarm clock should not be visible from bed.

CLINICAL PEARLS

1. Improving sleep hygiene is a part of most treatment programs for insomnia. However, used alone, this intervention has not been proven to be effective. However, persistent bad habits may reduce the potential effectiveness of behavioral treatments.
2. Some studies suggest that ingestion of alcohol in the early evening may still impair sleep quality many hours later. Although alcohol near bedtime may help some patients relax, it often is associated with awakenings and fragmented sleep later in the night.
3. Considerable individual variability exists in the effects of caffeine on sleep. Preliminary evidence suggests that genetic variation for the adenosine receptor may explain some of the differences. In some individuals, the half-life of caffeine is as long as 7 hours.

BIBLIOGRAPHY

American Academy of Sleep Medicine: *International classification of sleep disorders: diagnostic and coding manual*, ed 2, Westchester, IL, 2005, American Academy of Sleep Medicine.

Byrne EM, Johnson J, McRae AF, et al: A genome-wide association study of caffeine-related sleep disturbance: confirmation of a role for a common variant in the adenosine receptor, *Sleep* 35(7):967–975, 2012.

Geoghegan P, O'Donovan MT, Lawlor BA: Investigation of the effects of alcohol on sleep using actigraphy, *Alcohol* 47 (5):538–544, 2012.

Landholt HP, Roth C, Dijik DJ, Borberly AA: Late afternoon alcohol intake affects nocturnal sleep and the sleep EEG in middle aged men, *J Clin Psychopharmacol* 16:428–436, 1996.

Landolt HP: "No thanks, coffee keeps me awake": individual caffeine sensitivity depends on ADORA2A genotype, *Sleep* 35 (7):899–900, 2012.

Roehrs T, Roth T: Caffeine: sleep and daytime sleepiness, *Sleep Med Rev* 12:153–162, 2008.

Youngberg MR, Karpov IO, Begley A, et al: Clinical and physiological correlates of caffeine and caffeine metabolites in primary insomnia, *J Clin Sleep Med* 7(2):196–203, 2011.

A Woman with Sleepless Nights

A 50-year-old woman complained of severe sleep difficulty that she had suffered for over 10 years. She reported sleeping only 1 to 4 hours each night. She left the bed for variable periods but otherwise simply remained in bed awake for the majority of each night. On some nights, the patient felt that she had not slept at all. The bedroom was quiet and dark, but a clock with a lighted face was visible from her bed. The patient awakened feeling very fatigued but denied daytime sleepiness. She did not report naps. Her work performance was acceptable to her supervisor. The patient did admit to drinking about 4 to 5 cups of coffee over the day, including one cup after supper. The only medication the patient was taking was hydrochlorothiazide. The patient denied symptoms of depression. Actigraphy and a sleep log for the same period are shown in Figure P112-1.

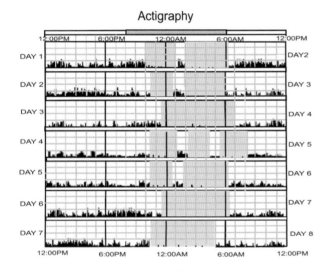

Actigraphy

Sleep Diary

	Time in Bed	Time trying to sleep	How long to fall asleep (min)	Number of Awakenings	Total Sleep (hrs)	Final awakening
Day 1	10P	10:30P	60 min	2	3	6A
Day 2	10P	10:30P	60 min	1	3	6A
Day 3	11P	10:30P	50 min	0	2	7A
Day 4	10P	10:30P	40 min	2	2	6A
Day 5	10P	10:30P	90 min	1	3	6A
Day 6	11P	10:30P	8 hrs	0	0	6A
Day 7	11P	10:30P	60 min	1	4	5A

FIGURE P112-1 ■ Actigraphy and a sleep diary for 1 week are shown. The light gray area in the actogram is defined as "rest" that is presumed sleep. The gray vertical lines are 1 hour apart. The actogram is a double plot with the information on the right half of each line repeated on the left half of the line below.

QUESTION

1. What is your diagnosis?

ANSWER

1. **Answer**: Chronic insomnia disorder—paradoxical insomnia subtype.

   Discussion: The severe degree of sleep disturbance reported in patients with paradoxical insomnia subtype (formerly called "sleep state misperception") is out of proportion to the relatively mild daytime impairment *and* the severity of sleep disturbance documented on polysomnography (PSG) or actigraphy. Patients often report little or no sleep on many nights, followed by days with relatively minimal dysfunction and no napping. In addition, patients with paradoxical insomnia often report hearing every noise in the house while in the bedroom, actively thinking for the entire night, or both. Daytime impairment reported is consistent with other types of insomnia but *is much less severe than expected*, given the severe level of sleep deprivation reported. For example, no intrusive sleep episodes or serious mishaps are caused by loss of alertness, even after nights reportedly without sleep.

   Sleep diary information is usually consistent with patient's complaints, but *not* consistent with objective evidence (from PSG or actigraphy data). On some nights little or no sleep may be reported, followed by days with no napping. PSG findings indicate lack of severe deficits in total sleep time (TST) or sleep latency. If abnormality in sleep latency or TST is present, they are much milder than the reported deficits. Usually, *the reported sleep latency and wakefulness after sleep onset (WASO) are at least 1.5 times the PSG values.*

   In the current patient, the sleep diary shows significantly reduced TST compared with actigraphy data. The estimate TST from actigraphy was almost 7 hours on average. One night the patient felt she had had no sleep at all (day 6). This was followed by a day without a nap. Actigraphy may overestimate the TST and underestimate sleep latency as patients with insomnia may lie very still (no movement) without sleeping. However, the very large difference between actigraphy data and the sleep diary is consistent with chronic insomnia disorder—paradoxical insomnia subtype. Another issue for this patient included excessive caffeine intake late in the day. The lighted clock being visible from the bed exacerbates the difficulty sleeping in many patients. Reduction in caffeine (after the morning cup of coffee) and moving the clock so that it was not visible from the bed were recommended. The patient was referred for cognitive behavioral treatment of insomnia. A combination of relaxation therapy, stimulus control, and sleep restriction were used. Over several months, her sleep improved. In particular, she seemed to respond to relaxation therapy.

CLINICAL PEARLS

1. Diagnosis of the cause of insomnia usually is made on the basis of a careful history and review of a patient sleep diary (log) and actigraphy, if possible.
2. PSG generally is not indicated in evaluation of insomnia. The exception is when a suspicion of sleep apnea exists or when the insomnia is severe and does not respond to empiric therapy.
3. Chronic insomnia disorder—paradoxical insomnia subtype—is characterized by report of a severe decrease in TST that greatly exceeds objective findings of sleep loss by actigraphy or PSG.
4. Patients with chronic insomnia disorder—paradoxical subtype—may report sleepless night followed by days without napping and minimal daytime sleepiness.
5. Actigraphy and the sleep diary provide complementary information.

BIBLIOGRAPHY

Agnew HW, Webb WB, Williams RL: The first night effect: an EEG study, *Psychophysiology* 2:263–266, 1966.

American Academy of Sleep Medicine: *International classification of sleep disorders: diagnostic and coding manual*, ed 2, Westchester, IL, 2005, American Academy of Sleep Medicine.

American Academy of Sleep Medicine: *International classification of sleep disorders*, ed 3, Darien, IL, 2014, American Academy of Sleep Medicine.

Buysse DJ: Insomnia, *JAMA* 309(7):706–716, 2013.

Chesson A, Hartse K, McDowell Anderson W, et al: Practice parameters for the evaluation of chronic insomnia, *Sleep* 23:1–5, 2000.

Littner M, Hirshkowitz M, Kramer M: Standards of Practice Committee of the American Academy of Sleep Medicine: Practice parameters for using polysomnography to evaluate insomnia: an update for 2002, *Sleep* 26:754–760, 2003.

Mai E, Buysee D: Insomnia, prevalence, impact, pathogenesis, differential diagnosis and evaluation, *Sleep Med Clin* 3:167–174, 2008.

Morgenthaler T, Alessi C, Friedman L, et al: Practice parameters for the use of actigraphy in the assessment of sleep and sleep disorders: an update for 2007, *Sleep* 30:519–529, 2007.

Sateia MJ, Doghramji K, Hauri P, Morin CM: Evaluation of chronic insomnia, *Sleep* 23:1–36, 2000.

Schutte-Rodin S, Broch L, Buysee D, et al: Clinical guideline for the evaluation and management of chronic insomnia in adults, *J Clin Sleep Med* 4:487–504, 2008.

Behavioral Treatment of Insomnia

The two major categories of insomnia treatment are (1) cognitive-behavioral treatment of insomnia (CBT-I) and (2) hypnotic medications. These treatments are not mutually. However, only one study has suggested that combination therapy is more effective than CBT-I alone.

COGNITIVE AND BEHAVIORAL THERAPY FOR INSOMNIA (CBT-I)

CBT-I is safe and effective for sleep-onset and sleep-maintenance insomnia as well as complaints of poor sleep quality.[1-4] The efficacy of CBT-I is equal to or better than results from pharmacotherapy.[5,6] Unfortunately, many locales do not have physicians, nurses, or psychologists skilled at this form of treatment. The 2006 update of the American Academy of Sleep Medicine (AASM) practice parameters for behavioral treatment of chronic insomnia state: "Psychological and behavioral interventions are effective and recommended in the treatment of chronic primary insomnia, secondary insomnia (due or associated with other medical or psychiatric disorders), insomnia in older adults, and chronic hypnotic users (Standard)."[2] In 2008, the *Clinical Guidelines for the Evaluation and Management of Chronic Insomnia in Adults*[1] recommended that CBT-I be utilized as initial treatment of insomnia if possible.

ELEMENTS OF CBT-I

Cognitive Therapy

Cognitive therapy is aimed at changing the patient's belief and attitudes about insomnia.[1,3] These dysfunctional cognitions are often identified by using questionnaires such as the Dysfunctional Beliefs About Sleep (DBAS) questionnaire.[7,8] Cognitive therapy uses a psychotherapeutic method to reconstruct cognitive pathways with positive and appropriate concepts about sleep and its effects. Common cognitive distortions that are identified and addressed in the course of treatment include "I can't sleep without medication," "I have a chemical imbalance," "If I can't sleep, I should stay in bed and rest," and "My life will be ruined if I can't sleep."[7,8]

CBT for Insomnia (CBTI): This technique combines cognitive therapy with behavioral techniques. The behavioral components usually include stimulus control therapy and sleep restriction therapy. Relaxation therapy may or may not be included. Sleep hygiene education is usually also included.

Sleep Hygiene: Up to 30% of patients evaluated for insomnia have inadequate sleep hygiene. Although education about sleep hygiene is a component of most CBT-I programs, no conclusive evidence suggests that education alone is effective treatment for insomnia.

Relaxation Therapy (RT): The term *relaxation therapy* (Table F38-1) is a generic term that encompasses a number of techniques. Progressive muscle relaxation (PMR) focuses on somatic arousal and was developed by Edmund Jacobsen.[1] Therefore, the technique is often called *Jacobsen PMR*. In this technique, the patient systematically goes through various areas of the body, initially tensing muscles, maintaining muscle tension, and relaxing the muscles. The patient is asked to concentrate on the sensations associated with tensing followed by relaxation. Guided imagery relaxation focuses on cognitive arousal and uses techniques of visualizing a relaxing setting or activity. RT is useful in patients who report or display elevated levels of arousal. The technique may be helpful with *both* sleep-onset and sleep-maintenance insomnia.

Stimulus Control Therapy (SCT) (see Table F38-1): This is a specific type of

TABLE F38-1 Behavioral Treatments for Insomnia

Technique	Evidence*	Brief Summary
Stimulus control therapy (SCT)	Standard	If not sleepy, get out of bed until sleepy Same wake time every day Bed is used only for sleep or sexual activity
Sleep restriction therapy (SRT)	Standard	Restrict time in bed so sleep ≥85% of time in bed
Relaxation therapy (RT)	Guideline	Progressive muscle relaxation Guided imagery
Biofeedback	Guideline	Reduce somatic tension
Paradoxical intention	Guideline	Passively remain awake and avoid any effort (intention) to fall asleep
Cognitive and behavioral therapy for insomnia (CBTI)	Standard	Cognitive therapy+one or both (SCT, SRT) With or without relaxation therapy
Sleep hygiene education	No recommendation	

*From Morgenthaler T, Kramer M, Alessi C, et al: Practice parameters for the psychological and behavioral treatment of insomnia: an update, *Sleep* 29:1415–1419, 2006 and Buysse DJ: Insomnia, *JAMA* 309(7):706–716, 2013.

BOX F38-1 **Stimulus Control Instructions**

1. Lie down with the intention of going to sleep only when sleepy.
2. Do not use the bed for anything except for sleep and sex. Do not use the bed for reading, television watching, eating, or thinking (worrying).
3. Do not watch the clock, but if you have not fallen asleep in 10 to 15 minutes, get out of bed, and go into another room. Stay up as long as you wish or until you feel sleepy, and then return to the bedroom.
4. If you cannot fall asleep, repeat rule 3 as often as needed.
5. Get up at the same time every morning irrespective of how much sleep you got during the night. *Goal:* Helps the body acquire a consistent sleep rhythm.
6. Do not nap during the day.

From Morgenthaler T, Kramer M, Alessi C, et al: Practice parameters for the psychological and behavioral treatment of insomnia: an update, *Sleep* 29:1415-1419, 2006; and Bootzin RR, Epstein D, Wood JM: Stimulus control instructions. In Hauri P, ed: *Case studies in insomnia*, New York, 1991, Plenum Press, pp 19-28.

---

behavioral therapy that is based on the idea that arousal occurs as a conditioned response to the stimulus of the sleep (bedroom) environment.[3,4,9] This technique is among the most effective behavioral treatments. The standard instructions are listed in Box F38-1. The goal of SCT is to extinguish the negative association between the bed and undesirable outcomes such as wakefulness, frustration, and worry. These associations become conditioned as a result of prolonged efforts to fall asleep and time in bed awake. SCT will replace these negative associations with positive associations between the bed and sleep.

Sleep Restriction Therapy (SRT): SRT limits the time in bed to the total sleep time (TST) (or 0.85 TST) as derived from sleep logs[3,10] (Box F38-2). The goal is to improve sleep continuity, thus enhancing sleep drive with sleep restriction. Sleep will become more consolidated when long periods in bed and napping are prohibited. As sleep continuity improves, the time in bed is gradually increased. When using this technique, the patient should be cautioned about sleepiness to prevent accidents or other mishaps.

Paradoxical Intention: This involves instructing the patient to passively remain awake and avoid any effort (intention) to fall asleep. The goal is to eliminate performance anxiety.

Biofeedback (Guideline): Biofeedback trains the patient to control some physiologic variable through visible or auditory feedback. The goal is to reduce somatic arousal.

Multicomponent Therapy (Without Cognitive Therapy): This form of treatment uses multiple behavioral techniques (e.g., SCT, SRT, RT) without cognitive therapy.

BOX F38-2	Sleep Restriction Instructions

1. A sleep log is kept for 1–2 weeks to determine the mean total sleep time (TST).
2. Set bedtime and wakeup time to achieve a mean TST with sleep efficiency >85%.
   - The minimum time in bed (TIB) is 5 hours.
   - If TST ÷ TIB = 0.85, then TIB = TST/0.85 0.85 = TST × 1.176.

Example: If TST = 310 minutes, then goal for TIB is (bedtime 11 PM, wake time 5:04 AM.)
3. Adjustments:
   A. If TST ÷ TIB >0.85 for 7 days, then add 15–20 minutes to TIB.
   B. If TST ÷ TIB <0.85, decrease TIB every 7 days.

Adapted from Morgenthaler T, Kramer M, Alessi C, et al: Practice parameters for the psychological and behavioral treatment of insomnia: an update, *Sleep* 29:1415-1419, 2006; and Speilman AJ, Saskin P, Thorpy MJ: Treatment of chronic insomnia by restriction of time in bed, *Sleep* 10:45-56, 1987.

Evidence for Behavioral Treatment

CBT-I for periods of 4 to 8 weeks has been proven to be effective by randomized, controlled trials.[11] Trials comparing CBT-I with standard care or pharmacotherapy[5,6] have found CBT-I to be at least as effective as pharmacotherapy (and in some studies better). In contrast to pharmacotherapy, the benefits persist (for up to 3 years) when treatment is stopped. CBT-I is effective for measures of sleep onset insomnia, sleep-maintenance insomnia, and nonrestorative sleep. Previous studies found no advantage of adding hypnotics to CBT-I. However more recently, Morin et al[12] found that initial combined behavioral therapy and pharmacotherapy, followed by CBT-I alone, produced the best long-term outcomes. CBT-I may be used in patients already on hypnotics, with the of weaning the hypnotic or reducing the dose or frequency of hypnotic use. Using structured programs, hypnotic tapering and withdrawal are facilitated by combining the process with CBT of insomnia.[13,14] In one study comparing supervised benzodiazepine (BZ) withdrawal, CBT alone, or supervised withdrawal and CBT-I, all groups significantly reduced BZ use. However, more patients were BZ free in the combined group, and both groups with CBT had better improvements in subjective sleep quality.[12] CBT-I has also proved effective in secondary (comorbid) insomnia caused by mental or medical disorders.[15] Although it is appropriate to optimize treatment of the underlying comorbid disorder, physicians should remember that CBT-I as well as hypnotics may help resolve insomnia complaints.

Brief Behavioral Therapy for Insomnia

CBT-I is usually delivered in 4 to 8 individual sessions. However, shorter interventions may be effective. Buysse et al[16] found that brief behavioral treatment of insomnia (BBTI) was effective compared with control (education about sleep only) in a group of older adult patients with insomnia. BBTI consists of a 45- to 60-minute individual intervention session, followed by a 30-minute follow-up session 2 weeks later, and 20-minute telephone calls after 1 and 3 weeks. BBTI emphasizes the behavioral elements of insomnia treatment rather than the cognitive components present in CBT-I. BBTI includes sleep education and discussion of homeostatic and circadian mechanisms of human sleep regulation. This education provides the rationale for the four main interventions of BBTI: (1) reduced time in bed; (2) getting up at the same time every day, regardless of sleep duration; (3) not going to bed unless sleepy; and (4) not staying in bed unless asleep. Napping is discouraged. These interventions derive from sleep restriction and stimulus control techniques, the efficacy of each technique has been well documented. Time in bed was limited to average self-reported sleep time plus 30 minutes, with a minimum of 6 hours. In the future, more interventions of this type may provide wider access to behavioral techniques. Insomnia interventions using the internet are also being developed.

Behavioral Treatment of Insomnia in Children

Behavioral treatment has also been used in children.[17,18] for sleep-association or limit-setting insomnia (Table F38-2). Unmodified and graduated extinction focus on removing reinforcement (parental attention) of unwanted behavior. Scheduled awakenings prevents reinforcement for unwanted behaviors following spontaneous awakening.

TABLE F38-2	Techniques Used for Behavioral Treatment of Insomnia of Childhood	
Technique	**Description**	**Rationale**
Unmodified extinction	Involves parents putting the child to bed at a designated bedtime and then ignoring the child until morning (parents continue to monitor for safety issues).	Reduces undesired behaviors (e.g., crying, screaming) by eliminating parental attention (reinforcer).
Graduated extinction	Involves parents ignoring bedtime crying and tantrums for predetermined periods before briefly checking on the child. A progressive (graduated) checking schedule (e.g., 5 minutes, then 10 minutes) or fixed checking schedule (e.g., every 5 minutes) may be used.	Enables a child to develop "self-soothing" skills and be able to fall asleep independently without undesirable sleep associations.
Scheduled awakenings	Involves parents preemptively awakening their child, prior to a typical spontaneous awakening, and providing the "usual" responses (e.g., feeding, rocking, soothing) as if child had awakened spontaneously.	Prevents nightly reinforcement for undesirable behaviors involved in waking.
Positive routines	Parents develop set bedtime routines characterized by enjoyable and quiet activities to establish a behavioral chain leading up to sleep onset.	Removes negative stimuli associated with bedtime.
Parental education and prevention	Involves parent education to prevent the occurrence of the development of sleep problems. Behavioral interventions are incorporated into these parent education programs.	Prevents problems before they occur.

Adapted from Mindell JA, Kuhn B, Lewin DS, et al: Behavioral treatment of bedtime problems and night wakings in infants and young children. An American Academy of Sleep Medicine Review, *Sleep* 29:1263-1276, 2006.

CLINICAL PEARLS

1. CBT of insomnia (also known as CBT-I) is as effective for insomnia (including sleep onset, sleep maintenance, and comorbid insomnia) as pharmacotherapy.
2. In the past it was believed that the combination of a hypnotic and CBT-I was not more effective than CBT-I alone. However, one study found that initial use of CBT-I with a hypnotic followed by CBT-I alone gave the best results. Additional studies are needed.
3. CBT-I is defined as cognitive therapy plus behavioral treatments (stimulus control and sleep restriction with or without relaxation therapy).

REFERENCES

1. Schutte-Rodin S, Broch L, Buysse D, et al: Clinical guideline for the evaluation and management of chronic insomnia in adults, *J Clin Sleep Med* 4 (5):487–504, 2008.
2. Morgenthaler T, Kramer M, Alessi C, et al: Practice parameters for the psychological and behavioral treatment of insomnia: an update, *Sleep* 29:1415–1419, 2006 and Buysse DJ: Insomnia, *JAMA* 309(7): 706–716, 2013.
3. Morin CM, Hauri PK, Espie CA, et al: Nonpharmacologic treatment of chronic insomnia, *Sleep* 22:1134–1156, 1999.
4. Morin CM, Bootzin RR, Buysee D, et al: Psychological and behavioral treatment of insomnia: update of recent evidence (1998–2004), *Sleep* 29:1398–1414, 2006.
5. Jacobs GD, Pace-Schott EF, Stickgold R, Otto MW: Cognitive behavior therapy and pharmacotherapy for insomnia: a randomized controlled trial and direct comparison, *Arch Intern Med* 164:1888–1896, 2004.
6. Smith MT, Perlis ML, Park A, et al: Comparative meta-analysis of pharmacotherapy and behavior therapy for persistent insomnia, *Am J Psychiatry* 159:5–11, 2002.
7. Morin CM: Dysfunctional beliefs and attitudes about sleep. Preliminary scale development and description, *Behav Ther* 163–164, 1994, Summer.
8. Morin CM, Vallières A, Ivers H: Dysfunctional beliefs and attitudes about sleep (DBAS): validation of a brief version (DBAS-16), *Sleep* 30:1547–1554, 2007.
9. Bootzin RR, Epstein D, Wood JM: Stimulus control instructions. In Hauri P, editor: *Case studies in insomnia*, New York, 1991, Plenum Press, pp 19–28.
10. Speilman AJ, Saskin P, Thorpy MJ: Treatment of chronic insomnia by restriction of time in bed, *Sleep* 10:45–56, 1987.
11. Edinger JD, Wohlgemuth WK, Radtke RA, et al: Cognitive behavioral therapy for treatment of chronic primary insomnia, *JAMA* 285:1856–1864, 2001.
12. Morin CM, Vallières A, Guay B, et al: Cognitive behavioral therapy, singly and combined with medication, for persistent insomnia: a randomized controlled trial, *JAMA* 301(19):2005–2015, 2009.
13. Morin CM, Bastein C, Guay B, et al: Randomized clinical trial of supervised tapering and cognitive behavioral therapy to facilitate benzodiazepine discontinuation in older adults with chronic insomnia, *Am J Psychiatry* 161:132–342, 2004.

14. Soeffing JP, Lichstein KL, Nau SD, et al: Psychological treatment of insomnia in hypnotic dependent older adults, *Sleep Med* 9:165–171, 2008.

15. Lichstein KL: Behavioral intervention for special insomnia populations: hypnotic dependent insomnia and comorbid insomnia, *Sleep Med* 7(S1):S27–S31, 2006.

16. Buysse DJ, Germain A, Moul DE, et al: Efficacy of brief behavioral treatment for chronic insomnia in older adults, *Arch Intern Med* 171(10):887–895, 2011.

17. Morgenthaler TI, Owens J, Alessi C, et al: Practice parameters for behavioral treatment of bedtime problems and night wakenings in infants and young children, *Sleep* 29:1277–1281, 2006.

18. Mindell JA, Kuhn B, Lewin DS, et al: Behavioral treatment of bedtime problems and night wakings in infants and young children. An American Academy of Sleep Medicine Review, *Sleep* 29:1263–1276, 2006.

PATIENT 113

Behavioral Insomnia of Childhood

Patient A: A 3-year-old male child born after normal gestation and with normal development was a good sleeper until the last 9 months. Now he refuses to go to his bedroom to sleep. Once carried in to his bedroom and placed in his bed, he does not fall asleep and will not stay in bed. Although placed in bed at 8:00 PM, he does not fall asleep until 11:00 PM. He repeatedly gets out of his bed and goes to his parents with multiple requests ("I can't sleep," "I'm thirsty," "There's something under my bed."). After the third trip to his parents' bedroom, he usually is allowed to stay up and watch TV. He falls asleep on the couch, and his parents move him to his room. When he awakens in the middle of the night, he repeats this behavior. His parents then give up and let him sleep in their bed. His parents report that he is irritable during the day and his behavior is difficult to control. During the clinic visit, he is running around the room, and his parents are unable to get him to behave.

Question 1: What is your diagnosis for Patient A?

Patient B: A 3-year-old girl is cooperative with getting into bed but will not stay in bed and fall asleep without a parent in the room. Despite 30 minutes of bedtime stories, she is wide awake at 8 PM. If she is left alone in her room, she cries loudly, so the parents return and must rub her back for her to go to sleep. After 9 PM, she falls asleep quickly if one of her parents is rubbing her back. Her parents then leave her room. Later, when she awakens in the night, she comes to her parents' bedroom and will not return to sleep unless the bedtime circumstances are reproduced. When they rub her back, she falls asleep quickly but she requires her parents' presence to return to sleep with subsequent awakenings. The child is cheerful and alert during her visit to your clinic, but the parents appear exhausted.

Question 2: What is your diagnosis for Patient B? What behavioral technique would you use?

ANSWERS

1. **Answer for Patient A:** Behavioral insomnia of childhood (BIOC)—limit-setting type.

   Discussion: The child refuses to go to bed or stay in bed because of lack of parental enforcement. The limit setting type of BIOC (Table P113-1), as defined in the *International Classification of Sleep Disorders*, Second Edition (ICSD-2) is characterized by (1) difficulty initiating or maintaining sleep, (2) refusal to go to bed or return to bed after awakening, (3) caregiver demonstrating insufficient limit setting to establish appropriate behavior. Many patients with BIOC have components of both types of BIOC (limit-setting type and sleep-association type). In the *International Classification of Sleep Disorders*, Third Edition (ICSD-3), BIOC is categorized under the heading "Chronic Insomnia Disorder." Many components of treatment the two types of BIOC have common elements. Some behavioral treatments for BIOC are listed in Table P113-2.

   It is important to establish what actual complaint the parents have to affect change. If the child's "sleep problem" is not really a problem for the parents, then they will not be motivated to change their approach at bedtime. If the child seems tired during the day or has behavioral problems that are linked to insufficient sleep or if the parents are suffering from insufficient sleep, behavioral management is more likely to be embraced by the family. The child's sleep–wake schedule should be evaluated to determine usual sleep-onset, sleep-offset, and napping behaviors. If the child is

TABLE P113-1 Behavioral Insomnia of Childhood

Sleep-association type	1. Falling asleep is an extended process. 2. Sleep-onset associations are demanding. 3. In the absence of associated factors, sleep onset is delayed.	Nighttime awakenings require the caregiver's intervention for return to sleep or for sleep onset conditions to be reproduced.
Limit-setting type	1. The child has difficulty initiating or maintaining sleep. 2. The child refuses to go to bed or return to bed after awakening. 3. The caregiver demonstrates insufficient limit setting to establish appropriate behavior.	

TABLE P113-2 Behavioral Treatments for Behavioral Insomnia of Childhood

Technique	Description
Unmodified extinction	Involves parents putting the child to bed at a designated bedtime and then ignoring the child until morning (parents continue to monitor for safety issues).
Graduated extinction	Involves parents ignoring bedtime crying and tantrums for predetermined periods before briefly checking on the child. A progressive (graduated) checking schedule (e.g., 5 minutes, then 10 minutes) or fixed checking schedule (e.g., every 5 minutes) may be used.
Scheduled awakenings	Involves parents preemptively awakening their child, prior to a typical spontaneous awakening, and providing the "usual" responses (e.g., feeding, rocking, soothing) as if child had awakened spontaneously.
Positive routines	Parents develop set bedtime routines characterized by enjoyable and quiet activities to establish a behavioral chain leading up to sleep onset.
Delayed (faded) bedtime	Involves temporarily delaying the bedtime to more closely coincide with the child's natural sleep onset time, and the fading is earlier as the child gains success falling asleep quietly.
Response cost	Involves removing the child from the bed for prescribed brief periods if the child does not fall asleep within a prescribed time.
Parent education and prevention	Involves parent education to prevent the occurrence of the development of sleep problems. Behavioral interventions are incorporated into these parent education programs.

napping excessively or late during the day, settling at bedtime will be more difficult. Constant sleep-offset (wake up) time should be constant each day. Sometimes, parental expectations are unrealistic, that is, putting the child to bed at 7 PM when the child's usual sleep onset is at 9 PM.

The family should be encouraged to develop a soothing and appropriate bedtime routine of 20 to 30 minutes' duration, including a last snack, bath, toothbrushing, and reading a book (positive routine; see Table P113-2). Bedtime should be 15 minutes before the child's usual sleep time; when the child begins to fall asleep quickly, bedtime may be advanced in small increments to achieve appropriate sleep duration. "Curtain calls" (repeatedly seeking parental attention after being placed in bed) at bedtime will be minimized if the child is put into bed closer to his or her natural sleep onset time. The family will need help in learning to set limits for the child during both sleep and wakefulness; that is, temper tantrums in the clinic are not rewarded with a promise to go to a favorite activity if the child will just "behave." Rewards should be given for desired behavior, and undesired behavior should be ignored. Curtain calls and awakenings should not be rewarded with extra attention during the night, as most toddlers view any attention as "good" attention. The family must deal with the child in a calm and matter-of-fact manner and not allow the child to stay up and watch TV with them or get into their bed. It is very important for all caregivers to be consistent with the bedtime routine, response to curtain calls, and dealing with nocturnal awakenings.

Unmodified extinction involves parents putting the child to bed at a designated bedtime and then ignoring the child until morning (parents continue to monitor for safety issues). *Graduated extinction* may be useful until the child learns to fall asleep quickly. One approach is to put the child into bed and have the parents visit him or her at progressively longer intervals between visits for reassurance and then quickly leave the room. This is difficult to enforce when the child is out of the crib. Another method is to gradually decrease adult intervention in the room; that is, the adult stays in room in a chair next to the child's bed but the child is not allowed to ask questions or engage the adult in conversation. After 3 days, the chair is moved 3 feet from the bed and further away after a subsequent 3 days until the chair is out of the room. It is important establish a reward system to reinforce desired behavior (sticker chart) and ignore undesired behavior. If the family situation does not improve with these interventions, if may be helpful to refer them to a behavioral specialist.

2. **Answer for Patient B:** BIOC—sleep-association type.

Discussion: In BIOC of the sleep association type the child requires parental presence in the bedroom to fall asleep either at the start of the night or following awakenings (see Table P113-1). Falling asleep is a lengthy process if the child's sleep onset needs are not met. In this case, the parents should allow the child to choose one or two books to read as part of the bedtime routine. The child should be put into bed close to their natural sleep onset time. Two approaches may be used. Unmodified extinction (see Table P113-1) may be tried if the parents are willing to endure the child's crying. However, if they give in after an hour, the patient will learn that if she cries long enough, she will get her way. Most parents these days are unwilling to stick to this routine. Another approach is to gradually reduce parental presence in the room as indicated above (graduated extinction). The parent should not get into bed with the child, but remain seated in a chair beside the bed and not touch the child (e.g., rub the back). The parent should not respond to any questions or demands by the child. The chair is then gradually moved away from the bed, to the doorway, and then out of the room. This should be repeated with nighttime awakenings. Desired behavior should be rewarded first thing in the morning (sticker chart), and undesired behavior should be ignored. If parents have difficulty with this technique, involvement of a clinical psychologist or behavioral specialist skilled in dealing with children may be helpful.

CLINICAL PEARLS

1. Children with bedtime refusal may have either sleep-association insomnia, limit-setting insomnia, or a combination of the two.

2. Behavioral management may effectively help parents deal with behavioral insomnia of childhood.

3. Pediatric clinical psychologists have expertise if helping families establish positive bedtime routines, limit setting, and independent sleep habits. If parental attempts at applying behavioral techniques are not successful, referral to a behavioral specialist is indicated.

BIBLIOGRAPHY

American Academy of Sleep Medicine: *International classification of sleep disorders: diagnostic and coding manual*, Westchester, IL, 2005, American Academy of Sleep Medicine.
Morgenthaler TI, Owens J, Alessi C, et al: Practice parameters for behavioral treatment of bedtime problems and night wakenings in infants and young children, *Sleep* 29:1277–1281, 2006.
Mindell JA, Kuhn B, Lewin DS, et al: Behavioral treatment of bedtime problems and night wakings in infants and young children. An American Academy of Sleep Medicine Review, *Sleep* 29:1263–1276, 2006.
Owens JA, Mindell JA: Pediatric insomnia, *Pediatr Clin North Am* 58(3):555–569, 2011.

PATIENT 114

Patient with Unfavorable Sleep Habits

A 65-year-old man complained of difficulty falling asleep and frequent awakenings (difficulty maintaining sleep). His sleep was unrefreshing. He had no history of snoring. His only medications included lisinopril (hypertension) and omeprazole (for gastroesophageal reflux disease [GERD]). He denied depression or anxiety. The sleep complaints worsened when he retired from his job. A sleep log is shown in Figure P114-1.

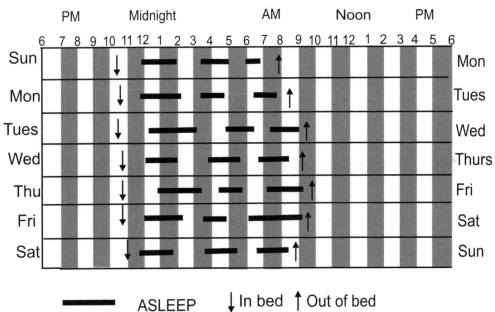

FIGURE P114-1 ■ Sleep log for the patient with insomnia.

QUESTIONS

1. Which behavioral treatment is most applicable to this patient?
   A. Stimulus control
   B. Sleep restriction
   C. Relaxation therapy
   D. Sleep hygiene education

2. Which of the following statements about cognitive behavioral treatment of insomnia is NOT true?
   A. It consists of cognitive therapy and one or more of behavioral treatments (stimulus control therapy, sleep restriction therapy with or without relaxation therapy).
   B. It continues to show benefits following the treatment period.
   C. It should never be combined with hypnotic treatment.
   D. It is effective for both primary and comorbid insomnia.

ANSWERS

1. **Answer:** Sleep restriction therapy.

2. **Answer:** C. CBT-I can be combined with hypnotic treatment. Conventional wisdom was that combination treatment was not more effective than CBT-I alone. However, a recent study found that CBT-I combined with initial use of a hypnotic may be more effective (at least in some patients).

   Discussion: The sleep diary of Patient A shows that he is in bed from around 10:30 PM to 9:30 AM (about 10 hours). The time the patient reported being asleep was much less. If time in bed greatly exceeds actual sleep time this tends to cause light and fragmented sleep. The actual estimate total sleep time (TST) of 5 to 6 hours was only mildly reduced from what could be considered normal. However, the sleep diary shows long sleep latency and frequent awakenings. Use of sleep restriction therapy should be one of the major treatments for patients who spend too much time in bed. Stimulus control techniques are also important in such a patient to address nocturnal awakenings or long sleep latency. In sleep restriction, the time in bed is restricted to approximately 1.2 times the actual estimated TST (Box P114-1). The goal is that TST should be about 85% of the total time in bed (sleep efficiency 85%). A simpler approach is a goal for time in bed to equal the estimated total sleep time plus 30 minutes. In the current patient, the estimated TST was about 5 hours. A total bed time of 6 hours was chosen (5 ×1.2) and a schedule of 11:30 PM to 5:30 AM was chosen. With the use of restricted time in bed, the nocturnal awakenings were reduced to one per night and sleep latency to 20 minutes. Sleep was more refreshing. When sleep efficiency was consistently over 85%, the time in bed was extended slightly by about 20 minutes each week until a time in bed of 10 PM to 6:00 AM was reached. The patient reported his estimated sleep time was 7 to 7.5 hours and that he was satisfied with the duration and quality of sleep.

   CBT-I consists of cognitive therapy and one or more behavioral treatments (stimulus control therapy, sleep restriction therapy with or without relaxation therapy). The benefits of CBT-I

| **BOX P114-1** | **Sleep Restriction Instructions** |

1. A sleep log is kept for 1 to 2 weeks to determine the mean total sleep time (TST).
2. Set bedtime and wake time to achieve mean TST with sleep efficiency >85%. The minimum TIB is 5 hours (hr). If TST ÷ TIB = 0.85, then TIB = TST ÷ 0.85.

Example: If TST = 310 minutes, then goal for TIB = 364 (bedtime 11 PM, wake time 5:04 AM.)
3. Adjustments:
   A. If TST ÷ TIB > 0.85 for 7 days, then add 15–20 minutes to TIB.
   B. If TST ÷ TIB < 0.85, decrease TIB every 7 days.

Adapted from Morgenthaler T, Kramer M, Alessi C, et al: Practice parameters for the psychological and behavioral treatment of insomnia: an update, *Sleep* 29:1415-1419, 2006; and Speilman AJ, Saskin P, Thorpy MJ: Treatment of chronic insomnia by restriction of time in bed, *Sleep* 10:45-56, 1987.

continue after the treatment period (in contrast to hypnotic treatment). CBT-I is effective for both comorbid insomnia (e.g., associated with a medical or mental disorder). Previously studies found no evidence to suggest that the addition of a hypnotic to CBT-I (combined treatment) offered an advantage to CBT-I alone. However, a study by Morin et al. in 2012 found that initial combined behavioral therapy and pharmacotherapy, followed by CBT-I alone, produced the best long-term outcomes. Additional studies to confirm the findings are needed. In any case, CBT-I is useful in assisting a patient to wean nightly hypnotic treatment. Some patients are able to wean hypnotics completely while others are able to reduce the frequency of hypnotic use.

CLINICAL PEARLS

1. If the total bedtime is greater than TST, sleep restriction is an essential behavioral technique to improve sleep consolidation.
2. Sleep restriction involves allowing a reduced time in bed so that the estimated TST is about 85% of the time in bed. When sleep efficiency increases, the time in bed is slowly increased.
3. CBT-I continues to improve sleep after active treatment sessions have stopped. This treatment is also effective in treating comorbid insomnia. The addition of a hypnotic to CBTI does not increase the effectiveness. However, CBT-I may help wean a patient off a hypnotic.

BIBLIOGRAPHY

Bootzin RR, Epstein D, Wood JM: Stimulus control instructions. In Hauri P, editor: *Case studies in insomnia*, New York, 1991, Plenum Press, pp 19–28.

Buysse DJ, Germain A, Moul DE, et al: Efficacy of brief behavioral treatment for chronic insomnia in older adults, *Arch Intern Med* 171(10):887–895, 2011.

Edinger JD, Wohlgemuth WK, Radtke RA, et al: Cognitive behavioral therapy for treatment of chronic primary insomnia, *JAMA* 285:1856–1864, 2001.

Lichstein KL: Behavioral intervention for special insomnia populations: hypnotic dependent insomnia and comorbid insomnia, *Sleep Med* 7S1:S27–S31, 2006.

Morgenthaler T, Kramer M, Alessi C, et al: Practice parameters for the psychological and behavioral treatment of insomnia: an update, *Sleep* 29:1415–1419, 2006.

Morin CM, Bastein C, Guay B, et al: Randomized clinical trial of supervised tapering and cognitive behavioral therapy to facilitate benzodiazepine discontinuation in older adults with chronic insomnia, *Am J Psychiatry* 161:132–342, 2004.

Morin CM, Bootzin RR, Buysee D, et al: Psychological and behavioral treatment of insomnia: update of recent evidence (1998–2004), *Sleep* 29:1398–1414, 2006.

Morin CM, Vallières A, Guay B, et al: Cognitive behavioral therapy, singly and combined with medication, for persistent insomnia: a randomized controlled trial, *JAMA* 301(19):2005–2015, 2009.

Schutte-Rodin S, Broch L, Buysee D, et al: Clinical guideline for the evaluation and management of chronic insomnia in adults, *J Clin Sleep Med* 4(5):487–504, 2008.

Soeffing JP, Lichstein KL, Nau SD, et al: Psychological treatment of insomnia in hypnotic dependent older adults, *Sleep Med* 9:165–171, 2008.

Speilman AJ, Saskin P, Thorpy MJ: Treatment of chronic insomnia by restriction of time in bed, *Sleep* 10:45–56, 1987.

Pharmacologic Treatment of Insomnia

GABA–BZ–CHLORIDE IONOPHORE COMPLEX

Gamma-aminobutyric acid (GABA) is the major inhibitory neurotransmitter in the central nervous system (CNS). The two major GABA receptor subtypes are GABA-A and GABA-B. The GABA-A receptor is associated with a chloride (Cl–) channel ionophore located in cell membranes. Ionophores are molecular complexes located in cellular lipid membranes that allow transport or passage of compounds across the membrane. The GABA-A receptor is the binding site for several drugs other than GABA, including agonists (muscimol, gaboxadol) and antagonists (bicuculline). The GABA-A receptor complex also contains a receptor for benzodiazepines (BZs) and related compounds, hence the complex is usually referred to as the GABA–benzodiazepine–chloride ionophore complex (GBC).[1-5] When GABA binds the GABA-A receptor on the complex, this allows passage of chloride ions through the membrane, resulting in hyperpolarization and reduced neuronal activity. When BZs and certain nonbenzodiazepine medications bind the BZ receptor on the GBC, the configuration of the GABA receptor changes to enhance the ability of GABA binding to the GABA-A receptor to open the associated chloride channel (increased frequency). The medications are, therefore, sometimes called *GABA-A receptor modulators.* Medications (including nonbenzodiazepines) that bind the BZ receptor and enhance the ability for GABA to open the chloride channel are called **benzodiazepine receptor agonists (BZRAs).** *Although BZRAs do not actually bind the GABA receptor (actually bind a BZ receptor on GBC complex), they are often referred to as* **GABA-A receptor agonists**.

The GBC is composed of five protein subunits surrounding the chloride channel (Figure F39-1). The subunits composing the GBC have different structure and are denoted as alpha, beta, gamma, epsilon, and rho units.[1-5] The receptor complex is usually composed of two alpha, two beta, and one gamma-subunit. In addition, the alpha, beta, and gamma-subunits have isoforms (e.g., alpha-1, alpha-2, alpha-3, etc.). The GABA-A binding site is located between the alpha and beta subunits and the BZ receptor site is located between the alpha and gamma-subunits (see Figure F39-1). The most common GBC receptor configuration is denoted as $alpha_1$, $beta_2$, $gamma_3$ (understood to mean two alpha-1, two beta-2, and one gamma-2 subunits), also known as a *BZ type 1 receptor.* The GBC also has receptors for barbiturates, certain inhaled anesthetics, and alcohol. The GBCs composed of alpha-1 subunits

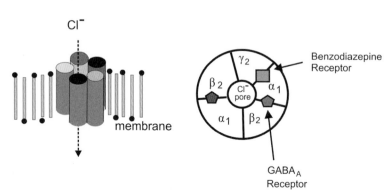

Cl⁻

membrane

γ_2
β_2 α_1
Cl⁻ pore
α_1 β_2

Benzodiazepine Receptor

GABA$_A$ Receptor

FIGURE F39-1 ■ *Left,* A schematic representation of the gamma-aminobutyric acid A (GABA$_A$)–benzodiazepine–chloride ionophore complex with five subunits arranged around the chloride pore. *Right,* A view from overhead shows the location of the GABA$_A$ receptors at the junction of the alpha-1 and beta-2 subunits and the benzodiazepine receptor at junction of alpha-1 and gamma-2 subunits.

mediate sedation (hypnotic effect), amnesia, and anticonvulsant effects. Those associated with alpha-2 and alpha-3 subunits mediate anxiolytic and myorelaxant effects. BZs tend to have high affinity for all these subtypes. The new nonbenzodiazepine BZRAs (zolpidem, zaleplon, eszopiclone), also known as the "Z" hypnotics, have preferential binding to GBCs containing certain subunits. Zolpidem and zaleplon selectively bind GBCs containing alpha-1 subunits and are often called *selective BZRAs*.[4-5] These non-BZ BZRAs have less anxiolytic and myorelaxant activity compared with BZs. However, the preferential binding is only relative, and at higher doses, these drugs bind to GBCs containing alpha-1, alpha-2, and alpha-3 subunits. Eszopiclone is another non-BZ BZRA with receptor binding more like traditional BZs but has many of the same effects on sleep as the other Z hypnotics. Eszopiclone does bind alpha-1 subunits with higher affinity than alpha-3 but also binds alpha-2 subunit receptors with only slightly lower affinity than alpha-1 subunits. The clinical importance of selective receptor binding is unclear. *The major property to consider in choice of a BZRA is the duration of action.* However, in general, zolpidem and zaleplon have minimal anxiolytic or muscle relaxant activity. If a patient's insomnia has a component on anxiety, these medications may be less effective. However, eszopiclone appears to have more affinity for GBCs with alpha-2 units than zolpidem and zaleplon and, therefore, possibly more anxiolytic effects.

BZRA Effects on Sleep

BZRAs have a number of important clinical effects including sedation (hypnotic), amnestic, anxiolytic, myorelaxant, and anticonvulsant (Table F39-1). BZRAs have a number of effects on sleep (Box F39-1). A decrease in sleep latency is common to all medications. Those with an intermediate or longer duration of action also may increase total sleep time (TST) and decrease wakefulness after sleep onset (WASO). BZRAs may increase sleep spindle activity and the amplitude of higher electroencephalography (EEG) frequencies. The BZs reduce stage N3 sleep with either no reduction or a mild reduction in rapid eye movement (REM) sleep. The major effect on stage N3 sleep is via a reduction in slow wave amplitude. Nonbenzodiazepine BZRAs (Z hypnotics) cause no or minimal decrease in the amount of stage N3 because they do not substantially reduce the amplitude of slow waves. The

TABLE F39-1	Benzodiazepine Receptor Agonists—Actions and Side Effects
Actions	**Side Effects**
Hypnotic	Sedation
Amnestic	Anterograde amnesia
Anxiolytic*	(learning new material)
Myorelaxant*	Tolerance[†]
Anticonvulsant	Dependence, abuse
	Rebound insomnia
	(especially triazolam)[†]
	Risk of falls
	Sleep walking, sleep sex,
	sleep violence
	Sleep-related eating
	Respiratory depression[†]

*Zolpidem and zaleplon have less myorelaxant and anxiolytic activity compared with BZs.
[†]Zolpidem, zaleplon, and eszopiclone has less tolerance, respiratory depression, and rebound insomnia compared to BZs.

BOX F39-1	Effects of Benzodiazepine Receptor Agonists on Sleep

1. Improved sleep continuity
   - Decreased sleep latency (short- and intermediate-acting BZRAs)
   - Increased total sleep time (intermediate acting BZs)
   - Decreased wake after sleep onset (intermediate-acting BZRAs)
2. Decreased stage N3 (BZs not Z drugs)
   - Reduced amplitude of slow waves (less with Z drugs)
   - Increased sleep spindles and faster activity
   - Decrease in REM sleep (mild effect, especially with Z drugs).

BZRAs, Benzodiazepine receptor agonists; *GABA,* gamma-aminobutyric acid; *REM,* rapid eye movement. Z drugs: zolpidem, zaleplon, eszopiclone

clinical importance of less reduction in stage N3 sleep is still unclear.

All three Z drugs are associated with less rebound insomnia or evidence of tolerance (decreased effect at the same dose) compared with the BZ BZRAs[4,5] (Table F39-2). Zaleplon has a very short duration of action (see Table F39-2) and may have less residual sedative effects especially after midnight dosing than longer acting Z drugs.[6] Zolpidem has a longer half-life compared with zaleplon but shorter compared with eszopiclone[7]. Zolpidem may not increase TST in some patients, and for this reason, zolpidem CR (continuous/extended release) was developed[8,9]. This is a two layered tablet, with one layer for rapid release and the other for slower release[8,9]. The half-life of zolpidem CR is that same as

TABLE F39-2 Benzodiazepine Receptor Agonist Hypnotic Medications (Nonbenzodiazepines)

Generic Name (Generic, If Available) [Brand Name] Dosage Forms Available	Dose	Onset of Action (T_{max})	Duration of Action (T½ half-life)	Indication	Selected Side Effects and Comments
Zaleplon (No generic available) [Sonata] (5, 10 mg capsule)	10 mg at bed time (qhs) (max 20 mg) 5 mg (hs) in women, older adults, debilitated, mild to moderate hepatic impairment, or concomitant cimetidine	10–20 minutes (min) (1 hour [hr])	Short-acting (T½ = 1 hr)	Sleep Onset Insomnia (SOI)	Rescue medication if 4 hr left for sleep
Zolpidem IR (generic available) [Ambien] (5, 10-mg tablets)	10 mg hs 5 mg in older adults, women, debilitated, hepatic impairment	10–20 min (1.6)	Short- to intermediate-acting T½ 1.5–4.5 hr	SOI > SMI	Sleep-related eating disorder and sleepwalking reported
Zolpidem CR (generic available) [Ambien CR] 6.25-, 12.5-mg layered tabs	6.25–12.5 mg qhs 6.25 mg qhs in women, older men	10–20 min (1.5)	Controlled-release, intermediate-acting similar half-life, higher drug level 4 hours after ingestion	SOI, SMI	Swallow whole not crushed, cut, or chewed Higher concentrations 3 to 8 hours after ingestion than zolpidem IR
Zolpidem SL (Buffered) (No generic available) [Intermezzo] 1.75-, 3.5-mg SL tablets	1.75 mg women, age > 65, hepatic impairment 3.5 mg in men < 65 yrs	10–20 min (0.6 hr)	T½ similar to IR zolpidem	MOTN awakening	At least 4 hours of sleep must remain
Zolpidem spray [Zolpimist] 5 mg per spray	Sprayed over the tongue 5 mg women 5 or 10 mg men < 65 yrs	10–20 min (0.9 hr)	Same as IR zolpidem	SOI, SMI	Slightly more rapid onset of sleep than immediate release zolpidem
Zolpidem SL [Edular] 5-, 10-mg per SL tablet	5 mg women 5 or 10 mg men	10–20 mg (1.4)	Same as IR zolpidem	SOI, SMI	Slightly more rapid onset of sleep than immediate release zolpidem
Eszopiclone (No generic available) [Lunesta] (1-, 2-, 3-mg tablets)	1 to 3 mg qhs (max 3 mg) 1 mg qhs starting dose in men and women those with hepatic impairment (max 1 mg)	10–30 min (1.5 hr)	Intermediate-acting T½ 6 hr	SOI, SMI	Unpleasant taste common side effect

Data from References 1-3.

IR, Immediate release; *MOTN*, middle of the night awakening and difficulty returning to sleep; *SOI*, sleep onset insomnia; *SOM*, sleep maintenance insomnia; *SMI*, sleep maintenance insomnia; T_{max}, time from administration to peak drug level.

Note: These medications are FDA approved as hypnotics (short-term indication, exception eszopiclone—indication not time limited) (Schedule IV Controlled Substances).

zolpidem, but there is a greater concentration of the medication 4 hours after drug administration (see Patient 115). Zolpidem CR, eszopiclone, and temazepam have an intermediate duration of action[2,7-9,12-14] (see Table F39-2) and may be more effective for treating sleep-maintenance insomnia compared with medications with a shorter duration of action. However, patients are quite variable in their responses to the different hypnotics, and some patients with sleep maintenance insomnia will respond to the non-CR preparations of zolpidem. Sublingual and spray preparations of zolpidem have been developed to speed the onset of action, although the difference in sleep latency compared with zolpidem IR (immediate release) is less than one half hour.[2] The only hypnotic approved for treating midnight awakening by the U.S. Food and Drug Administration (FDA) is Intermezzo (a buffered sublingual zolpidem preparation).[10,11] As noted above, zaleplon has a very short half-life and may also be used for midnight awakening. However, zaleplon is not FDA approved for this indication.

The BZ BZRAs used for insomnia are listed in Table F39-3. Temazepam is useful for treating sleep maintenance insomnia in patients in whom medications with a shorter duration of action are not effective. It has a delayed onset of action in some patients and may not be as effective as other medications for sleep-onset insomnia. Benzodiazepines that have NOT been approved by the FDA as hypnotics are listed in Table F39-4. Some patients have a combination of anxiety and insomnia that may respond to these medications better than other hypnotics FDA approved for insomnia treatment.

Side Effects of BZRAs

BZRAs have a number of side effects (see Table F39-1), including anterograde amnesia (decreased ability to learn and retain new information), ataxia (fall risk), as well as residual sedation during the day. Of note, eszopiclone is associated with an unpleasant (often metallic) taste in a significant number of patients ($\leq 25\%$).[7] BZRAs may also be associated with nausea in some patients. They are not recommended for use in nursing or pregnant women. In 2007, the FDA required packaging information on BZRA hypnotics to include a warning regarding several specific potential adverse effects. Current prescribing information notes that BZRAs have been associated with sleep behaviors, including sleepwalking and eating, driving, and sexual behavior during sleep. Patients taking BZRAs should allow for adequate sleep time and *not* take BZRAs in combination

with other sedatives, alcohol, or sleep restriction. Zolpidem is the BZRA most often associated with sleepwalking and sleep-related eating disorder, but these manifestations may occur with other BZRAs as well. Residual sedation is another important side effect of BZRAs. In general, shorter-acting medications are less likely to cause residual sedation. In 2013, the FDA mandated revised labeling that contained a warning that patients who take the sleep medication zolpidem extended-release (Ambien CR)—either 6.25 milligrams (mg) or 12.5 mg—are at risk for impairment of the ability to drive or engage in other activities that require complete mental alertness the day after taking the drug. Studies have shown that zolpidem levels may remain high enough the next day to impair these activities. Women metabolize zolpidem more slowly compared with men and are especially at risk for impairment.[15] This new recommendation has been added to the *Warnings and Precautions* section of the physician label and to the patient medication guide for zolpidem extended-release (Ambien CR). The FDA also recommended that the initial dose of immediate-release zolpidem products (zolpidem, Ambien) should be 5 mg for women (or geriatric men) and either 5 mg or 10 mg for younger men. The recommended initial dose of zolpidem extended-release (zolpidem CR, Ambien CR) is 6.25 mg for women (or geriatric men) and either 6.25 or 12.5 mg for younger men. The lower dose of zolpidem should also be used in patient's with hepatic dysfunction. If the lower doses (5 mg for immediate-release, 6.25 mg for extended-release) are not effective, the dose may be increased to 10 mg for immediate-release products and 12.5 mg for zolpidem extended-release. However, use of the higher dose may increase the risk of next-day impairment. The FDA has also lowered the recommended starting dose of eszopiclone (Lunesta) to 1 mg for both men and women. Respiratory depression caused by the BZRA hypnotics alone is uncommon. However, caution is advised with the use of hypnotics in patients with hypoventilation, obstructive sleep apnea (OSA), and severe lung disease. Respiratory depression is more likely when BZRAs are combined with other CNS depressants such as alcohol or narcotics.

The potential for dependence and abuse resulted in the BZRA hypnotics being classified as Schedule 4 medications. Drugs with high receptor binding affinity such as lorazepam, midazolam, and triazolam cause more side effects on withdrawal. Triazolam causes rebound insomnia and is no longer recommended as a first-line hypnotic. Significant rebound insomnia has *not* been noted in most studies of zaleplon, zolpidem,

TABLE F39-3 **Benzodiazepine Receptor Agonists (BZRAs) Used As Hypnotics (Benzodiazepines)**

Generic Name (Generic If Available) [Brand Name] Dosage Forms Available	Dose	Onset of Action (T_{max})	Duration of Action	Indication	Selected Side Effects and Comments
Benzodiazepines FDA Approved as Hypnotics					
Triazolam (Generic available) [Halcion] 0.125, 0.25 mg	0.125–0.25 mg at bedtime (qhs) 0.125 in older adults	10–20 minutes (min) (1.2 hours [hr])	Short acting T½ 2–5 hr	SOI	Rebound insomnia—not a first-line hypnotic
Estazolam (Generic available) [ProSom] 1-, 2-mg tablets	1–2 mg half strength (hs) 0.5 mg in older adults, debilitated	15–30 min (1.5 to 2 hr)	Intermediate-acting T½ 8–24 hrs	SOI > SMI	Residual daytime sleepiness
Temazepam (Generic available) [Restoril] 7.5-, 15-, 30-mg capsules	15–30 hs 15 mg in older adults, debilitated	45–60 min (1–2 hr)	Intermediate-acting T½ 8–20 hrs	SOI, SMI	Delayed onset of action in some patients
Flurazepam (Generic available) [Dalmane] 15, 30 mg capsules	15–30 mg hs 15 mg hs in older adults, debilitated	15–30 min (1.5 to 4.5)	Long-acting T½ 47–100 hrs	SMI	Residual daytime sleepiness active metabolites
Benzodiazepines Not FDA Approved as Hypnotics					
Clonazepam (Generic available) [Klonopin] 0.5, 1.0, 2.0 mg	0.25–0.5 mg qhs	20–60 min (Tmax 1–3 hrs)	Long-acting T½ 18–50 hr	SMI	Residual daytime sleepiness Potent BZRA Not FDA-approved as hypnotic
Lorazepam (Generic available) [Ativan] 0.5, 1.0 mg	0.5–1.0 mg qhs Max ≤2–4 mg	(1–3 hr)	Long-acting T½ 14 hr (range 10–20 hrs)	SOI, SMI	Not FDA-approved as hypnotic Wean slowly, can cause withdrawal side effects
Alprazolam (Generic available) [Xanax] 0.25, 0.5, 1, 2 mg	0.25 to 0.5 mg qhs	(0.6 to 1.4 hr)	Long acting T½ 11 hr (range 6–20 hrs)	SOI, SMI	Not FDA-approved as hypnotic Wean slowly, can cause withdrawal side effects

Data from References 1-3.
FDA, U.S. Food and Drug Administration; *SOI*, sleep onset insomnia; *SOM*, sleep maintenance insomnia.

and eszopiclone.[2] However, withdrawal side effects and rebound insomnia may potentially occur with all BZRAs, and slow withdrawal, if possible, is recommended.

Using BZRA Hypnotics

General Considerations

BZRA hypnotics are well studied and the medications listed in Tables F39-2 and F39-3 are FDA approved for treatment of insomnia unless otherwise noted. It is especially important to note the duration of action. The hypnotics are grouped into nonbenzodiazepines (see Table F39-2) and BZs (see Table F39-3). At this time, the only nonbenzodiazepine available in the United States in generic form is zolpidem. Brand-name Z hypnotics are generally quite expensive. Ideally, hypnotics should be used on a short-term or intermittent basis at the lowest effective dose. A lower dose and more caution is indicated in older

TABLE F39-4   **Sedating Antidepressants and Antipsychotics Used "Off-Label" as Hypnotics***

Generic Name (Generic Available or Not) [Brand Name] Dose Forms	Hypnotic Dose	Half Life/ Comments	Notable Side Effects
Trazodone (Generic available) [Desyrel] 50, 100 mg	25–100 mg at bedtime (qhs)	Less anticholinergic side effects than TCAs T½ 9 (7–15) hr	Priapism (1 in 8000) Postural hypotension
Mirtazapine (Generic available) [Remeron] 15, 30 mg	7.5–15 mg qhs	T½ 30 (20–40) hr	Weight gain Higher doses may be less sedating
Tricyclic Antidepressants (TCAs)			
Amitriptyline (Generic available) [Elavil] 10, 25, 50 mg	10–25 mg qhs	T½ 30(5–45) hr metabolite active (nortriptyline)	Very anticholinergic Dry mouth, constipation QT prolongation
Doxepin (Generic available) [Sinequan] 10,25,50 mg, 10 mg/mL	1–10 mg (elixir) 25 mg qhs	T½ 15 (10–30) hr	Dry mouth, constipation
Doxepin (Generic not available) [Silenor] 3, 6 mg	6 mg qhs 3 mg qhs older adults	T½ 15 (10–30) hr Less anticholinergic side effects At lower doses	FDA-approved for sleep maintenance insomnia Cimetidine increases drug levels— max dose of doxepin should not exceed 3 mg if cimetidine co-administered Sertraline may also increase levels of doxepin
Sedating Antipsychotic Medications			
Quetiapine (Generic available) [Seroquel] 25, 50, 100 mg	12.5–50 mg qhs	T½ 6 hr Intermediate-acting	Weight gain Headache, dizziness Neuroleptic syndrome Tardive dyskinesia Long QT Lens change

Data from References 1-3.
FDA, U.S. Food and Drug Administration; *TCAs*, tricyclic antidepressants.
*These medications not FDA-Approved as Hypnotics except for Silenor.

adults and in patients with impaired hepatic function because most BZRAs undergo hepatic metabolism. The FDA approved indication for most hypnotics is for short-term use. The exact treatment duration is not specified. The FDA indication for eszopiclone does not specify short term use. New studies have documented effectiveness of some hypnotic medications (eszopiclone, zolpidem CR) for 6 months or longer.[9,12-14] Clinical experience also has noted continued long-term effectiveness (at least by patient report) for a number of BZRA hypnotics. However, it is recommended that BZRA hypnotics be used in as low a dose as possible for as short a time as possible. The clinician should also remember that

cognitive behavioral treatment of insomnia is an effective alternative to hypnotics.

Choice of BZRA Hypnotic Medication

The major characteristic of BZRA medications to consider in choosing a hypnotic is the *duration of action*. Short-acting medications work in the treatment for sleep-onset insomnia but may not work for sleep-maintenance insomnia. Triazolam has a short duration of action and is associated with significant rebound insomnia. Zaleplon has a very short duration of action and may be useful as a "rescue medication" for middle of the night dosing (as long as 4–6 hours of potential sleep remain).[6] However, zaleplon is not FDA approved for middle of the night dosing.[6] However, only Intermezzo (a buffered sublingual zolpidem preparation) is FDA approved for middle of the night insomnia.[10,11] One study of experimental awakening during the middle of the night found morning effects with zolpidem but not with zaleplon. Zolpidem has a short to intermediate action and may work for some but not all patients as treatment of sleep-maintenance insomnia.

Intermediate-acting medications are indicated for sleep-onset and sleep-maintenance insomnia but may cause daytime sedation in some patients. Temazepam, eszopiclone, and zolpidem CR are in this category. As noted previously, temazepam has a long onset of action[2] in some patients (see Table F39-3) and may not be effective for treating sleep-onset insomnia in those individuals. However, the cost of temazepam is considerably lower than eszopiclone (Lunesta) and zolpidem CR (Ambien CR). Taking BZRA hypnotics with food delays the effect of these medications. Long-acting medications have an increased risk of daytime sedation and other residual effects. Flurazepam has a long half life and also has active metabolites. *It is important to note that sometimes patients who fail to respond to a given BZRA will respond to an alternate BZRA.* Lorazepam (Ativan) and clonazepam (Klonopin) are two BZ BZRAs that are not FDA approved for primary insomnia treatment. Lorazepam is approved for treatment of anxiety and may work better than approved hypnotics if insomnia coexists with anxiety. Although the standard dose for anxiety is 2 to 4 mg, lower doses (0.5–1 mg) of lorazepam may work as a hypnotic. The medication has a relatively long half-life and withdrawal symptoms may occur after long-term use. Clonazepam is a potent BZRA with a very long half-life and is commonly associated with morning grogginess. However, individual patients may respond to well to this medication and not report morning sedation. Starting with the lowest possible dose and having patients plan on a long sleep period is prudent. An occasional patient requires up to 2 mg of clonazepam for sleep maintenance insomnia. Alprazolam (Xanax) is FDA approved for the treatment of anxiety and panic disorder. Although the medication's half-life is fairly long, it is usually prescribed with dosing two or three times daily. If used as a hypnotic, the duration of effect may not last the entire night. An extended-release preparation is available. Alprazolam may also be associated with withdrawal symptoms.

RAMELTEON (ROZEREM)—A MELATONIN RECEPTOR AGONIST

Ramelteon is the first melatonin (MT) receptor agonist approved in the United States for treatment of insomnia.[16,17] It is an MT1/MT2 receptor agonist. The effects at MT1 are thought to inhibit neuronal firing of the suprachiasmatic nucleus (SCN), effectively turning off the alerting signal and allowing sleep to occur. In contrast, MT2 receptor effects are thought to mediate melatonin's phase shifting effects on circadian rhythms. Ramelteon is about 17 times more potent at the MT1/MT2 receptors than melatonin. Ramelteon is available as a 8-mg tablet and the dose is 8 mg taken 30 minutes before bedtime. Studies have shown an absence of next-day residual effects, withdrawal, or rebound effects. The medication lacks abuse potential. Randomized, placebo-controlled studies have demonstrated efficacy of ramelteon with most effects being on sleep latency. Ramelteon is FDA approved for sleep onset insomnia. The medication has a short half-life. One study by Mayer and colleagues[17] demonstrated that 8 mg of ramelteon 30 minutes before bedtime reduced subjective sleep latency over a 6-month trial. Ramelteon also decreased latency to persistent sleep by polysomnography (PSG) over the trial. TST was increased only during week one. Side effects of ramelteon include headache, nausea, dizziness, somnolence, nightmares, hallucinations, and rarely suicidal ideation. Arthralgia and myalgia may also occur. Because ramelteon has no dependence potential, it may be a good choice for patients with alcohol or drug dependency. Ramelteon undergoes hepatic metabolism and should be avoided in patients with severe liver disease. Use of ramelteon is contraindicated in patients taking luvoxamine because this antidepressant significantly increases the levels of ramelteon in blood.

SEDATING ANTIDEPRESSANTS AND ANTIPSYCHOTICS

Sedating antidepressants used in doses lower than used for antidepressant effects are widely used as hypnotics (Table F39-4). However, relatively little evidence has demonstrated their effectiveness as hypnotics in patients without depression. *Trazodone* is a sedating antidepressant with minimal anticholinergic activity that is frequently used as a hypnotic. The evidence for its efficacy as a hypnotic in patients without depression is very modest.[18-20] However, some patients seem to benefit from the medication. It is a reasonable hypnotic in comorbid depression, in patients with significant sleep apnea, or in patients with a history of medication dependence. Its main side effects are priapism (1 in 8000) and postural hypotension. The usual dose is 25 to 100 mg at bedtime. *Mirtazapine* (Remeron) is used in low doses as a hypnotic. Of interest, lower doses (7.5 mg and 15 mg) are sometimes more sedating than higher doses. The major side effect is weight gain. Mirtazapine antagonizes alpha-2 receptors and serotonin (5HT2) receptors. The sedative effects of trazodone are caused by its antihistamine activity. *Doxepin* (Sinequan, Silenor) and *amitriptyline* (Elavil) are sedating tricyclic antidepressants (TCAs) that have been used in low doses as hypnotics. Sedating TCAs have significant anticholinergic side effects (dry mouth, constipation, urinary retention). It is important to recall that TCAs are very dangerous in overdose. Recently, very low dose doxepin (1, 3, 6 mg) has been evaluated with randomized, controlled[21] trials for its utility as a hypnotic. Lower doses avoid significant anticholinergic side effects. In these studies, the major significant effect was a decrease in WASO. The mechanism of hypnotic action of doxepin is antagonism of histamine (H1) receptors. A preparation of doxepin (Silenor) is available as 3-mg and 6-mg tablets is approved by the FDA for treatment of sleep-maintenance insomnia. This is the only sedating antidepressant FDA approved for the treatment of insomnia. Silenor is fairly expensive. An alternative is to use a low dose of generic doxepin (10 mg or 5 mg using the elixir). Medications with substantial anticholinergic activity may cause urinary retention in patients with benign prostatic hypertrophy. Use of even low-dose doxepin in patients with severe urinary retention should be avoided.

Quetiapine (Seroquel) is a second-generation antipsychotic medications that antagonizes histamine, dopamine D2, and serotonin (5HT2) receptors. At low doses, the medication's main effect is as an antihistamine. Quetiapine is indicated for treatment of schizophrenia and bipolar disorder. Side effects include Q–T interval prolongation, weight gain, extrapyramidal symptoms, headache, lens changes or cataracts, and a decreased white blood cell (WBC) count. Even at low doses, quetiapine has been associated with significant weight gain. Because of its side effects, this medication is usually not used in patients without significant psychiatric disorders.

OTHER MEDIATIONS USED FOR INSOMNIA

Other medications associated with sedation have been used for treating insomnia. Gabapentin (an anticonvulsant structural analog of GABA that binds the alpha-2-delta subunit of voltage-gated calcium channels) is used for chronic pain and restless legs syndrome (RLS). The half-life of gabapentin is approximately 5 to 9 hours, and it is excreted by the kidneys unchanged. Because of the sedative properties of gabapentin, the medication may be used as an alternative hypnotic treatment in patients who do not respond to or tolerate traditional hypnotic medications. The usual dose is 300 to 900 mg at bedtime. Side effects include dizziness, ataxia, weight gain, and, less commonly, leukopenia. Gabapentin could potentially be useful in patients with insomnia associated with pain. Gabapentin may increase the amount stage N3 sleep.

Melatonin is a naturally occurring substance available as an over-the-counter (OTC) sleeping pill. According to a meta-analysis performed regarding the use of melatonin, it appears to have a small effect on sleep latency with little effect on WASO or TST.[2,22] As previously noted, Ramelteon is a melatonin receptor agonist (MT1, MT2) that is FDA approved for the treatment of sleep-onset insomnia. One problem with both ramelteon and melatonin as hypnotics is that the endogenous melatonin levels are already elevated during the dark hours. Melatonin also has a short half-life. The hypnotic dose of melatonin is 3 to 5 mg. Antihistamines (diphenhydramine and doxylamine) are the primary ingredients in OTC sleep aids. Some limited evidence exists for their efficacy. The main problem is that they have considerable anticholinergic activity (urinary retention) and may cause daytime sedation.

PHARMACOTHERAPY FOR PATIENTS WITH DEPENDENCE ISSUES

In patients with a history of past or current alcohol or BZ dependence, the use of BZRAs is problematic. For these patients, use of ramelteon (no abuse potential), a low dose of a sedating antidepressant, or cognitive-behavioral treatment of insomnia are the best treatment options.

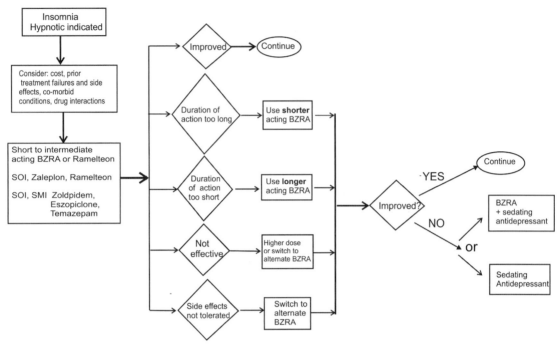

FIGURE F39-2 ■ Pharmacotherapy of insomnia. *SOI*, Sleep onset insomnia; *SMI*, sleep maintenance insomnia. (Adapted from Berry RB: *Fundamentals of sleep medicine,* Philadelphia, 2012, Saunders, pp 507.)

PHARMACOTHERAPY OF INSOMNIA: OVERALL STRATEGY

An algorithm for hypnotic therapy of insomnia is presented in Figure F39-2. The treatment of insomnia comorbid with depression is discussed in Patient 124. It is always important to ask patients about prior treatment failures and side effects. Drug interactions should also be considered. In patients with sleep-onset insomnia, treatment could be started with ramelteon or zaleplon. However, the cost of these medications may not be acceptable. A lower dose of a longer-acting medication could be tried. *The duration of action depends on both the dose and the elimination half-life.* If sleep-maintenance insomnia is a problem, use of zolpidem, zolpidem CR, eszopiclone, or temazepam could be considered. In older adult patients or those with impaired hepatic metabolism, a lower hypnotic dose is prudent. If the duration of action is not long enough, a switch to a longer-acting medication should be made, for example, a switch from zolpidem to eszopiclone. If the duration of action is too long (morning sedation), a switch to a shorter-acting medication or a reduction in dose of the current medication could be tried. If the medication is not effective, a switch to an alternative BZRA could be considered. Some patients will respond differently to alternative BZRAs. As noted above, temazepam may not work well for sleep-onset insomnia in some patients because of its longer onset of action. If anxiety is a major component of insomnia, use of a traditional BZ or eszopiclone with more anxiolytic activity might be more effective. If the current hypnotic medication is not tolerated because of side effects, a switch to an alternative BZRA could also be tried.

If treatment with standard BZRA hypnotics is not successful, a sedating antidepressant could be tried. Given the minimal anticholinergic effects associated with trazodone, most physicians would start with this medication when using a sedating antidepressant. However, low-dose doxepin or amitriptyline may be effective in some patients. If sedating antidepressants are not effective (or tolerated at an effective dose), the combination of a BZRA and a sedating antidepressant could be tried (e.g., zolpidem and trazodone). If a significant pain component to insomnia is present, gabapentin could be tried for its sedating as well as analgesic effects. If anxiety is a major component of the insomnia or the traditional BZRA hypnotics are not effective, use of lorazepam, alprazolam, or clonazepam could be tried. Lastly, a sedating antipsychotic (quetiapine) could be tried. These drugs have major side effects and are generally to be avoided unless a mental disorder is present or all other options have failed.

CLINICAL PEARLS

1. Hypnotics with a short duration of action are indicated to treat sleep-onset insomnia (e.g., zaleplon, ramelteon).

2. BZRAs with intermediate duration of action are indicated to treat sleep-onset and sleep-maintenance insomnia (zolpidem CR, eszopiclone, temazepam). Zolpidem is also effective for treating sleep-maintenance insomnia in some patients.

3. The most important property of a hypnotic medication is the duration of action.

4. An unpleasant taste is a distinctive side effect of eszopiclone.

5. Sleep-related eating disorder may occur with use of any of the BZRAs but is most often described with zolpidem.

6. The nonbenzodiazepine BZRAs (the Z drugs) tend to suppress stage N3 sleep less compared with benzodiazepines and are less commonly associated with rebound insomnia compared with benzodiazepine BZRAs.

7. Silenor (doxepin) is the only sedating antidepressant FDA approved for treating insomnia (sleep-maintenance insomnia).

8. Trazodone is a sedating antidepressant with minimal anticholinergic side effects. It is frequently used in low doses (25 to 50 mg) as a hypnotic. Priapism is an uncommon but serious side effect.

9. Rebound insomnia is less common with nonbenzodiapzepine receptor agonists (Z drugs) compared with the benzodiazepine hypnotics. However, it is best to wean the patient off all hypnotics to avoid rebound insomnia.

REFERENCES

1. Schutte-Rodin S, Broch L, Buysse D, et al.: Clinical guideline for the evaluation and management of chronic insomnia in adults, *J Clin Sleep Med* 4(5):487–504, 2008.
2. Buysse DJ: Insomnia, *JAMA* 309(7):706–716, 2013.
3. Mendelson W: Hypnotic medications: mechanisms of action and pharmacologic effects. In Kryger MH, Roth T, Dement WC, editors: *Principles and practices of sleep medicine*, ed 5, St. Louis, 2011, Saunders.
4. Olsen RW, Sieghart W: GABAA receptors: subtypes provide diversity of function and pharmacology, *Neuropharmacology* 56:141–148, 2009.
5. Nutt DJ, Stahl SM: Searching for perfect sleep: the continuing evolution of GABA-A receptor modulators as hypnotics, *J Psychopharmacol* 24:1601–1612, 2010.
6. Zammit GK, Corser B, Doghramji K, et al.: Sleep and residual sedation after administration of zaleplon, zolpidem, and placebo during experimental middle of the night awakening, *J Clin Sleep Med* 4:417–423, 2006.
7. Monti JM, Pandi-Perumal SR: Eszopiclone: its use in the treatment of insomnia, *Neuropsychiatr Dis Treat* 3:441–453, 2007.
8. Roth T, Soubrane C, Titeux L, Walsh JK: Zoladult Study Group: Efficacy and safety of zolpidem-MR: a double-blind, placebo-controlled study in adults with primary insomnia, *Sleep Med* 7(5):397–406, 2006.
9. Krystal AK, Erman M, Zammit GK, et al: Long-term efficacy and safety of zolpidem extended-release 12.5 mg administered 3 to 7 nights per week for 24 weeks in patients with chronic primary insomnia: a 6-month, randomized, double-blind, placebo controlled parallel-group, multi-center study, *Sleep* 31:79–90, 2008.
10. Greenblatt DJ, Harmatz JS, Roth T, et al: Comparison of pharmacokinetic profiles of zolpidem buffered sublingual tablet and zolpidem oral immediate-release tablet: results from a single-center, single-dose, randomized, open-label crossover study in healthy adults, *Clin Ther* 35(5):604–611, 2013.
11. Roth T, Krystal A, Steinberg FJ, et al: Novel sublingual low-dose zolpidem tablet reduces latency to sleep onset following spontaneous middle-of-the-night awakening in insomnia in a randomized, double-blind, placebo-controlled, outpatient study, *Sleep* 36(2):189–196, 2013.
12. Krystal A, Walsh JK, Laska E, et al.: Sustained efficacy of eszopiclone over 6 months of nightly treatment: results of a randomized, double-blind, placebo-controlled study in adults with chronic insomnia, *Sleep* 26:793–799, 2003.
13. Roth T, Walsh JK, Krystal A, et al.: An evaluation of the efficacy and safety of eszopiclone over 12 months in patients with chronic primary insomnia, *Sleep Med* 6:487–495, 2005.
14. Ancoli-Israel S, Krystal AD, McCall WV: et al.: A 12 week, randomized, double-blind, placebo-controlled study evaluating the effects of eszopiclone 2 mg on sleep/wake function in older adults with primary and comorbid insomnia, *Sleep* 33:225–234, 2010.
15. Kuehn BM: FDA warning: driving may be impaired the morning following sleeping pill use, *JAMA* 309(7):645–646, 2013.
16. Zammit G, Erman M, Wang-Weigand S, et al.: Evaluation of the efficacy and safety of ramelteon in subjects with chronic insomnia, *J Clin Sleep Med* 3:495–504, 2007.
17. Mayer G, Wang-Weigand S, Roth-Schechter B, et al.: Efficacy and safety of 6 month nightly ramelteon administration in adults with chronic primary insomnia, *Sleep* 32:351–360, 2009.
18. Mendelson W: A review of the evidence for the efficacy and safety of trazodone in insomnia, *J Clin Psychiatry* 66:469–476, 2005.
19. Walsh J, Erman M, Erwin CW, et al: Subjective hypnotic efficacy of trazodone and zolpidem in DSMIII-R primary insomnia, *Hum Psychopharmacol* 13:191–198, 1998.
20. Kaynak H, Kaynak D, Gözükirmizi E, et al: The effects of trazodone on sleep in patients treated with stimulant antidepressants, *Sleep Med* 5:15–20, 2004.
21. Roth T, Rogowski R, Hull S, et al.: Efficacy and safety of doxepin 1 mg, 3 mg, and 6 mg in adults with primary insomnia, *Sleep* 30:1555–1561, 2007.
22. Brzezinski A, Vangel MG, Wurtman RJ, et al.: Effects of exogenous melatonin on sleep. A meta-analysis, *Sleep Med Rev* 9:41–50, 2005.

Sleep-Maintenance Insomnia While Taking a Hypnotic

A 45-year-old woman has a long history of sleep-onset and sleep-maintenance insomnia. She is currently taking zolpidem 5 mg nightly. With this medication, the patient falls asleep rapidly but awakens at 4 AM and cannot return to sleep. The patient was switched to temazepam 15 mg but had difficulty falling asleep and was somewhat groggy in the morning.

QUESTION

1. What hypnotic treatment do you recommend?

ANSWER

1. **Answer:** Eszopiclone, zolpidem 10 mg, or zolpidem CR 6.25 mg.

   Discussion: The half-life (or duration of action) is the most important characteristic of benzodiazepine receptor agonists (BZRAs) to consider when choosing a hypnotic for treatment of insomnia. Therefore, familiarity with the duration of action of commonly used hypnotics is important to choose the best treatment for insomnia. In Table P115-1, commonly used hypnotics are listed, with sequentially longer half-life values in descending order. Of note, the duration of action depends on the dose, half-life, and potency of a medication. The higher the dose, the longer is the duration of action.

   Zaleplon has a very short half-life and is indicated for the treatment of sleep-onset insomnia. The medication may also be taken as a "rescue" hypnotic in the middle of the night if sufficient time remains for sleep (ideally 4 hours). However, zaleplon is not FDA approved for middle of the night dosing. Zolpidem, eszopiclone, or temazepam are each hypnotics that may be used for in the treatment of both sleep-onset insomnia and sleep-maintenance insomnia. If a patient taking zolpidem complains of early awakening, use of a longer-acting hypnotic (eszopiclone or temazepam) is an option. A modified release form of zolpidem (Zolpidem CR) is composed of one layer with rapid medication release and another with a slower release. The half-life of the medication once in serum is the same as that of zolpidem immediate release preparations. However, the effective serum level is maintained for a longer duration (4 to 6 hours) (Figure P115-1). Therefore, use of zolpidem CR 6.25 mg is a reasonable treatment option for the patient. Although a generic form of zolpidem CR is available, it is still relatively expensive. Eszopiclone has a longer half-life compared with zolpidem and might also be effective in this patient. Currently, no generic form of eszopiclone is available, so this medication is also relatively expensive. A generic form of temazepam is available and is

TABLE P115-1	Half-Life of Commonly Used Hypnotics
Medication	**Half-Life (hours)**
Zaleplon	1
Zolpidem	2.5–4
Eszopiclone	4–6
Temazepam	8–10

Note: Values vary between different references.

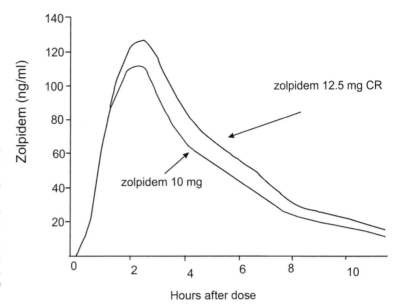

FIGURE P115-1 ■ Plasma level of immediate-release zolpidem 10 milligrams (mg) versus controlled-release zolpidem 12.5 mg. The half life is similar, but the level in serum is higher 4 to 6 hours after the dose. (Modified from Greenblatt DJ, Legangneux E, Harmatz JS, et al: Dynamics and kinetics of modified release formulation of zolpidem: comparison with immediate-release standard zolpidem and placebo, *J Clin Pharmacol* 46:1469-1480, 2006.)

inexpensive. This medication is useful for treating sleep-maintenance insomnia, but its onset of action may be slow in some patients. In the current patient, temazepam was not effective in treating sleep-onset insomnia. It is possible that a higher dose taken earlier might work (but the patient already complained of morning sedation). Finally, use of a larger dose of zolpidem immediate release may also prevent early-morning awakenings. As noted above, the duration of action of a medication depends both on dose and half-life. The disadvantage of the use of zolpidem 10 mg (or 7.5 mg) might be early-morning sedation. If none of the above options works, the addition of low-dose trazodone (25–50 mg) to zolpidem to assist with sleep maintenance could be tried. The patient should be warned about morning sedation and should try this medication combination when a long period is available for sleep. Another sedating antidepressant such as low-dose doxepin could also be added or substituted for the BZRA that is not effective for sleep maintenance. Of note, doxepin (Silenor) has been approved by the U.S. Food and Drug Administration (FDA) for sleep maintenance but is more expensive than generic trazodone or doxepin.

In 2013, the FDA mandated a change in labeling for immediate-acting and modified-release zolpidem. A dose of 5 mg of the immediate-acting and 6.25 mg of the modified-release formulation (6.25 CR) is recommended for women and older men. Higher doses (10 mg and 12.5 mg) are recommended only if the lower dose is not effective. A dose of 5 or 10 mg (6.25 or 12.5 mg CR) is now recommended for younger men. A dose of 5 mg or 6.25 mg (CR) is recommended for both men and women with hepatic impairment. Medication labeling also contains a warning about driving or performing tasks that require a high degree of coordination the next day following use of the CR preparations. It is also recommended that at least 7 to 8 hours should be available for sleep before taking a hypnotic. The FDA also recommends a starting dose of eszopiclone (Lunesta) of 1 mg in both men and women to avoid next day sedation. Of note, taking hypnotics with food (e.g., zolpidem) may delay the onset of action.

If a patient complains of morning grogginess with use of a hypnotic, a medication with a shorter half-life or the same medication at a lower dose could be tried. In dosing hypnotics, it is important to consider the increased risk of falls and slower metabolism in patients age ≥ 65 years, women, and patients with hepatic dysfunction. Of note, generally, cognitive behavioral treatment of insomnia CBT-I rather than a hypnotic, is considered the treatment of choice for insomnia. However, this therapy may not be available in some locales or acceptable to some patients. CBT-I has been used with structured programs to allow a patient to be slowly weaned off hypnotic use. The current patient was treated with zolpidem CR 6.25 mg and was able to maintain sleep until the desired wake time. She was referred for CBT-I with the goal of eventually being weaned off the hypnotic.

CLINICAL PEARLS

1. The duration of action in the most important characteristic of BZRAs to consider when choosing a hypnotic.
2. The duration of action of common hypnotics:
   Temazepam > eszopiclone > zolpidem > zaleplon
3. When the duration of the action of a hypnotic is not long enough, either a higher dose or a longer-acting medication should be used.
4. Longer-acting medications may cause significant daytime sleepiness in the morning.
5. The dose of zolpidem should be reduced in women and older men (5 mg immediate release or 6.25 mg modified release). The recommended starting dose of eszopiclone has been reduced to 1 mg for men and women.
6. Another option to increase the duration of a BZRA is to add a low dose of a sedating antidepressant (e.g., trazodone 25 mg).

BIBLIOGRAPHY

Buysse DJ: Insomnia, *JAMA* 309(7):706–716, 2013.
Greenblatt DJ, Legangneux E, Harmatz JS, et al: Dynamics and kinetics of modified release formulation of zolpidem: comparison with immediate-release standard zolpidem and placebo, *J Clin Pharmacol* 46:1469–1480, 2006.
Kuehn BM: FDA warning: driving may be impaired the morning following sleeping pill use, *JAMA* 309(7):645–646, 2013.
Roth T, Soubrane C, Titeux L, Walsh JK: Zoladult Study Group: Efficacy and safety of zolpidem-MR: a double-blind, placebo-controlled study in adults with primary insomnia, *Sleep Med* 7(5):397–406, 2006.
Schutte-Rodin S, Broch L, Buysee D, et al: Clinical guideline for the evaluation and management of chronic insomnia in adults, *J Clin Sleep Med* 4(5):487–504, 2008.
Stahl S: *Essential psychopharmacology*, ed 4, New York, 2011, Cambridge University Press.
Sullivan SS: Insomnia pharmacology, *Med Clin North Am* 94:563–580, 2010.

PATIENT 116

Middle-of-the-Night Awakening and a Patient with Drug Dependence and Insomnia

Patient A: A 45-year-old woman complained of middle of the night awakening that occurred about two times per week. After the awakening, it took 30 minutes to an hour for her to fall asleep. After such nights she felt very sleepy and fatigued the following day. She denied napping and had consistent bedtime and wake times. Her only medication was levothyroxine. She denied symptoms of depression. The patient did not want to take a nightly hypnotic.

QUESTION 1

1. What medications are suitable for Patient A with middle of the night awakening and difficulty returning to sleep?

Patient B: A 60-year-old obese man has a history of alcohol dependence, insomnia, and benign prostatic hypertrophy.

QUESTION 2

2. What is the most appropriate medication for treatment of insomnia in Patient B?
   A. Doxepin 25 milligrams (mg)
   B. Amitriptyline 25 mg
   C. Zolpidem 10 mg
   D. Trazodone 50 mg
   E. Diphenhydramine 25 mg

ANSWER

1. **Answer:** A medication with a rapid onset of action and a short half-life

   Discussion: A medication with a rapid onset of action and a short duration of action is needed for treatment of middle of the night awakening (MOTNA) with difficulty returning to sleep. Recall that the duration of action depends both on the elimination half-life and the dose. Zaleplon dosed at 5 to 10 mg in the middle of the night is one treatment option for middle of the night awakening and difficulty returning to sleep (Table P116-1). The elimination half-life of this medication is approximately 1 hour. In a study by Zammit et al, zaleplon 10 mg and zolpidem 10 mg effectively shortened sleep latency and lengthened sleep duration after dosing, when administered during experimental middle of the night awakening. Residual sedation was not detected as little as 4 hours after zaleplon 10 mg. Residual sedation was detected with zolpidem 10 mg up to 7 hours after treatment. These findings suggest that zaleplon may be an appropriate treatment for use when patients awaken during the night and have difficulty reinitiating sleep. However, zaleplon is NOT approved by the U.S. Food and Drug Administration (FDA) for treatment of awakening in the middle of the night.

   Buffered sublingual zolpidem tartrate (BSLZT) (Intermezzo) is FDA approved for treatment of middle-of-the-night awakening provided at least 4 hours remain for sleep. The medication should be taken when the patient is in bed and placed under the tongue. It should not be chewed or swallowed. The preparation is quickly absorbed, and the low dose allows minimal residual daytime effects, although the half-life of zolpidem has been shown to be up to 4 hours in some studies. The recommended and maximum dose of Intermezzo is 1.75 mg for women and 3.5 mg for men, taken only once per night, as needed, if a middle-of-the-night awakening is followed by difficulty returning to sleep. The recommended doses for women and men are different because women clear zolpidem from the body at a lower rate compared with men. The recommended Intermezzo dose for men and women who are taking concomitant central nervous system (CNS) depressants is 1.75 mg. The recommended dose of Intermezzo in men and women over 65 years old and patients with hepatic impairment is 1.75 mg, taken only once per night, if needed. As noted above, the duration of action depends on both dose and half-life. Some patients who are unable to afford Intermezzo take zolpidem immediate release tablets at a reduced does (e.g., 2.5 mg) during the middle of the night, but this is off-label treatment. Benzodiazepine receptor agonists (BZRAs) increase the risk of falls in older adults, and if taken without sufficient time for sleep, BZRA hypnotics can cause significant impairment in the morning.

   Some patients with sleep-onset insomnia also reported a delay in sleep onset with zolpidem. The onset of action is delayed if zolpidem is taken with food. New formulations of zolpidem have been developed to increase the speed of absorption (sublingual zolpidem, Edular 5 mg, 10 mg) and zolpidem spray (Zolpimist 5 mg, 10 mg). However, given the higher dose, these formulations are not recommended for middle-of-the-night use. The clinician should also remember that cognitive and behavioral treatment of insomnia (CBT-I) works for both sleep-maintenance and sleep-onset insomnia. Teaching patients techniques such as stimulus control may help them deal with middle-of-the-night awakenings and avoid medications.

   The current patient took BSLZT 1.75 mg following nocturnal awakenings when she was unable to fall asleep in 15 to 30 minutes. She was instructed to take the medication only if 4 hours of sleep time remained. The patient needed medications only about once a week. The knowledge that a medication was available also made her less anxious about the middle-of-the-night awakening.

TABLE P116-1	**Treatment Alternatives for Middle-of-the-Night Awakening**
Hypnotic Treatment	
Zaleplon (Sonata)*	5–10 mg
Buffered zolpidem sublingual (Intermezzo)	1.75 mg (women, men over age 65, when taken with other sedative mediations) 3.5 mg men
Only Intermezzo is FDA approved for treatment of middle-of-the-night awakening. Middle-of-the-night hypnotic use requires that at least 4 hours of sleep time remains.	

*Not FDA approved for middle-of-the-night dosing, CBT-I (is a non hypnotic treatment for this problem.

2. **Answer:** Trazodone.

Discussion: Doxepin (at 25 mg or higher), amitriptyline, and diphenhydramine all have significant anticholinergic activity and can cause urinary retention, constipation, dry mouth and cognitive dysfunction. These medications should not be used in a patient with urinary retention. Use of zolpidem is relatively contraindicated in a patient with current or prior substance dependence. In patients with drug dependence, BZRAs should be avoided, if possible. Trazodone is a sedating antidepressant with minimal anticholinergic activity and is used in a low does (25–50 mg) as a hypnotic. This is one treatment option for a patient with a drug dependence and urinary retention. Low-dose doxepin (3 mg and 6 mg, Silenor) has been FDA approved for treatment of sleep-maintenance insomnia. In low doses, the medication has minimal anticholinergic activity and thus might be another alternative. The hypnotic effect of doxepin and trazodone is thought to be mediated by their blockade of histamine-1 receptors. This effect is present at low doses, whereas the antidepressant effect requires considerably higher doses. Mirtazapine is another sedating antidepressant that may be used in low doses (7.5 mg) as a hypnotic. The medication also has minimal anticholinergic or sexual side effects but is commonly associated with weight gain. Quetiapine (a sedating atypical antipsychotic) may be used as a hypnotic when benzodiazepines are contraindicated. However, the medication is associated with hyperglycemia and rarely tardive dyskinesia. It is reserved for patients with significant psychiatric illness and prominent insomnia, but could potentially be used in a patient with a history of drug abuse or dependence. Ramelteon (Rozerem) is a melatonin receptor agonist that has been approved for the treatment of sleep-onset insomnia. The drug has no abuse potential but has a short half-life. The medication may also shift the circadian rhythms (see Fundaments 40). If a patient has mainly sleep-onset insomnia, this medication could be considered. Melatonin has been evaluated as a hypnotic at doses varying from 0.3 to 80 mg (most 1 to 5 mg) and meta-analysis has found a small but significant reduction in sleep latency but no effect on other sleep measures. Finally, cognitive behavioral treatment of insomnia (CBT-I) is a drug-free treatment option for insomnia.

CLINICAL PEARLS

1. Pharmacologic treatment of middle-of-the-night awakening and difficulty returning to sleep requires a hypnotic with a rapid onset of action and a short duration of action.
2. Buffered sublingual zolpidem is FDA approved for middle-of-the-night awakening. Another option is zaleplon, a medication with an ultra-short duration of action. However, this medication is not FDA approved for middle-of-the-night awakening
3. Hypnotic medications should not be taken in the middle of the night unless at least 4 hours remain for sleep. Residual impairment of coordination or cognition in the morning may be potentiated by coadministration of other sedative medications. Women, older adults, and patients with hepatic dysfunction are especially at risk given the slower clearance of medications such as zolpidem.
4. Patients with a history of substance or drug dependence or abuse are *not* candidates for treatment with BZRAs because of the potential for these drugs to result in dependence or abuse. Sedating antidepressants are an option.
5. In patient with urinary retention, treatment with sedative antidepressants or antihistamines with anticholinergic activity is relatively contraindicated. Trazodone or low-dose doxepin (3 mg, 6 mg) may be used in this situation, as prominent anticholinergic side effects are not present.

BIBLIOGRAPHY

Brzezinski A, Vangel MG, Wurtman RJ, et al: Effects of exogenous melatonin on sleep. A meta-analysis, *Sleep Med Rev* 9:41–50, 2005.
Buscemi N, Vandermeer B, Hooton N, et al: The efficacy and safety of exogenous melatonin for primary sleep disorders: a metaanalysis, *J Gen Intern Med* 20(12):1151–1158, 2005.
Buysse DJ: Insomnia, *JAMA* 309(7):706–716, 2013.
Greenblatt DJ, Harmatz JS, Roth T, et al: Comparison of pharmacokinetic profiles of zolpidem buffered sublingual tablet and zolpidem oral immediate-release tablet: results from a single-center, single-dose, randomized, open-label crossover study in healthy adults, *Clin Ther* 35(5):604–611, 2013.
Krystal AD, Lankford A, Durrence HH, et al: Efficacy and safety of doxepin 3 and 6 mg in a 35-day sleep laboratory trial in adults with chronic primary insomnia, *Sleep* 34(10):1433–1442, 2011.
Licata SC, Rowlett JK: Abuse and dependence liability of benzodiazepine-type drugs: GABA(A) receptor modulation and beyond, *Pharmacol Biochem Behav* 90(1):74–89, 2008.
Richardson GS, Zee PC, Wang-Weigand S, et al: Circadian phase-shifting effects of repeated ramelteon administration in healthy adults, *J Clin Sleep Med* 4(5):456–461, 2008.

Roth T, Hull SG, Lankford DA, et al: Intermezzo Study Group: Low-dose sublingual zolpidem tartrate is associated with dose-related improvement in sleep onset and duration in insomnia characterized by middle-of-the-night(MOTN) awakenings, *Sleep* 31(9):1277–1284, 2008.

Roth T, Krystal A, Steinberg FJ, et al: Novel sublingual low-dose zolpidem tablet reduces latency to sleep onset following spontaneous middle-of-the-night awakening in insomnia in a randomized, double-blind, placebo-controlled, outpatient study, *Sleep* 36(2):189–196, 2013.

Roth T, Rogowski R, Hull S, et al: Efficacy and safety of doxepin 1 mg, 3 mg, and 6 mg in adults with primary insomnia, *Sleep* 30(11):1555–1561, 2007.

Walsh JK, Erman M, Erwin CW, et al: Subjective hypnotic efficacy of trazodone and zolpidem in DSM-III-R primary insomnia, *Hum Psychopharmacol* 13(3):191–198, 1998.

Zammit GK, Corser B, Doghramji K, et al: Sleep and residual sedation after administration of zaleplon, zolpidem, and placebo during experimental middle-of-the-night awakening, *J Clin Sleep Med* 2(4):417–423, 2006.

FUNDAMENTALS 40

Circadian Rhythm Sleep-Wake Disorders

The word *circadian* means "about a day" and describes processes that vary over time with approximately a 24-hour period. In humans, many physiologic processes vary periodically on a nearly 24-hour schedule.[1,2] The major circadian pacemaker in mammals is the suprachiasmatic nucleus (SCN) in the anterior hypothalamus. The nucleus exists as paired structures on each side of the third ventricle above the optic chiasm.[2-4] The SCN controls the rhythms of core body temperature and sleep–wake propensity as well as the secretion of certain hormones (melatonin and cortisol). The alerting signal from the SCN increases during the day to counter the increasing homeostatic sleep drive (accumulated wakefulness since the last sleep). As the homeostatic sleep drive falls during the night, the alerting signal also decreases to help maintain sleep.

The SCN contains cells that oscillate independently with a period slightly longer than 24 hours. The period of the rhythm is called *tau* and the mean value in humans is about 24.2 hours.[3] For humans to maintain synchrony with the light–dark cycle, external stimuli must induce a slight daily advance (shift in circadian rhythms to an earlier clock time) to counteract the intrinsic tendency for phase delay caused by a period slightly longer than 24 hours. These external stimuli, called *zeitgebers* ("time givers"),

are said to "entrain" the SCN to the light–dark cycle (Box F40-1).

The most potent zeitgeber is light (sunlight). Other zeitgebers include exercise, food, and social activities. The light stimulus reaches the SCN via the retinohypothalamic tract (RHT) (Figure F40-1). The RHT is a monosynaptic pathway connecting the melanopsin-containing photosensitive retinal ganglion cells (pRGCs) to the SCN. The neurotransmitters of the RHT are glutamate and pituitary adenylate cyclase activating polypeptide (PACAP). The shorter wavelengths of light (blue) have the greatest effect on circadian rhythms.

The pineal gland secretes a hormone called *melatonin* during the dark cycle.[4-11] In the *absence of light*, certain dorsal parvocellular neurons in the autonomic subdivision of the paraventricular hypothalamic nucleus (PVH) provide tonic stimulation to the pineal gland via a circuitous pathway that passes through the spinal cord to the superior cervical ganglion and back to the pineal gland (see Figure F40-1). In the presence of light, some neurons of the SCN directly inhibit those neurons in the PVH that are responsible for stimulating the pineal gland to secrete melatonin. Thus, light inhibits melatonin secretion and the absence of inhibition (absence of light) allows secretion of melatonin. The melatonin

---

BOX F40-1 Circadian Physiology—Important Facts

- Circadian ("about a day") denotes processes with approximately a 24-hour (hr) period.
- The human period of circadian rhythms (tau) is about 24.2 hr.
- The suprachiasmatic nucleus (SCN) is the major circadian pacemaker in humans.
- The SCN function helps maintain alertness by producing an alerting signal during the day and maintaining sleep by a reduced signal at night.

- Human alertness:
  - Midday decrease in alertness 2–4 PM.
  - Alertness peaks in the early evening hours.
  - Lowest levels of alertness occur from 4–6 AM.
- Zeitgebers (time givers) entrain the SCN to the physical environment.
- Light (sunlight) is the major zeitgeber.
- Melanopsin-containing retinal ganglion cells are the major circadian photoreceptors and communicate the presence of light to the SCN via the retinohypopthalamic tract (RHT).

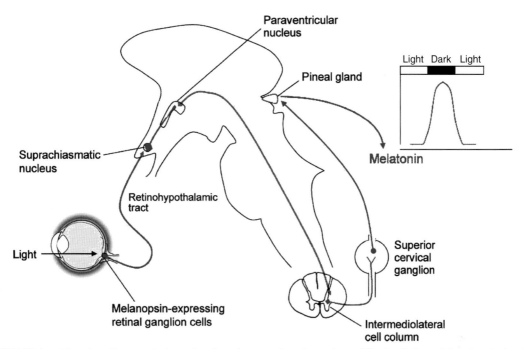

FIGURE F40-1 ■ The circadian regulation of melatonin secretion depends on (1) stimulation of the pineal gland to secrete melatonin by a circuitous pathway beginning in the paraventricular hypothalamic (PVH) nucleus and passing through the intermediolateral cell column of the spinal cord and then the superior cervical ganglion to the pineal gland. Via this pathway PVH neurons stimulate melatonin secretion (2) inhibition of melatonin secretion via light stimulating the photosensitive retinal ganglion cells with information reaching the SCN via the retinohypothalamic tract (RHT). In the presence of light, certain SCN neurons then inhibit neurons in the PVH that stimulate melatonin secretion (in the absence of inhibition). Thus during dark the SCN does not inhibit the PVH nucleus and melatonin is secreted by the pineal gland.

secreted by the pineal gland provides inhibitory feedback information to SCN neurons. Therefore, *the SCN and pineal gland are mutually inhibitory*. The SCN has a high density of two types of melatonin (MT) receptors, MT1 and MT2. *When melatonin binds the MT1 receptor on SCN neurons, it decreases the SCN alerting signal.* When melatonin binds the MT2 receptor, it induces a shift in circadian phase (direction depends on timing). Exogenous melatonin by oral administration may also affect the SCN. The half-life of exogenous melatonin is short (30–45 minutes) unless sustained-release melatonin preparations are used. As might be expected, the effects of exogenous melatonin are largest when no endogenous melatonin is being secreted.[8] Exogenous melatonin may decrease the SCN-alerting signal (hypnotic effects) and cause a phase shift of circadian rhythms (discussed in a later section).

MARKERS OF CIRCADIAN PHASE

The relationship of the internal rhythms to the external environment is the *circadian phase*. The minimum of the core body temperature (CBTmin) and the dim light melatonin onset

---

BOX F40-2 **Markers of Circadian Phase**

- CBTmin occurs 2–3 hours (hr) before awakening from unconstrained sleep (4–5 AM).
- DLMO occurs ~2 hr before habitual sleep onset.
- CBTmin = DLMO + 7 (CBTmin occurs about 7 hours later than DLMO).

CBTmin, Core body temperature minimum; *DLMO*, dim light melatonin onset.

(DLMO) are two useful markers of the position of an individual's circadian rhythms with respect to the external environment (i.e., time of day) (Box F40-2). The CBTmin occurs about 2 to 3 hours before *spontaneous awakening* from nocturnal sleep (4–5 AM in most individuals).[10–12] The reduction in core body temperature during the sleep period corresponds to the elevation in plasma melatonin. The DLMO occurs about 2 hours before habitual sleep onset.[10–17] The *CBTmin* can be estimated as *DLMO + 7 hours*. The DLMO is determined by interval measurement of salivary or plasma melatonin performed in dim light (5 lux; because light inhibits melatonin secretion) in the evening. A rise in melatonin levels detects the DLMO time The *melatonin*

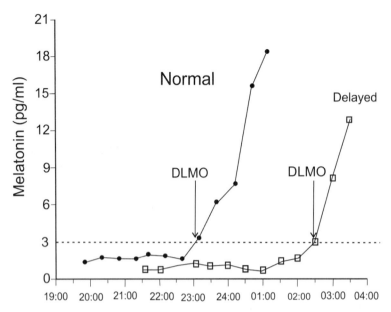

FIGURE F40-2 ■ Salivary melatonin measurements for a normal individual and one with delayed sleep-wake phase disorder (DSWPD). The dim light melatonin onset (DLMO) is taken as the time at which melatonin reaches 3 picograms per milliliter (pg/mL). This occurs around 23:00 in the normal individual but is delayed to around 02:30 in the morning in an individual with the DSWPD. (From Wyatt JK, Stepanski EJ, Kirkby J: Circadian phase in delayed sleep phase syndrome: predictors and temporal stability across multiple assessments, *Sleep* 29:1075-1080, 2006.)

midpoint may also be used as a circadian maker and occurs about 2 hours before CBTmin. When the circadian rhythm of the body (CBTmin or DLMO) moves to a later clock time, this is said to represent a *phase delay* in circadian rhythms and to an earlier clock time *phase advance*. The relationship between the timing of sleep and the circadian phase (as estimated by a circadian marker) may be quantified by the time interval (phase angle) between the two rhythms.

Use of the core body temperature as a marker of circadian rhythms is complicated by the fact that eating, activity, and sleep may affect the timing of CBTmin. Clinically, the most accurate way to determine the circadian phase is by monitoring melatonin in a dark environment to detect the DLMO. Plasma melatonin (threshold >10 picogram per milliliter [pg/mL]), salivary melatonin (>3 pg/mL), or urinary melatonin metabolite (6-sulfatoxymelatonin [aMT6s]) can be monitored. Figure F40-2 shows a DLMO onset in a normal individual and another with a delayed phase.

SHIFTING THE CIRCADIAN RHYTHMS

Phase Shifting by Light

Exposure to light *before* the CBTmin causes a phase delay and light exposure *after* the CBTmin causes a phase advance (Figure F40-3) in circadian rhythm.[15-19] Thus, normal light exposure during the early morning induces a daily phase advance in the circadian rhythms to compensate for the intrinsic tendency to phase delay because tau is

slightly longer than 24 hours. The amount of circadian rhythm shifting depends on the timing of light as well as the intensity and duration of light. Important facts concerning the phase shifting effects of light are presented in Box F40-3. For humans exposed to outside light daily (>10,000 lux) for a portion of each day, a relatively high light intensity is needed to shift circadian rhythms. Outside daylight is much more effective at shifting the circadian phase than indoor light. When outdoor light exposure is not practical or possible, light boxes are available (2500 lux) for therapeutic phase shifting by light. Natural light is composed of a spectrum from 380 nanometers (nm) (violet) to 760 (red). Blue light (460 nm) has greater phase shifting properties than the rest of the visible light spectrum.[20,21]

Phase-Response Curve for Light

The relationship between the timing of light exposure and the *amount of phase shift* is best presented using a phase response curve (PRC) (Figure F40-4). The curves are constructed by plotting the amount of phase shift versus the timing of the light stimulus (constant stimulus intensity).[15] By convention, the positive vertical axis represents phase advances (earlier clock time) and the negative axis phase delays (later clock time). The *magnitude* of phase shifting by light depends on the *proximity of the light stimulus to the CBTmin*. The closer the light stimulus is to the CBTmin, the larger is the phase shifting effect. Light in the middle of the day has minimal phase shifting effects. Figure F40-4 is a schematic of a PRC for light. The largest

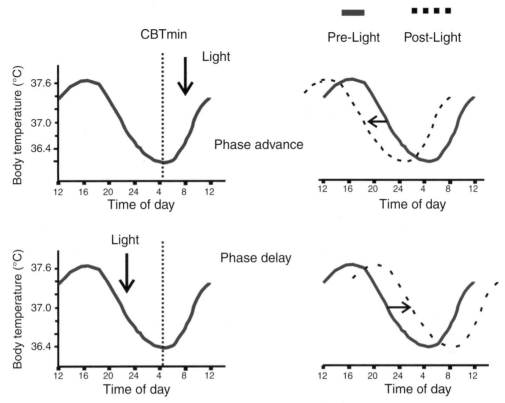

FIGURE F40-3 ■ Phase shifting of the core body temperature minimum (CBTmin) with light. Light after the CBTmin phase advances and light before CBTmin phase delays. (From Berry RB: *Sleep medicine pearls*, ed 2, Philadelphia, 2003, Hanley & Belfus, p 344.)

BOX F40-3 Phase Shifting with Light

COMMON LIGHT EXPOSURES

- Bright blue midday sky >100,000 lux
- Sunrise or sunset ~10,000 lux
- Commercial light boxes up to 10,000 lux
- Normal room light ~200 lux
- Moonlight 0.1 lux

PHASE SHIFTING WITH LIGHT

- Short wavelength light (blue ~460 nanometers [nm])—greatest effect

- Amount of phase shift depends on timing, intensity, and duration of light exposure
- Short pulses of light (intermittent) can also shift circadian rhythms
- Phase advance—light after CBTmin (about 3 hours after CBTmin greatest effect)
- Phase delay—light before CBTmin (about 3 hours before CBTmin greatest effect)
- Light in the middle of the day—relatively little effect

CBTmin, Core body temperature minimum.

---

phase advance is about 3 hours after CBTmin. Recall that CBTmin is about 2 to 3 before natural awakening. Therefore, light would have the greatest phase advance properties shortly after spontaneous awakening (ad lib sleep).

Phase Shifting by Exogenous Melatonin

Relatively small doses of exogenous melatonin (0.3–0.5 milligram [mg]) may shift the circadian phase if taken at the correct time (Table F40-1). As might be expected, the phase shifting effects of exogenous melatonin are minimal during the dark period when the endogenous plasma level of melatonin is high.[22–26] Melatonin in higher doses (3–5 mg) has a direct hypnotic effect[8] as well as a chronobiotic effect. However, the hypnotic effects of melatonin are limited by the drug's short half-life and the fact that if taken at night, the endogenous plasma melatonin is already high.

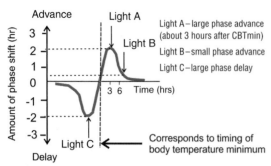

Schematic phase response curve to light

FIGURE F40-4 ■ Schematic of the phase response curve (PRC) for light. The direction of the phase change depends on whether light is applied before or after core body temperature minimum (CBTmin). The maximum phase advance (Light A) occurs about 3 to 4 hours after CBTmin. If light is applied 7 to 8 hours after CBTmin (Light B), the phase advance is much smaller. The maximum phase delay occurs 3 to 4 hours before the CBTmin. At midday to early evening, the effect of light on the circadian phase is insignificant. (From Berry RB: *Fundamentals of sleep medicine*, Philadelphia, 2012, Saunders, p 522.)

TABLE F40-1	**Phase Shifting with Melatonin**

- PRC approximately opposite to light PRC (12 hours [hr] out of phase).
- Reversal point (phase advance to phase delay) may be slightly before minimum of core body temperature but is always considerably after the DLMO.
- Dose-response curves may vary with dose (0.3 milligrams [mg] versus 3 mg).
- Note at larger doses, hypnotic effects are noted. Given closer to bedtime, melatonin may reduce SCN alerting signal (dampen wake maintenance zone).
- Exogenous melatonin half-life is about 30 to 45 minutes.
- Maximal phase *advance* for different melatonin doses (optimal timing).*

Dose	0.3–0.5 mg	3 mg
Before DLMO	2–3 hr	5 hr
Before habitual sleep onset	4.5–5 hr	7.5 hr
Before CBTmin	9 hr	12 hr

- Maximal phase delay—about 10 hours after DLMO

CBTmin, Core body temperature minimum; *DLMO*, dim light melatonin onset; *PRC*, phase response curve; *SCN*, suprachiasmatic nucleus.
*From Eastman CI, Burgess HJ: How to travel the world without jet lag, *Sleep Med Clin* 4:241-255, 2009.

The PRC curve for melatonin is roughly 12 hours opposite (out of phase) to the light PRC.[22,25,26] In displays of the melatonin PRC, the timing of melatonin is often expressed in relation to DLMO but may also be expressed in relation to the estimated CBTmin. Melatonin

when given in the early evening before the DLMO results in a phase advance. Melatonin given at the end of the subjective night–early subjective day causes a phase delay. As expected, the melatonin PRC has flat region (no phase shifting) between the DLMO and the CBTmin (endogenous melatonin already high). The cross-over point for melatonin (transition from phase advance to phase delay) is during the night but may not precisely coincide with CBTmin. In addition, the shape of the melatonin PRC appears to depend on the dose of melatonin studied and the method of determination of the PRC (see Figure F40-5). Note that the timing of the maximum phase delay induced by melatonin is several hours after the CBTmin. *Thus, taking melatonin 1 or 2 hours after spontaneous awakening causes the most phase delay.* However, melatonin administration is often not used in the early morning because any hypnotic effects would not be well tolerated outside of a research setting. An exception is when morning sleep is desired by a person working a night shift. Side effects of melatonin include headache, dizziness, nausea, and drowsiness. At high doses, melatonin may alter the sex hormones. For this reason, some clinicians are hesitant to use the medication long term in adolescents or children.

Summary of Effects of Light and Melatonin

The effects of bright light and melatonin are summarized in Figure F40-6 with illustrations of the use of these interventions in two circadian rhythm sleep–wake sleep disorders (CRSWDs). Bright light in the evening causes a phase delay and in the early morning a phase advance. Melatonin in the early evening causes a phase advance and in the early morning a phase delay. A simple description of the effects of light and melatonin is that *bright light pushes and melatonin pulls the circadian rhythms.* In this figure, it is assumed that the CBTmin lies within the initial sleep period in patients with advanced sleep–wake phase disorder (ASWPD) and delayed sleep–wake phase disorder (DSWPD).

Circadian Rhythm Sleep-Wake Disorders (CRSWD)

The International Classification of Sleep Disorders, Third Edition (ICSD-3),[1] lists general criteria for a CRSWD. The following must be present:

    A. A chronic or recurrent pattern of *sleep–wake disruption* due primarily to an *alteration of the circadian timing system or a misalignment*

Human Phase Response Curves to Different Doses of Melatonin

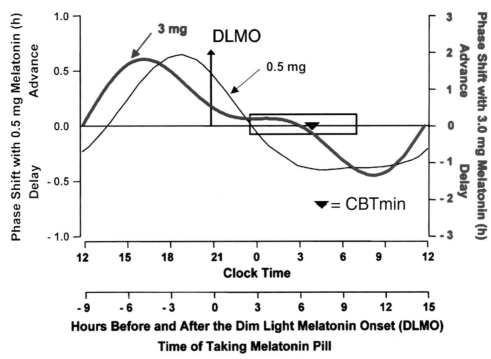

FIGURE F40-5 ■ Phase response curves (PRCs) for different doses of exogenous melatonin. Note that for the higher dose of melatonin, the maximal effect was noted at an earlier time than for a lower dose of melatonin (referenced to the dim light melatonin (DLMO) time). The rectangle illustrates a typical sleep period with core body temperature minimum (CBTmin) shown in the last half of the sleep period as an inverted triangle. (From Eastman CI, Burgess HJ: How to travel the world without jet lag, *Sleep Med Clin* 4:241-255, 2009.)

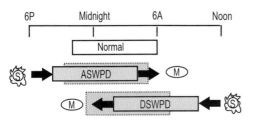

Light "pushes"   Melatonin "pulls"

FIGURE F40-6 ■ Summary of effect of light and melatonin on the circadian phase. In patients with the advanced sleep-wake phase disorder (ASWPD), melatonin in the late-night or early-morning phase delays and in patients with the delayed sleep-wake phase disorder (DSWPD), melatonin in the early-evening phase advances. For light, the effects are opposite with early-evening light phase delaying and early-morning light phase advancing the *CBTmin*, Core body temperature minimum. (Adapted from Barion A, Zee PC: A clinical approach to circadian rhythm sleep disorders, *Sleep Med* 8:566-577, 2007.)

between *internal circadian rhythm* and the *sleep–wake schedule* required by the physical environment or work schedule.
B. The circadian rhythm disruption leads to *excessive sleepiness, insomnia symptoms*, or both.

BOX F40-4   Circadian Rhythm Sleep–Wake Disorders

Delayed sleep–wake phase disorder (DSWPD)
Advanced sleep–wake phase disorder (ASWPD)
Non–24-hour sleep–wake rhythm disorder (Non24 SWRD)
Irregular sleep–wake rhythm disorder (IRSWRD)
Jet lag disorder
Shift work disorder (SWD)
Circadian rhythm sleep–wake disorder not otherwise specified

C. The sleep–wake cycle disturbances cause significant distress or impairment.
D. Sleep diary and actigraphy monitoring (the latter, if feasible) for at least 7 days (preferably 14 days) demonstrates disruption of the circadian sleep–wake cycle.

The CRSWDs are listed in Box F40-4 and summarized in Figure F40-7. The American Academy of Sleep Medicine (AASM) has published an evidence review[25,26] and practice parameters[27] for the evaluation of these disorders.

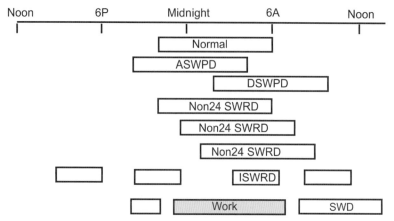

FIGURE F40-7 ■ Circadian rhythm sleep wake disorders shown schematically with the relationship to a normal sleep period (*rectangle*). *ASWPD*, Advanced sleep–wake phase disorder; *DSWPD*, delayed sleep–wake phase disorder; *ISWRD*, irregular sleep–wake rhythm disorder; *Non24 SWRD*, non–24-hour sleep–wake rhythm disorder; *SWD*, shift work disorder. Adapted from Lu BS, Zee PC: Circadian rhythm sleep disorders, *Chest* 130:1915–1923, 2006; and Barion A, Zee PC: A clinical approach to circadian rhythm sleep disorders, *Sleep* Med 8:566–577, 2007.

Evaluation of a patient for a suspected CRSWD includes history, sleep log (diary), actigraphy (at least 7 days; preferably 14 days), the Morning-Evening Questionnaire (MEQ), and circadian markers (DLMO).[27–29] In the ICSD-3, use of actigraphy for at least 14 days is recommended to be able to discern a pattern of non–24-hour SWRD. The MEQ was developed by Horne and Ostberg in 1976.[28] The MEQ contains 19 questions aimed at determining the natural propensity to perform certain activities during the daily temporal span. Most questions are framed in a preferential manner and require a response to specific times that individuals would prefer to do certain activities (as opposed to when they actually do them). Each question has answers 0 to 6. The sum ranges from 16 to 86. Lower values correspond to evening types. Patients with a delayed sleep period are usually evening types.

Sleep Logs and Actigraphy

The AASM practice parameters state that these are indicated for evaluation of patients with suspected or known CRSWD.[27] In Figure F40-7, a schematic of the changes in the sleep period with the different CRSWDs compared with normal is shown. In general, sleep logs or actigraphy documents a habitual sleep period compared with normal that is advanced (ASWPD), delayed (DSWPD) (Figure F40-8), progressively delayed (non–24-hour SWRD), irregular (irregular sleep–wake rhythm [ISWR]), or with a daytime major sleep episode (shift-work disorder).

Figure F40-8 shows an actigraphy recording of a patient with the delayed sleep–wake phase disorder. The actigraphy tracing shows a stable delay sleep onset. The patient gets up early on the weekdays (societal obligations) but sleeps late on the weekends.

CLINICAL PEARLS

1. In humans, the normal circadian period (tau) is *approximately 24.2 hours* (mean value). As the period is slightly longer than 24 hours, a slight phase advance is required daily to maintain entrainment with the light–dark cycle.

2. The major circadian pacemaker in humans is the SCN. The SCN is entrained to the light–dark cycle via light stimulation of melanopsin containing photosensitive retinal ganglion cells (pRGCs). The ganglion cells communicate via the RHT to the SCN. Blue light has the most potent effect.

3. The alerting signal from the SCN increases during the day to counter the increasing homeostatic sleep drive (accumulated wakefulness since the last sleep). The alerting signal falls during sleep, and the homeostatic sleep drive also falls.

4. Melatonin is secreted in darkness by the pineal gland. Light inhibits melatonin secretion by decreasing the activating influences of neurons in the hypothalamic PVH nucleus. The neural pathway from the PVH neurons to the pineal gland is circuitous passing through the spinal cord and superior cervical ganglion. *Melatonin is secreted in darkness and binds to receptors on the SCN decreasing the alerting signal during darkness (promoting sleep).*

5. The CBTmin occurs approximately 2 to 3 hours before the habitual wake time (natural, ad lib sleep).

6. The DLMO occurs about 2 hours before habitual sleep onset or about 7 hours before CBTmin (timing of CBTmin = DLMO + 7 hours).

7. CBTmin and DLMO may be used as markers of circadian phase. When the circadian rhythm of the body (CBTmin or DLMO) moves to a later clock time, this is said to represent a *phase delay* in circadian rhythms and to an early time *phase advance*.

8. Light *after* the CBTmin induces a phase advance and light *before* the CBTmin induces a phase delay.

9. Melatonin administered *before* the CBTmin induces a phase advance. Melatonin given *after* the CBT induces a phase delay.

10. Bright light "pushes" and melatonin "pulls" on the circadian phase (CBTmin, DLMO).

11. Sleep logs and actigraphy (for at least 7 days and preferably 14 days), circadian markers of phase (DLMO) are used to evaluate patients for circadian sleep–wake rhythm disorders. To evaluate a patient for the non24 SWRD actigraphy for a minimum of 14 days is recommended.

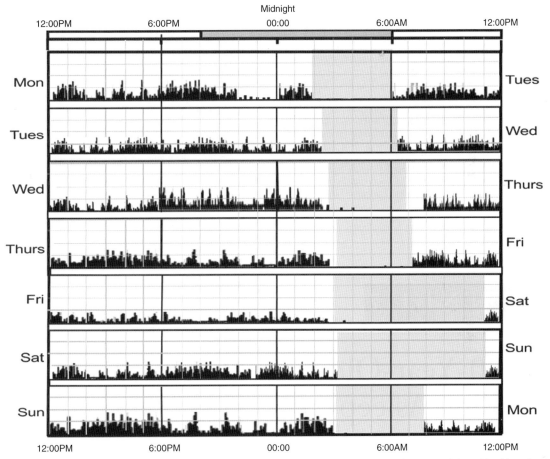

FIGURE F40-8 ■ Actigraphy of a patient with the delayed sleep wake phase disorder. Showing delayed bedtime (stable). The sleep onset time is usually 2 to 3 AM. The patient slept in on the weekend. Once asleep, the patient did not experience any awakenings.

REFERENCES

1. American Academy of Sleep Medicine: *International classification of sleep disorders*, ed 3, Darien, IL, 2014, American Academy of Sleep Medicine.
2. Zee PC, Manthena P: The brain's master circadian clock: implications and opportunities for therapy of sleep disorders, *Sleep Med Rev* 11:59–70, 2007.
3. Czeisler CA, Duffy JF, Shanahan TL, et al.: Stability, precision, and nearly 24 hour period of the human circadian pacemaker, *Sleep* 284:2177–2181, 1999.
4. Gooley JJ, Saper CB: Anatomy of the mammalian circadian system. In Kryger MH, Roth T, Dement WC, editors: *Principles and practice of sleep medicine*, 4th ed., Philadelphia, 2005, Saunders, pp 335–350.
5. Dijk DJ, Archer SN: Light, sleep, and circadian rhythms: together again, *PLoS* 7:3000145, 2009.
6. Benarroch EE: Suprachiasmatic nucleus and melatonin: reciprocal interactions and clinical correlations, *Neurology* 71(8):594–598, 2008.
7. Reid KJ, Zee PC: Circadian rhythm disorders, *Semin Neurol* 29:393–405, 2009.
8. Wyatt JK, Dijk D, Ritz-De Cecco A, et al: Sleep-facilitating effect of exogenous melatonin in healthy young men and women is circadian-phase dependent, *Sleep* 29:609–618, 2006.
9. Edgar DM, Dement WC, Fuller CA: Effect of SCN lesions on sleep in the squirrel monkey: evidence for opponent processes in sleep-wake regulation, *J Neurosci* 13:1065–1079, 1993.
10. Duffy JF, Dijk DJ, Klerman EB, Czeisler CA: Later endogenous circadian temperature nadir relative to an

earlier wake time in older people, *Am J Physiol* 275: R1478–R1487, 1998.

11. Fahey CD, Zee PC: Circadian rhythm sleep disorder and phototherapy, *Psychiatr Clin North Am* 29:989–1007, 2006.

12. Czeisler CA, Buxton OM, Khalsa SBS: The human circadian timing system and sleep-wake regulation. In Kryger MH, Roth T, Dement WC, editors: *Principles and practice of sleep medicine*, 4th ed, Philadelphia, 2005, Saunders, pp 375–394.

13. Wyatt JK, Stepanski EJ, Kirkby J: Circadian phase in delayed sleep phase syndrome: predictors and temporal stability across multiple assessments, *Sleep* 29:1075–1080, 2006.

14. Sack RK, Brandes RW, Kendall AR, Lewy AJ: Entrainment of free-running circadian rhythms by -melatonin in blind people, *N Engl J Med* 343:1070–1077, 2000.

15. Khalsa SBS, Jewett ME, Cajocen C, Czeisler CA: A phase response curve to single bright light pulses in human subjects, *J Physiol* 549:945–952, 2003.

16. Lu BS, Zee PC: Circadian rhythm sleep disorders, *Chest* 130:1915–1923, 2006.

17. Barion A, Zee PC: A clinical approach to circadian rhythm sleep disorders, *Sleep Med* 8:566–577, 2007.

18. Shirani A, St. Louis EK: Illuminating rationale and uses for light therapy, *J Clin Sleep Med* 5:155–163, 2009.

19. Zeitzer JM, Dijk DJ, Kronauer RE, et al: Sensitivity of human circadian pacemaker to nocturnal light: melatonin resetting and suppression, *J Physiol* 526:695–702, 2000.

20. Lockley SW, Brainard GC, Czeisler CA: High sensitivity of the human circadian melatonin rhythm to resetting by short wave length light, *J Clin Endocrinol Metab* 88:4502–4505, 2003.

21. Smith MR, Eastman CR: Phase delaying the human circadian clock with blue-enriched polychromatic light, *Chronobiol Int* 26:709–725, 2009.

22. Eastman CI, Burgess HJ: How to travel the world without jet lag, *Sleep Med Clin* 4:241–255, 2009.

23. Sack RL, Auckley D, Auger R, et al: Circadian rhythm sleep disorders: part I, basic principles, shift work and jet lag disorders, *Sleep* 30:1460–1483, 2007.

24. Sack RL, Auckley D, Auger R, et al: Circadian rhythm sleep disorders: part II, advanced sleep phase disorder, delayed sleep phase disorder, free-running disorder, and irregular sleep-wake rhythm, *Sleep* 30:1484–1501, 2007.

25. Lewy AJ, Bauer VK, Ahmed S, et al: The human phase response curve (PRC) to melatonin is about 12 hours out of phase with the PRC to light, *Chronobiol Int* 15:71–83, 1998.

26. Burgess HJ, Revell VL, Eastman CI: A three pulse phase response curve to 3 milligrams of melatonin in humans, *J Physiol* 586:639–647, 2008.

27. Morgenthaler TI, Lee-Chiong T, Alessi C, et al: Practice parameters for the clinical 27valuation and treatment of circadian rhythm sleep disorders, *Sleep* 30:1445–1459, 2007.

28. Horne JA, Ostberg O: A self-assessment questionnaire to determine morningness–eveningness in human circadian rhythms, *Int J Chronobiol* 4:97–110, 1976.

29. Wyatt JK: Delayed sleep phase syndrome: pathophysiology and treatment options, *Sleep* 27, 2004.

PATIENT 117

A 20-Year-Old with Difficulty Falling Asleep

A 20-year-old woman complains of difficulty falling asleep and inability to wake up for her classes in the morning. This problem has been present for at least 2 years. On school days, she gets in bed at 11 PM (in an attempt to get enough sleep) but does not fall asleep until 2 or 3 AM. She is awakened by an alarm clock at 6:30 AM to try to make it to an 8 AM class. Thus, she obtains only 4 to 5 hours of sleep per night during the school week and feels tired and sleepy throughout the day. She often drinks up to six cups of coffee to try to stay alert. On weekends, she usually sleeps until 10 to 11 AM and awakens feeling refreshed. Of note, once asleep, the patient reports having either a single or no awakening. Because she rarely feels sleepy at 11 PM, she sometimes takes either a drink of ethanol or an over-the-counter sleep-aid medication, both of which are only moderately successful at inducing sleep. She tried taking melatonin at 11:00 PM, but this did not help. Sleeping pills leave her feeling groggy in the morning.

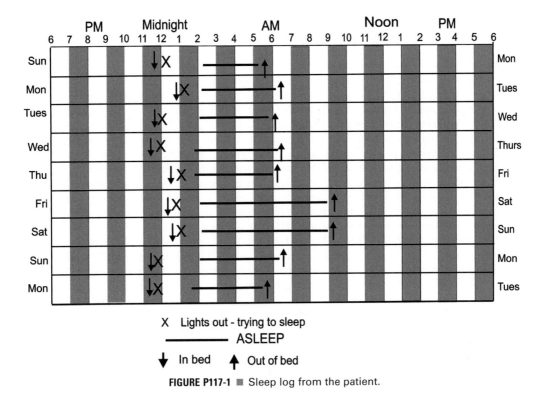

FIGURE P117-1 ■ Sleep log from the patient.

The physical examination is normal. Her sleep log (diary) is shown in Figure P117-1.

QUESTION

1. What is your diagnosis? If you were to use light therapy, would you apply this treatment at 10 PM, 5 AM, or 10 AM?

ANSWER

1. **Answer:** Delayed sleep–wake phase disorder (DSWPD; also known as the delayed sleep phase syndrome). Of the three choices, application of light at 10 AM is recommended.

   Discussion The DSWPD is classified as a circadian rhythm sleep–wake disorder (Box P117-1). In DSWPD, the timing of sleep onset is delayed relative to clock time (usually by 2 hours or more).

BOX P117-1	**Delayed Sleep–Wake Phase Disorder—ICSD-3 Diagnostic Criteria**

Criteria A-E must be met
A. There is a significant delay in the phase of the major sleep episode in relation to the desired or required sleep time and wake-up time, as evidenced by a chronic or recurrent complaint by the patient or a caregiver of inability to fall asleep and difficulty awakening at a desired or required clock time.
B. The symptoms are present for at least 3 months.
C. When patients are allowed to choose their ad libitum schedule, they will exhibit improved sleep

quality and duration for age and maintain a delayed phase of the 24-hour sleep-wake pattern.
D. Sleep log and, whenever possible, actigraphy monitoring for at least 7 days (preferably 14 days) demonstrate a delay in the timing of the habitual sleep period. Both work/school days and free days must be included within this monitoring.
E. The sleep disturbance is not better explained by another current sleep disorder, medical or neurologic disorder, mental disorder, medication use, or substance use disorder.

ICSD-3, International Classification of Sleep Disorders, Third Edition.

Attempts to initiate sleep by getting into bed at the desired sleep-onset time based on societal demands are unsuccessful at inducing sleep. Sleep-onset time tends to be regular, but delayed (2–6 AM). Usually, the patient has no problem maintaining sleep, and when sleep is undisturbed, the sleep period is of normal length. However, waking at a typical clock time (6 AM to 7 AM) to fulfill social, school, or work obligations results in a short duration of sleep.

The duration of DSWPD varies from months to decades. Adolescence is the most common age of onset; onset after age 30 is rare. True DSWPD must be differentiated from sleep-onset insomnia in individuals who delay sleep for social reasons and then experience difficulty falling asleep when they sporadically try to go to bed earlier. These individuals have a transient sleep–wake cycle disorder caused by a self-enforced phase shift. When they maintain a regular bedtime and wake time for several days, they quickly adjust to this schedule. Patients with bipolar affective disorder in the manic or hypomanic phase also may have sleep-onset insomnia. The sleep period is short in these patients, but they have no difficulty arising at a conventional time. The non–24-hour sleep–wake syndrome is characterized by a progressive, incremental phase delay in sleep onset and wake times. In the future, measurement of dim light melatonin onset (DLMO) will be more widely available and allow greater precision in diagnosis of DSWPD (see Figure F40-2 in Fundamentals 40). Salivary melatonin samples are obtained at intervals in dim light and processed later. The rise in melatonin is a circadian phase marker and is typically 2 to 3 hours before habitual bedtime (and 1-2 hours before habitual sleep time). In DSWPD, DLMO is delayed, instead of occurring at 10 PM, it often occurs at 1 AM to 2 AM or later. In some studies using DLMO, a number of individuals thought to have a delayed circadian phase did NOT have a delay in DLMO (behaviorally-induced delayed sleep period).

Treatment of the DSWPD is often difficult. Although hypnotics may be temporarily successful at inducing sleep at normal clock times, daytime grogginess typically results. Chronotherapy is one treatment option. This therapy is based on the fact that phase delay (delay the time of sleep onset) is easier than phase advance. Bedtime is progressively delayed by several hours on successive days. The sleep period is allowed to run its course with later and later wake times. Thus, the sleep period moves around the clock until sleep onset occurs at normal societal times. However, this therapy requires that the patient be free from societal constraints (e.g., job, child care) for the duration of the treatment, and the bedroom must be dark and quiet. Obviously, many patients are unable to commit to chronotherapy.

The application of bright light has been shown to shift the phase of the internal clock if applied at appropriate times. Therapy with bright light *following the temperature minimum will achieve phase advance in patients.* However, the timing of light exposure is critical. If light is applied before the temperature minimum, further phase delay will occur. It is often difficult to determine the timing of the patient's core body temperature minimum. This usually occurs at 2 to 3 hours before the unrestricted (unconstrained) wake time. That is, the wake time used to estimate the time of the minimum of core body temperature (CBTmin) should be the natural spontaneous wake time. It is best to estimate the habitual wake time (and CBTmin) using ad lib sleep on weekends (or holidays). If light is applied at 6 or 7 AM and the unrestricted wake time is 11 AM (estimated time of CBTmin at 9 AM), light may actually worsen the phase delay as light is applied before the time of the CBTmin. Patients should wear dark googles if they go outside before their estimated CBTmin (to avoid further phase delay). Starting treatment on the weekends may allow appropriate light exposure at a later clock time than permitted during the school or work week. Once, light treatment begins, the patient attempts to go to bed about half to 1 hour earlier each night. A typical schedule is listed in Box P117-2. The goal is to advance the bedtime by half hour per day. The most appropriate dose of light is not known. The suggested dose is either outdoor light or bright indoor artificial light of >2500 lux for 30 minutes to 2 hours. Commercial light boxes are available at many discount department stores for around $100.

Appropriately timed melatonin may also help with phase advance in patients. Melatonin must be applied *before* CBTmin. Various doses and timing of melatonin have also been used to treat the DSWPD. The goal is to give melatonin before DLMO to achieve phase advance. Mundey and colleagues used a dosage of 0.3 *and* 3 milligrams (mg) of melatonin and found the magnitude of phase advance correlated with the time of administration. A reasonable approach is to administer *0.3 to 5 mg of melatonin 2 to 3 hours before DLMO or 5 to 7 hours before habitual sleep time (DLMO occurs about 2 hours before habitual sleep time).* Small doses of melatonin (0.3 and 0.5 mg) have phase shifting effects but less hypnotic effect. The small doses may minimize hypnotic effects if sleepiness at the time of administration is not desirable. Larger doses of melatonin (1 mg and higher) are more likely to also have a hypnotic effect in addition to the phase shifting effect.

In the current case, the sleep diary shows that the patient had mainly sleep-onset insomnia (long sleep latency) with a stable but delayed sleep-onset time. Once asleep, the patient had little difficulty

BOX P117-2	Treatment for Delayed Sleep-Wake Phase Disorder
Chronotherapy	Progressive phase delay
Light therapy	2500–10,000 lux 30 minutes to 2 hours Timing—at or slightly after habitual wake time (ad lib sleep). Light should be applied following the time of the minimum core body temperature (CBTmin), which occurs about 2 to 3 hours before the habitual spontaneous (ad lib) wake time. Light is administered ½–1 hour earlier each day (use alarm if needed). Patient also goes to bed ½ to 1 hour earlier (see Table P117-1). Restrict light in the evening or in the morning before estimated CBTmin.
Melatonin	0.3–3.0 milligrams (mg) given 5–7 hours before habitual sleep-onset time 3–5 hours before DLMO Large melatonin dose has hypnotic effects

TABLE P117-1   Schedule for Phase Advance (Assuming CBTmin 8 to 9 AM)

Day	Bedtime (Sleep Time)	Wake Time–Start Light	End Light
Day 1	2:00 AM	9:00 AM	10:00 AM
Day 2	1:30 AM	8:30 AM	9:30 AM
Day 3	1:00 AM	8:00 AM	9:00 AM
Day 4	12:30 AM	7:30 AM	8:30 AM
Day 5	12:00 AM	7:00 AM	8:00 AM
Day 6	11:30 PM	6:30 AM	7:30 AM
Day 7 (Goal)	11:00 PM	6:00 AM	7:00 AM
Day 8 Maintenance	11:00 PM	6:30 AM	7:00 AM
Day 9 Maintenance	11:00 PM	6:00 AM	7:00 AM
Day 10 Maintenance	11:00 PM	6:00 AM	7:00 AM

Adapted from Wyatt JA: Circadian rhythm sleep disorders in adolescents and children, *Sleep Med Clin* 2:387-396, 2007.

maintaining sleep. Because of societal constraints, the wake time was set at 6 AM. Thus, during school days, a very short total sleep time, as well as symptoms of daytime sleepiness, was present. When unrestrained, the patient went to sleep at 11 AM. Using the ad lib wakeup time of 9 AM on the weekend the CBTmin could be estimated to occur around 6 AM to 7AM. Thus, administering bright light at 10 AM is the most appropriate answer to the question. A slightly earlier time of 9 AM could also be used. If light is administered at 6 AM there is a risk of being on the wrong side of the CBTmin. The patient was asked to wear dark glasses in the morning on school days if it was safe to do so (she took a bus to school) to avoid light earlier than her CBTmin. She also took 0.3 mg of melatonin about 5 hours before her actual sleep-onset time. The patient's habitual sleep time was around 2 AM and the patient took melatonin at 8 to 9 PM. On this treatment, a progressive advance in bedtime was noted, and the timing of light and melatonin were advanced about half hour per day (Table P117-1). Once sleep onset had reached a desired clock time, the patient continued maintenance light 3 days a week. She could usually fall asleep between 11 and 11:30 PM.

CLINICAL PEARLS

1. The delayed sleep–wake phase disorder (delayed sleep phase disorder) should be considered when a patient complains of primarily sleep-onset insomnia.

2. The DSWPD is the most common circadian rhythm disorder seen in sleep clinics. The onset is in adolescence or the early 20s.

3. Sleep log and actigraphy document a stable delayed sleep-onset time. Wake time may vary, depending on societal obligations.

4. Bright light at or soon after the spontaneous wake time may help with phase advance in patients. Care must be taken not to apply light on the wrong side of the CBTmin.

5. Melatonin given 5 to 7 hours before the habitual sleep-onset time (not taken at bedtime) may help with phase advance in patients.

BIBLIOGRAPHY

American Academy of Sleep Medicine: *International classification of sleep disorders*, ed 3, Darien, IL, 2014, American Academy of Sleep Medicine.

Barion A, Zee PC: A clinical approach to circadian rhythm sleep disorders, *Sleep Med* 8:566–577, 2007.

Bjorvatn B, Pallesen S: A practical approach to circadian rhythm sleep disorders, *Sleep Med Rev* 13:47–60, 2009.

Czeisler CA, Richardson GS, Coleman RM, et al: Chronotherapy: resetting the circadian clocks of patients with delayed sleep phase insomnia, *Sleep* 4:1–21, 1981.

Mundey K, Benloucif S, Harsanyi K, et al: Phase-dependent treatment of delayed sleep phase syndrome with melatonin, *Sleep* 28 (10):1271–1278, 2005.

Nagtegall JE, Kerkhof A, Smits MG, et al: Delayed sleep phase syndrome: a placebo controlled cross-over study on the effects of melatonin administered five hour before the individual dim light melatonin onset, *J Sleep Res* 7:135–143, 1998.

Paul MA, Gray GW, Lieberman HR, et al: Phase advance with separate and combined melatonin and light treatment, *Psychopharmacology (Berl)* 214(2):515–523, 2011.

Rosenthal NE, Joseph-Vanderpool JR, Levendosky AA, et al: Phase-shifting effects of bright morning light as treatment for delayed sleep phase syndrome, *Sleep* 13:354–361, 1990.

Watanabe T, Kajimura N, Kato M, et al: Effects of phototherapy in patients with delayed sleep phase syndrome, *Psychiatry Clin Neurosci* 53:231–233, 1999.

Wyatt JA: Circadian rhythm sleep disorders in adolescents and children, *Sleep Med Clin* 2:387–396, 2007.

PATIENT 118

A 60-Year-Old Man with Early-Morning Awakening

A 60-year-old man recently retired from his job that required him to get up very early in the morning. He had little success trying to adapt to the schedule followed by his wife who went to bed around 11 PM and woke up at 6:30 AM. In the evenings, it was difficult for him to stay awake past 8 PM, and he awoke reliably every morning between 4 and 5 AM. This caused him distress. He denied symptoms of depression or snoring. His sleep log is shown in Figure P118-1.

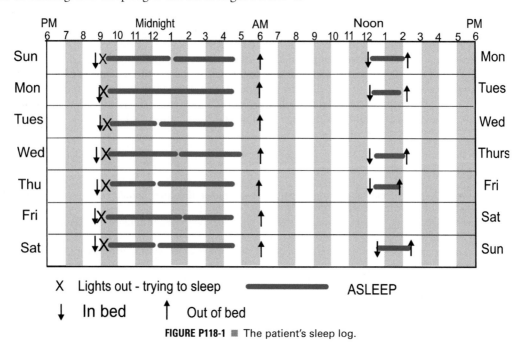

FIGURE P118-1 ■ The patient's sleep log.

QUESTION

1. What is your diagnosis?

ANSWER

1. **Answer:** Advanced sleep–wake phase disorder (ASWPD).

Discussion: ASWPD is thought to be uncommon if diagnostic criteria are strictly followed. Early morning awakening is a typical complaint. Often, patients are able to stay awake in the evening but are unable to stay asleep. As a consequence, classic ASWPD (inability to stay awake in the evening and stay asleep in the early morning) is less common than the complaint of early morning awakening. It may also be difficult to obtain a history of early onset of sleep as some patients consider the time of falling asleep outside the bedroom (e.g., falling asleep for an hour in the living room) as not counting as the start of sleep.

ASWPD is associated with aging, and non–aging-related ASWPD is rare. Early morning awakening may also be noted in depression. The prevalence of ASWPD is not well documented but is believed to be about 1% in the middle-aged population and increases with age. Men and women are equally affected.

Familial ASWPD has been described, with a mutation in the circadian clock gene *hPer2*. However, other familial cases do not show this pattern. Causes of ASWPD include a short endogenous circadian period or a dominant phase advance region to light. In older adults who take early morning walks, this behavior tends to cause phase advance. The habit of taking an afternoon nap may also shorten the nocturnal sleep duration.

The *International Classification of Sleep Disorders*, Third Edition (ICSD-3) criteria (Box P118-1) require that the sleep period be advanced with respect to the desired sleep time and wake time. The use of a sleep log or actigraphy for *at least 7 days* is required to document a stable advance in the normal sleep period. Patients with ASWPD demonstrate a stable advance in sleep period with sleep onset 6 PM to 9 PM and awakenings from 2 AM to 5 AM. Chronotype questionnaires [morningness-eveningness questionnaire [MEQ; Horne-Ostberg questionnaire] document a "morning type" and circadian markers such as dim light melatonin onset (DLMO) show an advance. The differential diagnosis includes poor sleep hygiene (evening or afternoon naps), caffeine abuse, alcohol, and depression (may cause early morning awakening).

Treatment of ASWPD may require only reassurance if the patient can adapt his or her life to their circadian rhythm. Chronotherapy (sleep schedule) may be used with a progressive phase advance around the clock (going the bed earlier and earlier) until the desired bedtime is reached. For most patients, this is not practical. Relatively few studies of treatment of the ASWPD exist. Generally, bright light in the evening from 7 to 9 PM is recommended. In one study, 4000 lux was administered for 11 consecutive days and then twice weekly for a 3-month period (maintenance). Unfortunately, patients have difficulty complying with this treatment plan. The American Academy of Sleep

---

BOX P118-1 | **Advanced Sleep–Wake Phase Disorder**

Criteria A-E must be met
A. There is an advance (early timing) in the phase of the major sleep episode in relation to the desired or required sleep time and wake-up time, as evidenced by a chronic or recurrent complaint of difficulty staying awake until the required or desired conventional bedtime, together with an inability to remain asleep until the required or desired time for awakening.
B. Symptoms are present for at least 3 months.
C. When patients are allowed to sleep in accordance with their internal biological clock, sleep quality

and duration are improved with a consistent but advanced timing of the major sleep episode.
D. Sleep log and, whenever possible, actigraphy monitoring for at least 7 days (preferably 14 days) demonstrate a stable advance in the timing of the habitual sleep period. Both work/school days and free days must be included within this monitoring.
E. The sleep disturbance is not better explained by another current sleep disorder, medical or neurologic disorder, mental disorder, medication use, or substance use disorder.

Medicine (AASM) practice parameters mention evening light as an "Option" for ASWPD. Another important form of light therapy is to *avoid* early morning light, which tends to cause phase advance. If light is administered 6 hours after the minimum core body temperature (CBTmin), it has minimal, if any, phase advancing effect. For example, if typical awakenings are at 5 AM, outside light 10 AM or later would be expected to have minimal phase advancing effect. Although early morning melatonin would be a potential treatment (phase delay), this is not practical and may not be safe if individuals have to function in the morning. Melatonin has sedative effects especially at higher doses and during periods when the endogenous melatonin is not elevated.

The current patient delayed his morning walks until late morning, stopped taking naps, and bought a light box to get early evening bright light. He was able to sleep until 5:30 AM, and this was satisfactory to him. He simply got out of bed and started his day earlier than his wife did. However, he avoided exposure to outside or bright light until late morning.

CLINICAL PEARLS

1. The ASWPD is usually noted in older adults. Patients are more likely to complain of early morning awakening than early sleep onset. Sleep onset may be resisted because of societal obligations.

2. Sleep logs and actigraphy show a stable advance of the sleep period. Patients are "morning" types.

3. Early morning light (e.g., early morning walks) worsen the problem by inducing a further phase advance. Bright light exposure in the early morning should be avoided.

4. Evening bright light could be tried to phase delay. Avoiding naps may also increase nocturnal sleep duration.

5. Early morning awakening may also be seen in patients with depression.

BIBLIOGRAPHY

American Academy of Sleep Medicine: *International classification of sleep disorders*, ed 2, Darien, IL, 2013, American Academy of Sleep Medicine.

Auger RR: Advanced related sleep complaints and advanced sleep phase disorder, *Sleep Med Clin* 4:219–227, 2009.

Horne JA, Ostberg O: A self-assessment questionnaire to determine morningness- eveningness in human circadian rhythms, *Int J Chronobiol* 4:97–110, 1976.

Jones CR, Campbell SS, Zone SE, et al: Familial advanced sleep phase syndrome: a short-period circadian rhythm variant in humans, *Nat Med* 5:1062–1065, 1999.

Lack L, Wright H, Kemp K, et al: The treatment of early morning awakening insomnia with two evenings of bright light, *Sleep* 28:616–623, 2005.

Moldofsky H, Musisi S, Phillipson EA: Treatment of a case of advanced sleep phase syndrome by phase advance chronotherapy, *Sleep* 9:61–65, 1986.

Morgenthaler TI, Lee-Chiong T, Alessi C, et al: Practice parameters for the clinical evaluation and treatment of circadian rhythm sleep disorders, *Sleep* 30:1445–1459, 2007.

Toh KL, Jones CR, Yan HE, et al: An hPer2 phosphorylation site mutation in familial advanced sleep phase syndrome, *Science* 291:1040–1043, 2001.

A Patient with Periods of Insomnia and Daytime Sleepiness

A 30-year-old individual suffered a blast injury to his face that resulted in the need for enucleation of both eyes. He slowly adjusted to the blindness but had severe difficulty maintaining a normal sleep schedule. He seemed to sleep well for a few days in a row, but within a few days, he began to experience insomnia at night and daytime sleepiness. The alternating periods of good sleep and poor sleep occurred periodically. He denied depression and was not on any medication. An actigram from the patient is shown in Figure P119-1.

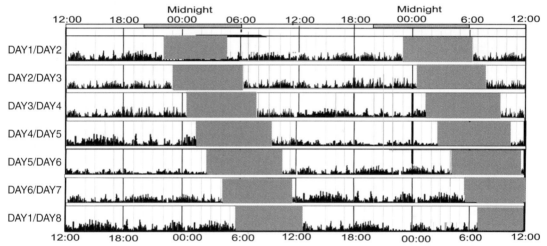

FIGURE P119-1 ■ A double plot, with each line showing 48 hours. The 24 hours on the right side of one line is repeated on the left side of the next line.

QUESTIONS

1. What explains the periodic severe insomnia and daytime sleepiness?

2. What treatment do you suggest?

ANSWERS

1. **Answer:** Non–24-hour sleep-wake rhythm disorder (Non-24-Hour SWRD).

2. **Answer:** Melatonin 0.5 milligrams (mg) at 10 PM (desired bedtime is 11 PM).

   Discussion: The Non-24-Hour SWRD, formerly called *free-running circadian disorder*, is characterized by a progressive delay in sleep onset and offset (Box P119-1; see also Figure P119-1). A steady drift of the sleep period by 1 to 2 hours occurs each day. When the circadian rhythm is out of phase with conventional sleep and wake times, symptoms occur. Patients may complain of periods of insomnia and daytime sleepiness (core body temperature minimum [CBTmin] during the day, e.g., noon), early morning awakening (core body temperature early evening, e.g., 10 PM), sleep-onset insomnia (core body temperature at 10 AM), and few symptoms (core body temperature in the middle of the night). The symptoms depend on the relationship of the internal circadian rhythms and external time. When the circadian phase is aligned with a normal sleep–wake period, complaints may not be present.

Up to 50% of patients with total blindness have nonentrained circadian rhythms. About 70% have chronic sleep complaints. Rarely, Non-24-Hour SWRD occurs in sighted individuals also. It has also been described after head trauma. For blind individuals, the tau (internal circadian period) may be normal, but they simply do not entrain to the dark–light cycle. Note that in some blind patients, the circadian system responds to bright light, even though they have no visual perception. Some nonvisual function is still present in patients with intact ganglion cells and retinohypothalamic tract (RHT). The etiology of Non-24-Hour SWRD in sighted individuals is unknown. The may have very long tau (long internal circadian period). The period is so long that it cannot be entrained by a half-hour phase advance from light.

Sleep logs and actigraphy (see Figure P119-1) demonstrate a progressive phase delay in the sleep period. Actigraphy monitoring for at least 14 days is recommended. The CBTmin and dim light melatonin onset (DLMO) also show a progressive delay. (Figure P119-2).

The treatment in blind patients includes melatonin of various doses 1 hour before desired bedtime. In one study, 10 mg of melatonin was given 1 hour before the desired bedtime (Figure P119-2) with subsequent use of a maintenance dose of 0.5 mg of melatonin. A few patients who failed to entrain on 10 mg of melatonin achieved success with a lower dose (Box P119-2).

BOX P119-1 | **Non–24-Hour Sleep-Wake Disorder—ICSD-3**

Criteria A-D must be met
A. There is a history of insomnia, excessive daytime sleepiness, or both, which alternate with asymptomatic episodes, due to misalignment between the 24-hour light-dark cycle and the non-entrained endogenous circadian rhythm of sleep-wake propensity.
B. Symptoms persist over the course of at least three months.

C. Daily sleep logs and actigraphy for at least 14 days, preferably longer for blind persons, demonstrate a pattern of sleep and wake times that typically delay each day, with a circadian period that is usually longer than 24 hours.
D. The sleep disturbance is not better explained by another current sleep disorder, medical or neurological disorder, mental disorder, medication use, or substance use disorder.

From American Academy of Sleep Medicine: International classification of sleep disorders, ed 3, Darien, IL, 2014, American Academy of Sleep Medicine.
ICSD-3, International Classification of Sleep Disorders, Third Edition.

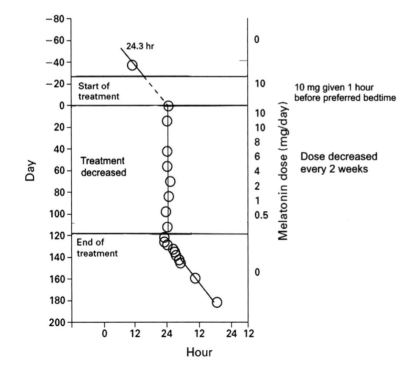

FIGURE P119-2 ■ A blind patient with Non-24-Hour circadian sleep-wake rhythm disorder (tau = 24.3 hours) was treated with 10 milligrams (mg) of melatonin about 1 hour before the preferred bedtime. The timing of dim light melatonin onset (DLMO) on sequential days is plotted (*circles*). Treatment was started when the DLMO occurred about 9 PM. Once entrained, the dose was slowly decreased every 2 weeks. Melatonin as low as 0.5 mg maintained entrainment. After treatment stopped, free running resumed in the patient. (Adapted from Lewy AJ, Emens JS, Lefler BJ, et al: Melatonin entrains free-running blind people according to a physiological dose response curve, *Chronobiol Int* 22:1093-1106, 2005.)

- Blind individuals:
  - Melatonin 0.5–10 milligrams given 1 hour before the desired bedtime.
  - Maintenance dose once entrained is 0.5 mg of melatonin.
  - If some light perception, may try morning light.
- Sighted individuals (recommendations are less clear):
  - Evening melatonin (phase advance).
  - Appropriately timed light exposure (most useful if begun when light will cause a phase advance (e.g., patient sleeping at night).
  - Keep regular sleep–wake schedule.

CLINICAL PEARLS

1. In the Non-24-Hour SWRD, a progressive delay of the sleep period occurs by 1 to 2 hours.
2. In blind individuals, this is caused by lack of the daily phase advance from light exposure (e.g., entrainment to day–night cycle). In sighted individuals, the syndrome is likely caused by a long tau or inadequate entrainment mechanisms.
3. The symptoms of Non-24-Hour SWRD include recurrent periods of fairly normal sleep followed by severe insomnia and daytime sleepiness.
4. Diagnosis is aided by the use of a sleep diary and actigraphy for at least 14 days.
5. In blind individuals, treatment is 0.5 mg of melatonin given 1 hour before the desired bedtime.

BIBLIOGRAPHY

American Academy of Sleep Medicine: *International classification of sleep disorders: diagnostic and coding manual*, ed 2, Westchester, IL, 2005, American Academy of Sleep Medicine.

Boivin DB, James FO, Santo BA, et al: Non-24-hour sleep-wake syndrome following a car accident, *Neurology* 60:1841–1843, 2003.

Hayakawa T, Uchiyama M, Kamei Y, et al: Clinical analysis of sighted patients with non-24 hour sleep-wake syndrome, *Sleep* 28:945–952, 2005.

Lewy AJ, Bauer VK, Ahmed S, et al: The human phase response curve (PRC) to melatonin is about 12 hours out of phase with the PRC to light, *Chronobiol Int* 15:71–83, 1998.

Lewy AJ, Bauer VK, Hasler BP, et al: Capturing the circadian rhythms of free-running blind individuals with 0.5 mg of melatonin, *Brain Res* 918:96–100, 2001.

Lewy AJ, Emens JS, Lefler BJ, et al: Melatonin entrains free-running blind people according to a physiological dose response curve, *Chronobiol Int* 22:1093–1106, 2005.

PATIENT 120

An Older Woman with an Irregular Sleep Schedule

The daughter of an 80-year-old woman seeks advice on improving her mother's sleep and alertness. Her mother has mild dementia (Alzheimer dementia) and is living in a structured living facility. Unfortunately, her mother has not been involved in the activities and is found by the staff to be frequently napping during the day and sometime awake, noisy, and confused at night. Her mother is taking donepezil 10 milligrams (mg) at bedtime nightly.

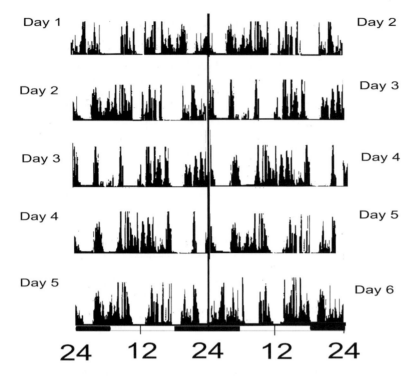

Day 1   Day 2

Day 2   Day 3

Day 3   Day 4

Day 4   Day 5

Day 5   Day 6

24   12   24   12   24

FIGURE P120-1 ■ Actigraphy data. At the bottom, above the times, the dark horizontal bar represents the night (typical dark time) and the light bar daytime hours. This is a double plot with the right half (24 hours) on one line repeated on the left half of the next line. (Reproduced from Berry RB: *Fundamentals of sleep medicine*, Philadelphia, 2012, Saunders, p 531.)

The mother's actigraph taken over a few days is shown in Figure P120-1. This is a double plot, with the 24 hours on the right half of one line repeated on the left half of the next line.

QUESTION

1. What is the problem affecting the mother's sleep? What treatment do you recommend?

ANSWER

1. **Answer:** Irregular sleep–wake rhythm disorder (ISWRD).

   Discussion: ISWRD, also known as *irregular sleep-wake rhythm (ISWR)*—is characterized by lack of a clearly defined circadian rhythm of sleep and wake behavior (Box P120-1). Typically, sleep and wake periods are interspersed throughout the day. The prevalence of ISWRD is unknown. The disorder occurs most frequently in institutionalized older adult patients with dementia or in institutionalized young patients with mental retardation. Precipitating factors include poor sleep

---

BOX P120-1	**Irregular Sleep–Wake Rhythm Disorder (ICSD-3 Diagnostic Criteria)**

Criteria A-D must be met

A. The patient or caregiver reports a chronic or recurrent pattern of irregular sleep and wake episodes throughout the 24-hour period, characterized by symptoms of insomnia during the scheduled sleep period (usually at night), excessive sleepiness (napping) during the day, or both.

B. Symptoms are present for at least 3 months.

C. Sleep log and, whenever possible, actigraphy monitoring for at least 7 days, preferably 14 days, demonstrate no major sleep period and multiple irregular sleep bouts (at least three) during a 24-hour period.

D. The sleep disturbance is not better explained by another current sleep disorder, medical or neurologic disorder, mental disorder, medication use, or substance use disorder.

From American Academy of Sleep Medicine: *International classification of sleep disorders*, ed 3, Darien, IL, 2014, American Academy of Sleep Medicine.

hygiene and limited exposure to synchronizing zeitgebers, including outside light, exercise, and social activities. Some patients may have a decrease in the circadian amplitude of the suprachiasmatic nucleus (SCN)–alerting signal. This may be caused by damage or deterioration of the SCN. In others, absence of zeitgebers (decreased light and activity) may be more important. Important risk factors for ISWRD include age, living in an institutional setting, and dementia or mental retardation.

The diagnosis requires a complaint of daytime sleepiness or insomnia (although the caregiver, rather than the patient, may complain). Actigraphy or sleep log for at least 7 days demonstrates multiple sleep periods (at least three) within 24 hours with approximately a normal total amount of sleep for age (see Figure P120-1). For most patients with ISWRD, the sleep log is problematic, and this is one setting in which actigraphy is especially helpful. Some actigraphy devices also record light exposure, and decreased light exposure may be a predisposing factor for ISWRD.

Treatment of patients with ISWRD aims at consolidating both sleep and wake periods. Daytime light has been tried with some benefit. Melatonin has not been found to be effective in most studies (especially when not combined with light treatment). A large randomized, controlled trial by Riemersma-ven der Lek and associates compared four groups including use of bright (1000 lux) or dim light (300 lux) with placebo melatonin or active melatonin (2.5 mg) in the evening in a group of older adult patients (87% had dementia). Light had a modest benefit in improving some cognitive and noncognitive symptoms of dementia. Melatonin decreased sleep latency and increased total sleep time but impaired mood when used alone. Bright light with melatonin did not impair mood but decreased sleep latency and increased total sleep time. Thus, melatonin should probably not be used alone in this group. A combination of light and melatonin might be effective. Conversely, melatonin has been shown to be of benefit in some populations of younger developmentally delayed or mentally impaired individuals. A study by Pillar and coworkers found that 4-week treatment with melatonin 3 mg improved sleep duration from 5.9 to 7.3 hours and sleep efficiency from 69.3% to 88% in a group of psychomotor-retarded children.

Interventions to treat ISWRD include bright light during the day, structured daytime activities (mixed modality treatment), and decreased noise and nighttime light. Hypnotics have also been used but are associated with side effects (falls or sedation) in older adults. The American Academy of Sleep Medicine (AASM) practice parameters recommended bright light during the day and mixed-modality therapy (societal activities). Melatonin is recommended only in younger patients with retardation but not for older nursing home patients (Option).

Alzheimer disease (AD) is the most common cause of dementia (>60% of dementias). The diagnosis is one of exclusion. The hallmark is a gradual onset of short-term memory problems. Patients with AD suffer from *sundowning*, which is defined as nocturnal exacerbation of disruptive behavior or agitation in older patients. This is likely the most common cause of institutionalization in patients with AD. Donepezil (Aricept), a cholinesterase inhibitor, is used to improve cognition in patients with AD but is often associated with insomnia. Although most often prescribed at night, morning dosing is suggested to minimize sleep disturbance.

In the current patient, actigraphy showed an irregular pattern of wakefulness and sleep. Note that much of the sleep occurred during the day. At least three episodes of sleep were noted each day. A structured plan of outside light during the day and structured activities every morning and evening were planned. The patient was encouraged not to sleep during the day. In addition, donepezil dosing was changed to morning dosing. On this regimen, nighttime sleep improved, with the need for fewer staff interventions at night. The patient seemed more alert during the day.

CLINICAL PEARLS

1. ISWRD is characterized by at least three sleep episodes scattered throughout the day. A complaint of insomnia or daytime sleepiness, either from the patient or caregiver, is required for the diagnosis.

2. Treatments include daytime light, structured social activities, and quiet and dark at night.

3. In young patients with mental retardation, melatonin at night has been shown to be useful in some studies.

4. If possible, administration of sedating medications should be avoided during the day and those causing insomnia avoided at night.

BIBLIOGRAPHY

American Academy of Sleep Medicine: *International classification of sleep disorders: diagnostic and coding manual*, ed 2, Westchester, IL, 2013, American Academy of Sleep Medicine.

Ancoli-Israek S, Martin JL, Kripke DF, et al: Effect of light treatment on sleep and circadian rhythms in demented nursing home patients, *J Am Geriatr Soc* 50:282–289, 2002.

Morgenthaler TI, Lee-Chiong T, Alessi C, et al: Practice parameters for the clinical evaluation and treatment of circadian rhythm sleep disorders, *Sleep* 30:1445–1459, 2007.

Pillar G, Shahar E, Peled N, et al: Melatonin improves sleep wake patterns in psychomotor retarded children, *Pediatr Neurol* 23:225–228, 2000.

Riemersma-ven der Lek RF, Swaab DF, Twisk J, et al: Effect of bright light and melatonin on cognitive and noncognitive function in elderly residents of group care facilities, *JAMA* 299:2642–2655, 2008.

Singer C, Trachtenberg RE, Kaye J, et al: A multicenter, placebo controlled trial of melatonin for sleep disturbance in Alzheimer's disease, *Sleep* 26:893–901, 2003.

Zee PC, Vitiello MV: Circadian rhythm disorder: irregular sleep wake rhythm, *Sleep Med Clin* 4:213–218, 2009.

PATIENT 121

A Patient with Night Shift Work

A 60-year-old man works the night shift 5 out of 7 days. His shift starts at 11 PM and ends at 7:00 AM. He typically returns home after his night shift and eats a light breakfast. He gets in bed about 9:00 AM and tries to fall asleep. His room is dark and quiet. He usually can only sleep until about 1 to 2 PM. He then gets out of bed and runs errands or works in his yard. He eats supper at 8:00 PM and leaves for work at 10:30 PM. During the shift, he is active, and the rooms he works in are well lit. He drinks about six cups of coffee through the shift. On his days off, he typically is able to sleep at night, although he does not sleep very well. The patient feels sleepy in the afternoon during the work week and considerably sleepy during the shift.

QUESTION

1. What set of interventions would be most helpful for this night shift worker (A, B, C, or D)?

A	Bright light start of shift	Dark glasses on the drive home	Nap before night shift
B	Bright light end of shift	Dark glasses on the drive home	Nap before night shift
C	Bright light start of shift	Delay bedtime until 11 AM	Nap before drive home in the morning
D	Bright light end of shift	Delay bedtime until 11 AM	Nap before night shift

ANSWER

1. Answer: A

Discussion: The correct answer is A. Bright light at the start of the shift, dark glasses on the way home (assuming he drives home in daylight), going to bed on arrival at home, and a nap before the shift are suggested interventions. Light at the end of the shift, on the way home, or during the first hours at home could cause phase advance in the patient. The goal is a phase delay so that his minimum core body temperature (CBTmin) is within the daytime sleep period. Shift work disorder (SWD) is characterized by excessive sleepiness or insomnia temporally associated with a recurring work schedule that overlaps the usual time for sleep (Box P121-1). The problem must last at least 1 month for a diagnosis of SWD. A sleep log or actigraphy for at least 7 days documents circadian and sleep time misalignment. The boundary between a normal and a pathologic response to circadian stress of unnatural sleep schedule associated with shift work remains unclear. SWD is a common problem in industrialized countries because of the need for some occupations and services to function continuously 24 hours per day.

Up to 20% of the population in industrialized societies works in an occupation requiring shift work. The total number of night shift workers is 2% to 5% of the population. About 5% to 10% of shift workers experience such significant insomnia or sleepiness during the shift (or day) to meet the criteria for a diagnosis of this disorder. Risk factors for this disorder include advancing age (possibly more in women than men) and morning light exposure (long commute home or morning social obligations). Light exposure on the drive home causes phase advance, moving the CBTmin toward

---

BOX P121-1 **Shift Work Disorder (ICSD-3 Diagnostic Criteria)**	
Criteria A-D must be met A. There is a report of insomnia and/or excessive sleepiness, accompanied by a reduction of total sleep time, which is associated with a recurring work schedule that overlaps the usual time for sleep. B. The symptoms have been present and associated with the shift work schedule for at least 3 months.	C. Sleep log and actigraphy monitoring (whenever possible and preferably with concurrent light exposure measurement) for at least 14 days (work and free days) demonstrate a disturbed sleep and wake pattern. D. The sleep and/or wake disturbance are not better explained by another current sleep disorder, medical or neurologic disorder, mental disorder, medication use, poor sleep hygiene, or substance use disorder.

From American Academy of Sleep Medicine: *International classification of sleep disorders*, ed 3, Darien, IL, 2014, American Academy of Sleep Medicine.

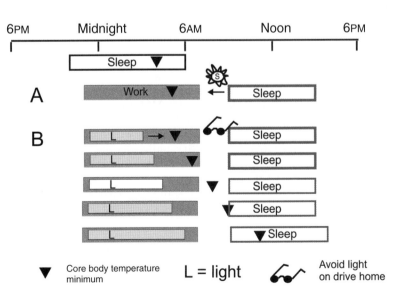

FIGURE P121-1 ■ Circadian problems and interventions for night shift work. **A,** Light on commute causes phase advance. The core body temperature minimum (CBTmin) is not within the desired daytime sleep period making daytime sleep difficult. **B,** minimum core body temperature (CBTmin) is shifted toward daytime sleep by using bright light at night during work during the first part of the shift (phase delay) and wearing dark goggles on the commute home (if driving in daylight). The goal is to shift the CBTmin into the daytime sleep period. Here the rectangle Sleep refers to the desired sleep period. (From Berry RB: *Fundamentals of sleep medicine*, Philadelphia, 2012, Saunders, p 539.)

Goal phase delay so CBTmin is within desired daytime sleep period

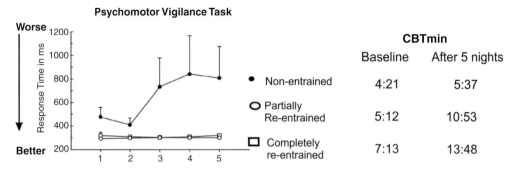

FIGURE P121-2 ■ Change in psychomotor vigilance task (PVT) (shorter reaction time better) over five consecutive simulated night shifts in nonentrained, partially entrained, and completely reentrained groups. The nonentrained group had a worsening in the PVT over 5 nights (increased response time). The other two groups did not show any deterioration over the five night shifts. The time of the minimum core body temperature (CBTmin) is illustrated for each group at baseline and after 5 nights. The CBTmin shifted to within daytime sleep in the two groups with better function. Subjects were given different combinations of bright light versus dim light during the simulated night shift, dark glasses or normal sunglasses in the morning, and melatonin or placebo before sleep time. (Adapted from Crowley SJ, Tseng CU, Fogg LF, Eastman CI: Complete or partial re-entrainment improves performance, alertness, and mood during shift-work, *Sleep* 27:1077-1087, 2004.)

the time of the nights shift and inhibiting adaptive phase resetting). A number of exacerbating factors exist, including long shifts (fatigue) and the common practice of resuming normal daytime activities and nighttime sleep on the weekends. It should be noted that in the early morning hours, the alertness of night shift workers is compromised by both sleep load (accumulated wake-sleep debt) and the fact that the alerting signal is at its minimum at the CBTmin, which, theoretically, is in the last part of the shift (Figure P121-1).

Available CBTmin data are limited. Sleep logs and diaries document the altered routine and the effect on sleep. Studies of dim light melatonin onset (DLMO) have suggested that night workers are quite variable in their circadian adaptation (some experience adaptive phase delay). Of note, symptoms do not always indicate whether or not circadian adaptation has occurred.

NIGHT SHIFT WORK: The daytime sleep in night shift workers is shorter than normal (5–6 hours [hr]). Most workers do not have circadian adaptation because of daytime societal obligations. They typically get light after their CBTmin of the drive home and, therefore, phase advance have occurred. As noted above, bright light during the start of the shift (before CBTmin) and avoiding light in the early morning (preventing phase advance) potentially move CBTmin to within the daytime sleep period. Scheduled naps before or in the early part of the shift may improve alertness. Two-hour naps during late afternoon before the evening shift are more effective than 2-hour naps during the shift. In a simulated night shift study over 5 consecutive nights, Crowley and colleagues studied the effects of different interventions and the effect on shifts in CBTmin and performance (Figure P121-2). The groups that shifted the CBTmin to within the normal sleeping hours had improved nocturnal functioning on the psychomotor vigilance task (PVT). The investigators used a combination of light during the simulated shift, dark glasses during simulated drive home, and melatonin before sleep. Of interest, the groups with the latest CBTmin at baseline were the ones able to completely entrain to the new schedule. Circadian phase was measured by DLMO, assuming CBTmin = DLMO + 7 hours. Melatonin given before morning sleep after a night shift resulted in minimal change in total sleep time and added little to circadian shifts induced by interventions with light.

Greater sleep loss occurs with rapidly rotating shifts than with slowly rotating shifts (slow = 3-week periods). Clockwise rotation is better tolerated than counterclockwise rotation because of the natural tendency for phase delay.

A number of complications of shift work have been proposed, including gastrointestinal disturbances (constipation or diarrhea), obesity, miscarriage, drug dependency, and social and family life disturbances.

TREATMENT OF SWD

The recommended treatments for SWD are listed in Box P121-2. The goals of treatments include interventions to (1) modify circadian rhythms to alleviate the symptoms of circadian rhythm misalignment, (2) decrease sleep load during the night (naps before the shift or hypnotics before daytime sleep), or (3) increase alertness during the shift (caffeine or modafinil).

Treatment interventions for the night shift include stimulants (coffee, modafinil, armodafinil) during the early shift to help counteract the tendency for sleep and bright light in the early part of the shift for its phase delaying properties and its direct stimulatory effect. A short nap either before

BOX P121-2	**Night Shift Recommendations**

- Bright light for 3 to 6 hours during the start of shift—phase delay
- Short scheduled naps (before or during shift)
- Avoidance of bright light on the way home in the morning (use dark goggles if driving in daylight to avoiding phase advances)
- Quiet dark sleep environment at home during sleep
- Melatonin administered in the morning at bedtime (hypnotic and phase delay effects)
- Going to bed as soon as possible after arriving at home

- Stimulants or alerting agents at the start of the shift
  - Caffeine (250–400 mg) during first 2 hours of night shift
  - Modafinil 200 mg (or armodafinil 150 mg) taken 30 to 60 minutes before start of the night shift (FDA approved for treatment of sleepiness in shift work to improve alertness during the night shift)
- Hypnotics before daytime sleep—may increase total sleep time but do not help alertness at night

FDA, U.S. Food and Drug Administration.

the shift or during the early part of the shift reduces sleep pressure and improved alertness. Avoiding bright light on the way home (avoids the phase advancing effects of light exposure after reaching CBTmin) and going to bed immediately make it possible to shift CBTmin into the daytime sleep period (see Figure P121-1). This is believed to improve sleep quality. As noted above melatonin could be tried before the early-morning sleep period to phase delay and for its hypnotic effect. However, light is, by far, the strongest phase-shifting influence. Hypnotics may be tried to increase the duration of the daytime sleep period. Walsh and colleagues found that use of triazolam increased daytime sleep duration by about 50 minutes but did not reduce circadian sleep tendency in the early morning hours (during the shift work hours).

CLINICAL PEARLS

1. Shift work (particularly night shift work) causes a misalignment between the circadian tendency for sleep and the need for alertness. The lowest alertness is usually at the last portion of the shift near CBTmin. At that time, the alerting signal is low, and sleep pressure is high (accumulated wakefulness).

2. Short naps before the night shift or in the early part of the shift improve alertness.

3. Bright light at the start of the shift will help phase advance the CBTmin toward the daytime sleep period and has direct stimulatory effects.

4. Caffeine, modafinil, armodafinil given in the early part of the shift increase alertness.

5. Avoiding light exposure on the drive home minimizes the tendency of light to cause a phase advance.

6. Going to sleep immediately after returning home may also be helpful. This avoids exposure to light in the phase advancing zone and makes it possible to shift the CBTmin within the daytime sleep period.

BIBLIOGRAPHY

American Academy of Sleep Medicine: *International classification of sleep disorders: diagnostic and coding manual*, Darien, IL, 2013, American Academy of Sleep Medicine.

Bjorvatn B, Stangenes K, Oyane N, et al: Randomized placebo-controlled field study of the effects of bright light and melatonin in adaptation to shift work, *Scand J Work Environ Health* 33:204–214, 2007.

Boivin DB, James FO: Circadian adaptation to night-shift work by judicious light and dark exposure, *J Biol Rhythms* 17:556–567, 2002.

Crowley SJ, Tseng CU, Fogg LF, Eastman CI: Complete or partial re-entrainment improves performance, alertness, and mood during shift-work, *Sleep* 27:1077–1087, 2004.

Crowley SJ, Tseng CY, Fogg LF, et al: Combinations of bright light, scheduled dark, sunglasses, and melatonin to facilitate circadian entrainment to night shift work, *J Biol Rhythms* 18:513–523, 2003.

Czeisler CA, Walsh JK, Roth T, et al: Modafinil for excessive sleepiness associated with shift-work sleep disorder, *N Engl J Med* 353:476–486, 2005.

Czeisler CA, Walsh JK, Wesnew KA, et al: Armodafinil for treatment of excessive sleepiness associated with shift work disorder: a randomized controlled study, *Mayo Clin Proc* 84:958–972, 2009.

Morgenthaler TI, Lee-Chiong T, Alessi C, et al: Practice parameters for the clinical evaluation and treatment of circadian rhythm sleep disorders, *Sleep* 30:1445–1459, 2007.

Sallinen M, Harma M, Akerstedt T, et al: Promoting alertness with a short nap during a night shift, *J Sleep Res* 7:240–247, 1998.

Schweitzer PK, Randazzo AC, Stone K, et al: Laboratory and field studies of naps and caffeine as practical countermeasures for sleep-wake problems associated with night work, *Sleep* 29:39–50, 2006.

Smith MR, Lee C, Crowley SJ, et al: Morning melatonin has limited benefit as a soporific for daytime sleep after night work, *Chronobiol Int* 22:873–888, 2005.

Walsh JK, Sugerman JL, Muehlback MJ, et al: Physiological sleep tendency on a simulated night shift: adaptation and effects of triazolam, *Sleep* 12:251–264, 1988.

Patients with Jet Lag

A business man travels from New York to Paris 6 hours eastward. Three questions concerning jet lag are presented below. The *International Classification of Sleep Disorders*, Third Edition (ICSD-3) diagnostic criteria for jet lag disorder are listed in Box P122-1.

QUESTIONS

1. What time should light be avoided in the new time zone?
   A. 7 AM – 10 AM
   B. Noon - 3 PM
   C. 3 PM - 6 PM

2. What interventions before the trip will allow more rapid adaptation in the new time zone?
   A. Pretrip phase advance
   B. Pretrip phase delay
   C. Avoid sun in the morning in Paris
   D. Melatonin in the evening in Paris

3. What direction of travel is the most difficult for adaptation?
   A. Westward travel
   B. Eastward travel

BOX P122-1　Jet Lag Disorder—ICSD-3 Diagnostic Criteria

Criteria A-C must be met
A. There is a complaint of insomnia or excessive daytime sleepiness, accompanied by a reduction of total sleep time, associated with transmeridian jet travel across at least two time zones.
B. There is associated impairment of daytime function, general malaise, or somatic symptoms (e.g.,

gastrointestinal disturbance) within 1-2 days after travel.
C. The sleep disturbance is not better explained by another current sleep disorder, medical or neurologic disorder, mental disorder, medication use, or substance use disorder.

From American Academy of Sleep Medicine: *International classification of sleep disorders*, ed 3, Darien, IL, 2014, American Academy of Sleep Medicine.

ANSWERS

1. **Answer:** Avoid light from 7 AM to 10 AM in Paris.

2. **Answer:** Pretrip phase advance.

3. **Answer:** Eastward travel is the most difficult as it requires phase advance.

   Discussion: Eastward travel across time zones requires phase advance for adaptation. Westward travel requires phase delay (easier for most individuals). It is easier to stay awake later than fall asleep earlier. In the person traveling from the United States to Paris, a phase advance is required. If the baseline minimum core body temperature (CBTmin) is assumed to be reached at 4 AM, this

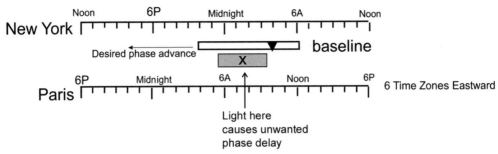

FIGURE P122-1 ■ Light should be avoided before the time of the minimum core body temperature (CBTmin) in the new time zone.

corresponds to 10 AM in the new time zone. Phase advance must occur for adaptation, and morning light exposure in Paris is before CBTmin, would cause, phase delay and should be avoided. Light for several hours *before the CBTmin* (10 AM in the new time zone) induces the most significant phase delay. Light exposure should be avoided before 10 AM and pursued from 11 AM to 2 PM to induce the maximum phase advancing effect. Light at 2 to 6 PM is so far away from the CBTmin that it has a minimal effect. The issues to consider are illustrated in Figure P122-1.

The ICSD-3 diagnostic criteria are listed in Box P122-1. Jet lag begins after travel across at least two time zones. Desynchrony between body and local time zone is known to cause problems with sleep, alertness, and performance. The degree of dysfunction depends on (1) the number of time zones crossed, (2) the direction of travel (westward travel better tolerated), (3) sleep loss during travel, (4) availability of local time cues (exposure to natural light at destination—depends on weather, business schedule, and other factors), and (5) ability to tolerate circadian misalignment (decreases with age). With westward travel, the internal circadian rhythms are phase advanced with respect to clock time in the new time zone. Adaptation requires a phase delay. Westward travel is better tolerated because it is easier to phase delay (stay awake) than to fall asleep. In eastward travel, the individual's internal circadian rhythms are phase delayed with respect to clock time in the new time zone. It is more difficult to undergo adaptation to the new time zone with a phase advance (falling asleep at an earlier tine with respect to the internal circadian rhythms). Sleep occurs normally on the rising phase of melatonin rhythm and the falling phase of core temperature rhythm. It is estimated that it takes about 1 day per hour of time zone change to adjust (maximum adaptation is a phase shift of ½–1 hour per day, depending on direction of travel).

Symptoms associated with jet lag may include (1) daytime tiredness or impaired daytime alertness, (2) inability to get to sleep at night (eastward flight), and (3) early awakening (westward flight). Other symptoms may include disorientation; gastrointestinal problems (poor appetite), inappropriate timing of defecation (gut lag), excessive urination, menstrual abnormalities (often experienced by flight crew), inappropriate metabolic responses (insulin and other hormones), and heart disease. Symptoms may be worsened by the stresses of air travel itself or the excessive consumption of caffeine or alcohol.

Travel over six time zones may result in phase shifting in the opposite direction of the direction of travel (i.e., adapting "the wrong way"), the so-called *antidromic reentrainment*. For example, an eastern flight requires phase advancing to acclimate to the new time zone. However, after an eastward flight across nine time zones, the traveler's CBTmin normally at 5 AM in the old time zone would occur at 2 PM in the new time zone. Thus, morning light in the new time zone would cause phase delay because light exposure occurs before CBTmin. Of note, some experts recommend that all flights that cross more than 8 to 10 time zones be treated as if they were westward travel (interventions target progressive phase delay).

Treatment of Jet Lag: A number of treatments for jet lag have been recommended according to the direction of travel (Table P122-1). Websites that allow the traveler to enter current and future locations are available. One difficulty with providing recommendations is in estimating the current CBTmin and also the fact that entrainment in the new destination may depend on societal demands in the new time zone that preclude following the prescription.

General sleep hygiene measures include a dark, quiet sleep environment with earplugs or eye shades, if needed. In overnight flights, some degree of sleep loss is inevitable. Flying first class (more room), wearing eye shades or ear plugs, and possibly a hypnotic may minimize sleep loss. If the

TABLE P122-1	**Recommendations for Jet Lag**	
	Eastward Travel	**Westward Travel**
	Internal rhythm is phase delayed. Adaptation—phase advance.	Internal rhythm is phase advanced. Adaptation—phase delay.
Before Travel		
Try to reset body clock to minimize necessary change.	Shift sleep 1–2 hours (*hr*) *earlier* before trip (bright light in the morning).	Shift sleep 1–2 hours *later* before trip (bright light in the morning).
During Travel		
During flight.	Sleep if possible—especially on long flights to avoid sleep loss.	Sleep if possible—especially on long flights to avoid sleep loss.
	Sleep during time corresponding to night in the destination, if possible.	Sleep during time corresponding to night in the destination if possible.
	Drink adequate water (H_2O); avoid alcohol.	Drink adequate H_2O; avoid alcohol.
On Arrival		
Anticipated changes in sleep.	Difficulty falling asleep. Difficulty waking up.	Difficulty staying asleep. Early awakening.
Appropriate light exposure.	Seek morning light (if after CBTmin).	Seek evening light (if before CBTmin).
If crossing more than eight time zones, avoid light when it may inhibit adaptation.	For the first 2 days after arrival, avoid bright light for the first 2–3 hr after dawn; starting on the third day, seek exposure to bright light in the morning.	For 2–3 days, avoid bright light in the late evening (at dusk), starting on the third day, seek exposure to bright light in the evening.
Melatonin	Take 0.5–3 mg at local bedtime nightly until you adjust (phase advance).	Take 0.5 milligrams (mg) during the second half of the night (after CBTmin to phase delay).
Hypnotics	Consider taking at bedtime for a few days.	Consider taking at bedtime for a few days.
Caffeine	Drink judiciously; avoid after midday.	Drink judiciously; avoid after midday.

Adapted from Sack RL: Jet lag, *N Engl J Med* 362:440-447, 2010.
CBTmin, Minimum core body temperature.

flight is long, sleeping on the flight during appropriate hours (destination nighttime) may be helpful. If this is not possible, a short nap on arrival at the new destination may help. In general, daytime naps should be avoided at the destination. However, napping may improve alertness for special demands (e.g., giving a talk). Napping removes photic stimuli, which may delay adaptation if napping occurs at a time when light exposure would shift circadian rhythms in the correct direction. Drinking adequate fluids and avoiding alcohol may also help. The availability of exposure to natural light in the new destination may be influenced by time of year, weather, and schedule (indoor meetings, societal obligations). The general recommendation is to eat on the destination schedule.

Eastward Flights: The patient is phase delayed (phase advance is required). One method is to phase advance 1 hour per day with bright light in the morning before travel begins. At the new destination, morning light should be sought (as long as it is after the CBTmin). Evening light should be avoided on arrival at the new destination (to avoid phase delay). Taking melatonin before the time of CBTmin might be useful if the hypnotic effects would not interfere with wakeful activities. Hypnotics may help with sleep but do not necessarily help with alertness the next day. Even if the individual gets adequate sleep, decreased circadian alertness will occur at the time of CBTmin. Stimulants (caffeine) may be helpful to maintain alertness during the day in the new locale. A study found that 150 milligrams (mg) of armodafinil (R enantiomer of modafinil) increased wakefulness after eastward travel through six time zones.

Westward Flights: The patient is phase advanced relative to local time (phase delay is required). Phase delaying could be tried before travel begins (go to bed later, get up later) using evening bright light for 1 to 3 hours. Light should be avoided in the morning in the new destination (if it occurs soon after CBTmin) to prevent phase advance. Exposure to light in the evening (if before CBTmin) may be helpful (phase delay). Melatonin at bedtime in the destination if taken before CBTmin may have hypnotic action but induces phase shift in the wrong direction (phase advance). If melatonin is used, it is recommended that a small dose (avoid prolonged hypnotic action) be taken during the last half of the night. Taking melatonin on awakening while at the correct time for phase delay may make the individual sleepy (counterproductive). Hypnotics at bedtime may help with sleep but do not necessarily help with alertness the next day. Even if the patients gets adequate sleep, decreased circadian alertness will occur at the time of CBTmin. Stimulants (caffeine) may be helpful to maintain alertness during the day in the new locale.

Crossing More Than Eight Time Zones: After eastward flights, very early light (inappropriate phase delay) should be avoided; on westward flights, light at dusk (inappropriate phase advance) should be avoided for 2 to 3 days. Thereafter, light at the usual times may help with adaptation. Conversely, as noted previously, some physicians recommend attempts at phase delay even if the direction of travel is eastward when more than eight time zones are crossed.

CLINICAL PEARLS

1. Symptoms of jet lag occur because of desynchrony between the internal rhythms and the external clock time. Difficulty falling asleep, staying asleep, or maintaining alertness are the major challenges.
2. Eastward travel is more difficult and requires a phase advance. It is much easier to phase delay. A phase advance in schedule in the home time zone before the trip may help make adaptation more rapid.
3. Westward travel requires phase delay. This is easier given the body's intrinsic tendency of phase delay. It is easier to stay awake later than to fall asleep earlier (with respect in internal circadian rhythm).
4. Decreased alertness will occur at the time of CBTmin even if a normal amount of sleep was obtained the night before. This is the low point of the suprachiasmatic nucleus (SCN) alerting signal.
5. Light on the wrong side of the CBTmin should be avoided and exposure to light on the correct side of the CBTmin sought to achieve the desired circadian shift.
6. In general, in takes about 1 day for each time zone crossed to entrain to the new time zone. The body's ability to shift is about 1 hour for westward travel and ½ hour for eastward travel.

BIBLIOGRAPHY

American Academy of Sleep Medicine: *International classification of sleep disorders*, ed 3, Darien, IL, 2013, American Academy of Sleep Medicine.

Eastman CI, Gazda CJ, Burgess HJ, et al: Advancing circadian rhythms before eastward flight: a strategy to prevent or reduce jet lag, *Sleep* 28:33–44, 2005.

Jamieson AO, Zammit GK, Rosenberg RS, et al: Zolpidem reduces the sleep disturbance of jet lag, *Sleep Med* 2:423–430, 2001.

Morgenthaler TI, Lee-Chiong T, Alessi C, et al: Practice parameters for the clinical evaluation and treatment of circadian rhythm sleep disorders, *Sleep* 30:1445–1459, 2007.

Revell VL, Eastman CI: How to trick mother nature into letting you fly around or stay up all night, *J Biol Rhythm* 20:353–365, 2005.

Rosenberg RP, Bogan RK, Tiller JM, et al: A phase 3, double-blind, randomized, placebo-controlled study of armodafinil for excessive sleepiness associated with jet lag disorder, *Mayo Clin Proc* 85:630–638, 2010.

Sack RL: Jet lag, *N Engl J Med* 362:440–447, 2010.

FUNDAMENTALS 41

Psychiatry and Sleep

Psychiatric disorders are among the most common health problems, with over 15% to 20% of Americans being treated for a significant psychiatric illness in any given year.[1,2] Almost one third of individuals with significant complaints of insomnia or hypersomnia show evidence of psychiatric disorders. Psychiatric disorders account for the largest diagnostic category for patients with sleep complaints. Conversely, sleep complaints are part of the diagnostic criteria for many psychiatric disorders and are a source of considerable morbidity. The psychiatric disorders commonly affecting sleep (or vice versa) are listed in Box F41-1. The diagnostic criteria presented in this chapter are adapted and abridged from the recently published *Diagnostic and Statistical Manual of Mental Disorders*, 5th edition (DSM-V). The reader is referred to that publication for comprehensive criteria.

MOOD DISORDERS

Mood disorders are the most common category of psychiatric disorders followed by anxiety disorders. The mood disorders include the major depressive disorder (MDD) and the bipolar disorders.

Major Depressive Disorder

The diagnostic criteria for MDD (adapted from DSM-V)[1] are listed in Table F41-1. To meet these criteria, a major depressive episode as defined by A–C and distress or impairment must be present, and the condition is not better explained by substance use, a medical disorder, or another psychiatric disorder. This diagnosis requires that *a manic or hypomanic episode has never occurred*. If so, a diagnosis of bipolar disorder is made. That is, the depressive episode is associated with a bipolar disorder (bipolar depression). The effects of MDD on sleep are listed in Box F41-2. A sleep complaint (insomnia or

---

BOX F41-1 **Psychiatric Disorders Commonly Affecting Sleep**

MOOD DISORDERS

Major depressive disorder
Bipolar disorder 1
Bipolar disorder 2

ANXIETY DISORDERS

Panic disorder
Posttraumatic stress disorder
Generalized anxiety disorder

TABLE F41-1 **Diagnostic Criteria for Major Depression Disorder**

A. Five (or more) of the following nine symptoms listed below have been present during the same 2-week period and representing a change from previous functioning; at least one of the symptoms is either (1) depressed mood or (2) loss of interest or pleasure.

  1. Depressed mood
  2. Markedly diminished interest or pleasure
  3. Significant unintentional weight loss or weight gain (or decrease or increase in appetite)
  4. **Insomnia or hypersomnia nearly every day**
  5. Psychomotor agitation or retardation nearly every day (observable by others, not merely subjective feelings of restlessness or being slowed down)
  6. Fatigue or loss of energy
  7. Feelings of worthlessness or excessive or inappropriate guilt
  8. Diminished ability to think or concentrate or indecisiveness nearly every day
  9. Recurrent thoughts of death (not just fear of dying), recurrent suicidal ideation without a specific plan, or a suicide attempt or specific plan for committing suicide

B. Symptoms cause distress or impairment in functioning.

C. Episode is not caused by a medical condition or substance.

D. The major depressive episode (defined as A-C) is not better explained by another psychiatric disorder.

E. A manic or hypomanic episode has never occurred.

BOX F41-2	Sleep and Major Depressive Episodes

- Symptoms:
  - 80% of depressive episodes are associated with insomnia
    - Early-morning awakening
    - Frequent awakening
  - 15%-20% hypersomnia
- Sleep abnormalities may persist after remission
- Persistent sleep abnormalities may be associated with a risk of recurrence (some but not all studies)

- PSG findings during depressive episodes
  - Prolonged sleep latency
  - Increased wake, early-morning awakening, frequent awakenings
  - Decreased stage N3 sleep
  - REM abnormalities
    - Short REM latency
    - Increased REM density
    - Increased REM early in the night
    - Increased REM (%TST)

MSLT, Multiple sleep latency test; *PSG*, polysomnography; *REM*, rapid eye movement; *TST*, total sleep time.

BOX F41-3	Diagnostic Criteria for Bipolar 1 Disorder

BIPOLAR 1 DISORDER

A. Criteria have been met for at least one manic episode is required (see below). One or more depressive episodes (as defined in Table F41-1 [A–C]) **may** be present.
B. The manic episode and depressive episodes are not better explained by another psychiatric disorder.
C. Mood disturbance is *sufficiently severe to cause marked impairment* in occupational function or in usual social activities or relationships with others or to *necessitate hospitalization to prevent harm to self or others*, or *psychotic features* are present.
D. The episode is not attributable to a medical condition or substance.

MANIC EPISODE

A. A distinct period of abnormally and persistently elevated, expansive, or irritable mood, *lasting at least 1 week (or any duration if hospitalization is necessary)*.

B. During the period of mood disturbance, *three (or more)* of the following symptoms have persisted *(four if the mood is only irritable)* and have been present to a significant degree:
1. Inflated self-esteem or grandiosity
2. Decreased need for sleep (e.g., feels rested after 3 hours of sleep)
3. More talkative than usual or pressure to keep talking
4. Flight of ideas or subjective experience that thoughts are racing
5. Distractibility (i.e., attention too easily drawn to unimportant or irrelevant external stimuli)
6. Increase in goal-directed activity (either socially, at work or school, or sexually) or psychomotor agitation
7. Excessive involvement in pleasurable activities that have a high potential for painful consequences (e.g., engaging in unrestrained buying sprees, sexual indiscretions, or foolish business investments)

Adapted from American Psychiatric Association: *Diagnostic and statistical manual of mental disorders*, ed 5, Arlington, VA, 2013, American Psychiatric Association.

hypersomnia) is one of the primary diagnostic criteria for major depression disorder. Nearly 80% of depressive episodes are associated with insomnia.[3,4] The insomnia complaints include early-morning and frequent awakenings. *However, up to 15% to 20% of patients complain of hypersomnia during depression.* Polysomnography (PSG) findings in patients during depression include prolonged sleep latency, increased wakefulness after sleep onset (WASO), decreased stage N3 sleep, and rapid eye movement (REM; stage R) abnormalities.[3,5] Stage R abnormalities include *short REM latency*, increased length of the first REM episode, and increased REM density in the early part of the night. Recall that REM density (number of REMs per time) is typically low during the first REM episodes. In depressed patients complaining of hypersomnia the MSLT (if performed) does not

demonstrate significant objective sleepiness (mean sleep latency >10 minutes).[6] Symptoms of insomnia or PSG abnormalities may persist after remission of depression.[1,3]

Bipolar 1 Disorder

A diagnosis of bipolar disorder 1 (BP-1) requires the presence of at least one manic episode (Box F41-3). One or more major depressive episodes may also have been present (not required). When the first manifestation of BP-1 disorder is a depressive episode, a diagnosis of MDD may be made initially. Often, the depression is "atypical" (Table F41-2). Manic episodes cause marked impairment, require hospitalization, or have psychotic features. In contrast, hypomanic mood disturbance does *not* cause marked impairment, does *not* necessitate hospitalization, and has *no* psychotic features. Manic episodes are associated with marked insomnia (Box F41-4), but the patient awakens refreshed after a few hours of sleep. PSG findings include reduced stage N3 sleep, short REM latency, and increased REM density. Of note, sleep loss may trigger a manic episode[7] as may treatment with an antidepressant.

Bipolar 2 Disorder

A diagnosis of BP-2 disorder requires the presence of at least one hypomanic episode and one or more major depressive episodes (Box F41-5). *A manic episode should never have occurred* (if so a diagnosis of BP-1 is made). Hypomanic episodes are similar to manic episodes but not

as severe. The patient may function, although the behavior represents an unequivocal change. BP-2 disorder should not be assumed to be a "milder" form of bipolar disorder as the recurrent episodes of depression may be very disabling. The effects of BP-2 on sleep depend on whether the current episode is hypomanic or depressive. Hypomania is associated with a complaint of insomnia (mainly short sleep duration) or decreased need for sleep. In general, patients with hypomania report similar sleep symptoms as mania, but the symptoms are not as severe and do not cause significant distress. In fact, patients may enjoy more energy and a lower sleep requirement. The depressive phase may be associated with hypersomnia (see Table F41-2). In most bipolar patients, it is the depressive phases of illness that are the longest and have the greatest negative impact on quality of life.

Summary of minimum episode durations:
– Major depressive episode: 2 weeks

TABLE F41-2 **Manifestations of Patients with Bipolar and Unipolar Depression**

Bipolar 1 Depression More Likely	Unipolar Depression More Likely
Hypersomnia	Prominent insomnia
Hyperphagia	Reduced appetite, weight loss
Psychomotor retardation	Normal activity levels
Earlier age of onset of first episode	Later age of onset of first episode
Psychotic features (pathologic guilt)	Somatic complaints
Lability of mood	No family history of bipolar
Family history of bipolar disorder	

From Mitchell PB, Goodwin GM, Johnson GF, Hirschfeld RMA: Diagnostic guidelines for bipolar depression: a probabilistic approach, *Bipolar Disord* 10:144-152, 2008.

BOX F41-4 **Manic or Hypomanic Episodes and Sleep**

MANIC EPISODES

1. Marked insomnia
2. Refreshed with only a few hours of sleep
3. Polysomnography (PSG) findings
   • Reduced stage N3 sleep
   • Short REM latency
   • Increased REM density
4. Sleep loss may trigger mania

HYPOMANIC EPISODES

1. Report of decreased sleep need
2. Similar PSG findings as in mania may occur

BOX F41-5 **Diagnostic Criteria for Bipolar 2 Disorder**

A. Criteria have been met for at least one *hypomanic* episode (see below) and one or more major depressive episodes (see Table F41-1, A–C).
B. No manic episodes have occurred.
C. The depressive and hypomanic episodes are not better explained by another psychiatric disorder.
D. The symptoms of depression or unpredictability caused by frequent alternation between hypomanic and depression cause distress or impairment.

HYPOMANIC EPISODE

A. A distinct period of abnormally and persistently elevated, expansive, or irritable mood, *lasting at*

least 4 consecutive days and most of the day nearly every day.
B. Same characteristics as for mania episode are present.
C. The episodes represent unequivocal change in the function of the individual.
D. Changes in mood or function are observable by others.
E. The episode is not severe enough to cause marked impairment or to require hospitalization. If psychotic features are present, it is a manic episode.
F. Episodes are not explained by use of a medication or substance.

Adapted from American Psychiatric Association: *Diagnostic and statistical manual of mental disorders*, ed 5, Arlington, VA, 2013, American Psychiatric Association.

- Manic episode: 1 week, or any duration with hospitalization
- Hypomanic episode: 4 days

Treatment of Mood Disorders

Major Depressive Disorder

The treatment of MDD includes psychotherapy and antidepressant medications. A detailed discussion of the use of antidepressants is beyond the scope of this chapter. The effects of some antidepressants on sleep are discussed below.[8-10] In some patients, treatment of comorbid insomnia must be addressed with separate medications or behavioral treatment. A discussion of treatment of comorbid insomnia is found in Patient 124. Treatment of comorbid insomnia[11,12] is often an essential part of treatment of depression. An example is the study by Fava et al[12] of a group of patients with both major depressive disorder and insomnia. The combination of fluoxetine (FLX) and placebo was compared with FLX + 3 milligrams (mg) of eszopiclone. Coadministration of eszopiclone resulted in improved subjective sleep latency, WASO, and total sleep time (TST) compared with FLX alone. Although this result was not unexpected, a surprising finding was that greater improvement in depression at 8 weeks also resulted with the combination of FLX and eszopiclone.

Bipolar Disorder

Treatment for bipolar disorder is often based on the different phases: manic phase, depressive phase, and maintenance phase.[13] Some of the typical medications used for each phase are listed in Table F41-3. In Patient 125, a discussion of the treatment of depression in bipolar disorder is presented. It is important to note that bipolar depressive episodes are usually treated differently than unipolar depressive episodes.

Antidepressants are not administered in BP-1 (if at all) without a mood stabilizer. The medications approved by the U.S. Food and Drug Administration (FDA) for bipolar depression include quetiapine extended-release (XR) (Seroquel, BP-1 and BP-2), a combination of fluoxetine and olanzapine, (Symbax, BP-1), and lurasadone (Latuda, BP-1). Olanzapine, quetiapine, and lurasadone are atypical antipsychotics (second-generation antipsychotics). Mood stabilizers, including lithium, divalproex, and lamotrigine, are also used for treating bipolar depression. In the treatment for BP-2, a traditional antidepressant is sometime added to a mood stabilizer. One concern with the treatment of bipolar depression with a traditional antidepressant is precipitation of a manic episode. Of note, despite maintenance medications, a significant number of patients with bipolar disorder relapse into manic, hypomanic, or depressive phases. A very high risk of suicide exists in patients with bipolar disorder.

Effects of Antidepressants on Sleep

In general, antidepressants increase REM latency and decrease the amount of REM sleep[8,9] (Table F41-4). Bupropion is one of the few medications that can actually increase the amount of REM sleep, although it increases REM latency (at least in some studies). Nefazodone is a sedating antidepressant that also tends to increase REM sleep. Mirtazapine also has been reported to be associated with no or only mild reduction is the amount of REM sleep. The monoamine oxidase inhibitors (MAOIs) are less commonly used but are the most powerful suppressors of REM sleep. In general, sedating antidepressants have a beneficial effect on sleep efficiency, whereas nonsedating antidepressants tend to decrease sleep efficiency. Of note, if patients respond to an antidepressant, their subjective

TABLE F41-3 **Commonly Used Medications for Phases of Bipolar Disorders**

Mania	Maintenance	Depression
Valproic acid/valproate* or lithium* ± SGAP[†] Aripiprazole (Abilify)* Risperidone (Risperdal)* Ziprasidone (Geodon)* Olanzapine (Zyprexa)*	Lamotrigine* Lithium* Valproic acid/ valproate Aripiprazole Olanzapine* Ziprasidone*	Olanzapine + Fluoxetine (Symbax*, BP-1) Quetiapine XR (Seroquel XR*, BP1, BP2) Lurasadone* (Latuda, BP-1) Lithium Lamotrigine

Note: The list does not include all medications.
SGAP, Second generation antipsychotic.
*FDA approved for this indication.
[†]Aripiprazole, Ziprasidone, Olanzapine are approved as adjuncts for mania.

TABLE F41-4 **Effects of Antidepressants on Sleep**

	Continuity	Stage N3	REM	REM Latency	Sedation
TCAs					
Amitriptyline	↑↑↑	↑	↓↓↓	↑	++++
Doxepin	↑↑↑	↑↑↑	↓↓	↑	+++
Imipramine	↑↔	↑	↓↓	↑	++
Nortriptyline	↑	↑	↓↓	↑	++
Desipramine	↔	↑	↓↓	↑	+
Clomipramine	↑↔	↑	↓↓↓↓	↑	↔
MAOIs					
Phenelzine	↓	↔	↓↓↓↓	↑↑↑↑	↔
SSRIs					
Fluoxetine	↓	↓	↓	↑	±
Paroxetine	↓↓	↓	↓↓	↑	+ to ++
Sertraline	↔	↔↓	↓	↑	+
Citalopram	↔	↓	↓	↑	+
Escitalopram	↔	↓	↓	↑	+
SNRIs					
Venlafaxine	↓	↔↓	↓↓	↑↑	+ to ++
Desvenlafaxine	Same				
Duloxetine	Same				
Atypical					
Bupropion	↓↔	↔	↔↑	↔ or ↓	↔
Trazodone	↑	↔↑	↔↓	↑	4+
Mirtazapine	↑	↔↑	↔↓	↔	3+

Adapted from Winokur A, Gary KA, Rodner S, et al: Depression, sleep physiology, and antidepressant drugs, Depress Anxiety 14:19–28, 2001 and Gursky JT, Krahn LE: The effects of antidepressants on sleep: a review, Harvard Rev Psychiatry 8:298–306, 2000.
MAOIs, Monoamine oxidase inhibitors; *REM*, rapid eye movement; *SNRIs*, selective norepinephrine reuptake inhibitors; *SSRIs*, selective serotonin reuptake inhibitors; *TCAs*, tricyclic antidepressants.
↑, increased; ↓, decreased; ↔, no or minimal change;
1 to 4 +, increasing amounts of sedation.

estimate of their sleep quality may improve, even if objective sleep quality does not as indicated by PSG. A study comparing fluoxetine and nefazodone by Gillin et al[10] showed subjective improvements in sleep quality with both medications, but only patients on the sedating nefazodone had objective improvements in sleep.

Panic Disorder

The diagnostic criteria for panic disorder are listed in Box F41-6. Recurrent unexpected panic attacks (PAs) must be present for the diagnosis. At least one of the PAs is followed by a minimum of 1 month of persistent concern about additional panic attacks or maladaptive change in behavior related to the previous PA, for example, difficulty falling asleep to avoid a nocturnal PA. A nocturnal PA is in the differential diagnosis of parasomnia, including night terrors. Up to 60% of patients with panic disorder have a least one

nocturnal PA. About one third of patients with panic disorder have recurrent nocturnal PAs. Of those panic disorder patients with nocturnal PAs, up to two thirds report insomnia often associated with fear of returning to sleep. The symptom of dyspnea appears to be more common in nocturnal panic attacks. The attacks occur from non–rapid eye movement (NREM) sleep, commonly at the transition from stage N2 to stage N3 sleep. In most patients, sleep architecture is normal (normal REM latency and sleep efficiency). However, some patients may develop sleep phobia—and this may be associated with findings consistent with insomnia. In Patient 126, nocturnal PAs, panic disorder, and treatment of panic disorder are discussed.

Posttraumatic Stress Disorder

Posttraumatic stress disorder (PTSD) is associated with symptoms (Box F41-7) that occur after

BOX F41-6 Panic Disorder Diagnostic Criteria

A. Recurrent unexpected panic attacks: A panic attack is an abrupt surge on intense fear or intense discomfort that reaches a peak with a few minutes, and during which time four or more of the following symptoms occur:
   1. Palpitations
   2. Sweating
   3. Trembling, shaking
   4. Sensation of shortness of breath
   5. Choking
   6. Chest pain or discomfort
   7. Nausea
   8. Dizziness
   9. Chills or heat sensations
   10. Paresthesia, numbness, or tingling
   11. Derealization, or being detached from one's self
   12. Fear of losing control
   13. Fear of dying
B. At least one of the attacks has been followed by 1 month or more of one or both of the following:
   1. Persistent concern about additional panic attacks
   2. Maladaptive change in behavior related to attacks (avoiding certain activities)
C. Disturbance not caused by effects of a medication, substance, or medial disorder
D. Disturbance not caused by another psychiatric disorder

Adapted from American Psychiatric Association: *Diagnostic and statistical manual of mental disorders*, ed 5, Arlington, VA, 2013, American Psychiatric Association.

BOX F41-7 Diagnostic Criteria for Posttraumatic Stress Disorder (Abridged)

A. Exposure to actual or threatened death, serious injury, or sexual violence in one or more of the following ways: direct experience, witnessing events, learning of an event involving a family member, experiencing repeated or extreme exposure to aversive details of traumatic events (first responder exposed to human remains)
B. Presence of one or more of the following intrusion symptoms:
   1. Recurrent, involuntary, distressing memory of traumatic events
   2. Recurrent distressing dreams in which the content is related to the traumatic events
   3. Dissociative reactions (flashbacks)—individual feels traumatic event is occurring again
   4. Intense psychological distress at exposure to clues that symbolize the traumatic events
   5. Marked reactions to external or internal clues the resemble the traumatic event
C. Persistent avoidance of stimuli associated with the traumatic event
   1. Avoidance of distressing memories, thoughts, or feelings about the event
   2. Avoidance of external reminders of the event
D. Negative alterations in cognition and mood associated with the traumatic event(s), as evidenced by inability to remember important aspects of the traumatic event, persistent distorted cognitions about the event, inability to experience positive emotions, markedly diminished interest in participating in significant activities, feelings of detachment
E. Alterations in arousal and reactivity associated with traumatic events, as evidenced by irritable behavior and outbursts, reckless behavior, exaggerated startle response, sleep disturbance, hypervigilance, problems with concentration.

The criteria are abbreviated for simplicity.
Adapted from American Psychiatric Association: *Diagnostic and statistical manual of mental disorders*, ed 5, Arlington, VA, 2013, American Psychiatric Association.

exposure to an extremely traumatic stressor involving (1) direct personal experience of an event that involves actual or threatened death, serious injury, or other threat to one's physical integrity; (2) witnessing an event that involves death, injury, or a threat to the physical integrity of another person; or (3) learning about unexpected or violent death, serious harm, or threat of death or injury experienced by a family member or other close associate. The person's response to the event must involve intense fear, helplessness, or horror. The characteristic symptoms resulting from the exposure to the extreme

trauma include persistent reexperiencing of the traumatic event, persistent avoidance of stimuli associated with the trauma, numbing of general responsiveness, and persistent symptoms of increased arousal.

Recurrent distressing dreams (i.e., nightmares) of the traumatic event are one of the diagnostic features of PTSD. For many patients with PTSD, the associated nightmares represent one of the most frequently occurring and problematic aspects of the disorder. Persistent nightmares may also be one of the most enduring symptoms in PTSD. High percentages of patients (70%–90%) describe subjective sleep disturbance. However, PSG studies of patients with PTSD have yielded variable and inconclusive findings with regard to abnormalities in REM sleep, and controlled studies have not found consistent abnormalities. More discussion of PTSD and nightmares is found in Patient 127.

CLINICAL PEARLS

1. A significant proportion of patients with a sleep complaint have a psychiatric illness, and a significant number of patients with a psychiatric illness have a sleep complaint.

2. Insomnia or hypersomnia nearly every day is one of the nine major criteria for a diagnosis of a major depressive episode.

3. During a major depressive episode, about 80% of patients complain of symptoms of insomnia (frequent awakenings, early-morning awakenings), and 20% complain of hypersomnia.

4. PSG during a depressive episode shows long sleep latency, reduced sleep efficiency, reduced stage N3 sleep, short REM latency, longer first REM period, and higher REM density early in the night. Early morning awakenings may also be present.

5. Insomnia may precede a major depressive episode and is often the last symptom of depression to resolve. Some, but not all, studies have suggested that the persistence of sleep complaints is a risk factor for relapse of depression.

6. During manic episodes, the patient reports a decreased need for sleep (feeling rested on a few hours of sleep). Sleep loss may precipitate a manic episode.

7. Hypomanic episodes have similar characteristics as manic episodes except for the following three conditions: (a) severe impairment is not present, (b) hospitalization is not necessary, and (c) no psychotic features are present. If any of the three are present, the episode is considered a manic episode.

8. BP-1 requires at least one manic episode with or without one or more depressive episodes. Note that unlike the diagnostic criteria for BP-2, the presence of at least one major depressive episode is not required.

9. BP-2 requires at least one hypomanic episode and one major depressive episode but *no* manic episodes.

10. Relapse rates in bipolar disorder patients even on maintenance medication are very high. Bipolar disorder is a significant risk factor for suicide. The depressive phases of BP disorders are more frequent than mania/hypomania and cause much of the morbidity of BP disorders.

11. Most patients with nocturnal PAs have similar episodes during the day. However, PAs may occur mainly at night and must be differentiated from NREM parasomnia types such as sleep terrors.

12. Most patients with PTSD have a high frequency of disturbed sleep. Recurrent nightmares are often a major cause of disturbed sleep.

REFERENCES

1. American Psychiatric Association: *Diagnostic and statistical manual of mental disorders*, ed 5, Arlington, VA, 2013, American Psychiatric Association.
2. Kessler RC, Demler O, Frank RG, et al: Prevalence and treatment of mental disorders, 1990 to 2003, *N Engl J Med* 352:2515–2523, 2005.
3. Peterson MJ, Benca RM: Sleep in mood disorders, *Psychiatr Clin North Am* 29:1009–1032, 2006.
4. Benca RM, Obermeyer WH, Thisted RA, et al: Sleep and psychiatric disorders: a meta-analysis, *Arch Gen Psychiatry* 49:651–668, 1992.
5. Rush AJ, Erman MK, Giles DE, et al: Polysomnographic findings in recently drug-free and clinically remitted depressed patients, *Arch Gen Psychiatry* 43:878–884, 1986.
6. Nofzinger EA, Thase ME, Reynolds CF 3rd, et al: Hypersomnia in bipolar depression: a comparison with narcolepsy using the multiple sleep latency test, *Am J Psychiatry* 148:1177–1181, 1991.
7. Wehr TA: Sleep loss as a possible mediator of diverse causes of mania, *Br J Psychiatry* 159:576–578, 1991.

8. Winokur A, Gary KA, Rodner S, et al: Depression, sleep physiology, and antidepressant drugs, *Depress Anxiety* 14:19–28, 2001.
9. Gursky JT, Krahn LE: The effects of antidepressants on sleep: a review, *Harvard Rev Psychiatry* 8:298–306, 2000.
10. Gillin JC, Rapaport M, Erman MK, et al: A comparison of nefazodone and fluoxetine on mood and on objective, subjective, and clinician-rated measures of sleep in depressed patients, *J Clin Psychiatry* 58:186–192, 1997.
11. Nierenberg AA, Adler LA, Peselow E, et al: Trazodone for antidepressant-associated insomnia, *Am J Psychiatry* 151:1069, 1994.
12. Fava M, McCall V, Krystal A, et al: Eszopiclone co-administered with fluoxetine in patients with insomnia coexisting with major depressive disorder, *Biol Psychiatry* 59:1052–1060, 2006.
13. Hilty DM, Leamon MH, Lim RF, et al: Diagnosis and treatment of bipolar disorder in the primary care setting: a concise review, *Prim Psychiatry* 13:77–85, 2006.

Patients with Fatigue and Abnormal Sleep

Patient A: A 40-year-old woman was evaluated for fatigue and disturbed sleep experienced over a period of 6 months. The patient went to bed at 11 PM and fell asleep in 15 to 45 minutes. She reported about three awakenings nightly and an earlier-than-normal wake time (5:00 AM). During the day, she felt extremely fatigued. No of history of cataplexy or sleep paralysis was present. The patient's husband reported that she frequently snored but never kicked or moved her legs during sleep. She denied feeling depressed but did admit to being under a lot of stress after a recent promotion and worrying that she was not spending enough time with her husband. Her usual recreation activities were no longer pleasurable to her. No history of prior treatment for depression or episodes of mania was present.

Physical Examination: Unremarkable **Polysomnography results:** Table P123-1.

TABLE P123-1 Polysomnography Results (Patient A)

Lights-Out	10:00 PM	Lights-On	6:00 AM	Final Awakening	4:17 AM
Total Recording Time	420 min	(419-464)	Sleep Stage	% TST	
Total sleep time	302 min	(402-449)	Stage N1	15	(3-7)
Sleep efficiency	72 %	(94-98)	Stage N2	55	(51-64)
Sleep latency	15 min	(2-14)	Stage N3	5	(5-17)
REM latency	40 min	(65-99)	Stage REM	25	(19-25)
WASO	103 min	(10-40)			
Arousal index (ArI)	10/hr				
Respiratory ArI	5/hr				
AHI	2/hr				
PLM index	0/hr				

REM, Rapid eye movement; ( ), normal range for age; *AHI*, apnea-hypopnea index; *WASO*, wake after sleep onset; *PLM*, periodic limb movement.

Question 1: What is causing the fatigue and sleep disturbance experienced by Patient A?

Patient B: A 45-year-old man was evaluated for a 6-month history of daytime sleepiness (Epworth Sleepiness Scale [ESS] score of 16/24). During this time, he had developed a tremendous appetite and had gained 20 pounds. He also had increased difficulty dealing with the stresses of his job. His wife reported that he was hypersensitive to criticism and that he seemed to believe she did not love him anymore. The patient usually retired at 10 PM and slept until the alarm clock awakened him at 6:30 AM. He had tremendous difficulty getting out of bed and was late to work on several occasions. On the weekends, he sometimes slept from 11 PM until 10 to 11 AM. The patient was reported to snore, but his wife had not noticed any pauses in breathing.

Physical examination: Height 5 feet 11 inches; weight 210 pounds; neck: 16 inch-circumference; HEENT: slightly edematous uvula; chest: clear; cardiac: normal; extremities: no edema **Polysomnography results:** (Table P123-2).

TABLE P123-2 **Polysomnography results (Patient B)**

Lights-Out	10:30 PM	Lights-On	6:00 AM	Final Awakening	4:17 AM
Total Recording Time	450 min	(419-464)	Sleep Stage	% TST	
Total sleep time	391.5 min	(343-436)	Stage N1	15	(3-7)
Sleep efficiency	87 %	(94-98)	Stage N2	60	(51-64)
Sleep latency	15 min	(2-18)	Stage N3	5	(5-17)
REM latency	35 min	(55-78)	Stage R	20	(19-25)
WASO	43.5 min	(0-40)			
Arousal index (ArI)	10/hr				
Respirtory ArI	5/hr				
AHI	1/hr				
PLM index	0/hr				

REM, Rapid eye movement; ( ), normal values for age; *AHI*,= apnea + hypopnea index; *WASO*, wake after sleep onset; *PLM*, periodic limb movement.

Question 2: What is causing this Patient B' hypersomnia?

ANSWERS

1. **Answer for Patient A:** Major depressive disorder with a short rapid eye movement (REM) sleep latency.

   Discussion: Approximately 90% of patients with major depression complain of sleep disturbance. If the patient reports feelings of sadness and despair, the diagnosis is obvious. However, a patient may emphasize loss of energy, change in appetite, or loss of pleasure in life (ahedonia). Therefore, depression should be considered in anyone complaining of sleep disturbance and fatigue. Rather than ask about depression, the question should be: "Do you find life less interesting or pleasurable?" A medical evaluation is essential to rule out anemia, hypothyroidism, vitamin D deficiency, and other causes of fatigue. Fifty percent of sleep studies performed in patients suffering from depression show objective abnormalities (Table P123-3). *Abnormalities of REM sleep are common and include reduced REM sleep latency (typically 40–60 minutes, but occasionally is in the range suggestive of narcolepsy [<15 minutes]), a longer first REM episode (20–25 minutes instead of the usual 10–15 minutes), and a higher REM density (number of REMs per time) than normal.* These alterations in REM sleep may persist even after successful treatment of depression or between depressive episodes. A short REM sleep latency may be seen with other psychiatric disorders, including schizophrenia and borderline personality disorder.

   In patients with unipolar depression, insomnia with early-morning awakening usually is the major sleep complaint (15% to 20% complain of hypersomnia). Sleep complaints tend to be more pronounced in older patients. Typical sleep study findings are increased sleep latency, decreased sleep efficiency, increased stage W (wakefulness) and stage N1, decreased stage N3, reduced total sleep, and early-morning awakening. The sleep of older patients with depression tends to be more disturbed than that of younger patients. *In the depressive phase of bipolar disorder, seasonal affective disorder (SAD), and atypical depression, hypersomnia typically is the major complaint, with a prolonged total sleep time and daytime sleepiness.* However, in research studies, sleep latency on the multiple sleep latency test (MSLT) was not found to be shortened.

   A sleep study for evaluation of possible depression is not indicated unless another sleep disorder is suspected. The finding of short REM sleep latency, of itself, is not specific for depression, but in the absence of other pathology, it is suggestive. Sometimes, it is difficult to determine if the major patient complaint is fatigue or daytime sleepiness. The major utility of a sleep study is to rule out other sleep disorders. Psychological questionnaires also may help uncover suspected depression.

In Patient A, a sleep study was ordered because of the history of snoring to rule out obstructive sleep apnea (OSA). The study (see Table P123-1) revealed a modestly shortened nocturnal REM sleep latency, early-morning awakening, and absence of evidence for sleep apnea and periodic limb movement disorder. Interestingly, the first REM period was quite long (25 minutes) and REM density (number of eye movements per epoch) was unusually high during this initial episode of REM. Recall that during the initial episode of REM sleep, only one or two bursts of eye movements are normally seen per epoch. The sleep study findings in Patient A suggested the possibility of depression. Subsequently, symptoms of depression were explored in more detail when the sleep study results were discussed with the patient. At that time, she admitted that she felt torn between her responsibilities to her employer and to her husband and was overwhelmed at times. The patient was referred to a psychiatrist so that she could explore these issues. Treatment with counseling and fluoxetine 20 milligrams (mg) every day resulted in improvement in symptoms and early-morning awakening. Of note, antidepressant treatment often improves the perception of sleep quality more that objective improvement. As discussed in Patient 124, treatment aimed specifically at insomnia complaints may be needed.

2. **Answer:** Atypical depression.

Discussion: Insomnia is the most common sleep complaint of patients with depression, and hypersomnia is commonly noted in patients experiencing the depressive phase of bipolar disorder, SAD (seasonal affective disorder, winter depression), or atypical depression. *Atypical depression is characterized by weight gain (hyperphagia), rejection hypersensitivity, hypersomnia, and leaden paralysis (heavy feeling in the extremities).* The classic treatment of atypical depression is a monoamine oxidase inhibitor (MAOI), as these medications increase serotonin, norepinephrine, and dopamine. Because of the required dietary restrictions, these medications are not commonly used unless other treatments fail. Selective serotonin reuptake inhibitors (SSRIs) are commonly used, as these have relatively few side effects and are not usually sedating. However, augmentation with another agent such as bupropion or aripiprazole is often needed. Aripiprazole (Abilify) is approved by the U.S. Food and Drug Administration (FDA) as adjunctive treatment for depression. The treatment of patients with bipolar depression is discussed in Patient 125. SAD is characterized by a regular temporal relationship between the onset of depression (fall or winter). Remission of depression occurs at a regular time (spring). Patients often complain of sleeping late and feeling tired all the time. SAD often responds to light therapy (usually in the early morning hours). For example, 10,000 lux for 30 minutes beginning about 3 hours after the sleep midpoint of spontaneous sleep has been recommended.

The differential diagnosis of hypersomnia with depression includes recurrent hypersomnia, sleep apnea, and idiopathic hypersomnia. Recurrent hypersomnia (Kleine-Levin syndrome) is characterized by episodes (at least once or twice yearly) lasting 3 to 21 days and featuring voracious eating, hypersexuality, and disinhibited behavior (e.g., irritability, aggression). Monosymptomatic forms (hypersomnolence only) also exist. This disorder typically affects males and starts in adolescence. Onset in adulthood and occurrence in women have been described. During intervals between periods of somnolence, individuals appear normal. Patients with idiopathic hypersomnia complain of sleep drunkenness and difficulty getting up in the morning. Although patients with idiopathic hypersomnia usually have a mean sleep latency (MSL) of ≤ 8 minutes on an MSLT, the MSL in atypical depression is usually ≥ 10 minutes. The depressive phase of bipolar disorder often has the characteristics of atypical depression, but the patient usually has a history of prior mania or hypomania.

In the present case, the history of snoring and weight gain prompted a sleep study to rule out OSA. The study (see Table P123-2) did not document obstructive sleep apnea. The REM sleep latency was moderately short—a characteristic of a variety of disorders, including sleep apnea, narcolepsy, and depression. However, no history consistent with narcolepsy was present. There was no history of mania or hypomania. Onset of recurrent hypersomnia is extremely unlikely at age 45. Given the weight gain, hypersomnia, and recent onset of problems dealing with criticism and rejection, the diagnosis of atypical depression was considered a likely possibility, and the patient was referred to a psychiatrist for evaluation. Treatment with fluoxetine produced considerable improvement within 4 weeks, but the patient remained fatigued and still had difficulty getting out of bed. Bupropion was added to fluoxetine for augmentation, and by 2 months, the patient had lost about 10 pounds. The symptoms of daytime sleepiness resolved.

TABLE P123-3 Polysomnography Findings in Mood Disorders

Mood Disorders	Complaints	Sleep Study Findings
Depression	Insomnia in about 80% and Hypersomnia in about 20% of those with sleep complaints Frequent awakening Early morning awakening Fatigue	Increased sleep latency Decreased rapid eye movement (REM) latency Increased REM density or long first REM period Normal or increased amount of REM sleep Decreased stage N3
Bipolar depression Season affective disorder Atypical depression	Hypersomnia	Decreased REM sleep latency Increased total sleep time

CLINICAL PEARLS

1. A moderately short REM sleep latency and a prolonged initial REM period with an increase in REM density is characteristic of depression. These findings may persist after successful treatment or be present between depressive episodes.

2. Depression may present with complaints of disturbed sleep and early-morning awakening (unipolar depression) or hypersomnia (bipolar depression, atypical unipolar depression, seasonal affective disorder).

3. Depression always should be considered when evaluating insomnia or excessive daytime sleepiness.

4. Consider depression when patients complain of fatigue and disturbed sleep.

5. Instead of asking "Do you feel depressed?" ask: "Do you find life less interesting or less pleasurable?" Many patients will not admit that they have depression, if asked directly.

6. Patients with atypical depression may gain weight (hyperphagia) complain of fatigue or sleepiness, and thus may trigger the suspicion of sleep apnea.

7. Atypical depression is characterized by hypersomnia, hyperphagia or weight gain, leaden paralysis (heavy feeling in the extremities), or rejection hypersensitivity.

BIBLIOGRAPHY

American Psychiatric Association: *Diagnostic and statistical manual of mental disorders*, ed 5, Arlington, VA, 2013, American Psychiatric Association.

Benca RM, Obermeyer WH, Thisted RA, et al: Sleep and psychiatric disorders: a meta-analysis, *Arch Gen Psychiatry* 49:651–668, 1992.

Kurlansik SL, Ibay AD: Seasonal affective disorder, *Am Fam Physician* 86(11):1037–1041, 2012.

Lam RW, Levitt AJ, Levitan RD, et al: The Can-SAD study: a randomized controlled trial of the effectiveness of light therapy and fluoxetine in patients with winter seasonal affective disorder, *Am J Psychiatry* 163(5):805–812, 2006.

Nofzinger EA, Thase ME, Reynolds CF 3rd, et al: Hypersomnia in bipolar depression: a comparison with narcolepsy using the multiple sleep latency test, *Am J Psychiatry* 148:1177–1181, 1991.

Pande AC, Birkett M, Fechner-Bates S, et al: Fluoxetine versus phenelzine in atypical depression, *Biol Psych* 40(10):1017–1020, 1996.

Peterson MJ, Benca RM: Sleep in mood disorders, *Psychiatr Clin North Am* 29:1009–1032, 2006.

Rush AJ, Erman MK, Giles DE, et al: Polysomnographic findings in recently drug-free and clinically remitted depressed patients, *Arch Gen Psychiatry* 43:878–884, 1986.

Terman JS, Terman M, Lo E, Cooper TB: Circadian time of morning light administration and therapeutic response in winter depression, *Arch Gen Psychiatry* 58:69–73, 2001.

A 45-Year-Old Man with Persistent Insomnia While on Treatment for Depression

A 45-year-old man was referred by his primary care physician for evaluation and treatment of insomnia. The patient had a long history of major depressive episodes, which generally responded to treatment with selective serotonin reuptake inhibitors (SSRIs). However, he had difficulty with the side effects of the medication. The current episode was under treatment with fluoxetine 60 milligrams (mg) daily, and although the patient's energy level and feelings of sadness were much improved, he continued to have difficulty initiating and maintaining sleep. Frequent awakenings during the night were a major problem. The patient felt tired in the morning. No history of snoring was present, and the patient's wife reported the absence of leg kicks and apnea.

Physical examination: Height 6 feet; weight 200 pounds; vital signs: normal; HEENT: Mallampati 2; neck: 16-inch circumference; chest: clear; cardiac: normal; extremities: no edema

QUESTION

1. What is your diagnosis? What treatment do you recommend?

ANSWER

1. **Answer:** Insomnia comorbid with depression or as a side effect of antidepressant therapy.

Discussion: Insomnia is a common complaint of patients with depression. Up to 60% of depressed patients complain of insomnia, including difficulty initiating sleep, maintaining sleep, or both and early morning awakenings. Although some characteristic findings on polysomnography (PSG) are present in patients with depression and insomnia (short REM sleep latency), the findings are not sufficiently sensitive or specific to make PSG a useful diagnostic test for depression. PSG is indicated mainly if sleep apnea is felt to be present.

Insomnia is also a well-known side effect of most antidepressants. The exceptions include sedating antidepressants (sedating tricyclic antidepressants (TCAs); amitriptyline, doxepin), mirtazapine, nefazodone, and trazodone. A unique property of nefazodone is that it may increase the amount of REM sleep. Most other antidepressants with the exception of mirtazapine, bupropion and possibly trazodone decrease the amount of REM sleep. Monoamine oxidase inhibitors (MAOIs) are sometimes used to treat refractory depression. They are the most potent inhibitors of REM sleep.

The two major treatment options for comorbid insomnia include cognitive and behavioral treatment of insomnia (CBTI) and pharmacotherapy (Table P124-1). CBTI may be an effective treatment, if available, and patients are motivated. Pharmacotherapy options include (1) full dose of a sedating antidepressant (e.g., mirtazapine), (2) nonsedating antidepressant + low-dose sedating antidepressant (e.g., escitalopram and low-dose trazodone), (3) nonsedating antidepressant + benzodiazepine receptor agonist (BZRA; e.g., fluoxetine and zolpidem), (4) full dose of a nonsedating antidepressant + low-dose sedating second-generation antipsychotic (e.g., fluoxetine + low-dose quetiapine). Most patients with mild-to-moderate depression are started on SSRIs such as fluoxetine, paroxetine, sertaline, citalopram, and escitalopram. SSRIs and selective norepinephrine

TABLE P124-1	**Treatment of Comorbid Insomnia and Depression**
1. Sedating antidepressant at an antidepressant dose	Full-dose sedating antidepressant: - Mirtazapine (15–45 mg) - Nefazodone (150-300 mg bid)[†]
2. Nonsedating antidepressant at an antidepressant dose + low-dose sedating antidepressant	Low-dose sedating antidepressant: - Trazodone (25–100 mg) - Doxepin 10–25 mg - Doxepin (Silenor)* 3 mg, 6 mg - Mirtazapine 7.5 mg
3. Nonsedating antidepressant at an antidepressant dose + benzodiazepine receptor agonist (BZRA)	BZRAs: - Zolpidem* (5–10 mg, 6.25 mg, 12.5 mg CR) - Eszopiclone* (2–3 mg) - Temazepam* (15–30 mg) - Lorazepam (0.5–2 mg) - Alprazolam (0.25–0.75)
4. Nonsedating antidepressant at an antidepressant dose + sedating atypical antipsychotic	Sedating atypical antipsychotic: - Quetiapine (25-50 mg)
5. Nonsedating antidepressant at antidepressant dose + cognitive behavioral treatment of insomnia (CBT-I)	

*FDA approved as a hypnotic. (Silenor approved for sleep maintenance insomnia).
[†]Rarely associated with hepatic failure (1 per 250,000 to 300,000 patient years), used if other medications not effective.

reuptake inhibitors (SNRIs; venlafaxine, desvenlafaxine, duloxetine), and bupropion (increases dopamine and serotonin) are also widely used. These agents have fewer side effects than the traditional TCAs. Unfortunately, insomnia is a common side effect of these medications.

The sedating antidepressants typically used at full antidepressant dose include mirtazapine and nefazodone. Nefazadone has been rarely associated with hepatic toxicity. The problem may have been related to the previous formulation. However, given the many other treatment options, nefazodone is rarely used.

Mirtazapine is an effective antidepressant that may be tried if patients have depression and refractory insomnia. This medication increases both serotonin and norepinephrine via central alpha-2 receptor blockade rather than reuptake inhibition. Like nefazodone, mirtazapine also blocks 5-hydroxytryptamine type 2 (5HT2) (serotonin type 2) receptors, and this may enhance sleep quality. Mirtazapine also blocks 5HT3 receptors and histamine type 1 receptors. The antihistamine activity is associated with sedation even at low doses. Unfortunately, the antihistamine activity is also frequently associated with weight gain. This is the side effect of mirtazapine that patients find most distressing. An advantage of nefazodone, bupropion, and mirtazapine is that they do not cause sexual dysfunction.

The sedating antidepressants used in combination with a full-dose antidepressant include low-dose trazodone (25–50 mg), mirtazapine (7.5 mg), and doxepin (3 mg, 6 mg). BZRA hypnotics such as zolpidem, eszopiclone, and temazepam may be added to an effective antidepressant medication. Other BZRAs not approved as hynotics by the U.S. Food and Drug Administration (FDA) for insomnia with anxiolytic activity (clonazepam, alprazolam, lorazepam) may also be added to a nonsedating antidepressant. Finally, a low-dose sedating second-generation antipsychotic such as quetiapine (25–50 mg) may be added to an antidepressant dose of a nonsedating antidepressant. The medication may cause hyperglycemia and tardive dyskinesia, so it is best reserved for refractory cases.

Trazodone was, at one time, the most commonly prescribed hypnotic, even though very little evidence for efficacy as a hypnotic in patients without depression is available. One reason for its popularity is that it has minimal anticholinergic side effects (constipation, urinary retention) compared with the sedating TCAs. Trazodone has no consistent effect on the amount of REM sleep but does prolong REM sleep latency. Men must be counseled about *priapism* (painful, persistent erection), a rare (1 in 8000), but significant, side effect. Priapism is a condition in which the erect penis does not return to its flaccid state within 4 hours despite the absence of both physical and psychological stimulation. Priapism may occur with trazodone doses in the range of 50 to 150 mg/day, with onset usually occurring during the first month of therapy. Cases of priapism have been reported after a single 100-mg dose of trazodone. Trazodone may rarely cause a female equivalent of priapism, *clitoral priapism*, which is associated with pain and discomfort. Priapism is believed to be cause by alpha-1 antagonism. Postural hypotension is another potential side effect of trazodone related to alpha-receptor blockade. Doxepin in low doses (Silenor: 3, 6 mg) is sedating without having the associated anticholinergic side effects noted at higher doses.

In some patients with depression, treatment with a nonsedating antidepressant may improve the subjective perception of sleep, even though minimal objective improvement occurs. For example, in a study by Gillin et al comparing nefazodone (sedating) and fluoxetine (nonsedating) in patients with depression, both were effective antidepressants, but only nefazodone improved *objective* sleep quality. Interestingly, the fluoxetine group also reported *subjective* improvements in sleep quality. Thus, the traditional SSRIs may actually improve a patient's perception of sleep by improving mood.

As previously mentioned, CBT-I is another treatment option in patients with comorbid insomnia and depression. If insomnia is a major concern in a patient with depression, CBT-I may be started along with antidepressant therapy.

In the current case, since the patient's depression had responded well to fluoxetine, trazodone 50 mg at bedtime was added to the fluoxetine regimen. The patient reported a slight improvement, and the dose was increased to 100 mg at bedtime. On this combination of medications, he reported improved sleep quality and felt rested on awakening in the morning.

CLINICAL PEARLS

1. Insomnia is a frequent complaint of patients with depression.

2. Insomnia in patients with depression may be exacerbated by treatment with SSRIs or SNRIs.

3. The addition of a low dose of trazodone (50–100 mg) or a BZRA at bedtime may improve sleep in patients having persistent or worsened sleep difficulty on SSRI, bupropion, or SNRI treatment.

4. Switching from an SSRI to nefazodone or mirtazapine may improve sleep quality in patients with depression and persistent insomnia.

5. Trazodone is associated with priapism (1 in 8000) and postural hypotension but does not have anticholinergic side effects. Low-dose doxepin (3, 6 mg) is also sedating with few anticholinergic side effects.

6. Mirtazapine is sedating at low or antidepressant doses. The major concern is weight gain.

7. Comorbid insomnia in a patient being treated for depression may improve with CBT-I.

BIBLIOGRAPHY

Edinger JD, Olsen MK, Stechuchak KM, et al: Cognitive behavioral therapy for patients with primary insomnia or insomnia associated predominantly with mixed psychiatric disorders: a randomized clinical trial, *Sleep* 32(4):499–510, 2009.

Gillin JC, Rapaport M, Erman MK, et al: A comparison of nefazodone and fluoxetine on mood and on objective, subject, and clinician-rated measures of sleep in depressed patients, *J Clin Psychiatry* 58:186–192, 1997.

Kent JM: SNaRIs, NaSSAs, and NaRIs: new agents for the treatment of depression, *Lancet* 355:911–918, 2000.

Neylan TC: Treatment of sleep disturbance in depressed patients, *J Clin Psychiatry* 56(Suppl 2):56–61, 1995.

Nierenberg AA, Adler LA, Peselow E, et al: Trazodone for antidepressant-associated insomnia, *Am J Psychiatry* 151:1069, 1994.

Sánchez-Ortuño MM, Edinger JD: Cognitive-behavioral therapy for the management of insomnia comorbid with mental disorders, *Curr Psychiatry Rep* 14(5):519–528, 2012.

Serretti A, Mandelli L: Antidepressants and body weight: a comprehensive review and meta-analysis, *J Clin Psychiatry* 71:1259–1272, 2010.

Watanabe N, Omori IM, Nakagawa A: Safety reporting and adverse-event profile of mirtazapine described in randomized controlled trials in comparison with other classes of antidepressants in the acute-phase treatment of adults with depression: systematic review and meta-analysis, *CNS Drugs* 24:35–53, 2010.

A 30-Year-Old Woman Who Has Difficulty Getting Out of Bed

A 30-year-old woman was referred for possible idiopathic hypersomnia. The patient had a sleep study that did not document obstructive sleep apnea (OSA). She has a 3-month history of severe sleepiness. She slept 9 to 10 hours a night and still had difficulty getting out of bed. The patient was not taking any medications but did admit to daily alcohol use and had gained 5 pounds over the last several months. She reported that "life is not fun anymore" and had no pleasure in any activity. Over the last 2 years, she reported at least two episodes, each lasting several weeks, during which time she had less need for sleep, with associated increases in mood, energy, and libido. During the last episode, she exceeded her credit-card limit and had sexual encounters with two married coworkers. This behavior was very atypical for her and almost resulted in her being fired from her job. Her Epworth Sleepiness Scale (ESS) score was 12/24. To evaluate the patient's daytime sleepiness a PSG and MSLT were ordered.

Laboratory findings: thyroid studies and vitamin D level are normal.

Polysomnography (PSG): total sleep time (TST): 420 minutes; sleep latency: 5 minutes; rapid eye movement (REM) sleep latency: 60 minutes; apnea–hypopnea index (AHI) 2 per hour

Multiple sleep latency test (MSLT): mean sleep latency (MSL): 10 minutes; no sleep-onset REM periods (SOREMPs)

QUESTION

1. What do you recommend?
   A. Escitalopram 10 milligrams (mg)
   B. Repeat PSG and MSLT
   C. Modafinil 200 mg every morning
   D. Psychiatric referral

ANSWER

1. **Answer:** D. Psychiatric referral for bipolar-2 disorder in depressive phase.

   Discussion: Depression is part of the differential diagnosis of excessive sleepiness. Patients may report sleepiness, but on close questioning, fatigue may be a better description of their problem. They often report not being able to get out of bed or function at work or school. Ahedonia (lack of pleasure) and depressed mood are usually reported. Although patients with typical depression often report insomnia and weight loss, patients with atypical depression report hypersomnia and often weight gain. Atypical insomnia may occur with unipolar depression, seasonal affective disorder (SAD), or the depressive phases of bipolar disorder. Some characteristics of bipolar depression versus unipolar depression are listed in Table P125-1.

   When patients present with bipolar depression, they are often incorrectly diagnosed as having major depressive disorder (e.g., unipolar depression). Unfortunately, the treatments for bipolar depression differ substantially from those for unipolar depression, so the treatment is often ineffective or precipitates an attack of mania or hypomania. The physician must carefully question the patient about prior episodes of mania or hypomania. Episodes of mania result in incapacitation, often resulting in hospitalization, inability to function, or psychotic behavior. Hypomania is more subtle, and the patient may continue to function but reports high energy level, less need for sleep,

TABLE P125-1   **Manifestations of Bipolar and Unipolar Depression**

Bipolar Depression More Likely	Unipolar Depression More Likely
Hypersomnia	Prominent insomnia
Hyperphagia	Reduced appetite; weight loss
Psychomotor retardation	Normal activity levels
Earlier age of onset of first episode (also peripartum depression)	Later age of onset of first episode
Psychotic features (pathologic guilt)	Somatic complaints
Lability of mood	No family history of bipolar disorder
Family history of bipolar disorder	

From Mitchell PB, Goodwin GM, Johnson GF, Hirschfeld RMA: Diagnostic guidelines for bipolar depression: a probabilistic approach, *Bipolar Disord* 10:144-152, 2008.

TABLE P125-2   **Diagnosis of BP-1 versus BP-2**

	Required	May occur
Bipolar (BP)-1	Mania— one or more episodes	Hypomanic episodes Major depressive episodes
Bipolar-2	One or more episodes of hypomania AND One or more major depressive episodes No episode of mania	

and impulsive behavior that is distinctly different from their normal functioning. The symptoms are similar to mania but less pronounced.

A diagnosis of bipolar depression 1 (BP-1) requires *at least one manic episode*. One or more major depressive episodes (MDEs) or hypomanic episodes may occur. Typically, patients have more MDEs than manic episodes during their lifetime. The depressive part of the illness is often the most debilitating. A diagnosis of BP-2 requires at least one hypomanic episode *and* at least one MDE. An episode of mania cannot occur (otherwise the diagnosis is BP-1). See Table P125-2.

Patients with BP-1 are typically symptomatic about 50% of the time, with time of depression being about three times that of mania. The illness is frequently associated with other coexisting conditions, most commonly anxiety disorders and substance use disorders. These disorders are associated with an increased risk of suicidal ideation and mood switches from depression to mania. Patients with BP-1 have an increased risk of suicide (about 5% completed suicide if never hospitalized). Patients with BP-2 do *not* have milder disease, and it is the episodes of depression that have the greatest negative impact on the patient's life.

A detailed discussion of the treatment of bipolar depression is beyond the scope of this book. However, a few important points will be emphasized. No selective serotonin reuptake inhibitors (SSRI) and selective norepinephrine reuptake inhibitors (SNRI) have been approved by the U.S. Food and Drug Administration (FDA)for the treatment of bipolar depression. The approved medications include quetiapine XR (Seroquel XR for BP-1 and BP-2) and a combination of fluoxetine and olanzapine, (Symbax for BP-1), and lurasadone (Latuda for BP-1). Olanzapine, quetiapine, and lurasadone are atypical antipsychotics (second-generation antipsychotics). Other medications used for the treatment of bipolar depression include lithium, lamotrigine, and valproic acid or divalproex (mood stabilizers). The addition of an antidepressant (except with Symbax) has not been shown to be beneficial. However, for treating BP-2, many psychiatrists add an antidepressant to a mood stabilizer if the patient is not responding. Paroxetine, fluoxetine, and sertraline have the best record of not inducing a switch to mania. Bupropion is also used. Of note, improvement in the symptoms of unipolar depression usually takes ≥4 weeks after starting an antidepressant. If a patient with depression responds very quickly to an antidepressant, this may actually be a switch to hypomania. Usually, the response wears off in a few weeks.

Sleep has a major role in BP disorders. In manic episodes, the patient reports sleeping little but not feeling sleepy. In hypomania also, the need for sleep is less but no sleepiness is present. Of note, sleep deprivation may also precipitate mania. During depressive episodes, patients complain of hypersomnia, but the MSL on a MSLT is usually ≥ 10 minutes. Patients with bipolar depression who have difficulty sleeping or have anxiety may require clonazepam, alprazolam, or a medication approved as a hypnotic (zolpidem, temazepam). It is important to note that although a stimulant or modafinil is sometimes used as adjunctive therapy for depression, these medications may on rare occasion precipitate an episode of mania.

In the present case, the patient was referred to a psychiatrist, who confirmed the suspicion of BP-2 disorder. The patient was started on quetiapine XR and referred to a dietician in an attempt to minimize weight gain. Unfortunately, weight gain and glucose intolerance prompted a change to lamotrigine (dose needs to be slowly increased to avoid skin reactions). After several months, the patient's condition improved. The patient continues on lamotrigine.

CLINICAL PEARLS

1. Bipolar depression is a part of the differential diagnosis of excessive daytime sleepiness. Patients do *not* usually have *objective* evidence of hypersomnia (MSL on a MSLT >10 minutes).

2. Bipolar depression is often misdiagnosed as unipolar depression.

3. The treatment of bipolar depression differs substantially from that of unipolar depression and is best directed by a psychiatrist.

4. A diagnosis of BP-1 requires at least one manic episode. Episodes of hypomania or depression may occur.

5. A diagnosis of BP-2 requires at least one hypomanic episode *and* one major depressive episode and the absence of any manic episode.

6. The major morbidity in BP disorders is actually from the depressive phases.

7. Use of an antidepressant without a mood stabilizer in BP disorders may cause a switch to mania or hypomania.

8. Hypomania and mania have similar characteristics. Mania is severe and results in severe impairment, psychosis, or hospitalization. Hypomania is *not* associated with severe impairment (but an abrupt change in functioning occurs), psychosis, or hospitalization.

9. Only three medications are FDA approved for the treatment of bipolar depression: quetiapine XR (Seroquel XR, BP-1 and BP-2), (fluoxetine+olanzapine, Symbax, BP-1), and lurasapride (Latuda, BP-1). Lithium, lamotrigine, and divalproex are also frequently used.

BIBLIOGRAPHY

American Psychiatric Association: *Task Force on DSM-V: Diagnostic and statistical manual of mental disorders*, ed 5, Arlington, VA, 2013, American Psychiatric Association.

Fountoulakis KN: An update of evidence-based treatment of bipolar depression: where do we stand? *Curr Opin Psychiatry* 23:19–24, 2010.

Frye MA: Clinical practice. Bipolar disorder—a focus on depression, *N Engl J Med* 364(1):51–59, 2011.

Geddes JR, Miklowitz DJ: Treatment of bipolar disorder, *Lancet* 381(9878):1672–1682, 2013.

Hilty DM, Leamon MH, Lim RF, et al: Diagnosis and treatment of bipolar disorder in the primary care setting: a concise review, *Prim Psychiatr* 13:77–85, 2006.

Mitchell PB, Goodwin GM, Johnson GF, Hirschfeld RMA: Diagnostic guidelines for bipolar depression: a probabilistic approach, *Bipolar Disord* 10:144–152, 2008.

Nivoli AM, Colom F, Murru A, et al: New treatment guidelines for acute bipolar depression: a systematic review, *J Affect Disord* 129:14–26, 2011.

Nofzinger EA, Thase ME, Reynolds CF 3rd, et al: Hypersomnia in bipolar depression: a comparison with narcolepsy using the multiple sleep latency test, *Am J Psychiatry* 148:1177–1181, 1991.

Phillips ML, Kupfer DJ: Bipolar disorder diagnosis: challenges and future directions, *Lancet* 381(9878):1663–1671, 2013.

Sachs GS, Nierenberg AA, Calabrese JR, et al: Effectiveness of adjunctive antidepressant treatment for bipolar depression, *N Engl J Med* 356:1711–1722, 2007.

Schaffer CB, Schaffer LC, Miller AR, et al: Efficacy and safety of non-benzodiazepine hypnotics for chronic insomnia in patients with bipolar disorder, *J Affect Disord* 128:305–308, 2011.

Patients with Terrifying Awakenings

Patient A: A 40-year-old woman was evaluated for episodes of awakening from sleep with intense anxiety and fear. These awakenings were first noted at age 38. Similar attacks sometimes occurred during wakefulness, but they did not seem as intense. The patient experienced shortness of breath, palpitations, diaphoresis, and chest pain during these episodes, which usually occurred within 1 to 2 hours of bedtime. During one of the episodes, she had been admitted to a hospital to rule out myocardial infarction. A subsequent evaluation for cardiac disease was negative. The patient denied having frightening dreams preceding the attacks and was able to remember the episodes the following morning. Previously, the patient was under the care of a psychiatrist for phobias related to elevators.

Physical examination: unremarkable

Question 1: What is your diagnosis for Patient A? What treatment do you recommend for Patient A?

Patient B: A 50-year-old male without any history of a psychiatric disorder began to experience weekly nocturnal attacks consisting of awakening from sleep followed by palpitations, fear, extreme shortness of breath and sweating. During these episodes, he was alert and remembers the episodes the following morning. No similar attacks were noted during the day. His primary care physician made a diagnosis of nocturnal panic attacks. However, the patient did not respond to alprazolam 0.25 milligrams (mg) at bedtime. A history of loud snoring was present for many years, but no history of witnessed apnea was present.

Question 2: What is the best initial approach to Patient B's complaint?

ANSWERS

1. **Answer for Patient A:** Nocturnal panic attacks (NPAs) and panic disorder (PD). Initial treatment with a low dose SSRI and antianxiety medication.

   Discussion: NPAs are characterized by abrupt waking with intense fear, diaphoresis, dyspnea, palpitations, and sometimes chest pain. The panic disorder (PD) is diagnosed in patients with recurrent PAs with at least one PA followed by 1 month or more of persistent concern about an additional PA or their consequences or a significant maladaptive behavior related to the PAs and designed to avoid future PAs (see Table F41-6). Patients with NPAs typically have attacks during the day as well. Up to 65% of patients with PD report at least one nocturnal PA. The duration of the attacks is usually <10 minutes. The symptom of dyspnea appears to be most common in NPAs. The attacks occur from non–rapid eye movement (NREM) sleep, commonly at the transition from stage N2 to stage N3 sleep. In most patients, sleep architecture is normal (normal REM latency and sleep efficiency). However, some patients may develop sleep phobia, which may be associated with findings consistent with insomnia.

   Diurnal PAs are similar to NPAs except that by definition they *occur during the day*. In one study of patients with PD, 41% experienced PAs during both wakefulness and sleeping, 56% during wakefulness only, and 2% only during sleeping. The differential diagnosis of NPA includes nightmares, arousal caused by sleep apnea, posttraumatic stress disorder (PTSD), NREM parasomnia (confusional arousal, sleep terrors), REM sleep behavior disorder, gastroesophageal reflux disease, nocturnal choking, nocturnal laryngospasm (stridor), and nocturnal paroxysmal dyspnea. In NREM parasomnia, the affected individual is not aware of his or her surroundings and does not remember the episodes in the morning. NREM parasomnia often occurs during N3 and, unlike NPA, is associated with amnesia about the event. In a PA, the patient is awake and aware of his or her surroundings. In a nightmare, the patient usually is aware of a frightening dream. In contrast, patients experiencing PAs remember the episodes, but typically do not report terrifying dreams. Polysomnography (PSG) is useful if obstructive sleep apnea (OSA) is a possibility (PSG may rarely document NREM sleep parasomnia). Of course, PAs may not occur during the sleep study.

The treatment of PAs includes behavioral psychotherapy or relaxation techniques and pharma-cotherapy. A selective serotonin reuptake inhibitor (SSRI) with or without an anxiolytic is the usual treatment for PD (or recurrent PAs). As SSRI may initially worsen symptoms, it is recommended to either start at a low dose or use the SSRI in combination with an anxiolytic. The medications approved by the U.S. Food and Drug Administration (FDA) for the treatment of PD include flu-oxetine, sertraline, paroxetine, alprazolam, and clonazepam.

An example of treatment would be paroxetine started at 10 mg daily (usual starting dose in adults is 20 mg) or sertraline 25 mg daily. The doses are slowly increased to 20 to 40 mg paroxetine or 50 to 150 mg sertraline as symptoms improve. Paroxetine is sedating in some patients and so may be given at bedtime. The medication has more anticholinergic side effects compared with other SSRIs. Because improvements may take 4 to 6 weeks or longer, many physicians add benzodiazepines dur-ing the early course of therapy. Alprazolam (Xanax) has a short half-life, and many psychiatrists prefer to use clonazepam (0.25–0.5 mg), which has a long duration of action. This is especially true for patients requiring antianxiety treatment during the day. Unfortunately, clonazepam may cause morning sedation in some patients. Alprazolam is available in an extended-release preparation (Xanax XR), which avoids repeat dosing.

In the current patient, sertraline 25 mg was started in the morning, with clonazepam 0.25 mg at bedtime. Over the course of a month, sertraline was increased to 75 mg every morning, and even-tually the clonazepam was discontinued. The patient reported resolution of the attacks.

2. **Answer for Patient B:** A PSG.

Discussion for Patient B: As noted above, PAs commonly occur during both day and night. PAs occurring only at night are rare. Therefore, other diagnosis should be considered. If any evidence suggests OSA, a PSG should be ordered. When OSA and nocturnal panic attacks (NPAs) are comorbid, one study suggests continuous positive airway pressure (CPAP) treatment may alleviate the frequency or severity of the NPAs. Of note, NPAs occur during NREM sleep, but nocturnal awakenings with shortness of breath may also occur in association with apneas during REM sleep. Some patients may wake up feeling extremely short of breath, which can be terrifying. Some patients report dreaming that they are drowning or struggling to breathe.

In the current patient with snoring and "possible PAs" confined to sleep, a diagnosis of OSA was considered likely. A PSG was performed and confirmed moderate OSA. The patient was started on CPAP, and the nocturnal episodes resolved.

CLINICAL PEARLS

1. Patients with sleep-related panic attacks usually have similar episodes when awake.
2. NPAs occur most commonly during the transition from stage N2 to stage N3 sleep.
3. Unlike sleep terrors, the patient is awake during nocturnal panic attacks and alert immediately after the attack begins.
4. PD is diagnosed when PAs are recurrent or are associated with dysfunction associated with fear of the attacks or avoidance of activities associated with the attacks (e.g., insomnia caused by NPAs).
5. Initial treatment is with low-dose SSRIs with or without an antianxiety benzodiazepine. As the dose of the SSRI is increased, the patient can often be weaned off the anxiolytic medication. If the usual starting dose of an SSRIs is used, PAs may worsen initially.
6. PAs isolated to the night (sleep) may occur but are uncommon. Other disorders such as OSA should be considered.

BIBLIOGRAPHY

American Psychiatric Association: *Diagnostic and statistical manual of mental disorders*, ed 5, Arlington, VA, 2013, American Psy-chiatric Association.
Benca RM: Sleep in psychiatric disorders, *Neurol Clin* 14:750–751, 1996.
Craske MG, Tsao JC: Assessment and treatment of nocturnal panic attacks, *Sleep Med Rev* 9:173–184, 2005.
Krystal JH, Woods SW, Hill CL, et al: Characteristic of panic attack subtypes: assessment of spontaneous panic, situation panic, and limited symptom panic, *Comp Psychiatr* 32:474–480, 1991.
Levitan MN, Nardi A: Nocturnal panic attacks: clinical features and respiratory connections, *Expert Rev Neurotherapeutics* 9:245–254, 2009.
Mellman TA, Ude TW: Patients with frequent sleep panic: clinical findings and response to medication treatment, *J Clin Psy-chiatry* 51:513–516, 1990.

Moroze G, Rosenbaum JF: Efficacy, safety, and gradual discontinuation of clonazepam in panic disorder: a placebo-controlled, multicenter study using optimized doses, *J Clin Psychiatry* 60:604–612, 1999.

Takaesu Y, Inoue Y, Komada Y, et al: Effects of nasal continuous positive airway pressure on panic disorder comorbid with obstructive sleep apnea syndrome, *Sleep Med* 13:156–160, 2012.

PATIENT 127

A 50-Year-Old Combat Veteran with Upsetting Dreams

A 50-year-old man was evaluated for recurrent awakenings with frightening dreams at night. These awakenings had been a frequent problem since his return from combat service. The dreams often were related to memories of combat, and when they occurred, he could not go back to sleep. The patient reported difficulty falling asleep on some nights, and he generally felt unrefreshed in the morning. His wife reported that he frequently thrashed about during the night while asleep. No history of snoring was present. Previous treatment with benzodiazepines had not improved his symptoms. He was started on sertraline for depression and anxiety, but this medication did not help resolve the nightmares.

Physical examination: unremarkable; a sleep study was ordered (Table P127-1).

TABLE P127-1	Polysomnography Results					
Lights-Out	**10:00 PM**		**Lights-On**	**6:00 AM**		
Total Recording Time	470 min	(419-464)	Sleep Stage	% TST	Normal Range	
Total sleep time	365.5 min	(402-449)	Stage N1	15	(3-7)	
Sleep efficiency	78 %	(88-96)	Stage N2	55	(51-64)	
Sleep latency	30 min	(1-22)	Stage N3	5	(5-17)	
REM latency	70 min	(65-99)	Stage REM	25	(19-25)	
WASO	64.5 min	(10-40)				
Arousal index (Arl)	10/hr					
Respirtory Arl	5/hr					
AHI	2/hr					
PLM index	20/hr					

AHI, apnea–hypopnea index, *PLM*, periodic limb movement; *REM*, rapid eye movement; *WASO*, wakefulness after sleep onset.
Normal values are age are shown in parentheses.

QUESTION

1. What is causing the patient's sleep disturbance? What medication do you recommend?

ANSWER

1. **Answer:** Posttraumatic stress disorder (PTSD); prazosin for nightmares.

   Discussion: PTSD is a disorder that occurs after exposure to an extremely traumatic stressor involving (1) direct personal experience of an event that involves actual or threatened death, serious injury, or other threat to one's physical integrity; (2) witnessing an event that involves death, injury, or a threat to the physical integrity of another person; or (3) learning about unexpected or violent death, serious harm, or threat of death or injury experienced by a family member or other close associate. The person's response to the event must involve intense fear, helplessness, or horror (see Table F41-7). The characteristic symptoms resulting from the exposure to the extreme trauma include persistent reexperiencing of the traumatic event, persistent avoidance of stimuli associated with the trauma, numbing of general responsiveness, and persistent symptoms of increased arousal.

   PTSD occurs in individuals who have experienced a traumatic event such as combat, physical attack, natural disaster, or traumatic injury. The disorder is characterized by reexperiencing the events in flashbacks, intrusive recollections, or recurrent dreams. Although it once was thought that complex dreaming is confined to rapid eye movement (REM) sleep, recent studies suggest dreams may occur in both REM and non-REM (NREM) sleep. Symptoms of PTSD may begin immediately after the event or have a delayed onset (up to years later). Patients with PTSD also report a heightened startle response. Given a common exposure to a traumatic event, PTSD appears to occur more frequently in women than in men. Patients with PTSD also may have depression and may abuse ethanol or other substances.

   Sleep disturbance is reported in up to 70% of patients with PTSD. Common complaints include sleep-onset and sleep-maintenance insomnia, as well as recurrent distressing nightmares. Patients often report waking up associated with anxiety and autonomic activation. The differential of awakening with anxiety includes nocturnal panic attacks (NPAs), REM sleep–related behavior disorder, and sleep terrors. Unlike patients with NPAs, patients with PTSD can recount a dream of a specific traumatic event. In contrast to night terrors, patients become alert quickly after awakening. The results of sleep studies in patients with PTSD have produced conflicting results. The duration of REM sleep latency and the amount of REM sleep have varied among studies. This may be a reflection of the fact that some patients with PTSD also are suffering from depression. Several studies have found an increase in REM density in patients with PTSD (as in depression), an increase in body movements during sleep, and the presence of periodic limb movements in sleep (PLMS). Some patients may have REM sleep without atonia (RSWA), but some are already on selective serotonin reuptake inhibitors (SSRIs), which can cause this finding. Studies have found high rates of sleep apnea in patients with PTSD (50%–90%). Some evidence suggests that continuous positive airway pressure (CPAP) treatment may improve sleep in those with PTSD. However, the presence of PTSD tends to worsen CPAP adherence.

   The treatment of PTSD includes behavioral counseling and medication. Although many patients with PTSD have anxiety, benzodiazepines have not been effective, and withdrawal of these medications may produce a flare-up of symptoms. Sertraline and paroxetine are the only antidepressants approved by the U.S. Food and Drug Administration (FDA) for treatment of PTSD. Sertraline was shown to be effective in a double-blind, placebo-controlled study. Open-label trials of paroxetine and escitalopram in PTSD have also been published. Other SSRIs may also be effective.

   For many patients with PTSD, the associated nightmares represent one of the most frequently occurring and problematic aspects of the condition. Persistent nightmares may also be one of the most enduring symptoms in PTSD. A high percentages of patients (70%–90%) describe a subjective sleep disturbance. A number of studies of patients with PTSD have found improvement in nightmares following treatment with prazosin. This medication and image rehearsal therapy were the only treatments that received a highest level recommendation in a systematic review of treatment of nightmares in PTSD. Image rehearsal therapy (IRT) is a modified cognitive behavioral technique that uses recalling the nightmare; writing it down; changing the story line, ending, or any part of the dream to a more positive one; and rehearsing the rewritten dream scenario so that the patient can displace the unwanted content when the dream recurs. Prazosin is a central and peripheral alpha-1 receptor blocker. Norepinephrine appears to play an important role in the pathophysiology of PTSD-related nightmares, arousal, selective attention, and vigilance. Norepinephrine levels in cerebrospinal fluid (CSF) and urine are elevated in patients with PTSD. CSF norepinephrine concentration appears to correlate with the severity of PTSD symptoms. It has been proposed that the consistently elevated central nervous system (CNS) noradrenergic activity may contribute to disruption of normal REM sleep and that agents that reduce this activity could be effective in the treatment of some manifestations of PTSD, particularly arousal symptoms such as nightmares and startle reactions.

Note that when prazosin is started, the drug should be initiated at a dose of 1 milligram (mg) at bedtime to avoid severe first-dose hypotension (often orthostatic hypotension). The drug may then be titrated upward slowly over several nights. A parallel placebo-controlled study of prazosin for treatment of nightmares in PTSD caused by traumatic combat experiences showed improvements in sleep and a reduction in nightmares with the medication. A relatively high dose (mean 13 mg) was reached over a protracted period of upward titration. Another study using a cross-over design and a dose of 2 to 6 mg at bedtime also found benefit in PTSD following civilian trauma.

If a suspicion for either sleep apnea or REM sleep–related behavior disorder exists, a PSG is indicated. As noted above several studies have found high rates of both sleep apnea and PLMS in patients with PTSD. It is often difficult to separate symptoms of thrashing about after dreams from the REM sleep–related behavior disorder.

The PSG in the current patient (see Table P127-1) was fairly unremarkable except for the prolonged sleep latency and reduction in REM sleep. The PLMS index was also mildly increased. The REM latency was not decreased (patient was on sertraline). Significant obstructive sleep apnea was not present. Prazosin was started at 1 mg at bedtime and slowly increased to 6 mg. On this dose, the patient noted a marked improvement in the number and severity of nightmares. The patient was also referred to a psychologist for counseling and assistance with image rehearsal therapy (IRT).

CLINICAL PEARLS

1. Sleep disturbance and awakenings with frightening dreams are common manifestations of PTSD.

2. Patients with PTSD have often have an increased REM density but variable amounts of REM sleep.

3. Increased body movements and PLMS also have been reported in PTSD.

4. A wide variety of medications are successful in different patient groups. Treatment must be individualized.

5. Anxiety is a major problem for many patients with PTSD, and antidepressants are usually more effective than benzodiazepines.

6. Recurrent distressful nightmares are a major problem for many patients with PTSD. Image rehearsal therapy and prazosin have both been effective for nightmares in patients with PTSD.

7. Several studies have reported high rates of sleep apnea in populations of patients with PTSD. Limited evidence suggests that CPAP treatment may improve PTSD if OSA is present. However, the presence of PTSD tends to worsen CPAP adherence. PTSD should be addressed if patients are to be started on CPAP.

BIBLIOGRAPHY

Aurora RN, Zak RS, Auerbach SH, et al: Best practice guide for the treatment of nightmare disorder in adults, *J Clin Sleep Med* 6:389–401, 2010.

Boehnlein JK, Kinzie JD: Pharmacologic reduction of CNS noradrenergic activity in PTSD: the case for clonidine and prazosin, *J Psychiatr Pract* 13:72–78, 2007.

Brown TM, Boudewyns PA: Periodic limb movements of sleep in combat veterans with posttraumatic stress disorder, *J Trauma Stress* 9:129–136, 1996.

Collen JF, Lettieri CJ, Hoffman M: The impact of posttraumatic stress disorder on CPAP adherence in patients with obstructive sleep apnea, *J Clin Sleep Med* 8(6):667–672, 2012.

Davidson JR, Rothbaum BO, van der Kolk BA, et al: Multicenter, double-blind comparison of sertraline and placebo in the treatment of posttraumatic stress disorder, *Arch Gen Psychiatry* 58:485–492, 2001.

Germain A, Richardson R, Moul DE, et al: Placebo-controlled comparison of prazosin and cognitive-behavioral treatments for sleep disturbances in US military veterans, *J Psychosom Res* 72(2):89–96, 2012.

Krakow B, Hollifield M, Johnston L, et al: Imagery rehearsal therapy for chronic nightmares in sexual assault survivors with posttraumatic stress disorder, *JAMA* 286:537–545, 2001.

Krakow B, Lowry C, Germain A, et al: A retrospective study on improvements in nightmares and post-traumatic stress disorder following treatment for comorbid sleep-disordered breathing, *J Psychosom Res* 49:291–298, 2000.

Maher MJ, Rego SA, Asnis GM: Sleep disturbances in patients with post-traumatic stress disorder: epidemiology, impact and approaches to management, *CNS Drugs* 20(7):567–590, 2006.

Mellman TA, Nolan B, Hedding J, et al: A polysomnographic comparison of veterans with combat-related PTSD, depressed men, and non-ill controls, *Sleep* 20:46–51, 1997.

Raskind MA, Peskind ER, Hoff DJ, et al: A parallel group placebo-controlled study of prazosin for trauma nightmares and sleep disturbance in combat veterans with post-traumatic stress disorder, *Biol Psychiatry* 61:928–934, 2007.

Raskind MA, Peskind ER, Kanter ED, et al: Reduction of nightmares and other PTSD symptoms in combat veterans by prazosin: a placebo-controlled study, *Am J Psychiatry* 160:371–373, 2003.

Ross RJ, Ball WA, Dinges DR, et al: Rapid eye movement sleep disturbance in posttraumatic stress disorder, *Biol Psychiatry* 35:195–202, 1994.

Taylor FB, Martin P, Thompson C, et al: Prazosin effects on objective sleep measures and clinical symptoms in civilian trauma PTSD: a placebo-controlled study, *Biol Psychiatry* 63:629–632, 2008.

Index

Note: Page numbers followed by "*f*" refer to illustrations; page numbers followed by "*t*" refer to tables; page numbers followed by "*b*" refer to boxes; page numbers followed by "*e*" refer to online only pages.